THE ENCYCLOPEDIA OF

NUTRITION AND GOOD HEALTH

Second Edition

Robert Ronzio, Ph.D., C.N.S., F.A.I.C.
Kennedy Associates

Checkmark Books®
An imprint of Facts On File, Inc.

The Encyclopedia of Nutrition and Good Health, Second Edition

Checkmark Books
An imprint of Facts On File, Inc.
132 West 31st Street
New York NY 10001

Library of Congress Cataloging-in-Publication Data

Ronzio, Robert A.
[Encyclopedia of nutrition & good health]
The encyclopedia of nutrition and good health / Robert Ronzio.—2nd ed.
p. cm.
Includes bibliographical references and index.
ISBN 0-8160-4966-1 (hc: alk. paper)—ISBN 0-8160-6227-7 (pb: alk. paper)
1. Nutrition—Encyclopedias. I. Title.
RA784 .R646 2003
613.2'03—dc21 2002035221

Checkmark Books are available at special discounts when purchased in bulk quantities for businesses, associations, institutions, or sales promotions. Please call our Special Sales Department in New York at (212) 967-8800 or (800) 322-8755.

You can find Facts On File on the World Wide Web at http://www.factsonfile.com

Text design by Cathy Rincon
Cover design by Pehrsson Design

Printed in the United States of America

VB FOF 10 9 8 7 6 5 4 3 2 1

This book is printed on acid-free paper.

To my family, Patricia, Lora, and Cynthia, for their love;

To Henry, Warren, Paul, and William,
who represent the next generation;

To the memory of Anthony R. and Roberta B. Ronzio;

And to people everywhere
who want to learn more about their health
and the fascinating world of nutrition.

CONTENTS

ACKNOWLEDGMENTS

To complete this encyclopedia, I drew on the support of many friends, colleagues, students, and family. The concept for the book originated from stimulating early morning conversations with Jeff Kelly, Ph.D., Lendon Smith, M.D., and Lisa Meserole, N.D., R.D., provided valuable suggestions in the early stages of this work. Denny Hannem; Loren Freeman; Amy Nystrom; Kathlyn Swann, L.Ac.; Gary Buhr, N.D.; Ralph Golan, M.D.; Nass Ordoubadi, M.D.; and John Hibbs, N.D., provided me with unwavering support. Jonathan Wright, M.D., generously offered the use of his extensive collection of reprints on nutritional medicine. Elizabeth Wales's advice during the evolution of this work proved to be invaluable. Patricia Ronzio, M.Ed., has been a constant source of inspiration throughout. Her enduring love and support made this book possible.

INTRODUCTION

The average American consumes an estimated 50 tons of food in a lifetime. This staggering amount of food represents the sum of daily choices each of us makes regarding the type, quality, and quantity of foods. These critical choices in turn reflect a complex interplay of many factors, including family upbringing, religious or philosophical beliefs, as well as practical matters, such as the cost and availability of foods and beverages. Importantly, Americans are increasingly selecting food for health reasons. They are increasingly aware that food choices profoundly affect health, the quality of life, and even longevity, and they realize that the explosive growth in medical costs requires attention to nutrition and food to prevent disease and even promote *optimal* health.

This change represents a "health revolution," based on advances in the science of nutrition. It is even changing the outlook of health professionals. The old model of curing disease and ameliorating symptoms is seen as incomplete. We now realize that disease prevention is the foundation of good health. This new model of health care emphasizes the importance of personal choices and lifestyle modification, especially the critical role of diet in maintaining health. Inadequate nutrition is linked to some of the most profound diseases of the last half-century. We now understand that incorporating specific nutrients and eating appropriate foods can reduce the risk of chronic degenerative diseases and, in some cases, treat or slow their progression. Arthritis, senility, cancer, obesity, coronary heart disease, high blood pressure, osteoporosis, and others were once believed to be inevitable consequences of aging.

The health revolution also has changed our thinking about how the body functions. There is less emphasis on distinct organ systems and more focus on integration—seeing the body as a whole. Extensive research has documented this mutual interdependence, particularly among the brain (nervous system), hormones (the endocrine system), and defenses (the immune system). For example, we cannot understand digestion without considering the effects of hormones, immune cells, and nerves of the digestive tract.

Americans face many challenges and opportunities to improve and maintain health. Overnutrition and excessive daily calories and, consequently, obesity and overweight are considered a major public health concern. We now realize that prolonged emotional and physical stress can deplete the body of critical protective nutrients and impair important functions of the body. Chronic exposure to potentially damaging chemicals in food, water, and air reduces the body's ability to fend off infections and cancer. The benefits of even modestly increasing regular physical exercise are well established, yet we are tugged in many directions by commitments that limit the time we can spend for self-care.

Healthy lifestyle choices, including eating wisely, can lead to a more productive and personally satisfying life. As one of my clients put it, "I can't change my job, I can't change my kids, and I can't change the way my spouse is, but I can change the way I eat and how much I exercise." By making informed choices about diet and lifestyles, we can level the environmental playing field so that we can feel better about ourselves and live more active and fulfilling lives.

Patients and consumers are increasingly more willing to ask questions. They want to be better informed, and they feel empowered when they take greater responsibility for their own health and the health of their families. Making wise choices requires facts, yet the amount of nutrition information available to consumers can be overwhelming. The basic issue lies in deciphering this mountain of information without becoming lost in the maze. We hear advice from talk shows, magazines and newspaper articles, a vast assortment of books, food advertisements, personal experience by family and friends, in addition to health professionals. The often expressed sentiment, "Since everything causes cancer (or is fattening), why bother?" reflects vast consumer frustration.

After working with many clients and teaching nutrition for many years in settings ranging from family programs to graduate school courses, I saw the need for a basic sourcebook to serve as a one-stop introduction to the world of nutrition. *The Encyclopedia of Nutrition and Good Health* can provide the keys to unlocking nutrition facts. My aim is to demystify scientific concepts without sacrificing accuracy, so you, the reader, can grasp the essential ideas quickly and easily. I have eliminated much of the scientific jargon that can hinder the understanding of fundamentals.

This encyclopedia is objective; it does not advocate particular vitamin or diet plan. It does not promote "cure-alls"; indeed, no single food or supplement can guarantee health or prevent disease. *The Encyclopedia of Nutrition and Good Health* is up-to-date and comprehensive. It provides current information on specific foods and nutrients such as vitamins, minerals, fats, carbohydrates, and proteins. I describe many herbs and plant products now being widely used, in addition to detailing each nutrient—how it works in the body and how it impacts health. The encyclopedia is more than a supplement guide. Here you will find a discussion of many food-related conditions, including eating disorders, obesity, addiction, weight loss and management, food sensitivities, diabetes, aging, cancer, and many other chronic degenerative conditions. Global issues such as world hunger are relevant.

I have sifted through thousands of scientific papers and carefully evaluated recent advances in nutrition, food technology, and pertinent medical breakthroughs. My analysis and synthesis of this information is based on 40 years of experience as a biochemist with a keen interest in human metabolism, nutrition, and clinical laboratory practice, and as a biomedical researcher and professor.

Why a second edition of *The Encyclopedia of Nutrition and Good Health?* The dramatic growth of nutrition research over the last decade has had a huge impact on health care and public health policy. I have incorporated much new information by expanding the number of entries to more than 1,800 and updating approximately 30 percent of the original text. For readers who wish to explore key topics, I have included dozens of up-to-date references to the medical and nutrition-related literature. Use of botanical preparations has increased dramatically, and, therefore, I have described more herbs and botanical preparations. In addition, the encyclopedia now provides a glossary of common medical terms and, as a further aid for consumers, I have included summaries of food labels and dietary guidelines.

Nutritionists and health care providers of many disciplines agree that diet and a healthy lifestyle are the mainstays of health. However, opinion is divided on amounts of specific nutrients needed for optimal health. Furthermore, because of research limitations, we still do not have a complete picture of the roles played by specific nutrients or supplements in use. For example, do results of animal studies extrapolate to humans? Do clinical observations based on a small population of white, middle-aged males extend to women, elderly persons, or to different ethnic groups? Sometimes there are differences of opinion among experts on how to interpret research findings when several different hypotheses can explain the observations. This is natural and inevitable as the science of nutrition progresses. Yet such controversy can be confusing and frustrating. Where there is disagreement in the scientific literature, I have taken the middle ground in describing pros and cons.

Only your physician is qualified to diagnose and treat health conditions. Please consult your physician for any medical problems you may have, rather than relying on self-diagnosis and self-medication, and before using any supplement. Supplements may alter prescribed treatments and could interfere with medications, so expert medical advice is essential.

Armed with new facts you will be able to ask more questions of your health care providers and become better informed about your specific conditions or health objectives—whether your concern is on lowering cholesterol levels, managing hypertension, preserving bone density, losing weight, boosting immunity, or combating the effects of environmental pollutants. Consider *The Encyclopedia of Nutrition and Good Health* your nutrition translator and stepping-stone on your pathway to wellness.

Yours in health,
Robert A. Ronzio, Ph.D., C.N.S., F.A.I.C.
Houston, Texas

A

absorption Generally, the passage of liquids into solid materials and of gases into liquids and solids. In terms of nutrition, absorption refers to the passage of substances into body fluids and tissues. Digestion is only the first step in the assimilation of nutrients. This chemical breakdown of food particles releases AMINO ACIDS, GLUCOSE, FATTY ACIDS, VITAMINS, and MINERALS, which must then be absorbed by the intestine in order to be used by the body. Nutrients enter cells lining the intestine (the intestinal mucosa) and then are drawn into underlying cells, where they may enter either the lymph or bloodstream for distribution to tissues throughout the body. Tissues absorb nutrients from blood via capillaries, the smallest blood vessels. Gases, too, are absorbed. Blood becomes oxygenated in the lungs by absorbing oxygen from inhaled air and releasing carbon dioxide that was absorbed from tissues.

Absorption requires a disproportionately large surface area to meet the body's needs. Consider the total area of the small intestine, which is a highly specialized absorptive organ. Though this tube is only about 20 feet long, it has a highly convoluted surface. Furthermore, the cells lining the surface, VILLI, are covered with microscopic, hairlike projections (MICROVILLI) that dramatically increase the absorptive area to a quarter the size of a football field. The microvilli move constantly, to trap nutrients and partially digested food, which is further digested. The upper regions of the small intestine, the lower DUODENUM, and upper ILEUM, are most active in absorbing nutrients. Other regions of the gastrointestinal tract carry out limited absorption: The stomach absorbs some ALCOHOL, glucose, ions, and water, and the colon absorbs primarily water and minerals. (See also DIGESTIVE TRACT; MALABSORPTION.)

Accent The trade name for MONOSODIUM GLUTAMATE (MSG). MSG, a common FOOD ADDITIVE, is used as a FLAVOR ENHANCER.

acerola (acerola cherry, acerola berry) Acerola fruit is a product from the Caribbean and is one of the richest natural source of VITAMIN C. Acerola juice contains nearly 40 times more vitamin C than orange juice. Acerola extract is sometimes added to natural vitamin C supplements. Because of its very limited availability, the amount added to supplements is usually very small; an acerola-enriched vitamin C preparation may contain as little as a tablespoon of acerola extract per barrel of vitamin C powder.

acesulfame-K (acesulfame potassium; Sunett) This non-caloric, ARTIFICIAL SWEETENER tastes approximately 200 times sweeter than table sugar (SUCROSE) and lacks the bitter aftertaste of SACCHARIN. The United Nations Food and Agriculture Organization endorsed acesulfame-K as a satisfactory artificial sweetener in 1983. Acesulfame-K was approved in 1988 by the U.S. FDA as a sugar substitute to be used in packets or as tablets and now is approved for use in chewing gum and in powdered drink mixes. Unlike ASPARTAME, acesulfame-K can be used in cooking because it does not break down at oven temperatures. Blending Sunett with other low-calorie sweeteners creates a beverage with a more sugarlike taste than one sweetened with any single low-calorie sweetener.

The Center for Science in the Public Interest has raised questions about Sunett's safety, saying a few tests on rats indicated a possibility of cancer, although this was not proof that the sweetener could cause cancer. The Calorie Control Council counters that the safety of acesulfame potassium has been confirmed by more than 90 studies, and it is endorsed by a committee of the World Health Organization. Theoretically, it would not be expected to be absorbed by the body. Nonetheless, some studies suggest that large doses raise blood CHOLESTEROL levels in diabetic laboratory animals and increase the number of lung and mammary tumors in other animals.

acetaminophen See ALCOHOL-DRUG INTERACTIONS.

acetic acid A fermentation product of wine. During fermentation, certain bacteria produce acetic acid by oxidizing alcohol when exposed to air. VINEGAR contains 4 percent to 6 percent acetic acid, which gives vinegar its characteristic sour taste. As vinegar, acetic acid is a common ingredient in food preparation.

One of the simplest organic acids, acetic acid contains only two carbon atoms. It is classified as a weak acid because it is only partially ionized, unlike strong mineral acids, such as hydrochloric acid.

Acetic acid plays a pivotal role in metabolism. To be metabolized, acetic acid must be activated as acetyl CoA, in which acetic acid is bound to a carrier molecule, COENZYME A, which is in turn derived from the B vitamin PANTOTHENIC ACID. Metabolic pathways that oxidize fatty acids, carbohydrate, and amino acids for energy, all yield acetyl CoA, the common intermediate by which carbons from these fuels enter the KREB'S CYCLE to be oxidized to carbon dioxide. Alternatively, acetyl CoA can be used as a building block. It forms saturated fatty acids, cholesterol, and ketone bodies. Nerve cells can use it to form the NEUROTRANSMITTER, ACETYLCHOLINE. Tissues combine acetic acid with amino sugars to form a family of sugar derivatives like N-acetylglucosamine and N-acetylgalactosamine that help define recognition sites on the surface of cells and blood group specificities, such as the A, B, O, and Lewis blood groups used in blood typing.

acetoacetic acid (acetoacetate) The most prevalent of the KETONE BODIES, which are acids produced by the liver. Acetoacetic acid is a useful fuel; it is readily oxidized by the heart and brain for the production of ATP, the energy currency of cells. Though small amounts of ketone bodies are normally produced by liver metabolism, an excessive buildup of acetoacetic acid and its derivative, BETA HYDROXYBUTYRIC ACID, in the blood (ketonemia) can occur during excessive fat breakdown, when the liver cannot completely oxidize massive amounts of fatty acids released from fat (ADIPOSE TISSUE). Conditions conducive to excessive acetoacetic acid production include STARVATION (prolonged FASTING), crash DIETING, uncontrolled DIABETES MELLITUS, and chronic ALCOHOLISM.

Ketone body production serves an important role in the physiologic adaptation to starvation. With prolonged starvation, the blood levels of ketone bodies rise, and more of them cross the BLOOD-BRAIN BARRIER to be taken up by nerve tissue, where they are burned for energy. Consequently, the brain requires less blood glucose (blood sugar) for energy at a time when this fuel is at a premium. The sustained build-up of acetoacetic acid in the blood (KETOSIS) can acidify the blood, leading to metabolic ACIDOSIS, and alter the acid-base balance of the body, a potentially dangerous condition. (See also ELECTROLYTES; FAT METABOLISM.)

acetone The simplest ketone. Ketones are an important class of organic compounds. Acetone is a volatile compound that forms spontaneously by the breakdown of the KETONE BODY, ACETOACETIC ACID. Unlike its parent compound, acetone is a metabolic dead end and cannot be metabolized for energy production. Its occurrence is a sign of severe and prolonged imbalanced carbohydrate and fat metabolism. Acetone has a characteristic sweet, ether-like odor, which accounts for the characteristic breath of individuals with uncontrolled DIABETES MELLITUS. Acetone and ketone bodies are excreted in urine under conditions promoting extensive mobilization of fat stores, as STARVATION and metabolic disorders. (See also ACETOACETIC ACID; FAT METABOLISM; KETOSIS.)

acetylcholine One of the best characterized NEUROTRANSMITTERS. This family of brain chemicals carries nerve impulses between individual nerve cells (neurons) and between neurons and muscle cells. Acetylcholine is involved in memory, in processes associated with thinking, in muscle coordination and in many other functions. Nerves that secrete acetylcholine are called cholinergic neurons. An electrical impulse traveling down such a neuron liberates acetylcholine, which then floods across the gap (synapse) separating the neuron from an adjacent cell, where it binds to its neighbor. A bound neurotransmitter in turn triggers an electrical impulse or other reaction in the receiving cell. Acetylcholine is destroyed by the enzyme cholinesterase, which clears it from the synapse and prepares it for the next impulse.

The brain synthesizes acetylcholine from CHOLINE, a nitrogen-containing ethanol derivative, and acetyl CoA, an activated form of acetic acid. Therefore, administering choline, or the phospholipid LECITHIN, a dietary source of choline, might be expected to increase brain acetylcholine levels. This strategy has been used in clinical trials to treat TARDIVE DYSKINESIA. Up to 50 percent of patients in mental hospitals suffer from this condition, characterized by uncontrolled twitches of muscles of the face and upper body. This is a side effect of certain tranquilizers and antipsychotic drugs, which may cause a deficiency of acetylcholine in critical regions of the brain. (See also SENILITY.)

acetylsalicylic acid The chemical name for ASPIRIN.

achlorhydria A condition resulting from the lack of STOMACH ACID. DIARRHEA, stomach discomfort, and bloating are common symptoms of achlorhydria, which has serious effects. It can lead to MALNUTRITION, even when the diet is well balanced, because achlorhydria drastically reduces the efficiency of DIGESTION. A chronic MALABSORPTION syndrome leads to deficiencies of VITAMIN B_{12}, CALCIUM, IRON, and other nutrients and sets the stage for chronic FATIGUE, OSTEOPOROSIS, ANEMIA, and serious infections. Although causes of achlorhydria are unknown, lowered stomach acid production is associated with anemia, stomach inflammation, CELIAC DISEASE, diabetes, lupus, myasthenia gravis, rheumatoid ARTHRITIS, and some forms of cancer.

Limited stomach acid production, not the absence of stomach acid, is termed HYPOCHLORHYDRIA. It is not as severe a condition as achlorhydria, although unless corrected, the ensuing malabsorption syndrome can have similar, detrimental long-range effects on health. In either situation patients may be advised to take supplemental hydrochloric acid in the form of BETAINE HYDROCHLORIDE or glutamic acid hydrochloride with meals to enhance digestion. These supplements should be used with medical supervision because of the danger of overdosing. (See also ACID; GASTRIC JUICE.)

acid A large family of compounds that taste sour and can neutralize bases to create salts. Strong acids like hydrochloric acid (STOMACH ACID) and sulfuric acid (battery acid) give up all of their protons in water and lower the pH, the effective hydrogen ion concentration. A pH of 7.0 is neutral, that is, neither acidic nor basic, while pH values less than 7.0 are considered acidic. Exposure to strong acids tends to damage cells and tissues. The stomach is the only organ normally exposed to strong acids, but it is protected from injury by a heavy mucous layer.

In contrast to strong acids, organic acids are classified as weak acids because they donate only a portion of their hydrogen ions, lower the pH to a lesser degree, and are less dangerous to tissues. Many compounds in foods are weak acids, including CITRIC ACID, ACETIC ACID, and TARTARIC ACID. Several weak acids are used as FOOD ADDITIVES, including benzoic acid, CARBONIC ACID, and alginic acid. As food additives and recipe ingredients, weak acids add tartness to foods. Weak acids are common intermediates, products of cellular processes that sustain life, including LACTIC ACID, KETONE BODIES, PYRUVIC ACID, acetic acid, FATTY ACIDS, SUCCINIC ACID, citric acid, even the nucleic acids DNA and RNA. GLUTAMIC ACID and ASPARTIC ACID (two common AMINO ACIDS) are classified as acidic amino acids, and are more acid than most.

In the body, weak acids characteristically have lost all their hydrogen ions and exist as a family of anions (negatively charged ions) classified as "conjugate bases" because they have been completely neutralized by the buffer systems of blood. In the blood, lactic acid exists as its anion, lactate; acetoacetic acid (a ketone body) as acetoacetate; citric acid as citrate, and so on. Often the names of acids and their anions are interchanged in nutrition literature. (See also ELECTROLYTES.)

acidemia The condition in which blood becomes acidic. (See also ACIDOSIS.)

acid-forming foods Foods that create acidic residues after they have been broken down by the body. Protein-rich food, such as EGGS, MEAT, and poultry, produce acidic residues when oxidized for energy. The combustion of sulfur-containing amino acids tends to acidify the body (acidic residue). In contrast, fruits and vegetables make the body more alkaline or basic. They contain magnesium, calcium, and potassium salts of organic acids, which yield an alkaline residue when oxidized. Fruits are accordingly classified as alkali-forming foods, even though juices and fruit taste acidic (sour). Excretion of organic acids (potential renal acid load) can be calculated for various foods based on their content of sodium, potassium, calcium, magnesium, chloride, phosphorus, and sulfur. Choosing more alkaline foods may ameliorate osteoporosis, autoimmune conditions such as rheumatoid arthritis, and chronic inflammation. (See also ACID.)

Remer, T., and F. Manz. "Potential renal acid load of foods and its influence on urine pH," *Journal of the American Dietetic Association,* 95, no. 7 (July 1995): 791–797.

acidifiers Common additives that increase the acidity (lower the pH) of foods and beverages. Acidifiers provide tartness and enhance flavors of processed foods. The increased acidity inhibits the growth of microorganisms; thus acidifiers act as preservatives. Certain acidifiers can also retard spoilage by acting as antioxidants, preventing chemical changes due to oxygen. This group of additives includes ADIPIC ACID (adipate), TARTARIC ACID (tartrate), benzoic acid (benzoate), and CITRIC ACID (citrate). (See also ACID; FOOD ADDITIVES.)

acid indigestion (heartburn, esophageal reflux, gastric reflux) A condition characterized by a burning pain near the stomach. Typically, this occurs an hour or so after a heavy (fatty) meal and is often relieved by taking ANTACIDS or by drinking MILK. Acid indigestion is the most common gastrointestinal complaint in the United States; one in 10 Americans suffer daily attacks. The pain associated with acid indigestion is caused by STOMACH ACID backing up into the ESOPHAGUS, the region of the throat connecting the mouth with the stomach.

Acid indigestion can be caused by air gulped when swallowing large bites of food, which can keep the passageway open. Some food allergies and food sensitivities may trigger acid indigestion by relaxing the sphincter muscles that normally seal off the stomach juices from the esophagus after eating. Although the stomach lining is protected from acid by mucus, the unprotected esophagus is irritated by repeated exposure to acid.

To prevent acid indigestion, patients should eat slowly and chew food thoroughly, avoiding foods and beverages that cause adverse reactions. Common examples include fatty foods, CHOCOLATE, COFFEE, CITRUS FRUIT, and alcoholic beverages. Also patients should consult a physician for any chronic stomach pain because what feels like acid indigestion may actually be inadequate stomach acid (HYPOCHLORHYDRIA). Patients should seek immediate medical attention if experiencing a crushing pain in the middle of the chest that extends to the left arm, since these symptoms could indicate a heart attack.

acidophilus (*Lactobacillus acidophilus*) A species of the bacterium *Lactobacillus* that produces lactic acid by fermenting LACTOSE (milk sugar). This organism in the upper intestinal tract forms a symbiotic relationship with its human host. Other acid-producing bacteria, including BIFIDOBACTERIA, are predominant in the lower intestine. Acidophilus is a member of the normal intestinal microflora, the so-called friendly bacteria that produce nutrients like BIOTIN and VITAMIN K. Acidophilus and other *Lactobacillus* species help balance the digestive system by maintaining conditions that inhibit the growth of yeasts like *CANDIDA ALBICANS*, as well as potentially dangerous bacterial species. Without beneficial bacteria to control them, such opportunistic microorganisms can multiply rapidly, leading to a full-blown infection.

A variety of conditions can drastically lower or eliminate the intestinal acidophilus population. Treatment with broad-spectrum antibiotics (such as tetracycline) imbalances gut microecology because these antibiotics destroy both benign and disease-producing bacteria. More generally, an unhealthful lifestyle and a diet high in SUGAR and PROCESSED FOODS also adversely affect beneficial intestinal bacteria.

Acidophilus is a common food supplement that may help repopulate the gut with beneficial bacteria to prevent hard-to-control yeast infections; to break down milk sugar for those with LACTASE DEFICIENCY; to control travelers' DIARRHEA; to relieve CONSTIPATION; to treat vaginitis (when administered as acidophilus douches); and to decrease the production of potential CARCINOGENS by certain bacteria populating the gut. (See also CANCER.)

Rosenfeldt V., K. F. Michaelsen, M. Jakobsen, et al. "Effect of Probiotic Lactobacillus Strains in Young Children Hospitalized with Acute Diarrhea," *Pediatric Infectious Disease Journal* 21, no. 5 (May 2002): 411–416.

acidophilus milk (sweet acidophilus milk) ACIDOPHILUS bacteria are sometimes added to low-fat MILK by the producer. Consumption of acidophilus milk and of yogurt may help lower blood cholesterol levels. Milk and yogurt labels should specify viable (active) acidophilus cultures, since PASTEURIZATION destroys acidophilus bacteria.

acidosis The acidification of the blood and other body fluids. This condition can be due to acid accumulation or to the loss of bicarbonate buffering capacity from kidney disease. The pH of blood is tightly regulated; the normal range is between pH 7.3 and 7.4. A drop in blood pH below pH 7.3, which corresponds to increased hydrogen ion concentration, could signal excessive acidity of the blood (ACIDEMIA). Homeostatic mechanisms (the body's regulatory system of checks and balances) help prevent acidosis. Bicarbonate and serum proteins take up hydrogen ions to neutralize excessive acid rapidly, while the kidneys more slowly compensate for acid production by excreting surplus hydrogen ions. Prolonged acidosis requires medical attention because it slows down many vital functions, including nerve transmission and heart muscle contraction. Symptoms of acidosis include nausea, vomiting, DIARRHEA, headache, rapid breathing, and, eventually, convulsions.

Two forms of acidosis are recognized: metabolic and respiratory. Metabolic acidosis can occur when metabolic acids accumulate excessively. For example, when the body burns FAT at a high rate, the liver converts FATTY ACIDS to KETONE BODIES, acidic substances. This condition may occur during crash DIETING and FASTING or in a person suffering from uncontrolled DIABETES MELLITUS or chronic ALCOHOLISM. Excessive ingestion of acids, such as in aspirin poisoning, also causes acidosis. Metabolic acidosis can also result from vomiting or diarrhea, which cause excessive loss of ELECTROLYTES like BICARBONATE and upset the acid/base balance. Renal disease may prevent the kidneys from adequately correcting acid production.

Respiratory acidosis can occur when breathing does not adequately remove carbon dioxide. Shallow breathing, associated with respiratory disease, can cause excessive CARBON DIOXIDE in the lungs, in turn causing carbon dioxide blood levels to rise and upset the bicarbonate buffer system of the blood. (See also BUFFER; FAT METABOLISM; KETOSIS; STARVATION.)

acidulant A food additive that acidifies prepared foods and beverages. Citric acid and sodium dihydrogen phosphate are examples. (See also ACIDIFIERS.)

acrylamide A chemical used in making plastics, textiles, and dyes and in purifying drinking water. Short-term exposure above safe limits (maximum contaminant levels) set by the Environmental Protection Agency (EPA) causes damage to the central nervous system. Long-term exposure can cause paralysis and possibly cancer. The chemical has been shown to cause cancer in laboratory animals.

In 2002 the World Health Organization (WHO) convened an emergency meeting of food safety and health experts after a team of Swedish scientists reported that some starch-based foods, like potato CHIPS, FRENCH FRIES, and some BREAKFAST CEREALS and BREADS, contain high levels of acrylamide. The amount of the chemical found in a large order of fast-food french fries was at least 300 times above EPA safe limits for drinking water. Additional studies in Norway, Great Britain, Switzerland, and the United States reached similar results.

Acrylamide apparently forms in some starchy foods when they are baked or fried at high temperatures. Raw or boiled samples of these foods, such as potatoes, test negative for the chemical. Research on the health effects of acrylamide in food is ongoing. For the time being, most health experts have stopped short of advising consumers to avoid the risky foods or change their cooking methods.

ACTH See ADRENOCORTICOTROPIC HORMONE.

addiction A chronic condition characterized by CRAVINGS for and uncontrollable use of a substance (often drugs or alcohol) despite negative physical, mental, or social consequences. People who suffer from drug or alcohol addiction are often malnourished and may be either overweight due to an increased consumption of foods high in refined CARBOHYDRATES or underweight due to a loss of APPETITE.

Nutrition offers a powerful adjunct to recovery and restoring the body's biochemical balance. A nutritional program for a recovering addict might advise:

- establishing new eating patterns, including eating frequent small meals to stabilize blood sugar (GLUCOSE) and prevent HYPOGLYCEMIA
- avoiding foods high in sugar or refined carbohydrates
- eating a varied, balanced diet of VEGETABLES, whole GRAINS, LEGUMES, FRUITS, lean MEAT, POULTRY, and FISH
- avoiding or eliminating foods that contain CAFFEINE
- taking daily supplements of certain VITAMINS and MINERALS, such as GLUTAMINE, VITAMIN C, and NIACINAMIDE.

(See also ALCOHOLISM; ADDICTION AND SUGAR.)

Markowitz, J. S., A. L. McRae, and S. C. Sonne. "Oral Nutritional Supplementation for the Alcoholic Patient: A Brief Overview," *Annals of Clinical Psychiatry* 12, no. 3 (September 2000): 153–158.

addiction and sugar Addiction to refined CARBOHYDRATES in general and to sucrose (table sugar) specifically is a controversial topic. Proponents believe that sugar has no effect on behavior, and that it has little effect on health other than promoting tooth decay. A government task force concluded in 1986 that typical sugar consumption does not generally pose a health hazard. Critics contend that sugar addiction is a common phenomenon. Preferring sugar and sweets seems to be programmed at infancy. A craving for sweets often develops later in life, and in this sense sugar may be psychologically addicting. Compounding the problem of defining sugar addiction is the general observation that related symptoms are rather vague, including a change in mood or feeling shaky when abstaining from sugary foods.

One hypothesis proposes that addicted persons have a drive to achieve a sense of well-being and to overcome depression. Some addicted persons seem to have an abnormal metabolism of NEUROTRANSMITTERS, chemicals that carry signals from one nerve cell to another cell. A primary example is the link between depression and low levels of the brain chemical serotonin and the correlation between high-sugar, high-fat diets, and high brain serotonin levels. Evidence suggests that eating certain sugary foods stimulates the production of brain peptides (ENDORPHINS), which trigger pleasant feelings. It has been hypothesized that the formation of endorphins may be abnormal in some individuals, possibly triggering compulsive eating behavior like BULIMIA NERVOSA. (See also APPETITE; BLOOD SUGAR; NATURAL SWEETENERS.)

additives See FOOD ADDITIVES.

adenine A building block of DNA, the genetic blueprint of the cell, and of RNA, the cell's messenger that directs protein synthesis. Adenine is also used to manufacture ATP (adenosine triphosphate), the energy currency of the cell, as well as several enzyme helpers (COENZYMES) required to produce energy. These include coenzyme A, derived from the B vitamin pantothenic acid; FAD (FLAVIN ADENINE DINUCLEOTIDE) from riboflavin; and NAD (NICOTINAMIDE ADENINE DINUCLEOTIDE) from niacin.

In DNA adenine constitutes one of the four bases that make up the alphabet of the genetic code and it stabilizes the unique double helix based on the attraction and complementary bonding between two parallel DNA chains.

Chemically, adenine is a cyclic structure belonging to the family of purines. Adenine is synthesized in the body from three amino acids (ASPARTIC ACID, GLUTAMINE, and GLYCINE). Therefore, adenine is not an essential dietary nutrient. (See also GOUT; GUANINE.)

adenosine triphosphate See ATP.

adipic acid (hexapedioc acid) A common FOOD ADDITIVE in vegetable oils, adipic acid prevents their oxidation and retards rancidity, thus acting as an ANTIOXIDANT. As an acidifier, adipic acid adds tartness to soft drinks, throat lozenges, gelatin desserts, and powdered, fruit-flavored beverages. Adipic acid is readily metabolized and is considered a safe food additive. (See also CHELATE.)

adipocyte FAT storage cell. The adipocyte is like a balloon; it expands in size when fat is added and it shrinks when fat is depleted. Adipocytes form ADIPOSE TISSUE, specialized for fat storage. The number of adipocytes increases during early childhood and adolescence as the amount of adipose tissue increases. At other stages in life, fat is deposited in, or released from, existing adipocytes. Stored fat comes from the diet or the liver adipocytes take up fatty acids from chylomicrons, which transport dietary fat in the blood, and from very low-density lipoprotein (VLDL), which transports fat synthesized by the liver. Adipocytes also synthesize fat from blood glucose in response to the hormone insulin. Conversely, many hormones initiate fat breakdown in adipocytes: EPINEPHRINE, GLUCAGON, GROWTH HORMONE, and ANDROGENS, among others. (See also LIPOGENESIS; LIPOLYSIS.)

adipose tissue (body fat, depot fat) Fat storage is a specialized function of adipose tissue, and it represents the major fuel depot of the body; it is as essential to normal function as any other tissue. Body fat serves other important functions: It insulates the body against low environmental temperatures and serves as a shock absorber. Typically, fat stored in adipose tissue represents 15 percent to 20 percent of men's weight and 20 percent to 25 percent of women's average weight. Women usually have more fat than men because fat is an important energy reserve during pregnancy and lactation.

Adipose tissue synthesizes fat after a high carbohydrate meal in response to the hormone INSULIN. During FASTING, STARVATION, or STRESS, a second hormone EPINEPHRINE (adrenaline) signals ADIPOCYTES (fat cells) to break down stored fat into FATTY ACIDS, which are released into the bloodstream. They are rapidly absorbed and oxidized for energy by muscles. In contrast, the brain relies on blood sugar to meet its energy needs.

The fact that an adult can consume approximately two pounds of food a day (or 700 pounds of food a year) with only small changes in body fat indicates how well the body regulates weight when the calorie intake matches the total body requirements.

Of course, common experience suggests that body fat can increase. For example, fat accumulation often accounts for the weight gain of middle-aged Americans. Older people tend to EXERCISE less and the metabolic rate slows with aging. An individual's optimal body fat at any age depends upon many factors, including inheritance, body build, sex, and age. Standard HEIGHT/WEIGHT TABLES or the BODY MASS INDEX can be used to estimate an appropriate body weight for an individual.

Excessive body fat is not healthy for many reasons. OBESITY carries with it the increased risk of CARDIOVASCULAR DISEASE, HYPERTENSION, and some forms of CANCER. It is interesting to note that the distribution of body fat plays a role in defining the risk for heart disease. Abdominal fat (the "spare tire" profile) carries a greater risk for cardiovascular disease than fat accumulated around hips and thighs (the "pear" profile).

The general approach to losing fat stored in adipose tissue is exercising and eating low-fat, high-fiber meals, while decreasing caloric intake. Dieting without exercise decreases muscle mass (not desirable) as well as the fat in adipose tissue, and the weight regained after a crash diet is mostly fat (also not desired). Cycles of dieting and not dieting also cause loss of muscle mass. Muscle burns more ENERGY per pound than fat, so DIET cycling may increase the difficulty of losing weight permanently. The number of fat cells in adipose tissue—the storage bags themselves—cannot be lost by dieting or exercise. The only way to lose fat cells of adipose tissue is by LIPOSUCTION, a surgical procedure. (See also FAT METABOLISM.)

adrenal glands Triangular-shaped glands attached to the kidneys that secrete two types of hormones that regulate tissue metabolism and blood composition. The body's two adrenal glands are each divided into two parts. The outer cortex secretes three classes of steroid hormones (adrenocorticosteroids), each with a different primary function. The GLUCOCORTICOIDS consist of CORTISOL and corticosterone. Their function is to develop a sustained response to stress. They increase blood GLUCOSE; stimulate the synthesis of liver GLYCOGEN; mobilize amino acids from protein; and stimulate ADIPOSE TISSUE to break down stored FAT and release free FATTY ACIDS into the bloodstream. MINERALOCORTICOIDS (mainly ALDOSTERONE) direct the kidney to conserve SODIUM and water, and therefore they play a key role in ELECTROLYTE and water balance. ANDROGENS (such as testosterone) are anabolic hormones that stimulate muscle protein synthesis and decrease the rate of protein breakdown, leading to an increase in growth rate. Androgens develop and maintain male secondary sex characteristics, such as genitalia, enlarged larynx, hair growth, and muscular development. Testosterone maintains the prostate gland, seminal vesicles, and sperm production of the testes.

The inner region of the adrenal gland, the medulla, is a major source of stress hormones. It functions independently of the cortex (outer layer). The medulla synthesizes a family of hormones (CATECHOLAMINES) that are derived from TYROSINE: EPINEPHRINE (adrenaline) and norepinephrine. Epinephrine is released when a threatening situation is perceived. The medulla increases the heart rate and the rate of breathing, constricts blood vessels, and relaxes bronchioles (the small air passageways of the lungs). It stimulates the release of free FATTY ACIDS from fat stored in ADIPOSE TISSUE and the release of glucose from glycogen. The effects of norepinephrine resemble those of epinephrine, described above, although it is less active. It, too, increases the liberation of free fatty acids, stimulates the central nervous system, and increases heat production. Norepinephrine increases blood pressure by constricting blood vessels in most organs.

The function of the adrenal glands is severely affected by sustained, long-term stress. In early stages of adaptation to chronic stress, the adrenal cortex produces large amounts of cortisol. This creates a highly catabolic state, in which muscle, fat, and glycogen are degraded, leading to chronic FATIGUE. Stressed adrenal glands may be linked to abnormal blood sugar regulation, to muscle protein breakdown, and to suppression of the immune system. In later, extreme stages of adaptation to chronic stress, cortisol production is depressed when the adrenal cortex can no longer be activated by signals from the pituitary gland. Inadequate cortisol in turn can lead to hypoglycemia (low blood sugar) and to chronic fatigue. (See also ENDOCRINE SYSTEM; HORMONE; HYPOGLYCEMIA, POSTPRANDIAL.)

adrenocorticotropic hormone (ACTH) A polypeptide HORMONE produced by the anterior lobe of the PITUITARY GLAND and secreted to activate and sustain the ADRENAL GLANDS. ACTH release from the pituitary gland is regulated by the HYPOTHALAMUS via a hormone, corticotropin-releasing factor (CRH). ACTH triggers the production of all steroid hormones of the adrenal gland, where it stimulates the conversion of CHOLESTEROL to steroid hormone precursors. ACTH also acts on ADIPOSE TISSUE to mobilize FAT and to increase blood levels of FATTY ACIDS. Inadequate ACTH leads to atrophy of the adrenal cortex, while excessive ACTH causes hyperplasia, the excessive growth of adrenal tissue. (See also CORTISOL; ENDOCRINE SYSTEM.)

adulterated food A food is classified as adulterated if it contains extraneous material, dangerous amounts of poisons or filth, or if it has been processed or stored under unsanitary conditions. In terms of food for interstate commerce, the U.S. Food and Drug Administration monitors environmental contaminants, toxins from microorganisms, bacterial levels, and potentially harmful substances. Since it is impossible for food to be 100 percent pure, tolerances have been set for each type of contaminant. Very hazardous materials can be ruled so dangerous that no amount should be detected (a "zero tolerance"). (See also RISK DUE TO CHEMICALS IN FOOD AND WATER.)

adult onset diabetes See DIABETES MELLITUS.

advertising Billions of dollars are spent each year on advertising food, and much of this is focused on specific markets. Food ads for breakfast cereals and junk food, for example, focus largely on the children's market. Toys, comic books, giveaways, and polished commercials can hinder young people from making independent judgments on how to eat a balanced diet. Instead, their choices may rely on the direction of advertisers. TV advertising plays a prominent role, where cartoons featuring food commercials dominate children's programming. Most of these emphasize PROCESSED FOODS—low in nutrients and high in CALORIES, SUGAR, SALT, and FAT. The American Academy of Pediatrics (AAP) discovered that less than 3 percent of advertising during children's programs focuses on healthful food, such as fruit and milk. The AAP concluded that there is a direct link between commercials promoting high-calorie food and health problems, and in 1991 recommended a ban on food commercials geared toward children.

The Better Business Bureau's Children's Advertising Review Unit was founded in 1972. Composed of representatives from the media, ad agencies, and others, its goal is to monitor truth in advertising in radio, TV, and the printed word for children up to the age of 12, according to self-regulating guidelines. It will review material before it is publicized upon request. The group provides a forum for information exchange and relies on a panel of academic professionals to provide expertise on the impact of images on children. (See also CONVENIENCE FOOD; EATING PATTERNS; FOOD ADDITIVES; OBESITY.)

Taras, Howard L., and Miriam Gage. "Advertised Foods on Children's Television," *Archives of Pediatric and Adolescent Medicine* 149, no. 6 (June 1995): 649–652.

aerobic A physiologic or cellular process requiring oxygen. Cellular RESPIRATION is the aerobic process by which oxygen diffuses into cells and is used in the oxidation of fuel to produce ENERGY. The waste product of respiration is carbon dioxide. Aerobic also refers to the ability to function only in the presence of oxygen. For example, aerobic bacteria that are potential pathogens (disease producers) do not flourish in the intestine when the availability of oxygen is limited. (See also ELECTRON TRANSPORT CHAIN; OXIDATIVE PHOSPHORYLATION.)

aerobic exercise Sustained physical EXERCISE involving moderate to high levels of exertion and characterized by increased heart rate and accelerated breathing. Vigorous activity associated with hard work and athletic sports can raise the pulse rate sufficiently to strengthen the cardiovascular system. Conditioning refers to increased physical endurance due to increased muscle mass and a strengthened oxygen delivery system, including heart, arteries, and lungs, as a result of aerobic exercise. (See also FITNESS.)

aerobic respiration See RESPIRATION, CELLULAR.

aflatoxin A mycotoxin, a family of toxic compounds derived from molds growing on foods and on grains used for animal feed. Aflatoxin is produced by ASPERGILLUS, a storage mold that often infests damp grains and nuts. Nuts such as PISTACHIOS, ALMONDS, WALNUTS, PECANS, and PEANUTS are susceptible to MOLD. Very low levels of aflatoxin often contaminate PEANUT BUTTER. Spot checks have shown that this contamination is usually below the U.S. Food and Drug Administration limit. In the 1970s and again in the 1980s, hot drought conditions caused outbreaks of mold in corn and, consequently, widespread aflatoxin contamination.

Concern has focused on aflatoxin because it is a potent liver CARCINOGEN. The amount of aflatoxin permitted by the U.S. FDA is 15 parts per billion, although levels as low as one part per billion can cause liver cancer in certain species of experimental animals. As yet there is no compelling evidence that aflatoxin consumption in the low amounts usually encountered in Western nations causes cancer. In regions of Africa where peanut consumption and consequently aflatoxin intake is very high, population studies suggest a correlation with liver cancer in humans. Recent epidemiological studies have shown that ingestion of aflatoxin B-1 increases the risk of developing liver cancer. The risk is even higher for people who are infected with hepatitis B. In addition to increasing the risk of chronic diseases such as cancer, ingestion of aflatoxin B-1 can cause acute symptoms of aflatoxicosis, including vomiting, abdominal pain, and even death.

Consumers should avoid moldy, discolored, or off-flavor nuts. Molds and fungi send out microscopic filaments beyond the immediate, visibly moldy area and cannot be easily removed. Furthermore, aflatoxin is not completely destroyed by cooking. Therefore moldy food (except cheese) should be discarded, rather than cutting out the mold. (See also CANCER-PREVENTION DIET; FOOD TOXINS; FUNGUS.)

agar An organic FOOD ADDITIVE that forms nondigestible gels. This extract from SEAWEED has no odor or flavor. It is used occasionally as a THICKENING AGENT in the manufacture of whipped cream, ICE CREAM, JELLY, JAM, and MAYONNAISE, and to prevent frosting on baked goods from drying out. In microbiology, agar gels in petri dishes are used extensively to culture microorganisms for identification purposes.

age-related macular degeneration A progressive impairment of the cluster of cells at the center of the retina (macula), which is responsible for central vision. This disease is the leading cause of irreversible blindness in the United States. About a quarter of people over age 65 have this condition, for which there is no cure.

However, the Age-Related Disease Study Research Group found that the combination of BETA-CAROTENE, vitamins C and E, and ZINC slowed the progression of age-related macular degeneration and vision loss. Smoking is considered to be a contraindication of beta-carotene supplementation.

Other studies have found that older men and women who ate the most dark green leafy vegetables were less likely to develop the condition than were those who ate the least amounts of those vegetables and carotenoids (a group of red, orange, and yellow plant pigments that includes beta-carotene). Two pigments in particular—LUTEIN and zeaxanthin—accounted for this reduction in risk of advanced age-related macular degeneration.

Scientists suspect that these carotenoids protect the retina by filtering out damaging light. Data from the Baltimore Longitudinal Study of Aging also suggests that vitamin E helps lower risk.

aging The progressive decline over time in physiologic function, including reflexes, vision, hearing, short-term memory and learning, physical strength and endurance, DIGESTION, cardiovascular function, and immunity. Although these changes often begin in the mid-twenties, heart functioning, memory, and reasoning need not drop significantly until very late in life.

Aging is commonly associated with chronic diseases. These include CANCER, diabetes, OSTEOPOROSIS, PERIODONTAL DISEASE, OBESITY, SENILITY, CARDIOVASCULAR DISEASE (STROKE, HEART ATTACK, ATHEROSCLEROSIS, and so on), and AUTOIMMUNE DISEASES (such as RHEUMATOID ARTHRITIS and SPRUE). A growing body of evidence indicates that chronic diseases are not inevitable, but are related to many controllable factors, including diet. The common expectation that decreased physical ability will accompany aging often leads to diminished exercise at mid-life or later, setting the stage for narrowed arteries, elevated blood CHOLESTEROL, and heart and kidney disease.

Possible Causes of Aging

Genetic research has confirmed that longevity is, in part, genetic. Scientists discovered a specific gene mutation in yeast, SIR2, that dramatically shortened the organism's lifespan. Researchers found that if the gene was doubled, the yeast's lifespan increased dramatically, but if a mutation was introduced that destroyed the gene, the yeast's lifespan was curtailed. Cellular molecular theories of aging are currently popular. According to these theories, genes limit a person's life span, and there may be genes for longevity and predisposition to ALZHEIMER'S DISEASE, cancer, and schizophrenia. The longevity determinant gene hypothesis predicts that a few key genes regulate the rate of aging of an organism. Aging may be the result of the improper readout of genes occurring during aging.

Accumulated oxidative damage is another molecular explanation of tissue aging; experts suspect that the body gradually loses the ability to repair damage caused by oxidation to genetic material, as well as to cellular machinery. The damaging agent is believed to be FREE RADICALS, highly reactive fragmented chemicals including extremely dangerous forms of oxygen. Free radicals bombard tissues and attack DNA, proteins, and cell walls.

Senescence could be linked to the structure of chromosomes. The tips of chromosomes are protected by structures formed of DNA and protein. With successive cell divisions, telomeres become progressively shorter, reaching a point at which they can no longer protect the chromosome and cell division ceases. Because senescent cells are no longer able to protect organs and blood vessels, they possibly contribute to aging.

Drastically limiting caloric intake may slow the age-related physiologic decline in experimental animals and increase their longevity dramatically. While this approach is a useful research tool, it is an impractical approach to slowing aging in humans. Few adults would volunteer to restrict their CALORIES by 20 percent or more for a lifetime. Investigators are trying to identify substances that will mimic the physiological effects of calorie restriction.

On the other hand, prevention seems a much more feasible approach to counteract aging. It is estimated that only about 30 percent of aging characteristics are genetically based. Consequently, how a person lives is the major key to a healthy old age. Regular physical activity, continued social relationships, the ability to recover from losses, and a feeling of control over life are predictors of successful aging.

Aging and Memory

Short-term memory functions and the speed of recall often decline with aging. Although it is annoying, forgetfulness need not be debilitating. Because memory is selective, it will usually serve the learning process throughout life. The mental faculties of most older people remain functioning when exercised and challenged by a commitment to lifelong learning and activity. Furthermore, research suggests that people may be trained to partially recover their mental function apparently lost during aging.

Forgetfulness can be caused by depression, by the use of alcohol, tranquilizers, and sleeping pills, by certain drug interactions and by any factor that decreases the supply of oxygen to the brain. Malnutrition can also cause mental deterioration. In this regard, antioxidants may be particularly important because free-radical damage may play a role in mental aging. Older experimental animals fed antioxidants dramatically improve their mental performance with a concomitant decline in oxidized brain proteins. Such experiments suggest the buildup of oxidized protein, the result of free-radical attack, may cause brain cells to age.

Preventive medicine proposes that making wise lifestyle choices sets the stage for health later in life. The following lifestyle choices increase the odds of living longer:

- Avoiding cigarettes. Smoking can lead to cancer, cardiovascular disease, and emphysema.
- Taking care of all emotional needs to reduce the stress of daily living and thus strengthening the immune system. Chronic stress leads to elevated CORTISOL, which suppresses the immune system.
- Keeping mentally active; individuals who use their reasoning power retain it longer.
- Exercising regularly to slow deterioration of sensory and physical abilities. AEROBIC EXERCISE can increase fitness and endurance throughout a lifespan.
- Eating wisely. A varied, balanced diet with minimally processed food is the foundation for lasting good health.

Nutrient Needs During Aging

Elderly persons are prone to MALNUTRITION for several reasons. They are more likely to eat alone and so take less interest in meal preparation, and they are more often disabled and immobile. Thus, they are less likely to eat properly. More than 30 percent of homebound older individuals may have difficulty in preparing their own meals. Low-fiber, high-carbohydrate meals typify the diets of many elderly persons. They use more LAXATIVES and medications for long periods. Furthermore, many elderly persons have periodontal disease and poor teeth. Their senses of smell, taste, and sight decline, making eating less appealing, and STOMACH ACID production gradually drops, decreasing nutrient uptake even with an adequate diet.

Evidence indicates that superior nutrition may prevent unnecessary illness and disability from shortening a productive life. Therefore, experts recommend the following health decisions:

- Avoiding excess calories and ALCOHOL. Surplus calories regardless of their source are converted to fat. Excessive body fat contributes to the risk of heart disease, hypertension, and some forms of cancer. Besides carrying a risk of addiction, excessive alcohol can damage the liver, pancreas, and brain, in addition to depleting the body of nutrients.
- Medical testing of stomach acid production. Low stomach acid production sets the stage for inadequate digestion of nutrients.
- Making informed choices regarding nutritional supplements. They can affect the quality of health of those who are nutrient deficient, though eating wisely.
- Choosing a diet based on DIETARY GUIDELINES FOR AMERICANS as a foundation. A BALANCED DIET, one that provides adequate amounts of all nutrients and FIBER from varied, minimally processed foods without excessive calories and FAT, is of paramount importance.

Relatively little is known regarding specific nutritional needs of people over the age of 65, although more research is being done in this area. Attention has focused on three classes of nutrients as being especially important in aging: minerals, vitamins, and antioxidants.

Minerals Diminished digestion and ABSORPTION can lead to deficiencies of MAGNESIUM, IRON, ZINC, COPPER, and CALCIUM. Older persons probably need more than the current calcium RDA of 800 mg because the ability of the intestine to absorb adequate calcium declines progressively with age. The common experience is that the bodies of elderly women and men remove calcium from their bones to meet their calcium needs. Supplementation with calcium and VITAMIN D, or calcium with low-dose ESTROGEN for post-menopausal women, seems to be more effective in slowing bone losses than supplementation with calcium alone. Normally, iron stores increase throughout adult life in men and in women after menopause. However, blood loss due to chronic ASPIRIN use and bleeding ulcers can cause iron deficiency; 5 percent of elderly men are iron deficient in the United States. CHROMIUM stores in the body decline steadily with age and this may contribute to the decline in the regulation of blood sugar. Chromium assists in insulin action and helps blood sugar regulation in some diabetics. Low chromium is correlated with elevated blood cholesterol levels.

Vitamins Research suggests there may be increased vitamin needs in elderly people; however, no definite proof that vitamin supplements increase the life span has been offered. Many elderly Americans obtain less than 50 percent of the Recommended Dietary Allowance of VITAMIN B_6. Medications such as penicillin, estrogens and antihypertensive drugs interfere with absorption of this vitamin. Folic acid and vitamin B_{12} are less well absorbed in elderly persons, and the RDAs should be higher. Inadequate diet and decreased uptake of fat-soluble vitamins probably account for the increased need for VITAMIN A and VITAMIN E with aging, and extra vitamin E may boost immunity, thus helping elderly persons resist disease. Vitamin E has also shown promise in slowing decline in mental functioning in the elderly. One study showed that people who took high amounts of vitamin E had a 70 percent reduction in the risk of developing Alzheimer's disease. In another study researchers followed more than 2,800 people over the age of 65 for three years. Those participants who had the highest amount of vitamin E consumption showed the slowest decline in mental alertness. Vitamin D requirements may increase during aging because the skin gradually loses its ability to manufacture the vitamin. Patients with hip fractures may be deficient in vitamin D.

Another problematic nutrient for elderly people is VITAMIN C, a versatile antioxidant. Consumption may be low with diets relying on processed, overcooked foods and lacking adequate fruits and vegetables. Vitamin C may protect against cataracts and atherosclerosis.

The RDA for RIBOFLAVIN is believed to be too low for elderly people. Geriatric outpatients can exhibit low-THIAMIN levels and evidence suggests that RDA of this critical nutrient is greater for older people than for middle-aged individuals.

Antioxidants Several nutrients seem to protect the body throughout life against damage by free radicals, highly reactive forms of oxygen that can attack cells. Trace minerals like copper, SELENIUM, and zinc, as well as vitamins C and E plus BETA-CAROTENE, function as antioxidants. Together with vitamin A they also keep the immune system balanced. The immune system protects the body against bacterial and viral diseases and defends against cancer.

Other ingredients in foods, especially fruits and vegetables, act as ANTIOXIDANTS. They strengthen the body's defenses and protect against cancer. These include FLAVONOIDS, PHYTOESTROGENS (ISOFLAVONES), and ISOTHIOCYANATES. Many more remain to be identified. From hundreds of studies, it is clear that diets that provide ample fruits, legumes, and vegetables protect against many of the degenerative diseases that commonly occur with aging. As an example, middle-aged men and women who eat plenty of fruits and vegetables are significantly less likely to experience cardiovascular disease and strokes.

More research is required to determine the optimal intake of anti-aging nutrients. Foods with anti-aging nutrients include orange vegetables (CARROTS, SQUASH) and dark green leafy vegetable (CHARD, KALE, SPINACH) for vitamin A and beta-carotene. Fresh fruit like ORANGES, frozen citrus juices, and BROCCOLI provide vitamin C. VEGETABLE OIL, WHEAT germ, and nuts supply vitamin E, while whole GRAINS, SEAFOOD, CABBAGE, ONIONS, and GARLIC provide selenium. (See also DEGENERATIVE DISEASES; DHEA; SENILITY.)

Gutteridge, John M. "Hydroxyl radicals, iron, oxidative stress, and neurodegeneration," *Annals of the New York Academy of Sciences* 738 (November 1994): 201–213.

agricultural chemicals See PESTICIDES.

Agricultural Marketing Service (AMS) A service-oriented arm of the U.S. Department of Agriculture (USDA) that provides marketing services to the agricultural industry. It facilitates marketing of agricultural products domestically and abroad while promoting competition and fair practices among U.S. food producers. Its six commodity divisions (cotton, DAIRY, POULTRY, FRUIT and VEGETABLE, livestock and seed, and tobacco) employ specialists who provide standardization, grading, and market news services for those commodities.

AMS also purchases a variety of foods that are in excess supply, including fruits and vegetables, meat, poultry, EGG products, and FISH, in support of the national SCHOOL LUNCH PROGRAM and other federal nutrition assistance programs.

AIDS (acquired immune deficiency syndrome) The last stage of a disease that diminishes the body's ability to fight off infections. The disease is caused by infection with the human immunodeficiency virus (HIV), which destroys the body's IMMUNE SYSTEM by attacking the white blood cells called T-cells. AIDS is diagnosed when HIV infection progresses to a point at which either the number of T-cells drops to dangerously low levels or the patient suffers a life-threatening condition or disease. A number of lifestyle factors have been implicated in increased physiologic susceptibility to HIV infection: overconsumption of refined foods; inadequate diet and malnutrition; malabsorption; use of recreational drugs; repeated infections, including sexually transmitted diseases; use of medications that weaken the immune system; blood transfusions; as well as STRESS and smoking. Relatively few carefully designed and controlled clinical studies of nutrition and HIV infections have been carried out to permit general conclusions.

As a result of increased susceptibility to disease due to lowered immunity, AIDS patients may develop pneumonia, Kaposi's sarcoma, and diseases due to infectious agents, including the yeast *CANDIDA ALBICANS*, Epstein-Barr virus, and herpes simplex virus. Poor nutritional status contributes to these diseases.

HIV-infected patients are more susceptible to parasites, such as CRYPTOSPORIDIUM, a contaminant in municipal water supplies. The recommendation is to avoid all public tap water and to drink water that has been boiled or filtered.

Weight loss characterizes HIV infection, but the causes remain ill-defined. In AIDS patients this may be due to MALNUTRITION or it may be due to the lack of appetite (anorexia) associated with the subsequent severe infections or cancer. Anorexia is worsened by DEPRESSION. Oral and throat yeast infections, early symptoms of depressed immunity, can also compromise food intake.

There is no cure for AIDS; however, several nutrients, food-related materials, and ENZYME preparations boost the immune system and may offer protection against the risk of CANCER and infection in some individuals with AIDS.

Trace Nutrients ZINC deficiency is common in patients with AIDS and may indicate trace mineral malnutrition or malabsorption. Zinc plays an important role in maintaining the immune system. Zinc inhibits an enzyme needed for HIV production. SELENIUM deficiency may be part of the malnutrition seen in AIDS patients. It is a COFACTOR for enzymes that serve as ANTIOXIDANTS. Selenium helps protect against liver and colon cancer in experimental animals, and clinical studies of the effects of selenium supplementation on cancer prevention are being carried out. Other vitamins and minerals, such as VITAMIN A, FOLIC ACID, VITAMIN B_{12}, and POTASSIUM, may be deficient in some AIDS patients.

Enzymes Megadoses of a variety of enzymes, including SUPEROXIDE DISMUTASE, are being used as antioxidants. There is no clear evidence that their use diminishes or prevents symptoms.

Antioxidants Evidence suggests that HIV-infected patients have lower levels of antioxidants, including VITAMIN C, CAROTENOIDS, COENZYME Q, GLUTATHIONE, and selenium. Such oxidative stress can promote HIV replication and decrease immunity. Antioxidant nutrients may lower the risk of cancer in the general population, and the same may be true for HIV-infected patients. BETA-CAROTENE and carotenoids may lower the risk of many cancers, including those of the lung, bladder, stomach, esophagus, and prostate. Beta-carotene can increase the numbers of T-helper cells. Significantly, the standard American diet is deficient in beta-carotene. Vitamin C boosts immunity, helps protect against viral and bacterial infections, and may decrease the risk of stomach, esophageal, and cervical cancer. It increases blood antibody levels and supports the function of the THYMUS GLAND and lymphocytes. Furthermore, vitamin C supports healthy connective tissue and assists in wound healing. FLAVONOIDS are associated with vitamin C in plants and enhance vitamin C therapy. Many flavonoids function as antioxidants and several types may stimulate the immune system. GLUTATHIONE supports the immune system and functions as a major antioxidant. N-acetylcysteine, a derivative of the sulfur amino acid CYSTEINE, can enhance glutathione levels.

Egg Lipids Mixtures of LECITHIN and other fatty materials from eggs have been used with some positive results in small clinical studies. Although there is a lack of strong evidence of its effectiveness, these mixtures are still being used. They are apparently nontoxic, though long-term effects are unknown.

Herbs Several herbs, such as GOLDENSEAL (*Hydrastis canadensis*), have been shown to enhance several aspects of immune function. The most active component of goldenseal is berberine, a broad-spectrum antimicrobial agent effective in treating the severe DIARRHEA that is typically seen in AIDS patients. Herbal treatment based on Chinese medicine is also being studied. Certain formulations inhibit viruses and boost the immune system. Some research suggests garlic may enhance immunity and help combat opportunistic organisms associated with AIDS, including Candida albicans, cryptococcus, herpes virus, and mycobacteria.

Gasparis, A. P., and A. K. Tassiopoulos. "Nutritional Support in the Patient with HIV Infection," *Nutrition* 17, nos. 11–12 (November–December 2001): 981–982.

Gramlich, L. M., and E. A. Mascioli. "Nutrition and HIV Infection," *Nutritional Biochemistry* 6 (1995): 2–11.

airline meals Over the years, airlines have revised the meals they serve in order to meet consumer expectations for more healthful choices. Changes include more chicken and less beef and fewer saturated fats, like coconut and palm oil.

On noncharter flights passengers can choose from up to a dozen special dietary meals. The requests must be made at least 18 hours ahead of the scheduled flight. Religious meals include kosher, Hindu, and Muslim. For medical conditions, bland, diabetic, GLUTEN-free, low-CALORIE, low-CARBOHYDRATE, low-CHOLESTEROL, low-fat, and low-SODIUM meals may be offered. Other options include a FRUIT plate, SEAFOOD, strict VEGETARIAN, ovolactovegetarian, and infant, toddler, and child meals. First-class meals follow the same nutritional standards.

Passengers on long flights, especially those who have been diagnosed as having phlebitis, inflammation of the VEINS in the leg, or who have a history of heart disease or stroke are considered at high risk of developing deep-vein thrombosis (DVT). A person suffering from deep-vein thrombosis has one or more blood clots in the body's deep veins, often those in the legs. Because constant air circulation in planes promotes DEHYDRATION, and this, coupled with prolonged sitting, increases the risk of DVT in even healthy people, passengers should drink plenty of fluids, including water and JUICE, and avoid ALCOHOL, COFFEE, and TEA on long flights. About 4 percent to 5 percent of high-risk patients may suffer DVT on flights of 10 hours or more.

A brown-bag, carry-on meal is always an option for those with special dietary needs or with food sensitivities.

alanine (Ala, L-alanine) One of the simplest AMINO ACIDS used to build PROTEINS. Alanine is readily formed in the body from PYRUVIC ACID, a direct product of GLUCOSE utilization; hence, it is classified as a non-dietary, essential amino acid.

In addition to serving as a protein building block, alanine plays an important role in transporting the toxic waste product, AMMONIA, out of muscle. Ammonia is produced when muscle cells break down amino acids for energy. Cells couple ammonia with a simple acid called pyruvic acid to form alanine, which is then released into the bloodstream. The LIVER next absorbs alanine and removes ammonia, which it rapidly converts to UREA, the ultimate nitrogenous waste of the body. The liver converts pyruvic acid back to glucose, which is released into the bloodstream. Blood glucose is taken up by the muscle, where it is broken down to pyruvic acid, which is then ready to accept ammonia and thus completes the cycle.

Alar (daminozide) A chemical formerly used to improve the color, yield, and storage qualities of APPLES. It is not a PESTICIDE. Until the late 1980s, Alar was used on an estimated 5 percent to 10 percent of the American apple crop. It was also used on CHERRIES and PEANUTS. Alar is a systemic pollutant, meaning it is distributed throughout the plant and cannot be washed off. Because alar has caused CANCER in experimental animals, experts worried that because young children drink more apple juice for their body weight than do adults, they are more susceptible to the potential risk.

In 1989 Alar was withdrawn by the manufacturer, Uniroyal Chemical Company. The following year it was formally banned by the EPA. Alar is still sold abroad, however. About 50 percent of apple concentrates for apple juice comes from foreign countries where Alar is widely used, and imports may be contaminated by Alar.

albacore (*Thunnus [germo] alalunga*) A type of tuna with white meat. Albacore is characterized by a large pectoral (side) fin. One of the smallest tuna, albacore usually weigh less than 40 pounds (18 kg). They are found near the surface of warm or temperate seas throughout the world, where they feed on ANCHOVIES, SARDINES, and other small fish. Albacore have been called the "chicken of the sea" because their white meat is comparable to chicken in flavor. Albacore is the highest quality canned tuna and is an excellent PROTEIN source. The food value of 3 ounces (85g) (packed in water): calories, 135; protein, 30 g; fat, 1 g; cholesterol, 48 mg; calcium, 17 mg; iron, 0.6 mg; sodium, 468 mg; zinc, 0.94 mg; vitamin A, 32 retinol equivalents; thiamin, 10.03 mg; riboflavin, 0.1 mg; and niacin, 13.2 mg (See also FISH OIL.)

albumin A class of water-soluble PROTEINS that are soluble in dilute salt solutions but are insoluble in pure water. Important members of this class are serum albumin and ovalbumin. The LIVER produces serum albumin, the most plentiful protein in serum. Serum albumin transports ions like CALCIUM, free FATTY ACIDS, and fat-soluble materials like BILIRUBIN through the blood. Serum albumin also helps buffer the blood. It is a highly charged molecule (polyelectrolyte) that cannot pass through cell membranes and thus helps maintain the electrolyte balance of body fluids.

Ovalbumin is one of the most abundant proteins of egg white. The Roman author Pliny recorded the name of egg white as albumen. Ovalbumin is an excellent source of sulfur-containing amino acids, such as CYSTEINE, and this accounts in part for the excellent food value of egg protein. (See also ELECTROLYTES; LIVER.)

alcohol (ethanol, grain alcohol, ethyl alcohol) A common term for the simple alcohol ETHANOL, the product of FERMENTATION. As a constituent of alcoholic beverages, ethanol is the most common, and longest used, sedative. To produce alcohol, special strains of yeast are incubated with CARBOHYDRATES of FRUIT juices and GRAINS together with other nutrients. Under ANAEROBIC conditions (in the absence of oxygen), these microorganisms ferment sugar to ethanol and CARBON DIOXIDE to obtain energy. The immediate product of the fermentation of grapes is WINE. When malted grains and hops are fermented, the product is BEER. Distillation, a process introduced in the Middle Ages, produces alcoholic beverages with a higher alcohol content. These include rum, whiskey, liqueurs, and the like. Beer and wine are perhaps the most popular beverages among moderate drinkers. A mug of beer (11 oz., 4.5 percent), a glass of table wine (4 oz.) and a shot (jigger; 1.5 fl.oz.) of liquor (80 proof) contain about the same amount of alcohol (9 to 13 grams.)

Excessive consumption of alcoholic beverages can cause MALNUTRITION because alcoholic beverages contain little else besides CALORIES. A glass of red wine contains 88 calories; a bottle of regular beer, 146; and a shot (1.5 fl. oz.) of whiskey (90 proof), 110 calories. VITAMIN, PROTEIN, and MINERAL content of alcohol is exceedingly low, though wine may contain a significant amount of IRON. For this reason, alcoholic beverages are classified as low-nutrient density or EMPTY CALORIES. To the extent they are consumed, they displace nutrient-dense foods.

The blood alcohol level is affected by the amount of alcohol ingested. Water and juice slow the absorption of alcohol, while carbonation increases the rate of uptake into the bloodstream. Alcohol taken with food is less intoxicating. How alcohol is metabolized is another factor. A portion of the ingested alcohol is destroyed by ENZYMES in the stomach that are more active in men than in women; consequently, women generally have a lower tolerance to alcohol. The liver's capacity to destroy alcohol in the blood is limited, and when the liver's metabolic system is saturated, a fraction of ethanol in the blood is destroyed each hour. The remaining alcohol readily penetrates the blood-brain barrier and interacts with the central nervous system. Alcohol can pass from maternal blood into breast milk; therefore, lactating mothers may wish to abstain from drinking.

Some studies suggest that a single alcoholic drink a day may slightly reduce the risk of heart attack and stroke in some individuals. Moderate alcohol consumption increases the level of HDL, the beneficial form of cholesterol that tends to protect against heart disease. Alcohol also inhibits platelet formation, which is required to form blood clots. Moderate alcohol use may also help prevent age-related decline in reasoning and problem-solving. The apparent benefits decline after more than one or two drinks, however. The American Heart Association does not recommend drinking alcoholic beverages to prevent heart disease because of the hazards of alcohol abuse.

Possible consequences of excessive alcohol consumption including the following:

Birth Defects and Mental Retardation in Infants Drinking during pregnancy can lead to FETAL ALCOHOL SYNDROME.

Addiction Alcoholism is one of the most common addictions.

Intoxication Excessive alcohol can lead to a progressive deterioration of mental functioning. Alcohol is a depressant and slows down the nervous system, especially the brain. While moderate drinking can be relaxing, being intoxicated means the control centers are blocked, which can lead to memory lapses, decreased coordination, loss of inhibitions, confusion, mood swings, and depression. Most individuals will be adversely affected when the alcohol content of the blood rises above a threshold value. Legal intoxication in the United States is often defined as having a blood alcohol content ranging from 0.01 percent to 0.02 percent, depending upon the state. (Normally, the alcohol content of the blood is negligible.) Drunk drivers contribute significantly to traffic fatalities in the United States.

Aggravated High Blood Pressure Excessive alcohol consumption can worsen hypertension.

Increased Risk of Disease Alcohol injures the liver (CIRRHOSIS), the pancreas (PANCREATITIS), and the brain. It causes intestinal inflammation, interferes with nutrient uptake and may increase uptake of toxins. Heavy drinkers have increased risk of heart failure, and alcohol causes a dangerous enlargement of the heart. For this reason some researchers do not recommend that anyone past the age of 50 drink alcoholic beverages. Alcohol increases the risk of cancer of the esophagus, mouth, larynx, liver, and breast. Women who drink two to five alcoholic drinks a day increase their risk of invasive breast cancer 30 percent to 40 percent, according to the American Medical Association. Invasive cancer is the type most likely to spread to other TISSUES or organs.

Surplus Calories One gram of ethanol provides seven CALORIES, almost as much as FAT. One beer is equivalent to 150 calories. One shot (1.5 fl. oz.) of 80 proof gin, vodka, or rye whiskey contributes about 110 calories that supply no other nutritional value. Alcohol even increases the body's need for vitamins.

Exposure to Sulfites Wine contains SULFITE, which can cause reactions in sensitive people. (See also ALCOHOL-DRUG INTERACTIONS; ALCOHOLISM.)

Holmberg, L., J. A. Baron, T. Byers, et al. "Alcohol Intake and Breast Cancer Risk: Effect of Exposure from 15 Years of Age," *Cancer Epidemiology Biomarkers Prev* 4 (1995): 843–847.

Menzano, E., and P. L. Carlen. "Zinc Deficiency and Corticosteroids in the Pathogenesis of Alcoholic Brain Dysfunction: A Review," *Alcoholism, Clinical and Experimental Research,* 18, no. 4 (July/August 1994): 895–901.

Smith-Warner, S. A., D. Spiegelman, et al. "Alcohol and Breast Cancer in Women: A Pooled Analysis of Cohort Studies," *JAMA* 279 (1998): 535–540.

alcohol-drug interactions ALCOHOL interacts with many medications. Drinking alcohol can alter the way the body metabolizes drugs. As an example, the LIVER adapts to alcohol consumption by increasing its battery of drug-destroying ENZYMES. Because a heavy drinker may metabolize a sedative rapidly, its effects could wear off sooner than in a non-drinker, leaving the heavy drinker undersedated. Patients should read prescription labels carefully before drinking, and inform dentists, physicians, pharmacists, and other health care providers if they drink.

Interactions include:

Analgesics Non-prescription pain killers, such as Tylenol, that contain acetaminophen can damage the liver of those who consume several drinks a day. ASPIRIN together with alcohol increases stomach bleeding.

Antidepressants Monoamine oxidase inhibitors, AMPHETAMINES, and tricyclic antidepressants such as imipramine cause severe reactions and increased sedation, if taken with alcohol. Taking any one of several antidepressant drugs called selective serotonin reuptake inhibitors (SSRIs), including Prozac, Paxil, and Zoloft, can increase the effects of alcohol, including drowsiness and impaired motor skills.

Antihistamines Drinking after taking drugs like benadryl can lead to excessive drowsiness.

Arthritis Medications Indocin and other drugs prescribed for arthritis taken with alcohol can irritate the gastrointestinal tract and may cause dizziness.

Barbiturates Alcohol should never be combined with drugs like amytal or phenobarbital, which is the most hazardous combination. The additive effects of taking the depressants can lead to respiratory failure and coma.

Diabetic Medications Individuals taking Diabinese, Orinase, and other sulfonureas to treat diabetes will probably not be able to tolerate alcohol because these drugs can make the user ill after drinking alcoholic beverages.

Niacin Large doses of niacin taken with alcohol can reduce blood pressure excessively.

Prescription Pain Killers Codeine and narcotics combined with alcohol cause increased sedation.

Sedatives and Tranquilizers Combining alcohol and tranquilizers such as Valium and Thorazine can lead to oversedation and extreme drowsiness.

alcoholism A condition characterized by an uncontrollable urge to drink, a tolerance to increasing quantities of ALCOHOL, blackout episodes, and withdrawal symptoms during abstinence. Alcoholics frequently deny that they have a problem.

The costs of alcoholism to society are enormous. Excessive alcohol is involved in one out of 10 deaths in America and typically shortens the life span by 10 to 12 years. Alcoholism contributes to accidental death, crime, violence, and abuse. According to the National Highway Traffic Safety Administration, half of all fatalities due to automobile accidents have occurred in crashes in which the driver or pedestrian had been drinking. Estimates of the total cost of alcoholism to society range from $65 billion to $117 billion. Alcohol abuse occurs among young people as well as the elderly, encompasses people of all social and economic backgrounds, and women as well as men. Children of alcoholics are more likely to abuse alcohol and drugs. Individuals may be born susceptible to alcoholism due to imbalanced body chemistry; however, the social environment obviously plays an important role.

Alcoholism leads to disturbances of the GASTROINTESTINAL TRACT: Excessive ethanol directly or indirectly increases chronic intestinal inflammation associated with MALABSORPTION, comprised digestion, and "leaky gut," in which the intestine more readily absorbs toxins and potentially harmful substances from food and microorganisms that the body recognizes as foreign (antigens). This can set the stage for FOOD INTOLERANCE and systemic effects. Alcohol affects the LIVER, where altered GLUCOSE and GLYCOGEN METABOLISM, fat formation, and fat export can lead to fatty deposits (FATTY LIVER). The ability of the liver to detoxify other potentially damaging materials can also be compromised.

The alcoholic individual faces profound health consequences in terms of MALNUTRITION, heart failure, high blood pressure, damage to pancreas, liver, stomach and brain, and increased risk of CANCER of the mouth and esophagus. Even moderate alcohol intake can cause birth defects if the mother drinks during pregnancy.

Alcoholism is treatable; however, recovery depends on the person's willingness to accept help. Individualized recovery programs work best and may incorporate family counseling, psychotherapy, support groups, rehabilitation programs, education, behavior modification, vocational guidance, and exercise. Nutritional and medical treatment is often recommended to remedy nutritional deficiencies and alcohol-related disorders and to speed detoxification. A number of clinics treat alcoholism by incorporating lifestyle changes affecting DIET and EXERCISE, while eliminating CAFFEINE and nicotine. Alcoholics Anonymous (AA) can provide a very strong support system for recovery. (See also ADDICTION.)

aldicarb (Temik; Carbamyl) A very toxic insecticide widely used on POTATOES, SOYBEANS, PEANUTS, and citrus crops for control of chewing and sucking insects. Aldicarb was assumed to break down rapidly after application. However, tests show that it can persist in soil for years and contaminate crops planted in the same soil later. Several instances of aldicarb poisoning indicate the potential hazard of using this pesticide.

Symptoms of aldicarb toxicity include seizures, disorientation, blurred vision, and gastrointestinal disorders. The EPA recently limited the use of aldicarb and directed states to determine areas susceptible to contamination and then to monitor them, to assure concentrations do not exceed the limits set by the EPA. Activated charcoal filters can remove aldicarb from drinking water. (See also PESTICIDES.)

aldosterone A hormone of the adrenal glands responsible for regulating SODIUM in the blood. It is classified as a corticosteroid, a group of hormones synthesized by the adrenal cortex. Aldosterone is the principal MINERALOCORTICOID, which directs the KIDNEYS to conserve SODIUM by reabsorbing sodium and water from urine. In the kidneys, aldosterone stimulates the renal tubules to release POTASSIUM and hydrogen ions in place of sodium, thus increasing urine acidity. Mineralocorticoids also increase sodium reabsorption from sweat, SALIVA, and GASTRIC JUICES. Other steroid hormones, deoxycorticosterone, corticosterone, and progesterone, can also cause sodium retention, though they are much less active.

Stimuli that increase aldosterone secretion include SURGERY, anxiety, physical trauma, high potassium intake, low sodium intake, and diseases of the heart, LIVER, and kidneys. The pituitary hormone ACTH stimulates steroid hormone release from the adrenal glands. Aldosterone is also regulated by the kidneys in response to low serum sodium levels. The kidneys produce an enzyme, RENIN, which forms the hormone ANGIOTENSIN in the blood that stimulates aldosterone release. (See also ADRENAL GLANDS; ANTIDIURETIC HORMONE; FLUID BALANCE.)

ale See BEER.

alfalfa (*Medicago sativa*) A LEGUME used primarily for fodder throughout the world. As a nutritional supplement, this plant is a rich source of TRACE MINERALS, BETA-CAROTENE, ESSENTIAL FATTY ACIDS, VITAMIN K, and the B COMPLEX vitamins. Alfalfa contains significant FIBER and is a rich source of PROTEIN (25 percent by weight). In Asia, alfalfa leaves are used in the form of greens as a VEGETABLE.

Claims that alfalfa boosts the IMMUNE SYSTEM may relate to its trace mineral content. It also has antibacterial activity, and there is some evidence that alfalfa can induce LIVER detoxifying enzymes that destroy toxins and pollutants. Alfalfa contains several classes of compounds, including SAPONINS, STEROLS, and FLAVONOIDS, which can affect the body. For example, alfalfa saponins decrease blood cholesterol levels in lab animals. Alfalfa may reduce damage due to radiation, perhaps due to the ANTIOXIDANTS it contains. Individuals who have heart disease, who are pregnant, who have a tendency to clot easily or take anticoagulants should avoid alfalfa supplements because their vitamin K content may promote blood clotting. Avoid consuming excessive amounts of alfalfa during pregnancy and when breast-feeding, because it contains substances with weak estrogenic activity.

Alfalfa sprouts are a healthful alternative to LETTUCE because it contains beta-carotene, VITAMIN C, and trace minerals at levels higher than those found in iceberg lettuce. In contrast with most lettuce, alfalfa sprouts are not treated with PESTICIDES. Alfalfa sprouts (100 g) provide 54 calories; protein, 6 g; carbohydrate, 9.5 g; fiber, 3.1 g; fat, 0.4 g; calcium, 215 mg; iron, 2.3 mg; thiamin 0.13 mg; riboflavin, 0.14 mg; niacin, 0.5 mg.

algae (seaweed) Simple plants found in fresh water and oceans throughout the world. Algae are largely undifferentiated and, unlike terrestrial plants, algal leaves and stems are composed of the same tissue. Edible species are either grown or collected along coastal intertidal zones. In Japan, six types are consumed, and together they account for an estimated 10 percent of the country's total food production.

Edible brown algae, which represent most of the edible seaweed harvested worldwide, include arame, hiziki, kelp, and kombu. Edible red algae include CARRAGEENAN (Irish moss), dulse, and nori. These "sea vegetables" are rich sources of MAGNESIUM, IRON, IODINE, and CALCIUM, and some are as rich in vitamins such as VITAMIN C, BETA-CAROTENE, VITAMIN E, and the B COMPLEX as the best cultivated sources. In addition, various algae are used commercially as sources of gums (AGAR, carrageenan, and ALGINATE). Carrageenan has the ability to form salt gels in milk products and is used to keep fats from separating, and to thicken ICE CREAM. Alginic acid (alginate) in brown seaweed can bind toxic metals in the body and speed their removal. These algae can be added to SOUPS, VEGETABLES, SALADS, BEAN dishes, and GRAINS to add zest and boost nutritional value. Their flavor is neither fishy nor salty.

There is little information on toxic metal contamination of any domestic or imported seaweed. One study found very low amounts of arsenic, cadmium, lead, and mercury in common imported varieties; the levels were well below limits set by the Food Chemicals Codex of the Food and Nutrition Board. Mercury levels were far below the limits set for fish.

alginate (ammonium, calcium, potassium, and sodium salts of alginic acid) A food additive obtained from the giant kelp, a brown algae commercially harvested off the coast of California. Alginate is a major constituent of the cell wall and consists of polymers of acidic sugars Alginate is used by the food industry as a thickening and stabilizing agent because calcium alginate forms very stable gels in water. It prevents jelly in pastries from melting during baking and provides smooth textures to ICE CREAM, YOGURT and CHEESE, CANDY, whipped cream in pressurized cans, and canned frosting. Alginate also helps keep cocoa butter dispersed in chocolate milk. The red PIMENTO stuffed in green OLIVES contains the most alginate (6 percent) of any food source. Alginate is not used in acidic foods and beverage such as salad dressings and SOFT DRINKS, because it forms sediment under these conditions.

Alginate is on the GENERALLY RECOGNIZED AS SAFE (GRAS) list of the U.S. FDA. Short-term animal testing indicates the alginate is not absorbed by the body and is not toxic. Because alginate forms highly charged gels in water, it remains to be determined whether it can limit the absorption of minerals and other nutrients by the body. (See also FOOD ADDITIVES.)

alimentary canal See DIGESTIVE TRACT.

alimentation The physiologic processes by which food nurtures and maintains the body. These include chewing (MASTICATION), swallowing, and digesting food. Alimentation also encompasses the ABSORPTION of NUTRIENTS (VITAMINS MINERALS, AMINO ACIDS, FAT, CARBOHYDRATES) by the intestine and their use in CATABOLISM (energy production) and in ANABOLISM (building cellular constituents). The term *alimentary canal* refers to the digestive cavity running from the MOUTH to the anus.

Artificial alimentation refers to feeding a patient artificially either by intravenous procedures or by a nasal tube. Forced alimentation is feeding a patient who is unwilling to eat. (See also DIGESTION; HYPERALIMENTATION.)

alitame A non-caloric ARTIFICIAL SWEETENER that is 2,000 times sweeter than sugar that has not yet been approved by the U.S. Food and Drug Administration. This sweetener was developed to be safer than ASPARTAME. Unlike aspartame, alitame does not contain phenylalanine and consequently would likely be safe for individuals with PHENYLKETONURIA (PKU), a genetic intolerance to this amino acid.

alkalemia A blood condition characterized by excessive alkalinity (excessively high pH). A blood pH greater than 7.4 is considered alkaline and represents an accumulation of hydroxide ions and depletion of hydrogen ions, CARBON DIOXIDE, and CARBONIC ACID. The body is exquisitely buffered to keep blood pH slightly alkaline, within a very narrow range, 7.35–7.45. However, this equilibrium can be shifted by loss of STOMACH ACID through vomiting; by the consumption of alkaline medications such as those used to treat ulcers; and by rapid breathing (hyperventilation), which rapidly decreases the body's stores of carbon dioxide.

The body compensates for alkalemia and reestablishes normal blood pH by slowing the respiration rate (breathing); this increases the level of carbon dioxide in the blood, which spontaneously forms more carbonic acid. The KIDNEYS can compensate for elevated pH by excreting alkaline urine. (See also ALKALOSIS; BUFFER; ELECTROLYTES.)

alkali-forming foods See ACID-FORMING FOODS.

alkaline A solution with a pH greater than 7.0, which is considered neutral. Alkaline solutions are also called basic, as opposed to acidic. MILK, BLOOD, and EGG yolk are examples of slightly alkaline solutions. Solutions of BAKING SODA (sodium bicarbonate) and AMMONIA form mildly alkaline solutions. In contrast, the corrosive metallic hydroxides such as sodium hydroxide (lye, caustic soda) are very strong bases and are very alkaline. They destroy TISSUE, create burns, and are considered toxic substances.

alkaline tide The slight rise in blood pH following a meal, when the BLOOD temporarily becomes more ALKALINE. When the STOMACH produces hydrochloric acid (STOMACH ACID) for use in DIGESTION, it removes a fraction of negatively charged CHLORIDE ions from circulation. Chloride is then replaced by BICARBONATE in the blood, which tends to raise blood pH. As the meal is digested, chloride ions are reabsorbed by the INTESTINE and again enter the bloodstream. In turn, bicarbonate is reabsorbed and the pH returns to normal. The URINE may become more alkaline during digestion as the body compensates for the change in blood pH.

alkaloids A large, diverse class of organic compounds prevalent in the plant kingdom that contain nitrogen and function as bases. Often alkaloids profoundly affect the body's physiology, and purified alkaloids are even more active. Examples of potent alkaloids include morphine, cocaine, quinine, strychnine, nicotine, CAFFEINE (COFFEE), and theobromine (CHOCOLATE). Depending upon the application and the dose, alkaloids may be used in therapy or they may cause toxicity. Socrates was killed by the alkaloid coniine that occurs in hemlock. Eating quail that have eaten poison hemlock can cause food poisoning in humans. Alkaloids such as nicotine and caffeine are addictive substances. Morphine and cocaine are controlled substances due to their addictive properties.

alkalosis Excessive alkalinity (elevated pH) of body fluids caused by either an accumulation of alkaline substances or a reduction in ACIDS. Alkalosis is thus more general than ALKALEMIA (alkaline blood). Respiratory alkalosis occurs with hyperventilation, aspirin poisoning, abnormal brain function, or inadequate oxygen supply, as may occur during exertion at high altitudes. Metabolic alkalosis occurs with severe VOMITING due to losses of hydrogen ions and chloride ions (STOMACH ACID); losses of POTASSIUM due to diuretic therapy; and ingestion of BAKING SODA (or other alkaline substances). Symptoms of both types of alkalosis include shallow breathing, a tingling sensation at fingertips and toes, muscular cramps, and convulsions. Like prolonged ACIDOSIS, alkalosis requires medical intervention. (See also BUFFER; ELECTROLYTES.)

allergen A substance or agent that causes an allergic reaction. Allergens provoke the IMMUNE SYSTEM when it senses an allergen as a foreign substance and overreacts. This "hypersensitivity" may be immediate, when symptoms appear within minutes to several hours after exposure, or it can be delayed, when symptoms appear hours after exposure or longer.

At the top of the list of food allergens are DAIRY products, PEANUTS, nuts (e.g., HAZELNUTS, CASHEWS), GRAINS (especially WHEAT and CORN), SOYBEAN products, CITRUS FRUITS, and SHELLFISH. The binders and other ingredients of vitamin supplements, as well as HERBS and SPICES, can cause reactions in susceptible individuals. Prescription drugs (including penicillin), antisera, and constituents of infectious agents (including bacteria and viruses, yeast, and parasites) can be allergens. Physical agents, including radiation, heat, and pressure may also provoke inflammation, an aspect of the immune response. In provoking an immune response, allergens typically react with ANTIBODIES, protective proteins formed by specialized cells of the immune system. (See also ALLERGY, FOOD.)

allergic rhinitis This condition refers to allergy symptoms associated with the chronic inflammation typical of hay fever: a perpetually stuffy, runny nose, sneezing, puffy bags and dark circles under the eyes, and a puffy face. Allergic rhinitis can lead to chronic earaches, especially in children, and to inflamed sinuses (sinusitis). It is more common among children, but can occur at any age. Allergic rhinitis is the result of a specific type of ANTIBODY, IgE, which binds to mast cells, defensive cells of the IMMUNE SYSTEM, to stimulate inflammation. Therefore allergic rhinitis can be measured by a skin test. Nasal symptoms occur immediately after exposure to common allergens, including pollen, animal dander, house dust, mites, insects, MOLD, and foods. Identification of the offending substance and reduced exposure are important; complete avoidance may be curative.

allergy, food An abnormal reaction of the IMMUNE SYSTEM to normally harmless foods. An allergic response involves two aspects of the immune system: circulating ANTIBODIES and specialized attack cells. Each branch of the immune system can react to foods as though they were foreign invaders. In contrast, other types of FOOD SENSITIVITY such as LACTOSE INTOLERANCE do not depend on antibody reactions, nor do they involve other aspects of the immune system.

Allergy patterns may change during a lifetime; old sensitivities may vanish, and new ones may appear according to the health of the immune system and to the amount of allergen exposure. Introducing solid foods before an infant's DIGESTIVE TRACT is fully developed carries an increased risk of the development of food allergies. Children are more likely to suffer from allergies than adults, though they often outgrow them. Individuals who have relatives with allergies are more prone to develop food allergies themselves. Food allergies are more likely to occur with inadequate nutrition, infections, and physical and emotional stress. Faulty DIGESTION and intestinal inflammation can allow food ALLERGENS to penetrate intestinal barriers and enter the bloodstream.

Depending on how food allergy is defined, estimates of the prevalence of food allergies range from 2 percent to 25 percent of the U.S. population. Opinion is also divided regarding the predominant form of food allergies. Those who consider food allergy an uncommon phenomenon focus on the readily observable, rapid systemic reactions to foods. These generate hay fever–like symptoms (immediate hypersensitivity). Other research indicates that typical food allergies are complex immune reactions resulting in delayed hypersensitivity. They frequently involve antibodies in the blood (IgG type), and symptoms develop over hours or days after consuming the problem food. This delay increases the difficulty in relating a specific food to sometimes vague symptoms.

The most common symptom of food allergy is FATIGUE. Other symptoms range from those typical of PREMENSTRUAL SYNDROME to HYPOGLYCEMIA, eczema, irritability, achy joints, puffy eyes with dark circles, or postnasal drip. Food allergies may produce asthma in the respiratory tract; in the brain, insomnia, mood changes, confusion, or fatigue; in the gastrointestinal tract, INDIGESTION, irritable colon, CONSTIPATION, or DIARRHEA.

A simple, proven method of coping with food allergies is abstinence. Avoiding the offending food for several days to several weeks may allow the immune system to return to normal. If symptoms recur when the questionable food is eaten again, that food is probably the culprit. ROTATION DIETS have been devised to minimize exposure to allergenic foods. Because allergy-restricted diets can be difficult to balance nutritionally, those who have multiple food allergies may wish to consult both a physician and a nutritionist. Individuals with food allergies often need to find substitutes for common foods. A wide variety of food allergy cookbooks are now available to help plan delicious, nutritious meals. The U.S. Government Printing Office publishes *Cooking for People with Food Allergies.* (See also ALLERGY, IMMEDIATE; ALLERGIC RHINITIS; CHALLENGE TESTING.)

Brostoff, Jonathan, and Linda Gamlin. *Food Allergies and Food Intolerance: The Complete Guide to Their Identification and Treatment.* Rochester, Vt.: Healing Arts Press, 2000.

Walsh, William E. *Food Allergies: The Complete Guide to Understanding and Relieving Your Food Allergies.* New York: Wiley, 2000.

allergy, immediate (immediate hypersensitivity) An inflammatory reaction responsible for the familiar hay fever, asthma, and hives due to exposure to an ALLERGEN. These symptoms seldom leave any doubt as to their cause. The key lies within mast cells, defending cells embedded in tissues, which carry a bound ANTIBODY (IgE) on their surfaces. Upon contact with an invader, mast cells release inflammatory agents such as histamine and leukotrienes that evoke swelling, itchiness, copious mucous secretion, and the spasm of muscles of the intestinal tract and of air passageways (bronchioles).

Common materials often trigger fast-developing reactions: dust, pollen, animal dander, medications, disease-producing microorganisms, and pollutants. Seafood, milk, sulfites, PEANUTS, and strawberries are a few of the food-related causes of immediate hypersensitivity. It may come as a surprise that immediate allergic reactions account for a small fraction of food allergies. Most food allergies are of the slow-reacting type.

Anaphylactic shock is the condition resulting from allergic reaction and affects the whole body quickly. It produces labored breathing, fever, erratic heartbeat, violent coughing, hives and edema, even convulsions. This severe response can be life-threatening. Individuals who are susceptible to severe allergy attacks may be advised to carry injectable medications ("bee sting" kits containing adrenalin or other drugs). (See also ALLERGY, FOOD.)

allspice (*Pimenta officinalis;* Jamaican pepper) A spice prepared from ground, unripened, reddish-brown berries of an evergreen tree found in the Caribbean, Central America, and Mexico. Its name derives from the observation that its aroma resembles a blend of cloves, cinnamon, nutmeg, and juniper berries. Allspice is used to season sausage, salt beef, pickle sauces, and marinades.

almond (*Prunus amygdalus*) A cultivated, elongated nut with white meat and a brown skin. The almond tree resembles the PEACH, to which it is related. The almond originated in Asia and was known to the Romans as the "Greek nut." There are two varieties: the sweet almond and the bitter almond, which has a stronger flavor.

Almond extracts are used to flavor cakes and pastries, and slivered or flaked sweet almonds are used in cakes, cookies, and pastry. Dried almonds are served raw or roasted and salted. Nuts roasted with coconut or palm oil dramatically increase their caloric content and increase their SATURATED FAT content. Almonds are also used as ingredients of stuffings and couscous, and they can accompany FISH or POULTRY dishes (the garnish is known as amandine). Almonds are a good source of CALCIUM and they are also rich in oil. Most of the oil is monounsaturated and more closely resembles OLIVE OIL than typical vegetable oils like SAFFLOWER oil, which are high in polyunsaturates. One ounce (28 g) of raw, sweet almonds provides 167 calories; carbohydrate, 5.7 g; fiber, 3 g; fat, 14.8 g; protein, 5.9 g; calcium, 75 mg; iron, 1.0 mg; niacin, 0.95 mg; thiamin, 0.06 mg; riboflavin, 0.22 mg.

aloe vera A succulent plant with long pointed leaves that produces a JUICE with medicinal properties. There are hundreds of different aloe species. Aloe extracts are a folk remedy, long used to treat mild burns, insect bites, abrasions, minor cuts and chafing, fever blisters, poison ivy, and to relieve joint inflammation and allergic reactions. Research has yielded mixed results. Most human studies have been uncontrolled. Evidence suggests that aloe vera may help heal ulcers and gastrointestinal inflammation and fight infections by boosting the immune system. Although a 1985 U.S. FDA study group concluded that aloe vera did not heal burns, recent clinical studies indicate burn healing is speeded up by aloe, possibly by improving collagen formation and by improving blood flow to damaged areas. There is preliminary evidence that aloe may help prevent severe conditions such as CANCER. Very rarely, aloe vera may cause a rash in sensitive people, and pregnant women should not take aloe internally. Aloe vera skin gel may slow the healing of infected surgical incisions.

alpha linolenic acid Chemically speaking, this FATTY ACID has 18 carbons and a pair of double bonds. It cannot be synthesized by the body and must be obtained from the diet. A POLYUNSATURATED FATTY ACID, it is classified as an essential dietary nutrient. Alpha linolenic acid is the smallest of the omega-3 family of polyunsaturated fatty acids, distinguished by subtle structural differences in which the double bonds begin at the third carbon from the end. It is the building block of larger omega-3 acids, including EICOSOPENTAENOIC ACID and DOCOSOHEXAENOIC ACID (DHA), which in turn form the PG_3 class of PROSTAGLANDINS, hormone-like substances that decrease inflammation, decrease blood clotting and lower blood CHOLESTEROL. PG_3 prostaglandins help return the body to equilibrium after physical stress or injury.

Omega-3 fatty acids are deficient in the standard American diet, and this deficiency may be linked to an increased risk of heart attacks and inflammation associated with degenerative disease. Chronic, severe deficiencies impair vision, increase inflammation, and diminish learning curves in experimental animals. The utilization of alpha linolenic acid may be limited in some disease states. The nervous system and brain contain high levels of the omega-3 fatty acids, and there is a positive relationship between the content of these fatty acids in the diet and vision and brain function. Pre-term babies need DHA because their livers are not mature enough to synthesize it from alpha linolenic acid.

Good dietary sources of the omega-3 fatty acids are limited. Breast milk contains omega-3 fatty acids, suggesting their importance in an infant's growth and development. Food processing destroys or removes the omega-3s, and there are none in FAST FOODS such as PIZZA, fried FISH sandwiches, fried chicken, or HAMBURGERS. The most common sources are fish and FISH OILS, FLAXSEED OIL, and pumpkin seeds; fish oil and flaxseed oil are sold as supplements. Because oils containing essential fatty acids readily oxidize and become rancid they need to be protected from oxygen and heat. They are usually packaged with ANTIOXIDANTS, such as VITAMIN E. Buying small quantities of these oils and refrigerating them in sealed containers after opening reduces the risk of rancidity. These oils should not be used for cooking.

alpha tocopherol See VITAMIN E.

aluminum A metallic ion that is widely distributed in water and soil. Drinking water often contains aluminum beyond levels leached from soil and clay because aluminum hydroxide is often added to municipal water supplies to clarify drinking water.

Aluminum is often added to food. Aluminum compounds make PROCESSED FOOD more creamy and pourable. They are quite versatile and are found in INFANT FORMULA, pickles, relishes, BEER, CREAM OF TARTAR, grated CHEESE, canned foods, BAKING POWDER, and self-rising FLOUR. Aluminum is also found in the medicine chest: A major source of aluminum is ANTACIDS (such as Maalox), which have a high aluminum hydroxide content. Antiperspirants, over-the-counter analgesics (pain relievers, such as buffered ASPIRIN for arthritis), and other pain medications contain aluminum. The average daily intake from all sources ranges from 10 to 100 mg. Most of this is not absorbed; of the fraction of aluminum that is absorbed by the body, most is subsequently excreted.

Although aluminum is not a heavy metal, accumulated evidence suggests that this substance may be harmful. Aluminum may cause dialysis dementia, SENILITY, and brain damage in young patients undergoing hemodialysis for kidney failure. Their increased aluminum intake is due to the use of antacids containing aluminum and to the elevated aluminum content of water used for dialysis. More generally, high levels of aluminum may inhibit phosphate uptake by the intestine and may increase CALCIUM losses by excretion by the kidneys. The imbalance may cause brittle bones and may disturb bone formation. Other evidence suggests that excessive aluminum impairs the body's immunity.

Aluminum seems to accumulate in the brain with age, and high levels of aluminum are found in the brains of victims of ALZHEIMER'S DISEASE. Whether this is a cause or an effect of the disease is not known.

Patients with kidney disease and anyone regularly consuming antacids that contain aluminum compounds should be aware of the risks. Patients should avoid taking medications containing aluminum with orange juice (CITRIC ACID); this combination can dramatically increase aluminum uptake in the body. Acidic foods like TOMATO sauce, applesauce, and SAUERKRAUT should not be placed in aluminum foil or in uncoated aluminum cookware because these foods dissolve aluminum, which can then be absorbed.

Alzheimer's disease A progressive, degenerative disease of the brain and the leading cause of SENILITY in the United States. About 4 million Americans have Alzheimer's disease, roughly 10 percent of the U.S. population over the age of 65 and nearly half of the population over 85. The disease can also strike younger adults (a small percentage of people in their 30s and 40s have Alzheimer's). On average, a person lives between eight and 20 years after the onset of symptoms, which include short-term memory loss, difficulty performing simple tasks, and disorientation to time and place. Alzheimer's disease results from the death of nerve cells in the forebrain and the hippocampus responsible for memory and learning. Patients also have a deficiency of ACETYLCHOLINE, a NEUROTRANSMITTER made by neurons that helps carry nerve impulses between cells. Currently, diagnosis of Alzheimer's disease is very difficult, yet a comprehensive diagnosis is critical in treating the senile patient.

Symptoms occurring before the age of 65 are designated early-onset Alzheimer's; after 65, it is called late-onset Alzheimer's.

Despite intensive research over the last decade, it is not known whether Alzheimer's disease is a function of AGING, or whether it is the result of a specific disease process. Alzheimer's seems to be a multifaceted disease, with environmental and genetic factors contributing. There is an association with Down's syndrome and thyroid disease. Smoking a pack of cigarettes a day increases the odds of developing Alzheimer's disease. Diet also plays a part. A healthy diet with low fat intake may reduce the risk of developing Alzheimer's disease; studies also suggest that a high-fat diet during early and mid-adulthood may be associated with an increased risk of developing Alzheimer's, especially in people with a genetic marker called apoE-4. In a retrospective study that examined food eaten by 304 men and women (72 with Alzheimer's disease and 232 healthy individuals), researchers found that people with the apoE-4 gene who also ate the most fat were seven times more likely to develop Alzheimer's than were people with the marker who ate lower-fat diets. In a separate 2000 study of Americans between the ages of 40 and 50, those who carried the apoE-4 gene and whose diet consisted of 40 percent fat calories had 29 times the risk for Alzheimer's compared to non-apoE-4 carriers on the same high-fat diet.

Some population studies have reported an association between low-fat diets and a lower incidence in Alzheimer's. For example, in China and Nigeria, where fat intake is low, the risk of developing Alzheimer's is 1 percent at age 65 compared to 5 percent in the United States. In the Netherlands researchers reported an association between dementia and diets high in total fat, saturated fat, and cholesterol.

Scientists have identified four genes that increase the risk of developing Alzheimer's. APOE-4 is implicated in late-onset cases. This gene can be passed down from one or both parents. Patients who have one copy of the gene have a three times greater risk of developing the disease than do patients who do not. Patients who inherit two copies have an eight times greater risk of developing Alzheimer's. The other three genes—presenilin 1, presenilin 2, and amyloid precursor protein—are associated with early-onset cases. Nearly everyone who carries one or more of these genes will develop early-onset Alzheimer's.

Another hypothesis for Alzheimer's links chronic CALCIUM deficiency to increased uptake of ALUMINUM and silicon by the brain. Aluminum concentrates in the brains of patients with the disease; whether this is a cause or an effect is unknown. In postmenopausal women, estrogen (hormone) replacement therapy may help prevent Alzheimer's. The importance of estrogen in brain health is gradually being recognized. Alternatively, there may be alterations in nerve cell membranes. Other evidence links immune system activation with the disease process.

Research points to the following possible causes of senility: exposure to toxins, oxidative damage due to FREE RADICALS, abnormal protein metabolism, slow viruses, the narrowing by cholesterol deposits of arteries feeding the brain, ZINC and VITAMIN B_{12} deficiencies, head trauma, and adverse drug reactions that decrease blood and oxygen supply to the brain.

Clinical trials of an experimental vaccine for the disease, called AN-1792, were halted abruptly in early 2002 when several participants developed brain inflammation after taking it. The drug was a form of beta-amyloid, a protein fragment found in the amyloid plaques that grow over the brain tissue of Alzheimer's patients. Researchers had hoped exposure to the protein would trigger participants' IMMUNE SYSTEMS to produce antibodies to the amyloid plaques.

Experiments in mice have shown that FOLIC ACID—a vitamin found in high amounts in dark green, leafy VEGETABLES, CITRUS FRUITS and JUICES, whole wheat BREAD, and dry BEANS—may help ward off Alzheimer's disease. Since 1998 the U.S. FDA has required the addition of folic acid to enriched breads, CEREALS, FLOURS, CORNMEAL, PASTA, RICE, and other GRAIN products.

There is limited evidence that antioxidants may help fight or prevent some of the brain cell damage in Alzheimer's disease that may be attributed to free radicals, thus slowing the progression of the disease. In particular, some evidence suggests that vitamin C or vitamin E supplements can slow the course of Alzheimer's over several years. In a National Institute on Aging study, the antioxidant vitamin E delayed by six months the progression of some symptoms of Alzheimer's disease.

In another National Institute on Aging study, people in the middle to late stages of Alzheimer's who took vitamin E at levels 70 times higher than the recommended daily dose noticed some beneficial effects. At a dose of 2,000 IU daily, vitamin E was able to slow the expected rate of decline compared to patients who did not take the vitamin.

Other studies suggest that taking antioxidants (vitamins C and E) might significantly lower the risk of developing Alzheimer's. In one preliminary

Massachusetts study, none of the 50 subjects who used either vitamin C or E developed Alzheimer's at follow-up studies. In a Dutch study of 5,000 people, a diet high in antioxidants reduced the risk of developing Alzheimer's.

Other antioxidants, such as GINKGO biloba and PHOSPHATIDYLSERINE, melatonin, flavonoids (chemicals found in many plants, including fruits and vegetables), and carotenoids (pigments found in plants such as carrots) also may help ease symptoms of Alzheimer's disease. Small studies of ginkgo did find slight improvement among patients with Alzheimer's who took the herb. Although German physicians have approval to use ginkgo to treat Alzheimer's, and it has been used for thousands of years in Chinese medicine, North American physicians disagree as to its benefits as a memory treatment.

According to several studies, eating plenty of dark-colored fruits and vegetables may slow brain aging. Extracts of blueberries and strawberries reversed age-related decline in lab animal brain function. Blueberries may be the best anti-Alzheimer's antioxidant of all. When Tufts University researchers analyzed more than 40 fruits and vegetables, they found that raw blueberries contained the highest level of antioxidants (nearly 60 times the recommended daily levels)—more than blackberries, beets, spinach, and garlic. Animals fed an antioxidant-rich blueberry extract diet showed fewer age-related motor changes and outperformed their study counterparts on memory tests.

Some studies on wine have reported a lower risk, but they have not been consistent. It might be that wine may increase even more risk of developing Alzheimer's for people who carry the apoE-4 gene that has been linked to Alzheimer's—while protecting people who do not carry the gene.

However, supplements containing high doses of antioxidants can cause adverse effects. In addition, high doses of vitamin E are potentially harmful if combined with blood-thinning drugs. No one should take these or any supplements without consulting a doctor.

It is safer to consume antioxidants as part of a healthy diet; antioxidants are found in most dark colored fruits and vegetables, whole grains, legumes, nuts, and wheat germ.

Nutritional approaches to treatment employ CHOLINE and LECITHIN (phosphatidylcholine) supplements. The rationale for their use is based on the fact that the brains of diseased patients do not make enough acetylcholine, and supplying this building block could boost acetylcholine production. Results of clinical studies have not shown consistent improvements. Researchers have used drugs that help maintain acetylcholine levels with mixed results. A growth promoter called nerve growth factor may enhance brain function in aged experimental animals. Preliminary research suggests that GINKGO biloba, a leaf extract, is known to have antioxidant and anti-inflammatory properties and to enhance NEUROTRANSMITTER function, alleviates the symptoms of Alzheimer's disease.

Scientists are currently studying whether a low-fat, high-fiber diet may reduce the risk of developing Alzheimer's disease just as it lowers the risk of other diseases associated with aging, like cardiovascular disease and cancer. Finnish researchers who studied 1,500 patients for 21 years found that subjects with high CHOLESTEROL and high blood pressure had a corresponding higher risk of developing Alzheimer's. French researchers noted a link between high blood pressure and Alzheimer's risk. (See also CARNITINE; SENILITY.)

Rogaeva E., A. Tandon, and P. H. St. George-Hyslop. "Genetic Markers in the Diagnosis of Alzheimer's Disease." *Journal of Alzheimer's Disease* 3, no. 3 (June 2001): 293–304.

Stramek, J., and N. Cutler. "Recent Developments in the Drug Treatment of Alzheimer's Disease," *Drugs and Aging* 14, no. 5 (1999): 359–373.

amanita A genus of MUSHROOM that includes many poisonous species, along with a few edible ones. Amanita species can be confused with edible mushrooms. The most common cause of mushroom poisoning is the ingestion of *A. phalloides* (death cap) and *A. virosa* (destroying angel). These species produce specific toxins called amatoxins and phallotoxins, compounds with cyclic AMINO ACID structures. A single mushroom may contain enough of these poisons to kill an adult. Eating the mushroom can cause LIVER, HEART, and KIDNEY damage, as well as symptoms of common shock and delirium.

amaranth (***Amaranthus cruentus;*** **grain amaranth)** A nutritious alternative to WHEAT. The tiny spherical seeds are the size of poppy seeds. Originally grown in Mexico as a staple food of the Aztecs, it was eaten in rituals of Native Americans until the Spanish conquest of Mexico, when its cultivation was outlawed. Amaranth is now cultivated in the United States, and its excellent nutritional qualities account for its present popularity. Amaranth possesses a higher PROTEIN content than most CEREAL GRAINS; the nutritional value of amaranth protein approaches that of MILK. Its protein contains a high percentage of the essential AMINO ACID lysine, which is low in other grain proteins like wheat. Amaranth does not contain typical wheat ALLERGENS, nor does it contain GLUTEN; therefore, people allergic to wheat can often eat amaranth because it belongs to an unrelated plant family. Amaranth is available in health food stores as a whole grain, a FLOUR, and as CRACKERS and breakfast cereals. Amaranth flour has a nutty flavor and can be used to supplement wheat flour. Popped amaranth seed is mixed with honey to make a Mexican confection known as alegria. Amaranth species have also been cultivated in Asia as a source of greens (*een choi* in China, *hiyu* in Japan, and CHAULAI in India). One hundred grams of amaranth provides protein, 15 g; carbohydrate, 66 g; fiber, 4.5 g; fat, 5.7 g; and fat, 4.5 g.

amine A very large family of basic organic compounds that contain nitrogen. Amines become positively charged ions (cations) in the blood. Physiologically important amines include the hormones EPINEPHRINE (adrenaline) and norepinephrine, and neurotransmitters such as ACETYLCHOLINE and SEROTONIN, chemicals released by activated nerve cells. CHOLINE serves as a raw material for both acetylcholine and LECITHIN, a common LIPID of cell membranes. All AMINO ACIDS used to build PROTEINS have properties of amines. Tyramine found in fermented foods is an amine that can cause headache and food sensitivities. A variety of amines in food can react with the food additive nitrite to produce cancer-causing substances (nitrosoamines).

amino acid metabolism Chemical processes by which amino acids are either synthesized or are broken down and are used for energy in the body. Amino acid synthesis is important because approximately half of the different amino acids used as PROTEIN building blocks can be made from CARBOHYDRATES. Amino acids such as ALANINE, GLUTAMIC ACID, and GLUTAMINE made by the brain and MUSCLE help transport NITROGEN waste products via the bloodstream to the LIVER for disposal. When amino acids are degraded, the first step (transamination) releases nitrogen with the help of VITAMIN B_6. The final nitrogen-containing waste product is UREA.

The second step of amino acid degradation requires the oxidation of the carbon atoms of amino acids to produce ATP, the energy currency of cells. The waste product is CARBON DIOXIDE. An alternative route permits the liver to convert most amino acids to blood sugar (GLUCOSE) when the diet does not provide adequate carbohydrates that can be digested to glucose to fuel the brain. This process is called GLUCONEOGENESIS. HEME (the pigment of red blood cells), neurotransmitters (brain chemicals that carry nerve impulses), purines (building blocks of RNA and DNA), and HORMONES represent important amino acid derivatives. (See also UREA CYCLE.)

amino acids (alpha amino acids) Small organic acids that serve as raw materials of PROTEINS. The 50,000 to 100,000 different proteins in the body are combinations of just 20 different types of amino acids. During protein synthesis, amino acids are linked together like beads on a string to form long chains (polypeptides). Each type of protein possesses a unique amino acid sequence, specified by the cell's genes.

As the name implies, each amino acid possesses an amino group and a carboxylic acid functional group, and therefore amino acids behave as both ACIDS and BASES. They also possess side chains with different properties. For example, certain amino acids, like ASPARTIC ACID and GLUTAMIC ACID, are acidic; others like ARGININE and LYSINE are basic; METHIONINE and CYSTEINE contain SULFUR. Another group repels water and has the branched chains: VALINE, LEUCINE, and ISOLEUCINE.

Just as hands and feet are mirror images of each other, amino acids occur as mirror-image forms (optical isomers). The left-hand forms are designated as "L," and the right-handed opposites are designated as "D." Only L-amino acids are supplied by food and synthesized in the body, and only the "L" forms occur in proteins. Therefore, unless indicated otherwise, an amino acid can be assumed to be the "L-" form when mentioned in nutrition literature. The only common amino acid that does not exist as optical isomers is glycine, the simplest of amino acids.

DIGESTION of food proteins releases amino acids, which are absorbed in the INTESTINE. Depending on the person's body size and the type of protein that is consumed, 55 g to 65 g of protein a day supplies adequate amino acids for an adult. Few Americans are likely to be protein-deficient, because the typical U.S. diet generally supplies twice as much protein as needed. With a varied diet, neither a meat eater nor a knowledgeable VEGETARIAN needs extra protein to obtain adequate amino acids.

MEAT, FISH, POULTRY, and DAIRY products like EGGS are the best sources of essential amino acids. Proteins that provide ample amounts of essential amino acids are said to be COMPLETE PROTEINS. Several plant proteins approach the quality of animal protein: soy, AMARANTH and QUINOA are examples. However, most plant proteins are deficient in at least one essential amino acid. For example, LEGUMES are low in methionine; CORN is low in lysine. These foods can be balanced during the day by eating "complementary" protein foods that provide ample amounts of those amino acids deficient in another food.

Surplus dietary amino acids may be used for energy, and amino acids from the breakdown of cellular protein can be important fuel sources when food intake is inadequate. After 12 to 24 hours without food, MUSCLE protein breaks down rapidly, releasing amino acids into the bloodstream and processing them in the LIVER. The liver removes NITROGEN and converts it to UREA, while converting the amino acids to GLUCOSE and releasing it into the bloodstream to maintain blood sugar levels. In this way, most amino acids can contribute to blood glucose; consequently, muscle protein can help fuel the brain during STARVATION when the glucose supply becomes critical.

Ten amino acids are designated as dietary "nonessential" amino acids because they are synthesized by the body and do not need to be supplied in food. On the other hand, the diet must provide the other eight amino acids to prevent malnutrition. These dietary "essential" amino acids are lysine, valine, PHENYLALANINE, TRYPTOPHAN, isoleucine, leucine, METHIONINE, and THREONINE. Two other amino acids may be conditionally essential. HISTIDINE may not be formed in adequate amounts by infants and growing children, and arginine may be inadequately synthesized by adults with liver disease and by BREAST-FEEDING mothers.

Amino acids like phenylalanine and arginine, thought to stimulate GROWTH HORMONE release and thus promote FAT loss, are neither safe nor effective methods for weight control. Large amounts (several grams per day) of single amino acids used as supplements or additives, can drastically affect the body and damage the KIDNEYS. The therapeutic use of amino acids is still in experimental stages. The U.S. FDA removed amino acids from the GENERALLY RECOGNIZED AS SAFE list of FOOD ADDITIVES, and it is prudent to consult a health care provider before supplementing with individual amino acids. (See also BIOLOGICAL VALUE; CHEMICAL SCORE; FOOD COMPLEMENTING.)

Cynober, Luc A., ed. *Amino Acid Metabolism and Therapy in Health and Nutritional Disease*. Boca Raton, Fla.: CRC Press, 1995.

amino sugars A family of nitrogen-containing sugars. Cells attach NITROGEN to the simple sugars GLUCOSE and GALACTOSE to produce GLUCOSAMINE and galactosamine, respectively. These and similar amino sugars are used to produce carbohydrate-containing proteins (GLYCOPROTEINS) that coat cell surfaces, and for structural materials (MUCOPOLYSACCHARIDES) that help form the matrix of cartilage for ligaments and joints.

ammonia (NH_3) The nitrogen waste produced primarily from AMINO ACID metabolism. Ammonia is highly toxic to the nervous system and the brain. It may interfere with metabolic processes required for energy production in the brain. Normally the brain transforms ammonia into GLUTAMINE, a safe, neutral amino acid released into the bloodstream. Next, glutamine is absorbed by the intestine, which releases the ammonia for disposal by the LIVER. Normally the liver very efficiently metabolizes ammonia to UREA, the ultimate nontoxic waste product, via the UREA CYCLE to keep the level of ammonia in the blood at very low levels. Urea is excreted safely in urine. Ammonia is also produced in the intestinal tract by bacteria. Ammonia is absorbed by the intestine and transported directly via the portal vein to the liver for disposal.

Liver disease, such as CIRRHOSIS, reduces urea production and leads to elevated blood levels of ammonia (ammonemia), which causes neurological abnormalities. Genetic defects in the ammonia-disposal mechanism of the urea cycle generally lead to brain damage.

ammoniated glycyrrhizin See GLYCYRRHIZIN.

amphetamines Prescription drugs that stimulate the central nervous system. Benzedrine sulfate, Amphaplex 10, Bexidrine and Biphetamine are examples of amphetamines that temporarily suppress APPETITE and were once prescribed for weight loss. Amphetamines are now used to control hyperactivity in children and to control bouts of uncontrollable sleepiness (narcolepsy). Amphetamine abuse can cause exhaustion, ADDICTION, suicidal depression during withdrawal, cardiac problems, insomnia, HYPERTENSION, and MALNUTRITION. (See also ALCOHOL-DRUG INTERACTIONS; APPETITE SUPPRESSANTS; DIETING.)

amygdalin See LAETRILE.

amylase (alpha amylase) The enzyme produced in the body that breaks down STARCH. Starch digestion begins in the mouth with amylase secreted in SALIVA, as saliva is mixed with food during chewing. Starch digestion is completed in the intestine by amylase secreted by the PANCREAS.

Amylase converts starch to a two-sugar fragment called maltose, which is too large to be absorbed. Therefore the intestinal enzyme MALTASE degrades maltose to GLUCOSE, which is readily taken up by the intestine and transported as blood glucose. (See also CARBOHYDRATE; DIGESTIVE TRACT.)

amylopectin The water-insoluble form of STARCH. Plants synthesize this very long chain of GLUCOSE units as a storage form of energy, often to nurture the future embryo, seedling or sprout. It is often the major form of starch and it possesses a highly branched, bushy structure resembling liver GLYCOGEN (animal starch). In contrast, AMYLOSE is made up of single straight chains of glucose units. Amylopectin forms a paste in hot water. Starch occurs in seeds, tubers, and root vegetables as both amylopectin and amylose, although the ratio of two forms varies with the source. Cooking softens starch granules, making them available to DIGESTION by AMYLASE. The ultimate product of amylopectin digestion is GLUCOSE. Commercial processing converts starch to glucose, then to HIGH-FRUCTOSE CORN SYRUP, a major sweetener. (See also COMPLEX CARBOHYDRATE; FRUCTOSE; POLYSACCHARIDE.)

amylose A water-soluble form of STARCH found in seeds, tubers, and root vegetables. It is made up of long chains of GLUCOSE units, and often contains a thousand or more glucose units. Amylose differs from the other prevalent form of starch, AMYLOPECTIN, which is highly branched. Amylose forms large spiral configurations when dissolved in water and can react with iodide to form a characteristic blue-purple pigment. Amylopectin and amylose occur together in starch, and the relative amounts vary depending on the plant sources. During digestion, AMYLASE breaks down amylose to maltose, a disaccharide composed of two glucose units. An intestinal enzyme, MALTASE, then hydrolyzes maltose to the simple sugar glucose, the ultimate product of starch digestion.

anabolic steroids A family of steroids related to the male sex hormone TESTOSTERONE. These are classified as prescription drugs used to make up for hormone imbalance and deficiencies. However, synthetic analogs of testosterone have been obtained illegally by athletes and by teenage males to build muscles, and the U.S. FDA has described steroid abuse as a drug epidemic. While testosterone stimulates growth during adolescence, the synthetic derivatives can cause many side effects. Athletes compound this unsafe practice by "stacking" anabolic steroids—taking a combination of brands at 10 to 100 times the recommended doses for weeks at a time.

In men, the side effects of anabolic steroid use include lowered sperm count, enlarged prostate gland, shrinking testicles, balding, and enlarged breasts. If taken before puberty, anabolic steroids can stunt growth. These effects seem to be reversible if anabolic steroids have been used for a short time. Some women body builders also use steroids to build muscle. Side effects in women do not seem to be reversible: masculinization, including increased muscles, increased size of clitoris, growth of facial hair, a deepening voice, shrinkage of breast size, uterine atrophy, and menstrual irregularities. Severe cases of acne and bouts of rage are signs of anabolic steroid use, especially in males. Anabolic steroid use can have more subtle, long-term detrimental effects; damage may show up years later as a HEART ATTACK, high blood pressure, CANCER, and LIVER damage in both men and women.

anabolism (biosynthesis) Processes involved in synthesizing the molecules needed for cellular growth and maintenance. Thus the formation of PROTEIN, DNA, RNA, LIPID, CARBOHYDRATE, FAT, and GLYCOGEN are anabolic processes. Anabolism consumes chemical energy in the form of ATP and NADPH (a reducing agent), which are supplied by CATABOLISM, the energy-yielding oxidative processes involved in degradation. Optimal function and health rely upon a balance of anabolic and catabolic processes (homeostasis). These two branches of metabolism are controlled by the ENDOCRINE SYSTEM, which in turn responds to external influences such as diet. Anabolic processes require small building blocks supplied by breaking down STARCH, PROTEIN, and FAT in foods to build larger molecules. GLYCEROL and FATTY ACIDS are the subunits of fat; AMINO ACIDS yield proteins; and glucose yields glycogen. Fat and carbohydrate degradation provides an energized form of ACETIC ACID (acetyl CoA) to synthesize fatty acids and cholesterol. Other specialized products are also assembled from several different types of smaller precursors. For example, heme, the iron-containing pigment of the oxygen transport protein HEMOGLOBIN, is synthesized from an amino acid (GLYCINE) and SUCCINIC ACID, a common intermediate in energy-producing pathways.

Growth and an anabolic state, seen as an increase in body mass and muscle mass, occur during childhood, adolescence, pregnancy, and strenuous physical activity, such as body building. The weight gained in these situations represents increased protein, bone, or fat, not fluids. Increased fat stores and accumulated body fat represent stored surplus energy in adults and can result from too little exercise, the over-consumption of FOOD, heredity, or a combination of the above factors. (See also ADIPOSE TISSUE; ANABOLIC STEROIDS.)

anaerobic Cellular processes that do not require oxygen. Energy can be produced in cells without oxygen. Anaerobic GLYCOLYSIS refers to an energy yielding process by which ATP, the energy currency of the cell, is produced from GLUCOSE without the participation of oxygen. As an example, skeletal muscle produces LACTIC ACID and ATP from glucose when oxygen supplied to muscle is inadequate to meet energy needs during strenuous physical exertion. Accumulated lactic acid is then converted back to glucose during the recovery period following EXERCISE when the oxygen supply is again adequate. Anaerobic processes are important for certain bacteria as well. Anaerobic bacteria in the intestine grow without oxygen and block the growth of potential disease-producing microorganisms. Anaerobic fermentation of SUGAR by yeast yields alcohol-containing products such as WINE and BEER. (See also AEROBIC; CATABOLISM.)

anaphylaxis An extreme reaction of the immune system in response to exposure to foreign substances. Insect bites, drugs, injected serum, and certain foods can create anaphylaxis. This abnormal response or immediate hypersensitivity is usually very rapid in susceptible individuals who may have been sensitized by previous exposure, and may produce shock ("anaphylactic shock"). The massive release of histamines and other inflammatory agents leads to spasming of smooth muscles, especially those of the air passageways, and to widespread swelling due to the increased water leaking out of capillaries. Symptoms range from asthma to fever, itching, hives, and flushed skin in mild cases, to chest constriction, irregular pulse, painful, labored breathing, and convulsions in severe cases.

Anaphylaxis can be life-threatening and may require emergency room care. (See also ALLERGIC RHINITIS; ALLERGY, FOOD; ALLERGY, IMMEDIATE.)

anchovy, European (*Engraulis encrasicholus*) A small, herringlike marine fish harvested mainly in the eastern Atlantic Ocean and the Mediterranean Sea. Anchovies are usually sold filleted, salted, and packed in oil. Their distinctly sea-salty taste is used in appetizers or as a garnish on pizza and in salads. Anchovies are a key ingredient in Caesar salad dressing. One anchovy packed in oil and salt provides calories, 111; protein, 17 g; iron, 2.7 mg; sodium, 88 mg; fat, 4 g; cholesterol, 51 mg.

androgen A class of steroid hormones that promotes secondary male characteristics (masculinization). Androgens function in the body to stimulate anabolic processes, such as deposition of muscle protein. Examples include TESTOSTERONE and androsterone, produced by gonads.

The synthetic ANABOLIC STEROIDS resemble testosterone. These drugs have been obtained illegally by male and female athletes and by those who wish to speed up or increase muscle mass and decrease body fat beyond the rate obtainable by training. The use of anabolic steroids causes physical and mental changes that may be irreversible and increase the risk of disease. (See also ANABOLISM.)

androstenediol (4-androstenediol, 5-androstenediol) An androgenic steroid that a certain liver enzyme converts to the male hormone testosterone. Androstenediol is one of several popular "prohormones" sold as DIETARY SUPPLEMENTS and taken primarily by athletes and bodybuilders, who believe these substances can increase muscle mass and strengthen much the same way as ANABOLIC STEROIDS. Other prohormones in the androstenediol family that are sold as dietary supplements include dehydroepiandrosterone (DHEA), androstenedione ("andro"), 19-norandrostenedione, and 19-norandrostenediol.

The bodybuilding attributes credited to androstenediol and related prohormones have not been substantiated by credible research. As dietary supplements they are not subject to the same rigorous government testing as are prescription drugs. Anabolic steroids do stimulate muscle growth, but use of these drugs solely for that purpose is illegal. Consequently, many athletes and bodybuilders see prohormones as a way to obtain the same fitness benefits that anabolic steroids confer without violating the law.

Little is known about the potential side effects of prohormones like androstenediol, but if they have the same testosterone-related body enhancing abilities as anabolic steroids, their side effects are probably similar. In men short-term side effects include lowered sperm count, enlarged prostate gland, shrinking testicles, balding, and enlarged breasts. Women may experience masculinization, increased size of clitoris, growth of facial hair, deepening voice, shrinking breasts, and menstrual irregularities. Long-term side effects for both sexes include increased risk of HEART ATTACK, high blood pressure, CANCER, and liver damage.

Blue, J. G., and J. A. Lombardo. "Steroids and Steroid-like Compounds," *Clinics in Sports Medicine* 18, no. 3 (1999): 667–689.

anemia A condition characterized by subnormal levels of HEMOGLOBIN, the oxygen-binding PROTEIN in blood. Half a million Americans are at risk for anemia, including 40 percent of pregnant women, pre-menopausal women, vegans (those who eat no animal products), adolescents relying on JUNK FOOD diets, infants, and children with inadequate diets. Anemia may result from either an inadequate number of RED BLOOD CELLS (erythrocytes) or an abnormally low hemoglobin content of red blood cells. With deficient functional red blood cells, the oxygen supply to tissues is inadequate for optimal RESPIRATION, causing shortness of breath, FATIGUE, weakness, pallor, headache, and lowered resistance to infection. There are two general types of anemia based on red blood cell size. Megaloblastic anemia is characterized by large red blood cells; their shortened life span results in a decreased number of cells. Microcytic anemia is characterized by small red blood cells with reduced hemoglobin content.

Many nutritional deficiencies lead to anemia. Inadequate dietary IRON, COPPER, FOLIC ACID, PROTEIN, VITAMIN B_6, vitamin B_{12}, VITAMIN C, VITAMIN A,

VITAMIN E, and RIBOFLAVIN can cause this condition. Each of these nutrients is required for the production of red blood cells (ERYTHROPOIESIS). Iron deficiency anemia is the most common diet-related anemia in the United States and it represents the last stage of iron deficiency. It is characterized by small, pale red blood cells (microcytic anemia), due to chronic blood loss or inadequate iron intake. Symptoms include FATIGUE, pallor, and shortness of breath. Studies of the nutritional status of developed nations have routinely found up to 30 percent of a population with iron deficiency. Groups that are at highest risk are children under the age of two years, teenage women, pregnant women, and the elderly. Pregnancy drastically increases the requirement of iron. In terms of blood loss the most common causes of iron deficiency are excessive bleeding during menstruation and intestinal bleeding due to parasites, ulcers, or malignancy. Iron deficiency can be caused by impaired iron uptake by the intestine, due to a lack of stomach acid (ACHLORHYDRIA) or from chronic DIARRHEA. With iron deficiency, the resulting anemia can be treated by iron supplementation.

Deficiencies of either folacin or vitamin B_{12} can cause anemia because each is essential for DNA synthesis and deficiencies impair erythrocyte production. Folic acid deficiency is much more common because folic acid stores in the body are small, yet folic acid participates in many biosynthetic reactions. On the other hand, vitamin B_{12} is stored in the LIVER, and only trace amounts are required daily for a few specific functions. Anemia due to inadequate folic acid and vitamin B_{12} produces large (macrocytic) cells with a short life span. This form of anemia can occur when intake of fresh vegetables is very limited, or when the need for folic acid outstrips intake, as may occur during pregnancy or in ALCOHOLISM. Treatment with folic acid can ameliorate megaloblastic anemia, yet mask an underlying vitamin B_{12} deficiency. This point emphasizes that treatment of anemia requires expert medical supervision.

Anemia can also indicate a serious condition unrelated to diet. Non-nutritional causes of anemia include chronic blood loss and congenital defects in red blood cell formation, such as thalassemia or sickle cell anemia, due to mutant hemoglobins, and spherocytosis (spherical red blood cells). Hemolytic anemia is the result of excessive hemolysis (destruction of red blood cells) in susceptible people exposed to bacterial toxins, toxic chemicals, or drugs that may produce JAUNDICE. Anemia also may result from reduced nutrient uptake due to the presence of parasites and chronic infections, gastrointestinal disease or bowel resection. (See also HEAVY METALS; HEMATOCRIT; LEAD; MALNUTRITION.)

Pruthi, R. K., and A. Tefferi. "Pernicious Anemia Revisited," *Mayo Clinic Proceedings* 69, no. 2 (1994): 144–150.

Viteri, Fernando E. "Iron Supplementation for the Control of Iron Deficiency in Populations at Risk," *Nutrition Reviews* 55, no. 6 (June 1997): 195–209.

anemia, aplastic A form of ANEMIA in which the numbers of RED BLOOD CELLS as well as white cells are reduced. This type of anemia is caused by exposure to chemicals (such as solvents), toxic heavy metals, some drugs like chloramphenicol, or ionizing radiation (like X rays). Radiation therapy, chemotherapy, and lead poisoning can damage bone marrow, thus reducing red blood cell production. Both the blood platelet count and immunity decline, with a concomitant increased susceptibility to infection. Destruction of the bone marrow is potentially life-threatening.

anemia, pernicious A form of ANEMIA caused either by a dietary deficiency of VITAMIN B_{12} or by inadequate B_{12} absorption. It is characterized by quite large red blood cells (macrocytic) that are overloaded in the hemoglobin (hyperchromic). Low vitamin B_{12} consumption is a concern for strict VEGETARIANS who avoid meat and meat products. Pernicious anemia is also caused by inadequate vitamin B_{12} uptake. Normally, the gastric lining secretes a PROTEIN called INTRINSIC FACTOR that's needed to specifically bind vitamin B_{12}. Because this protein is required for vitamin B_{12} absorption by the intestine, inadequate intrinsic factor production, even with adequate dietary B_{12}, can cause pernicious anemia.

Pernicious anemia affects the nervous system as well as the blood. Symptoms include memory loss, weakness, personality and mood swings, and numbness and tingling in the hands and feet. If this anemia continues unchecked, nerve damage may be irreversible. Pernicious anemia is most common in males between the ages of 40 and 65 years who have a family history of the condition. Treatment for intrinsic factor defect involves vitamin B_{12} injections. Oral doses of vitamin B_{12} can remedy dietary deficiencies when intrinsic factor production is normal. (See also FOLIC ACID.)

angiotensin A protein-like hormone formed in the blood that raises blood pressure. Angiotensin contracts the muscles of CAPILLARIES and ARTERIES (vasopressor), which increases resistance for blood flow. Angiotensin is liberated by the action of RENIN, an ENZYME formed by the kidneys, on a serum PROTEIN (angiotensinogen) produced by the liver. The release of renin by the kidneys is triggered when they experience lowered blood flow, for example, due to dehydration. Angiotensin also plays an important role in the regulation of blood pressure by stimulating the ADRENAL GLANDS to secrete ALDOSTERONE. Aldosterone, in turn, promotes SODIUM retention and water retention by the kidneys, to help regulate water balance. (See also ANTIDIURETIC HORMONE; HYPERTENSION.)

animal drugs in meat See ANTIBIOTICS; MEAT CONTAMINANTS.

anion A negatively charged ion. Anions are the opposite of CATIONS, which carry positive charges. Important anions are formed when weak acids ionize. Anions, together with their cation counterparts, occur in blood and are called electrolytes. They are required to maintain the appropriate effective concentration of ions and PROTEINS in the blood. Key anions in blood are chloride (Cl^-), phosphate ($H_2PO_4^-$), and bicarbonate (HCO_3^-). Chloride (Cl^-) is the predominant anion in body fluids. Neither chloride nor phosphate can be made by the body; they are essential nutrients to be supplied by the diet. Phosphate and bicarbonate ions help buffer blood at nearly a constant pH. These anions are examples of "conjugate bases," formed when weak acids ionize. (See also ELECTROLYTES.)

anise (*Pimpinella anisum*) An HERB belonging to the PARSLEY family that originated in India and was cultivated in ancient China and Egypt. The fruit, aniseed, is dried and used as a seasoning. The distinctive, licorice-like flavor of anise extract adds to the taste of shortbread cakes, such as *pizella* (Italy) and *pains á l'anis* (France). Anise is used in certain candies. Crushed aniseed together with cinnamon and coriander is used to make a liqueur, anisette. Chopped anise leaves have been used in pickled vegetables and soups.

annatto (*Bixa orellara*) A yellow-red, natural, vegetable food-coloring agent obtained from a small tropical tree that is native to Central America. Annatto is prepared from the pulp of the fruit and from the waxy layer around the seeds, and is used to give a yellow or orange color to several cheeses (Cheddar, Cheshire, Edam) and to smoked haddock, butter, and a variety of pastries and sweets.

anorexia nervosa An EATING DISORDER involving compulsive STARVATION, resulting in a loss of 25 percent or more of the body weight. Anorexia is characterized by a sudden or severe weight loss, a continued effort to lose weight, a refusal to maintain normal body weight, a failure to grow during adolescence, missed consecutive menstrual periods (amenorrhea), plus nausea, bloating, or constipation. Starvation symptoms include ACIDOSIS, KETOSIS, and ELECTROLYTE imbalance. Behavioral aspects include food hoarding, food phobia, ritualization of food preparation while eating very little, eating alone, phobia of being obese, and feeling fat when actually underweight. Anorexics seem to prefer PROTEIN over CARBOHYDRATE. A ZINC deficiency may be involved in the disease because zinc supplements (25 mg/day) have helped some patients gain weight.

Although boys and men can be anorectic, 90 percent to 95 percent of patients are girls and women. Anorexia and bulimia together affect 5 percent of young women in developed nations, although the disorder is absent from less developed nations. Anorexia usually begins with a desire to lose weight or to prevent weight gain. Extreme social pressure to be trim, an abnormal family environment, an imbalanced ENDOCRINE SYSTEM or nervous system can trigger this behavior. The typical patient is a white, female adolescent who is a bright overachiever, attempting to meet high parental expectations and wanting more control over her life. Low self-esteem may be an issue.

Anorexia is a multifaceted disorder and a broad-based treatment approach has been most successful. Therapeutic programs use nutrition counseling, individual psychotherapy, behavior modification, family counseling and medications when required. Such a multidisciplinary approach involves nutritionists and dietitians, nurses, physicians, social workers and counselors, and self-help groups. Their goals are to establish and maintain a desired body weight while resolving emotional issues and improving the home environment. Fundamental to nutritional care is a counseling program to help patients change their attitudes about food. Depending on the patient's nutritional status, a nutritional program might entail nutritionally balanced meals, adjusted for patient preferences, vitamin and mineral supplements to remedy deficiencies, slow refeeding with progressive increments in total daily CALORIES to reach the desired level of calories; and ongoing nutritional counseling. Anorexics will be managed by an outpatient treatment program or by hospitalization when weight loss has been severe, when there are serious metabolic problems, when the family is in crisis, or where the patient is suicidal. Nutritional rehabilitation programs vary according to the severity of the condition, but less restrictive approaches seem to have better results for weight gain. Psychotherapy usually focuses on feelings about body image, self-esteem, food, control of one's life and choices, and gaining independence from harmful family influences. Long illnesses, severe weight gain, a dysfunctional family background, late age of onset of the illness, and late occurring treatment make recovery more difficult.

The mortality rate is about 6 percent to 10 percent due to mineral imbalances. The National Association of Anorexia and Associated Disorders and the American Anorexia/Bulimia Association are among the resources available to anorexics. (See also DIET; MALNUTRITION.)

Woodside, D. B. "A Review of Anorexia and Bulimia Nervosa," *Current Problems in Pediatrics,* 25, no. 2 (1995): 67–89.

anorexigenic Capable of diminishing the APPETITE. Disease influences (DIABETES, OBESITY, CANCER) and certain drugs can diminish appetite. Certain substances produced by the body also modulate APPETITE, especially hormones. Somatostatin and corticotrophin-releasing factor (produced by the HYPOTHALAMUS to control secretions by the PITUITARY GLAND) and hormones of the gastrointestinal tract (vasoactive intestinal peptide) decreased feeding in experimental animals when trace quantities were administered directly to the brain.

antacid A substance that neutralizes STOMACH ACID used to relieve ACID INDIGESTION (heartburn), which manifests itself as a pain in the upper abdomen. Acid indigestion is very common; it affects one-third of Americans. Medications to relieve this condition are some of the most widely used over-the-counter drugs. Antacids are also used therapeutically to treat PEPTIC ULCERS. Stomach pain can be due to STRESS or emotion, and not simply the result of excess stomach acid. However, a severe pain could point to a more serious condition, such as a heart attack. Therefore, patients should seek medical attention for any severe chest pain accompanied by short breath, weakness, and sweating.

Antacid use poses potential problems, and antacids should be used only occasionally. They work best when taken one-half to two hours after a meal. Antacids may block the action of medications, such as tetracycline, digitalis, and anticonvulsants. Protracted use of antacids interferes with calcium METABOLISM and bone formation. CONSTIPATION or DIARRHEA are the two most common adverse reactions to antacid use. In particular, antacids that contain ALUMINUM hydroxide or calcium carbonate can lead to constipation. Regarding aluminum-containing antacids, there are indications that aluminum intake should be minimized because aluminum may cause calcium and phosphorus depletion. Aluminum hydroxide seems to have minimal complications when combined with magnesium hydroxide.

Calcium carbonate is a common antacid. Although it neutralizes acids effectively, it may cause acid overproduction later (rebound effect). Calcium carbonate can also block IRON uptake. Another option is sodium bicarbonate, a major ingredient of several popular antacids. However, it should be noted that the typical American diet provides excessive SODIUM, and sodium bicarbonate antacids could increase the burden for sodium-sensitive people. A further reservation: Bicarbonate-based antacids may promote alkaline blood (alkalosis) or they may alter KIDNEY or heart function.

Calcium carbonate is the major ingredient of several antacids. They have been recommended because they are inexpensive and calcium carbonate has a high content of calcium (40 percent of the weight). However, taking antacids as a calcium supplement can seriously lower stomach acidity and decrease the efficiency of digestion. Under normal conditions, most forms of calcium supplements (calcium aspartate, calcium carbonate, calcium gluconate, and calcium orotate) are absorbed about as well as the calcium in whole MILK. Remember that calcium uptake requires an adequate intake of VITAMIN D, MAGNESIUM, COPPER, and ZINC, while adequate physical EXERCISE promotes calcium deposition in bones. (See also ALUMINUM; BONE; OSTEOPOROSIS.)

anthocyanins A family of plant pigments responsible for red to blue-red colors in fruits such as BLACKBERRIES, RASPBERRIES, BLUEBERRIES, and CHERRIES. They belong to the family of FLAVONOIDS, plant substances that are nonnutrients but have beneficial effects. When eaten, these materials bind to connective TISSUE, where they crosslink and strengthen COLLAGEN, the primary structural PROTEIN of the body. Liberal consumption of flavonoid-rich foods may be appropriate for individuals subjected to oxidative STRESS and chronic inflammation. Flavonoids generally function as antioxidants to prevent tissue damage by FREE RADICALS, highly reactive molecules that can attack cells. They help counter inflammation and associated pain by blocking the production of proinflammatory agents including prostaglandins and leukotrienes. (See also PHYTOCHEMICALS.)

anti-aging nutrients See AGING.

antibiotics Chemicals that destroy or prevent growth of microorganisms including BACTERIA, MOLDS, and FUNGI. Natural or synthetic compounds are used extensively as antibiotics to treat infectious diseases in animals and plants as well as in humans. Sulfanilamides, penicillins, and erythromycins are examples of major families of these drugs. Antibiotics impact human health in several ways. The prolonged use of broad-spectrum antibiotics in treating disease drastically alters the intestinal microflora by destroying beneficial bacteria. The loss of beneficial bacteria can permit less desirable, opportunistic microorganisms like yeast to flourish, cause intestinal inflammation, and decrease production of nutrients important in maintaining health of the COLON.

Antibiotics can affect specific vitamin requirements; chloramphenicol blocks RIBOFLAVIN and VITAMIN B_6 and B_{12}, for example. Penicillin increases POTASSIUM requirements. Antibiotics can decrease nutrient absorption in general by altering the intestinal lining. Neomycin interferes with the uptake of FAT, AMINO ACIDS, CARBOHYDRATE, water-soluble and fat-soluble VITAMINS, CALCIUM, IRON, and VITAMIN K. Tetracycline decreases absorption of fat, amino acids, calcium, iron, MAGNESIUM, and ZINC, while increasing the rate of urinary excretion of RIBOFLAVIN, FOLIC ACID, and VITAMIN C.

Antibiotics can have a direct impact on the food supply. Half the antibiotics produced in the United States are applied to livestock. The benefits are more rapid growth and healthier animals. On the other hand the potential exists for generating drug-resistant pathogenic bacteria and persistent antibiotic residues in meat and dairy products. The application of antibiotics in animal husbandry and the permissible levels of antibiotic residues in animal products are regulated by the U.S. FDA. The following examples illustrate the dimensions of this food safety issue.

Chloramphenicol This drug can cause ANEMIA in humans due to damage to bone marrow. Though banned from use with food-producing animals, periodic spot inspections showed it was widely used in cattle and hogs in the 1980s. The degree to which chloramphenicol continues to contaminate meat through illegal application, and the degree to which such a contamination affects health, are unknown.

Penicillin This common antibiotic is used to treat dairy herds, among others. The allowable penicillin level in MILK is 0.01 units per milliliter (about 20 drops) of milk, but spot checks have found 10 times this level in commercial milk. Such high levels can cause allergic reactions in susceptible individuals.

Sulfamethazine This sulfa drug is a widespread contaminant in MEAT, POULTRY, and milk. One-fourth of milk sampled in the late 1980s was contaminated, despite the U.S. FDA ban on this drug in milk. Sulfamethazine is suspected of being a CARCINOGEN. (See also ACIDOPHILUS; MEAT CONTAMINANTS; PESTICIDES.)

antibodies A class of PROTEINS produced by the IMMUNE SYSTEM to combat viruses, bacteria, and FUNGI and to neutralize foreign substances. Antibodies are made in response to foreign substances by B cells, a type of lymphocyte or white cell found in bone marrow or the lymphatic system. The progeny of B cells are called plasma cells and are responsible for antibodies appearing in body fluids in COLOSTRUM and on mucosal surfaces.

The body produces millions of different antibodies and each type of antibody attacks a different foreign material (ANTIGEN). The basis of this diversity lies in antibody structure, which allows a close fit with the antigen, much like a lock fitting in a keyhole. Antigen-antibody binding then enables scavenger cells to engulf and degrade antigens. Long after exposure to the antigen, information for synthesizing it remains embedded in special lymphocytes called memory cells that enable the body to produce antibodies rapidly when again threatened by the foreign invaders.

Antibodies reacting to normally harmless materials may trigger overreactions of the immune system and may cause AUTOIMMUNE DISEASE, in which the body attacks its own tissues. Insulin-dependent DIABETES MELLITUS and rheumatoid ARTHRITIS are examples. Allergic reactions are another example of an overreaction of the immune system.

In nutrition, the most important classes of antibodies are IgE, IgG, and IgA. IgE antibodies are responsible for rapid allergic symptoms (immediate hypersensitivity) related to HISTAMINE release: red, runny nose; hives; asthma; swelling; itching; or, in extreme situations, shock (ANAPHYLAXIS). This class of antibody is important in TISSUES and is less prominent in the blood.

IgG (gamma globulin) is the major class of antibodies found in the blood. Elevated IgG is implicated in slow-developing food allergies (delayed hypersensitivity). After avoiding foods that cause such allergies, the immune system can return to normal as allergen-specific IgG gradually disappears from the blood. It may then be possible to tolerate allergenic foods if eaten infrequently.

Secretory IgA is the major antibody released by mucosal surfaces such as the mouth and the intestinal tract, where it binds potentially dangerous microorganisms and prevents their sticking to tissue and initiating infections. Secreted IgA is also an important antibody in COLOSTRUM and BREAST MILK that helps protect the nursing infant from infection until its own immune system is able to mount a vigorous defense. (See also ALLERGEN; ALLERGY, FOOD; ALLERGY, IMMEDIATE; BREASTFEEDING; IMMUNE SYSTEM; ROTATION DIET.)

anticaking agents A class of FOOD ADDITIVES used to maintain free-flowing powdered and granular materials. These useful additives are added to table salt, powdered sugar, malted milk powders, garlic and onion powders, powdered coffee whiteners, vanilla powder, BAKING POWDER, dried egg yolk, and seasoning salts. Examples include DEXTROSE and silicates (aluminum silicate, magnesium silicate, sodium calcium aluminosilicate, calcium silicate, and silicon dioxide). These agents are judged to be safe food additives. (See also ALUMINUM; SODIUM.)

anticancer diet See CANCER.

anticancer nutrients See CANCER.

antidiuretic hormone (ADH, vasopressin) A pituitary HORMONE that decreases urine output and conserves water in the KIDNEYS. ADH represents the body's primary water-conserving mechanism. The anterior PITUITARY GLAND releases ADH into the bloodstream in response to physiologic STRESS, DEHYDRATION, diminished blood volume, or high SODIUM concentration in the blood. The mechanism involves these steps: First, receptors located in the HYPOTHALAMUS detect increased osmolarity (ion concentration) of blood, then the hypothalamus stimulates the pituitary gland to release ADH. (See also ENDOCRINE SYSTEM; HOMEOSTASIS.)

antigen A foreign material recognized by the IMMUNE SYSTEM. Antigens stimulate the formation of specific antibodies, which bind the provoking antigens to neutralize them. Generally, a single type of antibody recognizes one type of antigen. Antigens may be PROTEINS, glycolipids, POLYSACCHARIDES, microorganisms, or cells. The body has the ability to neutralize a huge number of antigens because it can synthesize an immense variety of antibodies. Because some antigens may share common structural features, antibodies may cross-react. Thus, antibodies against cow's MILK may cross-react with goat's milk, and antibodies against WHEAT protein (GLUTEN) can cross-react with similar proteins in other grains. (See also ALLERGEN; ALLERGY, FOOD.)

antihistamine See HISTAMINE.

antimetabolite A drug that interferes with cell division. By mimicking an enzyme's usual nutrient reactant, an antimetabolite tricks the cell's machinery and prevents normal growth. Sulfa drugs are bacterial antimetabolites that block the bacterial synthesis of the B vitamin FOLIC ACID, required for bacterial growth. Because animal cells depend on folic acid in the diet and cannot synthesize it, they are immune to sulfa drugs. A somewhat different strategy underlies the use of the anticancer drug methotrexate. Methotrexate attacks cancer cells that have a high rate of growth, by blocking the activation of folic acid to its biologically active form (coenzyme). Without a ready supply of the coenzyme form, cancer cells stop growing rapidly.

antimycotic agents FOOD ADDITIVES used to prevent SPOILAGE. These PRESERVATIVES retard growth of YEASTS and MOLDS. Examples are sorbates, SODIUM BENZOATE, and CALCIUM PROPIONATE. Sorbic acid and POTASSIUM and sodium sorbates retard spoilage in CHEESE, syrup, JELLY, cake, MAYONNAISE, SOFT DRINKS, WINE, dried fruit, MARGARINE, and soft CANDY. Sorbates are readily broken down in the body and are considered safe additives. Sodium benzoate, which occurs naturally in FRUIT and VEGETABLES, prevents the growth of most microorganisms but requires acidic conditions for its antimicrobial action. Calcium propionate prevents the growth of mold and several bacteria and is a common additive in BREAD to be stored at room temperature. These too are safe food additives.

antineuritic An agent that is capable of relieving damaged nerve inflammations (neuritis). The inflammation of peripheral nerves of the whole body may be due to nutritional deficiency, toxic exposure, or metabolic imbalance. Neuropathy or nerve damage may result from long-term deficiencies of the B vitamins THIAMIN, NIACIN, VITAMIN B_6, VITAMIN B_{12}, or PANTOTHENIC ACID due to dietary deficiencies or to chronically poor absorption by the INTESTINE. As an example, thiamin counteracts neuritis, a typical symptom of severe thiamin deficiency. Alcoholics are prone to thiamin deficiency and neuritis because alcohol rapidly depletes the body's thiamin stores. (See also MALNUTRITION.)

antioxidant A compound that prevents or retards the oxidation of sensitive molecules found in the body or in foods. Antioxidants occur in many foods naturally as nutrients or non-nutrients, or as synthetic additives. Antioxidants typically block oxidation by preventing damage caused by FREE RADICALS, extremely reactive forms of oxygen and other molecules that lack an electron and tear electrons from molecules they meet. In the body, likely targets are DNA, PROTEINS, and LIPIDS (unsaturated FATTY ACIDS).

Free radicals form in the body by normal cellular processes. These include phagocytosis (engulfing viruses and bacteria) by immune cells; incomplete reduction of oxygen as mitochondria burn fuels; production of hydrogen peroxide by the breakdown of fatty acids and the generation of NITRIC OXIDE, a free radical that functions as a localized vasodilator, a defensive chemical and as neurotransmitter. Free radicals and reactive forms of oxygen occur by chemical modification of pollutants and toxic substances within the LIVER. Free radical damage may contribute to CANCER, CARDIOVASCULAR DISEASE, and AGING; consequently, antioxidants are a current focus of extensive medical research. It is intriguing that certain antioxidants are both anticancer nutrients and antiaging nutrients. Because there is such a large variety of reactive molecules and free radicals, the body requires a wide range of antioxidant defenses. A "pecking order" exists among antioxidants; some are more readily oxidized than others and will be consumed rapidly unless replenished or recycled in the body. Certain antioxidants are "preventive inhibitors," that is, they block the initiation of free radical attack. Preventive inhibitors include defensive ENZYMES like CATALASE and GLUTATHIONE PEROXIDASE (destroy hydrogen peroxide and lipid peroxides) and SUPEROXIDE DISMUTASE (destroys superoxide), chelating agents like CITRIC ACID that lock up metal ions, proteins that bind metal ions, including ALBUMIN, TRANSFERRIN, and FERRITIN. Other antioxidants, "chain breakers," convert free radicals to stable (safe) products. VITAMIN E and VITAMIN C are essential chain-breaking antioxidants. It is worth remembering that under certain conditions, an antioxidant may become an oxidant. If the antioxidant becomes a free radical, then it, too, must be disarmed and regenerated.

Antioxidants as Nutrients

VITAMIN A, BETA-CAROTENE, vitamin C, vitamin E, and SELENIUM are key antioxidant nutrients.

CAROTENOIDS, including beta-carotene, trap free radicals, while vitamin A helps guide normal tissue development. Inadequate carotenoid intake increases the risk of cancers of the lung, bladder, esophagus, stomach, colon, rectum, prostate, and skin. Studies indicate that when used alone, beta-carotene does not prevent cancer or heart disease. Indeed, there are hints that unless beta-carotene is protected by another antioxidant, such as vitamin E, it may actually increase damage. A multitude of studies indicates that the consumption of foods rich in carotenoids protects against cancer, cataracts, and cardiovascular diseases.

Vitamin C destroys water-soluble free radicals and protects against cancer. It is needed for a healthy IMMUNE SYSTEM and it also speeds wound healing. Vitamin C also protects LOW-DENSITY LIPOPROTEIN (LDL) cholesterol from oxidation. Evidence for the role of vitamin C in reducing the risk of coronary heart disease is weak. Ongoing clinical trials may help decide whether vitamin C supplementation is beneficial for preventing heart disease. There is some evidence that high dietary vitamin C may lower the risk of several cancers, such as breast cancer and stomach cancer. Evidence does not indicate that high doses of vitamin C decrease cancer risk, however.

Vitamin E acts as a fat-soluble, free radical trap that seems to protect the brain from free radical damage and to partially reverse age-related decline of the immune system in experimental animals. In addition, vitamin E promotes the normal function of smooth muscle cells and reduces platelet adhesion to arterial cells, factors which could reduce the risk of atherosclerosis. Many population studies have found a reduced risk of coronary heart disease with increased intake of vitamin E. However, most clinical studies of vitamin E supplementation for several years found no benefit in reducing heart disease risk.

Selenium works together with vitamin E by helping an enzyme system (glutathione peroxidase) block free radical attack and to disarm reactive lipids. Selenium is also required for a healthy immune system. Selenium deficiency increases the risk of cancer of the esophagus, stomach, and rectum.

Antioxidants as Nonnutrients in Food

In addition to vitamins, trace minerals, fiber, and carotenoids, vegetables and fruits provide many other ingredients important for long-term health. Vegetables and fruits contain orange-red and yellow pigments called carotenoids. They include carotenes such as beta-carotene and LYCOPENE (from tomatoes) and xanthophylls, oxygen-containing derivatives such as zeazanthin and lutein. Xanthophylls occur at high levels in dark green leafy vegetables. Though relatively few carotenoids serve as sources of vitamin A, they help protect the body as versatile antioxidants, and they enhance the immune system, complementing the actions of beta-carotene. Fruits, vegetables, seasoning, spices, and herbs (tea) possess a wide range of complex-molecules called polyphenols (FLAVONOIDS) and phenolic acids that are complex ring structures. Flavonoids include ISOFLAVONES (soybean), flavones (such as QUERCETIN from tea, berries, fruits) and flavonones (such as naringenin and HESPERIDIN from citrus), flavanonols (such as catechins, condensed and hydrolyzable TANNINS), anthocyanins (purple, red, and blue pigments of fruits and berries), coumarins (from citrus), ellagic acid (from GRAPES), and others. In general, flavonoids possess multiple properties; thus they can quench free radicals, inhibit inflammation, strengthen capillary walls, and reduce oxidative damage to serum cholesterol. The optimal intake of flavonoids and carotenoids is not known and the long-term effects of supplementation with large amounts of phytochemicals has not been studied. It should be pointed out that beta-carotene, vitamin C, and even vitamin E under the appropriate conditions can become oxidants (prooxidants). Certain flavonoids also exhibit prooxidant properties. Chelated (complexed) iron in the presence of vitamin C can generate free radicals spontaneously in the test tube and this could be a potential problem in the body with iron overload diseases. Finally, certain flavonoids can specifically block the thyroid hormone-generating enzyme in thyroid cells. As with many dietary constituents, a little may be beneficial, while a lot could be harmful.

Foods rich in vitamin A and beta-carotene and related carotenoids include orange-colored vegetables like CARROTS and SQUASH plus dark green leafy vegetables like CHARD, KALE, and SPINACH. Fresh fruit, frozen juice concentrate, and vegetables like green PEPPER and BROCCOLI supply vitamin C. Vegetable oil, wheat germ, and nuts provide vitamin E. Selenium occurs in whole grains, SEAFOOD, CABBAGE, ONIONS, and GARLIC. Fruits and vegetables also provide flavonoids.

Antioxidants Made by the Body

Glutathione is a sulfur-containing antioxidant present in very large amounts in the cytoplasm. Besides helping to keep proteins reduced, it assists amino acid transport, helps regulate the internal oxidation state of the cell, maintains vitamin E in a reduced state, and detoxifies potentially harmful substances.

COENZYME Q assists mitochondria to burn fat and carbohydrate for energy and it functions as a lipid soluble membrane antioxidant together with vitamin E, which it protects. Coenzyme Q production declines with age and the heart may become deficient in this nutrient.

URIC ACID is found in the blood. It is a nitrogen-containing waste product from the breakdown of DNA and RNA.

CITRIC ACID, succinic acid, and other complex organic acids generated by metabolism can bind iron and copper, preventing them from catalyzing of free radical-generating reactions.

MELATONIN, a hormone produced by the pineal gland, possesses strong antioxidant properties.

BILIRUBIN, a breakdown product of HEMOGLOBIN, acts as an antioxidant in blood.

Antioxidants as Food Additives

Antioxidants are extensively utilized to prevent or retard deterioration that produces off-flavors or color changes in foods, making them less appetizing or less nutritious. Oxidation can also be promoted by enzymes in foods when exposed to air. This explains why apples, bananas, pears, peaches, and potatoes darken after being sliced. The food industry often employs synthetic antioxidants, particularly butylated hydroxyanisole (BHA), butylated hydroxytoluene (BHT), ethylene diaminetetracetic acid (EDTA), and PROPYL GALLATE, as well as vitamin C, as preservatives to extend the shelf life of processed foods by preventing free radical damage.

Spontaneous oxidation of fats and oils in the presence of oxygen, sunlight, and metal ions causes rancidity unless blocked by antioxidants. (BHA) and BHT are used to prevent rancidity in fats and oils, particularly in baked goods like crackers and cookies. Their safety has been questioned. EDTA is a common additive in salad dressings, MARGARINE, MAYONNAISE, sandwich spreads, pureed fruits, and vegetables, as well as cured shellfish, BEER, and soft drinks. EDTA is judged to be a safe food additive. Propyl gallate retards spoilage of fats and oils and is often used with BHA and BHT to maximize their antioxidant effects. Several studies with experimental animals suggest that propyl gallate may cause tumors. A close relative of vitamin C, erythroboric acid, is a common antioxidant used in the preservation of processed meats such as bologna, frankfurters, and BACON. SULFITES are used as antioxidants to prevent discoloration of fruit and vegetables. Spices and herbs, including thyme, rosemary, and sage, are sometimes used as food additives to retard spoilage. (See also ATHEROSCLEROSIS.)

Fairfield, K. M., and R. H. Fletcher. "Vitamins for Chronic Disease Prevention in Adults." *Journal of the American Medical Association* 23, no. 287 (June 19, 2002): 3,116–3,126.

Singh, Ram B. et al. "Effect of Antioxidant Rich Foods on Plasma Ascorbic Acid, Cardiac Enzyme and Lipid Peroxide Levels in Patients Hospitalized with Acute Myocardial Infarction," *Journal of the American Dietetic Association* 95, no. 7 (July 1995): 775–780.

antipasto Cold hors d'oeuvres (from the Italian *ante,* meaning before, and *pasto,* for main course of the meal). A wide variety of foods is suitable for antipasto: marinated VEGETABLES and FISH; OLIVES; hard SAUSAGES like salami; ANCHOVIES; SARDINES; pickled onion, BEETS, PEPPERS, ARTICHOKE hearts, CHICKPEAS; and hard and soft cheeses.

antirachitic Refers to compounds related to VITAMIN D that are capable of preventing RICKETS, the disease that results from a severe vitamin D deficiency. Vitamin D is a family of 11 closely related sterols with similar activity; however, only two account for most of the vitamin D activity in foods. Ergocalciferol (vitamin D_2) is the commercial, supplemental form, and cholecalciferol (vitamin D_3) occurs in animal tissues and fish oils. The precursor of vitamin D_3, dehydrocholesterol, occurs in the skin where it is activated by sunlight. The body converts vitamin D to the active form, calcitriol, which is a hormone.

antiscorbutic Capable of preventing SCURVY, the disease caused by chronic VITAMIN C deficiency. Sources of vitamin C (ascorbic acid), usually fresh fruit and vegetables, relieve the symptoms of scurvy. Although scurvy has been known since the time of the ancient Egyptians, the antiscorbutic effect of limes and other fruit was not discovered in Europe until late in the 18th century, after experiments involving diets of British seamen. It was not until 1907 that scurvy was discovered to be caused by a nutritional deficiency. Though still prevalent in developing nations, scurvy in developed countries is usually associated with ALCOHOLISM and poverty. Sodium erythroborate, an antioxidant used with vitamin C in processed meats, has no antiscorbutic effects.

antivitamin (vitamin antagonist) A compound that diminishes the effect of a vitamin by specific mechanisms rather than by a general effect. Drugs can act as antivitamins, thus the anticancer drug methotrexate is a FOLIC ACID antivitamin. The drug prevents tumor cells from making tetrahydrofolate, the coenzyme or activated form of folic acid required for DNA synthesis. Another case is isoniazid, a drug employed to treat tuberculosis, which is an antagonist of VITAMIN B_6. This drug blocks the utilization of vitamin B_6 by the bacteria causing the disease. Dicumarol, a drug that prevents blood clots (anticoagulant), is an antagonist of VITAMIN K. Antivitamins occur in foods. For example, AVIDIN, a heat-sensitive PROTEIN in raw egg white, binds biotin, and prevents its uptake in the intestine. The viscera of raw FISH contain a THIAMIN antagonist, thiaminase, which breaks down this vitamin in the intestine. The ackee plum of Jamaica contains a RIBOFLAVIN antagonist and has caused an illness related to riboflavin deficiency. A vitamin or nutrient can become an antivitamin of another. For example, very high levels of VITAMIN A block the effects of vitamin K. (See also ANTIMETABOLITE.)

apoenzyme An inactive form of an ENZYME, lacking the appropriate small helper molecule (cofactor or coenzyme) required for activity. Apoenzyme thus refers to only the PROTEIN (polypeptide) portion of an enzyme. Enzymes that require coenzymes or metal ions to assist them in catalyzing reactions are entirely inactive unless they are combined with their non-protein helpers. Cellular protein-synthesizing machinery produces apoenzymes, and coenzymes and metal ion cofactors are added later to create a holoenzyme, which is active because it contains the required helper group.

apoferritin The iron-free PROTEIN required for IRON storage in TISSUES. Apoferritin must be first synthesized in cells before their iron atoms combine with apoferritin to form FERRITIN, the iron-storage protein. Ferritin, a large rust-red protein, contains a mixture of iron hydroxide and iron phosphate and accounts for most stored iron, especially in the intestinal lining, LIVER, spleen, and bone marrow. Apoferritin can be contrasted with another apoprotein of iron metabolism, TRANSFERRIN. Transferrin transports iron in the bloodstream to sites in the body that require iron, especially the bone marrow. Generally, transferrin is about 30 percent bound up with iron. Because 70 percent of its binding capacity is available for more iron, this apoprotein offers a reserve of iron transport capacity in the blood.

apolipoprotein A family of PROTEINS that are ingredients of serum LIPOPROTEINS, the lipid-protein complexes that transport FAT and CHOLESTEROL in the lymphatic system and bloodstream. There are at least nine different apoproteins associated with different lipoproteins, including Apo A, Apo B, Apo C, Apo D, and Apo E. Apo A is located on HDL (high-density lipoprotein), the desirable form of blood cholesterol, and serves as an analytical marker for this lipoprotein. Apo B and Apo E occur as LOW-DENSITY LIPOPROTEIN (LDL), the undesirable form of blood cholesterol. They guide LDL binding to TISSUES like MUSCLE so that cholesterol can be taken up. Apo C is a constituent of both VERY LOW-DENSITY LIPOPROTEIN (VLDL) and CHYLOMICRONS, which transport fat in the blood. Apo C activates an enzyme (LIPASE) in blood vessels that liberates FATTY ACIDS from these carriers to be absorbed by tissues. Apo D helps transfer cholesterol between lipoproteins in the blood. Genetic researchers have discovered that one allele of the Apo E gene (Apoe-E4) is a risk factor for ALZHEIMER'S DISEASE. Although the gene's role is still unclear, scientists suspect that the E4 allele promotes the growth of the amyloid protein plaques that grow on the brains of Alzheimer's patients.

appestat The hypothetical center in the brain that may regulate APPETITE and food intake. While the exact site of regulation of appetite is not yet defined, it probably involves the HYPOTHALAMUS, a part of the brain that regulates HUNGER and THIRST. Hunger may be regulated much like a thermostat to balance the body's energy requirements. Possibly one mechanism stimulates feeding and a second suppresses intake. Current research focuses on a complex array of factors that stimulate or inhibit appetite and feeding. Substances that decrease appetite include neurotransmitters, such as serotonin and norepinephrine; the peptide hormones, including cholecystokinin and peptide YY3-36, produced by the small intestine; and corticotrophin releasing factor from the hypothalamus. Leptin is released into the bloodstream by fat cells that signal the hypothalamus to stop sending signals that trigger eating fat and CARBOHYDRATE while increasing the metabolic rate of fat tissue. Factors stimulating appetite include the hormone ghrelin, produced by the gastrointestinal tract; galanin, a brain peptide; and neuropeptide Y, which acts as a transmitter in the brain.

appetite The learned desire to eat, often a specific food, for taste and enjoyment. Appetite is a pleasant feeling based on previous experiences with foods. Appetite can be triggered by association with aromas, meal time, memories, and certain food advertisements. In contrast, HUNGER relates to the innate need to eat and is associated with an unpleasant sensation coupled with a physiological need. A variety of foods may satisfy hunger.

Appetite is determined by many factors, including social influences (religion, philosophy, cultural taboos); taste and palatability; state of health; effect of medications; preferences and aversions learned by experience; environmental factors, such as climate; and metabolic factors (HORMONE levels, caloric requirements).

The physiologic basis of appetite and hunger is not completely understood. The HYPOTHALAMUS of the brain seems to be the interpretative center and clearinghouse for hunger signals. Anxiety, STRESS and psychological disturbances may cause the release of appetite-stimulating chemical signals from different regions of the brain.

Multiple chemical messengers including as many as 25 neuropeptides affect food intake. Appetite is regulated by a balance of signals that either stimulate or inhibit food intake. Several factors that stimulate appetite include neuropeptide Y, a brain protein that induces lab animals to consume more FAT and CARBOHYDRATE and acts as a neurotransmitter. It is produced by the hypothalamus and other regions of the brain. The levels of neuropeptide Y are modulated by hormones and by blood glucose levels. Another brain protein called GALANIN stimulates an appetite for fat. The hormone ghrelin, produced by the small intestine and stomach, acts as a powerful appetite stimulant. Blood levels of ghrelin increase in dieters and also generally increase just before meals. In contrast, another peptide hormone called leptin, produced by fat cells, regulates the hypothalamus to inhibit food consumption while increasing fat metabolism. In addition, when peptide YY3-36 (PYY) is released from the small intestine and travels to the hypothalamus, it turns off neurons that stimulate hunger. These various hormones, their receptors, and molecular mimics are the focus of intense current research on controlling obesity.

Appetite and Exercise

After beginning an EXERCISE program, appetite may increase during the first few weeks, then return to normal, while moderate exercise (15 miles per week of jogging or walking) may suppress appetite. Research suggests that exercise increases the intake of CALORIES by normal-weight men by an average of 200 calories, even when they burn an additional 600 calories. On the other hand, exercise does not seem to increase normal-weight women's caloric intake above the levels needed to make up for those burned by exercising. Regular exercise may not increase appetite or excessive eating in overweight women. (See also CRAVING.)

Bray, G. A. "Reciprocal Relation of Food Intake and Sympathetic Activity: Experimental Observations and Clinical Implications," *International Journal of Obesity and Metabolic Disorders* 24, supp. 2 (June 2000): S8–S17.

appetite suppressants A variety of drugs and plant products are used to curb appetite. In the past PHENYLPROPANOLAMINE (PPA) was used as an ingredient in many over-the-counter weight loss products, but following adverse reports of links to hemorrhagic stroke with these products, Yale University scientists discovered that PPA does increase the risk of hemorrhagic stroke in women (and possibly men). Consequently, the FDA recommended that consumers not use any products that contain PPA and ruled that PPA is not considered safe for nonprescription use. As a result the FDA is in the process of removing PPA from all drug products and has requested that all drug companies discontinue marketing products containing PPA. In addition, the FDA has issued a public health advisory concerning PPA. In response to the request made by the FDA in November 2000, many companies have voluntarily reformulated and are continuing to reformulate their products to exclude PPA.

Amphetamines (Dexedrine, Benadrine) are prescription drugs used to temporarily curb appetite, although appetite generally returns within two weeks. Bulking agents are forms of plant fiber that swell in water, filling the stomach and creating satiety. PSYLLIUM, GUAR GUM, and GLUCOMANNAN fall into this category. These bulking agents are often included in PROTEIN powders used in weight loss protocols to help satisfy hunger. Two appetite suppressants, fenfluramine and dexfenfluramine, were taken off the market by the FDA in 1997, when it was discovered that thousands of patients who took these drugs developed potentially deadly primary pulmonary hypertension and heart valve abnormalities. Dexfenfluramine was shown to cause these injuries when taken alone, and fenfluramine was linked to valve problems in patients who combined it with the drug phentermine in a mixture popularly known as "fen-phen." Both fenfluramine and dexfenfluramine helped patients lose weight by increasing serotonin levels in the blood stream, which provided a sense of well-being and satiety. The problem researchers discovered after the drugs were removed from the market was that the drugs destroyed the body's ability to control the amount of serotonin circulating in the blood. Excessive amounts of serotonin can cause cell damage to cardiopulmonary structures. (See also DIETING; DIET PILLS; FIBER.)

apple (*Malus pumila*) The rounded FRUIT of the apple tree; originated in Asia Minor. It has been grown for thousands of years and today is the most widely cultivated fruit tree in the world. Apples are one of the most popular fruits in North America and in Europe. Although there are an estimated 7,000 varieties, only 20 are available in the United States and just eight account for 80 percent of apple sales: Red Delicious, McIntosh, Golden Delicious, York, Rome Beauty, Stayman, Granny Smith, and Jonathan. Apples are typically 2.5 to 3.5 inches in diameter and range in color from russet red to yellow. The flesh can be white (Cortland) or yellow (Golden Delicious); the flavor may be tart (Winesap) or sweet (Grimes).

Apples are available year-round because they store well when refrigerated, although this decreases the content of VITAMIN C. Certain varieties like Red Delicious, McIntosh, and Rome Beauty store better than others. On the other hand, apples stored at room temperature become mealy and will turn mushy. Apples are used in a wide variety of desserts (turnovers, fritters, tarts, puddings, compotes, pies, strudels) and in JAMS, JELLIES, and apple butter. A significant percentage of the European and U.S. apple crop is used to produce apple JUICE and CIDER.

Goals of North American apple breeding programs include developing apples that will ripen before early August, when the first traditional red apples, the Jonathans, ripen. Another has been to develop apples that ripen in November. Eventually apples should be available that will extend the apple season (fresh picked apples) from early August to late October.

A typical unpeeled apple with only 80 to 125 calories can be served as a low-calorie, low-fat dessert or snack and can provide one of the recommended two to four servings of fruit per day. Unpeeled apples are an important source of FIBER; an apple can supply about 20 percent of the minimum of fiber recommended for daily consumption. Most of the fiber is soluble fiber (PECTIN). The sweeter the apple, the greater the sugar (FRUCTOSE) content. Commercial applesauce may contain added sugar. For comparison, a half-cup of apple butter provides 186 calories; a half-cup of sweetened applesauce, provides 92 calories; a half-cup of unsweetened applesauce, 50 calories. A typical 3.25-inch-diameter apple (212 g) provides calories, 125; protein, 0.4 g; carbohydrate, 32 g; fiber, 6.6 g; potassium, 244 mg; vitamin C, 12 mg; and traces of other vitamins. (See also ALAR.)

apricot (*Prunus armeniaca*) The oval FRUIT of a tree belonging to a member of the PEACH family. The ripened, fragrant fruit is golden yellow and has little JUICE, unlike the PLUM to which it is also related. Apricots originated in China, where wild apricots were harvested 7,000 years ago. Apricots were later cultivated in India and were introduced into the Mediterranean after the Greek conquest under Alexander the Great. The name is derived from the Latin term for early ripening. Apricots are best picked when ripe. They do not store well and can become grainy and soft. Canned apricots maintain their texture and are frequently used in desserts and fruit salads. Apricots are also used in JAMS, pastries, and cakes. Dried apricots are exported by California, Iran, Australia, and Turkey. Apricots are a rich source of POTASSIUM, BETA-CAROTENE, and FIBER. Three apricots (106 g) provide calories, 51; protein, 1.15 g; carbohydrate, 11.2 g; fiber, 2.23 g; potassium, 361 mg; vitamin A, 317 retinol equivalents; vitamin C, 8 mg; and small amounts of other vitamins.

arachidonic acid A long chain POLYUNSATURATED FATTY ACID that is the parent of important hormone-like agents called PROSTAGLANDINS and LEUKOTRIENES. It is a complex fatty acid, with 20 carbons and four double bonds. Arachidonic acid belongs to the omega-6 family of unsaturated fatty acids, which are derived from the ESSENTIAL FATTY ACID, LINOLEIC ACID. Because arachidonic acid can be made in the body, it is not classified as one of the essential nutrients. MEAT and DAIRY products are rich sources, and they contribute to the body's supply.

Arachidonic acid is processed by the "cyclooxygenase pathway," a series of ENZYMES that yield prostaglandins and related compounds. Prostaglandin PGE_2 and its relatives can increase BLOOD PRESSURE, induce BLOOD CLOTTING, and cause pain and inflammation. ASPIRIN and non-steroidal anti-inflammatory drugs are effective pain relievers because they specifically block the cyclooxygenase enzyme. Another prostaglandin from arachidonic acid, PGI_2, helps to counterbalance blood clotting, while still another derivative of arachidonic acid, prostacyclin, blocks blood clotting. Therefore, aspirin use carries the added risk of increased bleeding.

A second chain of reactions, the lipooxygenase pathway, converts arachidonic acid to leukotrienes, extremely powerful inflammatory agents linked to the allergic response including swelling and pain. FISH OILS are rich in the omega-3 family of unsaturated fatty acids, rather than the omega-6 fatty acids. Because they block leukotriene production from arachidonic acid, fish oils can reduce excessive chronic inflammation.

arame See SEAWEED.

arginine (Arg, L-arginine) A basic AMINO ACID. Arginine helps form the nitrogenous waste product UREA, as part of the chain of reactions called the UREA CYCLE, which disposes of the toxic waste AMMONIA in the LIVER. More generally arginine helps build PROTEINS. Arginine and LYSINE are classified as basic rather than acidic amino acids. Arginine is often considered a non-essential amino acid because of the capacity of the body to synthesize it. However, endogenous arginine formation may be inadequate in newborn infants and in adults with liver disease. Arginine is also converted to NITRIC OXIDE to regulate BLOOD PRESSURE.

Good dietary sources of arginine are nuts, CEREAL GRAINS, MEAT, FISH, and POULTRY. Arginine supplements have been used by athletes to increase GROWTH HORMONE production and increase MUSCLE mass. Whether growth hormone levels can be manipulated by diet is controversial. Oral doses of arginine can stimulate the production of anabolic hormones such as INSULIN and prolactin.

Animal studies of arginine supplementation have produced intriguing results. Arginine speeds up wound healing in lab animals and in patients. Arginine-rich diets also increase T-cell function in patients with traumatic injury or surgery. In experimental animals arginine activates the thymus gland and lymphocytes. It may enhance the release of growth hormone and prolactin, which indirectly stimulate the immune system. The estimated doses of arginine required to bolster immunity (up to 30 g daily) may cause bone disorders in children and adolescents. High doses of arginine may cause nausea and DIARRHEA. The use of large doses of individual amino acids is considered experimental and long-term effects on health are being worked out; therefore, their use therapeutically should be under the guidance of a physician.

Brittenden, J. M. B. et al. "L-arginine Stimulates Host Defenses in Patients with Breast Cancer," *Surgery* 115, no. 2 (1994): 205–212.

ariboflavinosis A disease arising from a chronic deficiency of the B vitamin RIBOFLAVIN. Symptoms characterizing this condition include sores on the TONGUE (bald tongue), sores at the corners of the mouth, skin irritation, and blood-vessel formation in the cornea. Oral doses of riboflavin rectify this deficiency. Typically, malnutrition produces a general deficiency of most B COMPLEX vitamins, rather than of a single vitamin like riboflavin because they occur together in foods. Furthermore, riboflavin is one of the enrichments of BREAD and BREAKFAST CEREALS in the United States and deficiency is uncommon. However, the dietary requirement for riboflavin increases under certain conditions. For example, riboflavin in MILK is destroyed by sunlight, thyroxine (thyroid medication) decreases riboflavin absorption in the INTESTINE, and boric acid increase urinary loss of this vitamin. There may be populations in America for whom riboflavin intake is a problem. A nutritional survey of the U.S. population (NHANES I) revealed that nearly 22 percent of African Americans could be riboflavin deficient.

aromatic compounds A family of organic compounds related to benzene. Typically, their ring or cyclic structures are composed of alternating single and double bonds. Benzene (one ring, an industrial solvent), naphthalene (two rings, an ingredient of mothballs), and BENZOPYRENE (four rings) are all carcinogens. Benzopyrene is a product of charcoal grilled or BARBECUED MEAT.

Aromatic rings are constituents of a wide range of physiologically important compounds. For instance, the amino acids PHENYLALANINE, TYROSINE, HISTIDINE, and TRYPTOPHAN contain aromatic ring structures. Important body regulators like EPINEPHRINE, norepinephrine, and SEROTONIN (nerve chemical neurotransmitters) and HISTAMINE (an inflammatory agent) are aromatic compounds, as are ESTROGENS (female hormones).

Aromatic compounds are made more water-soluble, hence excretable by the KIDNEYS, through ring oxidations carried out by LIVER detoxifying enzymes (oxidases). Unfortunately, these enzymes can transform the aromatic compounds into highly reactive ones during oxidation, and they can become CARCINOGENS. (See also CYTOCHROME P450.)

arrowroot (*Maranta arundinacea*) The STARCH or FLOUR from the underground stems or rhizomes of several Central American tropical plants. The name refers to its former use by Indians to treat wounds inflicted by poisoned arrows. As a food, pulped tubers produce a white fluid that is dried, powdered, and milled. Arrowroot flour can be used in wheat-free dishes. This thickening agent can replace CORNSTARCH in recipes for soups, cream sauces, pie fillings, puddings, and glazes that need to remain clear after cooking. Arrowroot thickens at a lower temperature than wheat flour and cornstarch. Sauces prepared with arrowroot should be served soon after thickening, because the consistency will not hold. Arrowroot has a neutral flavor and does not need to be cooked to remove residual taste. It is ideal for sauces that should not boil.

arsenic A toxic heavy metal. Arsenic as a pollutant occurs in smog and cigarette smoke. High doses are thought to interfere with neurological development in children and to increase the risk of some types of CANCER. As an ingredient in some pesticides, it can contaminate produce.

Arsenic may be an essential trace nutrient. In very low amounts it is a growth promoter in POULTRY and pigs. It plays an as yet unknown function in METABOLISM in animals and perhaps in humans as well. Traces of arsenic occur in common foods: FISH, SHELLFISH, POULTRY, and CEREAL GRAINS. (See also HEAVY METALS.)

arteriosclerosis A group of pathological conditions characterized by thickened, stiffened arteries. Alterations in the innermost or outermost vessel layers can cause arteries to lose their elasticity. Arteriosclerosis alters the function of TISSUES and organs, including the brain, where it can cause major pathological changes. ATHEROSCLEROSIS is a type of arteriosclerosis in which arteries accumulate waxy deposits called PLAQUE.

The cause of arteriosclerosis is unknown, although AGING, altered FAT METABOLISM, and family history have been implicated. DIABETES MELLITUS, HYPERTENSION, increased blood FAT and blood CHOLESTEROL levels, cigarette smoking, OBESITY, being male, an inability to cope with STRESS, and physical inactivity increase the risk of this disease. A typical treatment program entails regular EXERCISE; stress management; abstinence from smoking; control of diabetes, high blood pressure, and weight; and lowering dietary cholesterol and saturated fat. (See also CARDIOVASCULAR DISEASE.)

artery A vessel transporting oxygenated blood away from the heart. Most arteries carry oxygenated blood and nutrients to peripheral tissues like MUSCLE. Arteries lead to arterioles (minute arteries), which in turn lead to capillaries, the smallest vessels. In the capillaries, OXYGEN, GLUCOSE, and other nutrients are delivered to cells. In exchange, blood acquires waste products like AMMONIA and CARBON DIOXIDE. Because the vascular or blood circulatory system is a closed system (that is, blood returns to its starting point, the heart), blood flows out of capillaries to veins (vessels that lead blood back to the heart). Blood is pumped to the lungs to release carbon dioxide in exchange for oxygen. The pulmonary artery, carrying blood from the heart to the lungs, is the only artery that does not carry oxygenated blood. Several arteries are prone to PLAQUE accumulation. The arteries feeding the heart (coronary arteries) are prime candidates for disease in men. (See also CARDIOVASCULAR DISEASE.)

arthritis A family of inflammatory diseases of the joints, including chronic degenerative joint diseases such as osteoarthritis and rheumatoid arthritis. Thirty-seven million Americans suffer from various forms of arthritis; two-thirds of them are women. Many conditions are predisposing factors for joint inflammation, including viral infection (Lyme disease), some types of FOOD POISONING, disruption of the body's chemistry (GOUT), disruption of the

IMMUNE SYSTEM (AUTOIMMUNE DISEASE), certain bacterial infections (pneumococcus, staphylococcus, and streptococcus), certain parasitic infections (giardia), physical injury, OBESITY, and physical and emotional STRESS. Arthritis is associated with AGING, and heredity also plays a role.

Osteoarthritis is the most common form of joint degeneration. It affects weight-bearing joints, especially the hips and the knees. In this type of degeneration the affected joint may exhibit worn cartilage, with bone overgrowth and bone spurs. Osteoarthritis is related to abnormal CALCIUM metabolism and stress or injury to the joint. Symptoms include morning stiffness, pain that worsens with joint function, localized tenderness, creaking, cracking of joints during movement, and restricted mobility. In primary osteoarthritis, degenerative wear and tear often occurs after the age of 50, without trauma or previous inflammatory disease, because with aging there is a decreased ability to restore normal collagen and cartilage. Secondary osteoarthritis refers to a disease caused by a factor in the patient's medical history, such as a prior injury.

VITAMIN E and VITAMIN C seem to enhance the stability of cartilage constituents (chondroitin sulfate). The essential amino acid METHIONINE and MANGANESE are also needed to produce chondroitin sulfate. VITAMIN A and VITAMIN B_6, as well as ZINC and COPPER are needed for COLLAGEN, the structural protein that helps form cartilage. A deficiency of these nutrients can accelerate joint deterioration.

Rheumatoid arthritis refers to inflamed joints with overgrowth of joint tissue and swollen and stiff joints that often cripple the patient. Symptoms include FATIGUE, low-grade fever, joint stiffness, and pain, in addition to painful, swollen joints. Generally, small joints are first affected. Unlike osteoarthritis, rheumatoid arthritis is an autoimmune condition, in which the body attacks itself. Specifically, antibodies are launched against joint tissue. Although some medical opinion disclaims the effects of food on arthritis, accumulated clinical evidence indicates that certain foods can aggravate arthritis in susceptible individuals and that food allergies can increase joint pain. Common foods in this category are nuts, DAIRY products like MILK and CHEESE, grains like CORN and WHEAT, and BEEF. Vegetables of the NIGHTSHADE FAMILY may be implicated. Individuals who are sensitive to tomatoes, pepper, or eggplant may experience less joint pain when abstaining from these foods. VEGETARIAN diets may be beneficial in rheumatoid arthritis perhaps due to the decreased consumption of ARACHIDONIC ACID. This polyunsaturated fatty acid, found primarily in MEAT and dairy products, contributes to inflammation through its conversion to certain prostaglandins and LEUKOTRIENES, hormone-like compounds that stimulate the inflammatory process. FISH and FISH OIL benefit some patients. Fish oil also reduces the formation of these inflammatory substances, hence the overall effect of eating cold-water ocean fish is to reduce inflammation. (See also ALLERGY, FOOD; DEGENERATIVE DISEASES.)

artichoke (*Cynara scolymus*) The leafy, edible buds of a perennial plant resembling the thistle; the fleshy base is surrounded by scale-like leaves. The artichoke originated in Sicily and is now widely grown in other warm climates. In the United States, globe artichokes are cultivated in mid-coastal regions of California. The artichoke has diuretic properties and has a long folk history in treatment of LIVER complaints. Research supports its therapeutic effects. Artichokes contain cynarin, a substance that has significant regenerating effects and stimulates BILE flow from the liver.

The heart of the artichoke and the top layers of the inside scaly leaves are edible after cooking. Artichokes are used as a filling in omelettes and as fritters. Artichoke hearts can be stuffed, used as a garnish, or served cold with sauce. Canned artichokes are prepared from the hearts and leaves of young buds. When packed in oil, canned artichokes should be drained and rinsed to lower the CALORIE content. A medium-sized artichoke (120 g) contains 53 calories; protein, 2.8 g; carbohydrate, 12.4 g; fiber, 4.0 g; fat, 0.2 g; calcium, 47 mg; iron, 1.6 mg; potassium, 316 mg; niacin, 0.71 mg; and small amounts of other vitamins.

artificial flavors (flavoring agents) These flavors represent the largest group of FOOD ADDITIVES and are used to replace more expensive natural flavors and to improve the taste of manufactured or synthetic foods. Although approximately two-thirds of all food additives are flavorings and flavoring agents, they are used in very small amounts. Common examples include FUMARIC ACID, HYDROLYZED VEGETABLE PROTEIN, vanillin, and cinnamaldehyde. MONOSODIUM GLUTAMATE (MSG) is classified as a FLAVOR ENHANCER rather than a flavor.

The U.S. FDA does not require specific flavoring agents to be listed on the food label because they are consumed in small amounts. Consumption averages no more than several ounces a year per person. Substituting an artificial flavor for the natural food or flavor lowers the price; however, the consumer needs to be made aware that artificial ingredients have been used. The U.S. FDA permits the general term "artificial flavoring" to be used. Although nonspecific, this designation is still helpful to consumers because foods that list artificial flavorings on their food labels will probably contain little of the natural food that would normally provide that flavor.

The long-term safety of many synthetic or natural flavors has not been rigorously studied, although the review process has weeded out several natural and synthetic flavorings. Natural root beer flavoring (safrole) was shown to cause CANCER in animals and was withdrawn in 1960. The safety of cinnamon flavor, natural or synthetic, has been questioned. It is similar to cinnamyl anthranilate, which was used in grape and cherry flavors in ice cream and beverages until the FDA proposed in 1982 that it be banned because it causes cancer in lab animals. Benzylacetate, an artificial flavoring used in CHEWING GUM, puddings and CANDY, was found to cause cancer in rats and mice by the National Toxicology Program. On the other hand, many flavors, for example caramel, are safe. A major stumbling block in moving forward with assessing the safety of artificial flavors is that the most prevalent artificial flavors, which might pose a health threat, have not been prioritized for toxicological studies. (See also CONVENIENCE FOOD; FEINGOLD DIET; FOOD LABELING; PROCESSED FOOD.)

artificial food colors (food dyes, certified food colors, synthetic food dyes, FD&C colors, coal tar dyes) Synthetic colors account for 80 percent of food coloring agents used in the food industry, and these synthetic additives pose a greater potential health risk than any other class of food additive. Because manufactured and processed foods often lack the fresh colors of whole foods, synthetic dyes have been used for years to make such foods look more appetizing or more wholesome. They provide no nutritional benefits.

Certification of artificial food colors (indicated by the FD&C designation) implies the dyes meet standards of purity, but does not assure safety. The D&C designation stands for dyes permitted only in drugs and cosmetics, not foods. Most dyes need not be specified on food labels, and instead they can be grouped under the heading "artificial coloring." Consequently the consumer may not be able to identify the dyes used in a processed food or beverage. Six dyes can be used in any food: FD&C Blue No. 1 and No. 2, Green No. 3, Red No. 40, and Yellow No. 5 and No. 6. They are common additives in CANDY, SOFT DRINKS, desserts like ICE CREAM, baked goods, and SAUSAGES. Citrus Red 2 is used only to color ORANGE skins.

How safe are artificial food colors? Many studies with experimental animals suggest that artificial food dyes cause CANCER. Few safety studies were carried out before the DELANEY CLAUSE, forbidding the addition of cancer-causing agents to any food, became law in 1962. Examination of the safety of synthetic dyes in use before 1960 has been gradual. Debate centers on the issue of whether additives that slightly increase the risk of cancer represent a tolerable risk and can be used in food.

Safety concerns about approved synthetic dyes can be summarized as follows. FD&C Red No. 40 is a suspected cause of LYMPH tumors in experimental animals. It is widely used in soft drinks, sausage, GELATIN desserts, other desserts, and candy. A long controversy surrounds FD&C Red No. 3. It causes THYROID and lymph tumors in experimental animals. FD&C Yellow No. 5 (TARTRAZINE) is the only dye that must be specifically listed on food labels. Some asthmatics and individuals allergic to ASPIRIN are also allergic to this dye, which is used in soft drinks, sausage, baked goods, candy, and gelatin desserts. FD&C Blue No. 1 causes chromosomal damage, and FD&C Blue No. 2 may cause brain tumors in experimental animals. Both are used in candy and soft drinks. FD&C Yellow No. 6 has been placed on permanent approval by the U.S. FDA, although it may cause adrenal KIDNEY tumors in rats. FD&C Green No. 3 causes bladder tumors in experimental animals. (See also ALLERGY, FOOD; CARCINOGEN; CONVENIENCE FOOD; FEINGOLD DIET; FOOD LABELING.)

artificial sweeteners Very common FOOD ADDITIVES used in PROCESSED FOODS and low-CALORIE beverages. To satisfy consumers' desire for sweets without the surplus calories of sugary, fat-laden foods, food and beverage producers rely on artificial sweeteners. Only four artificial sweeteners are currently approved in the United States: ASPARTAME, SACCHARIN, ACESULFAME-K, and SUCRALOSE. These additives contribute few or no calories. CYCLAMATE, the first artificial sweetener, has been banned. Nutrasweet (aspartame) accounts for nearly 75 percent of the $1 billion artificial sweetener market. However, its instability to heat has restricted its use to powdered mixes, SOFT DRINKS, CHEWING GUM, and a sweetener for COFFEE. Saccharin is heat stable and contains no calories, but when used alone some users find a metallic aftertaste. Acesulfame-K (Sunett) and sucralose (Splenda) are the newest of the approved artificial sweeteners. They are both heat stable and may be used in baked goods. Sucralose, which is 600 times sweeter than sugar, cannot be digested and therefore adds no calories to the foods it sweetens.

Several lines of evidence suggest that artificial sweeteners probably do not assist with weight loss. A 1998 survey by the Calorie Control Council revealed that 144 million Americans consume low-calorie products that have been sweetened artificially. Nevertheless, the average American still eats about 20 teaspoons of sugar a day, of which about 60 percent is in the form of corn sweeteners. The use of artificial sweeteners has not lowered the incidence of OBESITY in the United States; just the opposite may be true. Obesity is a major health problem for many Americans. Women saccharin users were found to be more likely to gain, not lose, weight than non-users. No study suggests that artificial sweeteners diminish APPETITE. Artificial sweeteners may actually trigger a CRAVING for CARBOHYDRATES and increase appetite, especially after eating, and thus contribute to a craving for high-calorie desserts. (See also CONVENIENCE FOOD; DIET; NATURAL SWEETENERS.)

Henkel, John. "Sugar Substitutes: Americans Opt for Sweetness and Lite," *FDA Consumer* 33, no. 6 (November–December 1999): 14–16.

ascorbic acid See VITAMIN C.

ascorbyl palmitate A fat-soluble antioxidant FOOD ADDITIVE, derived from VITAMIN C (ascorbic acid). Ascorbyl palmitate helps retard rancidity in VEGETABLE SHORTENING by preventing the oxidation of unsaturated fatty acids. It is used to add vitamin C to fortified foods and to vitamin supplements as well. Palmitic acid, a common fatty acid, is linked to ascorbic acid to make it fat-soluble. (See also ANTIOXIDANTS.)

ashwagandha (*Withenia somnifera,* Indian ginseng) A plant in the pepper family that is native to India. The plant's roots have been used medicinally in India and Africa for thousands of years to treat a variety of ailments including inflammation, fever, infertility, and impotence. The roots are believed to contain withanoloids, naturally occurring oxygenated ergostane-type steroids that are similar to ginsenosides, the active components of ginseng. Ashwagandha is marketed in the United States primarily as a herbal remedy, an anti-inflammatory, a memory and energy enhancer, and an aphrodisiac. None of these benefits have been confirmed independently in the United States.

asparagine (Asn, L-asparagine) One of the 20 AMINO ACIDS employed as a building block for PROTEINS. It was the first amino acid to be isolated (from asparagus juice in 1806). Asparagine is formed in the body from the amino acid ASPARTIC ACID and thus is classified as a nonessential amino acid. Cells convert aspartic acid to aspargine by the enzymatic addition of AMMONIA. This process creates a neutral (uncharged) amino acid from an acidic one.

asparagus (*Asparagus officinalis*) A vegetable with succulent shoots and scale-like leaves, belonging to the lily-of-the-valley family. Asparagus was known to the ancient civilizations of Egypt and Rome. Although it still grows wild in Europe, it is widely cultivated. Asparagus is a perennial, and its underground stem produces white, purple, or green shoots or spears. Asparagus root has been used as a mild diuretic in folk medicine. Martha Washington and Mary Washington are the principal varieties grown in the United States.

Asparagus deteriorates quickly, unless refrigerated after harvesting. When kept at room temperature for two days, spears lose half their VITAMIN C content and they become tougher. Asparagus should be steamed or cooked before use in omelettes and scrambled eggs, in salads, served AU GRATIN or plain, hot or cold, with a sauce or pureed. Asparagus shoots supply vitamins and minerals and are quite low in CALORIES. Four medium-sized spears (cooked, 60 g) contain protein, 1.6 g; carbohydrate, 2.6 g; fiber, 1.1 g; iron, 0.4 mg; potassium, 186 mg; vitamin A, 50 retinol equivalents; niacin, 0.63 mg; vitamin C, 16 mg; and small amounts of other vitamins.

aspartame By far the most popular ARTIFICIAL SWEETENER in America, aspartame is nearly 200 times sweeter than SUCROSE. The patent for this sweetener expired in 1992 and several versions of aspartame are now marketed. Aspartame contains two amino acids, ASPARTIC ACID, and PHENYLALANINE, plus methanol (wood alcohol). Though a caloric sweetener, fewer aspartame calories are needed to obtain a degree of sweetness comparable to that of table sugar. Aspartame does not have a bitter aftertaste, nor does it contribute to tooth decay. It has been approved by the U.S. FDA for use in fruit juice-based drinks, MALT beverages with less than 3 percent ALCOHOL, baking mixes, and flavored beverages.

Aspartame was approved by the U.S. FDA as a safe substitute for table sugar for healthy people consuming up to 23 mg per pound of body weight. For reference, a can of diet SOFT DRINK typically contains 180 to 200 mg of aspartame. Aspartame is not safe for everyone. It can be unsafe for genetic reasons; people with the inherited disease of phenylalanine metabolism, PHENYLKETONURIA, cannot metabolize high levels of phenylalanine, and they must avoid aspartame because its digestion produces phenylalanine. Food labels must warn that the product contains phenylalanine, although products do not list the amounts of aspartame they contain.

Certain individuals may be sensitive to aspartame. There have been occasional reports of migraines, disorientation, ringing ears, and confusion after eating foods containing aspartame. Reactions occur in women three times more frequently than in men. Although an adult may tolerate the aspartame in six cans of diet soda, this might be too much for a child, because of the child's lower body weight. Aspartame is not recommended for pregnant and nursing women or for infants less than six months.

Wein, Debra. "Are artificial sweeteners safe? EN updates a sticky issue," *Environmental Nutrition* 18, no. 2 (February 1995): 1, 4.

aspartic acid (Asp, L-aspartic acid) An acidic AMINO ACID and one of the 20 amino acids incorporated into PROTEINS. Aspartic acid possesses an extra acidic functional group. Aspartic acid is readily formed from OXALOACETIC ACID, a KREB'S CYCLE intermediate that is produced during the conversion of CARBOHYDRATE to energy. Hence it is a nonessential amino acid.

In addition to serving as a protein building block, aspartic acid is the precursor of the amino acid ASPARAGINE. It also donates nitrogen atoms to create UREA, the main nitrogenous waste product of the body, and to synthesize PURINES, the raw materials of ATP, DNA, and RNA. During STARVATION, oxaloacetic acid can be converted to blood sugar (GLUCOSE) by the LIVER, and therefore aspartic acid is classified as a glycogenic amino acid.

aspergillus (*Aspergillus flavus*) A common MOLD known to produce AFLATOXIN B, the most potent, naturally-occurring CARCINOGEN for liver cancer. Aflatoxin was discovered in the early 1960s in England when thousands of turkeys consumed moldy groundnut meal and developed severe liver lesions. This mold is widespread and occurs in soil, air, and foliage throughout the world. Different strains produce varying amounts of mycotoxins (mold toxins). As "storage fungus," it develops when foods are stored. Aspergillus has long been studied by food technologists. Foods often contaminated with aspergillus after storage include PEANUTS, CORN, BARLEY, CASSAVA, cottonseed meal, peanut meal, RICE, SOYBEANS, and WHEAT. In addition, aspergilli can contaminate FRUITS, several MEATS, spices, cheddar CHEESE, and various prepared foods. Improper drying and storage, high humidity, and mechanical damage to grains or nuts favor mold growth and widespread contamination. Food contaminated by mold should be discarded. Its toxins cannot be washed off. (See also FUNGUS.)

aspic A gelatin-based salad with a clear body. Aspic jelly is prepared from the clarified broth of boiled MEAT, FISH, or POULTRY. SHELLFISH, VEGETABLES, or FRUIT can also be set in a molded jelly. Powdered GELATIN can be dissolved to prepare gels for DESSERTS and entrees. Aspics can be colored and flavored with WINE or sherry. Fresh PINEAPPLE juice contains a very powerful degradative enzyme that will break down gelatin. Therefore, cooked rather than fresh pineapple should be used.

aspirin (acetylsalicylic acid) One of the most widely used analgesics (pain relievers). More than 20 million pounds of this over-the-counter medication are sold in the United States each year. In addition to reducing pain, aspirin reduces fever and swelling associated with inflammation. Several grams daily are often prescribed to treat the symptoms of ARTHRITIS. At the cellular level, aspirin blocks the formation of PROSTAGLANDINS and thromboxanes, HORMONE-like compounds that promote pain, fever, swelling, and tissue reddening, from ARACHIDONIC ACID, their immediate FATTY ACID precursor.

Moderate aspirin use may combat a variety of diseases. Studies indicate that aspirin can reduce deaths from heart attack when given soon after the attack and that daily aspirin use lowers the risk of HEART ATTACKS in men and women. These observations are explained by aspirin's blocking prostaglandins that promote the clumping of small blood cell fragments called platelets. This is a critical step in the formation of blood clots that could be life threatening. The U.S. Preventive Services Task Force (USPSTF) strongly recommends that doctors discuss with their patients who are at an increased risk of coronary heart disease the benefits and harms of aspirin therapy. Studies have shown that regular use of aspirin reduced the risk of coronary heart disease by 28 percent in patients who had never had a heart attack or stroke but who were at increased risk. These patients included men over the age of 40, postmenopausal women, and all who smoked or suffered from diabetes or high blood pressure (HYPERTENSION).

Other potential benefits of aspirin include preventing dangerous high blood pressure during pregnancy; helping victims suffering from dementia due to minor STROKES; and reducing the risk of cancers of the ESOPHAGUS, STOMACH, and COLON, according to studies by the American Cancer Society. Most of these benefits are evident with low dosage—the equivalent of one tablet daily or every other day. Aspirin's long history of use has defined potential risks. Aspirin can cause water retention, decrease KIDNEY function, and promote allergic-like reactions in susceptible people. Asthmatics are more likely to react to aspirin. For the person with food allergies, aspirin can accentuate allergy symptoms. Some effects of aspirin can be observed after short-term usage. For example, aspirin use increases VITAMIN C loss after only four to five days.

Because aspirin thins the blood, it may cause bleeding in individuals who are prone to stomach irritation or ULCERS; who have a history of hemophilia, hemorrhagic stroke, uncontrollable high blood pressure, eye problems due to diabetes, liver or kidney disease; who are facing surgery; or who are in the last trimester of pregnancy. Aspirin increases gastric bleeding, especially in the elderly who drink alcoholic beverages. Aspirin should not be used by people taking other nonsteroidal anti-inflammatory drugs or drugs to thin the blood. Children and teenagers up to the age of 18 should not be given aspirin for viral infections because it increases the risk of Reye's syndrome (a serious condition affecting the central nervous system, liver, and heart). (See also ALCOHOL-DRUG INTERACTIONS; ALLERGY, FOOD.)

Hayden, M. "Aspirin for the Primary Prevention of Cardiovascular Events: A Summary of the Evidence for the U.S. Preventive Services Task Force," *Annals of*

Internal Medicine 136, no. 2 (January 15, 2002): 161–172.

as purchased (A.P.) Refers to untrimmed foods with inedible portions (bone, husk, rind) intact. This term describes food available from retail outlets. The term *as purchased* appears in tables describing the nutrient composition of foods, where it is important to indicate the form of a specific food that was analyzed.

assessment, nutritional status The use of objective data to determine an individual's nutritional status. Dietitians and nutritionists collect data from clients in order to develop appropriate individualized plans that assure that nutritional goals will be met. Typically an in-depth nutrition assessment includes four components: anthropometric measurements, laboratory tests, physical exam, and clinical evaluation and diet analysis. Anthropometric measurements provide basic data like height and weight. Commonly these measurements are used to calculate a BODY MASS INDEX (BMI), which is the weight in kg divided by height in meters. Body fat is often estimated from measurement of tricep skinfold thickness or midarm circumference. The major problem with interpreting anthropometric values is that there are no universally agreed upon standards for comparison. Additionally, human error can result in inconsistent measurements. Other means of assessing body fat and lean body mass such as measuring electrical conductivity of a region of the body (BIOELECTRIC IMPEDENCE ANALYSIS) are common in clinics.

Chemical laboratory tests can aid in detecting marginal nutritional deficiencies. However, interpretation depends upon the clinician's understanding of the many factors that may affect a given parameter. Typical markers include serum albumin, the most prevalent non-cellular protein in blood, which has been used to assess the adequacy of dietary protein. Serum transferrin, a blood protein that transports IRON, is affected by iron deficiency anemia, pregnancy, and by serum iron overload. Urinary creatinine, a waste product from MUSCLE, can help determine muscle protein stores, since the amount of creatinine excreted in the urine is proportional to a person's muscle mass. However, creatinine excretion decreases with age. Health of the immune system is compromised by nutrient deficiencies, and total lymphocytes (white cell) count is often used to assess the status of the immune system. Infections and steroid therapy can invalidate this as a nutrition parameter.

Physical Exam and Clinical Evaluation

Although clinicians can usually identify patients with moderate to severe malnutrition, they may be less experienced at identifying patients with mild nutritional depletion. A medical history evaluates health status and uncovers underlying health issues and factors that can affect nutrition, such as alcohol and drug use, chronic disease, disabilities, or use of medications. While some signs relate directly to nutritional deficiencies as noted above, further investigation may be needed to define the underlying cause. For example, a fatty stool may indicate pancreatic insufficiency or inadequate bile production, or impaired absorption as in celiac disease. Conditions such as shortness of breath, diarrhea, constipation, nausea, gingivitis, physical pain, poor-fitting dentures, and medications may interfere with food intake and digestion. Emotional stress can lead to anorexia or depression and dramatically affect nutrient consumption. Many lifestyle factors influence food intake, including income, family structures, eating habits, physical activity, accessibility to food, use of alcohol and drugs, and philosophical or religious beliefs.

Dietary history is an essential part of nutrition assessment. The simplest form is the 24-hour recall. An interview or a questionnaire is used to determine all foods eaten in the preceding 24 hours and to estimate the quantities by using plastic food models of typical serving sizes. Alternatively, food consumption frequency can be estimated using a food checklist (food frequency questionnaire), for weekly or monthly intake of 40 to 80 of the most frequently used foods. This is a descriptive, qualitative approach. In contrast, food records and diet diaries describe the individual's current food intake, recorded daily in terms of common household measures. To involve the client in behavior modification, she or he may also be required to record eating patterns, including locations, times, events, and feelings associated with a given meal. For evaluation, intake data are translated into nutrient intake. Food composition tables form the basis of detailed nutrient intake calculations, and extensive computer software is available to aid in dietary analysis. Food scoring systems can be based on identifying foods that are the main contributors to the elevation of blood cholesterol, that contribute saturated fat or that compose a major food group.

In the final analysis, dietary nutrient intake is compared to a standard for evaluation. Typically this is the RECOMMENDED DIETARY ALLOWANCE (RDA). Since the RDAs are derived for large populations, an individual's calculated nutrient intake that is somewhat lower than the RDA need not indicate a deficiency. Nutrient intake values less than two-thirds of the RDA are best interpreted as placing the individual at risk for undernutrition.

assimilation The process by which nutrients are incorporated into cells and TISSUES of the body. Assimilation is the culmination of DIGESTION and ABSORPTION. Food entering the body can be thought of as raw materials that first must be broken down to individual nutrients by digestion. The nutrients must then be taken up into the bloodstream by absorption, and then used by cells for growth and maintenance through a complex array of chemical reactions controlled by ENZYMES and categorized as METABOLISM. Therefore, interference at any stage—digestion, absorption, assimilation—can lead to malnutrition regardless of whether the individual is consuming a balanced diet.

astaxanthin A CAROTENOID found in algae in oceans around the world, astaxanthin is what gives the pinkish hue to the flesh of salmonids (SALMON and rainbow TROUT) and the shells of lobster, crab, and shrimp. Astaxanthin is added to the feed of farm-raised fish and crustaceans to compensate for the lack of it in their diet. Researchers have demonstrated that astaxanthin is a powerful ANTIOXIDANT, more effective than BETA-CAROTENE or VITAMIN E in slowing oxidative damage by FREE RADICALS to LOW-DENSITY LIPOPROTEIN (LDL) cholesterol (the good form of cholesterol), cell membranes, cells, and tissues. Unlike beta-carotene, astaxanthine is able to cross the blood–brain barrier. Because astaxanthin has been shown to provide potential health benefits in numerous tests using laboratory animals, it is the subject of extensive research to determine whether these results can be duplicated in humans. Scientists are currently investigating its ability to enhance IMMUNE SYSTEM function, prevent cancer, promote or restore vision, and prevent or treat neuronal damage associated with ALZHEIMER'S DISEASE, PARKINSON'S DISEASE, and spinal cord injuries.

Jyonouchi, H. et al. "Astaxanthin, a Carotenoid Without Vitamin A Activity, Augments Antibody Responses in Cultures Including T-Helper Cell Clones and Suboptimal Doses of Antigen," *Journal of Nutrition* 125, no. 10 (1995): 2,483–2,492.

asthma An inflammatory respiratory disorder with labored breathing, chest constriction, wheezing, and coughing. Asthma affects an estimated 10 million Americans of all ages, and the incidence is rising yearly. This respiratory condition occurs when muscles surrounding small air passageways spasm, thus restricting air flow in and out of the lungs. The inflammation of MUCOUS MEMBRANES and overproduction of mucus further obstruct air flow. It is the resistance to air flow that produces the wheezing sound so characteristic of asthma.

Asthma is an aspect of an allergy attack called immediate hypersensitivity because the effects appear within hours of an allergic reaction. A wide range of external factors can cause asthma, including inhaled ALLERGENS (pollen, mold spores, animal dander, dust); foods (EGGS, nuts, CHOCOLATE, SHELLFISH); and some drugs. Alternatively, internal causes like upper respiratory tract infections can cause persistent asthma.

There are five classes of medications used for chronic inflammation. For treatment of acute asthma attacks, EPINEPHRINE and bronchodilators, cromolyn sodium or glucocorticoids (anti-inflammatory steroids), can be used. However, steroids have been linked to bone loss and other problems. Antihistamines are often prescribed for the wheezing, sneezing, and itching associated with allergy attacks. Eliminating the offending allergens is a direct way of avoiding further distress when the allergens occur in the home or workplace.

Many asthmatic patients respond to nutritional approaches. Food allergies are related to an estimated 75 percent of childhood cases and to approximately 40 percent of adult asthmatics. ELIMINATION DIETS, in which allergenic foods are avoided for one to four weeks, may alleviate symptoms. CORN, WHEAT, CITRUS FRUITS, DAIRY products, FISH, and CHOCOLATE are often implicated. Certain additives can cause symptoms. FD&C Yellow No. 5 (TARTRAZINE) can trigger asthma. SULFITES, which are common preservatives, trigger asthmatic attacks in susceptible people. Sulfites appear in WINE and certain salad-bar vegetables that have been pickled or canned and in other processed foods. Eating apples and the mineral selenium may lower the risk of asthma, which suggests that certain antioxidants may protect the lungs from disease. Researchers have found that people who ate at least two apples a week faced a 22 percent to 32 percent lower asthma risk than did those who ate fewer apples.

Certain nutrient deficiencies are also associated with asthma, such as VITAMIN B_6 and MAGNESIUM. VITAMIN C serves as an anti-inflammatory agent and may be helpful. Sulfite sensitive people may benefit from VITAMIN B_{12} and MOLYBDENUM. In some asthmatics with low STOMACH ACID, supplemented hydrochloric acid may help reduce symptoms. (See also ALLERGIC RHINITIS; ALLERGY, IMMEDIATE; HISTAMINE.)

astragalus A Chinese herb derived from the root of the perennial *Astragalus membranaceus* used in traditional Chinese medicine for more than 4,000 years to strengthen the immune system. Regarded as a potent tonic for increasing energy levels and stimulating the immune system, astragalus has also been used as a diuretic, as a vasodilator, and as a treatment for respiratory infections.

Astragalus, also known as milk vetch root and huang-qi, is taken in China by cancer patients to boost immunity after drug or radiation treatment and is one of the most frequently used food supplements and remedies in China. It is available as a dry or powdered root, as an extract, or as the central ingredient in herbal tea. While some patients use only the root, others also use the leaves and flowers. It may be used as a decoction. (One teaspoonful of the root is boiled in a cup of water for 10 to 15 minutes and drunk three times a day. As a tincture 2 to 4 ml is taken three times a day.)

atherosclerosis (hardening of the arteries) A progressive, chronic CARDIOVASCULAR DISEASE characterized by thickening of arterial walls and deposits called atherosclerotic PLAQUE. Atherosclerosis is the major cause of heart disease, a widespread condition in the United States where an estimated 65 million people have a form of heart or blood vessel disease. Atherosclerosis occurring in arteries supplying oxygen to the heart causes coronary heart disease and contributes to HEART ATTACKS. Medical progress and changes in diet and lifestyle have significantly reduced the number of deaths from atherosclerosis in the last decade.

There are multiple causes for clogged arteries; some, like heredity, age, and gender, are risk factors that cannot be controlled. In an estimated 5 percent of cases, a genetic defect in the transportation and utilization of CHOLESTEROL is implicated. On the other hand, many factors can be controlled to reduce an individual's probability of developing atherosclerosis. HYPERTENSION (high blood pressure) and OBESITY contribute to atherosclerosis. Family history often accompanies these conditions, yet lifestyle choices can limit their impact. For example, the failure to cope adequately with STRESS can affect the course of hypertension and obesity, while excessive consumption of ALCOHOL or CALORIES contributes to obesity. A sedentary lifestyle contributes to obesity and elevated blood cholesterol. As other examples of personal choice and disease risk, cigarette smoking can cause hypertension and high dietary saturated fat often leads to high blood cholesterol.

The roots of atherosclerosis generally go back to childhood, when the inner surfaces of arteries first become rough; then "fatty streaks" develop as deposits of LIPIDS, fibrous TISSUE, CALCIUM, and blood components accumulate. During adolescence and early adulthood, further deterioration of the wall can lead to further accumulation of calcium and cholesterol in arterial walls. The body can respond to fatty streaks by forming tough and fibrous deposits called plaque. One form of plaque consists of proliferated cells and a second type consists primarily of accumulated lipids, especially of cholesterol and cholesterol linked to fatty acids. Thickening and hardening of plaque with calcium can progress throughout a lifetime and can ultimately narrow arteries sufficiently to restrict blood flow and cause clot formation. Often the blood clot blocks the already obstructed artery, preventing oxygen and nutrients from reaching tissues it would normally feed.

The initial events in plaque formation are not completely understood. However, a growing body of clinical evidence implicates an oxidized form of cholesterol called LOW-DENSITY LIPOPROTEIN (LDL). LDL transports cholesterol from the LIVER to all other tissues, and LDL is the most prevalent cholesterol carrier in blood. LDL cholesterol can be a target of FREE RADICALS, highly reactive and damaging forms of oxygen; in the process, LDL cholesterol becomes oxidized. Possibly an early event in atherosclerosis, phagocytic cells that patrol artery walls (macrophages and neutrophils, among others) ingest oxidized LDL at damaged arterial sites and in the process become transformed into "foam" cells that accumulate lipids. Muscle cells may migrate into the developing mass as it develops into a fatty streak.

Atherosclerosis has also been proposed to be the result of the tumor-like growth of arterial cells injured by oxidized cholesterol, CARCINOGENS, or other agents such as HOMOCYSTEINE, a degradation product of the amino acid METHIONINE. It is not known whether reducing blood levels of homocysteine will lower the risk of cardiovascular disease. Alternatively, mechanical injury to the arterial wall may induce clumping of platelets, cell fragments required in blood clot formation. Still others propose that localized overproduction of growth factors (platelet-derived growth factor) could stimulate underlying smooth muscle to proliferate. The detailed involvement of platelets, oxidized blood lipids, nitric oxides, circulating carcinogens, antioxidants, macrophages, and white blood cells in plaque formation and abnormal lipid metabolism is still being actively investigated. Sudden death, heart attacks and unstable angina are often caused by coronary blood clots (thrombosis), due to dislodged atherosclerotic plaque. Unstable sites are generally inflamed. Indeed, chronic inflammation plays an important role in the formation, progression, and disruption of atherosclerotic plaque.

Laboratory blood tests to measure an individual's risk of developing atherosclerosis have become increasingly sophisticated. Elevated blood lipids have often been regarded as a risk factor for atherosclerosis. However, elevated serum TRIGLYCERIDES (FAT) and elevated serum cholesterol levels are at best only crude indicators of risk of cardiovascular disease. A ratio of total serum cholesterol to HDL cholesterol is more useful. HDL (HIGH-DENSITY LIPOPROTEIN) helps remove cholesterol from tissues and returns it to the liver for disposal or redistribution, thus HDL serves a quite different role from LDL.

An even more accurate assessment of risk of atherosclerosis can be obtained from a determination of the ratio of specific marker proteins, apoprotein B, a marker for LDL cholesterol, to apoprotein A, a marker for HDL cholesterol. Another cholesterol carrier called lipoprotein (a), a close cousin of LDL, may be useful as a predictor of heart disease for children, especially for those whose parents or parent had suffered a heart attack before the age of 42. Elevated homocysteine is considered an independent risk factor. Vascular inflammation in coronary heart disease may be assessed by measuring a blood marker for inflammation called C-reactive protein.

Recent evidence suggests that atherosclerosis may be reversed. One protocol prescribes a near-VEGETARIAN diet supplying only 10 percent of total calories from fat and 5 mg of cholesterol a day; abstinence from smoking and alcohol; 30 minutes of EXERCISE daily at least six times per week; at least an hour daily of stress-reduction exercises, including yoga and meditation, with twice weekly meetings in a support group. The mental as well as the physical aspects of this program seem essential for its success in opening arteries partially blocked through disease. (See also HYPERCHOLESTEROLEMIA; VEGETARIAN.)

Brown, A. J., and W. Jessup. "Oxysterols and Atherosclerosis," *Atherosclerosis* 142, no. 1 (January 1999): 1–28.

Futterman, L. G., and L. Lemberg. "The Use of Antioxidants in Retarding Atherosclerosis: Fact or Fiction?" *American Journal of Critical Care* 8, no. 2 (March 1999): 130–133.

Ridker, P. M. "Inflammation, Atherosclerosis, and Cardiovascular Risk: An Epidemiologic View," *Blood Coagul Fibrinolysis* 10, suppl 1 (February 1999): S9–12.

Atkins diet A high-protein, low-carbohydrate weight loss program based on the book *Dr. Atkins Diet Revolution,* first published in 1972 by the late Dr. Robert Atkins, who described a theory that most people are overweight because they eat too many CARBOHYDRATES. Patients who follow the Atkins plan eat a diet of almost all protein and fat. Red meat, butter, cheese, eggs, mayonnaise, and similar high-fat, high-protein foods that are usually restricted on other weight-loss programs form the basis of the Atkins diet.

During the first two weeks of the plan—the "induction period"—patients are restricted to consuming no more than 20 g of carbohydrates a day. This induces the body to go into a state of fat-burning fasting called ketosis. During ketosis the body burns ketones, which is fuel created by the breakdown of fat cells. The theory is that instead of burning carbohydrates for fuel the body feeds on its stores of fat.

Use of this diet continues to be controversial. Ever since Dr. Atkins published his theory, nutrition and health experts have criticized it as unhealthy, and it has been denounced by the American Heart Association. The Atkins plan contradicts numerous studies that have demonstrated the significant correlation between diets high in saturated fat and increased heart disease risk, and it contradicts dietary recommendations set forth in the U.S. Department of Agriculture's (USDA) FOOD GUIDE PYRAMID, which recommends six to 15 daily servings of high-carbohydrate foods such as fruit, rice, bread, cereal, and whole grain products. There is little evidence that carbohydrates alone affect body weight. Being overweight reflects consuming too many calories.

Critics of the diet say the high levels of saturated fat in the food it recommends can elevate cholesterol levels and lead to cardiovascular disease and HEART ATTACK. Atkins supporters say blood cholesterol levels may rise initially but quickly return to prediet levels or drop to even lower levels with time. Because the diet recommends that patients restrict their intake of fruits and vegetables, some experts say it increases the risk of developing cancer. The National Cancer Institute recommends patients consume no fewer than five daily servings of fruits and vegetables, many of which contain cancer-fighting ANTIOXIDANTS, to minimize the risk of cancer. Recent research shows that patients who are most successful at losing weight and keeping it off do so by exercising regularly and lowering their daily caloric intake by eating foods low in sugar and fat and high in fiber. (See also WEIGHT MANAGEMENT.)

"The Truth About Dieting," *Consumer Reports,* June 2002.

Miller, B. V. et al. "Effects of a Low Carbohydrate, High Protein Diet on Renal Function," *Obesity Research* 8, suppl. 1 (2000): 82S.

atopic dermatitis See DERMATITIS.

ATP (adenosine triphosphate) A compound containing "high energy" phosphate bonds that function as the energy currency of cells. ATP contains chemical ENERGY and must be constantly replenished and recycled within cells. It is used for all energy-requiring processes including synthesis of all cellular constituents (PROTEINS, FAT, LIPIDS, POLYSACCHARIDES, DNA) and cell division, movement and MUSCLE contraction, nerve impulses, and even the maintenance of ELECTROLYTE balance in cells. ATP is not stored and it cannot be eaten to increase its level in the body.

ATP is produced by CATABOLISM, the summation of all chemical processes in the cell that convert energy stored in fat and CARBOHYDRATE to ATP. MITOCHONDRIA, subcellular structures that function as the cell's powerhouses, produce most of the ATP in many types of cells, except red blood cells, by the oxidation of fat and carbohydrate. The cellular mechanism coupling this oxidation with the trapping of about 40 percent of the released energy as ATP is called OXIDATIVE PHOSPHORYLATION. In this process, electrons obtained from fuel oxidation pass through a sequence of electron carrier proteins (CYTOCHROMES), which operate like a bucket brigade. Simultaneously, inorganic phosphate ions attach to ADP (adenosine diphosphate) to form ATP, while oxygen is reduced to WATER.

VITAMINS of the B COMPLEX assist the enzymic machinery of the mitochondrial engine in its energy conversions. Without B vitamins, fuel is not burned efficiently, curtailing ATP output. They do not create ATP nor are they burned as fuel, however. (See also CARBOHYDRATE METABOLISM; FAT METABOLISM; KREB'S CYCLE.)

atrophy A reduction in size and function of a tissue, organ, or structural element of the body. MALNUTRITION, decreased physical activity, a change in HORMONE balance, reduced cell proliferation, and diminished oxygen supply can cause atrophy of tissues. Emaciation characterizes extreme STARVATION, ANOREXIA, or disease processes preventing nutrient assimilation.

attention deficit-hyperactivity disorder (ADHD) Behavior disturbances characterized by overactivity and restlessness, aggressive behavior, poor self control, and short attention span. As many as 4 percent of children suffer from hyperactivity, which affects more boys than girls through adolescence. As many as 30 percent to 50 percent of individuals who had ADHD as children continue to have it as adults. Multiple factors have been implicated in hyperactivity and inattentiveness:

- Artificial FOOD ADDITIVES: Some experts believe that synthetic chemicals like ARTIFICIAL FOOD COLORS, PRESERVATIVES, and salicylates (compounds related to aspirin) affect the nervous system.
- Food allergies and FOOD SENSITIVITIES: Clinical studies indicate that elimination of offending foods from an allergic child's diet can sometimes improve scholastic performance dramatically.
- Abnormal CARBOHYDRATE METABOLISM: Some people with ADHD may be unable to metabolize SUGAR normally. Behavioral problems have been reported to be linked with excessive consumption in these individuals.
- Toxic exposure: Excessive aluminum, lead, and copper may be associated with hyperactivity.
- Nutritional deficiencies: Deficiencies of iron, calcium, magnesium, zinc, and essential fatty acids have been linked to fidgeting, restlessness, and learning difficulties. Occasionally, children respond to niacin, vitamin B_6, and thiamin supplementation.

Following the FEINGOLD DIET, which limits consumption of artificial colors and preservatives and eliminates sensitive food from the child's diet, can sometimes be beneficial. However, experience has shown that effective treatment involves the entire family in order to create a supportive environment. A high-protein, low-carbohydrate diet with limited refined sugar may be beneficial, but the role of sugar in behavior is controversial. The DIETARY GUIDELINES FOR AMERICANS state that sugar does not cause hyperactivity. Indeed, several clinical trials have not detected an association. On the other hand, excessive dietary sugar leads to nutrient deficiencies that contribute to hormonal imbalances affecting behavior.

Conventional treatment to regulate ADHD relies on psychological counseling, behavior modification and drugs (stimulants, tranquilizers, and tricylic ANTIDEPRESSANTS). (See also ADDICTION AND SUGAR; ALLERGY, FOOD.)

au gratin From the French term for a golden crust on the surface of a prepared dish. In the United States, this term usually refers to a food coated with grated, strongly flavored CHEESES or BREAD crumbs and melted BUTTER, therefore higher in CALORIES than baked or steamed foods. A scalloped or sauce dish can be lightly coated with bread crumbs, crushed corn flakes, ground nuts, or cracker crumbs and heated to form a golden brown crust. More generally, VEGETABLES, FISH, and PASTA dishes can be cooked so that a layer forms on the surface, thus protecting underlying food from drying out.

autoimmune diseases Disorders of the IMMUNE SYSTEM in which the body attacks itself. Normally, the body employs the immune system to discriminate very carefully between foreign invaders, which are attacked, and its own TISSUES. In autoimmune diseases, the immune system mistakenly produces ANTIBODIES against specific tissues. Such an attack can lead to crippling damage. Studies to define underlying causes suggest there is a major breakdown in the way the body discriminates between foreign cells and its own tissues. Monitoring self-recognition is a complex process involving many components of the immune system that are currently being studied:

- Normal controls (T-helper cells) that regulate B cells responsible for forming "self-directed" antibodies may be bypassed. T-cells and B cells are the two major types of lymphocytes (white blood cells).
- "Rheumatoid factor," antibodies present in 50 percent to 95 percent of patients.
- Defects in the production of cells regulating antibody production (T-helper cells or T-suppressor cells) due to genetic defects or defects caused by viruses.
- Specific antibody-binding sites. HLA antigens on cell surfaces are linked to a susceptibility to several autoimmune diseases, like insulin-independent diabetes and LUPUS ERYTHEMATOSUS.
- FOOD SENSITIVITY and ALLERGY are implicated in some cases.

Examples of different autoimmune diseases include the following:

Rheumatoid Arthritis A disease progressing from inflammation of the joint to a deterioration of cartilage. It is characterized by special antibodies, "rheumatoid factors" in the blood that can be measured clinically. Patients with rheumatoid arthritis have increased amounts of a specific type of "histocompatibility" (HLA) antigen. These antigens control transplantation reactions. In some cases food allergies are implicated.

Insulin-dependent Diabetes Glucose accumulation in the blood due to the destruction of insulin-producing cells of the PANCREAS. With the loss of the ability to make INSULIN, there is an absolute requirement for the hormone. This disease is also characterized by the presence of a specific kind of antibody recognition site (histocompatibility or HLA antigen). The best early marker of this disease appears to be an antibody against the insulin-producing tissue of the pancreas.

Lupus Erythematosus (Systemic) A chronic inflammatory disease that can attack many organs, especially their connective tissues. It is much less common than rheumatoid arthritis and occurs most frequently in women between the ages of 20 and 40. The rate of occurrence has steadily increased in the last 30 years, although its cause is unknown.

Multiple Sclerosis (MS) Characterized by blurred vision and a gradual loss of control of movement as nerve tissue is damaged. There is also spotty damage to the motor and sensory nerves. This disease apparently begins early in life. Early stages are characterized by feeling clumsy and heavy, with "pins and needles" sensations and feeling light-headed. Living in northern states increases the risk of getting MS. One or two people per thousand Americans have the disease. The cause of MS is unknown, and there is no proven cure. Abnormalities in the immune response have been detected in patients with MS, possibly triggered by a prior viral infection. Most nutrition research has focused on decreased dietary FAT and increased ESSENTIAL FATTY ACIDS. (See also NIGHTSHADE FAMILY.)

Harbige, L. S. "Nutrition and Immunity with Emphasis on Infection and Autoimmune Disease," *Nutrition and Health* 10, no. 4 (1996): 285–312.

avidin A protein in EGG white that binds to BIOTIN, making this B vitamin unavailable for intestinal absorption. Avidin in one of several nutrient binding proteins in egg white that help prevent bacterial growth, which could threaten the fertilized egg. Avidin binds biotin so tightly and selectively that it has been used to experimentally induce biotin deficiency in animals, which otherwise is difficult to study. There is no risk of biotin deficiency due to avidin when consuming cooked eggs because avidin is inactivated by heat. (See also ANTIVITAMIN.)

avitaminosis A vitamin deficiency disease. Such diseases can be caused by a dietary deficiency, by maldigestion or by the MALABSORPTION of a vitamin. Though rare in industrialized nations, acute vitamin deficiency diseases are all too common throughout developing nations, especially among children and elderly populations. Preclinical signs and symptoms usually precede the appearance of a full-blown deficiency disease such as SCURVY (VITAMIN C); PELLAGRA (NIACIN); BERIBERI (THIAMIN); RICKETS (VITAMIN D); and ANEMIA (various vitamins such as FOLIC ACID and VITAMIN B_{12}, among others). The MINIMAL DAILY REQUIREMENT was a standard operationally defined by the minimal amount of a nutrient that must be supplied to prevent deficiency disease. (See also MALNUTRITION.)

avocado (*Persea Americana*) A fruit native to Central and South America, and cultivated in the United States in California and Florida. Depending on the variety, avocados vary from bell-shaped and green to pear-shaped with a coarse, shell-like skin. This fruit is unusually high in FAT, ranging from 5 percent to 20 percent, although most of it is monounsaturated. A MONOUNSATURATED OIL derived from the avocado is rather expensive and resembles OLIVE OIL in FATTY ACID composition. Avocado oil contains 69 percent monounsaturated fatty acids and 14 percent POLYUNSATURATED FATTY ACIDS. The corresponding values for olive oil are 72 percent and 9 percent respectively. These monounsaturated oils are more healthful than saturated oils and polyunsaturates because they lower LDL CHOLESTEROL while maintaining HDL cholesterol levels with typical high fat consumption.

The flesh has a buttery consistency and a mild flavor. Fresh avocados may be used as hors d'oeuvres or in salads, mousses, and souffles. Sliced avocados darken rapidly when exposed to air and room temperature. The enzyme-catalyzed darkening can be reduced by refrigeration or by adding LEMON juice or VINEGAR. One half of an avocado, four inches long (100 g) provides calories, 160; protein, 2.0; fat, 15 g; carbohydrate, 7 g; potassium, 600 mg; iron, 1.0 mg; vitamin A, 60 retinol equivalent; vitamin C, 8 mg; niacin, 1.9 mg; thiamin, 0.1 mg; riboflavin, 0.1 mg.

azodicarbonamide A FOOD ADDITIVE used to age (condition) WHEAT flour. Aging is an OXIDATION process. During aging, FLOUR constituents, including PROTEIN, are chemically altered to yield an elastic dough that is lighter and easier to manage. Elastic doughs can rise more readily with the CARBON DIOXIDE released by LEAVENING AGENTS. Before the use of food additives, wheat flour was stored for several months in order to alter the properties of GLUTEN. Flour conditioning agents now accomplish the same result in a matter of days.

B

baby food Foods other than MILK and INFANT FORMULA fed to babies during their first year. Commercially prepared baby foods in jars (cooked or pureed food) and in packets (as dehydrated food) offer a large variety of wholesome and nutritious food, including MEATS, CEREALS, VEGETABLES, FRUITS, DESSERTS, and combination foods. Food consistency varies from strained to chunky according to the developmental age of the child.

No ARTIFICIAL FOOD COLORS or ARTIFICIAL FLAVORS are added. However, FOOD ADDITIVES may be included to inhibit MOLDS, increase texture, or soften foods. Until the 1980s, most bottled baby foods contained MODIFIED CORNSTARCH as a thickener. This questionable food additive is now seldom used in baby foods.

Salt and SUGAR were once common additives to manufactured baby foods. Ironically, these were often added to satisfy the parent's taste. Baby foods are now either unsweetened or contain low amounts of sugar, and manufacturers have eliminated salt. There is no health reason for adding SODIUM, SUCROSE, MONOSODIUM GLUTAMATE (MSG), or PRESERVATIVES to baby foods. Furthermore, tastes for salty and sugary foods can be acquired, which suggests a potential risk of establishing a child's preference for PROCESSED FOOD at an early age. Although all ingredients are listed on baby food labels, the labels can be misleading. For example, "high meat" dinners need be only 26 percent meat in baby food, and "chicken and rice" for babies need be only 5 percent chicken according to regulations. (See also BREAST-FEEDING; FOOD LABELING.)

Kurtzweil, Paula. "Labelling Rules for Young Children's Food," *FDA Consumer* 29, no. 2 (March 1995): 14–18.

Bacillus cereus A bacterium capable of causing FOOD POISONING. There are two forms of *B. cereus* food poisoning: In the diarrheal form, infection is associated with VEGETABLES, SAUCES, puddings, PASTRY, and MEAT dishes that have been improperly refrigerated after cooking, permitting bacterial spores to begin growing. The bacteria produce toxins (ENTEROTOXIN) in the intestine that cause symptoms including severe DIARRHEA and abdominal pain, and, occasionally, associated nausea. Symptoms generally appear 10 to 12 hours after consuming contaminated food and usually diminish within 24 hours.

A second food poisoning syndrome (EMETIC syndrome) is due to the production of a different toxin, which is produced in the food itself. Fried RICE is often a culprit in Asian restaurants. In the typical scenario, boiled rice is allowed to dry; then it may be stored overnight or longer before it is fried. Heat resistant bacterial spores may form. Symptoms generally appear within one to five hours and include nausea, vomiting, and malaise.

To minimize this source of food poisoning, freshly cooked food is best eaten hot. Food allowed to cool slightly and kept warm for extended periods may promote bacterial growth. Cooked food should be kept hot or cooled rapidly and refrigerated.

bacon Smoked and cured cuts from the back and rib area of the hog. Bacon is a high-fat food that is usually thinly sliced and fried or grilled. Bacon burns easily, and old bacon burns twice as fast as fresh. Bacon, 100 g or about three ounces, cooked and drained of FAT, represents 573 CALORIES, and most of this is due to SATURATED FAT. Canadian-style bacon resembles HAM and comes from a muscle in the eye of a pork loin; it should be cooked more like ham. It is a leaner meat than U.S. bacon; 100 g equals 183 calories.

NITRITES are added to bacon and other cured meats to retard bacterial growth and to maintain a brighter color. The legal limit of nitrite in bacon was set at 100 ppm (parts per million) in 1985. Cancer researchers are concerned that nitrite can react with nitrogen-containing compounds (AMINES) in foods to form a potent carcinogen (cancer-causing agent) called nitrosoamine. Among cured MEATS, levels of nitrosoamines were found to be highest in bacon because it is fried at high temperatures, which promotes nitrosoamine formation. The U.S. Department of Agriculture requires that VITAMIN C (ascorbic acid) or another ANTIOXIDANT be added to minimize the formation of nitrosoamine when the meat is cooked. (See also MEAT.)

bacteria, intestinal Microorganisms that normally grow in the human INTESTINE. In adults the intestine contains more bacteria than there are cells in the body. The colon contains most of the intestinal bacteria, weighing typically 4 to 6 pounds and including nonspore-forming anaerobic bacteria, anaerobic streptococci, and acid-forming bacteria. In this regard, lactobacillus species and bifidobacter species are most important. In a healthy person, the bacterial flora are relatively constant. This is remarkable, considering the many pounds of food ingested daily and the huge number of microorganisms in the environment.

"Friendly" gut bacteria are important in maintaining a healthy intestinal flora that benefit the body. Lactobacillus species occupy the lower portions of the small intestine, where they adhere to the intestinal wall and prevent potential pathogens (disease-producing microorganisms) from growing on the intestinal wall. The exclusion of potential pathogens from attachment sites on the intestinal wall where they might colonize in the presence of normal bacteria is referred to as microbial interference. Lactobacillus and bifidobacteria break down carbohydrate to produce LACTIC ACID, which helps create an acidic environment that is unfavorable for many potential pathogenic microorganisms. These bacteria also produce substances that limit the growth of undesirable organisms, including yeasts.

Intestinal bacteria ferment much of the FIBER an undigested carbohydrates, which are further metabolized by bacteria to short-chain fatty acids (ACETIC ACID, PROPIONIC ACID, and BUTYRIC ACID) and methane and hydrogen. The short-chain fatty acids may supply more than 10 percent of the body's energy needs, and butyric acid specifically promotes the health of the colon. Other useful bacterial products include VITAMIN K and BIOTIN in quantities usually adequate to meet most daily requirements.

A state of imbalanced intestinal bacteria is called dysbiosis, which is characterized by low levels of desirable bacteria and the appearance of harmful, opportunistic organisms. Many factors can cause dysbiosis. The most common cause is the chronic use of broad-spectrum antibiotics that destroy many types of bacteria, including the beneficial ones. A Western-style diet, characterized by high meat, high fat, and low fiber consumption, favors dysbiosis. STRESS, inadequate stomach acid to sterilize food in the stomach, and aging can imbalance gut bacteria.

Pancreatic insufficiency can lead to carbohydrate maldigestion and inflammation or other alteration of the intestine, which can limit carbohydrate digestion and uptake. Excessive undigested carbohydrate resulting from maldigestion and MALABSORPTION can promote bacterial proliferation leading to DIARRHEA, FLATULENCE, and bloating. LACTOSE INTOLERANCE, which is due to the inability to digest milk sugar, leads to intestinal discomfort when bacteria are able to ferment undigested lactose. Unusually rapid movement of food through the digestive tract (shortened transit time) and diarrhea change the amounts and the relative composition of intestinal bacteria. Lactic acid bacteria supplements are available to help repopulate the intestine and help relieve symptoms of diarrhea. (See also ACIDOPHILUS; *ESCHERICHIA COLI*.)

Gibson, Glenn R., and Marcel B. Roberfroid. "Dietary Modulation of the Human Colonic Microbiota: Introducing the Concept of Prebiotics," *Journal of Nutrition* 125, no. 6 (1995): 1,401–1,412.

bacterial toxins Complex substances produced by disease-causing bacteria. Toxins cause disease, especially FOOD POISONING. Enterotoxins represent one class of bacterial toxins. These substances irritate the lining of the intestines, causing diarrhea and intestinal muscle spasms.

The two most common toxin-producing bacteria that contaminate food and cause food poisoning are staphylococcus and clostridium. They produce protein enterotoxins and are a common cause of food poisoning in the United States and other countries. Other pathogenic bacteria, like SALMONELLA, cause illness by infecting the intestinal tract. Foods most likely to be involved in outbreaks of enterotoxin poisoning are contaminated, cooked foods such as HAM, POULTRY, BEEF, cream-filled pastry, FISH, SHELLFISH, potato salad, macaroni salad, and egg and milk products. Following contamination of a food, the staphylococcal bacteria require several hours of incubation at warm temperatures to form toxins. Sometimes large amounts of warm food placed in refrigeration cool so slowly that staphylococcal growth and toxin production occur. Brief reheating does not destroy enterotoxins.

Neurotoxins represent a second class of bacterial toxins. The most notorious neurotoxin causes BOTULISM, in a rare, potentially deadly form of food poisoning that occurs throughout the world. This disease is caused by the anaerobic, spore-forming bacillus *Clostridium botulinum,* which can produce a neurotoxin in inadequately canned or contaminated food. Botulinum toxins are heat-stable proteins that persist in cooked food. They are among the most poisonous natural toxins; only two micrograms can be lethal to an adult. Spores of clostridium botulinum are not killed at the temperature of boiling water, thus canning procedures must employ higher temperatures (230° F–250° F) for several minutes to assure destruction of this spore-forming bacteria.

Endotoxins are a third class of bacterial toxins. They represent a heterogenous group of products released from bacterial cell walls and protoplasm when bacteria die and disintegrate. They are normally excluded by the intestinal mucosal barrier and intestinal antibodies. However, with gut inflammation the intestinal lining becomes leaky and endotoxins may be absorbed to a limited extent. CYTOTOXINS are then capable of attacking cells of specific organs and causing disease. (See also FOOD TOXINS; LEAKY GUT.)

bagel A doughnut-shaped, dense roll made with high-protein flour. The basic ingredients are typical of most BREADS; FLOUR, water, YEAST, and salt. Recent trends are to add sweeteners like sugar or honey. Most of the CALORIES come from CARBOHYDRATE, not FAT. Egg bagels contain additional fat and CHOLESTEROL derived from eggs. Bagels are traditionally eaten with cream cheese and lox. A typical plain bagel weighing 68 grams (2.4 oz) supplies 200 calories; carbohydrate, 38.2 g; protein, 7.5 g; and fat, 1.75 g. Larger bagels may weigh three times as much and supply an additional 75 to 80 calories, and 1 to 2 grams of fat per ounce.

baker's yeast Strains of the yeast *Sacchromyces cervisia* used to leaven bread and other bakery items. The purpose of yeast is to metabolize carbohydrates and generate CARBON DIOXIDE, which when trapped as bubbles makes the dough rise. Yeast enzymes break down glucose released from the starch in dough. To maximize this leavening effect, strains of *S. cervisia* have been selected for their ability to ferment sugar with maximum carbon dioxide formation and minimal ALCOHOL production. Thus baker's yeast differs from BREWER'S YEAST, which maximizes ALCOHOL production from sugar. Dried, easy-blend baker's yeast is available in packets. It must be reconstituted in warm water before it is added to dough in order to activate yeast ENZYMES to generate carbon dioxide; the dehydrated yeast themselves cannot reproduce. Sugar fermentation is best carried out at 80° F to 95° F, the temperature recommended to permit dough to rise.

baking powder A mixture of chemicals that generates CARBON DIOXIDE in dough, both in the mixing bowl and in the oven and without the intervention of yeast. Bubbles of carbon dioxide create pockets in the dough that make leavened bread and baked goods lighter. Baking powders typically contain three types of ingredients to maximize their effectiveness: sodium bicarbonate, an acidic chemical, and an anticaking agent like CORNSTARCH or calcium silicate to prevent caking in high humidity. In the presence of water, the acidic ingredient reacts with the basic salt, sodium bicarbonate, to generate carbon dioxide bubbles. Sodium bicarbonate is considered a safe food additive. Baking powder (and baking soda) contribute approximately 25 percent of the typical American's SODIUM consumption, and typical dietary guidelines recommend cutting back on sodium to minimize the risk of high blood pressure in susceptible people.

Three types of baking powders are available that are classed according to their acidic ingredients. Tartrate baking powders contain sodium or calcium tartrate. These acidic salts reach quickly, and doughs containing them cannot be stored. Phosphate baking powders contain calcium acid phosphate, which can react in cold dough as well as releasing carbon dioxide during baking. Sodium pyrophosphate is sometimes added as an acidic ingredient. Studies suggest that pyrophosphate may harm fetal animals. Pregnant women may wish to avoid this particular food additive. Double-acting baking powders, designated (SAS), incorporate sodium ALUMINUM phosphate (or sulfate) and calcium acid phosphate. They generate carbon dioxide in cold dough, but they are most active when they contact the heated oven. A serving of cake prepared with these baking powders can contain 5 to 15 mg of aluminum. Aluminum was once thought to be a safe food additive, but its safety has been questioned because it has been shown to accumulate in the brains of senile patients. (See also ALZHEIMER'S DISEASE.)

baking soda (bicarbonate of soda, sodium bicarbonate) A common leavening agent used in baked goods. Baking soda can be used in place of baking powder when an acidic ingredient is also added. Sour milk, molasses, or CREAM OF TARTAR are sufficiently acidic to make dough and batter rise. The chemical reaction is the same as that occurring when baking powders are used, although baking soda produces more tender, lighter baked goods. Because bread and baked goods are a large part of the American diet, baking powder and baking soda are major dietary sources of SODIUM: They contribute one-quarter of the average person's sodium intake. Excessive sodium intake increases the risk of high blood pressure in susceptible people. To test the effectiveness of any baking powder, mix a teaspoon of baking powder with a half teaspoon of hot water. A fully active powder will bubble vigorously. Baking soda is classified as a safe food additive. (See also BAKER'S YEAST.)

balanced diet A diet that supplies all essential nutrients in the appropriate amounts for optional health throughout the life span. Food should provide VITAMINS, MINERALS, PROTEIN, CARBOHYDRATE, FAT, OILS, and FIBER to meet individual needs. The CALORIES consumed should match the amount used in order to stabilize body weight.

Variety characterizes a balanced diet, which emphasizes fresh, minimally processed, or whole foods. Exchange lists, which can be found in some nutrition books, simplify making healthful food choices by supplying a variety of options; for example, among different protein sources. While not specifically a low-fat, low-CHOLESTEROL diet, a balanced diet tends to have less saturated fat, refined carbohydrate and cholesterol. Diseases like CANCER, HYPERTENSION, OSTEOPOROSIS, diabetes, and CARDIOVASCULAR DISEASE have reached epidemic proportions and are linked to unbalanced diets. A balanced diet definitely plays a role in preventing these and other chronic diseases.

Those who rely on PROCESSED FOOD, high in fat, sugar, salt, and other FOOD ADDITIVES, run the risk of an unbalanced diet. Consumption of such foods increases the need for other foods in the diet that are nutrient dense. However, the temptation is to eat more of the same processed foods, which may also be less nutritious because of the way they were grown, stored, or processed. People who skip meals without replacing them with nutritious snacks, and who choose a weight loss diet, consuming less than 1,500 calories per day, are likely to have inadequate diets. Individuals at an increased risk include low-income, pregnant, or lactating women; low-income children and teenagers; elderly persons eating alone; and strict VEGETARIANS, who may not consume enough needed nutrients. Pollution and job-related chemical hazards may increase nutrient needs beyond those supplied by the usual diet. Limiting food choices because of income or strict religious or philosophical preference requires planning to assure adequate consumption of all essential nutrients.

Replacing EMPTY CALORIES and sugary foods with more nutritious options represents a major challenge in achieving a balanced diet. Variety simplifies the task. Vegetables supply low-fat energy in the form of starch, vitamins, beta-carotene, minerals, and fiber. Dark green leafy vegetables include

CHARD, KALE, and COLLARD, in addition to spinach. The cabbage family encompasses BROCCOLI, BRUSSELS SPROUTS, CAULIFLOWER, and Chinese cabbage. Winter SQUASH, summer squash, and YAMS represent yellow-colored vegetables. Whole grains are also important: WHEAT, CORN, MILLET, RICE, TRITICALE, RYE, and BUCKWHEAT for starch and minerals, vitamins, and fiber. LEGUMES supply fiber and protein: beans and peas, CHICKPEAS, lima beans, and LENTILS. A balanced diet includes low-fat dairy products: low-fat CHEESE, low-fat or skim MILK, YOGURT, KEFIR, and EGGS for protein and CALCIUM. Nuts and seeds provide plant oils: ALMONDS and SUNFLOWER and PUMPKIN seeds. Lean MEATS, POULTRY, FISH, and SHELLFISH provide trace minerals, vitamins, and AMINO ACIDS. A variety of fruits supply VITAMIN C, POTASSIUM, and fiber. (See also DIETARY GUIDELINES FOR AMERICANS.)

balm (*Melissa officinalis;* lemon balm, garden balm, balm mint) A lemon-scented herb native to Europe. Lemon balm is a perennial growing up to two feet in height with broad, dark green leaves. Its pale yellow flowers grow in clusters. Leaves and sprigs contribute a subtle lemon flavor to beverages (teas and lemonade), as well as to stuffings, sauces, fish, white meat dishes, soups, and salad dressing.

bamboo shoot (*Arundinaria, Bambusa, Dendrocalamus*) The young, tender, sprouting stems of several types of bamboo that are used in Asian cooking. This plant grows in tropical Asia. Edible shoots are white and conical in shape, averaging 25 inches in diameter and 4 inches in length. They are peeled and sliced into strips before cooking. Boiling bamboo shoots removes a toxin (hydrocyanic acid). Canned bamboo shoots are precooked. Precooked bamboo shoots are used in soups, stir fries, and hors d'oeuvres and can accompany MEAT and FISH. Salted, dried shoots are used as a seasoning. In Japan, bamboo shoots are a spring vegetable. The shoots have a high water content. Canned bamboo shoots (1 cup, 131 g) provide 25 calories; protein, 2.3 g; carbohydrate, 4.2 g; fiber, 3.3 g; iron, 0.42 mg; with traces of vitamins, minerals, and fat.

banana (*Musa paradisiaca*) A seedless fruit of the banana tree, the most popular fruit in the United States. Their popularity is based on the fact that bananas have a pleasant taste, are inexpensive, are easily chewed and are available year-round. The banana originated in India and is now cultivated in many tropical regions. The banana tree resembles a palm. Although there are many varieties of bananas, they fall into two major groups: Fruit bananas are eaten raw and occasionally cooked; plantains are cooked as vegetables. Yellow bananas are the most common variety sold in the United States. These bananas are harvested green to avoid damaged, overripe fruit at the market. Green bananas will ripen at room temperature in a few days, and ripened fruit (solid yellow flecked with brown spots) can be refrigerated to prevent further ripening. Refrigeration darkens the skin but does not affect the flavor. Overripe bananas are used in breads, muffins, and other baked goods. Bananas are a rich source of potassium. A single eight-inch banana (114 g) provides 105 calories; protein, 1.2 g; carbohydrate, 26.7 g; fiber, 3.3 g; iron 0.35 mg; potassium, 451 mg; thiamin, 0.05 mg; riboflavin, 0.11 mg; niacin, 0.81 mg.

barbecued meat/charcoal broiled meat MEAT that is cooked over a gas, electric, or charcoal grill. Cooking over charcoal is an ancient form of cooking, and most foods, including meat, FISH, and POULTRY, can be cooked on a grill. Foods acquire a distinctive flavor when grilled. Some meats are better flavored if they have been marinated beforehand. Vegetables like corn, potatoes, peppers, and mushrooms can be wrapped in aluminum foil and cooked on a grill. Barbecued food can be BASTED or served with any of a variety of traditional sauces. To prevent food poisoning, meat and poultry should be defrosted in the refrigerator. Leftover marinade should be discarded. Cooked food should never be put back on a plate that held raw food. Likewise, all surfaces and utensils touched by raw foods should be washed thoroughly with soap and hot water.

Barbecuing meat allows fat to drip on hot coals or hot metal, which forms CANCER-causing agents (BENZOPYRENES). These vaporize, adhere to soot, and deposit on the surface of the meat. To lessen the production of carcinogens, meat should be trimmed of all visible fat before cooking. Other methods to reduce fat drippings include wrapping meat in foil, placing foil under meat as it cooks, precooking meat to shorten grilling time, marinating meats before grilling, and cooking meat slowly at low temperatures.

barbiturates See ALCOHOL-DRUG INTERACTIONS.

barley (*Hordeum*) A CEREAL GRAIN, related to WHEAT and other grasses. Archaeological evidence suggests that barley was the earliest cultivated grain. Several varieties of barley are grown; the inedible husk must be removed from all of them. Whole kernels are available as scotch barley. Pearl barley is polished; that is, it is milled until it resembles small pearls. Pearl barley contains fewer nutrients; its COMPLEX CARBOHYDRATE content is high, its PROTEIN content moderate, and it is used primarily in soups, stews, and broths. Because it contains little gluten, the sticky protein prevalent in wheat flour, barley is not a chief ingredient of bread. Its major commercial use is as a malting agent in BEER, ale, and whiskey manufacture.

Barley is a good source of beta glucan, a water-soluble form of fiber. Several studies suggest that barley can lower cholesterol levels as much as 15 percent in individuals who have very high cholesterol levels; the viscous fiber seems to retard fat and cholesterol absorption by the intestine. The fiber tends to bind bile salts, thus increasing cholesterol removal from the body, and fat soluble substances, tocotrienols, appear to suppress cholesterol synthesis by the liver. Pearl barley (raw) supplies 349 calories per half cup (100 g); protein, 8.2 g; carbohydrate, 79 g; fiber, 8.2 g; fat, 1 g; iron, 4.2 mg; potassium, 160 mg; zinc, 2.23 mg; thiamin, 0.14 mg; riboflavin, 0.05 mg; niacin, 4.0 mg.

barley malt A natural sweetener derived from germinated barley. Barley malt tastes like blackstrap MOLASSES, which it can replace in a recipe. In the process of preparing barley malt, the grain is first sprouted. The sprouted barley supplies ENZYMES that then break down barley starch to the sugar, maltose. Although this sweetener contains a little THIAMIN (9 percent of the RECOMMENDED DIETARY ALLOWANCE per tablespoon) and lesser amounts of other B COMPLEX, it represents a refined CARBOHYDRATE, classified as EMPTY CALORIES because it contains little else.

basal energy expenditure (BEE) The increased energy requirements of patients recovering from disease or injury. In practice, BEE represents an estimate of the CALORIES needed to sustain physiologic functions while a patient is at rest. BEE is measured without intervening emotional stress or physical exertion, at least an hour preceding the measurement, and at a comfortable temperature several hours after a meal. The goal of recovering from illness, injury or surgery is to provide enough calories to meet energy needs and to maintain body weight and optimal metabolic function. In addition to BEE, a set of factors is used to predict the caloric needs required for healing various degrees of injury. An activity factor of 1.2 (for bedridden patients) or 1.3 (for ambulatory patients) is multiplied by injury factors: 1.2 for minor surgery, 1.35 for trauma, 1.6 for severe infection (sepsis), 2.1 for burns. Patients with burns have the longest period of increased energy needs.

basal metabolic rate (BMR) The energy expended to maintain the body at rest. The BMR is measured in the morning for an awake, resting individual 12 to 18 hours after the last meal. Oxygen consumption (in liters of oxygen) for a defined interval is multiplied by 4.8 calories per liter of oxygen to yield the BMR, the heat produced during the timed interval. In practice, it is easier to measure the resting metabolic rate (RMR), measured either sitting or lying down, in a comfortable environment several hours after a meal or significant physical activity. RMR does not require an overnight fast and is nearly equal to BMR. Normally this ranges from 1,200 to 1,800 CALORIES per day. The BMR represents a considerable energy expenditure, accounting for 60 percent to 75 percent of the calories. This energy is used for normal functions of the body, such as glandular secretions and maintenance of cellular metabolism, as well as activation of the autonomic nervous system, which maintains heartbeat, breathing and other involuntary activity.

Many factors influence an individual's metabolic rate: diet history; degree of activity of the sympathetic nervous system; physical and emotional stress; body temperature; menstrual cycle; sleep; adaptation to altitude; occupation; race; and even the season of the year. Differences in metabolic rates due to differences in body size, sex, or age largely disappear if the data are related to fat-free body mass. The decrease in basal metabolic rate observed with aging is primarily due to decreased lean body mass. A genetic component also contributes to the differences in BMR among individuals. BMR is partially controlled by the THYROID GLAND; thus low thyroid activity may promote weight gain. BMR decreases with illness, FASTING, and even stringent DIETING. This decrease is a temporary adaptation of the body to semi-STARVATION and accounts for the frequently observed decrease in the rate of weight loss a week into a dieting program. Recent studies indicate that after dieting, BMR rises to a new level that it is appropriate for the new body weight.

Physical conditioning is another factor. Calories are burned more rapidly after exercising than not. The duration and intensity of aerobic exercise needed to secure this benefit is an important question still being studied. If the individual is sedentary, moderate exercise seems to cause a 10 percent increase in basal metabolism for several hours. A moderately active individual needs to do aerobic exercise such as swimming, aerobic dancing, or jogging a total of six hours per week to increase the metabolic rate for several days afterward. In addition, exercise increases muscle mass, which burns more calories than fat does.

Nicotine seems to boost metabolic rates in proportion to the level of physical activity. This may be a reason why smokers often tend to weigh less than non-smokers, and why smokers tend to gain weight when they stop smoking. (See also DIET-INDUCED THERMOGENESIS.)

Felber, J. P., and A. Golay. "Regulation of Nutrient Metabolism and Energy Expenditure," *Metabolism* 44, no. 2, supp. 2 (February 1995): 4–9.

base A substance that can accept hydrogen ions (protons) and thus neutralize ACIDS. When added to water, bases raise the pH (the degree of a measure of acidity; a pH greater than 7.0 is considered to be basic). Typical mineral bases, such as sodium hydroxide (lye) and potassium hydroxide are caustic; they can cause severe burns and are classified as strong bases. Weak bases are much more common in foods and in the body. Ammonia and bicarbonate occur in the blood and body fluids and in other nitrogen-containing compounds. A very important weak base is BICARBONATE, which, in the blood and digestive juices, neutralizes acids, thereby increasing the pH. Bicarbonate plays an important role in buffering the blood. (See also BUFFER.)

basic food groups A simple guide for making food selections designed to help consumers plan a BALANCED DIET which has now been superseded by the FOOD GUIDE PYRAMID. This guideline emphasizes MEAT and dairy products to avoid undernutrition. It advises eating two servings of meat selections daily, two of MILK and dairy products, four of VEGETABLES and FRUITS, and four of GRAINS. There are several disadvantages. The Basic Four Food Group guidelines lack serving sizes and provide only the minimum numbers of servings. Overnutrition and nutritional imbalances are possible because they emphasize a diet high in animal FAT and lacking in FIBER. On the other hand, a diet with moderate quantities of low-fat dairy products, lean meat, poultry, and fish can easily meet the needs for CALORIES, and minerals like IRON and CALCIUM. (See also DIETARY GUIDELINES FOR AMERICANS.)

SUMMARY OF THE BASIC FOUR FOOD GROUPS

Food Group	Main Nutrient Contributions
Meat and meat alternatives	Protein, iron, riboflavin, zinc, vitamin B_{12}, thiamin
Milk and milk products	Calcium, protein, riboflavin, zinc, vitamin B_{12}, thiamin
Fruits and vegetables	Vitamin A, vitamin C, thiamin, additional iron and riboflavin, fiber, folic acid
Grains (bread and cereal products)	Additional amounts of niacin, iron, thiamin, zinc in whole grains; fiber

basil (*Ocimum basilicum*) A pungent herb; a member of the mint family. Its name is derived from the Greek *basilikos,* meaning "royal," because once the king alone was allowed to harvest it. Each variety of basil differs in height, color of foliage, and taste. Of the six common varieties of basil, sweet basil and dwarf basil are most popular in the United States. Basil can be used fresh or dried as a seasoning in seafoods, salads, potatoes, soups, and especially tomato-based dishes, and it is used extensively in Italian and Provençal cooking. In folk medicine, basil has been used to remedy flatulence.

bass (*Micropterus*) Refers to a number of different saltwater and freshwater species of spiny-rayed FISH. Bass is shaped like SALMON, but the flesh is white. Both freshwater and saltwater varieties occur in North America. Freshwater game fish varieties include white or silver bass and yellow bass. Saltwater varieties, like sea bass and striped bass, are among the best known. Striped bass caught in polluted offshore waters can be contaminated with industrial pollutants. Fish farms are a major source of bass. The flesh has a delicate flavor and is served poached, braised, or grilled. In order to keep the flesh intact during poaching, the scales are not removed.

basting Spooning or brushing sauces, cooking juices, or melted BUTTER over meat several times during cooking. This procedure keeps meat, particularly leaner cuts, moist during roasting or broiling. Basting brushes or a bulb-type baster simplify the operation. Roast turkey and meat cooked on a rotisserie are usually basted with fatty drippings or with butter to prevent them from drying out. If basting is performed with stocks or water, the resulting excess steam helps keep the meat moist. Prime cuts of meat contain so much fat that basting isn't necessary.

bay (*Laurus nobilis*) An evergreen shrub widely cultivated for its broad, aromatic leaves. The shrub is a species of laurel (bay laurel, true laurel). The edible bay should not be confused with the garden cherry laurel, *Prunus laurocerasus,* which is poisonous. Bay leaves are one of the most popular culinary herbs in North America. They can be obtained as dried leaves or in powdered form. Stews, soup stocks, marinades, and ragouts incorporate this versatile seasoning. Because it is so pungent, small amounts are recommended. Bay leaf, together with parsley, thyme, cloves, and celery are bound together as bouquet garni to flavor soups or stocks.

B complex (B vitamins) A group of eight water-soluble VITAMINS, required in very small amounts to convert FAT, PROTEIN and CARBOHYDRATE to ENERGY. The B complex is not stored in the body, unlike fat-soluble vitamins, and adequate amounts must be supplied daily.

The name originated from early nutritional research, when growth factors for organisms were designated as B_1, B_2, etc. As they were isolated and characterized chemically, each was found to serve as a parent of a specific enzyme helper (coenzyme): THIAMIN (vitamin B_1) forms thiamin pyrophosphate; NIACIN (vitamin B_3) forms NAD; RIBOFLAVIN (vitamin B_2) forms FAD; PANTOTHENIC ACID (vitamin B_5) forms COENZYME A; VITAMIN B_6 forms pyridoxal phosphate; VITAMIN B_{12} forms methylcobalamin; FOLIC ACID forms tetrahydrofolate; and biotin yields biocytin.

The amounts of vitamins required daily are quite low. Consider the REFERENCE DAILY INTAKE (RDI): folic acid, 400 mcg; niacin, 20 mg; riboflavin, 1.7 mg; thiamin, 1.4 mg; vitamin B_6, 2 mg; vitamin B_{12}, 6 mcg; biotin, 300 mcg; pantothenic acid, 10 mg. These amounts are so small that together they would weigh no more than a metal staple. Vitamins of the B complex work most effectively when all are present in the appropriate ratios. Common multivitamin supplements may not balance B complex vitamins when they provide small amounts of some B vitamins and large amounts of others.

On average, men require more of the B complex than women because their larger bodies need more nutrients. The daily requirement of thiamin increases as more food is eaten; drinking alcoholic beverages and eating SUGAR tend to deplete the LIVER's B vitamin supply. Populations with the greatest risk for B vitamin deficiency include those on weight-loss programs and who skip meals, infants and children, the elderly, and pregnant teenage girls. The daily intake of nutrients such as folic acid is frequently inadequate in diets relying on highly processed convenience foods. Junk foods with an excess of calories or fat and with refined carbohydrates (white flour and sugar) displace whole, minimally processed foods that are more nutritious and contain fewer calories.

As many as 30 percent of people over the age of 65 may not consume vitamin B_6, vitamin B_{12}, and folic acid in amounts adequate to prevent strokes and heart attacks, due to a buildup of a potentially harmful amino acid by-product called HOMOCYSTEINE. When homocysteine accumulates in the blood, there is an increased risk of damage to arteries. Only by consuming 400 micrograms of folic acid a day, twice the level specified by the RECOMMENDED DIETARY ALLOWANCES (RDA), do levels of homocysteine decline.

The richest sources of the B complex are organ meats such as liver and kidney. Low-fat options for folic acid include cooked lentils, chickpeas, kidney beans, and spinach; for thiamin, BREWER'S YEAST, extra-lean meat, wheat germ, enriched BREAKFAST CEREALS; for riboflavin, low-fat milk and other low-fat dairy products and enriched cereals; for niacin and vitamin B_{12}, fish, lean meat, poultry, and enriched cereals.

A diet that supplies adequate amounts of vitamins and minerals alone does not guarantee that a vitamin deficiency will not occur. There are several reasons for this. Foods must first be digested (broken down to amino acids, vitamins, sugars, fatty acids, and so on) in order to release individual nutrients, and DIGESTION may be incomplete if the production of STOMACH ACID or of DIGESTIVE ENZYMES is low. Second, the products of digestion must be absorbed by the small intestine to be of any benefit. An unhealthy intestine will be able to absorb individual nutrients effectively. (See also CARBOHYDRATE METABOLISM; CATABOLISM; MALABSORPTION; MALNUTRITION.)

"B Makes the Grade," *Consumer Reports on Health* 7, no. 6 (June 1995): 61–63.

beach plum (*Prunus maritama*) A member of the prune family that grows wild in North America. When ripe, the small fruit is dark purple with a tough skin. The flavor combines plum with cherry and grape flavors; its sour flavor usually limits its use to jams and jellies.

bean curd A highly nutritious source of plant PROTEIN, prepared from SOYBEANS. To prepare bean curd, soybeans are homogenized and the soy protein is coagulated by treatment with calcium sulfate or nigari, a mineral-rich liquid remaining after salt extraction of sea water. The precipitated protein is pressed into blocks for a low-fat, low-calorie alternative to meat. (See also TOFU.)

beans (*Phaseolus*) Seeds of trailing vines, as well as bushy plants belonging to the legume family. Beans can be divided into two groups: One yields edible pods, picked at an immature stage; another yields only edible seeds. In the former group are snap beans, yellow wax, and green beans. Bush varieties grow as short plants and pods at the same time. Pole beans grow like vines. Each stem grows a single pod, and pods mature at different times. They supply BETA-CAROTENE, FIBER, and some minerals, including IRON. Canned green beans contain a high level of SODIUM—340 mg per cup of drained beans as compared to 3 mg from raw beans. Green beans (one cup cooked, 125 g) provide 44 calories; protein, 2.4 mg; fat 0.4 mg; carbohydrate, 9.9 g; fiber, 3.1 g; calcium, 58 mg; iron, 1.6 mg; vitamin A, 583 retinol equivalents; thiamin, 0.09 mg; riboflavin, 0.12 mg; niacin, 0.77 mg; vitamin C, 12 mg.

Dried beans include navy, pinto, lima, kidney (red), and fava (or broad) bean. Dried beans are excellent PROTEIN sources; one cup of cooked beans supplies between 12 and 25 g of protein (25 percent to 50 percent of the RECOMMENDED DIETARY ALLOWANCE [RDA]). Shell beans are harvested halfway in their maturation to dried beans. They include SOYBEANS, BROAD (fava) BEANS, and lima beans.

Shell beans can be used interchangeably with dried beans in recipes. Bean protein, like most plant protein, is deficient in at least one essential amino acid. However, this "incomplete" protein is readily balanced by eating beans with whole grains, nuts, or small amounts of fish, poultry, meat, or dairy products. Dried beans contain STARCH, MINERALS (POTASSIUM, MAGNESIUM, iron, and calcium), and little fat. Dried beans are also excellent sources of fiber. For example, a cup of cooked pinto beans supplies 18.9 g fiber. One cup of cooked lima beans (190 g) provides 260 calories; protein, 16.1 g; carbohydrate, 49 g; fiber, 9.7 g; calcium, 55 mg; iron, 5.9 mg; potassium, 116.3 mg; thiamin, 0.25 mg; riboflavin, 0.11 mg; niacin, 1.34 mg. Navy beans (one cup cooked, 190 g) contain 225 calories; protein 15 g; carbohydrate 40.1 g; fiber, 16.5 g; and calcium 95 mg.

FLATULENCE after eating cooked dried beans is a common experience. The culprits in gas-producing foods are a family of carbohydrate (raffinose, stachyose, and verbascose) that cannot be digested but are broken down by gut bacteria that release excessive gas. This problem is reduced by soaking beans in water for several hours and discarding the water after soaking. Beans are then boiled in water, which is again discarded, rather than incorporated into soup or chili. Over-the-counter preparations of an enzyme (alpha galactosidase) that can degrade these sugars are now available. (See also COMPLETE PROTEIN; FOOD COMPLEMENTING.)

Guste, Roy F. *The Bean Book.* New York: Norton, 2000.

beef The flesh of steers, cows, and heifers representing the ruminant family, *Bovidae.* The Aberdeen, Angus, Brahma, Hereford, Santa Gertrudis, and Shorthorn represent typical breeds raised in North America for MEAT. Although beef consumption has declined significantly during the last two decades, beef is still America's most popular meat. The indirect costs of this preference are high, because the production of one pound of beef requires an estimated five pounds of GRAIN, and the energy equivalent of a gallon of gasoline.

Beef is an excellent source of PROTEIN, VITAMINS, and MINERALS (except calcium). On the other hand, beef is rather high in saturated fat. The high consumption of animal fat correlates with increased blood cholesterol and increased risk of heart disease and cancer. Traditionally, cattle were bred for a high degree of "marbled" meat, heavily laden with fat, and the animals were fattened in feed lots before slaughter. Due to the recent consumer demand for leaner meat, there is a trend toward producing leaner animals. A three-ounce (85 g) serving of round roast, which is about the size of a deck of cards, contains: calories, 205; protein, 23 g; fat, 12 g; cholesterol, 62 mg; calcium, 5 mg; iron, 1.6 mg; zinc, 4.7 mg; thiamin, 0.07 mg; riboflavin, 0.14 mg; niacin, 3 mg. Choice grades of several cuts of beef (cooked) provide the following calories per three-ounce serving: chuck roast (18 percent fat) = 257; rib roast (36 percent fat) = 400; sirloin steak (27 percent fat) = 240; canned corned beef (10g fat) = 185; trimmed round roast (8 g fat) = 175.

Beef as HAMBURGER is the most commonly eaten meat in the United States and is a major contributor of saturated fat to the standard American diet. A three-ounce serving of hamburger contains 18 g fat (21 percent fat). "Lean ground beef" is a designation that does not need to meet USDA standards. Therefore, the fat content can range from 20 percent to 30 percent. The average fat in "lean ground beef" is 21 percent. In contrast, meat labeled by the U.S. Department of Agriculture (USDA) as "lean meat" contains no more than 17 percent fat by weight, while "extra lean ground beef" contains 10 percent fat by weight. Supermarket brands of low-fat beef are designated as "light select" or "select" grades of beef and range from 5 percent to 15 percent fat.

Beef often contains chemical residues, such as growth promoters, ANTIBIOTICS like sulfa drugs, animal drugs, and pesticides. The health effects of low-level exposure to such compounds are unknown. Some of these residues are potential cancer-causing agents. In 1989 the European Community banned beef raised with growth hormones. Hormone-free beef is now commercially available in many areas of the United States. (See also FOOD LABELING; GRADED FOODS; MEAT CONTAMINANTS; BOVINE SPONGIFORM ENCEPHALOPATHY.)

beef tallow A hard FAT, high in saturated fatty acids and CHOLESTEROL, which is rendered from trimmed meat (usually beef). Rendering is the process of melting fat out of fatty tissue, then filtering and purifying the melted fat. Tallow is more saturated than pork fat (lard) and chicken fat.

Tallow is often used in fast-food restaurants to cook FRENCH FRIES because consumers seem to prefer the flavor of potatoes fried in animal fat. The practical advantages of beef tallow are that it is relatively inexpensive and it does not break down at the high temperatures needed for frying. However, the cholesterol becomes oxidized with prolonged heating at high temperatures, and oxidized cholesterol is known to be a factor in the buildup of plaque in arteries. Beef tallow finds other commercial uses, including the manufacture of candles and soap.

bee pollen The fertilizing element from flowering plants that is collected by bees and available as a food supplement. The composition of nutrients in bee pollen resembles that of legumes with varying amounts of B COMPLEX, such as thiamin, riboflavin, niacin, folic acid and pantothenic acid, PROTEIN, and

MINERALS. By weight it contains 50 percent CARBOHYDRATE and 25 percent protein. Bee pollen contains FLAVONOIDS, a type of plant pigment that helps normalize inflammation.

Bee pollen is widely marketed in health food stores as an aid in weight management and as an "energizer." There are no clinical studies that indicate bee pollen energizes the body, regulates weight, tones the skin, or protects against heart disease. The official position of the American Dietetic Association is that such claimed ENERGY-boosting supplements ("ergoneic") are ineffective. Those who are sensitive to pollen may have an allergic reaction to bee pollen. (See also ROYAL JELLY.)

beer An alcoholic carbonated beverage that is a product of FERMENTATION of grains such as WHEAT, MILLET, and BARLEY. U.S. breweries ferment barley, CORN, or RYE together with hops, with cultured yeast strains to provide the alcoholic content, carbonation, and characteristic flavor of this beverage. Lager beer, the most popular American beer, is aged to mellow its flavor. The ALCOHOL (ethanol) content is typically 3.2 percent.

Beer is the oldest known alcoholic beverage and has the highest consumption of any alcoholic beverage worldwide. Hops were cultivated in the 1200s by monasteries in Germany for use in brewing. Brewing beer follows well-defined steps. In order for the starch in cereal grains to ferment, the grains are first processed. In malting, grain is soaked long enough to initiate germination, then is kiln-dried. The color of beer is related to the extent to which malt is heated. The malt is next ground and the pigment, betalaine, mixed in hot water. Enzymatic degradation produces fermentable sugars from the starch. The insoluble material is separated and the resulting fermentable extract is called wort. Flowers of hops are added to the headed wort, then yeast is added after cooling. Most lager beer production far exceeds that of ale. Lager fermentation usually lasts seven days, to give a beer flavored by hops and malt. Ale fermentation is typically carried out for three days at a higher temperature. Directly fermenting roasted grains yields more strongly flavored (stout) ale.

One serving of regular beer (12 oz.) provides 116 calories (primarily alcohol), protein, 0.9 g; calcium, 18 mg; iron, 0.11 mg; niacin, 1.6 mg; and low levels of other B complex vitamins, indicative of its low nutrient density.

"Nonalcoholic" beers are not strictly alcohol-free because they may contain 0.5 percent alcohol. With less alcohol, non-alcoholic beverages contain fewer calories than their alcoholic counterparts. However, beer with 2.5 percent alcohol can still be called "low alcohol" beer because it contains less alcohol than the usual 3.2 percent alcohol. (See also ALCOHOLISM; BREWER'S YEAST; WINE.)

beet (*Beta vulgaris,* garden beet) A red root vegetable related to CHARD. Beets may be cultivated for their tops in addition to their roots. Common varieties include Crosby's Egyptian, Ruby Queen, and Detroit Dark Red. Red beetroot is a food coloring agent. Beets in general have the highest sugar content of all other vegetables. White-rooted sugar beets are a major source of domestic sugar (SUCROSE). Cooked, fresh red beets are a source of a red pigment, betalaine, a type of FLAVONOID, which is a class of plant products that have beneficial effects on the immune system, connective tissue, and cellular metabolism. One half cup (cooked, 85 g) provides 26 calories; protein, 0.9 g; carbohydrate, 5.7 g; fiber, 1.96 g; iron, 0.53 g; potassium, 266 mg; niacin, 0.23 mg; and low levels of VITAMIN C and B COMPLEX vitamins. Beet greens are an excellent source of fiber, beta-carotene, calcium, and iron. Cooked beet greens (one cup, 144 g) provide 40 calories; protein, 3.7 g; carbohydrate, 7.9 g; fiber, 3.0 g; calcium, 165 mg; iron, 2.74 mg; potassium, 1,308 mg; zinc, 0.72 mg; vitamin A, 734 retinol equivalents; vitamin C, 36 mg; thiamin, 0.17 mg; riboflavin, 0.42 mg; niacin, 0.72 mg.

behavior See FOOD AND THE NERVOUS SYSTEM.

behavior modification Considered a key to the successful treatment of EATING DISORDERS, OBESITY, and ADDICTIONS, this form of therapeutic intervention relies on the premise that eating behavior is learned and that undesirable eating practices can be unlearned. Strategies to change behavior permanently include specifying a written commitment to achieving a goal, rewards for accomplishments, exercises to assist building self-esteem, support groups, changes in the availability of certain foods, changes in the location in which meals are eaten, changes in the social environment, and increased physical activity. A major concern with many weight management programs is that fat can be lost without adequate commitment and training that are necessary to assure eating patterns are changed permanently. (See also DIETING.)

benomyl A post-harvest FUNGICIDE that reduces fruit spoilage by killing MOLDS and fungi. BANANAS, APRICOTS, PEACHES, CHERRIES, PEARS, PLUMS, and PINEAPPLES are among the commonly treated fruits. Benomyl has been linked to cancer and birth defects in experimental animals.

benzopyrene (benzo(a)pyrene) A multiringed organic compound related to benzene. Benzopyrene is classified as a polycyclic aromatic hydrocarbon, a member of a family of compounds that are potential mutagens (mutation-producing agents) and CARCINOGENS (CANCER-causing agents). The liver converts ingested benzopyrene to highly reactive intermediates (epoxides) that can attack the DNA in cells.

Traces of benzopyrenes occur in soil as the result of microbial activity. Plants can synthesize this hydrocarbon and may contain up to 10 mcg per kg of dry weight. However, far greater exposure comes from the incomplete burning (pyrolysis) of oil, fat, and organic material from cooking, cigarettes, exhaust from industrial combustion and automobiles, and home heating. BARBECUED MEAT contains benzopyrenes due to the FAT dripping on charcoal or heating elements. MEAT cooked in frying pans, griddles, or over open flames generates benzopyrenes. Benzopyrenes contaminate soot, which is deposited on meats on overlying grills.

benzoyl peroxide A bleach that is used to whiten FLOUR without necessarily aging it. Used at a level of 50 ppm (parts per million) with a mixture of aging agents, benzoyl peroxide bleaches most flours within 24 hours. However, along with destroying pigments, the peroxide destroys the vitamins in flour. The trade-off in producing white flour that makes excellent dough is decreased nutritional value. The breakdown product of benzoyl peroxide is benzoic acid, which remains in flour. This additive is classified as a FOOD ADDITIVE.

beriberi A condition, caused by chronic THIAMIN (vitamin B_1) deficiency, that affects peripheral nerves, the brain, and the cardiovascular system. Early symptoms of thiamin deficiency include FATIGUE, irritability, poor memory, anorexia, and sleep disturbances; with severe deficiencies, paralysis of limbs, cardiovascular abnormalities, and edema appear. Beriberi rarely occurs in North America because wheat products and flour are enriched with thiamin. It is more common in developing nations among populations subsisting on polished rice from which much of the vitamins and minerals have been removed. (See also CARBOHYDRATE METABOLISM; ENRICHMENT; MALNUTRITION.)

beta blockers Drugs used to control high blood pressure in salt-sensitive individuals, that may prevent fatal HEART ATTACKS. Beta blockers limit high blood pressure by preventing the kidneys from releasing angiotensin, a hormone that increases blood pressure. The drugs are also used to control migraine headaches and to reduce angina.

There are several precautions to be observed when using beta blockers. After years of use, they may promote heart repair, but they also may damage the kidneys. Beta blockers increase the risk of severe allergy reactions in patients taking allergy shots. Possible side effects include depression (in patients with a history of depression or mood disorders). FATIGUE, fuzzy thinking, impotence, mood swings, increased blood CHOLESTEROL, and diabetes-like symptoms. Use of alcoholic beverages while taking this medication can be fatal because the combination can cause a drastic drop in blood pressure. (See also ALCOHOL-DRUG INTERACTION; ALLERGY; IMMEDIATE; DIABETES MELLITUS; HYPERTENSION.)

beta-carotene (provitamin A) A yellow-orange pigment that is converted to VITAMIN A in the body. The yellow-orange coloring in fruit and vegetables is mainly due to the presence of beta-carotene. Commercially, beta-carotene is used as a safe FOOD COLORING. Beta-carotene is the most plentiful of the orange-yellow plant pigments (CAROTENOIDS) in foods, and it has the highest vitamin A activity.

Because of differences in uptake, storage, and chemical processing, only about one-sixth of the beta-carotene in a plant food ends up as vitamin A (retinol) in the body. For this reason the vitamin A content in plant foods is usually given as "retinol equivalents," that is, the amount of vitamin A that could be derived from the carotene content. One RE (retinol equivalent) is defined as 1 mcg of (trans) retinol (vitamin A), 6 mcg of (trans) beta-carotene, or 12 mcg of other carotenoids that can be converted to vitamin A. The other way of expressing the activity of carotenoids is in terms of international units, or IU. One IU of vitamin A is equivalent to 0.3 mcg and one IU of beta-carotene is equivalent to 0.6 mcg of beta-carotene. Thus 1 mg of beta-carotene represents 1,667 IU. Beta-carotene does not carry the risk of vitamin A poisoning because the body converts it to vitamin A only as needed. Some manufacturers of multiple vitamin supplements substitute beta-carotene for vitamin A in their formulations to reduce the danger of vitamin A toxicity.

Beta-carotene has a number of other functions that make it the most extensively investigated carotenoid. It is a very important ANTIOXIDANT as it can help prevent damage to tissues by FREE RADICALS—extremely reactive, damaging forms of oxygen and other chemicals. Beta-carotene helps boost the IMMUNE SYSTEM, and it affects lipid metabolism in important ways. It lowers LOW-DENSITY LIPOPROTEIN (LDL), the undesirable form of cholesterol, and raises HIGH-DENSITY LIPOPROTEIN (HDL), the desirable form. The U.S. FDA has approved the use of beta-carotene to treat a particular form of light sensitivity in patients who have a metabolic defect and overproduce pigments called porphyrins (erythropoietic porphyrias).

In exploring the role of carotenes in preventive health, attention has focused on the possibility of using beta-carotene and vitamin A to reduce the risk of HEART ATTACKS in men with coronary heart disease and CANCER. Regarding heart disease, the results of population studies have generally not shown a reduction in the risk of coronary heart disease with increased consumption of beta-carotene. Two studies found increased mortality in smokers who took beta-carotene supplements. Populations studies suggest that increased beta-carotene intake reduces the risk of cancer, especially breast, prostate, colon, and lung cancers. While many studies indicate that dietary beta-carotene from fruits and vegetables decreases the risk of lung cancer, two large studies—the Nurses Health Study and the Health Professionals Follow Up Study—reported lower lung cancer risk with increased consumption of foods rich in lycopene, alpha-carotene, and a variety of carotenoids, but not specifically beta-carotene. Clinical trials have examined the effects of beta-carotene supplementation on lung cancer. Smokers who take beta-carotene can increase their risk of lung cancer but nonsmokers do not appear to be at higher risk. The three studies include the Alpha Tocopherol, Beta-Carotene Cancer Prevention Trial (ATBC Trial), the Beta-Carotene and Retinol Efficacy Trial (CARET), and the Physicians' Health Study.

The ATBC Trial was conducted by the National Cancer Institute (NCI) in collaboration with the National Public Health Institute of Finland. The purpose of the study was to see if certain vitamin supplements would prevent lung and other cancers in a group of 29,133 male smokers in Finland. In the study 50- to 69-year-old participants took a pill containing either 50 mg of alpha tocopherol (a form of vitamin E), 20 mg of beta-carotene, both, or a placebo daily for five to eight years.

The CARET study is a large NCI-funded chemoprevention trial being conducted in six areas in the United States to see if a combination of beta-carotene and vitamin A supplements will prevent lung and other cancers in men and women aged 50 to 69 who are smokers or former smokers, and men aged 45 to 69 who have been exposed to asbestos. The 18,314 participants stopped taking the supplements before the completion of the trial.

The Physicians' Health Study was a study of 22,071 U.S. male physicians, of whom 11 percent smoked. The purpose of the study was to test whether a beta-carotene supplement reduced the risk of cancer and heart disease as well as whether low-dose aspirin reduced the risk of heart disease. The aspirin component was stopped in early 1988 because of a 44 percent reduction in risk of first heart attack among those taking aspirin. The beta-carotene component ended December 31, 1995, after more than 12 years of study.

In the ATBC study, 18 percent more lung cancers were diagnosed and 8 percent more overall deaths occurred in study participants taking beta-carotene. In CARET, after an average of four years of receiving supplements, 28 percent more lung cancers were diagnosed and 17 percent more deaths occurred in participants who took a combination of beta-carotene and vitamin A than in those who took placebos. Neither of these studies showed a benefit from taking supplements. Because the interim results of CARET were similar to the ATBC study, the intervention was stopped 21 months early. Both of these studies involved people who were specifically invited to participate because of their high risk for developing lung cancer.

The Physician's Health Study was completed at the end of 1995 and showed no benefit or harm in people taking beta-carotene supplements for more than 12 years.

CARET participants were told to stop taking the beta-carotene and vitamin A or placebos because the CARET and NCI safety committees saw that the interim results clearly showed no benefit from the supplements—and also showed there was a possibility they were harming participants.

The NCI has never made recommendations as to whether Americans should take supplements to prevent or treat cancer. For those who wish to reduce their risk of cancer, the NCI advises that it is prudent to adopt a low-fat diet containing plenty of fruits, vegetables, and grains. The best advice for smokers who want to reduce their risk of lung cancer is still the most direct: stop smoking. The results from CARET and the ATBC Trial suggest that smokers should avoid taking beta-carotene supplements.

The results of the Physicians' Health Study showed no benefit or harm to nonsmokers who took beta-carotene every other day for 12 years. The results from CARET and the ATBC study do not provide information about the effects of beta-carotene supplements on nonsmokers.

In both the ATBC Study and CARET, participants with the highest levels of beta-carotene in their blood, measured before the study began, went on to have fewer lung cancers. These results are consistent with the possibility that a different compound or compounds in foods that have high levels of beta-carotene may be responsible for the protective effect of dietary beta-carotene seen in epidemiological studies. Because these are studies of pills, not food intake, the NCI stresses that the study results do not change the results of studies that show that eating a variety of fruits and vegetables each day remains a good way to reduce the risk of some cancers and other chronic conditions. The overall impression from these studies is that beta-carotene needs to be part of a balanced antioxidant picture, including carotenoids, in order to protect the body against oxidation and chronic disease. Diets high in fruits and vegetables supply a rich mixture of PHYTOCHEMICALS in addition to beta-carotene that can be beneficial to long-term health. Natural, mixed carotenoids as found in whole, minimally processed foods appear to be better antioxidants than synthetic beta-carotene.

The optimal intake of beta-carotene and natural carotenoids to afford maximum protection is not known. According to guidelines to food choices published by the National Cancer Institute and the U.S. FDA, the beta-carotene intake should equal about 6 mg daily. Actual consumption is about 1.5 mg per day. This means most Americans should increase their daily intake of foods containing beta-carotene. One sweet potato contains 5 to 10 mg of beta-carotene, representing 2,500 retinol equivalents. About 15 milligrams daily may be recommended if the patient eats a lot of PROCESSED FOOD or has an infection or diabetes.

Many good sources of beta-carotene and carotenoids are eaten rarely in the typical U.S. diet although they are readily available. Good sources of beta-carotene include SQUASH, CANTALOUPE, sweet potatoes, YAMS, CARROTS, yellow-colored fruit like NECTARINES, and dark green, leafy vegetables like KALE, CHARD, greens (BEETS, COLLARD), spinach, and BROCCOLI. Although tomatoes, lettuce and sweet corn are relatively poor sources of beta-carotene, they contribute significantly to the nation's total intake of beta-carotene and carotenoids, because Americans eat so much of them. (See also DIETARY GUIDELINES FOR AMERICANS; HYPERVITAMINOSIS.)

Dietary Guidelines Advisory Committee, Agricultural Research Service, U.S. Department of Agriculture (USDA), "Report of the Dietary Guidelines Advisory Committee on the Dietary Guidelines for Americans,

2000." Available online. URL: http://www.ars.usda.gov/dgac.

Johnson, E. J. "The Role of Carotenoids in Human Health," *Nutrition and Clinical Care* 5, no. 2 (March–April 2002): 56–65.

Kritharides, L., and R. Stocker. "The Use of Antioxidant supplements in Coronary Heart Disease," *Atherosclerosis* 164, no. 2 (October 2002): 211.

Lee, I-Min et al. "Beta-Carotene Supplementation and Incidence of Cancer and Cardiovascular Disease: The Women's Health Study," *Journal of the National Cancer Institute* 91 (1999): 2,102–2,106.

Lee, K. W., and C. Y. Lee. "Vitamins, Diet, and Cancer Prevention," *American Journal of Clinical Nutrition* 75, no. 6 (June 2002): 1,122–1,223.

Pavia, S. A., and R. M. Russell. "Beta-Carotene and Other Carotenoids as Antioxidants," *Journal of the American College of Nutrition* 18 (1999): 426–433.

Sato,. R., K. J. Helzlsouer et al. "Prospective Study of Carotenoids, Tocopherols, and Retinoid Concentrations and the Risk of Breast Cancer," *Cancer Epidemiology and Biomarkers Prevention* 11, no. 5 (May 2002): 451–457.

beta-hydroxybutyric acid A simple acid produced by the liver's metabolism of fatty acids. Beta-hydroxybutyric acid belongs to the family of KETONE BODIES, which are derived from fatty acid degradation and accumulate in the blood during conditions that promote extensive breakdown of body fat, including STARVATION, crash dieting, uncontrolled diabetes, and ALCOHOLISM. Ketone body accumulation in the blood promotes KETOSIS (acid accumulation in body fluids.) (See also ACIDOSIS: ELECTROLYTES; FAT.)

betaine hydrochloride A common supplemental form of hydrochloric acid used to increase stomach acidity. Betaine hydrochloride contains 23 percent hydrochloric acid, by weight. As a supplement to be taken with meals, betaine hydrochloride bolsters STOMACH ACID to help improve digestion in patients with HYPOCHLORHYDRIA and ACHLORHYDRIA (inadequate stomach acid production). Excessive use of betaine hydrochloride can irritate the stomach wall.

Betaine is a nitrogen-containing compound related to CHOLINE. Its name comes from the fact that it occurs in *Beta vulgaris,* the common beet. Betaine helps to replenish the amino acid METHIONINE in the synthesis of compounds like the hormone epinephrine (adrenaline). (See also GASTRIC JUICE.)

betaline A system for the cold pasteurization of food products that uses electron-beam treatment, which reduces the risk of exposure to food pathogens such as SALMONELLA, *ESCHERICHIA COLI,* and CAMPYLOBACTER. Cold pasteurization of food using electron beams was approved by the U.S. FDA in 1997. Irradiation of food by electron-beam treatment does not affect the nutrient value of food. (See also FOOD IRRADIATION.)

beta-lipoprotein See LOW-DENSITY LIPOPROTEIN.

BHA (butylated hydroxyanisole) A common synthetic ANTIOXIDANT used in the United States since 1947 to retard RANCIDITY in vegetable oils and foods containing them. BHA destroys FREE RADICALS (highly reactive chemical species), before they can break down the fat. Therefore this antioxidant is extensively employed to extend the shelf life of many processed foods containing fat or oil, such as baked goods, CHIPS, BREAKFAST CEREALS, pork SAUSAGES, as well as active dry YEAST and some CHEWING GUMS. The average American consumes several milligrams of BHA daily from these sources.

BHA is relatively nontoxic. Most animal studies indicate it is safe, although a 1982 study suggested it may cause CANCER in experimental animals at very high dosages. A review committee concluded that the cancer risk is slight and recommended that BHA not be banned, pending further investigation. Huge amounts of BHA (0.25 percent to 0.5 percent of diet) cause abnormal development behavior in the offspring of treated animals. Rarely does it cause allergic reactions. (See also BHT; FOOD ADDITIVES.)

BHT (butylated hydroxytoluene) A synthetic ANTIOXIDANT in use in the United States since 1954. Like BHA, BHT helps prevent RANCIDITY in FATS, VEGETABLE OILS, and PROCESSED FOODS that contain them. Both BHA and BHT block the oxidation of POLYUNSATURATED FATTY ACIDS by reacting with FREE

RADICALS. These highly reactive forms of oxygen attack the double bonds of unsaturated fatty acids found in oils. They create off-flavor odors and break down products that are potentially damaging to cells. When included in the packaging material itself, BHT (and BHA) can migrate into the contents such as breakfast cereal, powdered milk, and mixes, in addition to baked goods and chips. The U.S. FDA allows BHT and BHA to be added to raw and cooked meat toppings for pizzas and meatballs.

A mixture of synthetic antioxidants is often more effective than single preservatives. Therefore many products contain BHA, BHT, and PROPYL GALLATE, a third, less safe antioxidant. BHT is less expensive than BHA but is unstable when heated during PASTEURIZATION and baking.

The average American consumes 5 to 10 mg of BHT daily. BHT accumulates in human tissues, although the long-term significance of this is unknown. The safety of BHT has been questioned, and some individuals are allergic to it. It is known that BHT induces production of certain liver detoxifying enzymes (mixed function oxidases). This is viewed as a mixed blessing because an increased level of these enzymes can destroy some toxic materials, but they also can transform others into carcinogens (cancer-causing agents). The relationship of BHT to cancer is murky. Several reports suggest that BHT prevents cancer in experimental animals. Other studies suggest it has no effect; still others conclude BHT can cause cancer. Rats fed 0.1 percent to 0.25 percent BHT diets (about 10 to 20 times the typical American diet) developed behavioral changes. The U.S. FDA proposed removing BHT from the GENERALLY RECOGNIZED AS SAFE (GRAS) list of FOOD ADDITIVES; however, it has not been classified as a regulated food additive. In view of the concern about safety, some companies omit BHT from processed foods. (See also CYTOCHROME P450.)

bicarbonate A common substance in the blood used to help regulate acid-base balance. Bicarbonate forms in the body when carbon dioxide dissolves in water or blood to form the weak acid CARBONIC ACID (H_2CO_3). Carbonic acid spontaneously yields bicarbonate. Together, bicarbonate and carbonic acid form an effective physiologic buffer system to maintain the blood at a very narrow range, pH 7.3 to 7.4. Thus bicarbonate can neutralize modest amounts of acid that might occur through ingestion or metabolism.

Bicarbonate also occurs in BAKING SODA as sodium bicarbonate. In the presence of acidic ingredients like CREAM OF TARTAR, bicarbonate forms carbonic acid, which spontaneously decomposes into water and carbon dioxide. It is this action that produces the gas bubbles that cause dough to rise.

bifidobacteria A type of nonspore-forming anaerobic (oxygen-sensitive) bacteria that ferments sugars to acids. Bifidobacteria ferment GLUCOSE, galactose, and FRUCTOSE to produce lactic and acetic acids. Bifidobacteria are often used in Japan during food preparation requiring the production of mild acids. In the United States, lactobaccilli are more widely used.

Bifidobacteria are normal, beneficial residents of the human colon. They acidify feces and produce antibacterial factors that limit the growth of undesirable bacteria and contribute to weight gain. Bifidobacteria get their start in the intestine, most readily through breast-feeding. Bifidobacteria are the predominant organisms in the large intestine of breast-fed infants; they can account for up to 99 percent of the microflora.

In adults, bifidobacteria populates primarily the lower regions of the intestine. In healthy individuals, the relative proportion of these bacteria remains rather constant. However, reduced gastric acidity, oral antibiotic therapy, and other conditions can disrupt the gut microflora. Furthermore, the levels of bifidobacteria can decline with age. Bifidobacteria are available as supplements. The major beneficial functions of bifidobacteria are:

- prevention of colonization of the intestine by potential disease-producing microorganisms with which they compete for nutrients and attachment sites;
- production of short-chain fatty acids, which nurture the colon, from fiber fermentation;
- production of vitamins like biotin.

(See also ACIDOPHILUS.)

bifidus factor A heat-stable factor in breast milk that promotes the growth of the bacterium *Bifidobacter infantis* in the intestinal tract of infants. None of a variety of nonhuman milks favor the growth of these strains. Successful implantation of this acid-producing bacterium helps to establish normal intestine flora and limit the growth of less desirable microorganisms. BIFIDOBACTERIA play an important role in balancing intestinal flora. (See also ACIDOPHILUS.)

bilberry (*Vaccinium myrtillus*) Variously known as whortleberry, blueberry, whinberry, or huckleberry, this wild berry is a rich source of vitamin C and a source of copper. Rarely cultivated, this species is the heather family, which also includes the CRANBERRY and the blueberry. The bilberry grows on the heaths and moors of Europe and northern Asia and is known for its round, juicy, bluish-black fruits. The raw fruit is too acid to be palatable without adding sugar. Quinic acid and tannin is found in the leaves.

The astringent fruit is especially valuable in diarrhea and dysentery. A decoction of the leaves or bark of the root may be used as a local application to ulcers and in ulceration of the mouth and throat. Positive results have been noted in studies that examined the effect of bilberry in a variety of eye problems, including pigmentary retinitis, diabetic and hypertensive retinopathy, retinal inflammation, macular degeneration, retinitis pigmentosa, glaucoma, and cataracts. The anthocyanidins in bilberry are the primary agents responsible for its ability to heal the eyes.

One serving provides 7.7 g of dietary fiber and supplies 60 kcal.

bile (gall) The juice secreted by the LIVER and temporarily stored in the GALLBLADDER to aid fat DIGESTION. The hormone CHOLECYSTOKININ, released during eating, triggers the contraction of the gallbladder, which expels stored bile into the small intestine. There, bile emulsifies FAT, permitting its digestion by a specific enzyme, LIPASE, secreted by the pancreas. The absorption of fat-soluble VITAMINS also requires bile emulsification.

Bile contains bile salts, natural detergents that are the principal emulsifying agents of fat. The liver synthesizes bile salts from CHOLESTEROL. Bile also contains the phospholipid LECITHIN to help dissolve fat and a small amount of free cholesterol, which is emulsified by bile salts and lecithin. If the ratio of water to lecithin to bile salt is altered, cholesterol can become insoluble in the gallbladder and form GALLSTONES in susceptible individuals. Bile also contains bilirubin, or BILE PIGMENT. Bilirubin is a waste product of hemoglobin metabolism from red blood cells and plays no significant role in digestion.

Once fat has been digested, bile salts are mainly reabsorbed by the intestine and recycled in the liver. A small amount is excreted in the feces. It is believed that some forms of fiber can lower blood cholesterol levels indirectly by binding bile salts so they cannot be reabsorbed. To compensate for this loss, the liver withdraws cholesterol from the blood to manufacture more bile salts, thus lowering blood cholesterol levels.

Bile salts may be decomposed by gut bacteria to potentially harmful products. A high FIBER diet helps to maintain a normal transit time to move waste out of the body. This action decreases both bile salt decomposition and exposure of the COLON to toxic materials. Such observations may explain why dietary fiber lowers the risk of colon CANCER. (See also ENTEROHEPATIC CIRCULATION.)

bile acids The primary FAT emulsifying agents of BILE. Bile acids and their derivatives, the bile salts, are powerful detergents. They are released from the gallbladder in order to dissolve fat prior to its digestion by the INTESTINE. They emulsify fat-soluble VITAMINS and promote their uptake as well. The liver synthesizes bile acids from cholesterol. In this process, the liver first oxidizes cholesterol to primary bile acids like cholic acid. The sterol ring structure that typifies cholesterol remains intact. Subsequent steps couple cholic acid to the amino acids TAURINE and GLYCINE to form the more soluble bile salts, taurocholate and glycocholate. These so-called conjugated products are even more powerful detergents than bile acids. Once in the intestine, bacterial metabolism can further modify bile salts to secondary bile acids, such as deoxycholic acid. Bile acids are partially reabsorbed by the intestine and are returned to the liver via the portal vein to be recycled. A small fraction, normally about 5 percent escapes in the stool. This fraction represents the primary pathway by which cholesterol can be metabolized to leave the body. (See also ENTEROHEPATIC CIRCULATION; FAT METABOLISM.)

bile pigment (bilirubin) A yellow-brown pigment that is the end-product of HEMOGLOBIN breakdown. Bilirubin serves no functional role in digestion, although in the blood it acts as an antioxidant. BILE pigment is derived from HEME, the red pigment of hemoglobin. Bilirubin is produced by the spleen, which breaks down heme. In the process, the heme ring is broken to form a chain, bilirubin. Iron is then released to be recycled. Bilirubin is next transported in the blood to the liver, where it is absorbed and converted to a water-soluble form called conjugated bilirubin, which can be secreted. This pigment, together with bile salts and lecithin, forms bile. Colon bacteria further modify bilirubin to stercobilin, which colors the stool brown. JAUNDICE is a condition characterized by excessive bilirubin accumulation. Jaundice itself is not a disease, but is an indication of abnormal metabolism or processing limited by the liver.

bilirubin See BILE PIGMENT.

bingeing See COMPULSIVE EATING.

bingeing and purging See BULIMIA NERVOSA.

bioavailability The degree to which NUTRIENTS are effectively absorbed and assimilated by the body. To ensure adequate nutrition, three events must occur: Enough food must be consumed to provide enough essential nutrients, the foods must be adequately digested, and the released nutrients must be absorbed efficiently. If food is not efficiently digested or if nutrients are not absorbed, an individual can eat a well-balanced meal and yet be undernourished.

Many factors limit bioavailability:

1. Antinutrients, chemicals occurring in some foods, bind nutrients and prevent their use. For example, acidic derivatives (oxalates in vegetables and phytates in grains) can limit the uptake of trace minerals such as IRON and ZINC; RUTABAGAS contain materials that bind iodine.
2. Nutrient uptake can be blocked by competition with pollutants in food and water. As an example, LEAD blocks the uptake of CALCIUM. On the other hand, a high calcium intake does limit lead absorption.
3. Excessive amounts of nutrients can block the uptake of others. Thus excessive zinc blocks the uptake of COPPER, and vice versa.
4. Inadequate DIGESTION may prevent the release of nutrients from food. Deficient STOMACH ACID (HYPOCHLORHYDRIA) reduces PROTEIN digestion. Inadequate BILE production limits FAT DIGESTION and uptake of fatty acids and fat-soluble vitamins.
5. A nutrient may not be in a suitably complexed form, for example, inadequate production of INTRINSIC FACTOR, a protein made by the stomach, limits VITAMIN B_{12} absorption in the intestine.
6. Inadequate intake of one nutrient can limit the bioavailability of another. Thus, too little VITAMIN D in the diet prevents the absorption of adequate calcium because vitamin D enhances the calcium uptake mechanism of the intestine.
7. An unhealthy intestinal lining limits nutrient absorption. The intestinal lining can be damaged by parasites (giardiasis). Allergy can cause intestinal swelling and thus reduce trace mineral uptake. An extreme example is CELIAC DISEASE, a severe reaction to the cereal grain protein, GLUTEN. This disease causes severe damage to the intestine, leading to MALNUTRITION, which is often associated with celiac disease. Food allergies can cause frequent spasms of the intestine, which can shorten the transit time of food through the intestine, thereby shortening the time available for nutrient uptake. (See also ANTIVITAMIN; GOITROGENS; SUBCLINICAL NUTRIENT DEFICIENCY.)

biochemical individuality The molecular differences that exist among individuals of a population. Each person's need for nutrients like VITAMINS and trace MINERALS to achieve optimal health varies from the norm of the population. Consequently, some people need lesser amounts of essential nutrients than the average intake for optimal health, while others, especially those affected by the standard American DIET of highly processed foods, or who smoke or who are pregnant, need larger amounts.

Tissue compositions differ in levels of ENZYMES, the metabolic machinery that operates cells, due to inherited differences, different medical histories and toxic exposures, diet, and age. Molecular genetics has uncovered a far greater degree of genetic polymorphism in people than previously known. There may be many variants of a given gene, thus variants of the protein it codes for. Most variant proteins support normal functioning. In certain cases, however, the variant form of an enzyme may operate normally only as long as there is an abundant supply of an essential vitamin helper (COENZYME). When the concentration of the vitamin falls below a critical threshold, function could be impaired.

For example, perhaps 10 percent of the U.S. population may not be able to process HOMOCYSTEINE, a by-product of the metabolism of METHIONINE, unless a sufficiently high level of folic acid is maintained in the diet. In other words, nutrition can affect genetic expression (the phenotype). In extreme cases, individuals may possess defective enzymes that cause genetic diseases such as phenylketonuria (PKU), an inherited inability to break down the amino acid PHENYLALANINE.

Differences in amounts of protective enzymes like antioxidant enzymes and detoxification enzymes of the liver can explain why some people are sensitive to environmental pollutants, while others can tolerate high exposures, and why individuals tolerate medications and anesthetics differently. A therapeutic dose effective for one person may be ineffective for the next. Biochemical individuality explains why only certain people experience side effects when exposed to a given food.

Individuals vary in their sensitivity to dietary salt, CHOLESTEROL, SUGAR, FAT, or ALCOHOL. About one out of five Americans is sensitive to SODIUM and will tend to develop high blood pressure with a high-salt diet; approximately one in five will respond to a high-sugar diet with elevated blood fat. An estimated one-third of Americans are sensitive to dietary cholesterol; their elevated serum cholesterol level puts them at high risk for developing clogged arteries. Biochemical individuality may explain, in part, why only a fraction of those who drink alcohol become addicted.

It is impossible to predict on an individual basis who will be sensitive to sodium, cholesterol, sugar, or alcohol. In some people with high blood cholesterol, clinical laboratory testing may provide clues, such as elevated blood fat or LOW-DENSITY LIPOPROTEIN, (LDL) the undesirable form of serum cholesterol. Family history often provides clues regarding susceptibility to illnesses like cancer, high blood pressure, heart disease, and diabetes that are affected by diet. With this information, prudent dietary and lifestyle choices can be made to lower the odds of chronic disease later in life. (See also ALCOHOLISM; ATHEROSCLEROSIS; CANCER; GENE; HYPERTENSION.)

Williams, Roger J. *Biochemical Individuality.* New Canaan, Conn.: Keats Publishing, 1998.

bioimpedance analysis meter (BIA meter) An electrical device sometimes used to check the amount of body fat. The BIA meter has been used in fitness centers and doctor's offices to adjust diets or to direct clinical treatment. The device attempts to measure body fat by measuring the flow of electricity between two electrodes attached at the ankle and the wrist when a very light current is applied. By gauging the resistance to the electrical current, the BIA meter can be used to estimate the water in tissues and thus fat content. There has not been an attempt to standardize measurements. Data are affected by body shape, moisture on the skin, the type of food or liquids consumed, muscle mass, and adjacent electrical appliances. In 1994, a panel assembled by the U.S. National Institutes of Health concluded that the BIA meter can give distorted values that have little bearing on measuring relatively small changes in fat.

biological value (BV) A measure of how efficiently the body uses dietary PROTEIN. The higher the biological value, the better the quality of food protein; that is, the more closely it supplies the optimal amounts of AMINO ACIDS for needed growth and maintenance. The intake of nitrogen for food protein is compared with loss of nitrogen under carefully controlled experimental conditions.

BV represents the percentage of food nitrogen retained by the body. It is defined as the amount of nitrogen from food protein retained by the body divided by the amount of nitrogen from food protein that was absorbed after digestion, expressed as a percentage.

Optimally, the BV could be 100 percent all the nitrogen that is absorbed is used in amino acids to build proteins. In practice, a protein with a BV higher than 70 (together with adequate calorie intake to meet energy needs) supports growth and represents a "complete" dietary protein. Most animal protein, except gelatin, has a high BV. A value less than 60 is considered low and represents "incomplete" protein. Many plant and grain proteins have low biological values because they are deficient in at least one essential amino acid. Typical CORN (maize) protein has a BV of 40 percent because it is low in the essential amino acid LYSINE, classified as a basic amino acid. High-lysine strains of corn have been developed that have a higher biological value. LEGUMES are low in sulfur amino acids (CYSTEINE and METHIONINE). Other plant sources (including AMARANTH, QUINOA, and SOYBEAN) provide protein that approaches the BV of meat.

The BV of plant protein can be improved by combining protein from different sources. When eating a variety of whole foods, VEGETABLES, GRAINS and grain products, BEANS, and other legumes daily, the body averages its daily protein intake. Thus, combining a food low in an essential amino acid with foods high in that amino acid raises the average for the day, and the net biological value is more than adequate. Knowledgeable vegetarians, or those on varied, high COMPLEX CARBOHYDRATE diets, can meet their protein needs with little or no meat. (See also DIETS, HIGH COMPLEX CARBOHYDRATE; DIETARY GUIDELINES FOR AMERICANS; FOOD COMPLEMENTING; NITROGEN BALANCE.)

biosynthesis The formation of molecules by cells generally from smaller, simpler raw materials. Chemical reactions in cells require protein catalysts, known as ENZYMES, and biosynthetic reactions are no exception. Those enzymes employed in biosynthesis require energy and are said to be "anabolic." Frequently, larger biomolecules are assembled from smaller building blocks. Thus biosynthetic reactions produce PROTEINS (polypeptides) from AMINO ACIDS; GLYCOGEN and STARCH (POLYSACCHARIDES) from GLUCOSE; DNA and RNA (polynucleotides) from simple nucleotides; FATTY ACIDS and CHOLESTEROL from acetic acid; FAT from fatty acids.

Biosynthesis requires an input of two forms of chemical energy: ATP, the "energy currency" of cells, and a reducing agent, reduced nicotinamide adenine dinucleotide phosphate (NADPH). ATP and NADPH are produced by the oxidation of fuels, especially CARBOHYDRATES and fat. Therefore energy production is coupled to biosynthesis (energy consumption). Biosynthetic pathways are localized within cells. Some, like fat synthesis and protein synthesis, occur exclusively in the cytoplasm. Others such as DNA and RNA synthesis are restricted to the nucleus. (See also ANABOLISM; CARBOHYDRATE METABOLISM; NICOTINAMIDE ADENINE DINUCLEOTIDE (NAD, NADH)/NICOTINAMIDE ADENINE DINUCLEOTIDE PHOSPHATE (NADP, NADPH).

biotin A member of the B COMPLEX and formerly designated as vitamin H, this water-soluble VITAMIN assists in energy production in the body. It is essential for synthesizing saturated fatty acids from CARBOHYDRATE and for synthesizing BLOOD SUGAR from non-carbohydrate precursors like lactic acid and pyruvic acid during STARVATION and FASTING. Biotin functions as a protein-bound COENZYME, assisting primarily in reactions in which enzymes transfer carbon dioxide to compounds to create carboxylic acids (carboxylation reactions). The oxidation of the short-chain fatty acid, propionic acid, requires biotin, as does the breakdown of the essential amino acid leucine. The safe and adequate daily intake for adults, except for pregnant women, is estimated to be 100 to 200 mcg.

Intestinal bacteria supply biotin. Furthermore, biotin is widespread in food, including egg yolk, liver, dark green leafy vegetables, and whole grains, so deficiencies are extremely rare. Deficiency symptoms include dermatitis, depression, pain, and weakness. Biotin supplements are very safe: These is no known toxicity even with high doses. Biotin does not cure baldness, nor does it cure dermatitis, two purported therapeutic uses of this vitamin. AVIDIN is a protein in raw egg white that functions as an antimicrobial agent to protect the yolk. Avidin binds biotin tightly, and it has been used to induce biotin deficiency in experimental animals. Because large amounts of raw egg white are very rarely consumed, avidin consumption is not an issue. (See also ACIDOPHILUS; FAT METABOLISM; GLUCONEOGENESIS.)

birth defects Abnormalities that are apparent at birth. They may manifest themselves as physiological, structural, or mental defects. The human embryo and fetus are sensitive to a wide variety of agents, ranging from chemicals, bacterial and viral infections, and radiation to the nutritional state of the mother and hence the fetus.

The type of birth defect and the degree of severity, depend upon the type of external factor, the dose, as well as upon the developmental stage at which the factor was taken up. The first three months of pregnancy (embryonic development) are particularly critical. Brain development and the formation of organs, the skeleton, and limbs occur in the embryo. Damage at this stage of human development may lead to severe structural birth defects. Agents that cause abnormal structural development in the embryo are known as TERATOGENS. They include maternal medications such as ESTROGENS, progestogens, certain anticancer drugs, some antibiotics, retinoic acid, VITAMIN D, and VITAMIN A (greater than 10,000 IU per day).

The terminal stages (the last six months) of pregnancy are also important. Fetal development involves integrating the ENDOCRINE SYSTEM and the elaboration of the nervous system. Certain medications may cause problems with the function of organ systems or with later development. These drugs are classified as "fetotoxic"; they include Neosporin, several cardiovascular drugs, certain sedatives and tranquilizers, excessive VITAMIN K, and the antibiotic tetracycline.

Maternal diet and nutrient status are critical for normal pregnancy and postnatal development. It is well established that nutritional deficiencies can lead to birth defects, mental retardation, and slowed development. If it is balanced throughout her life, the woman's diet before pregnancy can also enhance prenatal development. Maternal protein MALNUTRITION can lead to smaller brains in infants, premature birth, and difficulties after birth. ZINC is a key nutrient in maternal nutrition. Zinc deprivation can cause birth defects, delayed male sexual development, and, possibly, slow learning. Spina bifida and NEURAL TUBE DEFECTS (birth defects of the spinal chord) are linked to FOLIC ACID deficiencies. Repeated studies have shown that women who consume 400 mcg of folic acid daily before conception and in the early weeks of pregnancy reduce the risk that their babies will be born with neural tube defects by 70 percent. In 1998 the U.S. FDA required that folic acid be added to enriched grain products like BREAKFAST CEREALS, BREADS, and PASTA. A number of food-related agents affect embryonic and fetal development. Alcohol consumption during pregnancy can lead to mental retardation (FETAL ALCOHOL SYNDROME). CAFFEINE use by the mother during pregnancy can lead to abnormalities.

Many pollutants are implicated in birth defects and mental retardation. LEAD can affect mental development and learning. MERCURY can affect the nervous system of children, leading to mental retardation, seizures, and learning disabilities. The banana pesticide BENOMYL, FUMIGANTS (thiabenazole), and HERBICIDES (Dinoseb and dioxin) can cause fetal abnormalities in experimental animals. Women consuming PCB in FISH have a greater risk of having low birth weight babies and infants with developmental disorders. Pregnant women are advised to avoid fish caught in polluted waters. Trace amounts of industrial pollutants are commonly found in breast milk. Their effects on infant health are unknown. Chemical pollutants occur in freshwater BASS, TROUT, white fish, walleye pike, CATFISH, and fish from the Great Lakes and the Hudson River. Ocean fish caught from polluted waters, especially HALIBUT, MACKEREL, marlin, red snapper, sheepshead, TUNA, swordfish, BLUEFISH, and striped bass, are often contaminated by pollutants. (See also ALCOHOL; BREAST-FEEDING; HEAVY METALS.)

Cordero, Jose F. "Finding the Causes of Birth Defects," *The New England Journal of Medicine,* 331:1 (1994): 48–49.

biscuit A flat, sweetened, dry, baked food, usually containing a high percentage of fat. The term originated from the French and means "twice cooked." Heating fresh baked bread again in the oven dries it out. The hardened biscuit was a stable of military commissaries (sea biscuit, army biscuit) during the 19th century.

Biscuits contain varying portions of wheat flour, vegetable shortening, lard or butter, sugar, and flavorings. Ship biscuits are simply prepared from flour, salt, shortening, and water. Shortbreads are prepared from flour, butter or margarine, and sugar. Hot biscuits also contain milk and baking soda to create a tender dough. Biscuit flavorings vary with the menu, ranging from cinnamon and sugar to chives, parsley, cheese, fruit, or nuts.

bitters A family of aromatic beverages or tonics that have a bitter flavor. Bitters may or may not be alcoholic. Italian bitters are usually wine based. Bitters can be served as aperitifs, and peach and orange bitters are often used as flavoring in alcoholic mixed drinks (cocktails). Bitters can also refer to a dry ale tasting strongly of hops. Several plants used in herbal medicine are bitter "tonics," including GOLDENSEAL, DANDELION, CHAMOMILE, and gentian root. The physiologic actions include stimulation of glandular secretion to increase digestion, inhibition of inflammation, and antibacterial effects.

blackberry (genus *Rubus*) The conical fruit of a thorny shrub originating in Europe. A bramble of the rose family, the blackberry grows in Asia, Europe, and North America where it grows from Alaska to Mexico and from Newfoundland to Florida. In the 1800s, interest in blackberry cultivation led to the development of many varieties from wild stocks for commercial growers and gardens. Like the RASPBERRY, this fruit is composed of small seed-containing fruits called drupelets. Blackberries ripen from August through October, and the ripened fruit is purple-black. Many hybrids are now cultivated, including boysenberries, loganberries, and ollalieberries. Blackberries are used in jellies, tarts, pies, ice cream, syrups, and jam. They are an excellent source of FIBER and contain VITAMIN C. One cup (144 g, uncooked berries) provides 74 calories; carbohydrate, 18.4 g; fiber, 9.7 g; potassium, 282 mg; traces of protein and fat; iron, 0.8 mg; trace of B vitamins; and vitamin C, 30 mg.

black cohosh (*Cimicifuga racemosa;* American baneberry, black snakeroot, bugbane, bugwort, squawroot) A native North American plant that grows freely in shady woods in Canada and the United States. It is called black snakeroot to distinguish it from the common snakeroot (*Aristolochia serpentaria*). The root of this plant is used for many disorders, but particularly to treat symptoms of menopause and premenstrual syndrome (PMS). Many studies have been conducted to explore the medicinal benefits of black cohosh. It appears comparable to drugs used in hormone replacement therapy, but without the side effects. Black cohosh is popular in Europe, where most of the U.S. harvest is still shipped, but more and more Americans are becoming familiar with this plant.

black currant oil A seed oil used as a dietary supplemental source of essential fatty acids. Black currant oil is unusual because it provides both families of ESSENTIAL FATTY ACIDS, omega-6 and omega-3. It also contains a high level of GAMMA LINOLENIC ACID, a fatty acid that is converted to hormone-like substances, PROSTAGLANDINS, believed to counterbalance pain, elevated blood pressure, blood clotting, and inflammation. Gamma linolenic acid could help reduce blood clots and thus could potentially protect against STROKES and HEART ATTACKS. The conversion of gamma linolenic acid to prostaglandins may be inadequate when the diet contains excessive HYDROGENATED VEGETABLE OILS, excessive ALCOHOL, or if the individual is diabetic or elderly.

blackstrap molasses A semipurified, thick, dark-brown syrup made from concentrated sugar juice. The preparation of molasses involves several steps. Sugarcane is cut close to the ground, where it is richest in sugar. The stalks are shredded, then pressed to extract the juice, which is boiled down to concentrate it to the point of crystallizing sucrose (table sugar). The sugar crystals are removed; the remaining liquid (mother liquor) is blackstrap molasses—an important source of minerals. Light molasses is more purified and lacks the mineral content of blackstrap molasses. Two tablespoons (40 g) contain 85 calories; carbohydrate, 22 g; calcium, 274 mg; iron, 10.1 mg; manganese, 103 mg; and potassium 1,171 mg. (See also NATURAL SWEETENERS.)

bladder infections (urinary tract infections) Infections of the urethra or bladder, which increase the risk of a serious kidney infection. Cystitis refers to inflammation of the bladder. Ninety percent of patients with bladder infections are women; 20 percent of women have such infections at least once a year. Bladder infections are not uncommon in children; 2 percent of girls have excessive bacteria in their urine. The prevalence increases with age.

The problem generally occurs when fecal or vaginal bacteria are introduced into the urethra. If the bladder is not voided completely, especially if there is infrequent urination or during the last stage of pregnancy, the risk of infection increases.

Unsweetened CRANBERRY juice may lessen symptoms, but will not cure bladder infections; it contains hippuric acid, which retards bacterial growth, and a carbohydrate that prevents coliform bacteria from adhering to the bladder and urethra lining.

GARLIC has been shown to have antimicrobial activity, including activity against bacteria associated with urinary tract infections. The care of a physician is strongly recommended in the event of bladder infections because of the risk of kidney infections. (See also *CANDIDA ALBICANS*.)

blanching The process of exposing fruits and vegetables to boiling water or steam for a short time. Blanching both preserves color and inactivates ENZYMES that alter the texture and flavor of food. A typical procedure entails heating a vegetable up to three minutes in boiling water. Blanching CORN for two minutes before freezing helps preserve its flavor. Blanching TOMATOES and PEACHES simplifies peeling them. Blanched salad vegetables are softer than raw vegetables.

bleaching agents (flour) Chemical oxidizing agents used to whiten FLOUR. Milled wheat flour is initially yellowish and does not form an elastic dough. Oxidation of flour protein, GLUTEN, and pigments both whitens and matures flour so that it produces an elastic dough that is good for baking.

Consumer preference for white flour and white BREAD has led the baking industry to use an unusual list of food additives. Before World War II, agene (nitrogen trichloride) was used extensively to bleach flour. In wartime England, kennels increasingly used bread scraps to make up for the diminished supply of meat; dogs were observed to go into convulsions that mimicked epileptic fits. In severe cases, the animals became crazed. In 1946, Sir Edward Mellanby reported the correlation between neurological symptoms and bleached flour. Later research demonstrated that the sulfur amino acid METHIONINE was converted to a potent inhibitor of a brain enzyme by agene, and the modified methionine could itself cause seizures. As a result of these findings, agene was banned in 1946. After exhaustive testing, chlorine dioxide was found to be a safe bleaching and maturing agent. It is used mainly in the processing of fruit and vegetables. Instead of chlorine dioxide, the baking industry now uses powdered bleaching agents that are simpler and less expensive to use. Benzoylperoxide can bleach flour in 24 hours, for example. Such bleaching agents leave innocuous residues in flour.

blood The cell-filled liquid that circulates through the heart, arteries, and veins. A 70 kg adult has a blood volume of 5 liters. Blood is regarded as a tissue in which red and white cells are suspended in a liquid (plasma) in the ratio of 45 parts cells to 55 parts plasma. This vital fluid performs many tasks. Blood supplies all tissues with nutrients and oxygen, and it transports waste such as UREA to the kidneys, and CARBON DIOXIDE to the lungs, for disposal. Blood is the medium for integration and coordination of tissues of the body through hormonal regulation. It maintains the chemical equilibrium of the body in terms of ELECTROLYTES (ionic substances) and polyelectrolytes (serum proteins), which in turn regulate water distribution in blood versus tissues. Blood pH is buffered to maintain a very narrow range at 7.35 to 7.45. Circulating antibodies, gamma globulin, represent blood aspects of the immune system and thus are the first line of defense against foreign substances. Blood also contains special cells, platelets, and protein clotting factors to form clots and thus limit blood loss. Fats, cholesterol, and fat-soluble vitamins are transported in the blood by specialized structures (LIPOPROTEINS). Nutrients like vitamin A, iron, and copper are carried by their own transport proteins. In terms of mechanical function, the bloodstream assures an even temperature for all regions of the body.

Most cells in blood are RED BLOOD CELLS (erythrocytes), which are specifically designed to transport oxygen. WHITE BLOOD CELLS (leukocytes) represent a much smaller fraction; as part of the immune system they protect against infection. Lymphocytes, which represent 20 percent to 50 percent of white cells, are derived from either bone marrow or from the thymus gland. They mount a cellular defense against foreign cells and materials. Plasma, the fluid remaining once cells are removed, contains fibrinogen. This inactive protein can be activated to form fibrin clots to plug holes in blood vessels. The fluid remaining after blood has clotted is called serum which lacks cells and clotting factors, but contains GLUCOSE and minerals like POTASSIUM, SODIUM, and CHLORIDE, the most common electrolytes. These ions help maintain the appropriate ionic strength, pH, and FLUID BALANCE of the body. Serum contains ALBUMIN and other proteins that help maintain ion concentrations in the blood, and it contains transport proteins, such as VERY LOW-DENSITY LIPOPROTEINS (VLDL) for carrying fat and LOW-DENSITY LIPOPROTEINS (LDL) and HIGH-DENSITY LIPOPROTEINS (HDL) to transport cholesterol.

Several types of nutrients support the circulatory system. For example, VITAMIN K and CALCIUM support the blood clotting mechanism. ZINC, IRON, MANGANESE, MAGNESIUM, VITAMIN B_6, folic acid, vitamin B_{12}, and other nutrients support erythrocyte and leukocyte production. Vitamin C maintains strength and elasticity of capillaries. (See also BLOOD CLOTTING; ENDOCRINE SYSTEM; HEMOGLOBIN; IMMUNE SYSTEM.)

blood-brain barrier A structural barrier that limits the passage of a variety of substances, including certain drugs and nutrients, from blood vessels into the brain and the central nervous system. This barrier consists of cells lining capillaries (endothelial cells). The attachments between these cells are called "tight junctions." However, the nature of the physical barriers and biochemical mechanisms for transporting materials across the barrier are complex and are not completely understood. Very small molecules like water and oxygen simply diffuse through cells and capillaries. GLUCOSE, the major fuel of the brain, is an example of a substance that can penetrate the blood-brain barrier, passing freely across the barrier, though other sugars do not. During STARVATION or crash dieting, ketone bodies, small acidic compounds that accumulate in the blood during excessive fat degradation (a condition known as KETOSIS), can cross through capillary linings, pass into the brain and be burned for energy. In contrast, long-chain fatty acids that make up fat cannot penetrate the blood-brain barrier, and consequently fat cannot supply the brain with energy. Some nutrients rely on transport systems embedded in cell membranes to actively transport substances into the brain. Thus AMINO ACIDS enter by specific, energy-dependent processes (active transport) TYROSINE, PHENYLALANINE, LEUCINE, ISOLEUCENE, VALINE, and TRYPTOPHAN compete for the same transport sites. Different sites are specific for other types of amino acids. (See also FOOD; NEUROTRANSMITTER.)

blood cells See LEUKOCYTES; RED BLOOD CELLS.

blood clotting The formation of a semi-solid mass from blood constituents. Exposure of blood to air, to foreign substances or to substances released from injured tissues (thromboplastin) stimulates blood clotting. Blood clotting is a complex process requiring the sequential activation of a series of clotting factors, which are protein modifying (proteolytic) enzymes. It culminates in the activation of thrombin, the terminal enzyme that catalyzes the conversion of fibrinogen, a soluble blood protein, to insoluble FIBRIN. Fibrin forms fibers that create a sticky mass that enmeshes blood platelets, a very small type of white blood cell, and RED BLOOD CELLS. This mass of fibers and cells forms a plug that covers the injured region of a capillary. The platelets fragment and release serotonin, a compound that causes the capillary to contract and the blood clot to retract. The net result is that the hole is patched and blood flow is reduced at the site of injury.

Nutrition status affects blood clotting. The maturation of prothrombin, the parent molecule of thrombin, and of other blood clotting factors (proenzymes) further up the clotting sequence of reactions, requires VITAMIN K and CALCIUM. A calcium deficiency effectively slows the activation of clotting enzymes because a calcium-prothrombin complex must first form in order to be activated to thrombin. Vitamin K deficiency slows clotting because prothrombin cannot be modified to bind calcium. STARVATION and protein MALNUTRITION reduce clotting because the LIVER synthesizes lesser amounts of the protein clotting factors and fibrinogen.

blood lipids See CHOLESTEROL; TRIGLYCERIDES.

blood pressure The pressure maintained in arteries and veins by the heart. Blood pressure usually refers to an indirect measurement of pressure of large arteries at the height of the pulse. Blood pressure reflects the resistance of blood flow in the capillary bed and arterioles as well as the elasticity of arteries themselves. The heart exerts pressure throughout the circulatory system. Ventricles of the heart contract (the systolic phase of the heartbeat), creating systolic pressure in the cycle of heart pumping. Ventricular relaxation between heartbeats creates the lowest pressure between heartbeats, the diastolic pressure. Like a barometer for measuring air pressure, blood pressure is measured in units equivalent to the height of a column of mercury. A pressure of 120/80 represents a systolic pressure equivalent to 120 mm of mercury and a diastolic pressure of 80 mm of mercury. A systolic pressure persistently greater than 140 and a diastolic pressure persistently greater than 100 indicate stages of HYPERTENSION (high blood pressure), a potentially serious condition.

The following factors are linked to increased blood pressure: overweight, age, emotional STRESS, physical activity, and male gender. Quiet sleep and female gender are linked to with decreased blood pressure.

Dietary factors and heredity are risk factors for susceptible individuals. Approximately 20 percent of adults will be adversely affected by overconsumption of SODIUM. Unfortunately, these salt-sensitive individuals cannot be readily identified. Eating a large meal can lower blood pressure quickly in older people when the stomach fills with food, and experiments show that such people may feel faint or have an angina attack unless they lie down. (See also HEART DISEASE.)

blood sugar The level of GLUCOSE in the blood. RED BLOOD CELLS and most of the nervous system, including the brain, rely on this fuel to meet most of their energy requirements. The body strives to maintain blood sugar at a constant level. This reflects hormonal regulation and a delicate balance between diverse processes: CARBOHYDRATE DIGESTION and assimilation; tissue uptake of glucose; and release of glucose by the LIVER. During the fasting state, blood sugar levels remain relatively constant for an individual; the normal range of fasting blood sugar is 60 to 100 mg per 100 ml.

What Happens After a Meal?

Typically, blood sugar levels rise an hour or so after a meal containing carbohydrate, as the glucose produced by digestion of starch and complex sugars is absorbed by the intestine. Elevated blood sugar after a carbohydrate meal signals the endocrine PANCREAS to release INSULIN. This hormone lowers blood sugar by stimulating most tissues to take up glucose and metabolize it. The absorbed glucose is either stored as GLYCOGEN in muscle and liver, or it is converted to FAT by the ADIPOSE TISSUE and the liver. As a result, blood sugar levels return to base line values several hours after eating.

What Happens Between Meals (Fasting)?

Glucose is constantly being consumed by the brain and other tissues. In response to a drop in blood sugar or to stress, the ADRENAL GLANDS release CORTISOL and EPINEPHRINE and the pancreas releases GLUCAGON. These hormones signal the release of glucose from glycogen stores in the liver, and the synthesis of glucose from amino acids, by the liver, raising blood sugar levels to base line values.

HYPOGLYCEMIA refers to a sustained, abnormally low blood glucose level. If blood sugar drops too low, the brain does not function normally. This condition creates mood changes, irritability, fainting, and fatigue. Reactive hypoglycemia refers to a drop in blood sugar levels that can occur several hours after eating. This is usually due to the abnormal functioning of insulin (dysinsulism). Severe hypoglycemia due to profound metabolic imbalances can lead to coma.

HYPERGLYCEMIA (elevated blood sugar) is at the other extreme and is characterized by sustained, elevated blood glucose as observed in DIABETES MELLITUS. Chronic high blood glucose, frequent in uncontrolled diabetes, has many unfortunate ramifications. It can lead to the destruction of peripheral nerves and eye damage; lowered resistance to infections; toxemia during pregnancy; and heart and kidney disease. The excretion of excess sugar in the urine causes DEHYDRATION.

Lifestyle choices can help stabilize blood sugar levels and thus minimize wide swings in the changes brought about by the over- or underproduction of hormones. The body responds more efficiently to insulin with reduced intake of REFINED CARBOHYDRATES, COFFEE, and ALCOHOL. Specific nutrients may help the body regulate blood sugar. Dietary CHROMIUM can help insulin work more effectively; STRESS, coffee, and sugar consumption deplete the body of chromium. High levels of biotin seem to assist the liver with carbohydrate and fat metabolism. NIACINAMIDE, NIACIN, VITAMIN C, VITAMIN B_6, MANGANESE, MAGNESIUM, ZINC, and SELENIUM have been shown to improve glucose tolerance in some instances.

Eating frequent, light meals that are high in protein often helps to avoid swings in blood sugar levels, and balanced meals with whole foods high in STARCH and FIBER are effective time-released sources of glucose. Stress reduction with meditation, yoga or biofeedback, regular exercise, and maintaining optimal body weight, also helps minimize blood sugar imbalances. (See also DIETING; GLUCONEOGENESIS; GLYCOGENOLYSIS.)

Gold, Paul E. "Role of Glucose in Regulating the Brain and Cognition," *American Journal of Clinical Nutrition*, 61:supplement (1995): 987S–995S.

blueberry (*Vaccinium*) An edible, bluish berry related to the heath family of plants which includes American laurel, rhododendron, and broom. Varieties of blueberries include whortleberries and bilberries. They are an excellent source of fiber and anthocyanosides, blue-black pigments related to FLAVONOIDS. These pigments can help stabilize collagen structure. Blueberries also contain a carbohydrate that tends to prevent coliform bacteria from adhering to the walls of the bladder and urethra. (Attachment is the first step in infection.)

European bilberries are used in botanical medicine. Their FLAVONOIDS have many important effects on the body. They help decrease blood platelet aggregation; clumping of these small cell fragments of the blood is an essential step in blood clot formation, and excessive platelet aggregation increases the risk of strokes.

Bilberry flavonoids may benefit varicose veins by strengthening capillaries and vein structure. They also can strengthen the blood-brain barrier and limit uptake of harmful substances. They have been shown to help relieve day and night blindness and retinal degeneration. In folk medicine, bilberry leaf tea has been used to help normalize high blood sugar in diabetes.

Blueberries are eaten raw or cooked in pies, tarts, and muffins as well as in ice cream, compotes, and CHUTNEY. They are convenient to freeze. Frozen blueberries keep at least a year. One cup of blueberries (145g) provides 82 calories; carbohydrate, 20.5 g; fiber, 4.9 g; vitamin C, 20 mg; and small amounts of protein, fat, minerals, and vitamins.

bluefish (*Pomatomus saltatrix*) A silver and blue fish from the Atlantic Ocean neighboring the coasts of North and South America. This fish runs in schools that migrate north in spring along the eastern seaboard of North America and return southward in autumn. It is both an important game fish and a commercial food fish. The annual catch ranges from 3,000 to 4,000 tons in U.S. waters. Bluefish typically weigh 3 to 5 pounds and have a delicate flavor. Like most fish, it is an excellent protein source. The baked fish (100 g) provides 159 calories.

blue food colors Colors approved by the U.S. FDA for use in candy and soft drinks. Blue ARTIFICIAL

FOOD COLORS can be mixed with yellows (FD&C No. 5 and No. 6) to create shades of green. The safety of these dyes has been questioned. FD&C Blue No. 1 may cause chromosomal damage. FD&C Blue No. 2 may cause brain tumors in experimental animals. (See also DELANEY CLAUSE; FOOD ADDITIVES.)

body fat See FAT.

body fluids The water-based components of the body. Approximately 60 percent of the human body is water. Typically, 20 percent of body weight represents intracellular water, and in normal, healthy adults it accounts for about 55 percent of total body water; trained athletes have a higher percentage. Water outside the cells represents the sum of the lymph, blood plasma (the fluid of blood), the interstitial fluid (the water between cells and tissues), and the water bound to the skeleton and connective tissue. Plasma accounts for about 4 percent of body weight.

To function normally, cells maintain an appropriate osmotic pressure (the pressure generated by two solutions of different compositions separated by a partially porous membrane like the cell wall). Cells of the body generally maintain an osmotic pressure equal to that of blood. Cells are in danger of swelling and rupturing if too much water enters, and they will shrink and eventually collapse if excessive water moves out of cells. Cells regulate osmotic pressure by maintaining potassium ions inside and pumping sodium out. Water follows these ions, as well as the movement of chloride. Thus movement of these simple ELECTROLYTES plays a major role in water balance.

Circulating body fluids, the blood and the lymph, are protected against extreme variation in pH (a relative measure of the degree of acidity and alkalinity of a solution) by proteins, inorganic ions, bicarbonate, and phosphate, which bind an excess of acid (hydrogen ions) and neutralize bases. They help buffer the blood at a value of 7.3 to 7.4 A lower pH leads to acidosis (excessively low pH). A pH greater than 7.4 leads to alkalosis (excessively alkaline pH). Either imbalance can be dangerous.

body mass index (BMI) A standard for body weight based upon the measurements of height and weight. This is one of the most useful relationships: It can be used to assess health risks associated with overweight and it can be used as a therapeutic guide. There is a high degree of correlation between BMI and body fat determined from density measurements. The BMI for adults is based on surveys of lean adults between the ages of 20 and 29. To calculate this index of fatness, first divide the weight by the height in inches squared, then multiply the result by 703. A healthy BMI ranges between 18.5 and 24.9. A value of 30 or greater falls into the category of OBESITY. Nonetheless, there is no clear-cut, absolute standard for deciding if an individual is overweight or underweight. The interpretation of the BMI for children and adolescents aged two to 20 depends on the individual's age and sex. The typical American child's BMI declines after birth until the child is between four and six years old. It then gradually increases throughout the adult years. The point at which the increase begins is called the adiposity rebound. A child whose adiposity rebound begins at a young age is more likely to have a higher-than-average BMI as an adult. (See also ADIPOSE TISSUE; FAT; HEIGHT-WEIGHT TABLES; LEAN BODY MASS; OBESITY.)

bok choy (*Brassica chinensis;* Chinese mustard cabbage, pak-choi) A type of Chinese cabbage resembling celery, with dark green leaves that are smooth elongated, and generally 8 to 18 inches long. Bok choy does not form a heart, unlike pet-sai, another commonly used Chinese cabbage. Bok choy has a mild flavor. It can be eaten raw in salads and coleslaw or cooked in stir-fries and as a condiment for pork, fish, and shellfish. Bok choy is a good source of BETA-CAROTENE, FIBER, and VITAMIN C. One cup (170 g) provides 20 calories; protein, 2.6 g; carbohydrate, 3 g; fiber, 3.4 g; calcium, 158 mg; potassium, 630 mg; beta-carotene, 437 retinol equivalents; and vitamin C, 44 mg.

bologna A processed meat product. This large, seasoned sausage contains minced turkey, pork, beef, veal, or a combination of these meats packed into a casing and usually smoked. One slice contains 289 mg sodium. This high sodium content is typical of sausage.

Most bolognas can be considered high-fat foods. Two slices (2 ounces) of luncheon meat in a sandwich is the average serving, as determined by the U.S. Department of Agriculture (USDA). A rule of thumb is that 2 ounces of meat should supply no more than 2 grams of fat. Saturated fat accounts for most of the calories in bologna. The high level of fat, especially saturated fat, in the typical American diet is linked to an increased risk of heart disease. DIETARY GUIDELINES FOR AMERICANS recommends a diet with less saturated fat. The chemical sodium NITRATE is often added as a preservative to processed meats, including bologna, to prevent the growth of bacteria that can cause food poisoning. Nitrite can react in the stomach with nitrogen-containing compounds called amines to yield cancer-causing compounds called nitrosoamines. One slice of bologna (one ounce, [28 g]) contains 89 calories; protein, 3.3 g; carbohydrate, 0.55 g; fat, 8 g; cholesterol, 16 mg; calcium, 3 mg; iron, 0.4 mg; and small amounts of the B complex: vitamins.

bolus The mixture of food and saliva produced by chewing. To be digested efficiently, food must first be pulverized by teeth and mixed with saliva to ease swallowing. This disperses and lubricates food particles and eases their passage into the stomach and initiates starch digestion by the enzyme salivary amylase. The act of swallowing moves the food past the epiglottis and down into the esophagus, which transports it into the stomach. The downward movement of food is carried out by PERISTALSIS, waves of contraction of smooth muscles encircling the esophagus. In the stomach, the bolus becomes chyme, partially digested food mixed with GASTRIC JUICE. (See also DIGESTION; DIGESTIVE ENZYMES.)

bone A structure of hard tissue consisting of blood vessels, nerves, osteocytes (cells capable of bone synthesis), and a matrix of inorganic salts, protein, and mucopolysaccharides (acidic and sulfated carbohydrate chains).

Bones provide support and define the shape of the body. There are two structural arrangements in bone: external, compact bone is dense and hard; internal bone is porous and is found in most flat bones and at the ends of long bones of the arms and legs. Red bone marrow fills the cavities and the ends of some long bones and most flat bones. In adults, red marrow is the site of synthesis of red blood cells and certain white blood cells (lymphocytes of the immune system and blood platelets required for clotting).

The periosteum is the membrane covering the bone surface that supplies the bone with nerves and blood vessels.

Osteocytes absorb CALCIUM, MAGNESIUM, and other nutrients from blood, which is supplied by an exterior blood vessel and capillary system. These cells crystallize the ions as an insoluble matrix of hydrated calcium phosphate (hydroxyapatite) and calcium carbonate. In fact, bone accounts for 99 percent of the calcium in the body.

While mature bones have a fixed size and shape and are composed of crystalline materials, their chemical composition is constantly changing. Short-term changes occur when calcium is deposited in the bony matrix and is again released into the blood. Longer-term changes occur in both the chemical and the structural makeup during the aging process.

Several nutrients besides minerals play important roles in bone metabolism. VITAMIN D stimulates cells of the intestinal mucosa to take up calcium. A chronic deficiency of this vitamin leads to RICKETS (in children) and OSTEOMALACIA (in adults). VITAMIN C plays a role in collagen synthesis, required for bone deposition. A chronic deficiency leads to impaired calcification. VITAMIN K is implicated in bone formation also. Maturation of RED BLOOD CELLS and WHITE BLOOD CELLS, both critically important, requires vitamins (FOLIC ACID, VITAMIN B_{12}, VITAMIN B_6, VITAMIN A) and minerals (IRON, ZINC, BORON, MOLYBDENUM, among others). (See also OSTEOPOROSIS.)

bone disease See OSTEOMALACIA; OSTEOPOROSIS.

bone marrow in meat See MEAT.

bone meal Powdered bone obtained from livestock, long used as a supplemental source of CALCIUM and MAGNESIUM. Bone meal is no longer recommended. Analysis of many commercial products has revealed extensive LEAD contamination, probably because the livestock that supplied the bones were contaminated by lead. The fetus, infants, and children are especially sensitive to lead, which can retard growth and development.

A dose of three teaspoons of bone meal can result in a lead intake close to the acceptable maximum daily intake for infants and children between six months and two years. Pregnant and nursing women, and children, should not use bone meal; safer calcium supplements are available. (See also HEAVY METALS.)

bonito (*Thunnus*) Various medium-sized tuna, related to mackerel. A migratory fish, bonito inhabits both the Pacific and Atlantic Oceans and is harvested on a large scale and sold canned or fresh. Tuna is the most popular seafood in the United States and is an oily high-fat fish, rich in vitamins A and D. It is a relatively good source of omega-3 essential fatty acids, which help reduce the risk of blood clotting.

A 3 oz serving of tuna, packed in oil and drained, provides 140 to 200 calories; when packed in water it provides 90 to 110 calories. Both provide protein, 21 g; fat, 1 g; cholesterol, 40 to 60 mg, and calcium, 10 mg. Typically, salt added in processing contributes 300 to 500 mg of sodium per serving. The DIETARY GUIDELINES FOR AMERICANS recommends that salt and sodium be used only in moderation because of a risk of high blood pressure in susceptible individuals. Nutrient content is the same as ALBACORE tuna.

borage (*Borago officianalis*) A perennial herb whose beautiful flowers have been used in cooking and herbal preparations since Roman times. In folk medicine, borage is used to induce perspiration. The leaves are used to flavor salads and pasta or used as cooked greens and mixed with spinach. The flowers are used in salads as a garnish or in making a fragrant tea. Borage oil is one of the three major supplemental sources of GAMMA LINOLENIC ACID, the important polyunsaturated fatty acid that serves as a precursor of PROSTAGLANDINS (PG_1). The prostaglandins are hormone-like compounds that help regulate diverse physiologic processes. Due to lifestyle and dietary habits, production of this family of prostaglandins may be deficient in many Americans. The PG_1 prostaglandin family is a factor in widening blood vessels, reducing the tendency of blood to form clots, lowering cholesterol production, and regulating the immune system. Borage oil contains up to 26 percent gamma linolenic acid, more than is found in evening primrose oil or black currant oil. It also contains 40 percent linoleic acid, the omega-6 essential fatty acid from which gamma linolenic acid is derived.

boron An essential mineral nutrient found in trace amounts in most tissues. Although its precise role is unclear, boron may function in bone formation in both women and men and may also help prevent CALCIUM and MAGNESIUM losses in postmenopausal women. Boron seems to aid in the formation of steroid hormones (ESTROGEN) and VITAMIN D, and it improves COPPER metabolism. A magnesium deficiency accentuates the effects of boron. As yet there is no RECOMMENDED DIETARY ALLOWANCE (RDA) for boron because a requirement has not yet been quantified. An estimated safe and adequate daily intake is 1 to 3 mg for adults. Sources of boron include legumes, leafy vegetables, and fruit; APPLES, GRAPES, and PEARS are good sources. A varied diet would be expected to supply adequate amounts of this mineral. Excessive use of boron supplements can cause a dangerous overdose of boron.

Newham, R. "Role of Boron in Human Nutrition," *Journal of Applied Nutrition* 46 (1995): 81–85.

borsch (borscht) A traditional eastern European beet soup. Its characteristic red color derives from beets, a major ingredient. Recipes may specify adding white kidney beans, mushrooms, and various amounts of other vegetables such as shredded cabbage, carrots, parsley, and onions to beef or other stock and vinegar. Borsch may be served with diced stewmeat, sausage, and sour cream. It may be served hot or cold.

botanical extracts The extract of any part of a plant. Extracts may be produced "naturally" (by squeezing or crushing a plant) or by treating the plant with a solvent. The term *herbal* refers to the leaves and stems of a plant, while *botanical* refers to these parts in addition to roots, seeds, and fruits. Long-term safety and appropriate dosages have not yet been established for many botanical extracts. They are therefore not generally recommended for pregnant or breast-feeding women.

Safety and quality play an essential role when botanical extracts are used as supplements to enhance physical or mental performance. To guarantee safety many manufacturers are now standardizing their extracts. The goal in standardizing an extract is to control the complete chemical composition of the extract rather than one particular identified constituent or group of constituents. Standardization is obtained by determining a certain amount of its active principles, identified as typical "markers" or "active ingredients" that characterize every single plant species. Only high-quality standardized botanical extracts can be considered safe, with predictable, reproducible effects.

A number of standardized botanical extracts have been introduced into the United States. The heightened interest in standardized products is due to the belief that standardization is directly related to the potency of the extract. This is not necessarily the case.

All supplements, including herbs and vitamins, must conform to federal regulations that control production, labeling, and advertising. In order to sell an herbal supplement, a manufacturer must meet many different federal and state regulations and must also adhere to state and local health and business regulations. Because supplements are legally classified as a specifically defined type of food, all supplements are required to be manufactured to the same high standards that are required of all foods. These mandated good manufacturing practices establish basic guidelines to assure that supplements are manufactured under sanitary conditions and are fit for consumption. Any supplement that does not conform to these basic guidelines is subject to regulatory action by the FDA. In addition, all supplement products are required by law to provide certain information about their formulation.

Supplements must provide consumers with nutritional information and must also state the quantity of each of the contained ingredients or of the proprietary blends that make up a product. All herbal products are required to identify the parts used of each of the plant ingredients and to label them with their commonly accepted names.

The government is most interested in product claims of botanical extracts. The FDA prohibits the use of any statement that would brand the product as a drug, nor does it allow statements regarding prevention, cure, mitigation, or treatment of diseases. Claims are limited to statements that are legally defined as "statements of nutritional support" or "structure/function statements."

bottled water Commercially bottled drinking WATER that may or may not be carbonated. The sales of bottled water in the United States rose 9.3 percent in 2000 to $5.7 billion. This growth in bottled water consumption comes from the growing awareness of the widespread pollution of municipal water sources by pesticides, fertilizers, and industrial chemicals. Most bottled water comes from wells or springs. Bottled "drinking water" may be filtered water or distilled water with some minerals added. Bottled water is disinfected by ozone, not by chlorine treatment. Bottled water is classified as a food product by the U.S. FDA, but producers are not required to list the source.

Although bottled water may taste better than tap water, it may be no more healthful. The EPA sets water quality standards for most of the drinking water sources. However, there is no guarantee that a bottled water will be safer or more wholesome, because bottled water is less regulated than tap water. The issue of bottled water safety was publicized when analyses revealed a popular, imported brand was contaminated with the organic solvent benzene, a carcinogen. Spot checks have turned up traces of other organic solvents, NITRITES, and toxic HEAVY METALS in samples of bottled water, and the SODIUM content can be high. Consumers can request the latest chemical analysis of their preferred brand of water from the bottler.

The most common types of bottled water are:

- club soda: tap water that is filtered, carbonated with carbon dioxide, and treated with minerals to give it flavor
- distilled water: purified by condensing steam, it contains no minerals but may contain volatile

organic contaminants. Unless calcium and magnesium are added back, distilled water has a flat taste
- mineral water: any water containing minerals, although there is no federal standard to regulate them. California has a standard for the amount of dissolved minerals in its "mineral water"
- natural sparkling water: initially naturally carbonated, then reinjected with carbon dioxide to increase carbonation
- seltzer: carbonated water. Often seltzer is tap water that has been filtered to remove organic materials, and then treated with carbon dioxide to provide carbonation.

bottle feeding See INFANT FORMULA.

botulism (botulinus poisoning) A rare though deadly form of food poisoning caused by ingestion of a toxin produced by the anaerobic soil bacterium *Clostridium botulinum.* Several strains of *C. botulinum* produce one of the most deadly natural toxins. It is estimated that a few micrograms of the toxin could kill an adult. Botulinum toxins are neurotoxins, (nerve poisons) which trigger symptoms such as nausea, vomiting, sudden weakness, and difficulty in breathing, speaking, and swallowing; blurred vision, and headache. Paralysis and death can occur in two to 10 days. Early detection is a critical factor to assure timely treatment with botulinum antitoxin.

Infant botulism was first recognized in the United States in 1976, and it is now the most common form of botulism. In susceptible infants, the botulinum bacterium can propagate before the development of normal intestinal flora that would inhibit it. HONEY has been implicated as the probable source of botulism spores in some instances.

Botulism is becoming more common with the use of microwave cooking, which may not sterilize food completely. Botulism is usually associated with canned food, especially improperly home-canned nonacidic vegetables, such as string beans, sweet corn, beets, asparagus, spinach, and chard. Toxin production is favored when contaminated food is stored at neutral or slightly alkaline pH at room temperature for 12 to 24 hours away from air, and then not reheated before serving. Improperly stored restaurant foods (potato salad, pot pies, stews, turkey loaf, preserved meat, fish, and milk), have been reported as causes of outbreaks of botulism. Low-acid foods that are not canned, such as salami and other processed meats, depend upon a combination of treatments to inhibit germination of *C. botulinum* spores and bacterial growth: mild heat treatment, the addition of sodium nitrite and other additives, and refrigeration.

When in doubt about the safety of a food, it should be discarded. Commercially canned goods that are swollen and home-canned products that are bubbling, discolored, or are cloudy should also be discarded, because these are signs of improper canning. Cooked foods should be refrigerated, especially foods that are in a tight wrapping (such as a baked potato in foil or food coated with fat or batter, like sauteed onions). Food should be reheated thoroughly; 10 minutes of high heat destroys botulinum toxin. (See also AFLATOXIN; SALMONELLA.)

bouillabaisse A traditional fish stew from southern France. Freshly caught Mediterranean fish are cooked with tomatoes and herbs and served on a bed of vegetables. Originally, bouillabaisse was cooked by fishermen using the least suitable fish for market, such as rockfish, plus easily obtained shellfish like mussels and small crabs. According to legend, this fisherman's stew was divinely inspired and brought to humans by angels. A variety of whitefish and shellfish can be substituted for the traditional ones, including salmon, whiting, bass, lobster, crab, prawns, and eel. The seafood is marinated in olive oil, tomatoes, onions, garlic, parsley, thyme, bay leaf, shredded orange peel, saffron, and salt and pepper before boiling.

bouillon The clear broth obtained from boiling vegetables, meat, or poultry. Bouillon forms the base for a variety of dishes, soups, and sauces. Commercially prepared bouillons contain high levels of sodium. Although they possess appetizing flavors, they are not nutrient-dense foods: Beef bouillon concentrate (one package) provides 15 calories; protein 1 g; carbohydrate, 1 g; fat, 1 g; and sodium, 1,019 mg; and only very small amounts of other minerals and vitamins.

bovine growth hormone (bGH; bovine somatotropin) A genetically engineered hormone designed to increase MILK output from dairy cows. The U.S. FDA approved general use of bGH on cows; its assessment is that MEAT or milk from bGH-treated cows is nutritionally identical to milk from untreated animals.

Controversy surrounding the application of this synthetic drug focuses on several issues. Although all milk contains growth hormone, the synthetic drug differs from the natural bovine growth hormone in structure, by 49 amino acids added from human growth hormone. (Bovine and human insulin–like growth factors are very similar and are not destroyed by pasteurization.) Differences in the ability to cause an allergic reaction can be expected, even though bGH itself seems to be biologically inactive in humans. The hormone increases the level of an insulin-like growth factor (IGF-1) in cow's milk, higher than that found in breast milk, and its effects, if any, on children's upper GASTROINTESTINAL TRACT are unknown. Possible adverse effects in cows include infected udders; which would require treatment with antibiotics that could get into the milk. The FDA has issued assurances that milk is tested for antibiotic contamination. (See also BREAST-FEEDING; GENETIC ENGINEERING.)

bovine spongiform encephalopathy (BSE) The technical term for mad cow disease, a fatal brain disease in cattle that was first diagnosed in Britain in 1986. After an incubation period of three to five years characterized by normal behavior, BSE-infected cattle begin to stagger and become aggressive. The brains of such animals of autopsy look spongy; under the microscope nerve cells reveal protein fiber buildup. BSE is a member of a group of brain disorders characterized by chronic wasting that seem to be caused by a rogue protein called a prion. Prions appear to multiply in the brain, spinal cord, spleen, and thymus; they do not trigger an immune reaction in host animals. The possibility that the infection can be transmitted to other species raised the concern that beef or milk products from infected animals could transmit the disease to humans.

The source of the BSE outbreak is unknown, but evidence suggests it was spread, in part, by feeding to cattle meal that contained ground meat and bone from BSE-infected cattle. The British government took several steps to contain the disease, including slaughtering thousands of animals that were suspected of infection and banning the use of meat-and-bone meal. The measures were successful, reducing the number of confirmed cases in the United Kingdom from 36,680 in 1992 to fewer than 1,500 in 2000.

Then, in the 1990s, reports of people in Europe who developed a rare but deadly neurological disorder, variant Creutzfeld-Jakob disease (vCJD), raised public concerns about the safety of eating beef. In 1996 10 people in the United Kingdom began exhibiting unusual symptoms, including leg pain, difficulty walking, hallucinations, and slurred speech. Eventually, the patients could not walk, speak, or even feed themselves. Within two years they had all died. Autopsies revealed that the victims' brain tissue had disintegrated, giving it the spongelike appearance similar to the brains of cattle infected with BSE.

The patients' symptoms were like those seen in people who suffered from a rare, fatal neurological disorder called Creutzfeld-Jakob disease (CJD). Most victims of that disease die in their late 60s after years of suffering lingering dementia, but the patients diagnosed with variant Creutzfeld-Jakob disease were all in their 20s. Researchers decided these patients contracted vCJD after eating the flesh of cattle that had BSE.

By early 2002, 124 people in Europe had developed vCJD: 117 in the United Kingdom, five in France, one in Ireland, one in Italy, and three in Japan. There have been no confirmed cases of either BSE or vCFD in the United States.

No ruminants or ruminant products have been imported into the United States from countries known to have BSE. The World Health Organization has recommended that all countries ban the use of ruminant tissues in ruminant feed. A voluntary ban was instituted in the United States in 1996. A variety of marketed drugs are derived from cattle tissue, and many contain some amount of cow's blood. Gelatin, however, is believed to be safe because it is highly processed.

brain chemicals See ENDORPHINS; NEUROTRANSMITTER.

bran, oat The outer protective coating of the oat kernel. Oat bran is a good source of SILICON, a trace mineral needed for healthy joints and for normal bone growth. Oat bran supplies a water-soluble form of FIBER called beta glucan. Like cellulose, oat fiber is a POLYSACCHARIDE composed of glucose units. Because of the manner in which the glucose units are joined, the carbohydrate chain is not digestible, and because of its "kinks," it is water soluble and viscous. This differs chemically from water-insoluble fiber, like wheat bran, which is the kind of fiber usually found in bran breakfast cereals. Oat bran causes less bloating or diarrhea than is typical with an overdose of wheat bran.

Gel-like fiber often exerts physiologic effects. Soluble fiber reduces the rate of glucose absorption and insulin response after a meal, thus increasing glucose tolerance. Oat bran may help decrease blood FAT and blood CHOLESTEROL, especially the undesirable LOW-DENSITY LIPOPROTEIN (LDL) form, even in diabetics. Elevated LDL is associated with an increased risk of heart disease. Regular consumption of oat bran and oatmeal can lead to a modest reduction in blood cholesterol levels. Even a study purporting to show that oat bran lowers cholesterol by lowering fat intake suggested that a high oat fiber selectively lowered LDL, not HDL (the desirable form of cholesterol). The specific link between oat bran and lowered blood cholesterol has not been resolved. More generally, a diet high in fiber from vegetables, fruits, whole grains, and legumes, together with healthy lifestyle habits, forms a foundation for heart disease prevention.

The ability of oat bran to lower blood cholesterol launched a health food fad that dramatically increased sales of oat and bran cereals. Although the data continues to suggest that including oats in the diet is beneficial, oat bran is only one of a large number of sources of water-soluble fiber. Barley, for example, contains fat-soluble substances called tocotrienols that suppress cholesterol synthesis by the liver. Furthermore, most foods contain both soluble and insoluble forms of fiber. Even oat bran contains 60 percent insoluble fiber. What seems clear is that eating more COMPLEX CARBOHYDRATES such as whole grains and cereal products, beans, vegetables, and fruit, together with daily EXERCISE, can significantly lower blood cholesterol in most adults. (See also OATS.)

bran, wheat The outer coat of kernels of wheat. Although wheat bran contains vitamins, and minerals like CALCIUM and phosphate, most attention has focused on its FIBER content. Wheat bran represents a rich source of water-insoluble fiber that is mainly cellulose. Bleached flour is deficient in bran because bran is lost during milling and is not added back during ENRICHMENT. Wheat bran is typically included in bran BREAKFAST CEREALS. Bran flakes (wheat cereals) contain approximately 40 percent bran.

Insoluble fiber is implicated in maintaining the health of the gastrointestinal tract in several ways. Bran adds bulk and relieves constipation because it absorbs water, making the stool soft. It reduces the transit time (the time taken for the passage of material from the mouth through the gastrointestinal tract). Dietary fiber also normalizes rapid transit time caused by diarrhea due to IRRITABLE BOWEL SYNDROME.

Colon cancer is primarily a disease of developing countries. In searching for an explanation, investigations have shown that, in animals, diets high in fat and low in insoluble fiber are linked to colon cancer. Population studies indicate that countries whose populations are characterized by diets rich in grains and vegetables have lower cancer rates than does the United States. The standard American diet supplies only 30 percent to 50 percent of the soluble and insoluble fiber estimated to reduce the risk of diseases of the colon, including colon cancer. Nonetheless, the connection between colon cancer and fiber is not clear-cut. In some studies, bran offered protection from colon cancer; in others, it had no effect. Researchers propose that fiber can bind bile salts and toxic materials and speed up their passage, with wastes, through the intestine. The toxins would then have less time to damage the colon. Another explanation is that about 50 percent of cellulose is degraded by colon bacteria, producing SHORT-CHAIN FATTY ACIDS, which have anticancer properties.

Individuals who choose to supplement their diet with bran should add it slowly to allow the body to adjust. Suddenly increasing fiber intake can cause bloating, cramping, and diarrhea. Individuals with serious diseases of the digestive tract, such as ulcerative COLITIS, should not supplement with fiber without consulting a specialist. A fiber intake exceeding 35 to 40 g daily may bind essential mineral nutrients like calcium and limit their absorption. One-half cup (18 g) of wheat bran provides 38 calories; protein, 2.9 g; carbohydrate, 11.1 g; fiber, 7.9 g; fat, 0.83 g; calcium, 21 mg; iron, 2.0 mg; zinc, 2.3 mg; thiamin, 0.14 mg; riboflavin, 0.06 mg; niacin, 4.9 mg. (See also BRAN, OAT.)

branched chain amino acids A family of three essential dietary amino acids used as protein building blocks. LEUCINE, ISOLEUCINE, and VALINE are classified as branched chain amino acids because they possess a branched structure. All three are essential amino acids because the body is unable to synthesize these structures. Branched chain amino acids are largely absorbed from the bloodstream and broken down by skeletal muscle in response to insulin. In the first step of their metabolism, amino (nitrogen) groups are removed by transamination, a process dependent upon VITAMIN B_6, leaving the carbon skeletons as keto acids. The keto acids are then oxidized in the mitochondria for energy production. The multienzyme complex that oxidizes the carbon skeletons of all three amino acids is more active with high protein diets. It has been proposed that the branched chain amino acids may enhance skeletal muscle adaptation to exercise training. Blood levels of branched chain amino acids are low in patients suffering from chronic renal failure and encephalopathy, and supplemental amino acids have been used for critically ill patients.

Brazil nut (*Bertholletia excelsa*) The large edible seed of an evergreen tree that grows wild in the Amazonian rain forest of South America. The tree is considered a renewable resource of the rain forest. The hard-walled fruit is 4 to 6 inches in diameter with several inch-long seeds arranged around a center, like the sections of an orange. The shell of the nut is triangular, and the oily, creamy seed within has a rich flavor. Brazil nuts are available roasted in oil or dry roasted. One ounce (28 g, 7 nuts) provides 186 calories; fat, 18.8 g; protein, 4.1 g; carbohydrate, 3.6 g; fiber, 2.52 g; and small amounts of iron, zinc, thiamin, and niacin.

bread A baked food consisting of flour, water, or other liquid as the main ingredients. The many varieties available indicate the ethnic diversity of bread: bagels, baguettes, crumpets, matzo, pumpernickel, sourdough, tortillas, and whole wheat are a few of the varieties sold in the United States.

Unleavened breads like matzo and tortillas were the first breads. The invention of leavened bread is attributed to the ancient Egyptians. As a staple of the standard American diet, leavened bread is prepared with yeast or baking soda to make the dough rise before baking.

Bread is one of the best sources of complex CARBOHYDRATE. The carbohydrate in bread is starch, its main ingredient. Complex carbohydrate digests slowly to the simple sugar GLUCOSE. The slow rise in blood sugar requires a modest output of the hormone insulin to regulate blood sugar levels. The current recommendations specify obtaining 50 percent to 60 percent of daily CALORIES from complex carbohydrates. Contrary to popular opinion, breads are not "fattening" unless the consumer exceeds the daily limit of calories from all sources needed to equal those burned for energy. Bread is much less fattening than high-fat foods such as processed meats, cheese, and fried foods. However, spreading BUTTER, MARGARINE, or mayonnaise on a slice of bread doubles its calories. "Reduced calorie bread" contains half the usual calories, 20 calories a slice; bread may be made with powdered CELLULOSE as a noncaloric filler to lower calories.

Usually a bread is named after the grain from which the flour or meal is derived. An estimated 75 percent of Americans eat white bread and the remainder eat whole WHEAT and RYE. Wheat flour is ideal for leavened bread because wheat contains GLUTEN, a protein that becomes sticky when mixed with water. Dough made from wheat flour is elastic enough to rise, as bubbles of carbon dioxide become trapped, thus creating light-textured bread. In contrast, breads made with only low-gluten flour will tend to be heavy (dense).

The liquid used to prepare the dough affects the bread flavor and quality. Water produces bread with a stiff crust; milk produces a more tender crust and increases the nutritive value of bread. Added sugar helps brown the crust and helps yeast ferment, while fat may be added by bakers to make softer and lighter breads.

Bread is a major contributor of carbohydrate, SODIUM, NIACIN, THIAMIN, and IRON to the American diet, because so much of this enriched food is eaten. The sodium in bread comes from baking soda, the major ingredient of baking powder.

White bread is prepared from bleached flour, which is highly refined (purified). Milling and bleaching removes or partially removes more than 22 important materials such as FIBER, VITAMINS, and MINERALS. To make up for a portion of this depletion, bakeries replace only four: thiamin, niacin, riboflavin, and iron (ENRICHMENT). Other nutrients, such as vitamin B_6 zinc, manganese, and FOLIC ACID, are not added. Because flour is so widely used, producers add iron to increase the daily intake of this mineral, and because white bread contains only half a gram of fiber a slice, bakeries sometimes increase the fiber content by adding dates, raisins, or purified, powdered cellulose. Crystalline cellulose may not function in the body in the same way as the natural cellulose that occurs in the bran of whole wheat bread.

Whole-grain breads provide two to three grams of fiber per slice. Bread labeled "whole wheat" must contain 100 percent whole wheat as the first listed ingredient. Bread simply labeled as "wheat" or "cracked wheat" often contains white flour as the major ingredient; the brown color of such bread may be due to caramel coloring. Bread labeled "multigrain" may simply mean that the bread contains mainly refined wheat flour with small amounts of oatmeal, rye, or whole wheat. The label should indicate whether caramel coloring has been added to give the bread a more wholesome appearance. One slice of whole wheat bread typically provides 70 calories; protein, 3 g; carbohydrates 12.7 g; fiber, 3.17 g; fat, 1.2 g; iron, 0.96 mg; sodium, 180 mg; thiamin, 0.1 mg; riboflavin, 0.06 mg; and niacin, 1.07 mg. One slice of white, enriched bread typically provides 65 calories; protein, 2.1 g; carbohydrate, 12.2 g; fiber, 0.68 g; fat, 1 g; iron, 0.71 mg; sodium, 129 mg; thiamin, 0.12 mg; riboflavin, 0.08 mg; and niacin, 0.94 mg.

breadfruit **(*Artocarpus communis; A. altilis*)** The starchy fruit of a tree belonging to the mulberry family, which originated in southern Asia and Polynesia. Historically, breadfruit was a dietary staple among Asians and Pacific Islanders, and in Tahiti and other islands of the South Pacific breadfruit has a legendary importance. From its early origins in Southeast Asia it spread to Hawaii, and Europeans transported it to the Caribbean in the late 18th century. It is now grown from India to Jamaica. The closely related jackfruit is more widespread because it is hardier.

The egg-shaped fruit has a thick, pebbled skin and can weigh up to five pounds. The starchy flesh has a breadlike texture; its nutrient content is similar to that of wheat bread and it is eaten as a vegetable. The white to yellowish pulp sweetens as it ripens. When green, breadfruit tastes like potato. As it ripens, breadfruit resembles the sweet potato and is used similarly.

Canned or frozen breadfruit is available in markets catering to ethnic cuisines. Breadfruit with seeds can be eaten raw, or the seeds can be roasted like chestnuts. All seedless varieties must be cooked to be palatable. Breadfruit can be cooked like potatoes in recipes. It is boiled or roasted and can be added to stews and cooked as fritters. The ripened fruit can be baked as a pudding. Uncooked breadfruit (100 g) provides 114 calories; protein, 1.1 g; carbohydrate, 27.1 g; fiber, 1.5 g; fat, 0.23 g; thiamin, 0.34 mg; riboflavin, 0.17 mg; niacin, 2.1 mg; vitamin C, 26 mg.

breakfast The first meal of the day usually ends the six- to 10-hour fast due to sleep. During slumber, blood sugar levels are maintained by the liver through the breakdown of glycogen (the storage polymer of glucose) and the synthesis of glucose from amino acids. Breakfast provides energy and replenishes glucose stores.

Meal skipping is an emerging pattern; roughly a quarter of the U.S. population claims to never eat breakfast. Breakfast skipping is most prevalent among 19- to 34-year-olds, while consistent breakfast eaters seem to be older. For those who eat breakfast, often it is a high-calorie meal. Consider a typical American breakfast that provides more than 600 calories, with 40 percent of the calories from fat and more than 500 mg of cholesterol: two fried eggs (200 calories, 8 g fat), two slices of buttered white bread (220 calories, 9 g fat); coffee with 1 tablespoon cream with sugar (46 calories, 3 g fat); two slices of bacon (86 calories, 8 g fat)—rounded out with a glass of orange juice (90 calories). Such a breakfast can be converted to a low-fat meal with simple changes: two poached eggs (164 calories, 5.8 g fat); one cup of decaffeinated coffee with low-fat milk (12 calories); a large orange (58 calories); and two rice cakes (70 calories) or a slice of whole wheat toast without butter (70 calories)—total 304 calories, with 20 percent calories from fat. The cholesterol remains at 476 mg; this could be cut in half by eating a single egg.

The typical continental breakfast is a low-cholesterol meal: a cup of tea (no calories) or a cup of coffee with cream, 46 calories, 3 g fat; two buttered English muffins with honey or preserves, 373 calories, 7.6 g fat. Cholesterol from cream and butter amounts to 72 mg.

breakfast cereal A food prepared from grains, WHEAT, CORN, RICE, and OATS that is served hot or cold at breakfast. The basic ingredients of cold, ready-to-eat breakfast cereals have remained unchanged from the 19th century; only the processing of grain and the packaging has changed. Some brands may add other grains, such as barley, quinoa, or amaranth. Most flour used in breakfast cereals is bleached. Grain is processed by being pressed into feeders, shredded, and formed into biscuits, extruded into a shape that appeals to the consumer, or "pulped."

The label on breakfast cereals supplies nutritional information based on a serving size, usually 1 ounce or only a quarter-cup. When estimating the actual amounts consumed by individuals, it is important to multiply the SODIUM, fat, and sugar content by the number of servings actually eaten. Pouring half a cup of whole milk on a bowl of cereal adds 4 grams of fat and 75 extra calories. Skim milk adds 45 calories and no fat. Each adds 4 grams of protein.

Various additives are also used during processing, including sweeteners (including table sugar or corn syrup), salt, flavorings, preservatives, vitamins, or minerals. Nuts and raisins are other nutritious additions to breakfast cereals. There is no nutritional need to add sugar (sucrose) to cereals, and several varieties do not contain added sugar: puffed rice, puffed wheat, and shredded wheat. These same cereals are the lowest in FIBER. At the other extreme are cereals designed to appeal to children's attraction to sweets. Froot Loops and Apple Jacks (Kellogg); Count Chocula (General Mills); and Fruity Pebbles, Super Golden Crisp (Post) provide about 13 grams (2.5 teaspoons) of sugar per ounce of cereal. Many other cereals contain more than 300 mg of sodium per ounce (more than potato chips). Often cereals with the most sugar contain the least salt.

The fiber in ready-to-eat breakfast cereals is mainly wheat bran, which is essentially insoluble fiber. The body needs both the insoluble and soluble forms of fiber provided by a balanced diet. At the top of the list of high-fiber cereals are All Bran (Kellogg) with extra fiber and Fiber One (General Mills), which provide 12 to 13 g of fiber per ounce. Other bran cereals provide 5 to 6 g of fiber per ounce. Some bran-enriched cereals also contain sugar, however. The amounts of fiber in other typical cereals made with refined flour and without bran are: cold oat cereals, 0.9 per cup; crisp rice, 0.12 g; corn flakes, 0.4 g.

With the growing consumer awareness of the importance of whole grains, GRANOLAS have become popular. These typically contain vegetable oil to make them tastier. Thus a cup of commercially prepared granola can easily provide 600 calories or more. Such granolas often contain saturated fats and coconut and palm oils, although they can still be described as "100 percent natural cereal" on the label.

Hot breakfast cereals prepared from whole grains include oatmeal, creamed wheat, creamed rice, corn grits, and whole wheat cereals. Unless fortified, the levels of calcium, vitamin A, thiamin, riboflavin, and niacin in these cereals are generally less than in fortified, ready-to-eat cereals. On the other hand, hot cereals contain much less sodium, unless it is added during preparation. Only the quick cereals, which are simply added to hot water, contain substantial amounts of salt (240 to 260 mg sodium per packet). The fiber content varies depending upon the grain. Oatmeal or rolled oats provide 9.2 g of fiber per cup in a mixture of soluble and insoluble types of fiber. At the other end of the scale is creamed wheat, which provides much less fiber, 0.37 to 0.64 g per cup. (See also ACRYLAMIDE; BRAN, WHEAT; FOOD LABELING.)

Liebman, Bonnie, and Jayne Hurley. "How to Pick a Cereal," *Nutrition Action Healthletter* 22, no. 5 (June 1995): 11–13.

breast cysts Nodular breast cysts, usually affecting both breasts, are associated with premenstrual breast swelling and tenderness. Fibrocystic breast disease is the most common disorder of the breast and accounts for more than half of breast surgery in the United States. An estimated 20 percent to 40 percent of women under age 50 have breast lumps. Fibrotic cysts are not malignant, but the only way to positively identify a lump is with a biopsy. The cause of this condition is unknown, although apparently an increased ratio of estrogen to progesterone favors fibrocystic disease. The occurrence of cystic breast disease often correlates with premenstrual syndrome (PMS), family history, exposure to estrogens from drugs and birth control pills, early menstruation, late menopause, cigarette smoking, glandular imbalances, and a diet high in SATURATED FAT and calories.

Changing the diet may help prevent breast cysts. A COMPLEX CARBOHYDRATE diet, with reduced consumption of white FLOUR and SUGAR, reduced FAT (especially SATURATED FAT and animal products), and increased consumption of SOY products (ISOFLAVONES) may be advised. Eliminating CAFFEINE-containing beverages and foods (COFFEE, TEA, COLA SOFT DRINKS, CHOCOLATE, and COCOA) has been reported to reduce breast tenderness. Caffeine and related theophylline and theobromine ALKALOIDS stimulate production of fibrous tissue and cyst fluid. Vitamin E may relieve PMS symptoms, perhaps by helping to normalize blood levels of hormones. Thyroid hormone treatment may be helpful. High fiber normalizes bowel function, which may play a role in estrogen metabolism by increasing estrogen excretion. Vitamin B complex deficiency may also be linked to PMS and fibrocystic breast disease. More research is needed to draw firm conclusions regarding the efficacy of vitamins B_6 and E.

Love, Susan M., and Karen Lindsey. *Dr. Susan Love's Breast Book,* 3d edition. New York: Perseus Books Group, 2000.

breast-feeding Feeding an infant with breast milk. In general, health experts recommend breast-feeding for four to six months after an infant's birth, when breast milk can supply all the baby's requirements. The American Academy of Pediatrics recommends breast-feeding at least during the first one to two weeks after birth because the milk that is produced during this time, COLOSTRUM, contains the mother's antibodies, which protect the baby while the immune system develops. Consequently, breast-fed babies have a lower rate of diarrhea and respiratory infections. Colostrum also contains a unique blend of PROTEIN, FAT, and CARBOHYDRATE for the newborn infant. Furthermore, initial breast-feeding may enhance the return of the mother's uterus and body to the nonpregnant state.

Breast-feeding offers many advantages. Bonding between mother and child is strengthened by nursing, and studies indicate that this promotes the child's healthy development. Breast-feeding can help the infant's digestive system mature faster and take up nutrients more efficiently. Breast milk helps feed the infant's digestive tract with friendly bacteria to minimize intestinal infections. Breast-feeding and postponing the introduction of solid foods may decrease the risk of food allergies.

Breast-feeding affords advantages beyond infancy, including a decreased risk of childhood cancer, Crohn's disease, ear infections, and respiratory infections. ALCOHOL, nicotine, CAFFEINE, marijuana, and certain medications pass into breast milk and may affect a baby's development. Therefore, medications not approved by a physician should be avoided while nursing. Drinking more than a quart of cow's milk a day can introduce cow protein into the mother's own milk, causing an allergy. In some babies colic is caused by cow's milk proteins that pass through the mother's milk.

Breast-feeding also has advantages for the mother. Studies have shown that the longer a woman breast-feeds her children, the lower her risk for developing breast cancer. Studies suggest that a woman's breast cancer risk decreases by about 4.3 percent for every year she breast-feeds.

Milk production is a major metabolic burden to the mother. The nursing mother needs considerably more calories to produce milk composed of energy-rich nutrients, protein, fat, and carbohydrate than nonlactating women. Together, these nutrients represent an energy content of 670 to 770 calories per liter of human milk. Assuming a maternal efficiency conversion factor of 80 percent, and a daily milk production of 750 ml (0.75 l), approximately 600 extra calories per day are required by the lactating woman.

The mother's physiology changes during breast-feeding so she can use her fat stores gained during pregnancy to help provide the extra calories needed for lactation. Consequently an average of 500 calories per day is recommended during lactation for women whose gestational weight gain was normal. This metabolic shift may explain the typical problem of weight gain after pregnancy.

Certain nutrient needs increase from their pregnancy levels. The nursing mother needs more protein (65 vs. 60 mg daily); more vitamin A (1,300 vs. 800 mcg); vitamin E (12 mg vs. 10 mg); more vitamin C (95 mg vs. 70 mg); and other vitamins and minerals. From the B COMPLEX, the nursing mother needs thiamin, 1.6 mg; riboflavin, 0.8 mg; niacin, 20 mg; vitamin B_6, 21 mg; folacin, 280 mg; and vitamin B_{12}, 2.6 mcg. Also needed are vitamin C (95 mg) and the MINERALS calcium, 1,200 mg; phosphorous, 1,200 mg; magnesium, 355 mg; zinc, 19 mg; iodine, 200 mcg; and selenium, 75 mcg; and vitamin D, 10 mcg; and vitamin K, 65 mg. The diet should include MEAT, FISH, and POULTRY, dried beans and peas for protein, fat, and minerals; fruits and vegetables for fiber and vitamins A and C; complex carbohydrates like pasta, brown rice, and whole wheat bread for energy and trace minerals. Requirements for calcium may be too great to be met without supplements.

In spite of the clear benefits of breast-feeding and the recommendation of health experts, breast-feeding declined in the 1980s in the United States. Among African-American women the rate fell from 33 percent to 23 percent during that time. Rather than a reflection of a larger percentage of women in the workforce, public health officials propose that other factors are involved: Hospitals do not provide enough support for breast-feeding, and free formula is provided to low-income mothers under the Woman, Infants, and Children Program. However, extra food coupons are also issued to women who are breast-feeding, and consultants are available to breast-feeding clients. The choice to breast-feed involves different behavior and possibly changes in attitudes that can simplify the process. Resources are available for the expectant mother, including the La Leche League International, and she can enlist the support of her family and medical staff. Many health-care professionals do not know the basics of breast-feeding management. Limited evidence seems to indicate that breast-feeding is declining in low-income countries worldwide. For example, weaning seems to occur earlier in Latin America. In some countries, Jordan and Kenya among them, the levels of breast-feeding may be low enough to affect child health and mortality.

Regarding introduction of cow's milk, experts recommend that infants receive either breast milk or INFANT FORMULA for the first 12 months. When the baby is 12 months or older, whole milk may be used to substitute formula or breast milk, although optimally cow's milk could be withheld until the infant is two years old. The high casein content of cow's milk can increase gastrointestinal bleeding and lead to ANEMIA if introduced too soon.

Sears, Martha, and William Sears. *The Breastfeeding Book.* New York: Little, Brown, 2000.

breast milk Breast milk is optimally balanced to nurture the infant during the first months. It is rich in sugar lactose and has substantial fat (3.8 percent) for efficient energy production. Human MILK contains both essential fatty acids (linoleic and linolenic), easily digested protein, and a high level of free amino acids and other nonprotein nitrogen (25 percent of the total nitrogen). Special products like CARNITINE and TAURINE, believed to be important in infant metabolism, are present. The cholesterol content is relatively high, reflecting its importance in early development. Breast milk is relatively low in sodium and minerals, in accord with the limited capacity of the infant's immature kidneys to handle dissolved substances. The iron content, although low, is highly absorbable. Zinc, too, is better absorbed from breast milk. The calcium-to-phosphorus ratio is ideal for calcium absorption. The vitamin content (including vitamin C) to support infant growth is ample. Vitamin D content is low, although adequate for a normal-term infant.

The importance of omega-3 fatty acids in infant nutrition is suggested by the high level of the polyunsaturated fatty acid, DOCASOHEXAENOIC ACID (DHA), required in brain growth and development of the retina. DHA cannot be formed by preterm infants because their livers are not mature enough to synthesize it from essential fatty acids. Breast milk contains a complex mixture of hormones and growth factors, whose role in infant development is poorly understood. Thus milk contains unusually high levels of gonadotropin-releasing hormone, which could affect development of the newborn's sex organs. It also contains the hormone melatonin, possibly regulating the infant's internal clock; oxytocin, which could promote bonding between infant and mother; and thyroid hormones, which could stimulate the infant's immune system. Breast milk provides endorphins, which act as pain-killers and growth factors—nerve growth factor, epidermal growth factor, and insulin-like growth factor—that regulate development of the brain and digestive organs.

Pollutants in Breast Milk

Breast milk often contains traces of environmental pollutants, including pesticides and herbicides; industrial chemicals such as halogenated hydrocarbons (PBBs, PCBs, dioxin, cleaning solvents); and toxic heavy metals (cadmium, lead, mercury). These pollutants are insidious: They are odorless and colorless, they are not biodegradable, and they accumulate in animals and fish and in the people who eat them. Many pollutants slowly leave the body when there is no further exposure, while the body may accumulate halogenated hydrocarbons and toxic heavy metals (mercury and cadmium) throughout life.

The fetus and infant are very sensitive to halogenated hydrocarbons and toxic heavy metals. Significant exposure to these industrial chemicals increases the risk of cancer, abnormalities, and learning disabilities in children. The effects of chronic exposure to trace levels of these materials and whether there are any additive effects due to exposure to mixtures of pollutants, are not known. The UN's World Health Organization, the EPA and the La Leche League International argue that the advantages of breast-feeding outweigh any potential disadvantages. Concerned mothers can have their milk tested at their local health department.

Pregnant and nursing women may be advised to minimize exposure to toxic pollutants by avoiding certain ocean fish (shark, ocean perch, halibut, striped bass, bluefish, and swordfish) that are most likely to be contaminated. Among freshwater fish, catfish, brook and lake trout, freshwater perch and bass, walleye pike, and whitefish caught in polluted waters are likely to be contaminated. Washing vegetables thoroughly and consuming homegrown produce or certified organic produce reduce exposure to pesticides. (See also ACIDOPHILUS; BIFIDUS FACTOR; INFANT FORMULA.)

Angier, Natalie. "Mother's Milk Found to be Potent Cocktail of Hormones," *New York Times*, May 24, 1994.

brewer's yeast **(*Saccharomyces cerivisiae*)** A single-celled organism related to molds and fungi that ferments sugars to ethanol (ALCOHOL) under anaerobic conditions. Brewer's yeast is a by-product of BEER and ale production. It is used as a nutritional yeast when grown in the presence of VITAMIN B_{12} and other nutrients. This yeast is an excellent source of PROTEIN, B COMPLEX, IRON, and other nutrients, including organically complexed chromium in the form of GLUCOSE TOLERANCE FACTOR. Unlike BAKER'S YEAST, which is not a rich source of vitamins and minerals, nutritional yeast does not contain living cells. Yeast products are not recommended for those with yeast infections. One tablespoon of dry brewer's yeast provides 25 calories; protein, 3.1 g; carbohydrate, 3.1 g; calcium 6 to 60 mg; iron, 1.4 mg; zinc, 0.63 mg; thiamin, 1.25 mg; riboflavin, 0.34 mg; and niacin, 3.16 mg.

brine A concentrated solution of table salt (sodium chloride) used to preserve vegetables, FISH, and MEAT. A pickling brine can be prepared by dissolving 50 g table salt in 500 ml (1 pint) of water. Vegetables such as cauliflower and cucumber soaked overnight are usually stored in pickling spices and vinegar. (See also SODIUM.)

broad bean **(*Vicia faba;* fava bean, horse bean)** A large, flat bean resembling a lima bean that is cultivated as a staple food, as well as animal fodder, worldwide. Its origins can be traced to Africa, where broad beans were cultivated by ancient Egyptians perhaps 4,000 years ago. Ancient Greeks recommended broad beans for improved athletic performance. Broad beans are a part of traditional Mediterranean cuisine and are a very popular food in the Middle East.

Broad beans occur in flat pods that can be very large, up to 18 inches long. Fresh, shelled beans should be thoroughly cooked, and the outer layer or skin is often removed. Varieties of broad beans may be green, brown, or white after cooking. Young pods are cooked like green beans. Dried beans are usually soaked overnight and then cooked, with or without the skin. Broad beans are to be avoided by individuals who have an inherited sensitivity called FAVISM. This hemolytic syndrome (breaking down red blood cells) occurs in people of the Mediterranean regions (Sardinia, southern Italy, Greece, Turkey, Cyprus, and Egypt), in Iran and in China. In severe cases, ingestion of fresh broad beans can cause hemolytic anemia, an anemia caused by the rupture of fragile red blood cells. The toxic factors are apparently small, nonprotein compounds, vicine and convicine. The dried flat beans are rich in protein, fiber, B vitamins, and trace minerals. Uncooked broad beans contain (100 g): 76 calories; protein, 3.2 g; carbohydrate, 14.7 g; fiber, 1.7 g; fat, 0.5 g; calcium, 26 mg; vitamin A, 13.5 retinol equivalents; thiamin, 0.34 mg; riboflavin, 0.17 mg; niacin, 2.1 mg.

broccoli **(*Brassica aleracea*)** A dark-green vegetable with small, tight heads (curds) mounted on stemlike buds. A member of the cabbage (*Brassica*) family of CRUCIFEROUS VEGETABLES, closely related to CAULIFLOWER and BRUSSELS SPROUTS. Broccoli is one of the most popular vegetables of this group. Both stems and heads are edible. Broccoli originated in Italy, where the name is derived from the Italian word *broccolo,* meaning a cabbage sprout, and was first cultivated in the 17th or 18th century.

Broccoli and other cruciferous vegetables produce nitrogen-containing materials called indoles and ISOTHIOCYANATES that may reduce the risk of some forms of CANCER. Indoles seem to stimulate LIVER enzymes that modify the female hormone ESTROGEN, making it less active and possibly reducing the risk of breast cancer. Researchers recently discovered that sulforaphane killed *HELICOBACTER PYLORI,* a bacteria that causes stomach ulcers and stomach cancer, in mice. Scientists hope to duplicated these results in human studies. Broccoli and other cruciferous vegetables also contain sulfur compounds that stimulate the liver to produce detoxifying enzymes that help block the action of cancer-causing agents. Of particular interest is SULFORAPHANE, which specifically increases the level of so-called phase 2 detoxication enzymes, which attach highly water-soluble chemicals such as glutathione, taurine, glycine, and sugar derivatives to altered toxins so they can be more readily excreted. Broccoli is also an excellent source of FIBER, vitamin A precursor (BETA-CAROTENE), and vitamin C, and it contains ample amounts of folic acid, niacin, iron, and calcium. The most common kind in the United States is called Italian green broccoli. One cup chopped and cooked (156 g) provides 46 calories; protein, 4.6 g; carbohydrate, 8.7 g; fiber, 6.4 g; calcium, 178 mg; iron, 1.8 mg; vitamin A, 220 retinol equivalents; thiamin, 0.13 mg; riboflavin, 0.32 mg; niacin, 1.18 mg; and vitamin C, 98 mg.

bromelain A protein-digesting enzyme from pineapple. This enzyme occurs in the stems and fruit. Commercial sources come from Taiwan, Japan, and Hawaii. Because fresh pineapple contains this enzyme, neither fresh pineapple nor pineapple juice can be used in gelatin-containing desserts and salads; the gelatin would be broken down.

Bromelain is used as a MEAT TENDERIZER and as a digestive aid when taken with meals. Bromelain is an effective substitute for pancreatic enzymes when their production is inadequate. It may be more effective when combined with pancreatin, a preparation of digestive enzymes from hog pancreas, and bile. Bromelain can inhibit blood platelet aggregation and improve angina pain and several, inflammatory conditions. Orally administered bromelain seems to reduce swelling, bruising, pain, and healing time due to injuries. Bromelain inhibits platelet aggregation and increases fibromolytic activity ("clot busting" effect); consequently, it has been used to treat thrombophlebitis, a potentially dangerous condition due to blood clotting. In addition, it has been used to treat respiratory congestion and rheumatoid ARTHRITIS. Bromelain could possibly increase the risk of bleeding in patients taking blood thinning drugs and aspirin. (See also DIGESTION; DIGESTIVE ENZYMES.)

brominated vegetable oil (BVO) A FOOD ADDITIVE used by soft drink manufacturers to disperse flavoring oils in fruit-flavored beverages and to render them cloudy to create an illusion of thickness. Vegetable oils, including COTTON-SEED OIL, CORN OIL, and OLIVE OIL, can be chemically modified by bromine.

Long assumed to be safe, BVO was used extensively in North America until a Canadian report demonstrated that BVO has caused organ damage in experimental animals. BVO residues accumulate in human tissues, but the long-term effects are unknown. BVO is no longer classified as a GENERALLY RECOGNIZED AS SAFE food additive by the U.S. FDA, which had granted interim approval in 1970.

bronchi The two main branches of the trachea that form the major air passageways of the lung. Each bronchus joins to bronchial tubes, smaller branches further into the lung. Each bronchial tube in turn branches into bronchioles, even smaller subdivisions of the air passageway, where gas exchanges occur. Oxygen required by the body is absorbed, while the waste product of oxidation, carbon dioxide, diffuses from red blood cells into expired air.

Foreign objects such as seeds, nuts, or bran can lodge in the bronchi and cause diseases such as bronchitis or lung abscesses. ANAPHYLAXIS, shock due to a severe allergy attack affecting the entire body, can lead to labored breathing with spasming and contraction of smooth muscle surrounding the bronchioles. (See also ALLERGY.)

brown rice Unpolished rice after the husk has been removed. Brown rice retains bran and GERM, which provide most of the nutrients, as well as FIBER. Much of the fiber is cellulose and is found chiefly in the outer bran layer. Starch occurs in the internal portion (endosperm) of the GRAIN, which has much less fiber. The higher cellulose content is the major reason brown rice needs to be cooked about twice as long as white rice. Brown rice retains lectins, a class of protein that bind to cell surfaces. This protein may be the cause of allergic reactions to brown rice. Brown rice has a delicate, nutlike flavor. The cooking time is approximately 45 minutes. One cup cooked (195 g) provides 233 calories; carbohydrate, 49.7 g; protein, 4.9 g; fiber, 3.9 g; calcium, 23 mg; iron, 1.17 mg; niacin, 2.73 mg; thiamin, 0.18 mg; riboflavin, 0.04 mg.

brown sugar Table sugar colored with a little molasses or caramelized sugar. Classified as a refined CARBOHYDRATE, brown sugar supplies EMPTY CALORIES, like other purified sweeteners. Brown sugar is nutritionally equivalent to table sugar. The nutrient content of one tablespoon is 52 calories; carbohydrate, 15.6 g; calcium, 12 mg; potassium, 48 mg; and only traces of other minerals.

brussels sprouts (*Brassica oleracea*) A vegetable of the cabbage family (CRUCIFEROUS VEGETABLES), characterized by a stem with rows of small heads resembling miniature cabbages. Brussels sprouts are one of the seven vegetables developed from the wild cabbage native to northwestern Europe. The cruciferous vegetables in general possess cancer-inhibiting properties, as shown by experiments with animals and by population studies. This seems to be due to their content of materials that block cancer-causing agents; FIBER, VITAMIN C, and BETA-CAROTENE. In addition indoles, nitrogen-containing compounds occurring in cruciferous vegetables, seem to block the action of estrogen and reduce the risk of breast cancer, while ISOTHIOCYANATES, sulfur-containing compounds, stimulate liver enzymes that block the action of carcinogens. One cup (cooked, 156 g) contains 60 calories; protein, 6 g; carbohydrate, 13.5 g; fiber, 5.62 g; fat, 0.8 g; iron, 1.88 mg; beta-carotene, 112 retinol equivalents;

niacin, 0.95 mg; thiamin, 0.17 mg; riboflavin, 0.12 mg; vitamin C, 97 mg.

buckwheat A seed with a nutlike flavor used like a cereal grain. Buckwheat is not a true grain, nor is it related to wheat, which belongs to the grass family. Buckwheat is native to Siberia and Manchuria and was grown extensively in China for thousands of years. Three common varieties are Silverhead, Tartary, and Japanese. Regions of the former Soviet Union are major producers; other important producers include Poland, France, Canada, and the United States, where production has steadily declined.

Buckwheat can be a suitable wheat substitute for those sensitive to wheat protein (GLUTEN). However, for patients with CELIAC DISEASE (severe gluten sensitivity) buckwheat may be excluded from the diet, in addition to the cereal grains. Buckwheat has a high level of fiber and protein, though not of the quality of AMARANTH or QUINOA. Buckwheat flour has a distinctive flavor that can add variety to grain dishes. In the United States, buckwheat flour is often used in griddle cakes (pancakes). Buckwheat groats (kernels from which the hull has been removed) are roasted and served like rice in a traditional dish called kasha in the Soviet Union and Poland. Food value of 1 cup (175 g) has: calories, 586; protein, 20.5 g; carbohydrate, 128 g; fiber, 15.6 g; fat, 4.2 g; calcium, 200 mg; iron, 6.7 mg; zinc, 4.4 mg; thiamin, 1.1 mg; niacin, 7.7 mg; riboflavin, 0.26 mg.

buffer A substance that resists changes in the pH of a solution. A buffer system protects a solution against large fluctuations in hydrogen ion concentration by compensating for increased acidity (additional hydrogen ions that would normally lower the pH), as well as for increased alkalinity (due to bases that would raise the pH).

The constancy of the pH of body fluids is critically important for the normal functioning of enzymes. Small changes in hydrogen ion concentration (pH) can change the overall electrical charge on enzymes, alter their shape and thus usually inhibit their catalytic function. Other processes, such as the transmission of nerve impulses and ion transport across membranes into cells, are also exquisitely sensitive to changes in pH.

The major buffers in the blood are serum proteins, HEMOGLOBIN, BICARBONATE, and phosphate. They maintain the pH of blood and body fluids near neutrality (pH 7.4) and thus help regulate acid-base balance. The bicarbonate buffer system is constantly resupplied by the body from carbon dioxide produced by metabolism. Nonetheless, these buffers have limitations, and they can be overwhelmed by the excessive production of acid (ACIDOSIS) that accompanies STARVATION and uncontrolled diabetes or by excessively alkaline blood (ALKALOSIS) that accompanies hyperventilation (panting), for example. Persistent acidosis, alkalosis, and imbalanced electrolytes can pose long-term health hazards and require medical attention.

bulgur See WHEAT.

bulimia nervosa An EATING DISORDER characterized by repeated binge eating, usually in secret and often followed by purging. The number of cases of bulimia in the United States has increased dramatically since 1970. About 5 million Americans, and perhaps as many as 5 percent of adolescent women, binge and purge to some extent. Bulimics typically engage in repeated episodes of binge eating followed by self-induced vomiting, fasting, the use of LAXATIVES or DIURETICS and/or EXERCISE to lose weight. The use of laxatives or diuretics to lose weight is potentially life-threatening because these methods cause losses of ELECTROLYTES (SODIUM, POTASSIUM, CHLORIDE) and water that may severely affect brain and heart functions. A bingeing individual can consume the equivalent of three normal meals in an hour. The symptoms of bulimia include: bingeing and purging for months or years; a fear of not being able to stop eating; eroded tooth enamel and cavities from vomited STOMACH ACID; DEHYDRATION; antisocial behavior (such as eating alone); an obsession with food-related activities (like supermarket shopping or cooking); erratic eating; suppression of emotional vulnerability; chronic heartburn (from esophageal reflux); abdominal distension and gas; indigestion; undernutrition; and lower levels of body FAT.

There are about four times as many bulimics as there are anorexics. As in ANOREXIA NERVOSA, typical bulimic patients are young women obsessed with the fear of obesity. They fear being unloved, being judged in terms of their appearance and degree of success. Food, eating, and weight control become obsessions, dwarfing other areas of their personal lives. Bulimics often have low self-esteem.

Evidence suggests a biochemical component in some instances of this disorder. Bulimics often do not reach satiation after eating, and some bulimic women seem to make less of CHOLECYSTOKININ, a hormone that promotes a sense of satiation. Eating may also increase the level of DOPAMINE, a neurotransmitter in a region of the brain (nucleus accumbens) that triggers pleasure and satiation. High levels of the hormone vasopressin (ANTIDIURETIC HORMONE) are found in women with bulimia. This hormone is normally released in response to STRESS.

Bulimia can be controlled. Physical assessment and a return to a balanced diet are important in increasing a person's sense of well-being. As with any compulsive behavior, a person with an eating disorder needs supportive therapy from professional counselors in dealing with social, psychological, familial, nutritional, and physiologic factors. A nutritional program should include well-planned meals that are nutritionally balanced. Nutritional deficiencies may be remedied by supplementation as needed. In this regard, subclinical ZINC deficiencies have been associated with eating disorders. The program specifies ongoing nutritional counseling to help the patient control behaviors that could trigger binge-purge behaviors. The American Anorexia/Bulimia Association and the National Association of Anorexia Nervosa and Associated Disorders provide resources. (See also COMPULSIVE EATING.)

Fairburn, Christopher. *Overcoming Binge Eating.* New York: Guilford Press, 1995.

bulking agents See FIBER.

butter A saturated animal FAT (butterfat) obtained from MILK and cream. Butter is the fat from pasteurized cream and milk that has been solidified by churning. Butter contains 81 percent fat, 16 percent to 18 percent water, and other ingredients such as casein, lactose, and salt. The salt content varies with the brand. The yellow color of butter is due to BETA-CAROTENE, which comes from the plants eaten by the cow. In winter, fodder is more likely to be grain, which lacks beta-carotene, and butter is white; the yellow coloring agents, such as beta-carotene and ANNATTO seed extract, are added to maintain a yellow color year-round.

Butter is graded by the U.S. Department of Agriculture (USDA) according to its flavor, butterfat content, purity, and keeping quality, among other characteristics. U.S. Grade AA is a score of 93 and represents 80 percent or more butterfat.

Average annual consumption is about four pounds for each American, about a third as much as margarine, and is used in sauteing, frying, and baking. Like all oils, butter should be refrigerated to prevent rancidity (oxidation and decomposition). Sweet butter or unsalted butter are available for those on a salt-restricted diet. Whipped butter contains air as a filler, yielding only two-thirds of the CALORIES of regular butter. Spreadable butter was developed by the dairy industry as an alternative to margarine. Like regular butter, this product is made from cream and milk and with beta-carotene for coloring. However, it contains additional finely dispersed water. Because it has more water, spreadable butter has less fat, fewer calories, and less cholesterol than butter or regular margarine. Typically the content of one tablespoon (14 g) of regular butter is 101 calories; protein, 0.12 g; carbohydrate, 0.08 g; fat, 11.5 g; cholesterol, 31 mg; vitamin A, 825 retinol equivalents; sodium, 933 mg.

butter, clarified (ghee) A butter from which milk solids have been removed. Clarified butter is prepared by melting butter briefly to coagulate milk solids; the butter that floats to the top is clarified.

Clarified butter is a basic ingredient of Indian cooking; the term *ghee* or *ghi* is Hindustani for "clear butter." It is stable for extended periods at room temperature and in hot climates without refrigeration. Although some claim that ghee is more nutritious than butter, clinical studies to back this claim are lacking. Clarified butter is used when cooking at higher temperatures because it is less likely to burn or scorch than whole butter. On the other hand, clarified butter lacks much of the buttery flavor of casein, the protein component. One tablespoon contains 100 calories. Like butter, the fat is classified as saturated.

butterfat The FAT in cow's MILK and cream, which is classified as a SATURATED FAT because it contains 65 percent saturated FATTY ACIDS. It finds several uses in the food industry. Anhydrous butterfat, from which most of the water has been removed, is used commercially to reconstitute liquid dairy products and to prepare SHORTENING for special cooking purposes.

Fractional crystallization of butterfat can produce both a higher melting fraction and a lower melting fraction. The higher melting fraction is used to prepare ICE CREAM and CHOCOLATE, while the lower melting fraction is combined with whole butter to increase its spreadability.

butter-flavored granules Several products (sprinkles or granules) are available that supply a butter flavor to foods with even fewer calories than diet margarine. These products can be used with moist foods such as vegetables and cooked cereals, rather than dry foods. They cannot be used in sauteing because the granules break down when heated, and they contain very little oil. Typical ingredients include salt, partially hydrogenated vegetable oil, and butter flavor with annatto and turmeric as coloring agents. One half-teaspoon provides four calories.

buttermilk Originally, this was the sour liquid remaining after cream had been separated after churning. Modern preparation of buttermilk usually employs pasteurized skim milk to which lactic acid-producing bacteria are added to develop the characteristic flavor through fermentation. Lactic acid formed by fermentation precipitates milk protein, so buttermilk has a thicker consistency than regular milk. Cream or butter is added in commercial products. Buttermilk is often used in recipes in place of sour milk for BISCUITS, rolls, waffles, and the like, as well as in frozen desserts. One cup (245 g) provides 99 calories; protein, 8.1 g; carbohydrates 11.7 g; and butterfat, 2.16 g.

butylated hydroxyanisole See BHA.

butylated hydroxytoluene See BHT.

butyric acid (butyrate) An acid produced by the bacterial degradation of FIBER in the colon. Gut bacteria ferment undigested carbohydrate into a family of small saturated fatty acids, acetic acid, and propionic acid, in addition to butyric acid.

A small amount of butyric acid is present in the diet. Butyric acid occurs in MILK, and BUTTER contains 3.3 percent butyric acid. Butyric acid and other short-chain fatty acids are taken up by the intestine to be used for energy. It is estimated that the breakdown of short-chain fatty acids produced by colonic bacteria can satisfy 5 percent to 10 percent of the body's total energy requirements.

Butyric acid is an important energy source for the cells lining the COLON, where it seems to assist their normal development and maintenance. Butyric acid seems to reduce chronic inflammatory conditions of the colon, and high fecal levels correlate with decreased risk of colon cancer.

C

cabbage (*Brassica oleracea capitala*) A widely cultivated CRUCIFEROUS VEGETABLE with a compact head and overlapping leaves, related to BROCCOLI and BRUSSELS SPROUTS. There are hundreds of varieties of cabbage that differ in shape, color, and leaf texture, in either loose or firm heads. Colors range from white and green to purple. In the United States, the most popular varieties are green, red, Savoy, bok choy, and Napa.

Cabbage was originally cultivated 2,500 years ago in western Europe, where wild cabbage still grows. It was first used as a medicinal herb. Sauerkraut, or pickled cabbage, has been in use at least since 200 B.C. in China, when it was a staple of the diet for laborers building the Great Wall.

Cabbage and related vegetables contain compounds with potential anti-CANCER effects in experimental animals, such as ascorbic acid (VITAMIN C), an ANTIOXIDANT. A family of nitrogen-containing compounds called indoles may act as antioxidants; they also seem to speed the rate at which ESTROGEN, a female hormone, is inactivated. (Estrogen can stimulate the growth of breast cancer.) Cabbage also contains certain sulfur compounds called thiourea and thiocyanates, which may impede the assimilation of IODINE and THYROID hormone formation when consumed in excessive amounts. Raw cabbage juice has been used to heal ulcers.

Raw cabbage is used in coleslaw or cabbage salad. When prepared with mayonnaise, it can become high-fat fare. Cabbage can be cooked in many ways—baked, sauteed, stewed, and steamed—and the leaves can be stuffed with meat or grains and tomatoes. To preserve its vitamin and mineral content, cabbage should never be overcooked. To avoid the disagreeable odor sometimes associated with cooked cabbage, cabbage should be young and fresh and cooked rapidly. ALUMINUM cookware should be avoided as it promotes the release of pungent compounds; older cabbage and stored cabbage acquire stronger flavors. Raw cabbage (shredded, 1 cup, 70 g) provides 16 calories; protein, 0.8 g; carbohydrate, 3.9 g; fiber, 1.6 g; iron, 0.4 mg; thiamin, 0.04 mg; riboflavin, 0.02 mg; niacin, 0.21 mg; and vitamin C, 33 mg. (See also FOOD TOXINS; GOITROGENS.)

cacao (*Theobroma cacao*) An evergreen tree cultivated in tropical America that produces cacao beans, the source of COCOA and CHOCOLATE. Each pod contains 25 to 40 beans, which vary in shape and color, depending on the variety. Cocoa production begins when the harvested beans are stored in mounds to permit bacterial fermentation. This destroys the fruity pulp and germ and develops the characteristic color, aroma and flavor of the cacao bean. The beans are then washed, dried, and roasted. The raw material for cocoa products and chocolate is cocoa paste, prepared by grinding the fermented beans.

cachexia Severe wasting characterized by the progressive loss of body fat and lean body mass (skeletal muscle). Profound weakness, loss of appetite, and anemia accompany this wasting syndrome. Its causes are unknown. A fever-induced, increased rate of metabolism may account for some of the weakness. Internal bleeding from intestinal defects may account for anemia, and reduced food intake is associated with anorexia and a change in the sense of taste. (See also CATABOLIC STATE; CATABOLISM.)

cactus See PRICKLY PEAR CACTUS.

cadmium A toxic, HEAVY METAL pollutant. Cigarette smoke provides low levels of exposure. Drinking WATER can be contaminated when water leaches cadmium from galvanized or black polyethylene water pipes. Cadmium contaminates the food supply, a reflection of widespread low-level distribution from PESTICIDES, industrial waste, and tires, in addition to smoke from incinerator plants and coal-fired plants. Oysters contain unusually high levels of cadmium; three to four parts per million have been recorded. It is a natural contaminant of phosphate fertilizers and is easily taken up by plants. Livestock grazing on these plants become contaminated with cadmium, and humans eating BEEF accumulate cadmium because it is not readily excreted in urine or feces. This is a concern because trace amounts of cadmium cause HYPERTENSION, heart abnormalities, and toxic effects on reproductive organs in experimental animals. Severe symptoms (bronchitis, emphysema) develop in people exposed to cadmium at levels only 10 times more than the average daily exposure. Cadmium exposure may also increase bone loss in postmenopausal women, thus increasing the risk of OSTEOPOROSIS. The mechanism of cadmium toxicity is not understood, though it can block the use of the trace mineral nutrient, ZINC. (See also LEAD; MERCURY.)

caffeine A bitter ALKALOID (methylxanthine) occurring in more than 60 plants, including tea leaves, COFFEE beans, cocoa beans, and kola nuts. Up to 90 percent of the adults in North America consume caffeine regularly, provided mostly by coffee. Caffeine is the most widely consumed compound in the world that affects the nervous system.

Caffeine is water soluble and is rapidly absorbed by the body. During pregnancy, it enters the placenta and can affect placental function. Caffeine even enters breast milk. Caffeine stimulates the ADRENAL GLANDS to produce EPINEPHRINE (adrenaline), which normally gears up the body for action in response to a threatening situation (FIGHT OR FLIGHT RESPONSE) by increasing the heart rate, stimulating the nervous system, increasing STOMACH ACID production, raising BLOOD SUGAR, and increasing fat breakdown.

A cup of brewed coffee contains 80 to 115 mg of caffeine, while a cup of DECAFFEINATED COFFEE contains 2 to 3 mg. A cup of brewed tea contains 40 to 60 mg of caffeine. Per ounce, CHOCOLATE contains about 20 mg caffeine. In addition, cola beverages and some medications and over-the-counter drugs contain caffeine. Soft drinks can provide 30 to 72 mg caffeine per 12 oz serving.

Caffeine is classified as a GENERALLY RECOGNIZED AS SAFE food additive by the U.S. FDA, and moderate consumption of caffeine-containing foods does not seem to be harmful for the average adult. Most healthy individuals can tolerate 200 to 300 mg a day of caffeine as a mild stimulant. Side effects of excessive caffeine (800 mg or more) include anxiety, sleeplessness, agitation, shortness of breath, irregular heartbeat, nausea, HEARTBURN, and headaches. Caffeine usage is linked to most, though not all, attributes of ADDICTION (chemical dependency), including craving and withdrawal symptoms during abstinence. Withdrawal symptoms include irritability, vomiting, and headaches. To break a caffeine dependency, patients should reduce consumption gradually over four or five weeks.

Caffeine consumption may be linked to symptoms resembling PREMENSTRUAL SYNDROME. Caffeine can intensify symptoms of HYPOGLYCEMIA. It may interact with medications (ANTIDEPRESSANTS, tranquilizers, and antipsychotic drugs); aggravate arrhythmia (irregular heartbeat); and increase the risk of osteoporosis.

Studies of the effects of caffeine on miscarriage rates have had mixed results. One recent study showed that the risk increased only slightly in women who consumed as many as three cups of coffee a day, but another study showed that women who consumed between one and three cups of coffee daily increased their risk of spontaneous abortion by 30 percent. These researchers also noted that the more caffeine consumed, the higher the risk of miscarriage. Excessive caffeine consumption has caused birth defects in experimental animals.

On the other hand, a normal daily intake of caffeine in coffee does not seem to increase the risk of fibrocystic disease, or HYPERTENSION, as earlier believed. Recent studies show that consumption of coffee and caffeine does not contribute to CARDIOVASCULAR DISEASE, including STROKE, even in people who drink more than four cups of coffee a day. Researchers also have found no link between caffeine consumption and cancers of the bladder, breast, colon, lung, or prostate. At least nine studies have confirmed that regular coffee consumption over long periods of time may reduce the risk of developing Parkinson's disease. (See also ENDOCRINE SYSTEM; STRESS.)

Ross G. Webster et al. "Association of Coffee and Caffeine Intake With the Risk of Parkinson's Disease," *JAMA* 283, 20 (May 2000): 2,674'2–679.

Willet, Walter C. et al. "Coffee Consumption and Coronary Heart Disease in Women: A Ten-Year Follow-up," *JAMA* 275 (1996): 458–462.

calciferol (vitamin D_2, ergocalciferol, activated ergosterol) A synthetic form of VITAMIN D derived from a cyclic lipid from a yeast and mold, ERGOSTEROL, used to fortify MILK. Exposure to ultraviolet light converts ergosterol to calciferol. One cup of milk routinely contains 100 IUs of vitamin D as calciferol, which contributes most of the vitamin D ingested by children. Infant formulas are fortified with the same amount. Fortified prepared BREAKFAST CEREALS generally contain 40 IU of vitamin D per cup. (See also CALCIUM; ENRICHMENT.)

calcitriol See VITAMIN D.

calcium An essential mineral nutrient and the most abundant mineral in the body. Calcium represents approximately 2 percent of the total body weight; about 98 percent of this is found in the bones and teeth. The small amount of calcium in body fluids and cells plays an important role in nerve transmission, muscle contraction, heart rhythm, hormone production, wound healing, immunity, blood coagulation, maintaining normal blood pressure, and STOMACH ACID production. Calcium promotes blood clotting through the activation of the fibrous protein FIBRIN, the building block of clots. It lowers blood pressure in patients with spontaneous HYPERTENSION (not caused by KIDNEY disease) because it relaxes blood vessels, and it may also diminish the symptoms of PREMENSTRUAL SYNDROME (PMS).

High intake of saturated fat tends to raise LOW-DENSITY LIPOPROTEIN (LDL) cholesterol (the less desirable form) and to increase the risk of colorectal CANCER. On the other hand, calcium binds saturated fats, preventing their uptake by the intestine; consequently, calcium-rich diets may reduce LDL cholesterol. A high calcium intake also seems to reduce the risk of colon cancer.

If blood levels of calcium decrease in response to low calcium consumption, the body pulls calcium out of bones to use elsewhere. Thus, bones are dynamic tissues, constantly releasing calcium and reabsorbing it to maintain their strength. The level of calcium in the blood is carefully regulated by hormones. Parathyroid hormone from the parathyroid gland stimulates bone-degrading cells to break down bone tissue to release calcium and phosphate into the bloodstream (a process called bone resorption). Parathyroid hormone also stimulates calcium absorption from the intestines by activating VITAMIN D, and stimulates calcium reabsorption from the kidney filtrate back into blood. This effect is counterbalanced by calcitonin, released from the thyroid gland when blood calcium levels are high. Calcitonin triggers bone-building cells (osteoblasts) to take up calcium from blood to lay down new bone.

During growth spurts, more calcium is absorbed than lost. Therefore, adequate calcium intake in childhood and adolescence is critical for bone building. In addition, ZINC, manganese, fluoride, copper, boron, MAGNESIUM, calcium, and vitamin D, together with EXERCISE, minimize bone loss after the age of 35. Calcium absorption requires the hormone calcitriol, formed from vitamin D.

According to the U.S. Department of Agriculture (USDA), most Americans do not consume adequate amounts of calcium. The lack of calcium in the diet of children and adolescents is especially alarming because 90 percent of an adult's bone mass is established by the age of 19. Only 14 percent of girls and 36 percent of boys age 12 to 19 in the United States consume enough calcium daily to meet current requirements. Those who do not are at increased risk of developing osteoporosis and other bone diseases.

Symptoms of prolonged calcium deficiency include insomnia, heart palpitations, and muscle spasms, as well as arm and leg numbness. Chronic low calcium intake can lead to easily fractured bones due to bone thinning (OSTEOPOROSIS), and possibly hypertension. Severe deficiency symptoms are rare: convulsions, dementia, osteomalacia, rickets (bent bones and stunted growth in children), and periodontal disease.

In addition to age and heredity, many lifestyle and dietary factors increase the risk of developing calcium-related problems: age; heredity; chronic emotional STRESS; lack of exercise; dieting; excessive CAFFEINE, SODIUM, phosphorus (as found in processed foods and soft drinks), or dietary FIBER; high-fat foods; possibly high protein diets; low vitamin D intake; long-term use of corticosteroids; and cigarette smoking. Condition like INFLAMMATORY BOWEL SYNDROME, low stomach acidity, LACTASE deficiency, kidney failure, and diabetes increase the need for calcium, while mineral oil (laxative), lithium, and some DIURETICS (water pills) block calcium uptake.

Dietary Sources of Calcium

The DIETARY REFERENCE INTAKE for children between ages 4 and 8 is 800 mg; for children from 9 to 13, 1,300 mg; for adolescents between 14 and 18, 1,300 mg; for adults between 19 and 50, 1,000 mg; and for adults over 50, 1,200 mg. For calcium, the lowest observed adverse effect level is 2.5 g for adults. Milk products like yogurt and CHEESE represent rich calcium sources. They need not be high in fat. Low-fat dairy products like skim or low-fat milk and low-fat YOGURT contain about 300 mg calcium per cup. SARDINES and canned SALMON with cooked bones and high in calcium; plant sources include green leafy vegetables, COLLARD greens, CHARD, beet tops, BOK CHOY, spinach, and BROCCOLI, as well as various seeds and SOYBEANS. The calcium in spinach is less easily absorbed. Two very good plant sources are TOFU, prepared with calcium to curdle soybean protein, and corn tortillas, prepared with lime. The following are examples of low-fat, high-calcium food:

1% fat cottage cheese (half cup)	70 mg calcium
non-fat yogurt (half cup)	225
skim milk (1 cup)	300
cooked greens (1 cup)	100
cooked collard greens (1 cup)	280
cooked soybeans (1 cup)	450
tofu (1 ounce)	130
corn tortilla (1 ounce)	300
sardines (3 ounces)	370

Calcium Fortification

Calcium is added to foods and beverages. The food industry has responded to consumer fears of OSTEOPOROSIS (age-related thinning of bones) by adding calcium to a variety of foods and diet drinks, including some brands of orange juice, BREAKFAST cereals, whole milk, yogurt, cheese, sliced cheese, cottage cheese, white flour, bread, and cocoa. Fortified or enriched foods can supply 25 percent to 100 percent of the calcium RDA per serving. Individuals prone to kidney stones might have problems with excessive calcium, and excessive calcium from any source can cause milk-alkali syndrome, which damages the kidneys. A very high calcium intake can block the uptake of MANGANESE, another essential mineral. (See also ENRICHMENT.)

Calcium Supplements

The advantages of obtaining calcium from food are twofold. First, calcium is better absorbed, and second, it is almost impossible to overdose on calcium from food. However, the typical U.S. diet provides only 450 to 550 mg of calcium daily, and individuals who avoid dairy products may encounter difficulty in obtaining adequate calcium from foods alone. Certain groups are more likely to develop calcium deficiencies: dieters, smokers, women past menopause or who have had hysterectomies, and those who drink several cups of coffee or several alcoholic beverages daily. For those who have a marginal calcium intake, calcium supplementation with vitamin D is a responsible alternative.

Most types of calcium supplements are effective, and calcium carbonate is inexpensive. Orange juice can aid calcium uptake from calcium carbonate. It is generally believed that chelated calcium (calcium citrate, lactate, gluconate, orotate) may be more easily absorbed than calcium carbonate when stomach acid production is low, although this view has been challenged. Calcium tablets need to disintegrate in water for calcium absorption to occur. The best way to take calcium supplements is to combine them with vitamin D. Look for calcium supplements that are "essentially lead free" to minimize possible contamination with small amounts of lead.

Calcium supplementation can reduce depression, water retention, and pain related to premenstrual syndrome (PMS). Calcium supplementation reduces the risk of osteoporosis in postmenopausal women. Continuous supplementation with calcium after menopause can improve bone mass by 10 percent and reduce the risk of bone fractures by 50 percent. Moreover, drugs used to treat osteoporosis are most effective when calcium intake is adequate.

There are several precautions to be aware of in using calcium supplements. Excessive calcium supplementation (3,000 to 8,000 mg per day) increases the risk of ZINC and MAGNESIUM deficiencies. Calcium supplements taken with meals may block the uptake of other minerals like COPPER, IRON, and zinc. Overdosing with calcium supplements also increases the risk of kidney stones in susceptible people. Excessive calcium supplements can lead to vomiting, high blood pressure, DEPRESSION, excessive urination, muscle wasting, and CONSTIPATION. (See also ANTACIDS; BONE; CORTISOL; GASTROINTESTINAL DISORDERS; HYPERTENSION; LACTOSE INTOLERANCE.)

NIH Consensus Development Panel On Optimal Calcium Intake, "Optimal Calcium Intake," *Journal of the American Medical Association,* 272, no. 24 (December 1994): 1,942–1,948.

calcium blockers Drugs prescribed to help prevent HEART ATTACKS. CALCIUM blockers lower blood pressure by preventing calcium from entering smooth muscles around veins and capillaries, thus keeping them from contracting in response to high SODIUM. Calcium blockers also inhibit chemical signals from the brain that normally speed up the heart when the patient becomes excited.

calcium propionate The CALCIUM salt of PROPIONIC ACID, a short-chain fatty acid. This common, innocuous FOOD ADDITIVE is used in bread and rolls to prevent the growth of MOLDS and BACTERIA. The level of propionate in baked goods (0.1 percent to 0.2 percent) is sufficiently high to alter the growth of microorganisms like bacteria and mold, but it does not kill them. Sodium propionate is also used in pies and cakes to prevent the interference of calcium with BAKING SODA or powder.

Propionate is a harmless additive occurring naturally in foods. For example, Swiss cheese contains 1 percent propionate, which serves as a natural preservative. Metabolic processes produce propionate from AMINO ACIDS and certain FATTY ACIDS. Furthermore, propionate is easily oxidized for energy. This process requires VITAMIN B_{12}. (See also BREAD; FOOD PRESERVATION; FOOD SPOILAGE.)

California Certified Organic Farmers (CCOF) An agency that certifies organic produce and organic farms according to established standards in California. In particular, the CCOF label indicates the product has met limits of PESTICIDE residues lower than those set by the EPA. In general, unless organic produce is agency certified, there is no guarantee it has been grown without the use of pesticides, HERBICIDES, or chemical fertilizers. (See also ORGANIC FOODS.)

caloric value The maximum amount of CALORIES available from food. Caloric value refers to the number of calories released by completely oxidizing a gram of fuel nutrient, as FAT, CARBOHYDRATE, or PROTEIN. Metabolic processes oxidize fat and carbohydrate completely to CARBON DIOXIDE and water, the same combustion products as found in the laboratory. The caloric yield is the same whether fuel is burned in the body or in the test tube. The oxidation of GLUCOSE yields 3.7 calories per gram. STARCH yields 4.1 calories/gram; and SUCROSE, 4.0 calories/gram. Therefore an average yield of 4 calories per gram of carbohydrate is used by nutritionists. The oxidation of a monounsaturated fat like OLIVE OIL yields 9.4 calories per gram; of a more saturated animal fat like BUTTERFAT, 9.2 calories per gram. For simplicity an average value of 9 calories per gram of fat is used to approximate the caloric yield. AMINO ACIDS from protein contain nitrogen, which is not oxidized by the body but is excreted as UREA. Consequently the caloric yield of protein oxidized in the body is 4.1 calories per gram. This value is rounded off to 4 when used by nutritionists to calculate the caloric yield of food proteins. The key point is that fat contains more than twice as many calories as protein or carbohydrate.

calorie A standardized unit of heat. The caloric yield of nutrients and the body's energy requirements are expressed as large calories, "kilocalories" in the medical literature, or simply "calories" in common usage. One kilocalorie is the amount of heat required to raise the temperature of 1 kg of water by 1°C. Another unit of energy used in some scientific articles is the kilojoule. One large calorie equals 4.124 kilojoules (KJ).

Calories are a measure of the energy released when the body burns any fuel including FAT, PROTEIN, CARBOHYDRATES, and ALCOHOL. Calories from the oxidation of fuel nutrients maintain normal body functions such as the heart and circulation, as well as the (hormonal) endocrine system, nervous system, and digestive system. Energy from food supports reproduction, growth, physical work, the uptake of nutrients, and the repair of wear and tear in cells and tissues. The actual number of calories used depends on many factors, including body mass and the level of physical activity. A portion of the calories are released from food as heat to maintain body temperature. Women need fewer calories than men. Typically, women's needs range from 1,600 to 2,000 calories daily; men generally need 1,800 to 2,400 calories daily.

Caloric Balance

The relationship between caloric input and caloric expenditures is critical. Excessive calories, regardless of their source, may promote fat buildup because surplus calories are stored by the body rather than being destroyed. Contrary to popular belief, carbohydrates and STARCH are not high calorie NUTRIENTS; carbohydrates yield only 4 calories per gram. The distinction belongs to fat as a more concentrated source of calories (9 calories per gram). Calories derived from fat are linked to OBESITY because the conversion of dietary carbohydrate to body fat requires much more energy than the conversion of dietary fat to body fat. Consequently, it is harder to gain weight by eating large amounts of complex carbohydrates than by eating fat.

Common Sources of Excessive Calories

Popular high-calorie foods are cheeseburgers, soft drinks, processed and high-fat meats (SAUSAGE, BOLOGNA, and so on), FRENCH FRIES, doughnuts, cookies, cake, ice cream, fried food, cheeses, high-fat CRACKERS, CHIPS, and alcoholic beverages. PROCESSED FOODS and CONVENIENCE FOODS often also contain added saturated fat (which increases the risk of atherosclerosis) and sucrose (SUGAR), which provides no nutrients other than carbohydrates. To put this in perspective, consider that a person would need to walk one and a half hours to consume the calories provided by a single piece of pastry. Typical high-calorie items (HIGH-FAT FOODS) are easily replaced with low-calorie alternatives:

- one candy bar (500) vs. one cup of unbuttered popcorn (54)
- four pieces fried chicken (1,700) vs. one serving of broiled, skinless chicken (142)
- one slice of cheesecake (257) vs. one cup of strawberries (50)
- six ounces of potato chips (920) vs. one large salad, with a teaspoon of dressing (100)
- bread with two squares of butter (170) vs. one slice of bread (80)

Estimating Daily Caloric Needs

The following computation approximates daily caloric needs. Actual needs may differ depending upon age, gender, level of physical activity, personal METABOLISM, state of health, and STRESS level.

1. Divide body weight in pounds by 2.2 (to convert pounds to kilograms).
2. Choose appropriate energy factors: 1.0 for males, 0.9 for females, or 0.8 for those over 50 years old.
3. To calculate the calories needed to maintain body weight: Multiply weight in kilograms by the appropriate energy factor times 24 hours. For example, a 123-lb. woman weighs 55.9 kg. She needs 55.9 kg × 0.9 × 24 hr. = 1,207 calories per day just for maintenance.
4. To estimate the daily calories required for physical activity: Choose the best estimate of activity level. Very light (e.g., desk job) = 0.6; Light (e.g., teacher) = 0.8; Moderate (e.g., nurse) = 1.1; Strenuous (e.g., roofer) = 2.4. Multiply the hours per day spent on this major work activity by weight in kg. For example, for a woman with 7 hours of moderate work activity level: 55.9 kg × 7 hr. × 1.1 = 430 calories.

5. To calculate total calories, add Step 3 to Step 4. In our example, 1,207 calories plus 430 calories equals 1,637 calories, the estimate for a typical day.

Calorie Reduction Strategies

A knowledge of the calorie content of food is fundamentally important because a balanced diet must first provide adequate energy. Critical stages of life require more energy than usual. Pregnancy, lactation, growth during childhood and adolescence, and caloric restriction require medical supervision. Counting calories has long been a preoccupation of dieters. However, the most effective ways to lose weight require a change in behavior: Eating less high-fat food and exercising regularly. Specific dietary recommendations can be made to reduce calorie intake:

Dairy Products Replace cream CHEESE or sour cream with low-fat YOGURT. Replace Camembert, Cheddar, Cheshire, feta, Limburger, and provolone cheeses and cheese spreads, with lower-fat cheeses like mozzarella or low-fat COTTAGE CHEESE. Use skim MILK instead of whole milk or cream in recipes. Consume less ice cream, which can be 50 percent to 60 percent fat.

Meat and Poultry Bake MEAT and POULTRY on a rack to drain fat. Remove fatty skin from poultry before eating. Select lean cuts of meat instead of prime or choice. Trim off all visible fat.

Processed Foods Avoid processed foods. Often, convenience foods provide high levels of saturated fat as butter, lard, shortening, hydrogenated vegetable oils, coconut, and/or palm oils. Processed meats such as sausage, luncheon meats, and hot dogs usually contain large amounts of SATURATED FAT. Substitute VEGETABLES and FRUIT for high-salt, high-sugar, and/or high-fat snacks. Eat fewer fried foods, which contain 25 percent to 50 percent saturated fat. Drink less alcohol and sweetened soft drinks, which supply only calories. (See also DIETING.)

Sohal, R. S., and R. Weindruch. "Oxidative Stress, Caloric Restriction, and Aging," *Science* 273 (1996): 59–63.

campylobacteriosis A type of FOOD POISONING caused by the bacterium *Campylobacter jejuni.* The bacterium occurs in livestock and can contaminate MILK, raw MEAT, and POULTRY. Some 80 percent of poultry sold for human consumption is contaminated with the *Campylobacter* bacterium. More than 10,000 cases of campylobacteriosis are reported to the U.S. Centers for Disease Control and Prevention (CDC) each year.

Campylobacter is the leading cause of DIARRHEA from food in the United States. Diarrhea is potentially a serious condition because it can prevent nutrient uptake and cause dehydration, leading to electrolyte imbalance. Other symptoms are fever, stomach cramps, and sometimes bloody stools. Symptoms appear two to five days after eating contaminated food and can last a week. To avoid contamination during meal preparation, the utensils and cutting board used to prepare raw meat should not come in contact with VEGETABLES or cooked meat. Consumption of untreated water or unpasteurized milk is not advised because of the increased risk of bacterial contamination from these sources. (See also GASTRITIS; *HELICOBACTER PYLORI*.)

cancer A broad category of diseases characterized by an uncontrolled, virulent growth of cells. Cancer is classified according to the tissue of origin. The most common are carcinomas, which originate in epithelial tissues (tissues lining the body cavities and forming the outer surfaces of the body). Sarcomas develop from connective tissues, muscles, skeleton, circulatory, and urogenital systems. Myelomas originate from bone marrow; lymphomas from the lymph system; and leukemia from blood-forming cells. Many cancers typically invade adjacent tissues. Such metastasizing tumors spread throughout the body via the circulatory and lymphatic systems.

Cancer is the second leading cause of death among Americans. An estimated one out of every three or four adults will be diagnosed with cancer and about half of these patients will die of the disease. The chances of living longer once cancer is detected are better than ever, and the rates of new cancer cases and deaths from cancer in the United States are declining. However, the rates of some new cancers, including lung cancer in women and non-Hodgkin's lymphoma, have increased in recent years.

All cancers are caused by cell mutations that cause the cells to replicate over and over again. Most mutations are random and occur as an error during cells replication or as a response to injury from an environmental factor like radiation or chemicals. A small number of these mutations are inherited. Researchers involved in sequencing the human genome have identified about 100 of these inherited mutations, called genetic markers, that increase a patient's risk of developing cancer. Nearly three-quarters of these mutations are associated with somewhat rare cancers such as leukemias and lymphomas. The remaining markers have been linked to cancers of the breast, colon, prostate, lung, and ovary, which account for 80 percent of all cancer cases. A person who has one of these genetic markers will not necessarily get cancer; the mutation simply increases the risk.

Environmental factors such as nutrition, chemical exposure, and lifestyle choices can increase or decrease the risk of developing cancer whether or not a patient has a genetic predisposition for the disease. For example, cigarette smoking accounts for an estimated 25 percent to 40 percent of cancer cases, while flawed diets may cause roughly a third of cancer cases. Exposure to chemical pollutants (5 percent to 10 percent), infections (1 percent to 10 percent) and radiation are also significant causes.

Most adults have been exposed to cancer-causing agents, and their tissues already contain mutated genes, which can remain dormant for years. Cancer may not show up unless the precancerous state is stimulated by other agents called promoters. These may be viruses, chemicals, or agents in foods; excessive dietary fat is thought to be a cancer promoter. Consequently, carcinogens often manifest their effect many years after exposure. The body possesses powerful defenses. Efficient mechanisms repair DNA mutations; however, they can be compromised by a poor diet, disease, and age. The immune system wards off foreign cells, including cancer cells. Natural killer T-cells and anticancer factors (tumor necrosis factor) are produced to destroy altered cells, but this declines with age.

Cancer and Diet

Many experts believe that diet plays a role in the development of cancer—both by ingesting too many cancer-causing foods, such as broiled or preserved meats, and by not eating enough cancer-preventing foods, such as certain antioxidant-containing fruits, vegetables, and green teas.

Perhaps as many as one-third of all cancers are related to diet, and as many as 95 percent of colon cancer cases are diet related. Cancers of the prostate, breast, colon, and lining of the uterus (endometrium) are most common in affluent nations, while cancers of the liver, cervix, esophagus, and stomach are related to poverty. Although research and population studies suggest a correlation between specific nutrients and different types of cancer, most recommendations remain best guesses. Deficiencies of the following nutrients are linked to increased risk of cancer: AMINO ACIDS (CYSTEINE, METHIONINE, TRYPTOPHAN, ARGININE), B COMPLEX vitamins (riboflavin, FOLIC ACID, VITAMIN B_6), fat soluble vitamins (VITAMIN A, VITAMIN E), minerals (CALCIUM, ZINC, copper, iron, selenium), other nutrients (choline, BETA-CAROTENE), and other substances in foods that act as antioxidants or modify levels of liver detoxication enzymes (FLAVONOIDS, isothiocyanates, organosulfur compounds, PHYTOESTROGENS, and others).

Meat and fat are closely correlated in the Western diet, making the separation of these two variables difficult. Most animal studies show that meat per se does not affect carcinogenesis. Human population studies do not link meat consumption with colon cancer, although meat intake may increase the risk of pancreatic cancer.

Fat and energy intake may be correlated with cancer. Geographic correlations suggest that a high-fat diet is a risk factor for cancers of developed countries. To decrease cancer risk, some experts believe that fat should be cut back to 20 percent or less of daily calories. Diets high in fat enhance chemically-induced tumors in experimental animals. On the other hand, calorie restriction inhibits tumor growth even when the calorie-restricted animals ingest more fat than controls. One of the reasons animal studies have not strongly supported the link between fatty diets and colon cancer may be that human high-fat diets usually include cooked foods. Cooking seems to increase the cancer risk of meat cooked in beef fat.

Fiber has been the focus of intensive cancer research in recent years. In 1970 a British researcher published a study showing that in countries where the diets are high in fiber, the rates of gastrointestinal disease, including colon cancer, are low. Conversely, in countries such as the United States, where fiber consumption is low and protein and fat consumption are high, the rates of colorectal cancer are also high. This led health experts to assume that a high-fiber diet could reduce the risk of colon cancer, but a pair of studies published in 2001, one conducted by the National Cancer Institute and the other by the Arizona Cancer Center, both concluded that a high-fiber diet does not prevent the growth of the polyps that can lead to colon cancer. Nonetheless, diets supplying ample fiber are linked to a lower risk of many chronic degenerative diseases, including diabetes, heart disease, arthritis, and some forms of cancer.

Other studies have shown that dietary fiber can reduce the risk of cancers of the stomach and breast. These results, coupled with research showing a correlation between high-fat diets and cancer and studies showing that a high consumption of fruits and vegetables can decrease the risk of cancer generally, supports health experts' recommendation that patients eat a diet rich in vegetables, fruits, legumes, and whole grains, that provides between 20 and 35 grams of fiber each day. (For example, an apple provides 3 grams of fiber; a one-ounce serving of wheat bran, 8.4 grams; and one slice of whole wheat bread, 1.5–2 grams.)

Vitamin Deficiencies

Vitamin deficiencies are implicated in some forms of cancer and several vitamins may lower cancer risk. Animal studies indicate that NIACIN deficiency is linked to cancer. Niacin helps repair damaged DNA, known to occur in the action of several carcinogens. Studies indicate that megadoses of folic acid (25 times the RECOMMENDED DIETARY ALLOWANCE (RDA)) and vitamin B_{12} (160 times the RDA) can reduce precancerous lung tissue in some smokers. Folic acid has been used to treat cervical dysplasia (precancerous cervical tissue) in women taking oral contraceptives. Calcium deficiency is related to the risk of colon cancer. Vitamin A and beta-carotene therapy prevent the formation of precancerous areas in the mouth resulting from chewing tobacco.

Cancer Prevention

A diet rich in fruits, vegetables, and whole grains is believed to help reduce the risk of tumor development. While no single food or nutrient will remove the risk of cancer, following healthy guidelines can reduce a person's chances of developing certain types of cancer. To lower the risk of cancer, experts recommend people should eat a plant-based diet with plenty of roughage and a variety of natural, whole-grain foods. They should avoid high-fat diets, barbecued (burned) food, and smoked, pickled, salted, and cured food.

Cancer-protecting foods are rich in complex carbohydrates and fiber, factors that have been associated with a reduced risk of several types of cancer. They also contain substances that can inhibit tumor formation. For example, CRUCIFEROUS VEGETABLES contain sulforaphane as well as other plant chemicals such as dithiolthiones that may produce enzymes that help block damage to cell DNA. The cruciferous vegetables include broccoli, cauliflower, kale, brussels sprouts, and cabbage. Garlic and onions have sulfur compounds (allyl sulfides) that trigger enzymes that may help remove carcinogens from the body. Citrus fruits are rich in vitamin C and flavonoids, which may help inhibit cancer cell growth.

Soy foods are high in ISOFLAVONES, which block some hormonal activity in cells. Diets high in soy products have been associated with lower rates of cancers of the breast, endometrium, and prostate.

Tomatoes and tomato sauce are high in the phytochemical LYCOPENE, a powerful antioxidant. A diet high in tomatoes has been associated with a decreased risk of cancers of the stomach, colon, and prostate.

Saturated Fats Some evidence shows that people who have diets high in saturated fats (more than 10 percent of total calories) have a higher cancer risk than do those with lower-fat diets.

Plant-based Diet Many experts believe that adding more plant-based foods is the dietary cornerstone to prevent many types of cancer. Diets high in fiber, folic acid, polyunsaturated fats, vegetable protein, carotenoids, and vitamins B_6, C, and

E, are linked to a lower risk of certain cancers. Because fruits, vegetables, and other plant-based foods typically are low in saturated fats (the animal fats found in meats, butter, and cheese linked to an increased risk of cancer) and high in fiber, which may be associated with a lower risk of colon cancer. A plant-based diet is the best source of phytochemicals—natural substances in fruits and vegetables that seem to protect against certain types of tumors. A plant-based diet includes six to 11 servings of breads, grains, and cereals; two to four servings of fruit; and three to five servings of vegetables. The goal of "5 a Day" (five servings of fruits and vegetables each day) is the cornerstone of the NATIONAL CANCER INSTITUTE's (NCI) dietary guidelines for cancer prevention. According to the NCI, if everyone followed the "5 a Day" guidelines, cancer incidence rates could decline by at least 20 percent.

Roughage A high-fiber diet is a good way to reduce the risk of colorectal cancer. Fiber is found in all plant-based foods, including fruits, vegetables, grains, breads, and cereals, but is not available in meat, milk, cheese, or oils. White flour is not recommended because its refining process removes almost all the fiber from grains.

Fiber can be either soluble or insoluble. Soluble fibers dissolve in water and are found in highest amounts in fruits, legumes, barley, and oats. They generally slow down digestion time so that nutrients are completely absorbed. Soluble fibers also bind with bile acids in the intestines and carry them out of the body. Because bile acids are made from cholesterol, soluble fiber can lower a person's cholesterol levels. Studies linking high bile acid concentrations and colon cancer have led some scientists to suspect that binding bile acids may be one way fiber helps prevent colon cancer.

Insoluble fibers are found in vegetables, whole-grain breads, and whole-grain cereals, which increase the bulk of stool, help to prevent constipation, and remove bound bile acids. Insoluble fiber also increases the speed at which food moves through the gastrointestinal system. Some scientists believe a high-fiber diet reduces the risk of colon and other cancers because fiber can bind potentially cancer-causing agents in the intestines and speed the transit time so harmful substances do not stay in the body.

Both types of fiber are important for cancer prevention. Everyone should eat at least 25 grams of fiber each day (about twice the amount most Americans currently consume). A good way to achieve that amount is to eat the NCI's recommended five fruits and vegetables each day. It is possible to increase fiber intake by eating the skins of potatoes and fruits such as apples and pears and switching from refined foods (such as white bread and white rice) to whole-grain foods (whole-wheat bread and brown rice). Other good sources of fiber include legumes, lentils, and whole-grain cereals.

Low-fat A high-fat diet has been associated with an increased risk of developing cancer of the prostate, colon, endometrium, and breast. Low-fat foods are usually lower in calories than high-fat foods and are low in fat as well.

There are three types of dietary fats—saturated, monounsaturated, and polyunsaturated fats:

- *Saturated fats* are almost exclusively from animal products such as meat, milk, and cheese and have been linked to an increased risk of cancer.
- *Monounsaturated fats* are found in olive oil and canola oil.
- *Polyunsaturated fats* are found in vegetable oils.

While the latter two types of fat are less closely linked to disease, because overall fat intake is associated with cancer it is a good idea to limit all three kinds. Dietitians generally recommend tub margarine as a better choice than butter, because butter is rich in both saturated fat and cholesterol, and the hazards of saturated fats are better documented and appear to be more severe than do the hydrogenated fats in margarine. Most margarine is made from vegetable fat and has no cholesterol. The usual recommendation is that people get no more than 10 percent of daily calories from saturated fats and that total fat intake not exceed 30 percent of the day's calories.

Dietary fat can be reduced by limiting the amount of red meat, choosing low-fat or no-fat varieties of milk and cheese, removing the skin from chicken and turkey, choosing pretzels instead of potato chips, and decreasing or eliminating fried foods, butter, and margarine. Cooking with small amounts of olive oil instead of butter will significantly cut saturated fat intake.

Cancer Prevention Cancer prevention emphasizes proper nutrition, and increasing interest has focused on antioxidant nutrients in lowering the risk of FREE RADICAL damage and cancer. Free radicals are highly reactive molecules that lack an electron and attack cell components like DNA and proteins. Selenium, vitamin C, beta-carotene, and vitamin E are all logical candidates as protecting agents because they squelch free radicals. Fruits and vegetables provide a wide assortment of other substances that can reduce oxidative damage. These include FLAVONOIDS, such as TANNINS and ANTHOCYANINS (blue, red, purple pigments of berries), terpenes, coumarins, CAROTENOIDS (such as beta-carotene and lycopene), phytoestrogens (such as soy isoflavones), ISOTHIOCYANATES (found in cabbage family vegetables), organosulfur compounds (diallyl sulfide, others from oils, GARLIC), and diketones (curcuminoids from TURMERIC). Plant foods supply other materials that seem to bolster the body's ability to dispose of toxins and potential carcinogens or to repair damage they cause. Indeed, PHYTOCHEMICALS promise to play an increasingly important role in cancer prevention. Diets high in fiber, folic acid, polysaturates, vegetable protein, beta-carotene, vitamins C, B, and E are associated with a reduced risk of stomach and esophageal cancer.

Other cancer prevention guidelines emphasize stopping all use of tobacco because smoking is linked to many forms of cancer; minimal use of ESTROGEN, because estrogen increases the risk of breast cancer; moderate consumption of ALCOHOL, because alcohol increases the risk of breast, mouth, and esophageal cancer; practicing safe sex to minimize transmission of viruses that injure the immune system; reducing stress to bolster the immune system; avoiding sun exposure to minimize the risk of skin cancer; and minimizing exposure to carcinogens in cigarette smoke, toxic materials such as dust, solvents, industrial chemicals, PESTICIDES, and certain FOOD ADDITIVES like nitrates and artificial food colors.

The American Cancer Society notes that certain warning signs of cancer warrant medical attention: any unusual bleeding; a thickening lump, especially in the breast; a sore that does not heal; a persistent cough; hoarseness; a dramatic change in bowel movements or urination; indigestion; difficulty in swallowing; an unexplained weight loss; and a change in color or shape of a wart or mole.

Cancer-Preventing Agents in Food

Certain nutrients are being studied for their effectiveness in preventing cancer: vitamin A, VITAMIN C, vitamin E, beta-carotene, selenium, and fiber. Vitamin C, vitamin E, CAROTENOIDS (orange-red or yellow plant pigments like beta-carotene), and selenium are antioxidants. They help prevent chemical damage by free radicals, mainly highly reactive forms of oxygen, such as superoxide, which occur from cellular metabolism as well as from exposure to environmental pollutants and to oxygen. Free radicals are treacherous because they damage DNA, the genetic blueprint of a cell. Alterations of genes seem to convert some cells to cancerous types; thus, free radicals can function as carcinogens. Antioxidants are widely distributed in fruits and vegetables. Foods rich in carotenoids like beta-carotene are orange-colored vegetables like winter squash and dark-green leafy vegetables such as CHARD and broccoli. Fresh fruits provide vitamin C; vegetable oil, wheat GERM, and nuts supply vitamin E; whole grains, selenium; and fruit, vegetables, grains, and LEGUMES provide fiber.

A wide variety of other plant products seem to inhibit cancer formation, and their identification remains a very active area of research. These materials work in different ways. Flavonoids (complex multi-ring pigments found in many fruits and vegetables) serve as antioxidants, enhance the body's mechanisms for neutralizing toxic substances, and help regulate enzymes involved in malignancy. Ellagic acid, a flavonoid found in fruits, especially grapes, and in vegetables, seems to directly protect genes from chemical attack. Indoles (benzene-like compounds containing nitrogen) and flavones (flavonoids related to vitamin E) may serve as antioxidants. Certain phenolic compounds (oxygen-containing AROMATIC COMPOUNDS) also help neutralize carcinogens like NITROSOAMINES. Agents in the cabbage family may boost the liver's capacity to destroy CARCINOGENS. As an example, sulfur compounds in broccoli and cauliflower called dithiolthiones stimulate the transfer of GLUTATHIONE, the cell's major sulfur-containing detoxifier, to make cancer-causing agents more easily excreted in urine and feces. Other agents include saponins, garlic products, and fiber. Saponins and triterpenoids (unabsorbable carbohydrate derivatives) inhibit breast cancer in experimental animals. Soybeans contain isoflavones, plant substances that may decrease estrogen production in premenopausal women and thus apparently reduce the risk of breast cancer.

In 2001 the American Cancer Society adopted the following Nutrition and Physical Activity Guidelines for individual cancer prevention:

- **Eat a variety of healthful foods, with an emphasis on plant sources.** Eat five or more servings of a variety of vegetables and fruits each day. Choose whole grains in preference to processed (refined) grains and sugars. Limit consumption of red meats, especially those high in fat and processed. Choose foods that maintain a healthful weight.
- **Adopt a physically active lifestyle.** Adults should engage in at least moderate activity for 30 minutes or more on five or more days of the week; 45 minutes or more of moderate to vigorous activity on five or more days per week may further enhance reductions in the risk of breast and colon cancer. Children and adolescents should engage in at least 60 minutes per day of moderate to vigorous physical activity at least five days per week.
- **Maintain a healthful weight throughout life.** Balance caloric intake with physical activity. Lose weight if currently overweight or obese.
- **Limit consumption of alcoholic beverages.**

(See also AGING; BARBECUED MEAT; DELANEY CLAUSE.)

Albert, D. S. et al. "Lack of Effect of a Low-Fat, High-Fiber Diet on the Recurrence of Colorectal Adenomas," *New England Journal of Medicine* 342 (April 2000): 1,149–1,155.

Go, Vay Liang W. "Diet, Nutrition and Cancer Prevention: Where Are We Going From Here?" *Journal of Nutrition* 131 (2001): 3,121S–3,126S.

Kristal, A. R. "Diet and Trend in Prostate-Specific Antigen: Inferences for Prostate Cancer Risk," *Journal of Clinical Oncology* 20, no. 17 (September 1, 2002): 3,570–3,571.

Michels, K. B., and A. Wolk. "A Prospective Study of Variety of Healthy Foods and Mortality in Women," *International Journal of Epidemiology* 31, no. 4 (August 2002): 847–854.

Sporn, Michael B. "The War on Cancer," *Lancet* 347 (May 18, 1996): 1,377–1,381.

Candida albicans A disease-producing yeast belonging to the same family as MOLDS and FUNGI. *Candida* flourishes in warm, moist environments that supply a nutrient source: It can grow on moist tissues lining the body (mucous membranes). Traces of *Candida* and other yeasts may live in the intestine, but they are usually held in check by friendly gut bacteria and the immune system. *Candida* is an opportunistic organism that can spread when the immune system weakens and when secreted antibodies decline; when broad-spectrum antibiotics kill gut bacteria; and when the diet supplies excessive refined carbohydrate and sugar. *C. albicans* infection of the mouth (thrush) and esophagus occurs in infants and young children, and is also a sign of HIV (human immunodeficiency virus)-induced conditions. *Candida* presents up to seven different forms for the body to suppress. This may partially explain its ability to exploit weaknesses in the body's defenses. Laboratory tests can distinguish *C. albicans* from other pathogens. *Candida* resists typical antibiotics; therefore, treatment utilizes antifungal drugs like niastatin and botanical antifungal agents, such as berberine (goldenseal *Hydrastis*) and garlic extracts. (See also ACIDOPHILUS; CANDIDIASIS; FLORA, INTESTINAL.)

Chaitow, Leon. *Candida Albicans: Could Yeast Be Your Problem?* Rochester, Vt.: Healing Arts Press, 1998.

candidiasis A *Candida* (yeast) infection of the skin and mucous membranes of the body. Although *Candida albicans* is a common culprit, several *Candida* species produce disease. Typically candidiasis occurs in the colon, vagina, mouth, throat, lungs, or nails. However, a serious systemic (body-wide) infection may occur when *Candida* invades the bloodstream. The symptoms of candidiasis syndrome attributable to intestinal infection can be extremely variable, ranging from headaches, confusion, and loss of energy, to chronic fatigue, cramps, bloating, rectal itching, and gas. It can be associated with lowered immunity. Because these symptoms fit many clinical conditions, it is imperative that diagnosis be confirmed by specific clinical lab tests based on specimen culture and analyses of anticandida antibodies in the bloodstream.

Several factors promote candidiasis including use of oral contraceptives and steroid hormones (which can suppress the immune system), long-term use of antibiotics (which kill bacteria that normally hold *Candida* in check), nutritional deficiencies that weaken the immune system, chronic STRESS or viral (HIV) infection (which lowers immunity), low stomach acidity (which prevents sterilization of food and promotes maldigestion), high-carbohydrate diet, and diabetes (which increases sugar and support yeast growth).

In treating candidiasis, it is important to reduce the predisposing factors by:

- using digestive aids
- avoiding sugar and other refined carbohydrates
- eliminating exposure to known allergens, which can weaken the immune system
- bolstering the immune system with nutritional supplements
- correcting low stomach acid production
- repopulating the intestine with beneficial bacteria (lactobacillus species and BIFIDOBACTERIA) to reestablish normal microflora.

(See also ACIDOPHILUS; INTESTINAL; HYPOCHLORHYDRIA.)

Crook, William G. *The Yeast Connection Handbook.* Jackson, Tenn.: Professional Books, 1996.

candy A processed, sugar-based food first produced in Venice in the 15th century. The United States produces the most candy worldwide, reflecting its regional popularity. The average American consumption in 1990 was about 20 pounds per person, representing more than 2,000 different varieties of candy. The major ingredient is SUCROSE (table sugar), though candy may also contain MILK and milk products, GUMS, GELATIN, FAT and oils, STARCH, flavorings, fruit, and nuts. In the United States, CHOCOLATE is the major ingredient of the most popular brands of candy, the majority of which contain PEANUTS and peanut butter. Their high content of REFINED CARBOHYDRATES and SATURATED FAT indicates these are high-calorie, low-nutrient-density foods. Their EMPTY CALORIES are a concern for those who are attempting to improve their diet and eat more nutritious foods. Sugar-free candies are available to help satisfy a sweet tooth, which contain sugar derivatives such as SORBITOL and artificial sweeteners like ASPARTAME. Sugarless candies are not calorie free, however, because sorbitol and aspartame can be taken up and used for energy. (See also FLAVORS; NATURAL SWEETENERS; NUTRIENT DENSITY.)

canola oil A monounsaturated vegetable oil derived from a relatively new variety of RAPESEED. The composition of canola oil resembles that of OLIVE OIL. It contains 32 percent polyunsaturated FATTY ACIDS, 62 percent monounsaturated fatty acids, and only 6 percent saturated fatty acids. Monounsaturates are considered more healthful than saturated fats (animal fat, or COCONUT OIL and PALM OIL) because a diet high in monounsaturates and low in cholesterol tends to lower LOW-DENSITY LIPOPROTEIN (LDL), the less desirable form of blood cholesterol, while maintaining HIGH-DENSITY LIPOPROTEIN (HDL), the desirable form. Studies show that olive oil does not cause tumors in experimental animals, but long-term cancer studies have not been carried out with canola oil.

cantaloupe (*Cucumis melo cantalupensis*) A variety of muskmelon with orange pulp and a fragrant smell. Most melons originated in the ancient Middle East, then spread to the Egyptian and Roman empires. Cantaloupe is the most common melon in the United States; Arizona, California, and Texas are major domestic sources. Cantaloupe is an excellent source of BETA-CAROTENE, to which it owes its orange color, as well as ASCORBIC ACID. One cup of cubed melon provides calories, 60; protein, 1.4 g; carbohydrate, 13 g; potassium, 495 mg; vitamin A, 510 retinol equivalents; fat, 0.4 g; ascorbic acid, 65 mg. Cantaloupe contains only low levels of other minerals and B vitamins.

canthaxanthine A natural red food color belonging to the CAROTENOID family of plant pigment, which is related to BETA-CAROTENE. Used in foods such as candy, sauces, and margarines, canthaxanthine has no VITAMIN A activity, unlike beta-carotene. Since it is fat-soluble, canthaxanthine can accumulate in fat tissue and the skin, although food is a source for only small amounts of this food colorant. However, it is marketed as a tanning aid, and canthaxanthine pills can supply more than 20 times the amount normally consumed in the diet. Accumulation can lead to blurred night vision, allergic skin reactions, hepatitis, and in extreme cases, ANEMIA.

capillary A microscopic blood vessel that averages 0.008 mm in diameter, slightly larger than the diameter of a RED BLOOD CELL. A network of capillaries connects the arterial and venous systems. They connect with the smallest branches of the arteries (arterioles), and provide oxygenated blood and nutrients to cells within tissues. Capillary walls are sufficiently thin to permit rapid migration of oxygen and other nutrients from blood into surrounding tissues, and to permit waste products like CARBON DIOXIDE and LACTIC ACID to diffuse out of cells into the bloodstream. The total surface area provided by all capillaries for this transport function is huge: 6,300 square meters for an adult. (See also HYPERTENSION; PROSTAGLANDIN.)

caprylic acid An acid classified as a medium-chain FATTY ACID, found in BUTTER, goat and cow's MILK, and COCONUT OIL. Caprylic acid is classified as a saturated fatty acid because all carbon atoms are filled up with hydrogen atoms. Unlike the long-chain fatty acids typically found in fats and oils, medium-chain fatty acids are rapidly absorbed by the small intestine without the intervention of a special carrier (CHYLOMICRON) required to transport fats in the bloodstream. Medium-chain fatty acids can be readily used for energy by the LIVER and skeletal muscle. Oral caprylic acid products can combat intestinal yeast infections. Caprylic acid seems to block yeast cell-wall production. (See also CANDIDIASIS.)

capsaicin The spicy, pungent compound of CHILI PEPPERS, and the most fiery of the pepper alkaloids. Capsaicin probably evolved to protect the pepper from being eaten by predators. In humans, this substance can help digestion by stimulating salivation, STOMACH ACID production, and, perhaps, PERISTALSIS. Capsaicin has other potential benefits: It may also kill bacteria, reduce the risk of blood clots, and serve as an ANTIOXIDANT. It seems to boost the production of intestinal IgA antibodies produced to exclude foreign materials from the intestine.

Capsaicin also acts as a "counterirritant," that is, it is a mildly irritating substance that blocks pain sensations. It seems to do this by interfering with sensory nerves that relay pain messages from the skin to the brain. In particular, capsaicin can deplete a chemical messenger called substance P, which relays pain messages to the brain, short-circuiting pain signals. This effect can be anti-inflammatory as well, and capsaicin-containing creams have been developed to reduce the pain of shingles and chronic foot and leg pain. There are several precautions when using these creams: Capsaicin irritates membranes of the eye and nose, though it does not injure the stomach, and capsaicin supplements may interfere with the functioning of anticoagulants. (See also IMMUNE SYSTEM; NEUROTRANSMITTER.)

Altman Roy D. et al. "Capsaicin Cream 0.025% as Monotherapy for Osteoarthritis: a Double Blind Study," *Seminars in Arthritis and Rheumatism,* 23, no. 6, supp. 3 (1994): 25–33.

capsicum pepper See CHILI PEPPER.

captan A useful but potentially dangerous FUNGICIDE that retards the growth of MOLDS, yeasts, and fungi. Captan shows up frequently in GRAPES and is used generally for FRUIT (APPLES, PEACHES, STRAWBERRIES) and VEGETABLES (BEANS, PEAS, CARROTS, CORN, GARLIC, CABBAGE, LETTUCE, BROCCOLI). Traces of captan have been detected in FAT and cooking oils. In use since the 1950s, the legal limit for captan was set before the discovery that it can cause KIDNEY and intestinal CANCER in lab animals. Captan was named by the U.S. National Academy of Science as one of the most toxic PESTICIDES. The EPA has proposed banning captan because it is a suspected CARCINOGEN.

caramelized sugar A brown food coloring prepared by heating table sugar. As sugar turns brown, its sweetness is gradually replaced by a burnt flavor and aroma. Water is then added to create a brown syrup. Caramel provides a brown color to foods like pumpernickel bread, some partially whole wheat breads, and boeuf bourguignon. Vegetables like onion and carrots are glazed or lightly caramelized by being heated with sugar and water. The term *caramel* also refers to a type of brown, square-shaped CANDY with a chewy consistency. (See also ARTIFICIAL FOOD COLORS; FOOD ADDITIVES.)

caraway (*Carum carvi*) A small, seedlike herb used as an aromatic seasoning that is related to CARROTS and PARSLEY. Dried caraway seeds are used to season rye bread, as well as pastry, soups, vegetables, meats, and certain cheeses. It adds zest to potato salad and coleslaw. Caraway seed oil provides the distinctive flavor of kümmel, a liqueur. Fresh caraway leaves flavor soup, salad, cheeses, vegetables, and meat.

carbohydrate A large class of organic compounds that includes sugars, starches, and fiber. Carbohydrates contain two hydrogen atoms and one oxygen atom (H_2O) for each carbon atom, and the name *carbohydrate* relates to the apparent "hydrated carbons" in their chemical formulas. Carbohydrates represent such a variety of substances that they are grouped into several categories.

Nutritionally important carbohydrates are categorized as simple and complex, according to their size. SIMPLE CARBOHYDRATES are referred to as sugars. Simple carbohydrates in the form of NATURAL SWEETENERS are among the most common FOOD ADDITIVES. Examples are SUCROSE, DEXTROSE, FRUCTOSE, and CORN SYRUP, as well as any word on a food label that ends in "-ose." COMPLEX CARBOHYDRATES occur in plants as starch and fiber.

Nutritionists classify carbohydrates in foods according to their degree of processing. Refined carbohydrates, like sugar and white flour, are highly purified materials, containing little, if any, of the nutrients found in the whole food from which the carbohydrate was prepared; therefore, they supply mainly calories. Carbohydrates are also classified according to size: monosaccharides, dissacharides, oligosaccharides, and POLYSACCHARIDES. The simplest are monosaccharides, which include simple sugars. The family of HEXOSES are monosaccharides containing six carbon atoms; glucose and fructose are examples. PENTOSES are simple sugars with five carbon atoms; ribose, the raw material for RNA, is the most common example.

The predominant carbohydrate of the body is glucose. Glucose in the blood is called BLOOD SUGAR and is a major fuel source for most cells of the body. The brain relies on glucose to meet its energy needs.

Unless the diet supplies adequate carbohydrates, the body's metabolism switches to a STARVATION mode, in which body fat is burned to meet most energy needs. To fuel the brain during starvation, glucose is synthesized from AMINO ACIDS obtained by the breakdown of muscles.

Disaccharides contain two linked simple sugars. The most familiar is sucrose (table sugar). This disaccharide contains glucose and fructose. Fragments of complex carbohydrates are called oligosaccharides. As an example, food additives like maltodextrin are derived from starch and typically contain 3 to 10 glucose units. Because they are much smaller than starch molecules they are water soluble.

The largest carbohydrates are polysaccharides, which are polymers (long chains) and contain many simple sugars linked together. STARCH and GLYCOGEN ("animal starch") are polysaccharides important in nutrition and metabolism. Unlike sugars, complex carbohydrates do not taste sweet, and they are often insoluble in water. Starch is composed of long chains of 1,000 or more glucose units. The form of starch with many side chains or branches is AMYLOPECTIN; the unbranched form is called AMYLOSE. Starch functions as the plant storehouse of glucose. For example, when energy is needed during seed germination, the developing seed uses glucose from starch to grow into an embryonic plant. Starch is packed in granules that must be cooked to be edible. Digestion of starch yields glucose. Although glycogen is not an important food source of carbohydrate, it is the storage carbohydrate of tissues like muscle and the liver, and is broken down when fuel is needed.

Carbohydrates are classified as "macro nutrients" because they account for such a large part of the diet throughout the world. In the United States carbohydrates typically supply approximately 46 percent of the daily energy requirement. In Africa, carbohydrates constitute almost 80 percent of dietary calories. The prevalence of carbohydrate in the diet is due to its ready accessibility from plant sources, its low cost and its ease of storage. Major sources of starch include cereal GRAINS, such as WHEAT, RICE, RYE, MILLET, sorghum, and CORN. These grains contain 76 percent starch. Tubers, such as POTATOES and CASSAVAS, and root vegetables, such as parsnips, also supply starch. BEANS and seeds of legumes, rich sources of protein, also contain 40 percent of their weight as starch. Worldwide, wheat is the predominant crop source of dietary carbohydrate, followed by rice, corn, and potatoes, and then by barley and cassava.

Fiber refers to indigestible complex carbohydrates found in plant cell walls and structures. The major classes of fiber possess different sugars as building blocks. CELLULOSE, one of the most common fibers, contains only glucose. HEMICELLULOSES, PECTINS, GUM, and LIGNIN are other important types. Humans do not produce digestive enzymes that can break down fiber, though colon bacteria can feast on them. The soluble forms of fiber, such as pectins and gums, and insoluble forms like cellulose assure a healthy intestinal tract and reduce the risk of diverticulosis, hemorrhoids, constipation, colon cancer, and other intestinal disorders.

In the United States, there is a long tradition of avoiding starchy food for weight control, out of a mistaken belief that carbohydrates are calorie-rich, but the opposite is actually true. Bread and pasta can help a dieter because carbohydrates contain only 4 calories per gram, less than half the calories in fat based on weight. In addition, carbohydrate calories are less efficiently stored as fat, compared to dietary fat. But, in general, excessive consumption of calories from any nutrient—whether PROTEIN, fat, or carbobydrate—leads to fat accumulation. Every year, Americans eat more than 100 pounds of simple carbohydrates per person. This high sugar consumption contributes to excessive weight, promotes dental caries, and leads to poor nutrition. Current dietary guidelines recommend increasing the amount of complex carbohydrate while decreasing sugar consumption by eating whole, starchy foods like LEGUMES, grains, and fresh VEGETABLES to supply nutrients like MINERALS and FIBER, as well as plant substances that reduce the risk of cancer (isoflavones, ellagic acid, isothiocyanates, among others). (See also CARBOHYDRATE LOADING; CARBOHYDRATE METABOLISM.)

Asp, Nils-Georg. "Classification and Methodology of Food Carbohydrates as Related to Nutritional Effects," *American Journal of Clinical Nutrition* 61, no. 4 supp. (April 1995): 930S–937S.

carbohydrate, available The portion of dietary carbohydrate that can be digested to GLUCOSE and its storage form, GLYCOGEN. This fraction includes monosaccharides (such as glucose, FRUCTOSE, GALACTOSE, MANNOSE); disaccharides, which contain two sugars (LACTOSE, maltose, SUCROSE); starch fragments (DEXTRINS); and POLYSACCHARIDES (starches and glycogen, which contain hundreds of glucose units). Fiber is excluded from available carbohydrate because it cannot be digested. (See also DIETARY GUIDELINES FOR AMERICANS.)

carbohydrate digestion The conversion of starch and dietary carbohydrates to simple sugars that can be absorbed and used by the body. Many carbohydrates in food are too large to be absorbed by the intestine, which normally absorbs only simple sugars. Starch digestion yields the simple sugar, glucose, through a complex series of events: Starch digestion begins in the mouth with an enzyme in saliva called AMYLASE as food is chewed. In the intestine amylase secreted by the pancreas digests starch to maltose, a sugar containing two linked glucose units. Intestinal enzymes, MALTASE and dextrinase, carry out the final step, the breakdown of small starch fragments to glucose. Sugars composed of simple sugars are also digested to their simple building blocks. Sucrose (table sugar) yields glucose and fructose by the action of the intestinal enzyme SUCRASE, and lactose (milk sugar) yields glucose and galactose by action of LACTASE, also an intestinal enzyme. (See also CARBOHYDRATE METABOLISM.)

carbohydrate loading (glycogen loading) A procedure used by athletes who consume CARBOHYDRATES to force their muscles to increase the amount of stored carbohydrate (GLYCOGEN). Muscle glycogen represents emergency fuel because it is readily broken down to blood glucose, and increasing glycogen content in muscles delays exhaustion and increases endurance. A modified regimen, six days before competition would be: days 1–3, normal diet with 50 percent carbohydrate. Day 1, 90-minute aerobic workout; days 2 and 3, 40-minute workout. Days 4–6, high carbohydrate diet with 70 percent carbohydrate. Days 4 and 5, 20-minute workout. Day 6, rest.

Carbohydrate loading will not increase endurance when exercising less than 1.5 hours. However, eating high carbohydrate meals the night before an athletic event and the day of the event can assist individuals participating in short events lasting up to 1.5 hours.

Carbohydrate loading is not recommended for athletes over 40, for adolescent athletes, or for people with kidney problems, heart disease, or diabetes, nor is it recommended for anyone more than twice a year. After repeated episodes of loading, the glycogen in the heart increases. The additional water content of cells can adversely affect heart performance by altering the ability of those cells to perform work. (See also CARBOHYDRATE METABOLISM.)

Rauch, L. M., I. Rodger, G. R. Wilson, J. D. Belonje, S. C. Dennis, T. D. Noakes, and J. A. Hawley. "The Effects of Carbohydrate Loading on Muscle Glycogen Content and Cycling Performance," *International Journal of Sport Nutrition* 5, no. 1 (1995): 25–36.

carbohydrate metabolism Cellular reactions that convert carbohydrates to the simple sugar GLUCOSE, and subsequently break down glucose to produce energy or raw materials for cell synthesis. Lactose (milk sugar) contains galactose, and sucrose (table sugar) contains fructose (fruit sugar); both must be converted to glucose prior to their being used by cells.

Glucose After Digestion

Following digestion, simple sugars absorbed by the small intestine are carried via the bloodstream to the liver, which converts fructose and galactose into glucose. After a carbohydrate meal, blood glucose rises rapidly. In response to elevated blood sugar levels, beta cells of the pancreas release the hormone INSULIN, which promotes glucose uptake by most tissues like muscle and fat cells. The brain and the liver do not require insulin to use glucose.

Glycogen Metabolism

In muscle and in the liver, surplus glucose can be linked up to form long, branched molecules called GLYCOGEN, the major energy reserve in these two tissues. Two hormones, EPINEPHRINE (adrenaline) and GLUCAGON, stimulate glycogen breakdown when energy is needed. The liver's role is to maintain adequate BLOOD SUGAR levels; when the diet does not supply enough carbohydrate the liver releases glucose from liver glycogen by a process called GLYCOGENOLYSIS. The liver also produces glucose from noncarbohydrate materials like AMINO ACIDS and LACTIC ACID through a branch of carbohydrate metabolism called GLUCONEOGENESIS.

Glucose as a Source of Energy

Once in the cell, glucose can be used in many ways. It can be burned for energy; it can be converted to glycogen for storage; it can produce an agent to supply hydrogen atoms used for biosynthesis, NADPH (reduced nicotinamide adenine dinucleotide phosphate), an enzyme helper based on the B vitamin niacin. The carbon atoms of glucose can be used to synthesize lipids. All cells of the body can oxidize glucose to produce ATP, the energetic currency of the cell.

A collection of enzymes work together to carry out the first part of this process, called GLYCOLYSIS, to yield PYRUVIC ACID, a three-carbon acid. Pyruvic acid is shortened to acetic acid and the carbon atom is removed as CARBON DIOXIDE. An activated form of acetic acid called acetyl COENZYME A is used to synthesize FATTY ACIDS and CHOLESTEROL. Alternatively, acetic acid can be oxidized completely to carbon dioxide by mitochondria, the cells' powerhouses. The oxidation of pyruvate and of acetyl CoA requires the B vitamins NIACIN, RIBOFLAVIN, THIAMIN, and PANTOTHENIC ACID, which form key enzyme helpers (COENZYMES). The complete oxidation of each glucose molecule yields 38 ATP molecules. This is an excellent conservation of energy: it represents an overall efficiency of about 40 percent.

Glucose can also be oxidized by another route, a series of reactions called the pentose phosphate pathway, to produce the NADPH needed in the formation of lipids like cholesterol and in other compounds, and to produce ribose, a simple sugar needed for DNA and RNA synthesis. (See also CARBOHYDRATE DIGESTION; FAT METABOLISM.)

Flatt, Jeane-Pierre. "Use and Storage of Carbohydrate and Fat," *American Journal of Clinical Nutrition* 61, supp. (1995): 952S–959S.

carbohydrate sweeteners A variety of carbohydrates used in food production and home cooking as sweeteners. They include simple sugars (monosaccharides) such as FRUCTOSE and GLUCOSE, and the more complex disaccharides, like SUCROSE (table sugar).

Table sugar is highly purified from sugarcane or from beet roots. Other processed sugars are chemically prepared; corn sugar (glucose, "dextrose") yields high-fructose corn syrup. Syrup and molasses are partially purified mixtures. Even honey is considered a refined carbobydrate because it is processed by bees from nectar. Naturally occurring sweeteners are found in fruits, fruit juices, and some vegetables, such as beets and carrots.

Carbohydrate sweeteners account for about 25 percent of the total calories of the typical American diet. Regardless of their source, carbohydrate sweeteners are converted to glucose before they can be burned as fuels. Because they are purified substances, not whole foods, they supply only CALORIES.

Two-thirds of the sugar consumption in America represents sugar added by food and beverage manufacturers and processors. Sucrose and fructose (FRUCTOSE CORN SYRUP) are the two most prevalent sweeteners and are among the most common FOOD ADDITIVES. Sucrose is added to foods ranging from catsup to gelatin desserts. Current U.S. guidelines recommend decreasing sugar consumption while increasing consumption of complex carbohydrates (starches and fiber). (See also ARTIFICIAL SWEETENERS; CONVENIENCE FOOD; EMPTY CALORIES.)

carbonated beverages See CARBON DIOXIDE.

carbon dioxide (CO_2) A colorless gas produced by the complete oxidation of organic compounds through the release of energy. Carbon dioxide is the endproduct when CARBOHYDRATE, PROTEIN, and FATS are completely burned by the body to produce energy (respiration). This gas readily diffuses out of the cells where it is produced, dissolves in blood, and is transported to the lungs. There, carbon dioxide migrates out into air, contained in the lungs, while oxygen diffuses into the blood to replace that used in respiration. The distance between blood and air at the lung tissue lining is exceedingly small, only 0.0001 cm—too small to slow gas exchange. Shallow breathing and lung diseases lead to excessive carbon dioxide buildup, which can create acidic conditions (ACIDOSIS).

Carbon dioxide in the blood is more than a waste product. It combines with water to form CARBONIC ACID, which breaks down to BICARBONATE, a major pH BUFFER to neutralize acids. The kidney also forms bicarbonate to help maintain the acid-base balance.

Industrial Uses of Carbon Dioxide

Carbonated beverages contain carbon dioxide maintained under pressure. Carbon dioxide is responsible for the bubbles in BEER, mineral water, and SOFT DRINKS and contributes to their slightly sour (acidic) taste. Carbon dioxide is used as a refrigerant (dry ice), a foaming agent, and as a growth promoter of plants in greenhouses. (See also CARBOHYDRATE METABOLISM; FAT METABOLISM; HEMOGLOBIN.)

carbonic acid A weak ACID formed when CARBON DIOXIDE reacts with water in which it is dissolved. In beverages like champagne, BEER, carbonated SOFT DRINKS, and sparkling water, dissolved carbonic acid provides the fizz and the tart flavor.

Carbonic acid readily forms in the body when carbon dioxide, released as fuel, is burned and dissolves in the bloodstream. Carbonic acid breaks down to bicarbonate, and the mixture of bicarbonate and carbonic acid is maintained by RED BLOOD CELLS and the kidneys. Bicarbonate and carbonic acid buffer the blood at pH 7.35 to 7.45 by resisting changes in the hydrogen ion concentration. For example, bicarbonate neutralizes excess acids, while alkaline substances (bases) introduced into the bloodstream are neutralized by carbonic acid. (See also ACIDOSIS; ALKALOSIS.)

carboxylic acids A large family of acidic compounds found in foods and produced by metabolic reactions. Carboxylic ACIDS are capable of releasing hydrogen ions and neutralizing bases. Carboxylic acids are classified as weak acids because they release only a small fraction of their hydrogen ions.

When these acids are neutralized, they produce "conjugate bases," salt forms of the parent acids. Carboxylic acids in cells, including LACTIC ACID, CITRIC ACID, and FATTY ACIDS like PALMITIC ACID and OLEIC ACID, have been neutralized and exist in cells only as their conjugate bases. They are called, respectively, lactate, citrate, palmitate, and oleate.

The AMINO ACIDS can behave as acids, as the name suggests. Two amino acids possess extra carboxyl (acidic) groups and are classified as acidic amino acids: ASPARTIC ACID and GLUTAMIC ACID.

Many acidic compounds occur in foods as salts or conjugate bases. Common FOOD ADDITIVES include preservatives, SODIUM BENZOATE, potassium sorbate, and CALCIUM PROPIONATE; acidifiers, SODIUM, hydrogen phosphate, potassium tartrate, sodium citrate, FUMARIC ACID. (See also CARBOHYDRATE METABOLISM; FOOD ADDITIVES.)

carboxypeptidase A pancreatic enzyme that digests food PROTEINS in the intestine. Carboxypeptidase breaks down proteins by clipping the links between AMINO ACIDS in proteins and is classified as a proteolytic enzyme. Carboxypeptidase, like many other enzymes, requires ZINC as the cofactor.

Proteolytic digestive enzymes, including carboxypeptidase, are synthesized by the pancreas in an inactive form to protect the pancreatic cell from digesting itself. Only when it is released into the intestine does it become fully activated. (See also DIGESTION; PANCREAS; ZYMOGEN.)

carcinogen An agent or substance that causes CANCER in experimental animals or humans. Carcinogens occur in the environment as certain PESTICIDES, cigarette smoke, ozone, or mold toxins. Some industrial chemicals cause cancer. Four percent of the 10,000 tested chemicals have been shown to cause cancer in animals. Carcinogens may be various forms of ionizing radiation: X rays, ultraviolet light in sunlight, and emissions from radioactive materials like radon.

Carcinogens may be produced within the body by normal processes. The liver may convert a foreign compound into highly reactive oxides in an attempt to render it more water soluble, and hence excretable by the kidney. The BENZOPYRENE in cigarette smoke is such an example. Alternatively, carcinogens may form spontaneously in the body. The food preservative NITRITE reacts with amines, nitrogen-rich compounds in the digestive tract, to form NITROSOAMINES, which are carcinogens.

Trace amounts of carcinogens may inadvertently contaminate meat, dairy products, fruits, and vegetables. These include insecticides, like Heptachlor; FUNGICIDES, like O-phenylphenol; and HERBICIDES like Alachlor. Several chemicals used as feed additives for livestock and poultry are suspected carcinogens (such as gentian green). Whether or not exposure to multiple low-level residues poses a tolerable risk is still being debated.

Plants have evolved multiple chemical defenses to protect themselves against predators, and a variety of plant agents occur naturally in foods that, when isolated in pure form, have been shown to cause cancer in experimental animals. Americans eat an estimated 1.5 grams of natural pesticides daily. About half have been found to be carcinogenic in animals. It has been proposed that naturally occurring carcinogens pose a greater threat than synthetic chemicals and pollutants. On the other hand, there is little evidence that foods themselves cause cancer. To the contrary, plant foods are a rich storehouse of potential anticancer agents: VITAMIN C, CAROTENOIDS like BETA-CAROTENE and VITAMIN E. Substances like phenethyl isothiocyanate and indoles found in the cabbage family, and certain FLAVONOIDS such as ellagic acid, in strawberries and other fruits and vegetables, are powerful protective agents. More remain to be identified. Parsley, sage, oregano, and rosemary prevent toxin-producing MOLD from growing, and garlic, onions, cumin, cloves, and CARAWAY possess compounds that reduce the effects of cancer-causing agents.

Examples of common foods that contain possible cancer-causing substances include celery, parsley, and parsnips, which contain a chemical (5-methoxypsoralen) that can be a carcinogen when applied to the skin of experimental animals. It is unknown whether this causes cancer when consumed.

The common supermarket white mushroom (*Agaricus bisporus*) and the false morel, a wild mushroom, contain agartine. There is limited evidence that its breakdown products may cause cancer in experimental animals; however, agartine is destroyed by cooking.

Peels of oranges and other citrus fruits contain d-limonene. Studies of limonene are mixed: Some show that it did not cause cancer in lab animals, others that it acted as an anticarcinogen, and still others that it can cause cancer.

Beets, lettuce, radishes, spinach, and other dark-green leafy vegetables contain nitrate, which can be slowly converted to nitrite in the body, which can form carcinogenic nitrosoamines. The vitamin C and fiber present in these vegetables seem to counter this risk.

Identifying cancer-causing substances is complex. For example, a substance such as CAPSAICIN can pose a low-level cancer risk to the gut and at the same time may be an anticarcinogen elsewhere.

Natural carcinogens are often less powerful than synthetic carcinogens. More research is needed to evaluate the net effect of natural carcinogens and anticarcinogens together with fat, fiber, and others implicated in foods.

Overall, the predominance of evidence indicates that giving up smoking and improving the diet are the best defenses against cancer. The U.S. surgeon general and other experts recommend eating more fruits, vegetables, and legumes and less fat to reduce the risk of cancer. (See also ARTIFICIAL FOOD COLORS; FOOD TOXINS; MEAT CONTAMINANTS; PESTICIDES; RISK DUE TO CHEMICALS IN FOOD AND WATER.)

cardamom (*Elettaria cardamomum*) An aromatic spice native to tropical Asia that is a member of the ginger family. Cardamom seeds are sun-dried and marketed whole and cardamom is used as a seasoning in curry, stews, processed meats like FRANKFURTERS and sausages, pickling spices, and even pastries. Cardamom seeds contain several substances with cavity-fighting properties—contributing to a growing body of natural substances that potentially can fight disease.

cardiovascular disease (CVD) Chronic diseases of the heart and blood vessels associated with aging. CVD accounts for more than half of all deaths in the United States. The epidemic of CVD appeared in the 1920s, and mortality due to CVD increased until the 1960s, when the rate declined rapidly. In recent years the decline has slowed, yet this disease still affects nearly 66 million Americans; 1 million die each year, and most American men have a degree of arterial disease (clogged arteries).

The following are classified as cardiovascular diseases: ARTERIOSCLEROSIS (a general thickening or hardening of arterial walls), ATHEROSCLEROSIS (lipid accumulation on arterial walls), CORONARY ARTERY DISEASE (atherosclerosis of the arteries that supply blood to the heart), heart attack (damage to the heart muscle due to blocked arteries), STROKE (damage to the brain due to reduced blood flow because of blocked or damaged arteries), HYPERTENSION (elevated blood pressure), peripheral vascular disease (varicose veins, thrombophlebitis, atherosclerosis of extremities), and congestive heart failure. Several conditions cause arterial disease. Aneurysms are weakened segments of vessels that fill with blood, causing the vessel to balloon outward. Disorders of the muscle sheath may cause arteries to constrict or to dilate. In atherosclerosis, deposits (PLAQUE) on the inner arterial wall may cause blockage.

Major risk factors for CVD increase the odds of developing the condition, but they do not guarantee an individual will develop it, nor does the absence of risk factors guarantee that a person won't have a heart attack. Risk factors include high blood pressure, cigarette smoking, elevated serum cholesterol (or, more precisely, elevated LOW DENSITY LIPOPROTEIN (LDL) cholesterol), elevated serum TRIGLYCERIDES obesity, diabetes, stress, lack of aerobic exercise, a family history of cardiovascular disease, male gender, and increasing age. Recently, elevated blood homocysteine (an amino acid breakdown product) was found to be an independent risk factor for coronary heart disease. A reduced sensitivity to the hormone insulin (INSULIN resistance) is as great a risk factor for obstructive artery disease as high blood pressure or cigarette smoking.

These risk factors are more than additive; the combined effect of two or more risk factors is greater than it would be calculated by adding risks together. For an individual with three risk factors, the chances of heart disease are six times greater than when only one risk factor is present.

The Centers for Disease Control and Prevention found in 1992 that only 18 percent of Americans over age 18 were completely free of major risk factors for CVD. Among the least healthy were men between the ages of 50 and 64 and women over 65. Only 9 percent had no major risk factors.

Some risk factors can't be changed: heredity gender, and increased age, but many other risk factors are controllable. Diet and lifestyle play critical roles, and personal choices can profoundly alter the probability of CVD and many other chronic diseases associated with AGING. It is possible to prevent or improve heart disease through a varied diet of relatively unrefined foods, with many vegetables, whole fruits, brown rice, and whole grains that retain part of their original kernel structure. In addition, the ideal diet is high in fiber and some omega-3 oils (canola, flax, fish) but low in processed foods and hydrogenated hardened fats. The following steps have been recommended:

1. Stopping smoking. Smoking contributes to atherosclerosis, hypertension, cancer, and elevated blood cholesterol.
2. Controlling high blood pressure. Blood pressure above 120 (the larger number) increases the risk of heart attack.
3. Controlling DIABETES MELLITUS. Chronic elevated blood sugar and insulin predispose an individual to cardiovascular disease, in addition to cataract, infection, kidney disease, and nerve damage.
4. Exercising. Regular aerobic exercise is the cornerstone of prevention of CVD. A sedentary lifestyle increases the risk of obesity and high blood lipids. Walking 30 to 60 minutes a day affords significant benefits for cardiovascular health.
5. Losing weight to help prevent adult onset diabetes, to lower blood pressure, lower LDL cholesterol, and raise HDL cholesterol.
6. Consuming less fat, especially saturated (animal) fat to lower LDL cholesterol and blood triglycerides, and to lose or maintain desired weight. The content of unsaturated fatty acid is also important. A low polyunsaturated fat to saturated fat (P/S) ratio lowers blood cholesterol levels. Omega 6 polyunsaturated fatty acids (as found in most vegetable oils, such as safflower and soybean oil) and omega 3 fatty acids (as found in fish, fish oils, flaxseed oils) decrease the risk of plaque formation and of blood clots. Minimize transfatty acids as found in hydrogenated vegetable oils to lower LDL cholesterol.
7. Reducing alcohol consumption. Two drinks per day for men, one drink per day for women can raise HDL cholesterol. More than this increases the risk of hypertension, cancer, and abuse.
8. Cutting back on cholesterol-rich foods to lower LDL cholesterol and triglycerides, especially if there is a family history of CVD and elevated blood lipids.
9. Eating more potassium-rich foods and less sodium. Eating more vegetables and fruits and decreasing high-sodium convenience foods can lower or stabilize blood pressure.
10. Consuming at least five servings of fruits and vegetables daily. Choosing plenty of fruits, legumes, and vegetables provides FIBER and PHYTOCHEMICALS, including ANTIOXIDANTS that promote vascular health.
11. Taking vitamin supplements when needed. Supplements that provide folic acid and vitamin B_{12} may help decrease high levels of homocysteine to reduce the risk of stroke and heart disease. Consuming at least 100 IU of vitamin E seems to decrease the risk of heart attack, although the National Cholesterol Education Program believes the evidence so far is not strong enough to make a general recommendation.

One good heart-healthy diet is the DASH DIET, which is based on findings from the Dietary Approaches to Stop Hypertension study by the National Heart, Lung, and Blood Institute. This investigation found that high blood pressure can be lowered with an eating plan low in total fat, saturated fat, and cholesterol and rich in fruits, vegetables, and low-fat dairy products. More recently, another landmark study, DASH-sodium, showed that a combination of the DASH diet and sodium reduction can lower blood pressure even more. This combination benefits those with and without high blood pressure. The DASH diet is a healthy eating pattern that can be shared with the whole family. The DASH-sodium diet aims to reduce sodium to 1,500 mg a day.

A constellation of symptoms called METABOLIC SYNDROME (SYNDROME X) may appear in older people prone to cardiovascular disease. Syndrome X includes high blood pressure, insulin resistance, diabetes or prediabetic conditions, high serum triglycerides, low HDL cholesterol, and obesity. By controlling high blood pressure, making a lifelong commitment to being physically active, and consuming a semivegetarian diet (low in fat, high in fruits and vegetables), syndrome X can often be controlled.

It is now thought that the latest lipid deposits in arteries are those that are most likely to rupture and cause heart attacks. By eating less cholesterol and saturated fat, consuming a low-fat, mainly vegetarian diet with minimal animal protein, managing stress effectively, and exercising regularly, these deposits can shrink. It is never too late to change lifestyle patterns to lower the risk of CVD. (See also CHOLESTEROL.)

Heart Outcomes Prevention Evaluation Study (HOPE). "Vitamin E Supplementation and Cardiovascular Events in High-Risk Patients," *New England Journal of Medicine* 342 (2000): 154–160.

NHLBI editors. "Morbidity and Mortality: 2000 Chart Book on Cardiovascular, Lung, and Blood Diseases," National Heart, Lung, and Blood Institute, 2000. Available online. URL: http://www.nhlbi.nih.gov/resources/docs/00chtbk.pdf.

Ornish, D., L. W. Scherwitz, J. H. Billings et al. "Intensive Lifestyle Changes for Reversal of Coronary Heart Disease," *Journal of the American Medical Association* 280 (1998): 2,001–2,007.

Sanmuganathan, P. S., P. Ghahranani, P. R. Jackson, E. J. Wallis, and L. E. Ramsey. "Aspirin for Primary Prevention of Coronary Heart Disease: Safety and Absolute Benefit Related to Coronary Risk Derived from Meta-Analysis of Randomised Trials," *Heart* 85 (2001): 265–271.

carnitine (L-carnitine) A nutrient required for fat oxidation and energy production. Carnitine helps transport FATTY ACIDS into mitochondria, the cellular structure specialized for fuel oxidation. Carnitine also may be necessary for the oxidation of certain amino acids (VALINE, ISOLEUCINE, and LEUCINE) for energy.

The daily requirement for L-carnitine for health is unknown. The body synthesizes L-carnitine from two essential amino acids, LYSINE and METHIONINE. The rate may be inadequate for kidney patients on hemodialysis; patients with liver failure, strict VEGETARIANS, premature and low birth-weight infants, pregnant or lactating women, and children with genetic predisposition to carnitine deficiency or who experience infection or malnutrition. BREAST MILK contains a high level of L-carnitine to nurture the infant, and it may be an essential nutrient for the newborn.

Carnitine deficiency causes muscle weakness, severe confusion, angina, and high blood lipids, including CHOLESTEROL. Carnitine deficiency is also linked to cardiac enlargement and congestive heart failure. Fatty acid oxidation is a major source of energy for the heart muscle, and carnitine deficiency causes extreme metabolic impairment. The normal heart stores carnitine, but if it does not receive adequate oxygen, carnitine levels drop. Supplementation with carnitine raises heart carnitine levels, allowing the heart to use a limited oxygen supply more efficiently. Thus, carnitine has been used effectively to treat atherosclerosis, angina, and coronary heart disease. It has also been shown to improve exercise ability in people who have poor circulation in their limbs (peripheral arterial disease). Carnitine may reduce blood fat and LOW-DENSITY LIPOPROTEIN (LDL, undesirable cholesterol) and increase HIGH-DENSITY LIPOPROTEIN (HDL, desirable cholesterol). Carnitine also decreases blood fat. It may help patients with angina and CARDIOVASCULAR DISEASE, and with some types of muscle disease. A derivative of carnitine called acetyl L-carnitine appears to be neuroprotective. Supplementing with acetyl L-carnitine may improve cognitive defects associated with forms of senility and age-related depression. Low carnitine levels mav be linked to chronic fatigue symptoms.

Good sources of carnitine are red meats and dairy products like milk. Tempeh and avocados contain some carnitine; however, most vegetables, fruits, and grains are sources. Most soy-based infant formulas are supplemented with carnitine. The naturally occurring form of carnitine, (L-carnitine) appears to be safe. Safety data are inadequate for pregnant and breast-feeding women. High doses of synthetic carnitine (D, L-carnitine), a mixture of isomers, for many weeks can cause progressive weakness and atrophy of certain muscles. Symptoms disappear when supplementation with the mixture ceases.

Acetylcarnitine is a slightly different form of carnitine. Some studies suggest that acetylcarnitine is better than carnitine as an antioxidant because it improves coenzyme Q10 levels and protects mitochondria from damage. One of the roles of acetylcarnitine is to act as a shuttle for long-chain fatty acids to the mitochondria, where they are converted into energy. (See also FAT METABOLISM.)

Salvioli, G. and M. Neri. "L-acetylcarnitine Treatment of Mental Decline in the Elderly," *Drugs and Experimental and Clinical Research* 20, no. 4 (1994): 169–176.

carob (*Ceratonia siliqua;* St. John's bread) A CHOCOLATE substitute obtained from pods of a Mediterranean evergreen of the pea family. Carob pods contain many seeds, surrounded by an edible, fleshy pulp; a powder can be prepared from the pods of the carob tree.

Carob offers several advantages over chocolate: It is free of CAFFEINE-like stimulants and it contains only 1 percent FAT (0.18 calories per gram). In contrast, COCOA powder contains 23 percent fat. On the other hand, carob powder contains more sugar and TANNINS, bitter plant products, than chocolate. Carob CANDY may contain much more sugar and SATURATED FAT than chocolate bars, and may not be a low-calorie food. Carob candy provides an alternative for those with a chocolate allergy. (See also ALLERGY, FOOD.)

carob bean gum A food thickener prepared from the bean of the carob tree. The GUM prevents a granular texture when added to ICE CREAM. It is also added to thicken salad dressings, pie fillings, barbecue sauces, and doughs. Carob bean gum is classified as a safe additive. It is also a mild laxative. (See also CANDY; FOOD ADDITIVES; THICKENING AGENTS.)

carotene See BETA-CAROTENE.

carotenemia Elevated levels of carotene in the blood, a condition characterized by yellowed palms of the hands and soles of the feet. Carotenemia does not lead to coloration of the membranes that line eyes, unlike jaundice. The accumulation of BETA-CAROTENE is not associated with the toxicity characterized by excessive VITAMIN A. Consumption of excessive amounts of yellow vegetables, carrot juice, dark-green leafy vegetables, and beta-carotene supplements can cause carotenemia in susceptible individuals. Supplementation with high levels of beta-carotene when there is alcohol-induced liver damage can lead to toxic symptoms. (See also HYPERVITAMINOSIS.)

carotenoids Yellow, orange, and red pigments found in yellow and orange fruits and vegetables. Carotenoids also occur in dark-green leafy vegetables, where their color is masked by the green of chlorophyll. There are more than 500 carotenoids, all synthesized by plants; of these, 50 to 60 commonly occur in foods. Carotenoids are divided into carotenes and xanthophylls (oxygenated carotenes). The most famous carotenoid is beta-carotene. Though most abundant in nature, it does not stand alone; in dark-green leafy vegetables, xanthophylls can make up 90 percent of the total carotenoids.

Lobster and salmon are pink because they have ingested carotenoid-containing plants called asataxanthin; the pigments color their tissues. Egg yolk derives its yellow color from carotenoids eaten by the hen. Yellow oils like peanut and corn oil reflect their carotenoid content. Several carotenoids are manufactured for use as food colors: BETA-CAROTENE (orange to yellow); CANTHAXANTHINE (red); and apocaroenal (yellow). All three are approved food additives and are among the safest food colors. They are used in margarines, candies, and sauces.

About 38 carotenoids can be converted to vitamin A (provitamin A activity). Only a few of these such as alphacarotene and beta cryptoxanthin occur in sufficient amounts to be significant in the diet. The most important pro-vitamin is beta-carotene, followed by alpha and gamma carotene. Because of inefficiencies of absorption and conversion, beta-carotene is one-sixth as effective a source as vitamin A itself. Conversion of the other carotenes is less efficient. Pure beta-carotene used in supplements is the synthetic, all-trans form. Foods supply mixed carotenoids, including cis forms. The *cis* forms of beta-carotene rather than synthetic *all-trans* beta-carotene appear to be better antioxidants, suggesting that natural mixtures from foods may be more effective. Mild cooking generally improves beta-carotene utilization. The yellow food additive canthaxin is an oxidized form of carotenoid from mushrooms that has no pro-vitamin A activity.

Multiple recent population studies suggest that diets rich in carotenoid-containing foods decrease the risk of cancer and of cardiovascular disease. The beneficial effect of carotenoids in the prevention of cancer is believed to occur through protection against oxidative stress and enhanced immune function. In general, carotenoids act as versatile antioxidants to block cellular damage due to free radical attack. Free radicals are highly unstable molecules or molecular fragments with one electron. They avidly attack any cell component they meet, damaging proteins, membranes, and even DNA. Lycopene, the red carotenoid of tomatoes, red bell peppers, and pink grapefruit, has no vitamin A activity in the body, but it serves as an antioxidant. Lutein, lycopene, cryptoxanthin, and alpha-carotene complement the antioxidant activity of beta-carotene. These prevalent carotenoids occur chiefly in 50 commonly eaten fruits and vegetables. Various population studies and clinical trials have not supported the proposal that beta-carotene alone prevents cancer and cardiovascular disease. Rather, the emerging picture portrays beta-carotene as only one ingredient of multiple antioxidants found in plant foods that work together to protect the body. Increased carotenoid levels have been associated with decreased oxidation of LOW DENSITY LIPOPROTEIN (LDL), the less desirable form of cholesterol in the blood. Oxidized LDL is believed to play a key role in the initial events leading to clogged arteries. The only way to be sure of obtaining the full range of carotenoid antioxidants is to eat a variety of fruits and vegetables regularly. (See also FOOD ADDITIVES; FOOD COLORING, NATURAL.)

Pavia, S. A., and R. M. Russell. "Beta-Carotene and Other Carotenoids as Antioxidants," *Journal of the American College of Nutrition* 18 (1999): 426–433.

carrageenan A texturizer prepared from a SEAWEED (Irish moss) and classified as a dietary FIBER. This fiber has no nutritive value and is not absorbed. Irish moss, which grows along the shores of Maine and the Maritime Provinces of Canada, the British Isles, Scandinavia, and France, is often added to chocolate MILK. Carrageenan forms a mild gel with milk protein that prevents COCOA from settling. Carrageenan is used in frozen desserts like ICE CREAM, syrups, GELATINS, soups, jellies, YOGURT, and milk puddings. It is also added to some canned infant formulas to keep FAT and PROTEIN dissolved and to stabilize the BUTTERFAT suspended in evaporated milk. Carrageenan stabilizes the foam in BEER and gives body to soft drinks, and can be a replacement for gelatin in the diet of VEGETARIANS.

Unlike other plant polysaccharides, excessive carrageenan may be detrimental to health. Animal studies have shown that it can cause LIVER enlargement, birth defects, and ulcerated COLON. The United Nations World Health Organization concluded that it does not cause cancer. Carrageenan-containing products should not be given to premature infants because it may disrupt development of the gastrointestinal tract. (See also FOOD ADDITIVES.)

carrot (*Daucus carota*) A root vegetable belonging to the parsley family that has been cultivated for at least 2,000 years. The wild carrot is a native of Europe and Asia; orange-colored varieties were developed in the 19th century and owe their color to CAROTENOID pigment. Other varieties of carrots may have yellow, white, or purple roots that may be blunt or nearly round. Carrots contain more sugar than any other vegetable except beets.

Carrot juice is an excellent source of BETA-CAROTENE, the plant parent of VITAMIN A. There is no problem with moderate consumption of carrot juice, but too much carrot juice can saturate the body with beta-carotene and turn the skin yellow-brown (CAROTENEMIA.) If the body becomes saturated with beta-carotene, the individual should cut back to avoid possible problems with other plant materials in the carrot juice. Carrots are used as a salad vegetable, and in making stews and soup. Carrots (one-half cup, 55 g, grated) provide: 24 calories; protein, 0.6 g; carbohydrate, 5.6 g; fiber, 1.55 g; potassium, 178 mg; vitamin A, 1,547 retinol equivalents; niacin, 0.67 mg; and low levels of other B vitamins.

casaba (*Cucumis melo inodorus*) Large, smooth, pale-yellow winter melons that originated in Turkey, with a globular shape, resembling muskmelon. The ripe fruit has white or yellow flesh that is sweet and juicy and a characteristic cucumber-like flavor. Casabas are extensively cultivated in California, where they were first introduced late in the 19th century. One slice (245 g) yields 38 calories; protein, 1.7 g; carbohydrate, 9.1 g; fiber, 1.2 g; vitamin A, 40 retinol equivalents; potassium, 351 mg; vitamin C, 18 mg; thiamin, 0.06 mg; riboflavin, 0.04 mg; niacin, 0.8 mg.

casein (sodium caseinate) The principal PROTEIN of cow's MILK. When milk curdles, the curd is mainly casein. Casein is used to improve the texture of frozen desserts such as ICE CREAM, ice milk, frozen custard, and sherbet. In NONDAIRY CREAMERS, casein serves both as a whitener and as an agent used to suspend fat (emulsifier). Casein is added to boost the protein content of PROCESSED FOODS and is considered a safe FOOD ADDITIVE. It is a nutritious, high-quality protein because it contains large amounts of all essential AMINO ACIDS. In nutrient studies, casein is used as a reference for protein quality. For example, in calculating the Protein Efficiency Ratio (PER), the ratio of weight gained by young animals to the amount of protein consumed, the dietary protein is assumed to be adequate when it is equivalent to casein. In this case 45 grams of such protein provide 100 percent of the REFERENCE DAILY INTAKE (RDI) for protein.

cashew (*Anacardium occidentale*) A mildly flavored, kidney-shaped nut that is the fruit of a tropical evergreen native to South America. The world's leading producers of cashews are Brazil, China, East Africa, and India. Cashew apples (the pear-shaped fruit) are used in jams and jellies.

A double shell surrounds the kernel of the cashew nut, and between the two shells is a toxic oil that can blister the skin. The shell, acrid oil, and skin are removed before cashews are marketed. Because they contain 45 percent fat, cashews may become rancid and taste stale with prolonged storage at room temperature. The high fat content increases when the nuts are roasted in oil. Cashews yield a delicate table oil. Roasted as well as unroasted cashews are available and are used as snacks and in cooking. Ground cashews also make a pleasing nut butter. Cashews (per ounce, [28 g], dry roasted and salted) contain: 163 calories; protein, 4.3 g; carbohydrate, 9.3 g; fiber, 1.7 g; fat, 13.2 g; iron, 1.7 mg; potassium, 160 mg; sodium, 181 mg; thiamin, 0.06 mg; riboflavin, 0.06 mg; niacin, 0.4 mg.

cassava (*Manioc utilissima; Manioc dulcis aipi*) The tuber of a shrubby perennial of Central and South America that is widely cultivated in tropical regions. The two most widely grown varieties are the bitter manioc, *Manioc utilissima,* and the sweet, *M. dulcis aipi.* Manioc roots end in large reddish-brown tubers three feet long and nine inches in diameter, with a white pulp.

Tubers of the sweet manioc, which has a chestnut-like flavor, can be roasted and eaten plain. Cassava tubers contain compounds that break down to cyanide but are rendered harmless when cooked and yield a bland, high starch flour. Cassava is used like sweet potato in recipes. Traditionally, it is baked in thin cakes and combined with beans to make a balanced-protein meal. Cassava also can replace wheat FLOUR in the diet. TAPIOCA is prepared from cassava pulp that has been heated to form granules. Cassava root, raw (per 100 g), provides 124 calories; protein, 3.1 g; carbohydrate, 27 g; fiber, 2.5 g; fat, 0.39 g; calcium, 91 mg; iron, 3.6 mg; thiamin, 0.23 mg; riboflavin, 0.10 mg; niacin, 1.4 mg; and vitamin C, 48 mg.

catabolic state A physiologic condition characterized by rapid weight loss, associated with losses of body fat and muscle mass. A catabolic state often occurs when food intake does not provide enough calories to meet the body's energy needs. Conditions favoring the breakdown of the body's own stores of PROTEIN, FAT, and CARBOHYDRATE for energy production frequently occur during STARVATION, CRASH DIETING, FASTING; uncontrolled diabetes; ALCOHOLISM; and recovery from severe burns, surgery, illness, and radiation or chemotherapy treatment for cancer. The average weight loss after surgery is about 10 percent of body weight, and typical weight loss during a week in the hospital amounts to 5 percent of body weight. Chronic STRESS can also place the body in a catabolic state.

Nutritional support is important when the catabolic state is prolonged and the patient has diminished nutritional reserves and lowered immunity. Body protein breakdown can be slowed by administration of calorie-rich foods and adequate protein. Specific nutrients may benefit the seriously ill patient.

Supplements of ZINC, IRON, VITAMIN A, VITAMIN C, VITAMIN K, and the B COMPLEX may be recommended to help speed wound healing, to rebuild red blood cells quickly, to assist in blood clotting, and to build up the immune system. Specific amino acids may be used therapeutically. GLUTAMINE is usually classified as a nonessential amino acid, but the postoperative administration of glutamine decreases the rate of muscle loss and supports rapidly growing tissues like the mucosal lining of the intestine. In the kidney, glutamine serves as a donor of ammonia to help regulate acid-base balance, and it is produced in muscle to help dispose of ammonia, a by-product of amino acid degradation. ARGININE can also benefit seriously ill patients by enhancing wound healing and increasing the activity of T-cells, thus increasing the immune response; it may also increase growth hormone and insulin levels. Supplemental essential fatty acids may modify the immune response and thus limit inflammation by stimulating the formation of regulatory substances (thromboxane A_3, leukotrienes B_5) that restrict inflammation. However, even aggressive nutritional support may not prevent body protein loss during severe catabolic illness, where there is utilization of body fat and breakdown of skeletal muscle protein. (See also CATABOLISM; FATTY ACIDS; OMEGA-3 FATTY ACIDS.)

catabolism The processes of METABOLISM by which FAT, CARBOHYDRATE and PROTEIN fatty acids, glucose, and surplus amino acids are oxidized to release energy measured as CALORIES.

The body requires vast amounts of energy each day. For example, every day the kidneys filter the equivalent of 425 gallons of fluid and the heart beats more than 4,000 times. Most usual energy needs are met by carbohydrate and fat in the diet. Oxidation of these fuels occurs by increments with a series of ENZYMES that trap energy released in fuel oxidation as ATP. This energy "currency" is used by cells for growth and maintenance. Most untrapped energy is released as heat. ATP production occurs in MITOCHONDRIA, small subcellular structures that function as the cell's powerhouses where fuel is burned for energy. The ultimate breakdown products of catabolism are CARBON DIOXIDE and WATER.

Catabolic enzymes work together to catalyze reactions (speed up chemical reactions without being destroyed in the process). A series of functionally linked enzymes is called a enzymatic pathway. The following represent typical catabolic pathways: GLYCOLYSIS oxidizes glucose to a simple acid, pyruvic acid, which yields acetic acid. KREB'S CYCLE oxidizes acetic acid to carbon dioxide. Muscle and liver GLUCOSE is stored as a polymer, GLYCOGEN. In GLYCOGENOLYSIS, glycogen is broken down when glucose is needed to supply energy. Fatty acid oxidation yields the most ATP; consequently, fat is the most efficient form of energy storage. When insufficient calories are consumed, muscle protein is also broken down for many tissues. Muscle protein breakdown yields amino acids whose carbon atoms are either shunted into blood glucose by the liver or are oxidized by many tissues. In this case, the catabolic end products are carbon dioxide, water, and UREA (nitrogenous waste).

The B complex supports catabolic processes. NIACIN, RIBOFLAVIN, THIAMIN, PANTOTHENIC ACID, FOLIC ACID, VITAMIN B_6, and VITAMIN B_{12} are key players in catabolic pathways. These vitamins form specific enzyme helpers (COENZYMES). They do not provide energy; instead they help catalyze energy production, much as the spark plugs of a car engine activate gasoline combustion without themselves being consumed. (See also CARBOHYDRATE METABOLISM; CATABOLIC STATE; FAT METABOLISM.)

catalase A highly active ENZYME that destroys HYDROGEN PEROXIDE. Catalase is considered an antioxidant. Hydrogen peroxide is a powerful oxidizing agent occurring naturally in cells as a by-product of metabolism that can damage cells. It is formed by specialized oxidative structures within cells called peroxisomes. Catalase is widely distributed among tissues and fluids such as SALIVA, and it is concentrated in the lens of the eye, where it serves a protective function. Commercially, catalase is applied in food processing to degrade excess hydrogen peroxide that is added as an oxidizing agent. (See also CATARACT.)

cataract An opacity of the lens of the eye and/or of its capsule that impairs vision. Cataracts and macular degeneration are the leading causes of blindness in older people. AGE-RELATED MACULAR DEGENERATION refers to the age-related degeneration of a tiny area of the retina responsible for seeing fine detail. Cataracts affect about 60 percent of Americans over the age of 75.

The cause of mature onset cataract formation is unknown. According to a recent hypothesis, age-related deterioration of the lens is the result of oxidative damage due to sunlight's UV light. The lens is particularly vulnerable to cigarette smoke and other forms of air pollution that contribute to oxidative damage. Damaged lens proteins cannot be replaced and they tend to clump and scatter light, rather than staying transparent. In animal models, cataracts can be caused by oxidative stress, and can be prevented or delayed by ANTIOXIDANTS. The level of the general cellular antioxidant GLUTATHIONE decreases in the lens in aging animals and humans. Cataracts are linked to increased risk of ATHEROSCLEROSIS, and they can be classified as a degenerative disease associated with aging. Cataracts can also be the result of DIABETES MELLITUS and congenital defects in infants.

Current cataract research emphasizes the role of nutrition in prevention. A wide variety of clinical studies have shown that a CAROTENOID-rich diet decreases the risk of cataracts.

In one Australian study, researchers found that the nucleus of the lens is particularly sensitive to nutrient deficiencies; protein, vitamin A, niacin, thiamin, and riboflavin all protected against cataracts in this study. Data from the Physicians' Health Study suggested a 27 percent decrease in the relative risk among doctors taking multiple vitamin supplements. The Nurses' Health Study found that women with the highest intake of VITAMIN C, VITAMIN E, and carotenoids had 40 percent fewer cataracts. Those who supplemented with vitamin C for 10 years or more decreased their cataract risk by half.

According to statistical data from the World Health Organization (WHO), most cases of cataract and glaucoma throughout the developing world stem from poor diet and lack of hygiene. There are approximately 50 million people in the world who have very poor vision; 85 percent of these live in Asia and Africa. WHO reported that many of these cases could be prevented by improved hygiene and nutrition.

In terms of prevention, experts recommend a diet rich in fruits and vegetables, with restricted sugar usage. Sugars such as excessive glucose and galactose derived from milk sugar (LACTOSE) diffuse into the lens and are converted to sugar alcohols, such as sorbitol, that do not leave the cells as readily. Accumulation can cause water imbalance in the cell, and eventual damage. Lactose can increase the risk of cataract for those with genetic defects in galactose metabolism. Folic acid, vitamin C, vitamin E, carotenoids, selenium, and zinc may decrease the risk of oxidative damage, particularly with deficiency of these nutrients. FLAVONOIDS, complex substances that protect plants form oxidation, such as QUERCETIN, inhibit the enzyme that converts glucose to sorbitol.

Varma, S. D., P. S. Devamanoharan, and S. M. Morris. "Prevention of Cataracts by Nutritional and Metabolic Antioxidants," *Critical Reviews in Food Science and Nutrition* 35, nos. 1 & 2 (1995): 111–129.

catecholamines An important family of AMINES (nitrogen-containing compounds) derived from TYROSINE, an AMINO ACID. Dopamine, EPINEPHRINE (adrenaline), and norepinephrine constitute this family of amines whose functions depend upon their tissue of origin. Dopamine functions as a NEUROTRANSMITTER and serves as a raw material of norepinephrine, a HORMONE produced by the adrenal gland, which increases blood pressure by constricting blood vessels. Elsewhere norepinephrine functions as a neurotransmitter. Norepinephrine is a precursor of epinephrine, itself a key adrenal hormone released in response to stress and to stimulation of the sympathetic NERVOUS SYSTEM.

catfish (*Ictalus punctatus;* channel catfish) A large group of mainly freshwater FISH without scales. It gets its name from the appearance of its feelers which resemble a cat's whiskers. Of the 2,500 or so species of catfish, only a small number are used for food. Originally a mainstay of Southern cuisine, catfish now ranks fifth in consumption in the United States, behind TUNA, shrimp, COD, and Alaskan pollock. It was previously caught in rivers, but fish farms now supply 75 percent of catfish consumed. The farm-raised fish grow on a diet of soy protein, grains, fish meal, and potatoes. In the wild, the catfish may become contaminated with industrial pollutants as it feeds from the bottom of streams and rivers. This tasty fish is sold fresh and frozen throughout the United States. Because the skin is hard to remove most people prefer fillets. While traditionally fried, catfish can also be poached, baked, or grilled. A 3 ounce (100 g) serving provides 103 calories; protein, 15.5 g; fat, 3.6 g; calcium, 34 mg; thiamin, 0.038 mg; riboflavin, 0.09 mg; and niacin, 1.84 mg. (See also SEAFOOD.)

cat's claw (*Uncaria tomentosa*) A woody vine that grows in the tropical rain forests of Peru. The plant gets its name from small thorns, which look like cat's claws, that grow where leaves sprout from the vine. It has been used for medicinal purposes by Peru's Ashanica Indians for nearly 2,000 years.

The active substances in cat's claw, ALKALOIDS, TANNINS, and PHYTOCHEMICALS, are credited with helping the body fight infections, lowering, blood pressure, and reducing inflammation. The alkaloids have antimutogenic and antioxidant properties, and studies are being conducted on the herb's ability to prevent CANCER and fight infection in patients who test positive for the human immunodeficiency virus (HIV). The herb also has been used for years as a homeopathic remedy for gastrointestinal illnesses, including CROHN'S DISEASE, COLITIS, GASTRITIS, and LEAKY GUT syndrome. It has also been used to treat female hormone imbalances, colds, joint and muscle pain, cirrhosis, and urinary tract disorders, among other illnesses and conditions.

The safety of cat's claw has not yet been established. Until further research is completed, it should be avoided by children and pregnant or breast-feeding women. Cat's claw is usually sold in powdered or liquid form and is commonly available as a tincture or cream or in capsules or tablets. It is also available as a tea.

Keplinger K. et al. "*Uncaria Tomentosa* (Willd.) DC.—Ethnomedicinal Use and New Pharmacological, Toxicological and Botanical Results," *Journal of Ethnopharmacology* 64 (1999): 23–34.

cauliflower (*Brassica oleracea*) A vegetable closely related to broccoli. Cauliflower, a true flower belonging to the CABBAGE family, was originally grown in Cyprus. The white head, called a curd, represents immature buds and stems that form slightly rounded, compact flower buds. The head of white cauliflower is surrounded by blue-green leaves that protect it from light so that it doesn't turn green.

The hybrid cauliflower-broccoli looks like cauliflower, but its head is pale green. It cooks more quickly and has a less marked taste than white cauliflower. Cauliflower and BROCCOLI are cruciferous vegetables, believed to contain anticancer substances, like phenethyl isothiocyanate, which activate enzyme systems in the liver that can potentially destroy dangerous substances. Population studies suggest that consumption of cauliflower and its relatives decreases the risk of some forms of CANCER.

The strong odor associated with cooking cauliflower can be minimized by cooking it for a short time. Cooking this vegetable in an aluminum or iron pan will turn it off-color. Cauliflower can be used in soups, purees, cold salad, and vegetable fondue, and it can be sauteed, braised, or fried after it has been blanched. Food value of a cup of cooked cauliflower (180 g) is 34 calories; protein, 2.9 g; carbohydrate, 6.8 g; fiber, 3.9 g; ascorbic acid, 56 mg; calcium, 31 mg; iron, 0.74 mg; thiamin, 0.07 mg; riboflavin, 0.1 mg; niacin, 0.56 mg. (See also CANCER PREVENTION DIET.)

caviar The roe of sturgeon and other fish that has been salted and pressed. Sturgeon of the Caspian Sea yield 90 percent of the world's caviar, although this source is endangered by overfishing and pollution.

To prepare caviar, washed, sieved eggs are placed in brine, and then drained and packed. Less expensive versions of caviar are made from the roe (eggs) of SALMON, whitefish, HERRING, and COD, among others. Various types of caviar differ in taste, color, and texture. Caviar generally contains high levels of sodium, 300 to 700 mg per tablespoon (16 grams). A tablespoon of caviar also contains 94 mg of CHOLESTEROL (one-third the recommended daily dose) plus 40 calories; protein, 4 g; carbohydrate, 0.64 g; and fat, 2.9 grams.

cayenne (*Capsicum frutescens* and *c. anum.;* long pepper) A perennial derived from red pepper and a member of the nightshade family. Peppers were domesticated 5,000 years ago in South America, and some two dozen varieties are now cultivated. The long, dried fruit is ground to produce a pungent red seasoning. This very hot pepper is used in seasoning SAUSAGE, curry, soups, and pizza. CAPSAICIN is the predominant ingredient that accounts for the hot taste. This plant compound is an ALKALOID, an aromatic compound chemically related to vanilla, and has a history of use as a pain reliever. Cayenne is used as a salve to relieve chronic pain due to arthritis or shingles, apparently by upsetting the chemical balance inside sensory cells that relay pain messages to the brain.

celeriac (*Apium graveolens var. rapaceum,* celery root) A dark variety of CELERY with a bulbous root. Celeriac originated in Europe, where it is still a popular vegetable. Like true celery, it is related to parsley. The cooked root is eaten in salads, soups, and stews; it can also be marinated or eaten raw. Like celery, it is a low-calorie food. One half-cup (100 g, raw) provides 44.5 calories; protein, 1.5 g; carbohydrate, 9.2 g; fiber, 1.3 g; fat, 0.3 g; calcium, 43 mg; potassium, 300 g; thiamin, 0.03 mg; riboflavin, 0.03 mg; niacin 0.03 mg; vitamin C, 6.3 mg.

celery (*Apium graveolens var. dulce;* true celery) A biennial stalk vegetable grown in temperate regions that is a member of the parsley family. Celery is native to Europe, northeastern Africa, and western Asia. It was used by the ancient Chinese as a medicinal plant, and the Greeks and Romans used it as a flavoring. First cultivated in its modern form in France early in the 18th century, this popular vegetable is now grown commercially in the United States in California, Florida, and Michigan. The Pascal variety does not have the characteristic stringiness of other varieties.

Celery leaves, stalk, and root are edible and are used raw in salads. They are cooked as a vegetable in soups, and celery leaves and seeds are used as a seasoning. Part of celery's popularity rests in its classification as a low-calorie food because of its high water content. Diced celery (raw, one half-cup, 60 g) contains 10 calories; protein, 2.2 g; carbohydrate, 2.2 g; fiber, 1.2 g; calcium, 22 mg; potassium 326 mg; vitamin C, 4 mg; thiamin, 0.03 mg; riboflavin, 0.03 mg; and niacin, 0.3 mg.

celiac disease (nontropical sprue, gluten-induced enteropathy) A severe ALLERGY to cereal GRAINS, especially WHEAT. It is estimated that in the United States one person in 2,000 to 3,000 has celiac disease. Patients with celiac disease react strongly to GLUTEN, a grain protein common to wheat, OATS, RYE, and BARLEY. Repeated exposure to gluten injures the cells lining the intestine, which are required to completely digest and absorb carbohydrates and sugars like table sugar (sucrose) and milk sugar (lactose), as well as FAT and protein. Consequently, celiac disease drastically reduces the uptake of fat, glucose, and AMINO ACIDS, as well as IRON,

ZINC, and water-soluble vitamins, including VITAMIN B_{12}, and fat-soluble vitamins like vitamin A.

Symptoms of celiac disease include weight loss, diarrhea associated with fatty stools (STEATORRHEA), MALNUTRITION, LACTOSE INTOLERANCE, ANEMIA, skin disorders, OSTEOMALACIA, sore tongue, abnormal bleeding, and bleeding gums. Children with celiac disease grow poorly. Symptoms generally appear within the first year of life, when grains are introduced into the infant's diet. The cause of celiac disease is unknown. Family history plays a role, and breast-fed babies have a decreased risk.

Gluten is the major protein fraction of wheat, composed of GLIADENS and glutenins, two protein fractions. Only gliaden is associated with the disease. Closely related proteins in other cereal grains cause similar symptoms. The closer a grain is related to wheat, the greater is its ability to activate celiac disease. Thus, rice and corn are not closely related to wheat and seldom activate the disease. Completely predigested gliaden does not activate the disease in susceptible individuals because it can no longer be recognized by the immune system as foreign.

Treatment programs specify a gluten-free diet devoid of all wheat, rye, barley, and oat products. Ninety percent of patients respond to this diet within two months. However, the problem of avoiding gluten is compounded by the fact that wheat and wheat products are so prevalent in food products, appearing in baked goods, CRACKERS, gravy, soy sauce, many PROCESSED FOODS, salad dressing, and extenders used in ICE CREAM. Gluten-free flours are available: QUINOA, AMARANTH, RICE, CORN, and POTATO. At the beginning of treatment, vitamin and mineral supplements can remedy deficiencies and rebuild nutrient stores. It is important that there be no underlying zinc deficiency, which will cause the disease to be unresponsive to diet therapy. Vitamin B_{12} and FOLIC ACID are not well absorbed by patients with celiac disease if administered orally; they may be administered by injection. (See also ALLERGY, FOOD; GASTROINTESTINAL DISORDERS.)

cellulite A pseudomedical term for FAT stored under dimpled skin of the thighs, hips, and buttocks. Subcutaneous tissue that binds the skin to underlying tissue contains fat cells, and this basic thigh tissue structure differs between women and men. The layer beneath the epidermis is thinner in women, and their fat cells are arranged in chambers, which have a vertical orientation not seen in men.

As women age, this layer thins as fat cells migrate into it. Subsequently, the connective tissue structure breaks down, allowing alternating depressions and protrusions to form; the number of supporting elastic fibers also decreases. Dimpled skin is more likely to occur in women with loose skin. Dimpled thighs are common in obesity and after menopause, while slim women and female athletes have little or no cellulite

EXERCISE and normal body weight are the best way to prevent cellulite; gradual weight loss permits gradual change in skin and connective tissue. Massage may be helpful in increasing circulation.

While it is often claimed that cellulite can be broken up by physical methods, body fat cannot be shaken, sweated, or rubbed off. It must be burned by the body's metabolism. This requires an exercise regimen and diet management. (See also ADIPOSE TISSUE.)

cellulose An insoluble form of dietary FIBER and a building block of plant cell walls and the woody parts of plants. Cellulose is the major ingredient of BRAN, the outer coating of seeds of cereal GRAINS. Cellulose is a linear polysaccharide (very long carbohydrate chain) in which glucose units are bound to each other in such a way that digestive enzymes cannot break down the chains.

Cellulose binds water. Thus, when wheat bran is consumed, the cellulose it contains softens stools, reduces pressure on the colon, and can improve symptoms of constipation and diarrhea. Bran slows down carbohydrate digestion, thus aiding BLOOD SUGAR regulation. Cellulose does not seem to lower blood cholesterol levels, and excessive amounts may bind minerals like CALCIUM and limit their absorption. Cellulose and other dietary fiber is broken down extensively by colon bacteria to produce short-chain fatty acids, the preferred fuel of the gut lining.

Processed cellulose (microcrystalline cellulose) is a common FOOD ADDITIVE. It gives liquids a creamy consistency and improves the spreading properties of foods such as syrups and peanut butter. (See also COMPLEX CARBOHYDRATE; STARCH.)

cellulose, carboxymethyl (CMC, cellulose gum) A chemically modified CELLULOSE that is the most widely used form of cellulose added to foods. Cellulose from wood pulp and cotton is treated with acetic acid to form CMC, which is neither digested nor absorbed. CMC is added to ICE CREAM in conjunction with GELATIN or CARRAGEENAN; to BEER; to pie filling and jellies and to cake frosting. It holds moisture in bread doughs and prevents the sugar in CANDY from crystallizing. In diet foods, CMC adds bulk and helps to create a feeling of satiety without added CALORIES. It adds body to artificially sweetened soft drinks. Other types of modified cellulose improve the clarity of pie fillings, thicken foods, and partially substitute for eggs in cake batter. (See also GUMS.)

ceramics and pottery See LEAD.

cereal grains The edible seeds of cultivated members of the grass family (*Gramineae*). They include RICE, RYE, WHEAT, BARLEY, CORN, and OATS of the *Festucoideae* subfamily. MILLET belongs to a separate subfamily, *Panicoidacea;* it is more distantly related to wheat. BUCKWHEAT, AMARANTH, and QUINOA are unrelated to wheat, though they are considered cereals. Cereal grains contain 7 percent to 14 percent protein and 70 percent to 80 percent carbohydrate in the form of STARCH. The protein from these sources is generally deficient in essential AMINO ACIDS, typically LYSINE. Millet is deficient in TRYPTOPHAN. Consequently, the BIOLOGICAL VALUE, the nutritional score that rates protein quality, for cereal protein is low. However, when cereal grains are eaten together with other foods containing ample levels of amino acids, which are low in grains, the overall quality of the combined protein increases and satisfies daily protein requirements. In wheat FLOUR, gluten becomes sticky when moistened and creates resilient dough that can be used with leavening agents. Other types of flour are less suitable for baking because they contain little gluten. Gluten-containing foods, particularly wheat, must be avoided by patients with CELIAC DISEASE.

Worldwide, rice, wheat, and corn are major dietary staples. Cereal grains are also used as feed for livestock and poultry. Industry uses grains to produce GLUCOSE, ALCOHOL (ethanol), and oils. Americans currently consume half as much cereal grains as they did in 1900. Grains provide about 20 percent of the daily calories of a typical American diet, primarily as starch (COMPLEX CARBOHYDRATE).

Cereal grain kernels possess a tough outer coat (BRAN), associated with FIBER and MINERALS, the nutrient-rich GERM (embryo of the seed), the innermost part of the kernel, and the starchy ENDOSPERM. Milling and refining remove the bran and germ, thus removing much of the fiber, minerals, and vitamins, and leaving the starch. To replenish partially lost nutrients, wheat flour and products like BREAKFAST CEREALS are enriched with NIACIN, THIAMIN, and RIBOFLAVIN, and are fortified with IRON. (See also BREAD; DIETARY GUIDELINES FOR AMERICANS; FLOUR.)

cereals See BREAKFAST CEREAL.

certified food colors See ARTIFICIAL FOOD COLORS.

certified organic vegetables Vegetables certified to have been grown without pesticides and chemical fertilizers. Each U.S. state can set its own limits for levels of PESTICIDES in ORGANIC produce. For example, California permits up to 10 percent of the U.S. Environmental Protection Agency (EPA) tolerance levels. Several state departments of agriculture offer organic certification programs. However, there is currently no uniform standard for organic farms, nor is there agreement on the best way to certify inspection of farms or to test produce for pesticide residues. Certification agencies, formed by regional trade associations, define standards for organic growers and certify farms that meet the standards. There are about 40 certification agencies in the United States and Canada, including the CALIFORNIA CERTIFIED ORGANIC FARMERS (CCOF), Independent Organic Inspectors Association (IOIA), and the Farm Verified Organic (FVO).

Commercial testing labs may be used by markets and growers to test their fresh vegetables and fruit for pesticide residues.

In 1990, Congress passed the Organic Foods Production Act, requiring the U. S. Department of Agriculture (USDA) to create national standards for food labeled "organic." The National Organic Program (NOP), a division of the USDA's AGRICULTURAL MARKETING SERVICE, enforces the Organic Foods Protection Act.

The new standards

- prohibit the use of genetic engineering, irradiation, and sewage sludge in the production of organic foods
- address organic crop production, wild crop harvesting, organic livestock management, and processing and handling of organic agricultural products
- include production and handling requirements, including recommendations by the National Organic Standards Board concerning items on the national list of allowed synthetic and prohibited natural substances
- prohibit antibiotics in organic meat and poultry
- require 100 percent organic feed for organic livestock

With few exceptions, if the word "organic" appears on food produced in the United States, this means the ingredients and production methods have been verified by an accredited certification agency as meeting or exceeding the USDA standards. Farms and food-handling operations that sell less than $5,000 annually of organic agricultural products are exempt from certification. (See also FOOD TOXINS; MEAT CONTAMINANTS.)

ceviche A raw fish dish typical of Peruvian and Mexican cuisine in which various fish are marinated in lemon juice and served with LIMES, ONIONS, or CORN. The acid content produced is strong enough to chemically soften the soft flesh of fish. However, to correctly soften the fish, adequate marinating time must be allowed. Like other raw fish dishes such as sushi, ceviche carries with it a risk of infection by parasitic worms. (See also SEAFOOD.)

challenge testing A strategy used to identify chemical and FOOD SENSITIVITIES. Sensitivities to foods are often difficult to pinpoint. A generally accepted way of identifying an offending agent in a food is to first eliminate exposure to suspected agents in order to permit the body's chemistry to reequilibrate. This may require several days to several weeks. After this time, suspected agents can be introduced one by one, and any response is noted. If symptoms reappear, the inference is that a particular food or agent is the culprit. (See also ALLERGY; ROTATION DIET.)

chamomile (*Matricaria chamomilla*) A medicinal plant with a long history in folk medicine. Chamomile contains several physiologically active ingredients, among them chamazulene, an anti-inflammatory agent that has been used to treat ulcers. In animal studies, chamomile infusions act as a mild central nervous system depressant, perhaps explaining the effectiveness of chamomile tea as a soothing relaxant. In addition, chamomile has antibacterial effects and has been used to stimulate LIVER function. Chamomile tea is obtained from the flowers of the plant and has a pleasing fragrance. However, people who are allergic to ragweed and its relatives (aster and chrysanthemum) may react to drinking chamomile tea with hay fever–like symptoms and hives. (See also HERBAL MEDICINE.)

champagne A sparkling WINE named for the region in France where it originated that is used in celebrations throughout the world. For champagne, pinot noir and chardonnay GRAPES are most often used.

In the 1600s, a Benedictine monk developed the technique for producing and bottling champagne to maintain its effervescence. Wines in general release small amounts of CARBON DIOXIDE during a secondary FERMENTATION carried out in vats. For champagne, after the initial fermentation, a little sugar (GLUCOSE) is added and the wine is bottled before the second fermentation begins. Carbonation requires about three months. Substantial pressure builds up in the bottle during this time; therefore, care should be taken in uncorking the bottle. (See also ETHANOL.)

charcoal-broiled meat See BARBECUED MEAT/ CHARCOAL BROILED MEAT.

chard (Swiss chard; *Beta vulgaris cicla*) A dark-green leafy vegetable that is a variety of beet. Chard is a common garden vegetable because it is hardy, prolific, and tolerates both heat and cold. The leaves and stalks are well defined, in contrast to the root, which is small and inedible. This biennial provides leaf stalks that can be boiled or steamed like spinach. Varieties of chard have either white stalks or beet red stalks. Unlike most cooking greens, the stalks can be sliced and cooked like asparagus. Chard is an excellent source of BETA-CAROTENE (pro-vitamin A) and other CAROTENOIDS and a good plant source of IRON and CALCIUM. A half-cup, boiled (70 g), provides calories, 15; protein, 1.5 g; carbohydrate, 2 g; calcium, 55 mg; iron, 1.3 mg; vitamin A activity, 390 retinol equivalents; and small amounts of other vitamins.

cheddar See CHEESE.

cheese A solid food prepared from coagulated MILK PROTEIN. Cheese is a popular food; the average annual consumption in the United States in 1998 was 28 pounds per person, twice that in the late 1960s. As is typical of dairy products, cheese is a high-FAT, high-calcium food. The flavor and texture of cheeses depend upon the source of the milk, the types of microorganisms used to ripen the cheese, and the ripening conditions. In cheese manufacture, the enzyme RENNET is used to clot milk. The precipitate (curd) is then separated from the liquid (whey), salted, and pressed into a block. Specific strains of MOLDS and BACTERIA are added to ferment (ripen) the cheese.

Unlike MEAT, which can be trimmed of fat, the fat in cheese is hidden. Ten pints of whole milk typically make a pound of cheese, which retains most of the original fat. This mainly SATURATED FAT accounts for 65 percent to 75 percent of the CALORIES of most cheeses. In other words, two slices of cheese contain as much fat as 3.5 pats of BUTTER. Also unlike meat, cheese is an excellent source of CALCIUM. A slice of cheddar provides 204 mg, or 20 percent of the calcium in the REFERENCE DAILY INTAKE (RDI). A half-cup of ricotta made from part-skim milk provides 700 mg of calcium, 70 percent of the RDI. Cheese is also a high-sodium food, typically containing 200 to 400 mg of SODIUM per slice. Certain processed cheeses contain even more.

Food Labels for Cheese

A food label that states "made from partially skim milk" does not indicate how much cream has been added to make the final product. Most hard and soft cheese made from whole milk is quite high in fat. As an example, three ounces of cheddar cheese (18 grams fat or two slices) provides more fat than the same size sirloin steak. Fat contributes 70 percent of the calories of Muenster, blue, Parmesan, American, provolone, Swiss, Roquefort, Monterey Jack, and Colby cheeses, all of which contain 7 to 9 calories per ounce. Havarti provides 11 g fat per ounce. For reference, one ounce is equivalent to a one-inch cube of cheese. Fat accounts for 90 percent of the calories in cream cheese.

Using lowfat or nonfat milk allows cheese makers to produce cheese with less fat than usual (4 to 6 g of fat per ounce). Fat contributes 66 percent of the calories of part-skim mozzarella, whole milk ricotta, feta, and creamed cottage cheese. The fat content of a food label "reduced fat" or "less fat" must be reduced by at least 25 percent per serving compared to the reference food.

"Low fat" cheese products are slightly lower in fat than the usual cheeses. For example, two slices of part-skim mozarella cheese provide 7 g of fat (55 percent calories as fat), while regular mozzarella contains 9 g per two slices. "Low fat" indicates that a food provides a maximum of 3 g of fat per serving if the serving size is over 30 g (1.07 oz). If the serving size is the typical one-ounce slice (28 g), then the lowfat food must contain no more than 3 g of fat per 50 g (1.78 oz) of that food.

"Light" or "lite" cheese is a nutritionally modified food containing 33 percent fewer calories or at most 50 percent of the fat of the reference food when 50 percent or more of its calories come from fat. Most light cheese is labeled "cheese product" and contains 7 to 9 g of fat per ounce. Light cheese may contain more sodium than natural cheese.

Low-fat options include cottage cheese with 1 percent fat, dry curd cottage cheese, several kinds of processed cheeses, part-skim ricotta, and yogurt cheese. Some "reduced fat" and "part-skim" cheeses can also be low-fat options. (See also DIETARY GUIDELINES FOR AMERICANS; FOOD LABELING; LACTOSE INTOLERANCE.)

cheese imitations Products with less butterfat than natural CHEESE, as defined by a standard formulation (STANDARD OF IDENTITY). Cheese substitutes made from vegetable oil and milk protein alone do not contain CHOLESTEROL. However, they may have just as much fat as real cheese because of added vegetable oil. The following terms are used on the food label if the product does not conform to the Standard of Identity for cheese: "cheese product," "cheese food," and "imitation cheese." "Lite" or "light" means that the cheese substitute represents a 50 percent reduction of its fat CALORIES when 50 percent or more of its calories come from fat. "Low SODIUM" versions of imitation cheese may mean the product contains only reduced sodium with the same high-fat calories.

cheese powders An additive used to create a CHEESE flavor in baked goods, chips, and other convenience foods, salad dressings, and soups. The desired cheese is dispersed in skim MILK or in a whey slurry. The suspension is homogenized, emulsified, and spray-dried. Food manufacturers can select the flavor intensity, saltiness, and blend of whey or other milk protein in cheese powders. (See also PROCESSED FOOD.)

cheilosis Cracks at the corners of the mouth and reddened lips and mouth, due to a deficiency of the B COMPLEX vitamins, particularly RIBOFLAVIN. Acute riboflavin deficiency is also accompanied by a glazed, shiny tongue (GLOSSITIS) and DERMATITIS. This condition often accompanies PROTEIN deficiency as well. In industrialized nations, cheilosis is more likely to occur in alcoholics and in patients with chronic infection, CANCER and other serious illnesses. Cheilosis can also be caused by VITAMIN A overdose or by an allergic response to food. Short-term, mild deficiencies and subsequent cheilosis may occur during pregnancy and lactation and during adolescence, when there is an increased vitamin requirement. (See also ARIBOFLAVINOSIS.)

chelate Usually an organic compound capable of binding metal ions by forming a very stable ring or cage-like molecular structure. Although chelated ions remain in solution, the chemical and biological properties of chelated metal ions differ from unbound ions. For example, ETHYLENEDIAMINETETRAACETIC ACID (EDTA) is a highly efficient chelate added to PROCESSED FOOD to trap metal ion impurities—ALUMINUM, COPPER, IRON, MANGANESE, and nickel. Trace amounts of metals are inevitable because of the metal plumbing, grinders, and processors used in food preparation. Chelating agents scavenge these metal contaminants, preventing reactions that would detract from the appearance and nutritive quality of the food. Large excesses of EDTA would trap CALCIUM, iron, ZINC, and other essential mineral nutrients and prevent their assimilation.

Chelates are used therapeutically; desterrioxamine, a chelate specific for iron, removes excess iron in HEMOCHROMATOSIS and HEMOSIDEROSIS, diseases of excessive iron accumulation, while British anti-Lewisite, a chelator of LEAD, is used in cases of lead toxicity. Many products of cellular metabolism like CITRIC ACID are chelating agents.

Chelated Minerals

Mineral nutrients like calcium, copper, iron, MAGNESIUM, manganese, and zinc can be converted to water-soluble forms by combining them with chelating agents. In supplements, minerals are often chelated with citric acid (as citrate), ASPARTIC ACID (aspartate) and other AMINO ACIDS, orotic acid (as orotate), gluconic acid (as gluconate), and picolinic acid (as picolinate). These chemicals form stable complexes with positively charged metal ions. Chelated minerals often are more easily absorbed in the intestine; thus they are more "bioavailable." HEME is one of the most important iron chelates in the body because it functions in HEMOGLOBIN to transport oxygen in the blood. The uptake of iron in heme found in meat is about 30 percent efficient, while the uptake of non-heme iron, as supplied by vegetables, may only be 1 percent to 5 percent. Because the organic chelates contribute a larger percentage of the weight of the mineral compound than carbonates, for example, more milligrams of the chelated forms are needed to provide the equivalent amounts of minerals in a tablet compared to those containing a simple nonchelated form like carbonate. Chelation may increase mineral absorption in some individuals when stomach acidity is low, as is often the case for elderly people. For individuals sensitive to iron supplements, chelated iron is less likely to cause an upset stomach. (See also BIOAVAILABILITY; HEAVY METALS; TRACE MINERALS.)

chemical imbalance The shift of chemical processes in the body away from equilibrium states. Imbalanced body chemistry underlies many disease processes, and a return to health entails a return to normal functioning. Acid-base balance, water balance, electrolyte balance, and GLUCOSE sugar are carefully regulated by mechanisms involving the brain and the endocrine system. They assure that combined systems will first maintain a relatively constant internal environment. The following examples of possible imbalances highlight the importance of nutrition.

Water The body's main constituent. The cytoplasm of cells, the fluid between cells and the circulation, are watery environments. The normal functioning of cellular processes and waste disposal requires an adequate water supply at all times.

Minerals Sodium, potassium, chloride, and bicarbonate are required to maintain the appropriate ionic strength within cells and the circulation. Processes ranging from nerve transmission and kidney resorption to heart muscle contraction require the right balance of minerals. Excesses or deficiencies cause toxic symptoms.

Acid-base (pH) Balance Because enzymes are exquisitely sensitive to their ionic environment and require a limited range of hydrogen ion concentration to catalyze reactions, excessive acids or bases will alter enzyme function and, in the extreme cases, denature (irreversibly damage) them.

Blood Sugar Imbalance A wide variety of foods can imbalance the body's chemistry. For example, excessive consumption of REFINED CARBOHYDRATES may trigger postprandial HYPOGLYCEMIA (low BLOOD SUGAR after a meal), when the pancreas releases the hormone insulin into the blood rapidly to compensate for the surge in blood sugar. Overcompensation by insulin causes blood sugar to plummet below normal levels until other hormonal compensating mechanisms take over.

Amino Acids Blood levels of certain AMINO ACIDS are linked to mood, thus affecting behavior. The brain and nervous system convert several amino acids to NEUROTRANSMITTERS, chemicals for nerve transmission. Low neurotransmitter production is believed to affect brain function. For example, DEPRESSION has been linked to low levels of the neurotransmitters dopamine and norepinephrine, formed from the amino acid TYROSINE. SEROTONIN is linked to decreased sensitivity to pain and to sleep and relaxation. This neurotransmitter is synthesized from the amino acid TRYPTOPHAN. The levels of dopamine, norepinephrine, and serotonin in the brain also depend on the levels of precursor amino acids in the bloodstream, and this in turn depends to an extent on the type of foods consumed.

Trace Minerals A wide range of mineral imbalances are possible. Excessive COPPER and inadequate ZINC consumption correlates with periodic violent behavior in some individuals. Excessive zinc intake can suppress immunity temporarily and can block copper absorption. Excessive CALCIUM consumption can block IRON uptake, leading to FATIGUE.

Vitamin Deficiencies Deficiencies of most vitamins will affect behavior. Thus VITAMIN B_{12} deficiency is linked to memory loss in susceptible individuals; a classical symptom of NIACIN deficiency is DEMENTIA; severe THIAMIN deficiency is linked to nervous disorders.

Food Allergies In addition to rapid responses like asthma, hive, and runny nose, food allergies can cause slow-developing symptoms. Inappropriate immune responses can cause a large variety of symptoms ranging from headache to joint pain. The subsequent inflammation of the intestine can lead to the "leaky gut" syndrome, in which normally excluding antigens (foreign materials) can penetrate the body, setting the stage for multiple food allergies and malabsorption of nutrients.

Food Sensitivities This broad term refers to any negative physiologic response to food. A common example is LACTOSE INTOLERANCE, which does not involve the immune system. It can cause diarrhea, bloating, and intestinal upset. However, avoiding milk because of lactose intolerance can lead to calcium malnutrition.

Pollutants As an example of HEAVY METALS toxicity, LEAD poisoning is associated with a shortened attention span, slowed learning and development in children, ANEMIA, and chronic fatigue. Toxic heavy metals also interfere with the uptake and the function of many trace mineral nutrients. PESTICIDES, flame retardants (PBBs), and transformer insulation (PCBs) can adversely alter METABOLISM, and in extreme cases cause chronic illnesses such as cancer.

Drugs Many prescription drugs can create imbalances profoundly affecting mood and behavior. VITAMIN B_6 deficiency can be caused by drugs used to treat tuberculosis, high blood pressure (hydralzaine), Parkinson's disease (L-dopa), and oral contraceptives. Folacin deficiency may be caused by cancer chemotherapy (methotrexate). Vitamin B_{12} deficiency can be caused by drugs used to treat diabetes, tuberculosis, and high blood CHOLESTEROL. Tardive dyskinesia is a frequent side effect of antipsychotic drugs. ALCOHOL modulates many physiologic processes and excessive use leads to malnutrition. Alcohol imbalances liver metabolism, and over time, alcohol abuse will irreversibly damage the liver, as well as the brain. (See also ALLERGY, FOOD; CARBOHYDRATE; FOOD; MALNUTRITION; METABOLISM.)

chemical score A measure of the quality of a food PROTEIN based on its amino acid content. The chemical score relies on a comparison of a food protein with a reference protein, rich in all ESSENTIAL AMINO ACIDS, such as egg protein. Specifically, the chemical score is the percentage of the essential amino acid found in the lowest concentration in the food protein, divided by the percentage of that same amino acid that occurs in the reference food protein. For example, a chemical score of 65 indicates that the limiting (less abundant) essential amino acid in the food protein is only 65 percent of the amount found in egg protein.

The World Health Organization has published tables of chemical scores for food proteins used throughout the world that permits a simple assessment of whether a particular protein source needs to be complemented. The data are easily obtained and amino acid analyses are inexpensive and convenient in comparison with the animal studies required to measure the BIOLOGICAL VALUE and PROTEIN EFFICIENCY RATIOS, other measures of protein quality. Hence nutritionists frequently use chemical scores to express the adequacy of protein in a food. However, the chemical score does not assess the degree of digestion and assimilation of a particular food protein source, and suffers from this important limitation. Amino acid analysts cannot detect toxins or other materials in food that could limit protein bioavailability.

chemical sensitivity Also known as multiple chemical sensitivity (MCS), this is a sensitivity to environmental chemicals. An estimated 15 percent of the U.S. population may experience symptoms when exposed to chemicals. Susceptible individuals can react to food and FOOD ADDITIVES, drugs and medications, tobacco smoke and other particulate pollutants, plastics, formaldehyde, perfume and scents, detergents, solvents, hydrocarbons (auto and natural gas), PESTICIDES, animal dandruff, pollen, molds, mildew, synthetic fabrics, and polyurethane insulation.

Chemical sensitivity can cause behavioral changes, learning disorders, FATIGUE, muscle pain, headaches, irritability, mood swings, breathing problems, irregular heartbeat, and even chronic antisocial behavior.

ENVIRONMENTAL MEDICINE is a branch of medicine dealing with people and factors in the environment causing illness. Clinical ecologists are physicians who deal with MCS. After consultation with a qualified health care provider, a personal strategy for hypersensitive individuals might entail avoiding contact with materials that provoke a response; avoiding highly processed food and allergenic foods (to improve digestion and absorption of nutrients); and taking VITAMIN and mineral supplements to remedy deficiencies and to normalize the body's chemistry and immune system. An immunologic treatment (desensitization) by an allergist also may be required. (See also CHALLENGE TESTING; FOOD POISONING; FOOD SENSITIVITY; ROTATION DIET.)

Matthews, Bonnye L. *Defining Multiple Chemical Sensitivity.* Jefferson, N.C.: McFarland & Co., 1998.

chemoprevention The policy supporting the dietary supplementation of specific nutrients in cancer prevention. The American Association for Cancer Research supports chemoprevention, which differs from chemotherapy (the use of drugs to destroy parasites, bacterial or virus, or cancer cells).

Potential anticancer dietary supplements are being clinically tested worldwide. They include VITAMIN A and its progenitor BETA-CAROTENE and other CAROTENOIDS: CALCIUM, VITAMIN B_6, VITAMIN B_{12}, VITAMIN C, and VITAMIN E; plus FOLIC ACID, SELENIUM, and wheat bran. One of the largest studies involved more than 22,000 male physicians who consumed 50 mg beta-carotene or placebo for 10 years (the Physicians Health Study).

After four years, researchers concluded that taking an aspirin tablet could lower the risk of first-time heart attacks, but after 10 years, investigators found no evidence that synthetic beta-carotene alone prevented cardiovascular disease mortality or cancer.

In general, studies of beta-carotene and carotenoid-rich foods suggest that beta-carotene must be protected by other ANTIOXIDANTS like vitamin E to be maximally effective, and that rather than acting alone, the combination of beta-carotene with other carotenoids and plant substances as supplied in a diet well stocked with fruits, vegetables, and legumes can lower the risk of cancer and heart disease. In addition, plant-derived antioxidants appear to be more effective in preventing the early stages of cancer induction, rather than in blocking later stages of tumor growth. (See also CANCER PREVENTION DIET; CLINICAL TRIAL.)

Greenwald, Peter, and Sharon S. McDonald. "Cancer Prevention: The Roles of Diet and Chemoprevention," *Cancer Control Journal* 4, no. 2 (1997): 118–127.

cherry (*Prunus*) A small, long-stemmed red fruit. More than 600 varieties are cultivated for edible fruit or as ornamental trees and shrubs worldwide. Cherry trees are native to many temperate regions of the world. Leading producers of edible cherries are Germany, Italy, France, Turkey, and the United States (Washington, Oregon, Utah, and Michigan). Most edible cherries are hybrids of European varieties. There are two main types, sweet and sour. Sweet cherries, the most common type grown, belong to the species *P. avium*. Common sweet cherries include Bing, Black Tartarian, Coe, Elton, Giant, Lambert, Royal Ann, Seneca, Schmidt, Windsor, and Yellow Spanish. Colors range from deep red (Bing) to yellow-red (Royal Ann). Most sour cherries (*P. cerasus*) are either canned or frozen commercially, for use in pies and pastries. Morellos (Morello, Olivet) have a red juice, while anarellos (Montmorency, Early Richard, Carnation, and English) have a colorless juice. Duke cherries are hybrids of sweet and sour varieties (May Duke, Late Duke, Royal Duke).

Cherries contain red-blue pigments known as anthocyanins. The FLAVONOIDS (plant pigments) function as ANTIOXIDANTS, to prevent oxidative damage and help reduce inflammation. In terms of their nutrient content, cherries contain fruit sugar (FRUCTOSE). Sour cherries provide more vitamin C and less sugar than sweet varieties. However, the addition of sugar in sweetened cherries increases their calories. Ten sweet cherries (68 g) provide 49 calories; protein, 0.8 g; carbohydrate, 11.3 g; fiber, 1.25 g; fat, 0.7 g; potassium, 152 mg; vitamin C, 5 mg; thiamin, 0.03 mg; riboflavin, 0.04 mg; niacin, 0.3 mg; and low levels of other vitamins and minerals.

chervil (*Anthriscus cerefolium*) A delicate herb with small leaves. Chervil resembles PARSLEY with lacy leaves. An annual with small white flowers, chervil is used to season stews, soups, or salads. It has a delicate parsley flavor and can be used in the same way as parsley. Turnip root chervil, *Chaerophyllum bulbosum,* is used as a root vegetable.

chestnut (*Castanea dentata*) A dark-brown nut with a shiny shell that pops out of a spiny burr when ripe. Chestnuts were used as food by ancient Greeks, Chinese, and Japanese and are today considered one of the most important tree crops. Almost all commercial chestnuts in the United States are now supplied by Europe. The chestnut

(*C. sativa*) native to southern Europe, northern Africa, and western Asia) is fungus resistant. The American chestnut, belonging to the beech family, was essentially destroyed by a European blight that began in 1904. The trees now grown in the eastern United States are blight-resistant crossbreeds of Chinese and Japanese chestnuts. (The horse chestnut is unrelated and is inedible.) Fresh chestnuts, in brown shells, are called roasting chestnuts and may be roasted, boiled, or dried. They provide more CARBOHYDRATE, less PROTEIN, and less fat than many other nuts. Roasted chestnuts (3.5 oz, 3/4 cup) provide 245 calories; carbohydrate, 53 g; protein, 3 g; fat, 2 g; potassium, 592 mg; thiamin, 0.2 mg; riboflavin, 0.2 mg; niacin, 1.4 mg; vitamin C, 26 mg.

chewing gum A flavored product for chewing, usually made with synthetic gums. Chewing gum bases provide no nutritive value, although added sweetness may contribute calories (four to six calories per stick). Gum bases include natural gums (such as chicle and natural rubber); synthetic gums (including butyl rubber, paraffin, polyethylene); and synthetic softeners (glycerated gum resin). MANNITOL is used to "dust" chewing gum sticks. It prevents gum from absorbing moisture and becoming sticky and is poorly absorbed by the body.

Sugarless gum is not calorie-free unless the label specifies "non-caloric." Most sugarless gum contains as many calories as sugared gum. Instead of sugar, SORBITOL may be used as a sweetener. This sugar derivative yields as many calories as sugar. Sugarless gum may also contain glycerol, hydrogenated glucose syrup, ASPARTAME, ARTIFICIAL FOOD COLORS, and BHA. Nicotine gum can lessen the craving for tobacco when abstaining from smoking. However, overcoming a nicotine addiction requires abstaining from all forms of nicotine, whether in cigarettes or gum.

Chewing gum can reduce the risk of tooth decay. Chewing any gum seems to lower the amount of acids produced in the mouth because chewing increases saliva flow, which neutralizes acids produced by bacteria living on carbohydrates in the mouth. Neutralization prevents the acids from dissolving tooth enamel. (See also CANDY; NATURAL SWEETENERS; TEETH.)

chicken The most popular type of poultry in the United States, and a dietary staple worldwide. Domestic chicken consumption has steadily increased since 1940 to about 73 pounds per person annually, partly because of changes in breeding and production that have made chicken more affordable and plentiful.

The increased popularity of chicken since the 1960s also reflects the shift away from BEEF, as consumers have become more concerned with SATURATED FAT and its correlation with high blood cholesterol and heart disease. A three- to four-ounce serving of cooked chicken provides half the adult protein requirement. Chicken is a good source of B vitamins and trace minerals, but has less IRON than red meat.

The modern chicken is fatter than in the past (80 percent of calories from fat), but much of the fat is associated with the skin. Trimming off visible fat and discarding the skin will reduce the fat content by up to 50 percent. Dark meat (thighs, wings) contains more fat (10 grams per 3.5-oz serving) but is more moist than breast meat. Roasting chicken at low temperatures melts away much of the fat. Chicken without the skin can be low-fat fare: A roasted, skinless chicken breast gets 19 percent of its calories from fat, well below the recommended guidelines of 30 percent of calories from fat. By comparison, the leanest steak gets about 37 percent of its calories from fat.

Yellow chicken has been fed more yellow corn than a pale chicken. Some suppliers add yellow materials like marigold petals, which give chicken flesh an appealing golden color, although it does not improve the nutrient content of the meat.

Chicken is graded by the U.S. Department of Agriculture (USDA) on a voluntary basis, as is beef. USDA grade A represents higher quality, while lesser grades are used in processed meat products. The grading system for chicken is based on appearance—a lack of tears or blemishes rather than on fat content—unlike the grading system for beef, which relies on fat content.

Fast-food chains have capitalized on consumer interest in chicken by offering more options, such as "nuggets" or "chunks"; their tastiness lies in their high fat and sodium content. A typical 4.4-ounce nugget provides 290 calories, of which 50 percent comes from fat. Ground chicken skin and breading used for frying are often major fat contributors. The sodium level can be as high as 500 mg per serving. Producers of convenience foods have followed suit by offering chicken "patties" and "rondelets," which contain ground chicken skin. They are breaded and fried and their fat content ranges from 50 percent to over 60 percent of calories.

With mass chicken production has come the increased risk of bacterial contamination. An estimated 25 percent to 33 percent of chickens and turkeys contain salmonella, a disease-producing bacterium. According to the U.S. Centers for Disease Control and Prevention, most of the chicken sold in the United States is contaminated with *Campylobacter jejuni,* a bacterium that is the leading cause of bacterial diarrhea in the United States. Conveyor lines in slaughterhouses have speeded up, leaving federal inspectors with only seconds to observed each bird. "Free range" chickens have been allowed to run more freely on farms, in contrast to mass-produced chickens raised in cages. However, both types of chicken are processed the same way, and both are subject to bacterial contamination by fecal matter on the production line.

Although thorough cooking kills bacteria, the burden is on the consumer to minimize the risk of food poisoning. Poultry should be refrigerated or frozen as soon after purchase as possible to avoid bacterial growth. To avoid contaminating other foods, chicken juice should not touch other foods. Everything that comes into contact with uncooked poultry and its juices should be washed, including cutting board and knife. Rubber gloves should be worn if the preparer has a cut. The skin should be removed before cooking; it is likely to be fatty and dirty. Cook poultry thoroughly—180°F to 185°F in the thickest part of the meat—to assure sterilization. Nutrient content: dark meat, 1 cup roasted (140 g) provides 286 calories; protein, 38.3 g; fat, 13.6 g; cholesterol, 130 mg; calcium, 21 mg; iron, 1.86 mg; thiamin, 0.1 mg; riboflavin, 0.32 mg; niacin, 9.2 mg.

Hurley, E. C. "The Skinny on Cooking Chicken," *Journal of the American Dietetic Association* 95, no. 2 (1995): 167.

chickpea (*Cicer arietinum,* garbanzo bean, Spanish bean, ceci pea) A tan-colored legume the size of a small hazelnut. Pods grow on a small, bushy plant and produce one or two edible peas; different varieties produce white, black, or red peas. Chickpea is native to Asia and has been cultivated since ancient times. Chickpea is now extensively cultivated in California, Latin America, and the Middle East. Chickpeas are a rich source of FIBER and PROTEIN and are often used in soups. They are a major ingredient of Middle Eastern, Latin American, and Indian cuisine; hummus and falafel are typical Middle Eastern dishes that include chickpeas. Soaking overnight before cooking softens chickpeas and shortens the cooking time. One cup cooked beans (163 g) yields 270 calories; protein, 15 g; carbohydrate, 45; fiber, 8.63 g; fat, 4.0 g; calcium, 90 mg; iron, 4.9 mg; potassium, 749 mg; zinc, 1.72 mg; thiamin, 0.25 mg; riboflavin, 0.13 mg; niacin, 1.3 mg. They do not contain vitamin C.

chicory (*Cichorium intybus*) A curly-leafed member of the endive family. Chicory is native to Europe and was cultivated by the Greeks and Romans. It can grow up to six feet high and possesses feathery leaves with dark-green edges. Chicory is now widely cultivated for its nutritious greens. The foliage is blanched to decrease the bitter taste and is used in salads. Plants given growth stimulants produce a crown of leaves (witloof); the greens are used as pot herbs. Chicory is an excellent source of BETA-CAROTENE. Several varieties yield edible tap roots, which are roasted, ground, and used as coffee extenders and coffee substitutes. The nutrient content of 100 g raw is 28.8 calories; protein, 1.7 g; carbohydrate, 4.7 g; fiber, 0.8 g; fat, 0.3 g; calcium, 100 mg; iron, 0.9 mg; potassium, 420 mg; thiamin, 0.06 mg; riboflavin, 0.1 mg; niacin, 0.5 mg; vitamin C, 24 mg.

chief cells Specialized cells in the stomach lining (gastric mucosa) that produce a digestive enzyme called pepsin. Pepsin initiates protein DIGESTION in the stomach. Pepsin is secreted as an inactive precursor called pepsinogen, which is converted to pepsin by stomach acid. Glands of the main body of the stomach contain both chief cells and PARIETAL CELLS, which secrete hydrochloric acid (stomach acid) and INTRINSIC FACTOR required for intestinal uptake of VITAMIN B_{12}. These secretions mix with mucus and are released as gastric juices. (See also DIGESTIVE ENZYMES.)

children's vitamins Supplements designed to help meet the growth requirements of children. The RECOMMENDED DIETARY ALLOWANCES (RDA) for children are usually, although not always, lower than for adults because of their smaller body size. However, children grow rapidly, and their requirements for nutrients remain proportionately higher. As examples, the RDA for vitamin A for a typical five-year-old (500 mcg of vitamin A) is half the adult's RDA (1,000 mcg). The RDA for niacin is 12 mg for children (four to six years), while the RDA for an adult is 19 mg.

An estimated 10,000 children in the United States under the age of six mistakenly swallow large amounts of VITAMINS each year. This statistic reflects the need to educate children that vitamin pills are not snacks. When they look and taste like candy, chewable vitamins are a temptation for small children. The most serious consequence of overdosing on children's vitamins is an IRON overdose, the symptoms of which are vomiting and diarrhea. (See also HYPERVITAMINOSIS.)

chili pepper (*Capsicum frutescens;* capsicum pepper) A spicy, hot PEPPER related to red bell peppers and the tomato. Hot peppers are unrelated to seasoning pepper, which comes from ground peppercorns.

Chili peppers were first used 5,000 years ago in the Americas. Some two dozen varieties are available in the United States, including poblano, Anaheim (long-lobed, either green or red), cayenne (a very hot chili used as a spice), habanero (lantern-shaped and the hottest domestic pepper), and jalapeño (a very hot pepper that is canned, pickled, and used in a wide variety of processed foods). Chili pepper is a good source of VITAMIN C, VITAMIN A, and POTASSIUM. The hot ingredient, a family of chemicals called CAPSAICIN, is very concentrated in the white tissue of the pepper, not the seeds. Apparently capsaicin evolved to shield pepper plants against animal predation.

Research suggests that consuming chili pepper can lower the risk of heart disease by decreasing the risk of blood clots. Chili pepper also increases APPETITE and the production of digestive juices and it may help relieve congestion in the GASTROINTESTINAL TRACT. Capsaicin may stimulate the production of endorphins, brain chemicals responsible for the so-called eater's high. Chili doesn't injure the stomach of most people, nor does it cause ULCERS. It can cause skin redness (a rubefacient), and chemically purified capsaicin has been used topically to reduce painful conditions like shingles and arthritis. Chili oil (hot oil), prepared from red chili pepper and sesame oil, is used in Asian cooking, including Thai and Szechuan Chinese dishes. (See also DIGESTION.)

China Project, The A six-year study of diet and health in the People's Republic of China that was one of the most comprehensive studies of its kind. More than 6,000 Chinese in 130 villages in rural areas of the eastern half of China took part in this survey, which generated more than 100,000 correlations among diet, lifestyle, and disease. In China, each region has retained traditional dietary patterns and generally relies on locally grown foods.

The study highlighted significant differences between the U.S. population and the Chinese. The average Chinese blood CHOLESTEROL level is 127, much lower than an American's average of 212. The average Chinese eats three times as much FIBER as Americans, consumes many more FRUITS, GRAINS, and vegetables, and eats MEAT only once a week. In countries such as the United States, where meat is frequently eaten, rates of CARDIOVASCULAR DISEASE are higher. For the Chinese, FAT accounts for an average 15 percent of daily CALORIES, while in the United States about 37 percent of calories come from fat. Although the Chinese consume 20 percent more calories than Americans, OBESITY is not a major health problem in China, as it is in the United States. The results suggest that a diet with 80 percent or more vegetables, grains, and fruits—and low in fat—may be optimal for health and longevity.

Patterns of Chinese mortality also differ from those in Western nations. The rate of colon CANCER is 50 percent that of Americans, while the rate of heart disease among Chinese men is one-seventh that of their U.S. counterparts. The rate of breast cancer is five times higher in the United States than in China. However, the leading cancer in China is stomach cancer, now rare in the United States.

In addition to diet, clearly heredity, exposure to environmental pollutants, quality of medical care, and other factors influence health. The Chinese in general are more physically active: They seldom depend on cars for transportation, bicycles are common, and the Chinese perform more physical labor throughout their lives. (See also AGING; DIETARY GUIDELINES FOR AMERICANS.)

chips A baked convenience food often prepared from corn or other grains or potatoes. These snack foods include corn chips, tortilla chips, and potato chips. Fruit and vegetable chips are gaining in popularity. Chips are generally high-fat foods. The best way to judge the fat content of a particular chip is to examine the percent of total calories that are derived from fat. Governmental agency guidelines recommend no more than 30 percent of calories from fat. Fat accounts for 60 percent of the calories in regular potato chips and 52 percent in corn chips.

"Light" chips, including fruit chips, generally get about 40 percent of their calories from fat and oils. Often manufacturers add "natural grains" to increase the nutritional value of chips. However, the main ingredients are often the same as that in the regular chip, with only a slight increase in fiber content. Chips are also high-salt foods; regular potato chips contain 133 mg sodium per 1-oz serving; regular corn chips, 233 mg; and regular tortilla chips, 140 mg. Some varieties are available with reduced sodium. (See also ACRYLAMIDE; DIETARY GUIDELINES FOR AMERICANS.)

chitosan Chitosan is derived from chitin, one of the three most abundant polysaccharides in the world and found in especially concentrated amounts in the exoskeletons of shellfish such as shrimp, lobster, and crabs. Chitosan is produced by grinding the shells of these sea animals into powder. The powder is then treated with chemicals (deacetylated) to produce chitosan, which is similar in chemical structure to the plant fiber cellulose.

Chitosan has been used commercially for years as a water purifier and to clean up oil and toxic chemical spills. When it is spread over the surface of water, chitosan binds to toxic substances, forming a scum that can be easily skimmed from the surface.

Chitosan has recently been successfully marketed as a "fat magnet," a dietary supplement that can speed weight loss. Producers claim that the same properties that make chitosan effective against oil slicks make it the perfect weight-loss pill. According to these claims, chitosan binds to fats in the stomach, preventing them from being digested and absorbed and consequently reducing levels of LOW-DENSITY LIPOPROTEIN cholesterol, the bad form of cholesterol.

Studies show that chitosan does prevent the absorption of some fat by the body but that the amount contained in the daily doses of dietary supplements is too small to significantly affect cholesterol levels. There is no evidence that chitosan can help patients maintain or lose weight. Moreover, because chitosan prevents absorption of fat, this reduces the body's uptake of the fat-soluble CAROTENOIDS and VITAMINS A, D, E, and K. Less serious side effects include gas, bloating, and diarrhea. Safety data are inadequate for pregnant and breastfeeding women.

Pittler, M. H. "Randomized, Double-Blind Trial of Chitosan for Body Weight Reduction," *European Journal of Clinical Nutrition* 53 (May 1999): 379–381.

chive (*Allium schoenoprasum*) An HERB that bears thin, hollow green shoots and is a small, hardy relative of onions and garlic. Chives are easily grown in a flower pot for a ready supply of fresh seasoning as an ornamental plant. The slender, tubular leaves, fresh or dried, provide a mild onion flavor to meat, stews, eggs, salads, soups, and vegetable dishes.

chlordimeform A common contaminant of COTTONSEED OIL. Chlordimeform was classified as one of the 10 most dangerous PESTICIDES by the National Academy of Sciences. Since the cotton plant is not grown as a food, permitted treatment with pesticides is less restrictive than for crops. Partially hydrogenated cottonseed oil is a frequent FOOD ADDITIVE in baked goods like corn chips and smoked oysters. (See also FAT; PROCESSED FOOD.)

chloride A major mineral NUTRIENT that occurs in body fluids. Chloride is prominent negatively charged ion (anion) and a predominant ion (ELECTROLYTE) of blood, where it represents 70 percent of the anions. Its negative charge balances positive charged ions (cations), SODIUM and POTASSIUM ions, to maintain osmolarity (total concentration of ions). For example, in serum the number of cations and anions both equal 155 milliequivalents per liter (MEq/L). The exchange of chloride and BICARBONATE between RED BLOOD CELLS and plasma, the cell-free fluid, helps regulate the pH and CARBON DIOXIDE transport by the blood. Chloride also functions with sodium and potassium in nerves to transmit electric impulses. Chloride is converted to stomach acid (hydrochloric acid) to maintain the acidity of the stomach; when stomach acid is neutralized, chloride is reabsorbed by the intestine and recycled.

Most dietary chloride comes from table salt (sodium chloride), which occurs both as a FOOD ADDITIVE and as a natural ingredient in food. Chloride is nontoxic, and a safe and adequate daily intake ranges between 1,700 and 5,100 mg. Chloride deficiency is rare because it is so plentiful in food. However, a chloride deficiency can occur with excessive perspiration, vomiting, or diarrhea. Chloride deficiency symptoms resemble those of ALKALOSIS (alkaline blood): apathy, irritability, and DEHYDRATION. Chloride is an essential nutrient for infants. Chloride inadvertently omitted from baby formula in 1978 led to poor muscle control, delayed speech, and slowed growth in affected infants. (See also ELECTROLYTES; INFANT FORMULA.)

chlorinated hydrocarbons A family of very stable organic compounds that have become widespread food contaminants. This class includes PESTICIDES (DDT, heptachlor, aldrin, diedrin); a wood preservative (pentachlorophenol); contaminants of processed paper products (DIOXIN); transformer coolants (PCB or partially chlorinated biphenyls); and cleaning solvents (carbon tetrachloride). Many are linked to cancer and chronic disease.

Chlorinated hydrocarbons in general are stable compounds due to their composition of carbon, hydrogen, and chlorine. Because they are fat soluble and are not effectively broken down in tissues, chlorinated hydrocarbons concentrate in fatty tissue. Chlorinated hydrocarbons gradually spread up through the FOOD CHAIN. Humans, carnivorous fish, and birds of prey, which occupy the top of the food chain, possess relatively high levels in their tissues. Though many chlorinated hydrocarbons have been banned or their use drastically limited by the EPA, they persist in the environment and are detected in fish caught in polluted waters, in MILK, and in livestock.

Most Americans carry trace amounts of the modified forms of DDT and dioxin in their fatty tissues. Traces occur in BREAST MILK because this is one way the body can remove fat-soluble materials. Women are encouraged to breast-feed, however. The benefits to babies are greater than the small risk of their ingesting these contaminants. BEEF TALLOW (fat) often contains traces of chlorinated and brominated hydrocarbons due to contaminated animal feed and pastures. Exposure to chlorinated hydrocarbons in the home and workplace should be minimized; the cumulative effects of low exposure and the long-range effect of mixture of residues on human health are unknown. (See also BREAST-FEEDING.)

Scheele, J., M. Teufel, and K. H. Niessen. "A Comparison of the Concentrations of Certain Chlorinated Hydrocarbons and Polychlorinated Biphenyls in Bone Marrow and Fat Tissue of Children and Their Concentrations in Breast Milk." *Journal of Pathology, Toxicology and Oncology* 14, no. 1 (1995): 11–14.

chlorine dioxide A BLEACHING AGENT used to produce white FLOUR. This agent works by releasing oxygen, which attacks pigments in flour. Concomitantly, it modifies AMINO ACIDS of PROTEIN and destroys much of the VITAMIN E content of flour. The use of chlorine dioxide was instigated after World War II to replace a bleaching agent found to cause convulsions in animals. By the 1980s powder bleaching agents had largely replaced chlorine dioxide because they are less expensive and are easier to manage than this toxic gas. The low level (14 ppm) of chlorine dioxide used to treat flour causes no adverse effects in laboratory animals, and it is considered safe as a bleaching agent. Since 1975, chlorine dioxide has been used in processing vegetables and fruits. (See also FOOD ADDITIVES.)

chocolate The extract of the cocoa bean of the CACAO tree, which grows within 20 degrees of the equator. To make chocolate, the beans are roasted, the shells are removed, and the meat of the bean is ground and extracted to obtain cocoa flavor, which is quite bitter. This extract represents the main ingredient of baking chocolate. Chocolate was consumed by the Aztecs in Mexico and the Mayans of Central America.

Chocolate CANDY originated in 1847. The candy contains 50 percent sugar, roasted cocoa, and cocoa FAT, which is a saturated fat. Usually the darker the chocolate, the more fat it contains. The total amount of fat in chocolate is higher than in BEEF. Milk chocolate was developed in 1876. It contains BUTTERFAT, SUGAR, and VANILLA, among other ingredients. The slight differences in very low concentrations of flavor compounds like aldehydes and other compounds give distinctive flavor to various types of chocolate candy.

Chocolate is generally the food most frequently craved in those countries where it is available. It is a complex food with more than 400 different compounds. Chocolate also contains stimulants, 20 to 30 mg of CAFFEINE and theobromine per ounce of dark chocolate. These stimulants can appear in BREAST MILK. In susceptible individuals, chocolate may cause irregular heartbeat. Chocolate contains TYRAMINE and phenylethylamine, substances that increase alertness and a sense of well-being. Chocolate contains significant MAGNESIUM (82 mg per oz.), which is frequently low in the typical U.S. diet. These factors, together with fat and sugar, may account for chocolate's widespread popularity. Chocolate consumption has been linked to BREAST CYSTS, food allergies, and heartburn. Despite notions to the contrary, chocolate does not cause ACNE, though psoriasis can be a symptom of an allergy to chocolate.

Chocolate sometimes develops a white discoloration ("bloom") due to improper storage, which could represent cocoa fat that has risen to the surface when stored too long at room temperature or sugar that has been drawn to the surface by condensation.

One ounce of plain milk chocolate (28 g) provides 45 calories; protein, 2 g; carbohydrate, 16 g; fiber, 0.3 g; fat, 9 g; calcium, 50 mg; thiamin, 0.02 mg; riboflavin, 0.1 mg; niacin, 0.1 mg. (See also ACID INDIGESTION; ALLERGY, FOOD.)

chocolate substitute See CAROB.

cholecalciferol (vitamin D_3) The most common form of VITAMIN D, occurring naturally in MEAT and DAIRY products. (See also CALCIUM.)

cholecystitis Inflammation of the GALLBLADDER. Chronic infection can change the lining of the gallbladder, altering its ability to keep CALCIUM and CHOLESTEROL in solution. Lowered bile acids or less water promotes cholesterol stone formation. Chronic cholecystitis is far more common than acute disease. It is usually associated with GALLSTONE formation and occurs most often in middle-aged and older obese women. The cause is poorly understood, but bacterial infection may be involved. Crohn's disease, cystic fibrosis, and parasitic infection of the gallbladder increase the risk of gallbladder disease. Acute cholecystitis, although rare, is more likely to involve a medical emergency. In most cases it is caused by the impaction of a gallstone in the neck of the gallbladder or the duct.

cholecystokinin (pancreozymin) A HORMONE produced by the upper segment of the small intestine. Cholecystokinin is released into the bloodstream as food moves into the intestine from the stomach. This hormone also stimulates the gallbladder to release BILE and the PANCREAS to release DIGESTIVE ENZYMES. Cholecystokinin also causes the feeling of SATIETY after a meal; it directs the hunger center of the brain, located in the region known as the HYPOTHALAMUS, to stop sending "hunger" signals. This process requires about 20 minutes. Bulimia (binge eating) is linked in some bulimic women to abnormally low levels of cholecystokinin after eating. Nonetheless, APPETITE and CRAVING are complex phenomena, unlikely to be controlled by a single chemical signal. (See also BULIMIA NERVOSA.)

cholesterol A waxy LIPID derived from food and from liver synthesis. Cholesterol is the substance from which all steroid hormones are obtained. Both cholesterol and FAT are classified as lipids because they do not dissolve in water. However, cholesterol differs from fat because it does not contain fatty acids and cannot be oxidized in the body for ENERGY. Fat represents the body's major energy reserve.

Although cholesterol has the reputation of an unwanted, even dangerous substance, all cells of the body require cholesterol because it is an essential constituent of all cell membranes. Cholesterol forms sex HORMONES and hormones of the adrenal cortex, which regulate water and ELECTROLYTE balance, as well as the METABOLISM of CARBOHYDRATE, fat, and PROTEIN. In addition, the skin converts cholesterol to VITAMIN D, while the liver converts cholesterol to BILE salts, to digest and absorb fat. Bile salts are the primary way in which cholesterol leaves the body.

Cholesterol is not an essential nutrient because the body makes most of the cholesterol it needs. Liver synthesis produces approximately 50 percent of the cholesterol manufactured in the body. Cholesterol is constructed from a much smaller material, ACETIC ACID, used as an activated form (acetyl COENZYME A). INSULIN increases glucose utilization by tissues and stimulates cholesterol synthesis in the liver after a high-carbohydrate meal.

Cholesterol Transport

Because cholesterol does not mix with water, specific carriers are required to transport cholesterol in blood, which is mainly composed of water. The liver exports cholesterol to tissues by a carrier known as LDL (LOW-DENSITY LIPOPROTEIN), which accounts for 60 percent to 70 percent of the cholesterol in serum, the clear liquid remaining after blood has clotted. LDL is considered the undesirable form of cholesterol because elevated levels have been linked to clogged arteries. LDL originates from VLDL (VERY-LOW-DENSITY LIPOPROTEIN), a carrier of fat synthesized by the liver. Peripheral tissues such as muscle absorb LDL at specific sites on cell surfaces. HDL (HIGH-DENSITY LIPOPROTEIN), the so-called good cholesterol, plays a unique role in cholesterol metabolism. HDL acquires cholesterol from peripheral tissues and thus acts as a scavenger. HDL can exchange cholesterol with other lipid carriers, and it also transports cholesterol to the liver for disposal.

Cholesterol and Diet

Cholesterol occurs in animal products such as liver, EGGS, CHEESE, animal fat (BUTTER, lard), and in fatty meats like PORK and BEEF. Contrary to popular opinion, updated analysis indicates that SHELLFISH like shrimp do not contain unusually high amounts of cholesterol. Vegetable oil, peanut butter, GRAINS, and VEGETABLES do not contain cholesterol because plants don't make it. In 1993, the U.S. FDA approved the following definitions of cholesterol content on food labels: "Cholesterol free" implies the product contains less than 2 mg of cholesterol per serving. SAFFLOWER oil is an example of a cholesterol-free product. "Low cholesterol" implies the product contains less than 20 mg per serving. Low-calorie MAYONNAISE is such a product. "Reduced cholesterol" simply means that the product contains 75 percent less than that in the original version.

In recent decades the average daily cholesterol intake in the United States has dropped significantly. Since 1978 average total cholesterol levels among U.S. adults have fallen from 213 mg/dL to 203 mg/dL. Nonetheless, consumption of saturated fat remains high. While increased dietary cholesterol tends to raise cholesterol levels, the type of dietary fat also has a strong influence on the blood cholesterol level. SATURATED FAT, including hard fats like SHORTENING, lard, butter, and hard MARGARINE, tend to raise LDL levels dramatically. Fats with a high content of saturated FATTY ACIDS, especially PALMITIC ACID, seem to stimulate cholesterol production. On the other hand, unsaturated vegetable oils tend to lower LDL and blood cholesterol levels.

In 1995 a survey of 38 clinical studies of the effects of soy protein concluded that eating soy protein significantly reduces moderate to high levels of blood cholesterol. For people with the highest cholesterol levels, the reduction averaged 24 percent with the consumption of an average of 31 to 47 g daily. Rather than simply adding soy protein to the diet, the recommendation is to replace animal protein with soy protein to decrease fat consumption.

LDL Cholesterol and Cardiovascular Disease

Elevated blood cholesterol is considered to be a widespread public health problem in the U.S. An estimated 40 million Americans have high blood cholesterol. People with high blood cholesterol are susceptible to heart disease due to clogged arteries (ATHEROSCLEROSIS). Furthermore, susceptible middle-aged American men may be prone to heart disease and colorectal cancer if their blood cholesterol is above 250. Since 1960, blood cholesterol levels, which represent predominantly LDL cholesterol, have dropped nearly 8 percent in the United States, most of this occurring since 1976 when public education programs geared toward lower dietary fat and cholesterol were initiated.

Whether elevated blood cholesterol increases the risk of coronary heart disease in older adults is not certain. Some reports have found a correlation between high cholesterol levels and increased risk of heart disease in elderly women but not in elderly men. For men over the age of 70, there is a progressive decline in cholesterol levels, more so than in women. There is also an age-related drop in HDL, a beneficial form of cholesterol, and this is a better predictor of heart disease and death.

Although high LDL cholesterol may increase the risk of cardiovascular disease in middle-aged men in the United States and northern Europe, increased HDL levels in the blood lower the risk. Apparently, high LDL cholesterol can promote fatty deposits within arteries (PLAQUE) and, over time, plaque buildup can block arteries, causing coronary heart disease, HEART ATTACK, and STROKE. The actual culprit in damaging arteries may be rancid (oxidized) cholesterol and lipids in LDL, not fresh cholesterol in whole foods. Cholesterol in tallow used in some fast-food cooking, powdered eggs, and FRENCH FRIES is oxidized. Oxidized cholesterol is also found in pancake mixes, powdered custards, and powdered whole milk. LDL is a primary target of FREE RADICAL attack. Free radicals are highly reactive forms of oxygen that damage molecules by stealing their electrons. Therefore, ANTIOXIDANTS, such as vitamin E, may lower the risk by preventing the oxidation of LDL lipids. (Many other factors increase the risk of cardiovascular disease, including inheritance, smoking, OBESITY, HYPERTENSION, and DIABETES.)

Current guidelines advise reducing saturated fat consumption so that fat accounts for less than 30 percent of daily CALORIES. This translates to cutting back on fats and oils by one-quarter to one-third for the typical American diet. In addition, exercise may be recommended. The last line of defense is anticholesterol drug treatment, which needs to be carefully monitored. The long-term effects of these drugs are not known.

Cholesterol Measurements

Monitoring total serum cholesterol is frequently used to screen high-risk people. It has generally been assumed that the higher the cholesterol, the greater the risk of dying from heart disease. However, other indices such as LDL/HDL ratios or ratios of proteins that characterize each of these carriers, such as APOLIPOPROTEIN B/apolipoprotein A, correlate much better with risk. Serum cholesterol is measured as milligrams per deciliter (a deciliter is equivalent to 100 ml or 3.3 oz.) of blood. Regarding "normal" levels, the upper limit for normal is 180 for individuals under the age of 30; a cholesterol value below 200 is considered desirable for individuals over 30. Cholesterol between 200 and 239 is considered a "borderline-high" risk. Above 240, there is a high risk of coronary heart disease. An estimated 50 percent of American adults have elevated blood cholesterol by this criterion. For people with coronary artery disease, the total cholesterol value should be less than 160.

A single measurement of blood cholesterol is not reliable for diagnosis because of biological and test variation. Repeated tests help assure accuracy. Although the permitted uncertainty in cholesterol tests is currently 5 percent the American Heart Association reported appreciable variation among different testing laboratories. Factors affecting serum cholesterol levels include the time of day, the meal time, the month (January and February are highest), and whether the patient is sitting or lying down. Generally, blood is drawn before breakfast, with the patient seated. Finger-stick cholesterol values are higher than the usual test in which a blood sample is taken from a vein.

According to federal guidelines, a simple total cholesterol reading does not provide enough information for diagnosis and treatment; a complete serum lipid analysis provides a more accurate assessment. This involves measuring high-density lipoprotein (HDL), low-density lipoprotein (LDL), and blood fat (triglyceride) levels in serum, the cell-free fluid remaining after blood has clotted. An average of several tests may provide more accurate assessment than a single test. LDL should be below 130 for people with fewer than two risk factors and without coronary heart disease. If the LDL value is between 130 and 159 (borderline high), the situation needs to be watched, while LDL above 160 is considered a high risk for people without coronary heart disease and who have fewer than two risk factors. With coronary artery disease, LDL levels should be below 100. HDL is an important indicator of the risk of heart disease, and HDL levels of 35 or less increase the risk of heart disease. Values of 60 or more confer protection.

A complete lipoprotein analysis, which measures HDL to obtain a ratio of total cholesterol to HDL, is prudent for those whose cholesterol is 240 or above, and for those with several risk factors for heart disease. A ratio above four increases the risk of heart disease. The most discriminating cholesterol tests to assess the risk of heart disease measure the ratio of serum Apoprotein A-1 to Apoprotein B. This ratio correlates highly in the degree of coronary artery blockage. Apo A-1 is a specific protein marker for HDL and Apo B a specific for LDL. High levels of another cholesterol carrier called lipoprotein(a), a close relative of the LDL-cholesterol, are a risk factor for children who may develop heart disease later in life.

National Cholesterol Education Program (NCEP)

Sponsored by the National Heart, Lung, and Blood Institute, this program is designed to alert Americans to the presumed link between blood cholesterol and coronary heart disease. The message is that people over 20 should have their total blood cholesterol and HDL levels measured at least every five years. A person with a high blood cholesterol (240 or more), with coronary artery disease, or with borderline high cholesterol and two or more risk factors for heart disease, should get a complete blood lipid profile (total cholesterol, HDL, and triglycerides). Heart disease risk factors are considered to be age, a family history of heart attacks, current smoking, high blood pressure, diabetes, and HDL below 35. Even when total cholesterol is normal, a complete lipid profile is recommended when the HDL level is below 35 for women over 55 and men over 45. The desirable level of triglycerides is less than 200.

Adults with high blood cholesterol should change their diet and lifestyle as their first line of defense. Cutting back on saturated fat and avoiding excess calories are priorities.

Cholesterol and Children's Diets

American children have significantly higher blood cholesterol levels than children in other industrial countries. About 30 percent of U.S. children have high blood cholesterol and 5 percent of children between the ages of five and 14 years have very high blood cholesterol levels. Experts generally agree that atherosclerosis begins in childhood with the appearance of "fatty streaks" (fat deposits) in arteries that are thought to lead to clogged arteries in adult life. Clogged arteries can lead to heart disease, and one-third of U.S. adults will have a heart attack by the age of 60. Family history increases the odds of clogged arteries. Therefore, high-risk children (those from families in which the father or grandfather has had heart disease at the age of 55 or younger, or the mother or grandmother has had heart disease at the age of 65 or younger, or in which a parent has high blood cholesterol) should have their cholesterol levels tested.

In 1991, the National Cholesterol Education Program (NCEP) recommended that children older than two (but not younger) adopt a low-fat, low-cholesterol diet, with a maximum of 30 percent of calories from fat and only 10 percent of the calories coming from saturated fat. Many cardiologists, the American Heart Association, and the National Heart, Lung, and Blood Institute recommend limiting a child's fat intake to less than 30 percent of calories from fat after the age of two, while providing a balanced diet with enough calories to support rapid growth. Only one-third of their dietary fat would come from saturated fat sources (palm kernel and coconut oils, fat fried foods, cheese, fatty meat like hamburger, and ice cream). The American Academy of Pediatrics agrees with the cholesterol limits recommended by the NCEP but adds that children's fat consumption should be at least 20 percent of total calories over several days.

A specialist should be consulted before any child is placed on a diet. Dietary changes should be moderate because severe, fat-restricted diets create the risk of slowed growth in children who do not have enough fat, cholesterol, vitamins, and minerals to develop normally. Nutrition educators emphasize that parents can assist children in developing healthful, lifelong habits by providing nutritious meals and low-fat snacks and by supporting a healthful lifestyle.

Cholesterol-lowering Strategies

"Heart healthy" or cholesterol-lowering diets are designed to reduce LDL cholesterol. The underlying assumption is that eating foods excessively high in cholesterol can increase blood cholesterol, leading to an increased risk for cardiovascular disease. Only about one-third of Americans are sensitive to cholesterol in their diets. These "responders" experience an increase in blood cholesterol levels when they eat large amounts of cholesterol as found in eggs, butter fat, or meat. Another 25 percent respond to elevated saturated fat in their diets by increasing the level of blood cholesterol. There is no simple way to screen individuals unable to cope with high dietary cholesterol or fat.

The American Heart Association's Eating Plan for Healthy Americans recommends the following cholesterol-lowering nutrition strategies:

- Eating a variety of fruits and vegetables (five or more servings per day)
- Eating a variety of grain products, including whole grains (six or more servings per day)
- Choosing fat-free and low-fat milk products, fish, legumes (beans), skinless poultry, and lean meats
- Choosing fats and oils with 2 g or less saturated fat per tablespoon, such as liquid and tub margarines, canola oil, and olive oil
- Balancing the number of calories consumed with the number used each day. (To find that number, patients should multiply their weight by 15 calories. This represents the average number of calories used in one day by a moderately active person. Patients who are sedentary should multiply their weight by 13 instead of 15. Less-active people burn fewer calories.)
- Keeping physically active; walking or doing some other physical activity at least 30 minutes on most days
- Limiting consumption of foods high in calories or low in nutrition, including foods like soft drinks and candy that have a lot of sugars
- Limiting foods high in saturated fat, trans fat, and/or cholesterol, such as full-fat milk products, fatty meats, tropical oils, partially hydrogenated vegetable oils, and egg yolks
- Eating less than 6 of salt (sodium chloride) per day (2,400 mg of sodium)
- For women, consuming no more than one alcoholic drink per day; for men, no more than two. "One drink" means it has no more than 1/2 ounce of pure alcohol. Examples of one drink are 12 ounces of beer, 4 ounces of wine, 1–1/2 ounces of 80-proof spirits, or 1 ounce of 100-proof spirits.

(See also DIETARY GUIDELINES FOR AMERICANS.)

"Cholesterol in Food: Tempest in an Eggcup?" *Consumer Reports on Health* 7, no. 4 (April 1995): 42–43.

"Lowering Blood Cholesterol to Prevent Heart Disease," National Institutes of Health Consensus Development Conference Statement, 5:7.

cholesterol-lowering drugs Prescription drugs used to lower CHOLESTEROL levels in the blood. Very high blood cholesterol levels, together with a family history of HEART ATTACKS, greatly increase the risk of heart disease. In only 1 percent to 5 percent of persons with high blood cholesterol is the basic cause FAMILIAL HYPERCHOLESTEROLEMIA, a genetically determined high blood cholesterol. To lower blood cholesterol in these cases, medication may be prescribed, together with weight loss, EXERCISE, and low-fat diet plans. The drugs of first choice for elevated low-density lipoprotein (LDL) cholesterol are statin drugs, which are very effective for lowering LDL cholesterol levels and have few immediate short-term side effects. These include the HMG CoA reductase inhibitors such as lovastatin, pravastatin, and simvastatin.

Some studies have shown that these drugs can reduce arterial plaque buildup even in patients who do not have high cholesterol levels. Researchers also discovered that statins might also reduce the occurrence of ALZHEIMER'S DISEASE.

Statins work by blocking a liver enzyme that is necessary in the body's production of LDL cholesterol. However, one brand of this category of cholesterol-lowering drugs, Baycol, was voluntarily recalled in 2001 after more than 30 people who were taking it died of complications related to severe muscle breakdown.

The most common side effects of statins are gastrointestinal, including constipation and abdominal pain and cramps. These symptoms are usually mild to severe and generally subside as therapy continues.

Another class of drugs for lowering LDL cholesterol is the bile acid sequestrants—cholestyramine and colestipol—and nicotinic acid (niacin). These drugs have been shown to reduce the risk of coronary heart disease in controlled studies.

Both classes of drugs appear to be free of serious side effects, but they can have annoying side effects. Nicotinic acid is preferred in patients with triglyceride levels above 250 mg/dL because bile acid sequestrants tend to raise triglyceride levels.

Other available drugs include gemfibrozil, probucol, and clofibrate. Gemfibrozil and clofibrate are most effective for lowering high triglyceride levels; they moderately reduce LDL cholesterol levels in hypercholesterolemic patients, but the U.S. Food and Drug Administration (FDA) has not approved them for this purpose. Probucol also moderately lowers LDL levels and has been approved for this purpose.

If a patient does not respond adequately to single-drug therapy, combined drug therapy may further lower LDL cholesterol levels. For patients with severe hypercholesterolemia, combining a bile acid sequestrant with either nicotinic acid or lovastatin can markedly lower LDL cholesterol. For hypercholesterolemic patients with high triglycerides, nicotinic acid or gemfibrozil should be considered as one drug for combined therapy.

choline (trimethylaminoethanol) A nitrogen-containing substance that functions as a building block of an important lipid, LECITHIN, and an important brain chemical, ACETYLCHOLINE. Lecithin is a phospholipid and a primary component of all cell membranes. As a membrane constituent, lecithin helps insulate nerves. As a NEUROTRANSMITTER, acetylcholine is one of the chemicals that carries impulses for cholinergic nerves. Choline is synthesized by most tissues from the essential AMINO ACID, METHIONINE.

Choline occurs in foods as a component of lecithin. Good sources of lecithin are egg yolk (1.5 percent); SOYBEANS (0.35 percent); beef liver (0.6 percent), as well as CAULIFLOWER, BEANS, LEGUMES, GRAINS, and WHEAT germ. The typical Western diet supplies adults with 500 to 900 mg daily. A deficiency disease has not been demonstrated in humans, and it is not clear whether a dietary source of choline is required for optimal health.

Proponents believe that choline and lecithin supplements may improve short-term memory in normal and in senile people, since the brains of Alzheimer's disease patients are deficient in acetylcholine and choline. However, these supplements do not reverse or arrest Alzheimer's disease. Diet doesn't boost the level of choline in the brain very much.

Choline may help the liver mobilize fat deposits (fatty liver) that accompany a decline in normal liver function; it is used in IV formulas to correct liver problems. Fatty liver occurs during STARVATION and ALCOHOLISM. Choline has been used to treat tardive dyskinesia, a twitching of muscles that can develop as a side effect of treatment with antipsychotic drugs. High doses of choline can cause dizziness, vomiting, and a strong fishy odor.

Canty, D. J., and S. H. Zeisel. "Lecithin and Choline in Human Health and Disease," *Nutrition Reviews* 52, no. 10 (1994): 327–339.

chondroitin (chondroitin sulfate; CS) Long molecular chains composed of sugar units found in the body's connective tissue. This complex CARBOHYDRATE acts like a sponge, drawing nutrient-filled fluids into tendons, ligaments, and cartilage. This helps make the cartilage more shock absorbent.

As a dietary supplement chondroitin can reduce joint pain and inflammation and may help maintain or repair cartilage. It is still unclear how this is achieved; however, patients who have taken chondroitin supplements show increased levels of hyaluronic acid, a primary component of the synovial fluid that lubricates joints. These benefits seem to increase when chondroitin is taken in combination with glucosamine, an AMINO ACID needed by the body to form connective tissue. Patients suffering from osteoarthritis who took chondroitin and glucosamine supplements showed reduced pain and improved joint mobility. There is also some evidence that suggests that chondroitin may reduce the risk of myocardial infarction in those with previous heart attacks and those with unstable angina.

Oral CS has been used safely in studies lasting from two months to six years. There is inadequate safety data regarding use during pregnancy and breast-feeding, so CS should not be used during these times. There are some indications that glucosamine can increase blood sugar levels, so people with diabetes should avoid taking supplements that mix chondroitin with glucosamine, unless this is done under a doctor's supervision. Because supplements are derived from cow's trachea there is some concern regarding associated risks of contamination.

McAlindon, Timothy E. et al. "Glucosamine and Chondroitin for Treatment of Osteoarthritis: A Systematic Quality Assessment and Meta-Analysis," *Journal of the American Medical Association* 283 (2000): 1,469–1,475.

chromium A trace mineral nutrient, needed only in minute amounts to help increase the body's sensitivity to the HORMONE insulin for efficient utilization of surplus GLUCOSE. Its role in metabolism was discovered in 1969. Chromium is converted in yeast and in tissues to GLUCOSE TOLERANCE FACTOR, in which chromium is complexed with nutrients like AMINO ACIDS and niacin. In this form, chromium can assist insulin. As a supplement, chromium may be effective in treating high blood sugar (hyperglycemia) in some elderly patients, and in some diabetics, as well as in healthy non-diabetic people. It may protect against a form of non-insulin-dependent diabetes. However, clinical studies of this aspect have yielded mixed results. Chromium may protect against CARDIOVASCULAR DISEASE by helping to regulate FAT and CHOLESTEROL synthesis in the liver and by raising HDL ("desirable" cholesterol) and by lowering LDL ("undesirable") in the blood.

Only the less oxidized form of chromium (Cr^{3+}) is biologically active and can be used by cells. The more oxidized form (Cr^{+6}) is a toxic industrial waste product, which is not formed in the body. The human body contains only very low levels of chromium (an estimated 6 mg or less). Chromium in food is poorly assimilated and only 1 percent to 5 percent of dietary chromium is absorbed. It is estimated that 90 percent of Americans consume less than 40 mcg of chromium daily, and many people may be chromium deficient, especially elderly persons, pregnant or lactating women, athletes, and healthy people who rely on PROCESSED FOOD. Chromium loss increases with injury, STRESS, AGING, and strenuous EXERCISE. Consuming excessive SUGAR increases chromium losses from the body and lost chromium is slow to be replaced. Consequently, chromium levels decline with age.

Chromium deficient animals exhibit weight loss, lowered male fertility, elevated blood sugar, ATHEROSCLEROSIS, and nerve degeneration. Deficiency symptoms in humans include intolerance of ALCOHOL and a decreased ability to use insulin to help metabolize blood sugar, a prediabetic condition. Chromium supplementation, either as chromium chloride or chromium picolinate, did not increase strength or improve body composition (in terms of increased muscle mass or decreased body fat) in male volunteers participating in an eight week weight-training program. Possibly, the beneficial effects of chromium can occur when people are deficient in chromium. Chromium supplementation can lower iron transport and distribution in the body, possibly placing the individual at risk for iron deficiency.

The chromium intake for optimum health isn't known. A safe and adequate dose is thought to be 50 to 200 mcg daily. BREWER'S YEAST is the best food source. Other sources are liver, oysters, whole potatoes, egg yolks, prunes, mushrooms, WINE, BEER, MEAT, and BEETS. Fruits are low in chromium; so are polished rice and bleached flour. Chromium levels in GRAINS and vegetables depend on the amount of chromium in the soil in which they were grown; however, chromium in vegetables isn't well absorbed. Surprisingly, calcium-fortified BREAKFAST CEREALS are often good sources of the mineral because added calcium contains chromium as a contaminant. Supplemental chromium is available as chromium chloride. When taken together with niacin, its effect on lowering blood lipids is significantly improved, and the combination is as effective as taking yeast glucose tolerance factor. Several organically complexed forms of chromium such as chromium picolinate may be more readily absorbed than chromium chloride as supplements. (See also GLYCEMIC INDEX.)

chronic fatigue syndrome (CF) A complex syndrome with persistent flulike symptoms with fever, lymph node swelling, joint and muscle pain, often with mood swings and other psychological symptoms. Although controversial, a clinical diagnosis of CFS may be confirmed by the following CDC criteria: fatigue causing a 50 percent reduction in activity for at least six months, exclusion of other illnesses that can cause chronic fatigue; presence of at least four of several symptoms, including recurrent sore throat; painful lymph node; muscle weakness; prolonged fatigue after exercise; recurrent headaches; joint pain; neurological symptoms (forgetfulness, confusion); and sudden onset of the above symptoms.

CFS is a major public health concern in the United States and several other Western countries. The cause or causes of CFS remain unknown. Attention has focused on the possibility of a viral infection. Possible candidates include Epstein-Barr virus (EBV), herpes virus HHV-6, and enteroviruses (polio, Coxsackie, and Echo) since these have been shown to be active in some patients. Evidence for the presence of an RNA-containing virus (HTLV), and the fact that the antiviral drug seems to benefit at least some patients, argues for the involvement of a virus as an infectious agent in CFIDS. Another hypothesis suggests that an immune disorder is the underlying cause of symptoms. A variety of immune system abnormalities have been observed in patients with CFIDS, including depressed natural killer T cell and white cell activity. FIBROMYALGIA, a chronic musculoskeletal pain, is a closely related syndrome.

Fatigue is often the result of preexisting conditions, including DIABETES MELLITUS, ANEMIA, CANCER, chronic pain, RHEUMATOID ARTHRITIS, prescription drug use (such as tranquilizers, antihistamines, birth control pills), DEPRESSION, liver conditions, toxic exposure, and HYPOTHYROIDISM. STRESS may also be involved in CFIDS and often patients are deficient in the adrenal steroid hormones, CORTISOL and DHEA. Many patients with CFIDS have food allergies, which can worsen fatigue symptoms. There is also a well-established connection between chronic fatigue and HYPOGLYCEMIA. LEAKY GUT SYNDROME, in which persistent intestinal inflammation leads to the uptake of potentially harmful substances, is sometimes implicated in CFIDS.

Although there is no published scientific evidence that CFS is caused by a nutritional deficiency, enhancement of the immune system is likely to be one of the most vital steps in achieving resistance and reducing susceptibility to viral infection. Nutritional support of the immune system includes trace minerals, particularly zinc, selenium, chromium, and manganese; and vitamins, especially B_6, B_{12}, pantothenic acid, and FOLIC ACID. BETA-CAROTENE is a potent antioxidant and is an effective booster of the immune system. Vitamin C helps increase the immune response. Magnesium deficiency has been suggested as a possible factor in CFIDS. Injections of this mineral, as well as vitamins, may be beneficial. A diet that eliminates allergenic foods and simple and refined carbohydrates can help balance the body's defenses. Alternatively, chelated minerals (such as potassium, magnesium aspartate) may help alleviate fatigue. Siberian ginseng has a reputation for enhancing stamina. COENZYME Q and ANTIOXIDANTS can help support efficient energy production. Branched chain amino acids (VALINE, LEUCINE, and ISOLEUCINE) are preferred fuels of muscles and have been prescribed. Certain supplements, including N-acetyl CYSTEINE and GLUTATHIONE, support liver disposal of toxic substances. Glutamine and folic acid can help normalize gut function. Anti-inflammatory drugs and antidepressants may help. Therapeutic doses of steroids, hormones such as DHEA, and cortisol may be beneficial when these hormones are low. Whole, minimally processed food including garlic and onions and fresh fruit may also assist in normalizing the immune system.

Mawle, A. C. et al. "Immune Responses Associated with Chronic Fatigue Syndrome: A Case–Control Study," *Journal of Infectious Diseases* 175 (1997): 136–141.

chutney A sweet-sour condiment prepared from a wide variety of fruit and vegetables. Chutney is cooked in vinegar and sugar and has the consistency of jam. Chutneys originated in Britain as an attempt to reproduce Indian recipes for a relish made of vegetables, sweet fruits, and hot pepper. PLUMS, APPLES, raisins, and unripened tomatoes are other examples of foods that can be used. More exotic fruit like mango and tamarind can also be used. Chutneys can be seasoned with GINGER, GARLIC, or CHILI PEPPER.

chylomicron A lipid-protein particle that transports dietary FAT and fat-soluble vitamins to the liver, muscles, and fat tissue via the lymph and the bloodstream. Chylomicrons keep water-insoluble lipids suspended in body fluids, which are mainly water. In this sense they can be considered emulsifying agents. Normally chylomicrons disappear from the blood within a few hours after a meal, as the fat they carry is consumed.

Chylomicrons demonstrate a complex metabolic history. After cells lining the small intestine (intestinal mucosa) absorb fatty acids from fat digestion, they convert them back to fat before packaging them as chylomicrons, to be released into the lymph. The lymph carries chylomicrons into the bloodstream. When chylomicrons reach the capillaries, they encounter an enzyme that breaks down the fat molecules in chylomicrons to free fatty acids. Released fatty acids are quickly taken up by cells for energy or fat storage. The deflated chylomicron remnants carry vitamins and cholesterol to the liver for storage or processing. (See also HIGH-DENSITY LIPOPROTEIN; LOW-DENSITY LIPOPROTEIN; VERY LOW-DENSITY LIPOPROTEIN.)

chyme The homogeneous, semiliquid mixture of masticated food and digestive juices found in the stomach. GASTRIC JUICE provides hydrochloric acid and PEPSIN to initiate protein digestion of chyme. PERISTALSIS, the rhythmic contraction of the stomach, and the periodic opening of the valve between the stomach and intestine move chyme from the stomach into the small intestine for complete DIGESTION and absorption of nutrients. (See also DIGESTION; STOMACH ACID.)

chymotrypsin A potent digestive ENZYME secreted by the PANCREAS for protein digestion. Like other proteolytic (protein-degrading) enzymes, chymotrypsin is synthesized and secreted as an inactive form (ZYMOGEN) to prevent the pancreas from digesting itself. Pancreatic zymogens are activated only when they reach the intestine where their powerful digestive action breaks down food. An intestinal enzyme called enteropeptidase triggers this activation. Proteins are chains of amino acids linked together by peptide bonds, and chymotrypsin breaks bonds next to the amino acids PHENYLALANINE, TYROSINE, and METHIONINE within protein chains. Other proteolytic enzymes clip protein chains at other amino acid links, so that food proteins are reduced to single amino acids. Therefore, chymotrypsin complements the activity of other major proteolytic enzymes. (See also DIGESTIVE ENZYMES.)

cider (apple cider) The juice from pulped, pressed APPLES. Sweet cider refers to unfermented juice, while fermented or hard cider contains ALCOHOL and is carbonated; in Europe, the term *cider* refers to fermented apple juice. In the United States and Canada, homemade cider is unprocessed, with a sweet flavor. It will eventually ferment and turn into a vinegar. Basic cider preparation has changed little over the years: Whole apples are grated in a mill and the juice is extracted with a press. Preservatives are often added to commercially prepared cider, which is then pasteurized before being bottled. Frozen apple concentrate, first introduced in the 1960s, is a common household substitute for cider. Mulled cider has been heated with cloves and cinnamon sticks. Applejack refers to cider brandy, prepared by distilling hard cider. Cider VINEGAR is a mild, yellow vinegar, prepared from hard cider, containing between 5 percent and 6 percent ACETIC ACID; it is comparable to wine vinegar.

ciguatera poisoning An illness caused by eating fish contaminated with a toxic substance, ciguatoxin, that is produced by algae. This toxin is carried through the food chain from the algae to certain fish that eat the algae. Ciguatera poisoning has been most frequently associated with amberjack, grouper, goatfish, barracuda, and snapper caught in Hawaii, Puerto Rico, the Virgin Islands, Florida, and Guam.

Symptoms appear within six hours after eating contaminated fish. They include headache, dizziness, blurred vision, joint and muscle pain, a metallic aftertaste, and sensations of alternating hot and cold. Very rarely does it cause death. The toxin is not destroyed by cooking. (See also FOOD POISONING; SEAFOOD; SEAFOOD INSPECTION.)

circulatory system The cardiovascular system (veins, arteries, CAPILLARIES, the heart) and the lymphatic system devoted to transporting fluids though the body. The cardiovascular system is a true closed system because blood returns to its starting point, the heart. Pulmonary circulation refers to circulation of blood from the heart to the lungs and back to the heart in order to oxygenate the blood and to remove carbon dioxide loaded into the blood by tissue metabolism. Systemic circulation refers to blood circulating through the rest of the body. Arteries carry blood away from the heart to other tissues, and veins carry blood back to the heart. Capillaries carrying oxygenated blood from the smallest arteries (arterioles) distribute blood to cells; blood then flows into the smallest veins (venules). Blood pumped out of the heart follows this sequence: from arteries, to arterioles, to capillaries, to venules, then to veins and back to the heart.

The cardiovascular system contains about 5 liters of blood in the average adult. It provides nutrients and OXYGEN to every tissue. Waste products are removed from tissue; generally they are processed by the LIVER and excreted by the KIDNEYS. Hormones are released into the bloodstream where they are transported to their target tissues, to regulate physiologic processes and maintain the internal environment of the body. The IMMUNE SYSTEM relies on circulation to effectively defend the body from invaders via ANTIBODIES and defensive cells. The circulation system assures an even temperature regulation for the entire body. With circulating hormones and nutrients, blood provides an avenue for communication between the endocrine system and the brain. In addition, the bloodstream contains a system to plug leaks in blood vessels (clotting factors).

The heart beats an average of 70 times per minute; this is equivalent to pumping about 4 liters of blood per minute. At this rate, the heart pumps 260 liters or 85 gallons an hour. Considering that the heart beats an average of 36 million times a year, it is capable of an astonishing amount of work in a lifetime.

The circulatory system is subject to disease, such as hardening of the arteries and CORONARY ARTERY DISEASES. The coronary arteries, two small branches of the aorta that deliver oxygenated blood to the body, supply the heart with nutrients. Two diseases of the coronary arteries are prevalent. Angina pectoris causes severe pain in the upper left portion of the chest when insufficient quantities of oxygen are carried by the coronary arteries. Nitroglycerine dilates these arteries and provides temporary relief. Myocardial infarction (heart attack) occurs when the heart does not receive enough oxygen, for example when a blood clot or cholesterol deposits (PLAQUE) clog arteries. Blockage of coronary arteries by plaque is a leading cause of heart disease.

The lymphatic system collects fluid that has leaked into tissues and body cavities. It serves a unique transport function by returning water, serum proteins and electrolytes, and by transporting dietary fat to the bloodstream. Unlike the cardiovascular system, the lymphatic system is not a closed circuit: Skeletal muscles contract and relax to propel lymph through the lymphatic ducts. This fluid enters lymphatic capillaries and moves into larger lymphatic ducts and finally returns to the blood in veins in the neck region. The lymphatic system also plays a key role in the body's defenses. Lymph nodes house bacteria and virus-destroying cells as part of the body's immune defense. (See also ATHEROSCLEROSIS; CARDIOVASCULAR DISEASE; RED BLOOD CELLS.)

cirrhosis (liver) A serious LIVER condition involving extensive scarring and reduced liver functions. Scarring extends throughout the liver, altering tissue structure. This degeneration seems irreversible.

ALCOHOLISM is the leading cause of liver cirrhosis. Other causes include MALNUTRITION, chronic HEPATITIS, rare metabolic disorders leading to the deposition of IRON or COPPER, exposure to toxic chemicals and certain drugs, and a blocked bile duct. Destruction of liver tissue results in nausea, FATIGUE, low energy, susceptibility to bleeding, frequent infections, and OSTEOMALACIA (soft bone disease). Liver failure can lead to death. Treatment entails abstinence from the damaging agent and nutritional strategies, including vitamin supplements to bolster the liver (lipotropic agents). The prescription drug cholchicine has recently been used. Milk thistle (silymarin) is an herbal preparation reported to have a beneficial effect on liver metabolism.

A healthy liver is critically important to overall health. It produces most of the blood proteins like clotting factors (FIBRIN and prothrombin) and serum ALBUMIN as well as FAT, CHOLESTEROL, and their LIPOPROTEIN carriers; BILE for DIGESTION; UREA to dispose of the toxic nitrogenous waste AMMONIA; KETONE BODIES to fuel the body during starvation; and carrier proteins for iron, copper, steroid hormones, and others. The liver processes steroid hormones, drugs, and toxic chemicals for excretion, and it maintains BLOOD SUGAR levels between meals so that the nervous system is adequately nourished. (See also CARBOHYDRATE METABOLISM; DETOXIFICATION.)

Britton, R. S., and B. R. Bacon. "Role of Free Radicals in Liver Diseases and Hepatic Fibrosis," *Hepato Gastroenterology,* 41 (1994): 343–348.

citric acid (citrate) A common organic acid occurring in high concentration in CITRUS FRUITS and berries. For example, LEMON juice contains up to 8 percent citric acid. Commercially, citric acid is produced by the mold *Aspergillus niger* during the FERMENTATION of MOLASSES from sugar beets. Citric acid is a key to energy production in plants and animals. Citric acid is the starting point of the KREB'S CYCLE, the final energy-producing pathway of CARBOHYDRATE, FAT, and PROTEIN metabolism. Once citric acid is formed, a series of enzymic reactions converts it to CARBON DIOXIDE and OXALOACETIC ACID, a smaller acid that initiates the Kreb's cycle.

Citric acid efficiently binds or traps metal ions. This process is called chelation, and citric acid acts as a chelating agent. When ZINC and CALCIUM are chelated as citrates, these minerals are more efficiently absorbed by the intestine. Citric acid is used therapeutically to chelate heavy metals in the body and to prevent recurrent kidney stones.

Citric acid is one of the most common FOOD ADDITIVES. It adjusts acidity and contributes a tart flavor to fruit juice drinks and carbonated beverages. It also serves as an ANTIOXIDANT. It is often used with synthetic antioxidants which trap FREE RADICALS, highly reactive and damaging forms of oxygen. Citric acid traps metal ion contaminants that could promote SPOILAGE, RANCIDITY, or discoloration of many processed foods. It helps preserve fresh FISH, instant potatoes, and CHIPS. Citric acid is added to ice cream, sherbet, jellies, jams, canned fruit and vegetables, and CHEESE. Citric acid is used in wine making to react with traces of iron, which could precipitate TANNINS and make the wine cloudy. Citric acid, citrate salts, and citrate esters are considered safe food additives. (See also CARBOHYDRATE METABOLISM; CHELATE; FAT METABOLISM.)

citric acid cycle See KREB'S CYCLE.

citrus fruit Fruits of the genus *Citrus,* including LEMONS, LIMES, ORANGES, TANGELOS, TANGERINES, GRAPEFRUIT, PUMMELO, UGLI, and KUMQUATS. They all share a flavorful rind that is sometimes used in flavorings and teas. Citrus fruits contain many juicy wedges and their tart flavor is due in part to the high amount of citric acid. Citrus fruits originated in southern Asia and are now cultivated throughout the world, especially in California and Florida and in Mediterranean regions (Spain, Italy, Israel). Citrus fruits are used extensively by the fruit juice industry. They are consumed as fresh fruit or as preserves or in baked goods. Oranges, lemons, and limes are the most popular. The rind of lemon and grapefruit provides a commercial source of FLAVONOIDS, plant substances that enhance the effects of vitamin C. Citrus fruits are good sources of VITAMIN C and POTASSIUM. As an example, a medium-sized orange contains 80 mg of vitamin C; half a grapefruit, 47 mg; a tangerine, 26 mg. Several citrus fruits are more unusual. The Jamaican ugli is a hybrid of grapefruit and Mandarin oranges and is a popular citrus in Canada. It is more tender and juicy than other citrus fruits and has a sweet, unique flavor. Citron is used mainly for its very thick rind, which is often candied. Kumquats are the smallest of commercial citrus. They are the size of grapes with a bright orange rind. Blood oranges are closely related to Valencia oranges and other common oranges, except their pulp is scarlet red. Popular in Mediterranean countries, blood oranges are flavorful and have a sweet rind. The pummelo is quite large and resembles a grapefruit. It has a soft texture.

clam A mollusk with two equal shells that is a member of the invertebrate class, *Bivalvia.* More than 12,000 species are known, many of which are edible. The hard-shell clam or quahog is an edible clam found in North America. The northern quahog (*Mercenaria mercenaria*) is found from the Gulf of the St. Lawrence to the Gulf of Mexico and is the most important food clam in those waters. The southern quahog (*M. campechiensis*) is found from Chesapeake Bay to the West Indies. One of the larger edible clams on the West Coast is the geoduck (*Panopea generosa*), which grows along beaches lying between low tide and high tide from Alaska to Baja California. It can weigh up to 11 pounds and grows up to 20 cm in length. The soft-shell clam (*Mya arenaria,* steamer clam), found in oceans throughout the world, is used in soups and chowders. Other edible varieties include the donax or coquina clam (*Donax*). The northern species (*Donax fossot*) is found from Long Island to Cape May, New Jersey. The southern coquina (*D. variabilis*) lives in sandy beaches from Virginia to the Gulf of Mexico, while the razor clam is found on both the Atlantic and Pacific beaches of the United States. The Atlantic razor clam is *Ensis directus.*

In the United States the majority of seafood-related illnesses are caused by eating raw or partially cooked mollusks, including clams, which may be contaminated by harmful bacteria and viruses from seawater. For this reason, thorough cooking of mollusks is very important for anyone with LIVER, stomach, or immune disorders.

Red tides, caused by the overpopulation of microorganisms called dinoflagellates, can contaminate clams and their toxin can cause shellfish poisoning. Therefore, shellfish harvests may be banned at certain times of the year. Clams (mixed species, 100 g, raw) provide 74 calories; protein, 12.8 g; carbohydrate, 2.6 g; fat, 0.97 g; calcium, 46 mg; iron, 14.0 mg; sodium, 56 mg; riboflavin, 0.213 mg; niacin, 1.77 mg.

clarifying agents A class of FOOD ADDITIVES added during processing to react with contaminants that would otherwise turn cloudy or coagulate. Examples of clarifying agents include enzymes and chelating agents, such as citric acid and EDTA, materials that remove minerals such as iron and copper from liquids. (See also PROCESSED FOOD.)

clay eating See GEOPHAGIA.

clinical ecology See ENVIRONMENTAL MEDICINE.

clinical trial A carefully planned experiment, involving human subjects, to investigate the effects of a therapeutic agent or treatment. The experimental design typically incorporates a PLACEBO-controlled, double-blind procedure. In this case, neither physician nor subject nor patients know who has received a test material and who has received an innocuous substitute called a placebo until the study is completed. Those who receive the placebo are the control group and are used as a basis for comparison. Independent review boards must approve these studies, and participants are required to give their informed consent, based on the risks and benefits of the treatment. Selection of subjects for either the control group or the test group is random.

Group studies, such as large clinical trials, have several important limitations. They generally ignore individual differences due to each person's unique genetic makeup (BIOCHEMICAL INDIVIDUALITY). Treatment protocols that are effective in group studies rarely apply to all individuals; some may actually be harmed by the treatment. In addition, treatments that are effective for a small subgroup will often be ignored and the treatment be judged ineffective in such clinical trials. Nutritional therapies usually required long periods of time, possibly years, in order to detect an effect. Chronic conditions such as degenerative diseases of AGING may have developed over decades. Therefore, studies must be performed over a sufficient period of time for an observable effect. On the other hand, when studies are carried out over many years, study groups may no longer be homogeneous and the therapeutic approach may become outdated (different dosage, different treatment substance may be more effective).

In addition, epidemiology notes a variety of possible pitfalls in clinical studies. It may be difficult to establish which factor is a cause and which is an effect after linkage has been demonstrated. For example, low serum cholesterol and cancer are linked, but it seems that cancer can lead to a drop in cholesterol, rather than low cholesterol being a cause of cancer. Often, there are confounding factors, that is, many variables may be involved. Elaborate statistical procedures with their own limitations are used to sort out the contribution of each. The fact that a diet rich in fruits and vegetables is associated with a lowered risk of CANCER and CARDIOVASCULAR DISEASE may be due to increased consumption of fiber, trace minerals, ANTIOXIDANT nutrients such as VITAMIN C, FLAVONOIDS, CAROTENOIDS, or any of a huge array of PHYTOCHEMICALS typical of these foods. People who eat more fruits and vegetables may also smoke less, exercise more, and generally be more health conscious. Chance is another pitfall the researcher needs to be aware of. Typically, a result is called significant if the odds of it being due to chance are one in 20. The odds of a finding being a fluke can be quite low, but not 100 percent eliminated. Bias can also influence the result. As an example, a patient's preexisting health condition can be the major determining factor governing food choices.

Results obtained from this type of study are considered more reliable for groups of people than studies of single individuals or anecdotal information in which physician and patient know of the treatment and may have an expectation of its outcome. Knowing what treatment is being used and what results should be obtained to support an hypothesis can bias the evaluation by a physician or a patient. Clinical trials have been used to investigate the effectiveness of single drugs such as vaccines against polio, measles, and rubella; food allergies; and the effects of CHOLESTEROL-LOWERING DRUGS. However, clinical studies are less appropriate for examining nutrients and ANTIOXIDANTS, which often function synergistically as members of complex interacting systems.

In contrast with the large-scale intervention study of a group of people, clinicians sometimes employ "N of 1" studies to examine the effectiveness of a nutritional treatment on single patients. The N of 1 study features the patient serving as his or her own control. According to one design, the patient randomly receives either an active substance or an inactive treatment. Optimally, neither the patient nor the physician knows the sequence of treatment until after the study is completed. Each treatment period needs to be long enough to establish an active response, and the intermediate period needs to be long enough to establish baseline values during the inactive period. N of 1 studies can be generalized to groups by repetition with many subjects. (See also RISK DUE TO CHEMICALS IN FOOD AND WATER.)

"Clinical Trials: Help Yourself by Helping Others," *Consumer Reports on Health* 7, no. 2 (February 1995): 18–19.

Clostridium botulinum See BOTULISM.

Clostridium perfringens An anaerobic bacterium that is a potential source of FOOD POISONING. Strains of this bacterium produce toxins (enterotoxins) that can cause diarrhea, severe abdominal pain and flatulence 8 to 24 hours after eating. The symptoms usually end within a day, although older individuals can become seriously ill. *C. perfringens* occurs widely in raw and processed foods, and it can grow in food sealed in containers that are slowly cooled or kept warm for extended periods of time. Therefore, consumers should keep hot food hot, and cold food cold. Cooked foods should be kept above 60° C (100° F) or cooled to below 10° C (50° F) within two to three hours after cooking. As an added precaution, chilled foods can be heated to a minimum of 75° C (170° F) immediately before serving to destroy toxin-producing bacteria. (See also FOOD TOXINS.)

clove (*Eugenia aromatica*) An aromatic SPICE that is the dried flower bud of the clove tree. Clove is a member of the myrtle family and originated in the Molucca Islands. Cloves have been used since antiquity to season food. Cloves were used in ancient China for their medicinal properties and as a spice. They were introduced into Europe during the fourth century A.D. Whole or ground cloves find use in meat loaves, pork and ham, chili sauce, pickles, and in combination with other sweet spices, in baked goods like gingerbread, spice cake, and pumpkin pie. In mulled wine, cloves are often combined with cinnamon. Cloves enhance the flavor of bean soups, baked beans, and barbecue sauces. Clove oil has long been used to relieve the pain of toothaches and tooth extractions. The oil contains 60 percent to 90 percent eugenol, an analgesic (painkiller). (See also HERBS.)

coagulated protein Protein that has been cooked or otherwise treated to form curds or clumps. Soluble proteins in food often clot when exposed to heat, extreme pH, enzyme action, organic solvents, or extreme changes in concentration of the medium in which they are dissolved. Denatured or inactivated proteins are easier to digest because their AMINO ACID chains are more accessible to attack by digestive enzymes. Cooked eggs and meat juices are visible examples of coagulation by heat. Whey is a coagulated milk protein produced by acids of fermentation and by rennet during CHEESE manufacture. A protein such as egg albumin in egg white is soluble before cooking because the protein molecule is folded tightly into a ball whose outer surface is negatively charged so that individual protein molecules repel each other. When the egg is cooked, heat breaks the tenuous links holding the globular structure together, exposing sticky regions that permit protein chains to bind randomly, forming a sticky mass. (See also COOKING; DENATURED PROTEIN.)

coal tar dyes Synthetic dyes used to color processed foods, fabrics, and cosmetics. Originally these dyes were synthesized from compounds isolated from coal tar, itself prepared by heating coal in the absence of oxygen. Modern manufacture prepares artificial dyes from compounds obtained from various sources including petroleum, rather than from coal tar. However, this descriptive name persists. (See also ARTIFICIAL FOOD COLORS; CANCER.)

cobalamin The generic chemical name for VITAMIN B_{12}. As it occurs in supplements and many foods, it is called cyanocobalamin and contains a single cyanide ion bound to cobalt in cobalamin. The level of cyanide supplied by vitamin B_{12} supplements is entirely safe because the dosage is minuscule. In the body, a water molecule displaces the cyanide of vitamin B_{12} to form aquocobalamin, which is then converted to enzyme helpers (coenzymes). Methylcobalamin is an example of a coenzyme containing a bound single carbon atom. Cobalamin concentrate (USP grade) is used to treat vitamin B_{12} deficiency. (See also ANEMIA; INTRINSIC FACTOR.)

cobalt A TRACE MINERAL nutrient for bacteria. Its only established role in animals is as a component of VITAMIN B_{12}. Animals like ruminants that depend on bacteria for vitamin B_{12} require inorganic cobalt as a nutrient. Only microorganisms are capable of incorporating cobalt into vitamin B_{12}. The body cannot use unattached cobalt, and cobalt supplements are therefore ineffective. Though cobalt has a low order of toxicity, overdosing with cobalt could lead to goiter and overproduction of red blood cells in susceptible individuals.

Low concentrations of cobalt salts were once added to beer as an antifoaming agent. However, cobalt was incriminated in several epidemics of cardiac failure among beer drinkers. The typical American diet provides low levels of cobalt. Green leafy vegetables are the richest source, while dairy products and refined grain products are among the lowest. For example, spinach provides 0.4 to 0.6 mcg per gram, and white flour contain 0.003 mcg per gram. The oral intake of cobalt necessary to produce toxicity is many times greater than can be obtained by normal consumption of foods and beverages. (See also HEAVY METALS.)

cocoa A powder prepared from cocoa beans that is the raw material for CHOCOLATE and chocolate-flavored beverages. The name *cocoa* is derived from the Aztec word *caca huatl,* meaning "the beautiful tree of paradise." The Aztecs attributed to cocoa the power to convey wisdom and to heal. Cocoa reached Europe in the 16th century; but it was not until the following century that cocoa became a popular beverage.

To prepare cocoa, cocoa beans are dried, roasted, shelled, and ground to yield cocoa paste, the starting material for cocoa and chocolate. Cocoa paste contains 45 percent to 60 percent FAT or cocoa butter; the fat (cocoa butter) is partially removed to produce cocoa. The remaining cocoa cake is ground to obtain cocoa powder, which contains 8 percent to 20 percent fat. Treatment of cocoa with an alkaline solution yields "Dutch process" cocoa with a dark color and rich flavor. Instant cocoa contains SUGAR, flavorings, and an EMULSIFIER to suspend cocoa butter, in addition to cocoa powder. A cup of instant cocoa drink prepared with water contains 133 calories; protein, 4.8; carbohydrate, 30.2 g; fiber, 0.19 g; fat, 1.43 g; calcium, 118 mg; potassium, 300 mg; thiamin, 0.04 mg; riboflavin, 0.22 mg; niacin, 0.24 mg. Chocolate contains more sugar and more cocoa butter.

coconut (*Cocus nucifera*) The fruit of a palm tree. A coconut has an outer husk and a tough brown shell that encases a layer of white meat. The coconut probably originated in Polynesia, and it is now grown in tropical and subtropical regions worldwide.

Coconuts mature in a year. The hollow center of the coconut contains a sweet liquid called coconut milk. Coconut meat is a high-fat food, and COCONUT OIL is one of the most highly SATURATED FATS. Western recipes usually call for dried, shredded coconut meat when used in cakes, cookies, and candy. In many regions of the world, fresh coconut is used in condiments to season raw vegetables, and as an ingredient in stews. Coconut milk gives characteristic flavor to curries, sauces, and rice. The coconut is an important ingredient in African, Indian, Indonesian, and South American cooking. The nutrient content of 1 cup (80 g, shredded) of fresh coconut meat is 283 calories; protein, 2.7 g; fat, 34 g; carbohydrate, 12.2 g; fiber, 11.2 g; fat, 26.8 g; calcium, 12 mg; potassium, 285 mg; thiamin, 0.05 mg; riboflavin, 0.02 mg; niacin, 0.43 mg.

coconut oil A TROPICAL OIL obtained from coconut meat and used extensively as an additive in PROCESSED FOODS. Dried coconut pulp, called copra, is refined to produce this oil. Coconut oil is especially common in commercially prepared cookies, CHIPS, and baked goods, as well as in NONDAIRY CREAMER. A food label listing only "100 percent VEGETABLE OIL" will likely be high in coconut, palm, or palm kernel oils—all classified as SATURATED FAT. Coconut oil is 92 percent saturated, one of the most saturated of dietary fats and oils. By comparison, BUTTERFAT is 65 percent saturated. (See also FOOD ADDITIVES.)

cod (*Gradus morrhua;* codfish) A large food fish from the North Atlantic, the adult cod averages three to four feet in length and weighs up to 10 pounds. Cod is classified as a very lean fish with a relatively low-fat oil content. Roe (fish eggs), which can account for half a female's weight, are a source of caviar. Cod is among the top five fish eaten in the United States. Haddock and pollack also belong to the cod family. Cod is a versatile fish and can be broiled, baked, or used in chowder. A 3.5 oz. (100 g) portion, poached, represents 94 calories; protein, 20.9 g; fat, 1.1 g; cholesterol, 60 mg; calcium, 29 mg; iron, 0.5 mg; zinc, 0.75 mg; and niacin, 3 mg. (See also SEAFOOD INSPECTION.)

cod liver oil An important FISH OIL and dietary supplement of VITAMIN A and VITAMIN D. Cod liver oil also contains polyunsaturated FATTY ACIDS, EICOSAPENTAENOIC ACID, docosahexaenoic acid, and other omega-3 acids, that may help protect against CARDIOVASCULAR DISEASE and some CHOLESTEROL. A tablespoon of cod liver oil provides vitamin A, 12,000 IU; vitamin D, 1,200 IU; vitamin E, 3 mg; and cholesterol, 85 mg. Excessive consumption of cod liver oil can lead to vitamin A and vitamin D toxicity; these fat-soluble VITAMINS are stored and it is difficult for the body to rid itself of excessive amounts. The Recommended Dietary Allowance for vitamin A is 800 to 1,000 mcg (2,667–3,333 IU). Doses 10 to 100 times greater than this over a period of months lead to nausea, cracked skin, headache, and abdominal pain. Symptoms disappear when supplementation is stopped. (See also HYPERVITAMINOSIS.)

coenzyme An organic compound required by an ENZYME in order for it to function as a catalyst. Coenzymes are low molecular weight, often heat-stable substances, while enzymes are hundreds of times larger and are usually heat sensitive. As enzyme activators, coenzymes combine with the inactive PROTEIN (APOENZYME) to form the active enzyme (HOLOENZYME). Vitamins of the B COMPLEX form coenzymes that are essential in metabolizing FAT and CARBOHYDRATES for energy production. Each coenzyme serves a unique role in the body so that a surplus of one vitamin cannot correct for a deficiency of another. NICOTINAMIDE ADENINE DINUCLEOTIDE (NAD from NIACIN) transfers electrons in oxidations and reductions. FLAVIN ADENINE DINUCLEOTIDE (FAD, from RIBOFLAVIN) also transfers electrons. THIAMIN pyrophosphate (from thiamin) helps catalyze oxidations that create carbon dioxide from carbohydrate breakdown. COENZYME A (from PANTOTHENIC ACID) is used to carry fatty acids in metabolic pathways. BIOTIN attaches carbon dioxide to key intermediates while tetrahydrofolate (from FOLIC ACID) transfers single carbon fragments especially important in DNA synthesis. Pyridoxal phosphate (VITAMIN B_6) transfers amino groups ($-NH_2$) in the first step of amino acid degradation, while coenzymes of VITAMIN B_{12} transfer carbon atoms and alter carbon chains of several compounds.

coenzyme A An enzyme helper based on the B vitamin pantothenic acid that prepares FATTY ACIDS and ACETIC ACID to participate in biosynthetic and degradative reactions of cells. For example, when fatty acids are oxidized as fuel, they are first attached to coenzyme A. The enzymatic breakdown of AMINO ACIDS, FAT, and CARBOHYDRATE ultimately produces acetic acid, bound to coenzyme A (acetyl coenzyme A). In turn acetyl CoA is used to create new fatty acids, fat, CHOLESTEROL, and other important lipids. Alternatively, acetyl CoA is shunted to the KREB'S CYCLE, the central oxidizing process used by tissues to produce energy. (See also CARBOHYDRATE METABOLISM; FAT METABOLISM.)

coenzyme Q (ubiquinone, coenzyme Q_{10}, vitamin Q_{10}) A lipid oxidation-reduction agent found in MITOCHONDRIA, the powerhouses of the cell. Coenzyme Q helps mitochondria oxidize fuels like FAT and CARBOHYDRATE to produce cellular energy (ATP) in a process known as OXIDATIVE PHOSPHORYLATION.

Because most cellular processes require energy, coenzyme Q is essential for health. Coenzyme Q can be viewed as a collector of hydrogen atoms removed during cellular oxidations. Coenzyme Q is liberally distributed in membranes of the cell and possibly serves as a membrane ANTIOXIDANT. A protective role for coenzyme Q in mitochondrial membranes appears likely. The body can synthesize coenzyme Q and therefore it does not have vitamin status. However, deficiencies can occur in patients with heart disease such as angina and congestive heart failure, as well as in older people with high blood pressure. There is as yet no simple clinical test to measure coenzyme Q deficiency.

Coenzyme Q has been prescribed as a supplemental treatment for cardiovascular conditions, and it is a promising treatment for angina. Coenzyme Q supplements can aid cardiac patients, especially those with congestive heart failure who are deficient in coenzyme Q, and their use lowers high blood pressure. Coenzyme Q also bolsters the IMMUNE SYSTEM and may improve immune function in patients with AIDS or HIV-infection. Coenzyme Q helps protect against the side effects of radiation and chemotherapy in cancer treatment.

Promising results in animal studies showing that coenzyme Q might be effective against cancer prompted researchers in Denmark to conduct similar studies on small groups of women who had breast cancer. In many cases the women in these studies responded positively, sometimes experiencing complete remission. However, the results are not conclusive because many of the women were taking other supplements and receiving standard cancer therapy while they were taking coenzyme Q. No results of randomized clinical trials of coenzyme Q as a cancer treatment have yet been published in peer-reviewed scientific journals. No side effects have been reported for moderate doses. However, the issue of long-term safety of this supplement has not been explored. (See also CARBOHYDRATE METABOLISM.)

Overvad K. et al. "Coenzyme Q_{10} in Health and Disease." *European Journal of Clinical Nutrition* 53 (October 1999): 764–770.

Portakal O. et al. "Coenzyme Q_{10} Concentrations and Antioxidant Status in Tissues of Breast Cancer Patients," *Clinical Biochemistry* 33 (April 2000): 279–284.

cofactor A heat-stable enzyme activator. Most trace metal nutrients, including COPPER, IRON, ZINC, MANGANESE, SELENIUM, MOLYBDENUM, and MAGNESIUM, function as enzyme cofactors. Many enzymes carrying out oxidation-reduction reactions require iron. An example is catalase, which degrades HYDROGEN PEROXIDE to water and oxygen. The mitochondrial enzyme complex that ultimately uses oxygen to burn fuels, CYTOCHROME oxidase, requires copper, while SUPEROXIDE DISMUTASE, an antioxidant enzyme that destroys a toxic form of oxygen, requires manganese, zinc, and copper. Manganese is also required to operate the KREB'S CYCLE, the central enzyme system for oxidizing fat and carbohydrate for energy. The enzyme that destroys SULFITE preservatives (sulfite oxidase) and the enzyme that produces the nitrogenous waste URIC ACID (xanthine oxidase), require molybdenum as the cofactor. Magnesium and zinc are cofactors for hundreds of enzymes, including those for the synthesis of RNA and DNA required in cell division. (See also ANABOLISM; CATABOLISM.)

coffee A popular, mildly stimulating beverage prepared from coffee beans. Coffee ranks as the second most popular beverage in the United States after soft drinks. As many as 54 percent of U.S. adults drink coffee daily and among coffee drinkers, the average annual consumption is about 70 gallons per person.

Coffee beans are imported from Central and South America. They are cured either by air-drying or FERMENTATION. The dried, hulled beans are then roasted and ground. The beverage is prepared by extracting ground coffee with hot water (brewing). Brewed coffee is a complex mixture of more than 300 chemicals; CAFFEINE is perhaps the most notorious. A cup of coffee contains approximately 100 mg of this stimulant. Caffeine increases EPINEPHRINE (adrenaline) release, which stimulates the central nervous system, increases states of alertness and increases heartbeat.

Drinking coffee carries with it several risks. Coffee beans are grown abroad where fertilizer and PESTICIDES are not required to meet U.S. regulations; consequently there is an increased risk of contamination. In addition, caffeine can be habit forming; even a single cup of coffee a day contains enough caffeine to create the risk of withdrawal if it is suddenly eliminated. Coffee also can cause heartburn by relaxing the muscle between the stomach and esophagus, allowing stomach acid to rise into the esophagus. Although coffee does not cause ulcers, it boosts stomach acid production, which can exacerbate ulcers.

On the other hand, drinking coffee does not seem to lead to high blood pressure, pancreatic CANCER, or bladder cancer. The caffeine in coffee can block calcium and IRON absorption; coffee drinkers who avoid milk and dairy products need more calcium to minimize the risk of OSTEOPOROSIS.

Recent studies show that consumption of coffee and caffeine does not contribute to CARDIOVASCULAR DISEASE, including STROKE, even in people who drink more than four cups of coffee a day. Researchers also have found no link between coffee consumption and cancers of the bladder, breast, colon, lung, or prostate. At least nine studies have confirmed that regular coffee consumption over long periods of time may reduce the risk of developing Parkinson's disease.

Research shows that there does seem to be some correlation between coffee consumption and rates of miscarriage. One study showed that the risk increased only slightly in women who consumed as much as three cups of coffee a day, but another study showed that women who consumed between one and three cups of coffee daily increased their risk of spontaneous abortion by 30 percent. These researchers also noted that the more caffeine consumed, the higher the risk of miscarriage.

It is best to use a common-sense approach to coffee. Drink it in moderation—which, according to the U.S. FDA, is one to two cups a day. People with high blood cholesterol levels, coronary diseases, heart arrhythmias, and hypertension, and pregnant women may want to cut back on high coffee consumption and consumption of other beverages containing caffeine. Those who drink boiled coffee may want to switch to drip-filtered coffee. (See also ADDICTION.)

Ross, G. Webster et al. "Association of Coffee and Caffeine Intake With the Risk of Parkinson's Disease," *JAMA* 283, no. 20 (May 2000): 2,674–2,679.

Willet, Walter C. et al. "Coffee Consumption and Coronary Heart Disease in Women: A Ten-Year Follow-Up," *JAMA* 275 (1996): 458–462.

cola soft drinks Beverages based on cola extract. The cola tree produces a fruit with many seeds (cola nuts). These seeds yield a brown extract that contains CAFFEINE and is a mild stimulant. Typical ingredients of cola SOFT DRINKS include: cola extract, caramel as additional coloring, carbonated water, additional caffeine, high-FRUCTOSE CORN SYRUP or ASPARTAME as sweeteners, and PRESERVATIVES. (See also EATING PATTERNS.)

cold-pressed vegetable oil Vegetable oils that have been extracted from seeds under mild conditions. Consumers often assume that cold-pressed oils contain more essential nutrients like VITAMIN E and polyunsaturated FATTY ACIDS than more typical hot-pressed oils. This may not be true.

To prepare oils, seeds are first crushed and then pressed to expel oil. With the exception of olive oil, all vegetable oils are heated to varying degrees to increase their efficiency of extraction. Cold-pressed oils may be heated between 120° F and 150° F. Subsequently these oils are often purified, bleached, and deodorized. These processes can involve further heating, possibly as high as 450° F, and such products possess compositions similar to hot-pressed oil. Seed oils containing high levels of the essential polyunsaturated fatty acids (such as evening primrose oil, borage oil, and flaxseed oil) need to be prepared under mild conditions that exclude air, heat, and light in order to minimize rancidity. Vitamin E and BETA-CAROTENE are often added to help stabilize these oils. (See also ESSENTIAL FATTY ACIDS; VEGETABLE OIL.)

colitis (ulcerative colitis) A condition characterized by chronic inflammation and/or ulcers of the colon and rectum. Colitis is one of the two forms of INFLAMMATORY BOWEL DISEASE, affecting 1 to 2 million Americans. Colitis is more common in whites than in other groups and occurs more frequently between the ages of 15 and 35. The occurrence of colitis is increasing in Western societies while it is rare in populations consuming less refined, less PROCESSED FOODS. Symptoms include rectal bleeding, severe DIARRHEA, painful cramping, FLATULENCE, stomachache, and weight loss. The immune system is often imbalanced, and colitis is considered an autoimmune disorder. The causes of colitis are unknown, though stress and viral or bacterial infections are implicated. FOOD SENSITIVITY may also be involved because many patients improve with intravenous nutrition and elemental diets (containing only pure nutrients), and symptoms can reappear when foods are reintroduced. Patients may be allergic to household dust and MOLDS and they may be low in the steroid hormone DHEA.

For most people, colitis lasts for years and requires persistent medical attention. Patients are often malnourished due to a lack of appetite and inadequate nutrient uptake because of damage to the intestinal lining. Zinc, calcium, magnesium, and iron, as well as B vitamin intake, may be low. Persistent diarrhea can upset the ELECTROLYTE balance. Inflammation and scarring can narrow the intestinal lumen, raising the possibility of obstruction. Colitis and similar diseases can increase the risk of colon and rectal cancer.

Recommendations for colitis include eliminating common food ALLERGENS, like WHEAT, CORN, CITRUS FRUIT, YEAST, or dairy products including EGGS, as well as eliminating refined sugar and alcohol while emphasizing vegetables and other FIBER-rich foods. Traditional medical treatment includes steroid hormones to reduce inflammation. The chronic use of steroids carries additional risks, however. Sections of the bowel may be removed surgically but the disease may flare up even after surgery. Butyrate (BUTYRIC ACID) enemas have proven effective in treating colitis. Butyrate is a short chain fatty acid naturally produced in the colon by bacterial fermentation of FIBER and undigested carbohydrate. Colonic cells use butyrate as a major fuel and it promotes normal structure and function of the intestinal lining. (See also MALNUTRITION.)

collagen A fibrous, structural protein of connective tissue, skin, cartilage, and BONE matrix, and the most prevalent PROTEIN of the body. The stability of collagen fibers requires the amino acids HYDROXYPROLINE and hydroxylysine. Hydroxyprotein synthesis from the amino acid proline requires VITAMIN C. Similarly, LYSINE is converted to hydroxylysine. With prolonged vitamin C deficiency, neither hydroxyproline nor hydroxylysine may be formed in sufficient amounts for optimal collagen fiber formation. One consequence is weakened capillary walls, slow wound healing, bleeding gums, and loose, painful joints—the symptoms of SCURVY.

Connective tissue and collagen content influence the toughness of meat. The more connective tissue, the tougher the meat. Slow moist-heat cooking, like braising and stewing, tenderizes flesh by breaking down connective tissue and converting collagen to GELATIN. Food processors prepare gelatin by boiling collagen in cartilage. High temperature has the opposite effect on muscle fibers and toughens meat. Two or three hours of moist heat at 180° F strikes a balance between softening connective tissue and minimizing muscle hardening.

MEAT TENDERIZERS soften tough meat by breaking down collagen with enzymes. Most powdered meat tenderizers use the plant enzyme PAPAIN as the tenderizing agent. This papaya product breaks down proteins of muscle, fibers, and connective tissue to small fragments. Tenderizers generally work on the surface of the meat. As proteins, they are inactivated along with meat during cooking. (See also AMINO ACIDS; BIOLOGICAL VALUE.)

collard (*Brassica oleracea*) A dark-green leafy vegetable of the cabbage family. Like KALE, collard forms tall, broad leaves on long stalks but no head. Of the cabbage family, kale and collard have been cultivated the longest. In the southern United States, collard greens are boiled with bacon or salt pork. Collard greens are relatively good sources of FIBER, BETA-CAROTENE, IRON, and CALCIUM. A cup of collard, cooked (145 g), provides 20 calories; protein, 1.6 g; carbohydrate, 3.8 g; fiber, 4.1 g; calcium, 113 mg; iron, 0.59 mg; zinc, 0.93; vitamin A, 322 retinol equivalents; folic acid, 55 mg; ascorbic acid, 14 mg; thiamin, 0.03 mg; riboflavin, 0.06 mg; and niacin, 0.34 mg.

colloidal minerals (glacial milk) Herbal supplements reputed to contain nutrients that have been filtered from mined shale containing the mineral remains of ancient rain forests. Colloids are small particles ranging in size from 1 to 1,000 nm that can remain suspended in another substance (such as liquid). The particles may be single molecules or aggregates of molecules or ions. Promoters of so-called colloidal minerals claim that unlike minerals derived from other sources, the minerals harvested from the leachate of the shale deposits are so small they are more readily absorbed by the body. These minerals, the promotions say, are more powerful than those derived from modern plant and animal sources.

Colloidal mineral marketers claim that most of Americans' health problems—including male-pattern baldness, leukemia, cystic fibrosis, and impotence—are caused by eating food deficient in minerals and that these problems can only be resolved by supplementing the diet with "plant-based" colloidal minerals rather than "metal-based" minerals in standard daily supplements.

The health benefits of colloidal minerals have never been substantiated by reliable studies in reputable medical or science publications. Furthermore, no government agency has determined the safety of taking these dietary supplements.

colon (large intestine) The lower part of the digestive tract, beginning with the end of the small intestine, the ileocecal valve, and ending at the rectum. The length is approximately 1.3 meters or 4 feet. Its divisions are the cecum, a pouch at the beginning of the colon, and the ascending, transverse, descending and sigmoid colon, which lies close to the anus. These sections form an inverted "U" surrounding the small intestine. The sigmoid is a common site of polyp formation and of colon cancer. Examination of this region is called a sigmoidoscopy. However, examination of the entire colon (colonoscopy), can reveal polyps and lesions that would be missed by a sigmoidoscopy. Colonic conditions affect millions of Americans. They include: bulges (DIVERTICULOSIS), inflamed pockets (DIVERTICULITIS), CONSTIPATION, ulcerated colon (COLITIS), and hemorrhoids. All are influenced by diet.

The ileocecal valve regulates the flow of food remnants from the small intestine into the colon. The colon is filled by the gastrocolic nerve reflex, by which food entering or leaving the stomach causes a discharge of contents of the ILEUM into the colon. The colon also fills four to five hours after a meal. Feces solidify in the colon during the next 24 hours. No digestion occurs during passage through the colon. The colon absorbs CALCIUM and electrolytes like sodium and potassium, as well as water and microbial products.

The colon secretes mucus, which provides lubrication to ease the movement of fecal material and to serve as a physical barrier between the epithelial cells lining the colon and fecal matter. Pouch-like segments of the colon slow the movement of fecal material through the colon. Nonetheless, peristaltic movement gradually pushes feces through the colon where fecal material is squeezed and mixed to permit more efficient absorption. When malfunctions do not allow adequate reabsorption of water, the feces appear watery, a condition known as DIARRHEA. If excessive amounts of water are removed from the feces, constipation results. The distal end of the colon is the rectum, and the valve keeping the fecal matter within the colon is the anal sphincter. Bowel movements are triggered by involuntary responses; however, muscles of the anal sphincter can be consciously contracted to delay bowel movement.

The colon houses a vast amount of bacteria and other microorganisms. Typically, the amount in an adult is about 4 to 6 pounds, and the total number of bacteria exceed the cells that exist in the body. This intestinal microflora forms a symbiotic relationship with the host. While deriving nutrients from undigested food supplied by the host, the beneficial bacteria supply the host with vitamin K, B complex vitamins, BIOTIN, and SHORT-CHAIN FATTY ACIDS from the fermentation of fiber and undigested carbohydrate. These can supply several hundred calories daily. The beneficial bacteria limit the growth of potentially pathogenic bacteria and yeasts as well. (See also ACIDOPHILUS; CROHN'S DISEASE; IRRITABLE BOWEL SYNDROME.)

color additives See ARTIFICIAL FOOD COLORS.

colostrum (pre-milk) A thick, milk-like secretion produced by mammary glands, especially during the first two or three days after birth and before true lactation. This high-calorie fluid contains PROTEIN and FAT to nurture the infant. In comparison to mature milk, it contains more protein and less milk sugar and fat. Its yellow color reflects a high content of BETA-CAROTENE. Colostrum provides maternal ANTIBODY (IgA) and lymphocytes (white blood cells) to assist in protecting the infant's GASTROINTESTINAL TRACT. Some of the antibodies leak into the infant's bloodstream and provide additional protection. Colostrum provides BIFIDUS FACTOR, which helps beneficial bacteria populate the infant's intestine. Colostrum is sterile so the baby cannot contract bacterial infections, although the mother may have one. Colostrum changes to transitional milk between the third and sixth day after birth. By the 10th day, the major changes in milk composition are complete. (See also ACIDOPHILUS; BIFIDOBACTERIA; BREAST-FEEDING.)

combining See FOOD COMBINATION.

comfrey (*Symphytum officinale*) An herbal ingredient of teas, used in folk medicine as an astringent to close wounds or sores and a tonic for asthma, coughs, and disorders of the gastrointestinal tract. This is an example in which a "natural" product is not necessarily safe. The comfrey leaves and roots contain substances including allantoin, consolidine, and pyralizidine alkaloids, that can injure the LIVER. Though symptoms may not show up until several months after use, liver damage can occur in a week. Infants are more susceptible to side effects. This herb is unsafe when taken internally. Comfrey leaves can cause CANCER in experimental animals. (See also HERBS.)

complete protein A food PROTEIN that contains all AMINO ACIDS in amounts adequate for normal growth and maintenance. Such proteins possess a high BIOLOGICAL VALUE (BV). Thus all protein building blocks are supplied simultaneously for optimal protein synthesis. If the diet does not supply adequate amounts of the dietary essential amino acids (that is, amino acids the body cannot make), then protein synthesis will be limited. Animal protein (DAIRY PRODUCTS, MEAT, POULTRY, SEAFOOD) are excellent sources of complete proteins. In contrast, most plant proteins are deficient in one or more essential amino acids. Consuming a variety of protein from different plant sources helps the vegetarian meet the daily requirements for all essential amino acids. Certain plant proteins approach the quality of meat: They include AMARANTH, QUINOA, and SOYBEAN. (See also FOOD COMBINATION.)

complex carbohydrate Long-chained CARBOHYDRATES (POLYSACCHARIDES) that occur in plant-derived foods like FRUITS, VEGETABLES, and LEGUMES. Nutritionists recognize two major classes of complex carbohydrate: STARCH and FIBER. Starch is the plant storage form of glucose, and it may be unrefined, as found in unprocessed foods such as brown RICE, whole WHEAT flour, fresh vegetables, tubers, and root vegetables. Whole foods provide VITAMINS, MINERALS, and fiber that are removed more or less completely by refining, milling, and other food processing. Refined starch appears in bleached FLOUR, white rice, and PASTA and lacks other nutrients.

Eating starch, particularly in minimally processed foods, offers many advantages. Starch digestion yields GLUCOSE, an excellent energy source. The digestion of starch in unprocessed foods generally yields blood glucose more slowly than from simple SUGARS. This diminishes the burden of the pancreas to produce INSULIN; thus, whole foods are conducive to better GLUCOSE TOLERANCE. Glucose from carbohydrate digestion is converted to body FAT more slowly and with a greater expenditure of energy than are dietary fats and oils. Therefore, surplus starch calories are not as fattening as fat calories. Starch does not promote CHOLESTEROL build-up, unlike saturated fat. When following dietary recommendations for achieving a more healthful diet, the increased consumption of complex carbohydrates simplifies reducing fat intake.

The second type of complex carbohydrate is fiber, a diverse family of polysaccharides made up of various sugar constituents that serves as the other protective layers of plant cells. Digestive enzymes do not attack fiber as they do starch. Although fiber is not digested, intestinal bacteria may break it down more or less completely, according to the type of food ingested. For example, short-chain fatty acids released by microbial metabolism can supply between 5 percent and 25 percent of daily energy requirements. Fiber can be divided into two general classes. Water-soluble fiber like PECTIN and GUMS form gels. Insoluble fiber, like CELLULOSE, HEMICELLULOSE, and LIGNINS, provide bulk. They absorb water and soften stools. Research indicates that both soluble and insoluble fibers are essential for a healthy digestive tract. Abundant dietary fiber helps with weight management; reduces the risk of constipation, diarrhea, hemorrhoids, diverticulosis, or pouching of the colon; reduces the risk of colon cancer and cardiovascular disease; and assists in the regulation of blood sugar and diabetic control.

Canadian and U.S. guidelines agree that increased consumption of foods containing more complex carbohydrates, and decreased consumption of concentrated sweets and fat, would be beneficial in most cases. Typically, Americans derive 25 percent of their calories from sugar. U.S. guidelines advise decreasing this to 10 percent while increasing complex carbohydrates to meet 50 percent of total energy intake. These additions would represent major additions to the DIET in terms of vegetables, grains, fruits, and legumes. Americans generally need to increase their fiber intake. (See also BRAN, OAT; BRAN, WHEAT; BUTYRIC ACID; CEREAL GRAINS; DIETARY GUIDELINES FOR AMERICANS; GLYCEMIC INDEX; GLYCOGEN.)

Chinachoti, P. "Carbohydrates: Functionality in Foods," *American Journal of Clinical Nutrition* 4S (1995): 922S–929S.

compulsive eating Episodes of excessive eating. Compulsive binge eating, BULIMIA, and ANOREXIA NERVOSA are considered to be the three major eating disorders in America. Though most normal-weight individuals periodically overeat, compulsive behavior indicates an underlying problem.

Often compulsive eating is triggered by unresolved emotional issues. Like ADDICTION, abstaining from food may cause symptoms of distress. The failure to acknowledge personal feelings and to resolve personal pain may underlie compulsive eating. Identifying the feelings that are being shunned and working through alternative ways of dealing with emotions represent powerful first steps in recovery. Available programs provide a framework for change and a strong support system. One example is the 12-step program of Overeaters Anonymous, patterned after Alcoholics Anonymous. Individualized programs assist the client in feeling safer and more in control of eating behavior. Programs usually involve psychological counseling, providing emotional support, BEHAVIOR MODIFICATION, education about addictions, nutrition counseling, a BALANCED DIET, and regular EXERCISE.

Behavior modification involves learning to eat only when hungry and to stop eating when hunger is satisfied. Counseling can help with attitudes toward food and self-nourishment. Affirming that the client has the choice of eating or not, without judgment, and that the client is in control at every bite, are valuable steps forward. During a binge, identifying underlying feelings may clarify whether food is being substituted for a deeper need, such as love and acceptance. Counseling also emphasizes a return to eating normally after bingeing and self-forgiveness in order to break patterns of guilt and self-defeat. A diet diary can reveal eating patterns and the accompanying feelings. Eating more whole, fresh foods and eating less highly processed CONVENIENCE FOODS moves the individual to a more balanced diet. As an added benefit, avoiding sugar and sweets may stabilize BLOOD SUGAR levels and moderate mood swings that can trigger a bout of bingeing.

condensed milk A mixture of whole MILK and sugar (SUCROSE), concentrated by evaporation. Approximately 60 percent of the water is removed by heating. It is enriched with VITAMIN D (400 IU per pint). Sugar accounts for 40 percent to 45 percent of condensed milk. Because the high sugar content slows bacterial growth, condensed milk will keep somewhat longer than whole milk. Condensed milk is used in custards and pumpkin pies.

condiment An extra flavoring for meat and vegetable dishes including relish, pickled fruit, and vegetables. Condiments are used to heighten natural flavors and to stimulate the appetite. Unlike seasonings, which are added to foods during preparation, condiments are chosen to complement the main serving. They may be fresh (ONIONS, fresh herbs, CRESS, or PARSLEY) or they may be prepared (sweet and sour sauces, purees, MUSTARDS, CHUTNEYS, catsup, and capers). *Condiment* also can refer to natural coloring like beetroot and caramel, as well as extracts such as aniseed, almonds, some flowers, and even cheeses.

conditioning See FITNESS.

conjugated linoleic acid (CLA) A variant of the ESSENTIAL FATTY ACID linoleic acid. Like linoleic acid, conjugated linoleic acid has 18 carbon atoms and two double bonds holding the chain together. However, the double bonds in conjugated linoleic acid are adjacent to each other. Low levels of CLA occurs naturally in the fat of animals that eat grass (ruminants). It can be found in dairy products such as MILK, CHEESE, and BUTTER and in the meat of cattle and lamb.

This so-called good fat has been shown in animal studies to inhibit the three stages of cancer: initiation, promotion, and metastasis. In these studies CLA was shown to block proliferation of malignant melanoma and colon, breast, and lung cancer cells. Researchers have also discovered that CLA lowered CHOLESTEROL and reduced arterial plaque build-up in rodents. It also appears to have antioxidant properties. ANTIOXIDANTS may help prevent chronic diseases such as heart disease and cancer by inhibiting FREE RADICALS (molecules or ions that possess a single electron and that attack other molecules, removing an electron to make up for their own deficiency). In experiments mice that received CLA supplements had 60 percent lower body fat and 15 percent increased lean body mass than did mice that did not receive CLA. These positive results have not yet been duplicated in human studies.

Cordain L. et al. "Fatty Acid Analysis of Wild Ruminant Tissues: Evolutionary Implications for Reducing Diet-Related Chronic Disease. [Review]," *European Journal of Clinical Nutrition* 56 (2002): 181–191.

constipation Infrequent or incomplete bowel movements with firm stools. One out of every ten Americans is constipated and 20 percent of those individuals over the age of 65 are chronically constipated. Chronic constipation is the cumulative result of a faulty DIET and inadequate fluid intake. Straining during bowel movements weakens muscles of the colon; they lose their tone (DIVERTICULOSIS) and, over time, pouches, or bulges may develop in the walls of the colon. Many medications cause constipation. These include codeine; a CALCIUM BLOCKER (verapamil); ANTIDEPRESSANTS (Elavil and Tofranil), especially in elderly persons; ANTACIDS containing aluminum or calcium; and some CHOLESTEROL-LOWERING DRUGS (Questran and Colestid). Some FOOD SENSITIVITIES, for example, to milk and dairy products, may cause constipation in sensitive people.

Constipation may be alleviated by drinking enough water and consuming more fiber-rich food like WHEAT bran, VEGETABLES, PRUNES, FIGS, PEARS, and BEETS. GUAR GUM and PSYLLIUM powder are other types of fiber that have been used as BULKING AGENTS to soften stools. Individuals need to consult their physicians before supplementing with fiber. Some people do not respond to dietary fiber because they have a slow rate of movement of waste through the intestine. Magnesium salts are traditional LAXATIVES and may help these persons. However, the long-term use of any laxative can lead to dependence on it. Soapsud enemas are not recommended because they irritate the rectum and colon. (See also DIGESTION; GASTROINTESTINAL DISORDERS; GASTROINTESTINAL TRACT.)

convenience food Foods that have been precooked or processed to minimize meal preparation at home. Convenience foods include cold BREAKFAST CEREALS, powdered soft drinks, prepared foods to be heated at home, canned foods, and frozen foods (FROZEN ENTREES like pizza, tacos, and TV dinners). Consumers may choose among gourmet microwave dinners; foods in pouches that need only to be mixed with water, warmed, and served; snack foods; and a plethora of fast-food restaurants.

The number of different foods carried by a typical supermarket ranges between 15,000 and 40,000 and the variety continues to grow. Presently about 1,000 new food products are introduced each month. The abundance of convenience food does not necessarily mean that it is easier to make healthful choices among these products. Convenience foods are often highly processed and so are not as nutrient-dense as whole, minimally processed foods. The increased consumption of convenience foods has raised concerns because of the increased consumption of food additives like FAT and oils, salt, and SUGAR. For example, frozen pizza, chips, and snack foods often contain fat and oil, sugar, salt, and other additives not present in whole foods and recipes prepared at home.

The basis for increased consumption of convenience foods lies in the changing attitude toward meals and meal preparation. Marketing surveys reveal that shoppers desire convenience in preparing tasty meals and snacks. More people are eating meals away from home, and busy work schedules dictate shorter meal preparation times. These desires have spawned a huge variety of foods that require a minimum of preparation and/or eating time. The degree to which consumer demand for convenience food has been shaped by ADVERTISING is debatable. Certainly children who watch TV commercials have a different attitude toward meals than their grandparents did. Home environments continue to change. Increased numbers of households in which both parents work, and of single-parent families, reflect important trends affecting family meal choices and meal preparation. (See also BALANCED DIET; EATING PATTERNS; FOOD ADDITIVES; PROCESSED FOOD.)

cooking Heating food to increase its nutritional quality and/or flavor. Accessibility to nutritive foods has played a dominant factor in human evolution. The use of fire for cooking preceded the domestication of plants and animals by perhaps 40,000 years. The importance of cooking cannot be overemphasized because cooking causes profound changes in a food. The chemical changes soften, coagulate, break down, or dissolve PROTEIN, ENZYMES, and meat fiber. CELLULOSE and PECTIN fibers in plant materials are softened, thus increasing the digestibility of starch and other nutrients trapped within cell walls. All plant foods now used as staples require cooking for human consumption. These include grains, tubers, legumes, and plants such as BREADFRUIT. FLOUR becomes edible when cooked because starch granules are made accessible to digestive enzymes. Cooking is no less important for MEAT. COLLAGEN is the main protein constituent of connective tissue. In a hot, moist environment collagen is gradually transformed to GELATIN as the connective tissue gradually dissolves. This makes the meat both more tender and more easily digested. Extensive cooking can also toughen meat as muscle fibers harden. Two or three hours of slow moist heat at 180° F is recommended to balance the softening of connective tissue, minimizing the hardening of muscle fibers and destroying bacterial contamination.

Cooking sterilizes foods; disease-producing viruses, parasites, yeast, and bacteria are generally destroyed with adequate cooking times. Cooking often destroys "antinutrients," proteins that can block nutrient uptake (goitrogens) or inhibit enzymes (soybean trypsin inhibitor, an inhibitor of kidney beans). Cooking also can destroy toxic substances that are common in raw foods. Uncooked BROAD BEANS (fava beans) can induce hemolytic ANEMIA in susceptible individuals. OXALIC ACID crystals in RHUBARB, BEETS, and SPINACH are broken down during cooking. Carbohydrate derivatives that release cyanide occur in the CABBAGE family, raw LIMA BEANS, and CASSAVA. These are destroyed or reduced by cooking, especially by boiling.

Basic cooking techniques include frying (cooking in hot oil, which dramatically raises the fat content); poaching (simmering in hot water, a gentle technique for eggs and fish); pressure cooking (cooking with steam at high pressure); sauteing (a rapid pan-frying method); baking (a dry heat method); boiling (water method, best for potatoes, beets, and cabbage, rather than for green leafy vegetables); braising (slow moist-heat method for fish and poultry); broiling (oven-heated from the top, or grilled from the bottom, to provide a crisp outer layer on the cooked item while maintaining juices); steaming (an ideal way of cooking vegetables because foods are not immersed in water and nutrient loss is minimized); and microwaving (a rapid method that relies on generating microwaves to heat foods with little or no water, thus minimizing nutrient loss).

Cooking develops flavors that can be enhanced by HERBS and SPICES or marinating (treating the food before cooking with ingredients that permeate the food). Cooking also enhances the appearance of food, making it more palatable and appetizing. Glazing of vegetables is an example. (See also ACRYLAMIDE; FOOD POISONING; MICROWAVE COOKING.)

copper An essential TRACE MINERAL. The body of an adult contains 100 to 150 mg copper. Although copper is present in all tissues, including RED BLOOD CELLS, the LIVER is the main site of copper storage. Most of serum copper is bound to ceruloplasmin, the copper transport PROTEIN synthesized by the liver. Ceruloplasmin also aids in IRON transportation and storage. Like most trace minerals, copper functions as an enzyme COFACTOR by activating certain key enzymes required to strengthen the structural protein COLLAGEN, which in turn strengthens cartilage, tendons, BONES, and blood vessels. Copper also serves as a cofactor of a protein in the blood that helps maintain lung tissue and prevent emphysema; and it is essential for insulating (mylination) nerve cells. As a cofactor for the enzyme superoxide dismutase, copper helps prevent oxidative damage by a highly reactive form of oxygen and thus is classified as an ANTIOXIDANT. Copper functions as a cofactor for CYTOCHROME oxidase of MITOCHONDRIA, the enzyme complex that ultimately transfers electrons from the oxidation of fat, carbohydrate and protein to oxygen for energy production. Copper also serves as a cofactor in the synthesis of norepinephrine, an important NEUROTRANSMITTER and adrenal hormone.

The estimated safe and adequate daily intake of copper for normal adults is 2 to 3 mg. About 30 percent of dietary copper is assimilated. Good sources of copper include LIVER, KIDNEYS, SHELLFISH, nuts, seeds, FRUIT, and dried LEGUMES. Cow's MILK is low in copper. The standard American diet is copper-deficient, and between 66 percent and 75 percent of the U.S. population do not consume enough copper. Dieters, elderly persons, and chronic alcoholics are especially vulnerable. The following factors increase the need for copper: excessive dietary FIBER, high zinc supplements (50 mg or more daily), CADMIUM, excessive VITAMIN C, and excessive sugar (fructose) intake (at least in rats).

Low copper consumption increases the risk of high blood CHOLESTEROL and coronary heart disease, lowered immunity, GOUT, diabetes, high blood pressure, ANEMIA, nervous disorders, decreased pigmentation of skin, fragile bones, and erratic heartbeat. Low dietary copper is linked to an increased risk of HEART ATTACK. Evidence also links copper deficiency with increased oxidative damage to cell membranes. Levels of norepinephrine in the brain are decreased with copper deficiency but may be restored by supplemental copper. There are certain precautions to keep in mind for copper supplements. Consumption of 10 to 15 mg of copper daily can cause side effects. Patients with a rare copper accumulation disease (Wilson's disease) should not use copper supplements. An excessive copper overload has been linked to various psychiatric syndromes. A green stain in the sink from a faucet drip, or in a tea kettle, suggests excessive copper in drinking water, leached from copper plumbing. (See also FERRITIN; ZINC.)

Klevay, L. M., and D. M. Medeiros. "Deliberations and Evaluations of the Approaches, Endpoints and Paradigms for Dietary Recommendations About Copper," *Journal of Nutrition* 126 (1996): 2,419S–2,426S.

corn (*Zea mays;* maize) A high-carbohydrate CEREAL GRAIN. Corn originated in Central America 5,000 to 6,000 years ago and its cultivation spread throughout the Americas. After its discovery by Europeans, corn spread throughout the world. Americans eat about 25 pounds of corn per person annually. Although it is often considered a vegetable, corn is actually a grass. *Field corn* refers to nonsweet varieties with a high STARCH content. Dried kernels are used as livestock feed, and are processed to yield CORNSTARCH, high-FRUCTOSE CORN SYRUP, whiskey, and nonfood products ranging from paper to plastics. Popcorn is a type of field corn with thick kernels. When heated, steam is generated within dried kernels, which causes them to pop.

Recent research at Cornell University indicates that cooking sweet corn (creamed, steamed, or on the cob) unleashes beneficial nutrients including carotenoids that can substantially reduce the chance of heart disease and cancer. Cornell researchers recently reported that cooking sweet corn significantly boosts the grain's health-giving antioxidant activity.

Despite popular opinion that processed fruits and vegetables result in a lower nutritional value than does fresh produce, cooked sweet corn retains its antioxidant activity despite the loss of vitamin C. In fact, cooking increased the antioxidants in sweet corn by up to 53 percent. In addition to its antioxidant benefits, cooked sweet corn releases ferulic acid, an aromatic compound, which provides health benefits such as battling cancer.

Ferulic acid is a unique phytochemical found mostly in grains and in very low amounts in fruits and vegetables. It is found in very high levels in corn. Cooking sweet corn increases the amount of ferulic acid significantly quite a bit.

Corn is closely related to millet and cane sugar. Sweet corn is the most popular variety of corn and has a high sugar content. Super-sweet varieties with even higher sugar content have now been bred. The sugar, GLUCOSE, begins to be converted to starch as soon as it is harvested. However, cold storage retards this process. In addition to sweet corn, hundreds of varieties of corn have been developed that may be yellow, white, or multicolored. Those with yellow color contain a small amount of BETA-CAROTENE. Corn is considered a significant source of this important antioxidant because so much of it is consumed. Corn contains ample amounts of protein; however, corn PROTEIN is low in the essential AMINO ACID, LYSINE. This contributes to the low protein quality of this grain. New high-lysine strains have been bred to remedy this deficiency.

PELLAGRA, the NIACIN deficiency disease, occurs among low-income people on inadequate corn-based diets that provide very little niacin or the essential amino acid TRYPTOPHAN. Inclusion of high quality animal protein, an excellent source of tryptophan, or of niacin supplements, abolishes the disease. Under normal conditions, the body converts some tryptophan to niacin. Niacin is not easily released from corn protein unless premixed with alkaline substances. For example, in Mexico, corn flour is traditionally treated with slaked lime (calcium hydroxide, an alkali) in the preparation of tortillas. This procedure releases protein-bound niacin, and pellagra does not occur. One half-cup, as kernels (cooked, 82 g), provides: calories, 67; protein, 2.5 g; carbohydrate, 16.8 g; fiber, 3.9 g; fat, less than 0.1 mg; vitamin A, 20 retinol equivalents; thiamin, 0.11 mg; riboflavin, 0.04 mg; niacin, 0.96 mg. (See also BIOLOGICAL VALUE; CORNMEAL; CORN OIL; CORN SYRUP.)

Dewanto, V., X. Wu, and R. H. Liu. "Processed Sweet Corn Has Higher Antioxidant Activity," *Journal of Agriculture and Food Chemistry* 50 (August 2002): 4,959–4,964.

corn chips See CHIPS.

cornmeal Ground corn kernels. Corn kernels consist of bran or hull, hominy or ENDOSPERM, and GERM, which contains oil. Traditionally, dried whole kernels were ground to prepare cornmeal. This cold-processed cornmeal contains more oil and BETA-CAROTENE than in the "new process." In this latter procedure, both the hull and germ of the kernel are removed before milling. New-process cornmeal keeps better because it contains less fat. Corn flour represents more finely ground corn. Both yellow corn and blue corn are available as meal and flour; neither contains GLUTEN, the sticky protein occurring in WHEAT, oats, and, to a lesser extent, in RYE. Corn does contain protein that may cause food allergies in susceptible people. Cornmeal: whole-ground, 1 cup (122 g), provides 435 calories; protein, 11 g; carbohydrate, 90 g; fiber, 9 g; fat, 5 g; potassium, 346 mg; vitamin A, 62 retinol equivalents; thiamin, 0.46 mg; riboflavin, 2.4 mg; and niacin, 2.4 mg. (See also CEREAL GRAINS.)

corn oil A polyunsaturated vegetable oil. Corn oil is often used in deep-fat frying and in the preparation of margarine. To prepare corn oil, the germ is first separated from the starchy endosperm by steaming, milling, and sifting and is then heated and pressed to yield oil. Corn oil is rich in unsaturated fatty acids, that is, fatty acids whose carbon atoms are deficient in hydrogen atoms. It contains 59 percent polyunsaturated FATTY ACIDS and 24 percent monounsaturated fatty acids. Corn oil has a high level of LINOLEIC ACID, an ESSENTIAL FATTY ACID, but lacks ALPHA LINOLENIC ACID, the other essential fatty acid. This issue becomes relevant in powdered INFANT FORMULAS that are corn oil-based and lack DHA (DOCASAHEXAENOIC ACID), an omega-3 fatty acid derived from alpha linoleic acid and believed to be essential for normal brain and nervous system development.

cornstarch A form of starch purified from corn kernels and used as a food additive. Cornstarch thickens gravies, sauces, and puddings. Cornstarch is a more effective thickener for acidic fruits than wheat FLOUR. However, overcooking breaks down this thickening agent. New varieties of corn yield waxy cornstarches that are used to stabilize frozen sauces and fillings. Nonfood uses of cornstarch include incorporation in laundry starch.

Starches in general are long chains of GLUCOSE, and cornstarch is no exception. Starch breakdown yields glucose syrup, a NATURAL SWEETENER. Glucose syrup in turn is enzymatically converted to high-FRUCTOSE CORN SYRUP, a popular sweetener that is sweeter than table sugar. (See also CARBOHYDRATE; THICKENING AGENTS.)

corn syrup A sweetener prepared by digesting corn starch with acid to yield the simple sugar building block, glucose. Corn syrup is an inexpensive sweetener, used extensively in PROCESSED FOODS like PEANUT butter, catsup, NON-DAIRY CREAMER, imitation fruit drinks, and mixes. Corn syrup has replaced maple syrup as the main ingredient in most commercial syrups. Together with its derivative, high-FRUCTOSE CORN SYRUP, it is rapidly replacing sucrose (table sugar) as the major carbohydrate sweetener in processed foods and beverages. As with other refined sugar sweeteners, corn syrup represents EMPTY CALORIES. It lacks important nutrients found in unrefined foods. The dramatic increase in the consumption of sweeteners in the United States during the 1980s was mainly due to the increased use of corn sweetener additives. (See also CALORIE; FOOD ADDITIVES; NATURAL SWEETENERS.)

coronary artery disease (CAD) A pathologic condition caused by the narrowing of coronary arteries, the major arteries feeding heart muscle, to the point where they cannot adequately supply the heart with blood. CAD is a major health concern because it causes more deaths in the U.S. than any other disease. HEART ATTACK is the leading cause of death in the United States accounting for 20 percent of death in people over 65. A frequent cause is ATHEROSCLEROSIS, where fatty deposits and cellular buildup containing CHOLESTEROL (PLAQUE) create arterial thickening and partial blockage of blood flow. Such constrictions can close off the artery completely or they can trigger the formation of blood clots that can lodge in such constrictions. Blockage of coronary arteries in either case causes heart attacks in which a lack of oxygen damages heart muscle.

Coronary Heart Disease (CHD)

This disease is the result of damage to the heart muscle (myocardium) due to an inadequate blood supply. A heart attack refers to the sudden blockage of an artery supplying blood to the heart. Diseased arteries can be blocked by blood clots (thrombosis) or by accumulated cholesterol (plaque buildup) or by a combination of both processes.

Risk Factors for CAD and CHD

As with any chronic disease, the incidence of CHD is the product of dietary, environmental, and inherited risk factors. Risk factors simply increase the odds of developing CAD; they do not guarantee a person will have a heart attack. Likewise, the absence of known risk factors is no guarantee a person will not have a heart attack. The cumulative effect of risk factors is greater than if individual risks were simply added together. Thus, a person with three risk factors has a sixfold increase in his or her risk of heart attack.

Major risk factors for CAD have been identified. They include lifestyle factors such as smoking; lack of physical exercise; chronic emotional stress, and certain personality traits that relate to coping with stress; overeating, weight gain, and high-fat diet.

Medical history can dramatically increase the risk of heart disease: high blood pressure (HYPERTENSION), DIABETES MELLITUS, GOUT, OBESITY, high LDL cholesterol (the less desirable form of blood cholesterol), and low HDL cholesterol (the more desirable form of cholesterol). Premature menopause without hormone replacement therapy is another risk factor related to medical history. Elevated levels of HOMOCYSTEINE, a breakdown product of the amino acid METHIONINE, has been shown to be an independent risk factor for heart attacks and strokes.

Low vitamin C levels may be a risk factor for CHD in women, since increased vitamin C levels are linked to increased HDL (the "good" cholesterol). Other risk factors relate to inheritance and cannot be altered:

- Gender. Men are more likely than women to develop heart attacks before the age of 55. After 75 or 80, the rate of developing CAD is the same for both men and women.
- Racial background. Certain groups face greater odds for heart attacks, including African Americans, who are more at risk for developing hypertension, and Pima Indians, who are more likely to develop diabetes.
- Aging. The occurrence of CAD increases dramatically after the age of 65.
- Family history of premature or coronary heart disease. A heart attack or sudden death in father, brother, or son before the age of 55 or a heart attack or sudden death in a mother, sister, or daughter before the age of 65.

Effect of Diet on CAD and CHD

A high-fat DIET, especially one with large amounts of animal or saturated fat, is linked to diseases of arteries and heart. Certain saturated FATTY ACIDS seem to promote plaque buildup, including lauric acid (with 12 carbons), myristic acid (with 14 carbons), and PALMITIC ACID (with 16 carbons). Palmitic acid is the most common saturated fatty acid in animal fat and it is the most atherogenic (promoting plaque accumulation). In addition, the lauric, myristic, and palmitic acids seem to promote blood clot formation. Diets high in the longer fatty acid, STEARIC ACID (with 18 carbons, a common saturated fatty acid in animal fat), do not raise serum cholesterol. Nonetheless, foods are mixtures of nutrients, and fats consist of both stearic acid and palmitic acid. A second point to consider: fats and oils contribute more than twice as many calories as carbohydrate and protein; therefore, the total number of fat calories consumed per day is a determining factor for risk of obesity, CHD, and cancer. Meat consumption alone, especially red meat consumption, shows no apparent correlation with CHD among individuals in 26 European countries.

Other dietary factors that may protect against CAD and CHD include unsaturated oils. Most vegetable oils contain polyunsaturated fatty acids related to LINOLEIC ACID, an ESSENTIAL FATTY ACID, and classified as omega-6 fatty acids. These oils are called "polyunsaturates" because their fatty acid structures possess several double bonds and are deficient in hydrogen atoms. (Saturated fats are filled up with the maximum number of hydrogen atoms.) In a reduced-fat diet, in which less than 30 percent of calories come from fat, polyunsaturates reduce serum cholesterol levels when the polyunsaturates account for more than 10 percent of calories. However, they also lower HDL cholesterol, an undesirable effect. Polyunsaturates reduce platelet aggregation (blood clotting) thus reducing the risk of dangerous blood clots. Monounsaturates contain monounsaturated fatty acids with a single double bond and are much less susceptible to oxidation (lipid peroxidation) than are polyunsaturates. Olive oil and related monounsaturated oils may lower LDL without lowering HDL when total fat consumption is high. TRANS FATTY ACIDS in hydrogenated vegetable oils such as stick margarine and vegetable shortening may increase the risk of cardiovascular disease, even though consumption of trans fatty acids is estimated to be approximately 15 g/day.

Cold water ocean fish in the diet are important because they provide omega-3 polyunsaturated fatty acids, DHA (DOCOSAHEXAENOIC ACID) and eicosahexaenoic acid, which are related to a lowered risk of heart disease. These omega-3 fatty acids seem to lower blood fat and LDL cholesterol levels when blood cholesterol is high, while increasing HDL levels. They also lower mildly elevated blood pressure and reduce the risk of blood clot formation.

People with high blood levels of HOMOCYSTEINE, an amino acid byproduct, often do not consume enough B vitamins, especially FOLIC ACID, VITAMIN B_{12}, and VITAMIN B_6. Eating enough foods rich in folic acid—including beans, green leafy vegetables, and liver, to obtain 400 mcg of folic acid daily—may reduce the risk of heart disease and, incidentally, this may lower the risk of BIRTH DEFECTS.

Fiber consumption is another important consideration. Reports of the effects of dietary fiber on CAD and CHD are conflicting. Oats and oat bran can lower serum cholesterol in men with raised cholesterol levels. In middle-aged American men, fatal and nonfatal heart attack were found to be 41 percent less common among those who consumed at least 28 g of fiber per day, as compared to those eating the level typically found in the standard diet (12 to 13 g per day). These effects may pertain to women as well. The benefits of fiber lie beyond increasing satiety and reducing fat intake. Diets rich in fiber from fruits and vegetables provide antioxidants and other important nutrients. Wheat bran cereals, which supply mainly insoluble fiber, reduce the risk of heart disease. Other sources of mixed fiber include legumes like kidney BEANS, PEAS, APPLES, GRAPEFRUIT, BROCCOLI, and leafy vegetables.

ANTIOXIDANTS protect against heart disease by squelching free radicals, which are highly reactive forms of oxygen and other chemicals that lack a single electron. Free radicals attack cells indiscriminately and can damage genetic material, DNA, and even proteins. Dietary antioxidants include: vitamin C; vitamin E; BETA-CAROTENE and related orange-red plant pigments (CAROTENOIDS); trace minerals like COPPER, SELENIUM, and MANGANESE; and FLAVONOIDS (complex plant substances), together with certain compounds made by the body like GLUTATHIONE, bilirubin, and uric acid. Vitamin E and selenium may also be important in regulating platelet aggregation and clot formation as well as serving as important antioxidants. Current attention focuses on the possibility that free radicals oxidize LDL cholesterol which in turn induces plaque deposits and clogged arteries. Thus, inadequate antioxidants can promote the development of CHD by increasing LDL oxidation. Many population studies have observed a reduced risk of coronary heart disease and related events, such as heart attacks, with increased intake of dietary vitamin E. However, most clinical studies of vitamin E supplementation for several years found no benefit in heart disease risk. Consequently, vitamin E in foods, rather than vitamin E supplements, seems to offer protection. Vitamin E promotes normal function of smooth muscle cells and it reduces platelet adhesion to arterial cells, factors that could reduce the risk of atherosclerosis. Increased consumption of vitamin C, another potent antioxidant vitamin, may lower the risk of ischemic heart disease and the risk of death as the result of cardiovascular disease. It has not been proven that vitamin C supplements offer the same protection, however. Soy protein has been shown to reduce the risk of CHD according to the FDA, which concluded that foods containing soy protein as part of a diet low in saturated fat and cholesterol may reduce the risk of CHD by lowering blood cholesterol levels.

Clinical trials have shown that consuming soy protein compared to other proteins such as those from milk or meat can lower total and LDL cholesterol levels. Soy protein foods include soy beverages, tofu, tempeh, soy-based meat alternatives, and some baked goods. Studies show that 25 g of soy protein daily in the diet is needed to show a significant cholesterol-lowering effect. Because soy protein can be added to a variety of foods, it is possible for consumers to eat foods containing soy protein at all three meals and for snacks.

The "French Paradox" refers to the observation that some European populations such as the French who consume plenty of animal fat (saturated fat) and large amounts of red wine have a lower prevalence of cardiovascular disease than seen for the U.S. Moderate alcohol consumption (one or two drinks per day) can raise the levels of HDL cholesterol, the most beneficial form, regardless of the source of alcohol, thus the paradox may be more apparent than real. Drinking to reduce cardiovascular risk is not recommended, because the risks of addiction and alcohol abuse are so great.

Recommendations to Modify Controllable Risk Factors for CAD

A comprehensive program that entails very low-fat diets, providing ample fruits, vegetables, grains, and restricted amounts of animal protein and used in conjunction with exercise, stress reduction, and group support have caused a decrease in plaque accumulation (atherosclerotic lesions) in some coronary patients. For healthy coronary arteries, consumers should eat more whole-grain breads and pasta; brown rice; fruits and vegetables. Other heart-healthy choices include steamed, baked, or fresh foods; 1 percent or fat-free milk, fish, skinless poultry, lean meat, soy products, egg whites or egg substitutes, and olive oil or canola oil in small amounts.

Fatty foods to avoid include potato chips; french fries; vegetables cooked in butter, cheese, or cream; fried food; whole milk; bacon; sausage and organ meats; egg yolks; pastries; doughnuts; ice cream; and butter or margarine.

An optimal lifestyle can retard the progression of CHD and possibly prevent heart disease.

- Stopping smoking. This is perhaps the single most important preventive action a person can take.
- Preventing hypertension, or control existing hypertension. With each drop in one point in the diastolic blood pressure reading (the larger of the two blood pressure measurements), the risk of CAD declines by 2 percent to 3 percent.
- Making a lifelong commitment to stay physically fit. Sedentary people can decrease their risk of CAD by an estimated 35 percent to 55 percent. Even walking or other low intensity exercise, when done regularly for years, can lower lifetime risk.
- Maintaining a healthy body weight. Being overweight doubles or triples the risk of CAD for adults at any age. Fat accumulation around the waist is more risky than fat around the thighs.
- Preventing diabetes, or control existing diabetes. Non-insulin dependent diabetes increases the odds of CAD in men by a factor of two or three, and in women, by three to seven.
- Eating plenty of fruits, vegetables, and foods rich in soy protein, while getting plenty of antioxidants, including vitamin E, vitamin C, and beta-carotene and carotenoids. Population studies in Europe suggest that a high intake of antioxidants from foods reduces the risk of CAD. Consuming enough B vitamins, especially folic acid, vitamin B_{12} and vitamin B_6 is also prudent.
- Managing stress effectively. Suppressed anger, hostility, and a sense of lack of control at work can increase the risk of heart attack. Emotional support is an important factor.

For Those with High Blood Cholesterol

Perhaps as many as one-third of Americans are extremely sensitive to dietary cholesterol; their blood levels rise significantly when they eat cholesterol-rich foods. These individuals should limit their dietary cholesterol to no more than 300 mg per day. Particularly those with a family history of early heart disease or high cholesterol levels need to be watchful. The following step program outlines an approach to modifying the diet.

Step 1: Dietary fat should account for less than 30 percent of total daily calories. Less than 10 percent of total calories should come from saturated fat and daily consumption of cholesterol should not exceed 300 mg per day. If a patient is already on a Step 1 diet, and the response is inadequate, the patient may be advised to incorporate Step 2 recommendations.

Step 2: While dietary fat should account for less than 30 percent of calories, less than 7 percent of total calories should come from saturated fat, and cholesterol consumption should be less than 200 mg per day. (See also AGING; CARDIOVASCULAR DISEASE; DEGENERATIVE DISEASES; DIETARY GUIDELINES FOR AMERICANS.)

Hooper, Lee et al. "Dietary Fat Intake and Prevention of Cardiovascular Disease: Systematic Review," *British Medical Journal* 332 (2001): 757–763.

Schaefer, E. J. et al. "Lipoproteins, Nutrition, Aging and Atherosclerosis," *American Journal of Clinical Nutrition* 61, supplement (1995): 726–740S.

cortisol (cortisone, hydrocortisone) A steroid hormone produced by the inner portion of the ADRENAL GLANDS in response to stress. Unlike EPINEPHRINE, which is released by the outer region of the adrenal gland as a rapid response to stress, cortisol alters METABOLISM over a period of hours and days, rather than minutes. Cortisol stimulates the body's catabolic processes, such as increasing protein degradation and fat breakdown. It stimulates the LIVER to build GLUCOSE from AMINO ACIDS (GLUCONEOGENESIS), which appears as BLOOD SUGAR. Cortisol also reduces inflammation. Cortisol levels in the blood normally follow a circadian rhythm, reaching a maximum concentration in the morning before breakfast and reaching a nadir in the evening.

Chronic stress, which may cause excessive cortisol production, can suppress the immune system. This, in turn, may increase the risk of chronic infections and promote FOOD SENSITIVITIES. Higher than normal cortisol production could also increase blood cholesterol and cause blood sugar fluctuations. With prolonged stress, the precursor steroid, pregnanolone, can be diverted to cortisol synthesis, rather than to sex hormones and DHEA. Subsequently, DHEA levels in blood can drop, leading to increased insensitivity to insulin and decreased ability to maintain normal blood sugar levels.

In late stages of adaptation to chronic, severe stress, the fatigued adrenal glands no longer respond adequately to stimuli or follow the normal circadian rhythm. With lowered cortisol output, the body becomes even more prone to inflammation, excessive fatigue, and HYPOGLYCEMIA.

Aerobic exercise and stress reduction strategies such as meditation are keys to normalizing adrenal function. Nutritional support for adrenal glands includes VITAMIN C, pantothenic acid, niacinamide, COENZYME Q, as well as the minerals magnesium, manganese, zinc, and potassium. For low cortisol output, thiamin, CARNITINE, and OCTOCOSANOL in addition to the above may be beneficial. In general, essential fatty acids from flaxseed, borage, or black currant seed oils may help reduce inflammation, and ANTIOXIDANTS such as FLAVONOIDS may be effective. Sulfur amino acids, methionine, and taurine may help the liver detoxify accumulated waste products. It is also important to avoid sugar, CAFFEINE, and nonsteroidal anti-inflammatory drugs. The diet should favor whole grains and fresh vegetables. (See also CATABOLISM.)

cottage cheese A high-PROTEIN, low-fat CHEESE prepared from curdled milk (curds). The curdling process leaches CALCIUM from the curds into the liquid, called whey, which is removed. Consequently cottage cheese retains only 25 percent to 50 percent of milk calcium. Cottage cheese is prepared with varying amounts of FAT. It is highest in creamed small curd cheese (4.2 percent fat), while low-fat cottage cheese contains 1 percent or 2 percent fat, and dry curd cottage cheese has 0.5 percent fat. Cottage cheese is usually salted, but unsalted versions are available. One cup (210 g) of small curd, 1 percent cottage cheese, provides: calories, 164; protein, 28 g; carbohydrate, 5.6 g; fat, 2.3 g; calcium, 138 mg; sodium, 850 mg; vitamin A, 101 retinol equivalents; cholesterol, 31 mg; thiamin, 0.04 mg; riboflavin, 0.34 mg; niacin, 0.27 mg. For comparison, one cup of creamed cottage cheese (210 g) provides: calories, 215; protein, 26.2 g; carbohydrate, 5.6; fat, 8.93 g; calcium, 126 mg; cholesterol, 31 mg; sodium, 1,850 mg; vitamin A, 101 retinol equivalents; thiamin, 0.04 mg; riboflavin, 0.34 mg; niacin, 0.23 mg.

cottonseed oil A polyunsaturated oil derived from cotton. Cotton is not classified as a food, therefore pesticide use in its cultivation is not as restricted as for vegetables, and cottonseed oil may be contaminated. This oil contains 52 percent polyunsaturated FATTY ACIDS, 18 percent monounsaturated fatty acids and 26 percent saturated fatty acids. The ratio of unsaturated to saturated fatty acids is 2.7:1. The higher degree of saturation makes cottonseed oil less prone to oxidation and rancidity than soybean, corn, or safflower oils. It is thus a useful additive in salad dressings and in processed foods such as CHIPS, where shelf life stability is important. Like all oils and fat, cottonseed oil provides 9 calories/gram. (See also CHLORDIMEFORM; FOOD ADDITIVES; PROCESSED FOOD.)

cow's milk See MILK.

crab A broad-backed crustacean related to lobster and shrimp, with five pairs of legs. One pair is enlarged for foraging. The head and thorax are fused and are covered by a hard armor-like plate called a carapace. True crabs can be divided into two categories: swimming crabs (the blue crab) and walking crabs (rock crab). They represent 4,500 species although only a few types are common. Edible crabs that are important commercial seafoods are found in Europe (*Cancer pagurus*); along eastern coasts of the United States (*Callinectes sapidus,* blue crab or soft-shell crab; and the Florida stone crab); and along the Pacific Coast of the United States (*Cancer magister,* Dungeness crab). The largest crab is the Alaskan king crab.

Crab meat is delicate and is available fresh, cooked, canned, or frozen, and is used for crab salad, stuffed crab, aspics, and soufflés. Because this seafood is so expensive, imitation crab is sometimes substituted. This fish-based product (SURIMI) has been processed to have the same consistency as crab meat and flavored by small amounts of crab products. Alaskan king crab (100 g, edible portion) provides 84 calories; protein, 18.3 g; fat, 0.6 g; iron, 0.59 mg; calcium, 46 g; potassium 204 mg; sodium, 836 mg; thiamin, 0.043 mg; riboflavin, 0.043 mg; niacin, 1.10 mg. (See also CHITOSAN.)

cracked wheat See WHEAT.

cracker A thin, flat biscuit usually made of wheat flour. Chips and crackers are popular processed snack foods. Unless the food label specifically states "whole wheat" as the first and only wheat ingredient, the cracker contains between 50 percent and 90 percent bleached flour. Words like "stone ground" do not guarantee whole wheat. Crackers often contain substantial FAT or vegetable oil such as the highly saturated tropical oils (COCONUT or palm kernel oils). The fat content in crackers can vary by a factor of 10. For example: wheat wafers contain 1.1 to 2 g of fat per ounce; cheese-flavored, fat-rich crackers, 8.0 g; and corn chips and potato chips, up to 10.0 g. The typical fat content of cheese-flavored crackers is 40 percent to 55 percent. If the cracker leaves a grease spot on a paper napkin, it has a high fat content. A sense of fat content can be obtained from the list of ingredients on the food label. The lowest in calories are crispbreads and matzo-type crackers.

Rye crisp or rye flatbread may provide 2 to 4 g of fiber per half-ounce serving, equivalent to one or two peaches, with 40 to 70 calories. By comparison, a whole wheat cracker can provide only half a gram of fiber for the same serving size. Note that "unsalted" crackers still contain some sodium. "Low sodium" or "low salt" means that the food cannot contain more than 140 mg of sodium per serving, while "sodium free" can appear on food labels that contain less than 5 mg of sodium per serving.

cranberry (*Vaccinium*) A tart, bright red berry produced by a shrub that is a member of the heath family. Both American and European varieties are cultivated in the United States. Cranberries are used in relish, canned sauce, pies, and preserves. Because cranberries are so sour, sugar is usually added to these products. One cup (95 g) of fresh cranberries provides 46 calories; protein, 0.37 g; carbohydrate, 12 g; fiber, 1.14 g; potassium, 67 mg; thiamin, 0.029 mg; riboflavin, 0.019 mg; niacin, 0.095 mg; and vitamin C, 44 mg.

cranberry juice Cranberry juice has been recommended for BLADDER INFECTIONS because it contains a carbohydrate that inhibits the growth of disease-producing bacteria. This material prevents the bacteria from binding to the lining of the urinary tract, a preliminary step in infection. Because it limits bacterial growth, cranberry juice is considered "bacteriostatic" rather than "bactericidal," which refers to agents that kill bacteria. Used by itself, cranberry juice doesn't prevent or cure urinary tract infections. Often the infection flares up when the juice is no longer used. Cranberry juice is a DIURETIC and promotes urine production. Cranberry juice is so sour that juice producers add large amounts of sweeteners, and consequently it is high in CALORIES. One cup of cranberry juice cocktail provides 145 calories; carbohydrate, 36.6 g; fiber, 0.76 g; fat, 0.1 g; potassium, 45 mg; thiamin, 0.02 mg; riboflavin, 0.02 mg; niacin, 0.09 mg; and vitamin C, 90 mg.

Lee, Yee-Lean et al. "Does Cranberry Juice Have Antibacterial Activity?" *Journal of the American Medical Association* 283 (April 5, 2000): 1,691.

crash dieting See DIETING.

craving A strong desire for a food that is stronger than HUNGER and specific for a particular food. Though craving food may suggest a dependency, usually the desire to eat a specific food declines once it has been eaten. Women generally experience more food craving than men; however, by middle age this difference disappears. There probably is no single mechanism underlying food craving. Social factors are involved since taste and appearance of food are learned and profoundly influence food choices. It is also possible that craving sweets represents a desire for gratification.

Food craving by women may be hormonally driven. Studies have shown that cravings for sweets and fatty foods are associated with PREMENSTRUAL SYNDROME, DEPRESSION, and seasonal mood changes.

A biochemical imbalance may promote food craving. This model focuses on the NEUROTRANSMITTER SEROTONIN, a chemical that helps in the transmission of nerve impulses. Brain serotonin is lowest before menstruation. Brain centers requiring serotonin regulate APPETITE, as well as thirst, mood, and sleep. Certain individuals may produce abnormally low serotonin due to their unique genetic makeup or dietary imbalance. Thus, craving sweets could be a form of self-medication. According to one hypothesis, carbohydrate consumption stimulates the brain to increase synthesis of the serotonin from its raw material, the amino acid TRYPTOPHAN, and that low serotonin levels can trigger the urge to eat sweets. However, brain serotonin levels may not influence carbohydrate food choices on an ongoing basis.

Alternative explanations have been offered for food craving. Craving may be based on ENDORPHINS that decrease pain perception. Endorphin production increases during ovulation and drops during menstruation. Endorphin formation and release are stimulated when fat and carbohydrate are eaten together. The craving for chocolate associated with premenstrual syndrome may be explained by chocolate's high content of phenylethylamine, a compound that can promote relaxation and affect mood. Food craving is a possible sign of a FOOD SENSITIVITY, in which the body may gradually tolerate an allergy-producing food to the extent that omitting that food from the diet could create a craving (withdrawal) similar to a physical dependency. A disturbance in the body's HOMEOSTASIS could create biochemical imbalances in the brain and in the endocrine system. Thus, changes in hormone levels, nutritional deficiencies, disease states, and addictions can be predisposing factors to these imbalances. For example, it is known that low blood-sugar levels can trigger cravings for carbohydrates and sweets. There could also be a link with the consumption of junk food: CONVENIENCE FOOD is high in sugar and fat, which slows down digestion, slowing signals to the brain to shut off hunger signals, which could in turn induce people to eat more junk food than they would normally. Food craving increases the risk of cigarette smoking and alcohol and drug abuse. (See also ADDICTION; BULIMIA NERVOSA.)

creamer See NONDAIRY CREAMER.

cream of tartar (potassium tartrate) A widely used food additive that serves many roles. As an ingredient in BAKING POWDER, tartrate provides an acidic environment that converts the BICARBONATE in baking powder to CARBON DIOXIDE, which creates bubbles in dough of leavened baked goods. Cream of tartar serves as an anticaking agent to keep powdered materials from clumping. Sodium tartrate and sodium potassium tartrate are added to stabilize emulsified foods and to control pH in such foods as cheese, jam, and jelly. Cream of tartar also provides tartness to beverages, CANDY, ice cream, baked goods, and gelatin desserts. Tartaric acid is a natural ingredient of fruits such as GRAPES and is a by-product of wine production. (See also BUFFER; FOOD ADDITIVES.)

creatine (creatine monohydrate) A synthetic compound related to creatine phosphate, which is found naturally in muscle tissue and a few organs, including the brain. Creatine phosphate plays an important role in nerve function and in the body's ability to produce energy during short bursts of intense exercise. It is produced by the liver, pancreas, and kidneys, but most of the body's natural stores are obtained from foods that contain creatine, such as fish or meat.

The primary energy currency of cells is ATP (adenosine triphosphate). When energy is released, ATP loses a phosphate atom and breaks down to ADP (adenosine diphosphate). Because the body only maintains enough ATP for short bursts of activity, it must be replenished. This is done when ADP combines with creatine phosphate, borrowing that molecule's phosphate group to become ATP again.

Creatine supplementation with the synthetic version, creatine monohydrate, has become popular among athletes and bodybuilders who often use massive doses. Several studies appear to support the theory that providing more than the average daily consumption of creatine can increase muscle strength during short periods of intense activity, such as sprinting and weightlifting. Other studies indicate creatine supplementation may slow the effects of muscle degeneration associated with diseases like amyotrophic lateral sclerosis and muscular dystrophy.

Because creatine monohydrate is classified as a dietary supplement and not a drug, its safety and efficacy as a strength enhancer has not been confirmed by the Food and Drug Administration (FDA). Nevertheless, that agency has received some reports of serious negative side effects from taking creatine supplements, including seizure, irregular heartbeat, vomiting, and even death. Safety data are inadequate for pregnant and breast-feeding women.

Juhn, M. S. et al. "Oral Creatine Supplementation in Male Collegiate Athletes: A Survey of Dosing Habits and Side Effects," *Journal of the American Dietetic Association* 99 (1999): 593–594.

Snow, R. J. et al. "Effect of Creatine Supplementation on Sprint Exercise Performance and Muscle Metabolism," *Journal of Applied Physiology* 84 (1998): 1,667–1,673.

cress A green leafy vegetable of the mustard family. The most popular is watercress (*Nasturtium officinale*), a hardy perennial native to Europe and now widespread in the fresh running water of many regions. Watercress's pungent leaves are used as seasoning, garnish, and as a salad green. Garden cress or pepper cress (*Lepidium sativum*), native to western Asia, is cultivated and is used as a garnish like parsley. As a member of the CRUCIFEROUS VEGETABLES, cress supplies nutrients and plant substances with anticancer properties. Cress (100 g, raw) provides: calories, 32; protein, 2.6 g; carbohydrate, 5.5 g; fiber, 1.10 g; fat, 0.70 g; calcium, 81 mg; potassium, 606 mg; thiamin, 0.08 mg; riboflavin, 0.26 mg; niacin, 1.0 mg; vitamin C, 69 mg.

Crohn's disease (ileitis) A chronic inflammatory condition in which the intestinal tract is ulcerated, characterized by deep sores in the lower part of the SMALL INTESTINE, the COLON and other regions of the digestive tract. The inflammatory condition often involves all layers of the bowel wall, and granular growths often occur. Crohn's disease is one of two forms of INFLAMMATORY BOWEL DISEASE, which collectively affect 1 to 2 million Americans. Crohn's disease is most prevalent in developed, Western societies. This disease most often affects people between the ages of 12 and 40, and the incidence is highest among teenagers.

Symptoms include low-grade fever, cramps, gradual weight loss, anorexia, flatulence, weakness, MALNUTRITION, persistent bouts of DIARRHEA, possibly ARTHRITIS, skin inflammation, abdominal tenderness, vaginal and urinary inflammation, and rectal bleeding. Crohn's disease causes malabsorption, and nutrient deficiencies can delay development in children. Diarrhea accompanying Crohn's disease upsets ELECTROLYTE balance and also limits nutrient availability, while abdominal pain may limit food intake.

Whether infectious agents are involved is still debated. Viruses like Epstein-Barr, rotavirus, and cytomegalovirus and bacteria are candidates. Family history is a risk factor. Possibly this is an AUTOIMMUNE DISEASE, in which antibodies attack the mucosal lining of the lower intestinal tract. Processes regulating immune activation of the intestine seem to be imbalanced in Crohn's disease, creating an exaggerated inflammatory response. Crohn's disease may also be associated with increased intestinal permeability, thus increasing the penetration of foreign materials into the body leading to increased inflammation and tissue injury.

Crohn's disease patients typically consume more refined SUGAR and eat less raw fruit, vegetable, and FIBER than healthy individuals. Deficiencies of minerals (CALCIUM, MAGNESIUM, IRON, ZINC, SELENIUM), of water soluble vitamins (VITAMIN B_{12}, VITAMIN C, FOLIC ACID), and of fat-soluble vitamins (VITAMIN A, VITAMIN D, VITAMIN K) may cause some of the symptoms of this disease. It is important to rule out FOOD SENSITIVITIES; which may be a contributing factor. Food allergies contribute to increased gut permeability. A variety of nutrients support healing of the small intestine. They include the amino acid GLUTAMINE, zinc, and folic acid. Improving DIGESTION can help absorption, decrease the burden of food antigens, and help decrease intestinal inflammation. Other dietary modifications include avoiding seeds, nuts, greasy food, CAFFEINE, and sugar. If lactose intolerance has developed, the patient may be advised to avoid milk and milk products. Eliminating allergenic foods has been an effective approach in treating inflammatory bowel disease.

Crohn's disease is a serious condition and treatment requires a broad-based approach. Emotional support is needed by patients with Crohn's disease, especially if the person is young. Hydrolyzed protein formulas and ELEMENTAL DIETS, which combine simple nutrients rather than protein or starches, are more easily absorbed and have been used during acute phases of the disease. Oral intake of food may be withheld temporarily while IV feeding is used in order to normalize the bowel. As the client progresses, an oral diet that is nutrient-rich and well-balanced may gradually be tolerated. Smoking should also be avoided, as this aggravates the condition.

There is presently no drug available to cure Crohn's disease. Medical treatments have included surgery and steroid treatment. Surgery does not necessarily impede the progress of the disease, and it can contribute to weight loss and malabsorption. Steroids reduce inflammation, but their side effects include increased risk of bone loss, high blood pressure, BLOOD SUGAR fluctuations, and suppressed immunity—all limiting their effectiveness. (See also CATABOLIC STATE; COLITIS; GASTROINTESTINAL DISORDERS; LEAKY GUT SYNDROME.)

Gomez, Joan. *Positive Options for Crohn's Disease: Self-Help and Treatment,* Alameda, Calif.: Hunter House, 2000.

Wu, Scott et al. "Intense Nutritional Support in Inflammatory Bowel Disease," Digestive Diseases and Sciences 40, no. 4 (April 1995): 843–852.

cruciferous vegetables A large family of vegetables that help protect against some forms of CANCER. Members include BOK CHOY, BROCCOLI, BRUSSELS SPROUTS, CABBAGE, CAULIFLOWER, Chinese cabbage, COLLARD greens, horseradish, KALE, KOHLRABI, mustard greens, RADISH, RUTABAGA, turnip greens, and watercress.

Population studies show that consumption of cruciferous vegetables lowers cancer risk. Cruciferous vegetables are very good sources of VITAMIN C, FOLIC ACID, and BETA-CAROTENE, in addition to FIBER—all of which inhibit certain cancers. Furthermore, vegetables of this group also contain protective substances called dithiothiones, indoles, and isothiocyanates. These seem to help activate the liver to destroy cancer-causing agents. An example is sulforaphane, which increases the levels of detoxification enzymes of the liver. These enzymes attack highly water-soluble chemicals to altered toxins so they can be more easily excreted. Cruciferous vegetables contain ANTIOXIDANTS that can inhibit oxidative damage to DNA. It is probable other substances with anticancer activity remain to be characterized as members of this versatile group of vegetables.

To avoid the possible off-taste and odor of cruciferous vegetables when cooked, they should be cooked for as short a time as possible. Acids in lemon juice and VINEGAR turn the rich green color of cabbage-family vegetables to an unappetizing olive drab.

crude fiber See FIBER.

cucumber (*Cucumis sativus*) A long, cylindrical, crisp green vegetable produced by a vine related to squash. Cucumbers have a shiny skin with a watery, crisp flesh. The cucumber once grew wild in the foothills of the Himalayas and was domesticated at least 3,000 years ago in India. Used in ancient times by Egyptians, Hebrews, Greeks, and Romans, it has had a long history in the West. The larger, "slicing" varieties are eaten fresh, while smaller, lighter varieties are pickled. The European cucumber tends to be smooth-skinned, long (1 to 2 ft.) and seedless.

If the skin has a sheen, it has probably been waxed. All waxed cucumbers should be peeled. Although it has a low nutrient content, cucumber's characteristic flavor makes a useful addition to salads. The skin can be bitter and is often peeled before eating in salads. Sometimes raw cucumbers are salted and drained to remove bitterness. Cucumbers are cool and crisp because their water content is high (96 percent). Cucumbers can be sauteed, cooked au gratin, or stuffed. Gazpacho (cold tomato soup) incorporates grated cucumber.

Several varieties of cucumbers like the Kirby (dill pickles) and gherkins are pickled in salt. Pickling incorporates pickling salt, white vinegar, and pickling spices. Grape and cherry leaves help maintain the firmness of pickled cucumber. A cup of fresh sliced cucumber (104 g) provides 14 calories; protein, 0.56 g; carbohydrate, 3.0 g; fiber, 0.62 g; vitamin A, 46 retinol equivalents; thiamin, 0.032 mg; riboflavin, 0.02 mg; niacin, 0.32 mg.

cumin (*Cuminum cyminum*) A seasoning that is the principal ingredient of curry powder, a blend of powdered Indian spices. Cumin is a member of the PARSLEY family, and cumin seeds resemble caraway seeds. The aromatic seed has a characteristic strong, slightly bitter taste. Traditionally, cumin has been used to flavor cheese, sauerkraut, unleavened bread, marinades, chili, and tomato sauce.

curcumin See TURMERIC.

cyanocobalamin See VITAMIN B_{12}.

cyanogen (cyanogenic glycosides) A family of sugar derivatives found in many plants that can break down to cyanide in the intestines. Cyanogens occur in varying amounts in lima beans, sweet potatoes, YAMS, peas, and fruit (seeds of apricots, cherries, plums). Usually, the levels are so low as to pose no hazard, and these foods contribute significantly in creating a balanced diet low in fat and high in complex carbohydrate. Furthermore the content varies with the strain, and most cultivated strains contain little cyanogen; for example, American strains of lima beans contain little cyanide. CASSAVA, which does contain cyanide, is traditionally prepared in a manner that destroys cyanogens. Small, nonfatal doses of cyanide lead to headaches, a sensation of tightness in the throat, palpitations, and weakness. (See also COOKING; FOOD TOXINS.)

cyclamate (sodium, calcium cyclamate) An ARTIFICIAL SWEETENER used until 1970 as a food and beverage additive. Cyclamate is 30 times sweeter than table sugar (SUCROSE) but does not contribute calories. Cyclamate also lacks the aftertaste commonly experienced with SACCHARIN.

Cyclamate was banned because evidence linked it to bladder CANCER in rats and mice. Its safety was reexamined in 1985 and the National Academy of Sciences/National Research Council concluded that cyclamate by itself does not cause cancer, but it could still be a tumor promoter, that is, it could enhance the effect of cancer-causing agents. The evidence that it causes genetic damage and testicular atrophy continues to be examined. (See also DELANEY CLAUSE; FOOD ADDITIVES.)

cysteine (cys, L-cysteine) A sulfur-containing AMINO ACID that serves both as a building block of proteins and as an ANTIOXIDANT to prevent oxidative damage within cells. Most people manufacture ample amounts of cysteine from METHIONINE, an essential sulfur-containing amino acid; thus, cysteine is not generally essential when the diet provides ample, high-quality protein. However, cysteine may become a conditionally essential amino acid for the newborn infant when its synthesis by the immature liver is limited. Cysteine is the only amino acid with a free sulfur group, and in proteins sulfur groups from neighboring cysteines link up to stabilize the protein structure to enhance biological activity; for example, cysteine links stabilize the hormone INSULIN, the digestive enzyme CHYMOTRYPSIN and the protective protein keratin, found in hair, nails, and skin.

Cysteine is a raw material for the important cellular antioxidant, GLUTATHIONE, made in large amounts by most cells. Glutathione represents a key in the defense against FREE RADICALS, highly reactive molecules that are suspected culprits in the initiation of CANCER. Both cysteine and glutathionine lessen tissue damage due to radiation therapy, perhaps through their antioxidant activity. Glutathione also helps boost immunity.

Cysteine seems to reduce chemical toxicity: In experimental animals, cysteine reduces toxicity to certain anticancer drugs, ACETAMINOPHEN (a common analgesic drug), certain PESTICIDES, industrial compounds (acrylonitrite), and even ALCOHOL (ethanol). A derivative, N-acetyl cysteine, can decrease abnormal thick mucus (mucolytic activity) and has been used to raise glutathione levels in the liver. It may be a therapeutic agent for cardiovascular disorders and AIDS. There is evidence that cysteine stimulates B cells, a part of the IMMUNE SYSTEM that is responsible for antibody production. Cysteine should be used only with medical supervision. Excessive cysteine may interfere with insulin, a critical hormone for regulating blood sugar in diabetics. More generally, very little is known about safe doses and long-term effects of cysteine supplements. There is a possibility of causing kidney stones when cysteine is oxidized; VITAMIN C may counteract this effect. (See also CYSTINE; HOMOCYSTEINE.)

cystine The oxidation product that forms spontaneously from the sulfur-containing AMINO ACID, CYSTEINE. Cystine itself is not a protein building block and is not considered one of the 20 basic alpha amino acids. Cystine is quite insoluble and can precipitate (crystallize) in the urine, forming stones in the kidneys and the bladder.

cystitis An inflammation of the bladder and one of the most common ailments of the urinary tract. (See also URINARY TRACT.)

cytochrome P450 A family of iron-containing enzymes, primarily responsible for the ability of the LIVER to modify potentially dangerous chemicals and to neutralize normal products of metabolism. Unlike cytochromes found in MITOCHONDRIA, cytochrome P450 occurs as part of the membranous system (ENDOPLASMIC RETICULUM) of liver cells, as well as intestinal and kidney cells, which help detoxify chemicals.

Repeated exposure to pollutants and drugs stimulates the liver to form high levels of cytochrome P450. While the increased activity allows the liver to dispose of a greater toxin load, it also increases the likelihood that the liver will produce highly reactive by-products and FREE RADICALS that are potential MUTAGENS and CARCINOGENS. Thus pollutants can increase the oxidative damage associated with AGING, CANCER, and DEGENERATIVE DISEASES such as ATHEROSCLEROSIS.

The levels of cytochrome P450 enzymes in the liver vary greatly among individuals. Low levels or high levels of certain cytochrome P450s can reflect the inherited ability of the body to synthesize certain of these enzymes. A person with high levels of these detoxifying enzymes may process toxins quickly, creating free radicals and potentially damaging compounds in the process and creating a drain on antioxidant defenses. Alternatively, those who produce very low levels may be very sensitive to environmental toxins due to their limited ability to clear them from the body. "Rapid detoxifiers" may need a higher dosage of drug or anesthetic; slow detoxifiers may need less. Riboflavin, niacin, VITAMIN B_6, phospholipids like lecithin, as well as FLAVONIDS, support the function of the cyctochrome

P450 detoxication. (See also ANTIOXIDANT; CHOLESTEROL; FOOD TOXINS.)

cytochromes A family of iron-containing PROTEINS that function in important oxidation reactions of cellular chemistry (METABOLISM). Cytochromes possess a helper compound, HEME, a red oxidation-reduction pigment containing IRON. Cytochromes play a key role in cellular RESPIRATION, in which FAT and CARBOHYDRATE are burned (oxidized). Cytochromes belong to a group of electron carriers, the ELECTRON TRANSPORT CHAIN, that function in MITOCHONDRIA, the energy-producing particles of cells. Electrons pass sequentially from one cytochrome to another, like a bucket brigade, and simultaneously energy released from burning metabolic fuels is harnessed as ATP, the energy currency of cells. Other cytochromes are key constituents of the liver's battery of drug-destroying enzymes. These enzymes attack drugs, pesticides, pollutants, and other foreign chemicals to inactivate them and to make them water soluble so they can be excreted. (See also CYTOCHROME P450; DETOXIFICATION.)

cytolithiasis The formation of stones (calculi) in the urinary bladder and kidneys. The occurrence of kidney stones is steadily increasing worldwide, paralleling the occurrence of CARDIOVASCULAR DISEASE, diabetes, and HYPERTENSION. More than 5 percent of males and 10 percent of females experience a kidney stone during their lifetime. Kidney stones account for one out of every 1,000 hospital admissions in the United States. There are usually no apparent symptoms of cytolithiasis until a stone blocks the urinary tract, when the pain can become excruciating as the stone passes down the urinary tract. In the first half of the 20th century, stone formation occurred almost exclusively in the bladder. Presently in the United States, stones form more often in the upper urinary tract or kidney.

Conditions for the formation of kidney and bladder stones include increased rate of excretion of CALCIUM, OXALIC ACID, and URIC ACID in the urine. With DEHYDRATION, the concentration of excreted calcium oxalate can increase to the point where calcium oxalate crystallizes. To prevent all types of stones, dilution of urine is critical; this is best accomplished by drinking 2 liters of fluids daily. The formation of calcium-containing stones, the most prevalent kind, is associated with consumption of low-FIBER, highly REFINED CARBOHYDRATE, high-FAT, high-SODIUM, and high-CALCIUM foods. A high VITAMIN D intake, excessive MILK consumption, and ALUMINUM salts, in addition to kidney disorders and glandular conditions like hyperthyroidism, may also play a role. Many patients with GOUT have a higher risk of kidney stones due to their excessive buildup of uric acid. A high oxalic acid intake from black tea, COCOA, SPINACH, BEET greens, and RHUBARB promotes stone formation. Poor fat absorption, possibly excessive VITAMIN C, and VITAMIN B_6 deficiency, increase the risk of stone formation, and ANTACIDS containing calcium carbonate, when overconsumed, can lead to kidney stones in susceptible people.

Prevention of Gallstones

Vegetarians have a lowered risk of developing kidney and bladder stones, suggesting that diet plays a role in the etiology. To the extent this is true, most kidney stones may be preventable. Eating more FRUITS and VEGETABLES, controlling weight, and minimizing SUGAR intake helps avoid high urinary calcium. Adequate MAGNESIUM in the diet limits the crystallization of calcium oxalate as kidney stones. VITAMIN K is required to form a urinary glycoprotein that inhibits calcium oxalate crystallization in the bladder, while VITAMIN B_6 reduces the production of oxalates. Furthermore, many patients with recurring stones show abnormal B_6-dependent enzyme levels. CITRIC ACID binds calcium and retards stone formation; consequently, citrate supplementation may prevent recurrent kidney stones. (See also GALLSTONES.)

cytoplasm The gel-like liquid that fills all cells, excluding organelles like the nucleus and MITOCHONDRIA. The cytoplasm is surrounded by the cell's outer boundary, the plasma membrane, and consists primarily of WATER, in which ions (especially POTASSIUM and CHLORIDE) and ENZYMES are dissolved. The cytoplasm houses all of the protein synthesizing machinery including messenger RNA,

AMINO ACIDS, and ribosomes, as well as enzymes of carbohydrate metabolism (GLYCOLYSIS) and fatty acid synthesis. An elaborate array of subcellular protein fibers, such as actin, myosin, microfilaments, and microtubules, assist in cell movement and help direct the flow of materials to the cell membrane. HORMONES affect cellular function via cytoplasmic messenger molecules. Embedded in the cytoplasm is a system of smooth membranes, called the ENDOPLASMIC RETICULUM, which, in the liver, completes FATTY ACID synthesis, synthesizes steroid hormones and destroys drugs and pollutants. (See also FAT METABOLISM; FATTY ACIDS.)

cytosine A nitrogen-containing compound that is a building block of DNA and RNA. Cytosine is one of the four nitrogen-containing compounds used by DNA to define the genetic code. Cytosine is synthesized by all cells with nuclei from the amino acids aspartic acid and GLUTAMINE, together with BICARBONATE, and therefore is not an essential nutrient.

Cytosine is degraded to CARBON DIOXIDE, AMMONIA, and smaller fragments, all of which are water soluble and do not contribute to the URIC ACID load in the bloodstream. Therefore cytosine breakdown does not promote GOUT. (See also PURINE.)

cytotoxins (cytotoxic agents) A diverse family of chemicals capable of destroying cells and tissues. Cytotoxins can be antibodies or they can be toxic agents from BACTERIA, MOLD, or MUSHROOMS that attack a particular organ. Examples include AFLATOXIN, a liver carcinogen from grain mold; BOTULINUM TOXIN, a bacterial neurotoxin responsible for BOTULISM, a deadly form of food poisoning; and toxins in shellfish that accumulate during "red tides," a brownish-red coloration of tidal water resulting from the growth of huge numbers of microscopic organisms. Other cytotoxic agents include by-products of lipid oxidation, for example in rancid FATS and oils, as well as oxidized CHOLESTEROL formed when animal fat is heated at high temperature. Foods fried in lard contain oxidized cholesterol, as do powdered whole MILK and powdered EGG products. Oxidized cholesterol may damage cells lining arteries (ATHEROSCLEROSIS).

Cytotoxic agents also include a family of drugs developed to kill cancerous cells. The strategy of chemotherapy lies in selecting cancerous, diseased cells as targets, while sparing other normal, rapidly dividing cells such as cells of the IMMUNE SYSTEM. As an example, methotrexate and aminopterin, drugs that resemble the B vitamin FOLIC ACID, are used to inhibit cell division in leukemia cells. (See also ANTIOXIDANTS; CANCER; VEGETABLE OIL.)

D

Daily Reference Values (DRVs) A set of dietary reference values established for nutrients for which no standards have previously existed. This includes FAT, SATURATED FAT, CHOLESTEROL, total CARBOHYDRATE, PROTEIN, FIBER, and POTASSIUM. The DRVs for nutrients that produce energy, including fat, protein, carbohydrate, and fiber, are based on a 2,000 CALORIE-a-day diet, unless listed otherwise for a 2,500 calorie diet.

DRVs are calculated according to the following guidelines:

- fat: 65 g, based on 30 percent of calories and saturated fat 20 g, based on 10 percent of calories
- total carbohydrate: 300 g, based on 60 percent of calories
- fiber: 25 g
- protein: 50 g, based on 10 percent of calories. (This DRV for protein is for adults, except for pregnant women and nursing mothers, and children over the age of 4 years: The DRV for infants under 1 year is 14 g; for children between 1 and 4 years, 16 g; pregnant women, 60 g; and nursing mothers, 65 g.)

The DRVs for cholesterol, sodium, and potassium do not change with the calorie level because they do not yield energy:

cholesterol: 300 mg
sodium: 2,400 mg
potassium: 3,500 mg

Daily Values (DVs) A set of reference values designed to help consumers use food labels and assist them in planning a healthful diet. They appear on food labels and are comprised of two sets of nutrient reference values, the Daily Reference Values (DRVs) and the REFERENCE DAILY INTAKES (RDIs), as the basis for declaring the nutrient content on a food label. Food labels now provide the amount of key nutrients as percentages of the DVs for each nutrient provided by one serving. DVs also provide a basis for thresholds in such descriptions as "high FIBER" or "low FAT." Thus the term "high fiber" designates the fiber content in a serving of food providing 20 percent or more of the daily value for fiber, that is, 5 g or more. (See also DIETARY REFERENCE INTAKES.)

dairy-free frozen desserts Ice cream substitutes that contain no MILK, cream, lactose (milk sugar), or cholesterol. TOFU and soy-milk frozen DESSERTS, frozen natural fruit confections, and even frozen rice desserts are now marketed. Usually these desserts lack CALCIUM, ARTIFICIAL FLAVORS, and artificial colors, artificial stabilizers, preservatives, or the SATURATED FAT found in ice cream. On the other hand, frozen desserts generally contain large amounts of SUGAR or other sweeteners (FRUCTOSE CORN SYRUP, FRUCTOSE, or HONEY). Rice-based frozen desserts may contain maple syrup and fermented rice sweetener in addition to rice.

Some brands of frozen desserts also contain VEGETABLE OIL. Tofu-based frozen desserts are usually high-calorie, high-fat foods. The calories in dairy-free desserts range from 128 to 247 per half-cup serving, and the fat or oil content of soy-derived desserts ranges from 6 to 14 g per serving, which is equivalent to ice cream. The amount of tofu varies from brand to brand and can be less than 10 percent of the ingredients.

Fruit-based frozen desserts are prepared from whipped fruit juices and fruit purees. Some brands contain only 9 percent fruit and fruit juices and may contain GUMS and PECTIN. Sugar or fat are not usually added, so fruit-based desserts are lower in fat and total calories than the tofu frozen desserts or ice cream. They generally provide 63 to 80 calories per 4 oz. serving. Sorbet and fruit ices are almost fat free, but they contain more sugar, including corn syrup.

Sometimes people who are sensitive to cow's milk react to foods labeled as "nondairy" or "pareve" (containing neither milk nor milk products). Traces of milk protein have been found in samples of frozen soy and rice desserts. This is an important consideration because an estimated 0.1 percent to 7.5 percent of children have adverse reactions to cow's milk. (See also BALANCED DIET; PROCESSED FOOD; SOYBEAN.)

dairy product MILK or a food that is derived from it, including CHEESE, BUTTER, ICE CREAM, and YOGURT. Consuming dairy products, which are typically high in CHOLESTEROL and SATURATED FAT, can increase the risk of CARDIOVASCULAR DISEASE and OBESITY. Dairy products make up about 15 percent to 20 percent of the American diet. Dairy products are generally good sources of calcium.

dandelion (*Taraxacum officinale*) A green leafy plant that is a member of the sunflower family. Though gardeners have long confronted the dandelion, dandelion greens are a nutritious food. Like other vegetable greens they are a rich source of IRON and CALCIUM. The BETA-CAROTENE content of dandelion greens exceeds that of CARROTS. Dandelion greens also provide INULIN and PECTIN (soluble FIBER). Herbalists throughout the world use dandelion to improve liver function and bile flow and for liver conditions such as hepatitis and jaundice. Dandelion also seems to act as a diuretic (increases water loss).

Cultivated dandelion greens are more tender than wild greens. Wild dandelions may have been sprayed with a weed killer or fungicide, and plants growing next to roads with a high volume of traffic may have been contaminated by exhaust pollution. A cup of chopped, cooked dandelion greens contains 35 calories; protein, 2.1 g; carbohydrate, 6.7 g; fiber, 1.4 g; calcium, 147 mg; iron, 1.89 mg; vitamin A, 1,229 retinol equivalents; and vitamin C, 19 mg.

DASH diet (Dietary Approaches to Stop Hypertension) A clinical study sponsored by the National Heart, Lung, and Blood Institute that tested the effects of diet on patients with elevated blood pressure (HYPERTENSION). Participants ate a diet rich in FRUITS, VEGETABLES, and low-fat DAIRY PRODUCTS. They avoided red MEAT, sweets, and SUGAR-rich drinks. The DASH diet provides high amounts of FIBER, POTASSIUM (4,700 mg), CALCIUM (1,240 mg), and MAGNESIUM. Study participants exhibited lowered blood pressure and LOW-DENSITY LIPOPROTEIN (LDL) cholesterol (the less desirable form of cholesterol). High blood pressure and cholesterol levels are major risk factors for CARDIOVASCULAR DISEASE.

In a second clinical study, participants reduced their consumption of dietary SODIUM. Some participants followed the DASH diet while the remainder ate a typical American diet. Results showed that lowered sodium intake reduced blood pressure levels in both groups, but the group that followed the DASH diet had the most significant results.

Svetkey, Laura P. et al. "Effects of Dietary Patterns on Blood Pressure: Subgroup Analysis of the Dietary Approaches to Stop Hypertension (DASH) Randomized Clinical Trial," *Archives of Internal Medicine* 159, no. 3 (February 8, 1999): 285–293.

date (*Phoenix dactylifera*) The fruit of the date palm tree. Dates are actually a single-seeded berry. They have been cultivated in North Africa and regions of the Middle East since 2,000 B.C. or earlier. The Middle East still supplies most of the world's date crop, although Arizona and California supply U.S. domestic needs. Unripened dates are green. When ripened, they are yellow or red with a thick, syrupy flesh. Dates are harvested, ripened, and dried before shipping. Dates are good sources of dietary FIBER and IRON; although, unlike most fruits, dates do not contain significant amounts of VITAMIN C. The most common variety of date produced in the United States is the Deglet Noor, which is semisoft. Semisoft dates can be stored up to eight months if refrigerated. Dry dates contain little moisture and are often pasteurized to inhibit MOLD growth. Dates are a very sweet fruit, they can contain up to 70 percent SUGAR. Ten pitted dates provide 228 calories; protein, 1.6 g; carbohydrate, 61 g; fiber, 7.23 g; potassium, 540 mg; iron, 1 mg; niacin, 1.83 mg; thiamin, 0.07 mg; riboflavin, 0.08 mg. Most of the CARBOHYDRATE is in the form of sugar.

DDT (dichloro-diphenyl-trichloroethane, chlorophenothane) One of the first powerful, synthetic PESTICIDES to be used worldwide. DDT has been used against a wide range of insects, especially Japanese beetle and European cornborer, as well as louse, mosquito, bedbug, fly, flea, and cockroach. DDT is classified as a CHLORINATED HYDROCARBON, a type of compound that is neither easily degraded in the environment, nor readily broken down in the body. The first pesticides were designed to persist in the environment in order to control pests longer. This has had profound ramifications. First, the widespread use of DDT rapidly led to DDT-resistant insects. Second, DDT and other chlorinated hydrocarbons accumulate in the FOOD CHAIN because they are not readily biodegradable. Birds, including the American eagle, and fish suffer well-documented toxic effects from DDT, and in 1972 the United States banned DDT except for public health use (to control insects that can spread disease) and for crop protection where no alternative pesticide was available. In spite of the ban on DDT, high levels were reported in fish caught off California coastal waters nine years after its manufacturing was terminated. Individuals eating polluted fish have more DDT in their blood.

DDT causes CANCER in mice, but the effects that chronic exposure to small doses have had on human health are unknown. Breast cancer rates in the United States have risen steadily, and an increased environmental exposure to pollutants has been implicated. A Kaiser Foundation Research Study of 57,000 women did not find a link between DDT exposure and increased risk of breast cancer. In the United States a woman's breast milk can contain DDT at a level that is one-and-a-half times more concentrated than in the woman's blood. For an average infant, this represents a daily intake of about 50 mcg of DDT—on a weight basis, equivalent to about 10 times the average adult intake. The long-term effects on childhood development of this exposure are unknown. (See also GREEN REVOLUTION.)

Snedecker, Suzanne M. "Pesticides and Breast Cancer Risk: A Review of DDT, DDE, and Dieldrin," *Environmental Health Perspectives* 109, suppl. 1 (March 2001): 35–47.

decaffeinated beverages Drinks, especially COFFEE, TEA, and SOFT DRINKS, from which most of the caffeine has been extracted. The process of decaffeination causes a small loss in flavor and aroma. Decaffeinated coffee is not caffeine free; it contains low levels of caffeine, 1 to 5 mg per cup, compared to 100 to 150 mg for a cup of regular. This level may be enough to trigger cravings in those attempting to overcome caffeine addiction. Some producers extract caffeine from roasted ground coffee with organic solvents, either methylene chloride or ethyl acetate. Following solvent extraction, the decaffeinated beans are steamed to remove residual solvent. The excess moisture is removed and the decaffeinated beans are roasted. Ethyl acetate seems to be a safe solvent for caffeine extraction, though concern was raised about the use of methylene chloride because it is a weak carcinogen. The U.S. FDA has ruled that the trace amounts of these solvents present in some decaffeinated coffee pose no health threat.

To avoid organic solvents altogether, caffeine can be extracted with water, followed by charcoal filtration. In this process, beans are first steamed, then soaked in water for long periods to remove 97 percent of the caffeine. They are then dried and roasted to develop aroma and flavor. Tea can also be decaffeinated. Typically, solvent extraction either with ethylacetate or with carbon dioxide at high temperature and pressure can remove most of the caffeine from tea. Decaffeination affects the flavor of tea more than coffee.

decalcification The removal of CALCIUM from BONES. A deficiency of calcium or inadequate VITAMIN D required for calcium uptake, and an imbalance of certain HORMONES (parathyroid hormone and calcitonin), can cause mineral loss from bone (dissolution). Calcium usage in the body and bone loss depend upon complex interactions. If calcium levels in the blood begin to decrease, the parathyroid glands secrete parathyroid hormone, parathormone, which increases calcium levels by activating osteoclasts (cells that break down bone) while decreasing calcium excretion by the kidney and increasing calcium uptake by the intestine. Parathormone stimulates the kidneys to convert vitamin D to the hormone, CHOLECALCIFEROL.

It is believed that a deficiency of the female sex hormone ESTROGEN after menopause causes osteoclasts to be more sensitive to parathormone, resulting in increased bone breakdown and elevated blood calcium levels. Elevated blood calcium in turn would decrease parathormone output, decrease vitamin D activation and thus further increase excretion of calcium. Estrogen replacement therapy is ultimately aimed at maintaining bone mass in postmenopausal women.

Calcium losses are influenced by the diet. High protein intake, high phosphate intake (from SOFT DRINKS), and excessive sugar consumption increase calcium loss in the urine. Calcium is also lost when excessive dietary FIBER is ingested. MAGNESIUM, VITAMIN B_6, FOLIC ACID, VITAMIN B_{12}, BORON, and STRONTIUM have been shown to stabilize bone calcium and bone density. Boron seems to increase estrogen levels in postmenopausal women; it may also help activate vitamin D. (See also HORMONE; OSTEOMALACIA; OSTEOPOROSIS.)

decoction The extraction of water-soluble materials and flavors from meat and vegetables by boiling in water for varying times. BOUILLONS are prepared in this way. In botanical medicine, essences may be extracted from plant material by boiling in water. Decoction differs from an infusion, in which boiling water is poured on a plant material; extraction continues without further boiling. A common example of infusion is TEA steeped in hot water. Because the act of boiling is more vigorous and occurs at a higher temperature, decoction extracts more material than infusion.

deficiency, subclinical The state of being marginally nourished. In contrast with overt malnutrition, which causes identifiable diseases, mild or moderate nutrient deficiencies need not reveal obvious signs of illness. Nonetheless, subclinical deficiencies lead to lowered immunity and decreased resistance to viral, bacterial, and fungal infections; difficult pregnancies, low birth-weight infants, and delayed growth and development; learning problems; short-term memory loss; and a host of vague symptoms ranging from fatigue to depression.

A marginal nutrient deficiency can lead to inadequate reserve to meet emergencies. For example, a woman who diets, especially a teenage woman whose body is growing, may not have enough IRON reserves to support a pregnancy adequately. Subclinical malnutrition can have long-term consequences. Subclinical deficiencies can set the stage for DEGENERATIVE DISEASES that include CANCER, HEART DISEASE, high blood pressure, diabetes, OSTEOPOROSIS, ARTHRITIS, PERIODONTAL DISEASE, AUTOIMMUNE DISEASES, and SENILITY.

For optimal health, the body needs more than minimum amounts of vitamins and minerals to prevent full-blown disease. However, the nutrient requirements for optimal health are unknown for most nutrients. The RECOMMENDED DIETARY ALLOWANCES (RDAs) are standards designed to maintain health for a healthy population and do not define the optimal amount for each of the nutrients for individuals. As a general guideline, an intake of a given nutrient that is consistently two-thirds of the RDA or less increases the risk of malnutrition. When several nutrients fall substantially below the RDA, there is a much greater risk of malnutrition and its consequences.

Problem Nutrients

Surveys in the United States and Canada indicate the most common nutrient deficiencies are: CALCIUM, IRON, MAGNESIUM, ZINC, VITAMIN A, VITAMIN C, VITAMIN B_6, and FOLIC ACID, among certain groups. In developing countries, protein-calorie malnutrition is the major nutritional disorder, followed by vitamin A deficiency. In developed countries, the most obvious cause of subclinical nutrient deficiency is an inadequate diet. Reliance on highly processed foods can lead to inadequate intake of key nutrients beyond those used as food enrichment or fortification.

Causes of Subclinical Deficiencies

Historically, poverty, illiteracy, and malnutrition are intertwined. Infants and children in low-income families, pregnant teenagers, elderly persons, and institutionalized clients are most likely to be inadequately nourished in the United States. Nutritional deficiencies can occur even with an adequate diet. Inadequate stomach acid and DIGESTIVE ENZYMES limit nutrient assimilation. A diseased or inflamed intestine will not be able to complete DIGESTION, nor will it absorb individual nutrients effectively, especially if transit through the gastrointestinal tract is too rapid for efficient absorption, as during diarrhea.

Strategies to Correct Marginal Nutrition

Even if the amount of each nutrient needed for optimal health were known for the average person, the amounts needed by individuals would still differ, due to the unique biochemical makeup of each individual. Variations in nutrient needs reflect different genetic compositions, overall health, diet histories, lifestyles, ages, and exercise patterns. Therefore, individualized nutrition counseling is a most effective strategy to overcome nutritional deficiencies. Nutrition counseling relies on evaluating how well the body is stocked with nutrients and on dietary planning to correct nutritional imbalances. Optimally, the physician and nutritionist work as a team in evaluating results of diagnostic tests, comprehensive physical examinations and medical history, as well as assessment of nutrient intake, to work out an individualized program that meets the client's needs, including patient education. (See also BIOCHEMICAL INDIVIDUALITY; DIETING; MALABSORPTION.)

deficiency disease A disease state caused by inadequate nutrient uptake and assimilation. Modern nutrition has its origins in the repeated demonstration that severe diseases can be the result of severe, chronic nutrient shortages and are treatable with the appropriate VITAMINS and minerals. In this respect, the importance of vitamins to human nutrition was well established before 1940. Most outright nutrient deficiency diseases have vanished in the United States, though worldwide they are all too prevalent. It is worth noting that nutritional deficiencies can occur with maldigestion and MALABSORPTION even if the diet supplies adequate amounts of vitamins and minerals. Foods must be digested and nutrients must be absorbed to be effective.

Conditions related to severe vitamin deficiencies are listed below.

- NIACIN deficiency causes PELLAGRA.
- THIAMIN deficiency causes BERIBERI.
- VITAMIN B_{12} deficiency leads to PERNICIOUS ANEMIA.
- VITAMIN A deficiency promotes NIGHT BLINDNESS.
- VITAMIN D deficiency causes RICKETS and bone disease.
- VITAMIN B_6, VITAMIN E, vitamin A, and FOLIC ACID deficiencies can cause ANEMIAS.
- VITAMIN C deficiency causes SCURVY.

The following conditions are related to mineral deficiencies:

- CALCIUM deficiency leads to bone disease and bone malformation (OSTEOPOROSIS, OSTEOMALACIA, RICKETS).
- Zinc deficiency causes BIRTH DEFECTS.
- IRON and COPPER deficiencies cause deficiency anemia.
- IODINE deficiency causes GOITER.
- ESSENTIAL FATTY ACID deficiencies cause skin conditions and can contribute to heart disease.

Conditions Related to Protein-Energy Malnutrition

An inadequate intake of protein and energy is the most important nutritional problem in developing nations. Protein and energy deficiencies cause STARVATION syndromes, KWASHIORKOR, and MARASMUS, as extremes. Children bear the brunt. The World Health Organization has suggested that close to 500 million people suffer from nutritional deficiencies. The effects of starvation and semi-starvation on children are profound: anemia, infections due to depressed immunity, chronic DIARRHEA, stunted growth, and failure to thrive. Growth retardation may be irreversible. (See also BALANCED DIET; DIETARY GUIDELINES FOR AMERICANS.)

degenerative diseases Diseases commonly associated with aging in Western, developed countries. They include CARDIOVASCULAR DISEASE (ATHEROSCLEROSIS or clogged arteries; ARTERIOSCLEROSIS or hardening of the arteries, coronary heart disease, STROKE, HEART ATTACK); OSTEOPOROSIS (brittle bones); SENILITY (dementia, ALZHEIMER'S DISEASE); adult diabetes; PERIODONTAL DISEASE; AUTOIMMUNE DISEASES (rheumatoid ARTHRITIS, SPRUE, insulin-dependent diabetes); and CANCER. Several of these diseases are now epidemics of industrialized nations. Cardiovascular disease, cancer, diabetes, and others are linked to OBESITY, itself a potential harmful condition characteristic of affluent societies.

Although a history of inherited tendencies plays a role, degenerative diseases are not necessarily inevitable because lifestyle choices profoundly affect susceptibility to chronic diseases. Often many can be prevented, or at least reduced in their intensity, with a lifelong commitment to EXERCISE, wise food choices, emotional well-being, and avoiding exposure to harmful substances.

Many degenerative diseases respond to nutritionally sound practices. Moderate CALORIE intake and WEIGHT MANAGEMENT help prevent obesity, diabetes, and hypertension, while adequate CALCIUM, trace minerals, VITAMIN D, and exercise help prevent later bone loss. Moderate SODIUM consumption lowers the risk of hypertension and related heart and kidney diseases, and adequate FIBER intake helps maintain the health of the digestive tract and lowers the risk of colon cancer. ANTIOXIDANTS found in fruits and vegetables, like VITAMIN C, VITAMIN E, BETA-CAROTENE, and CAROTENOIDS may decrease the risk of some forms of cancer, cataracts, mental aging, and heart disease. Moderation is a key. Moderate sugar consumption lowers the risk of dental caries; moderate alcohol consumption helps prevent liver disease; and moderate fat consumption lowers the risk of obesity, heart disease, and some forms of cancer. (See also AGING.)

deglutition The process of swallowing, especially foods. Deglutible refers to a substance that can be swallowed. In the first stage of swallowing, chewing pulverizes food and mixes it thoroughly with SALIVA. The tongue forces the BOLUS (wad) of food back into the mouth and into the upper part of the throat. In the involuntary or automatic stage of swallowing, the bolus moves into the ESOPHAGUS, the tube leading to the stomach. The bolus triggers nerve signals to the deglutition center in the brain stem. In turn, the brain signals the palate to close the nasal passage. Breathing is interrupted for about two seconds and the palate again reopens. PERISTALSIS, rhythmic contractions, conducts the bolus through the esophagus to the stomach.

Gulping food can lead to swallowing an excessive amount of air, which in turn can cause an excessive air buildup in the stomach, which is one cause of heartburn. Chewing food thoroughly not only eases swallowing but also aids digestion because pulverized food is more easily broken down. Furthermore, up to 20 minutes may elapse before the stomach senses that food has entered the stomach itself and relays that signal to the brain. The brain responds by triggering the release of hormones that stimulate the release of stomach acid and digestive enzymes. (See also DIGESTIVE TRACT.)

dehydrated food Refers to a wide range of dried foods. The removal of most of the water content of foods is an ancient form of preservation. Modern dehydration methods employ freeze-drying technology to remove the water rapidly and to preserve nutrients and food quality. Microbial breakdown and many chemical reactions are minimized in dehydrated foods. However, light-induced reactions and lipid oxidation can still occur. Therefore, dehydrated foods are generally sealed both from air and from light, as well as from moisture.

Freeze-drying works best with foods that can be frozen quickly and can be spread in thin layers. For example, soups, vegetables, and stews are quick-frozen at very low temperature, then subjected to a vacuum (reduced pressure). Under reduced pressure, ice evaporates (sublimes), leaving behind the powdery residue minus the weight of water.

On the other hand, sliced fresh fruit, like pears, plums, apples, apricots, and other watery fruit, can be dried in an evaporator that blows warmed air over the food. Dates, figs, currants, and raisins are traditionally sun-dried. Modern production of dried vine fruit employs blown hot air over the fruit on racks.

Dehydrated milk, powdered eggs, and cheeses are commercially dehydrated. They are first blown through a nozzle to create a mist of fine droplets, which is sprayed into a heated chamber for drying. Studies indicate such processes create oxidized forms of CHOLESTEROL, which promotes PLAQUE buildup in arteries in experimental animals. (See also ATHEROSCLEROSIS.)

dehydration A condition resulting from excessive WATER loss. The importance of adequate water for health cannot be overemphasized. The body is a watery environment containing 60 percent water, and blood is 90 percent water. The internal environment of the cell, the cytoplasm, is primarily water. Water also functions in digestion and absorption. Water helps maintain the ELECTROLYTE balance, the balance of dissolved ions in body fluids. Water is the medium for acid-base balance, so that the appropriate pH can be maintained. Water helps the body dispose of wastes. The kidney requires water to filter wastes out of the blood, and the liver requires water to remove toxic materials and waste products. Water evaporation helps regulate body temperature.

During dehydration, the kidneys do not filter out wastes efficiently, and toxic products such as AMMONIA can accumulate in the blood. Extreme dehydration can lead to coma, and even death.

COFFEE, TEA, BEER, and COLA SOFT DRINKS can increase water loss through increased urination. People with busy lifestyles often do not drink enough water. THIRST may not be a good indicator of how much water is needed because the sensation of thirst lags behind real need. Consumption of eight to 10 glasses daily of water and other beverages will replace water lost through urine, sweat, and wastes. Food supplies the equivalent of about four glasses of water daily.

Many situations can lead to dehydration. Dehydration can affect athletes (especially during prolonged exertion in hot weather); individuals working in a hot environment; elderly people who gradually lose their sense of thirst; and institutionalized patients. Other situations causing dehydration are prolonged vomiting or DIARRHEA; use of DIURETICS (water pills) that cause excessive urination; and excessive sweating. (See also ANTIDIURETIC HORMONE; EXERCISE.)

dehydrocholesterol (7-dehydrocholecalciferol) A substance formed by the skin that can be converted to VITAMIN D. As the name implies, dehydrocholesterol is closely related to its parent compound, CHOLESTEROL. The skin and other tissues convert cholesterol to dehydrocholesterol. Exposure to ultraviolet light in sunlight converts this cholesterol derivative into vitamin D. In northern latitudes (Scandinavia, Canada, northern United States) winter skin exposure to sunlight may be inadequate for vitamin D formation. Institutionalized patients who are not exposed to sunlight and who do not drink vitamin D-fortified milk are also prone to the effects of vitamin D deficiency because of inadequate formation of vitamin D from dehydrocholesterol. (See also CALCIUM; MALNUTRITION.)

Delaney Clause An amendment to the Federal Food, Drug and Cosmetic Act banning the addition of CANCER-causing additives to processed food, cosmetics, and drugs. This legislation reflected the belief that there is no safe limit of exposure to a cancer-causing material (CARCINOGEN). Controversy has surrounded the Delaney Clause since it was enacted in 1958.

In the 1980s reinterpretation of the existing law directed the U.S. FDA to permit the low-level use of known carcinogens. The Food Quality Protection Act of 1996 supersedes the Delaney Clause and it amends the Federal Insecticide, Fungicide, and Rotenticide Act by establishing a single health-based standard for PESTICIDE residues in all foods. The new safety standard is defined as "a reasonable certainty that no harm will result from aggregate exposure to the pesticide chemical residues." This act will allow the use of additives that present a negligible risk. The EPA will have authority to require chemical manufacturers to disclose information about their pesticides. All existing tolerances for pesticides will be reviewed within 10 years. Provisions to ensure the safety of children are included. When the evidence for safety is questionable, then the allowable levels will be lowered to permit up to 10-fold more protection for children. The act also requires distribution of health information about pesticides in foods by food stores nationwide.

Only a fraction of chemicals cause cancer. Identifying the risks of cancer due to new additives and chemicals, as well as to food additives introduced before the legislation in the 1960s, are major goals of medical research. A fundamental issue lies in the estimated number of cancer-related deaths that are tolerable when balanced against the benefits of using a given additive. An additional complication is a result of modern technology. Chemical analytical techniques are now ultrasensitive so that carcinogens at extremely small concentrations, a few molecules in a billion or less, are routinely measured. The consequences of exposure to such minute amounts of carcinogens, pollutants, and possible additive effects, are areas of active research. (See also EPIDEMIOLOGY; CHEMICALS.)

Degnan, Frederick H., and Gary W. Flamm. "Living With and Reforming the Delaney Clause," *Food and Drug Law Journal* 50 (1995): 235–256.

dementia A permanent mental deterioration characterized by impaired judgment, memory loss, orientation problems, poor intellectual functioning, and changeable emotional response. General mental deterioration often occurs after the age of 70 with a gradual onset. Dementia occurs more often in women than in men. Typically, dementia brings short-term memory lapses, loss of interest in life, fitful sleep, mood swings, and confusion. It can progress to tantrums, paranoia, severe depression, and refusal to eat. The patient may become incontinent and unable to feed herself.

Dementia may be caused by decreased blood supply to the brain, hardening of the arteries (cerebral ARTERIOSCLEROSIS), high blood pressure, and nutrient deficiencies, including severe deficiencies of VITAMIN B_{12} and NIACIN.

Certain illnesses can create apparent dementia: heavy metal poisoning (such as lead poisoning); alcoholism; high fever due to infections; disorders of the liver and kidney; hormonal imbalances.

Many common medications can produce apathy, weakness, depression, and mental confusion; this is an increasing problem among the elderly, who often take multiple medications. (See also AGING; AIDS; ALZHEIMER'S DISEASE; PELLAGRA; SENILITY.)

denatured protein A PROTEIN that has lost its biological function or activity. Typically, ENZYMES become inactive and no longer serve as catalysts. Proteins are fragile molecules; their biological function depends upon the maintenance of a single shape or conformation, which can be altered by a wide variety of agents, including heat; extreme acid or alkaline conditions; foaming; oxidation; and removal of ions from solution. Organic solvents and detergents are also denaturing agents. BLANCHING vegetables denatures enzymes that cause changes in texture, color, and flavor of food. Cooking protein-rich foods like MEAT, EGGS, and legumes denatures the protein, making it more accessible to DIGESTIVE ENZYMES and speeding DIGESTION. Stomach acid (hydrochloric acid) also serves as a protein denaturant, significantly increasing digestion. (See also COAGULATED PROTEIN.)

dental caries See TEETH.

dental fluoridosis A light brown mottling of tooth enamel due to excessive FLUORIDE consumption during tooth maturation and before the tooth has erupted from the gum. The mottling of teeth is not considered a health risk. Continued exposure to high levels of fluoride may be related to a risk of bone fractures later in life. (See also FLUORIDATED WATER.)

dental plaque Transparent deposits of BACTERIA and debris adhering to tooth surfaces. Dental plaque precedes tooth decay and PERIODONTAL DISEASE.

Diet has an important role in the formation of plaque, and sugar remains the leading dietary cause of tooth decay because it is a particularly effective food for the bacteria. Bacteria responsible for dental plaque, such as *Streptococcus mutans*, ferment sugars in food to organic acids, which dissolve the minerals in teeth. Tooth enamel cannot repair itself. Bacteria can then infect pockets in enamel, leading to cavities. In addition, several strains of bacteria can infect gums. Plaque buildup and periodontal disease may be prevented by proper flossing, brushing, and periodic cleaning by a dental hygienist and by limiting consumption of sugar-rich foods like candy and sweets. Brushing immediately after eating such foods limits plaque formation. (See also CANDY; CARBOHYDRATE.)

deoxycholic acid See BILE ACIDS.

deoxyribonucleic acid See DNA.

deoxyribose A simple SUGAR building block of DNA, the genetic material of cells. The DNA molecule consists of very long chains with a "backbone" of deoxyribose. Deoxyribose is not an essential nutrient because the body makes ample amounts from ribose, a common sugar containing five carbon atoms. (See also CARBOHYDRATE METABOLISM; GLUCOSE.)

depression A prolonged feeling of overwhelming sadness, with an inability to feel pleasure, loss of appetite, weight loss or weight gain, excessive guilt, diminished ability to concentrate, sense of hopelessness, lethargy, insomnia, suicidal thoughts, and persistent headaches. Chronic and severe depression can lead to psychosis and suicide. Depression is a serious health problem; an estimated 25 percent of Americans suffer from clinical depression at some time in their lives. Depression may indirectly increase the risk of clogged arteries by increasing the risk of cigarette smoking, which raises levels of a clotting protein (fibrinogen).

Causes

Depression has no one specific cause but is the result of a complex interaction among genetics, biochemistry, and psychological factors that leads to abnormally low levels of several important brain chemicals related to emotions.

Food allergy and environmental sensitivities as causes of psychological symptoms remains controversial. However, in some cases, food allergies or chronic exposure to toxic chemicals, solvents, and toxic metals may cause mental disturbances. Nutritional deficiencies, hormonal imbalances, and reactions to medications can contribute to depression.

Many nutrient deficiencies can influence the onset of depression. A deficiency of the essential amino acid TRYPTOPHAN, and several mineral deficiencies, including calcium, iron, magnesium, and potassium, lead to depression. Certain vitamins are specifically associated with behavioral changes: These include VITAMIN C, BIOTIN, VITAMIN B_{12}, FOLIC ACID, NIACIN, RIBOFLAVIN, PANTOTHENIC ACID, VITAMIN B_6, and THIAMIN. Folic acid and vitamin B_{12} status are low in some patients suffering from depression; 31 percent to 35 percent of patients suffering from depression in the United States may be deficient in folic acid. In the brain, folic acid and vitamin B_{12}, together with the essential amino acid methionine, seem to raise levels of the neurotransmitter SEROTONIN, which acts as an antidepressant.

Circumstantial evidence links thiamin deficiency and depression. Thiamin deficiency alters brain chemistry, and thus, on admission, psychiatric patients are frequently found to be thiamin deficient. Depression is one of the symptoms of chronic niacin deficiency (PELLAGRA).

Other Causes

Imbalances of the PITUITARY, HYPOTHALAMUS, THYROID, and/or ADRENAL GLANDS have been implicated in depression. Depression is an early symptom of hypothyroidism (low thyroid output), and adrenal gland malfunction can lead to excessive cortisol production, which can produce depression, nervousness, and insomnia. The brain is very dependent upon blood sugar (glucose) for energy, and severely emotionally disturbed patients are prone to HYPOGLYCEMIA (low blood sugar). A gradual onset of hypoglycemia can lead to depression, blunted mental functioning and emotional instability.

Pharmaceutical Causes

Depression can be induced by corticosteroids, betablockers, and blood pressure medications that disrupt the normal balance of neurotransmitters, the chemicals that convey nerve impulses. Oral contraceptives can induce deficiencies of VITAMIN B_6, presumably resulting in lowered serotonin production in the brain, which can affect mood.

Nutritional Approaches to Treatment

Normalizing swings in blood sugar levels may help treat depression. Small, frequent meals that are high in protein and complex carbohydrates, while eliminating sweets and refined carbohydrates are useful strategies. Nutritional supplements can help ameliorate depression associated with nutrient deficiencies.

Much research has focused on neurotransmitter imbalances associated with depression, especially serotonin. Supplementing nutrients that are raw materials for neurotransmitters, particularly the amino acids tryptophan, PHENYLALAMINE and L-TYROSINE, together with vitamin B_6, have been used therapeutically with inconsistent results. Most likely to benefit are those with bipolar disorder. These nutrients may enhance the effects of antidepressants in some cases. The use of gram amounts of amino acids requires the supervision of a physician skilled in nutrition. In 1990, the U.S. FDA withdrew tryptophan as an isolated nutritional supplement. St. John's wort (*Hypericum perforatum*) has been used historically to elevate mood in cases of mild depression.

Alpert, J. E., and Fava. M. "Nutrition and Depression: The Role of Folate," *Nutrition Reviews* 55, no. 6 (May 1997): 145–149.

Elkins, Rita. *Solving the Depression Puzzle,* Pleasant Grove, Utah: Woodland Publishing, 2001.

dermatitis A range of skin conditions involving inflammation, with redness and swelling, itching, and other abnormalities. Contact dermatitis is caused by exposing the skin to an irritating substance. Poison ivy and poison oak are classic examples of agents causing contact dermatitis. Regular exposure to mild irritants can cause the skin to become red, dry, scaly, cracked, or flaking. Cosmetics (hair care products, colognes, antiperspirants), antibiotics, and kitchen chemicals like detergents and cleansers can be causes of contact dermatitis in susceptible people.

ATOPIC DERMATITIS is associated with more severe symptoms, such as ECZEMA, with skin eruptions, blisters, and crusts. This condition runs in families. About 3 percent of infants have atopic dermatitis, which often clears up by 18 months of age. Food allergy is often implicated as a possible cause. In adults, itchiness, redness, and swelling may worsen with STRESS and FATIGUE. An allergy to wool, excessive exposure to oils and soaps, and a deficiency of any vitamin of the B COMPLEX can cause atopic dermatitis. (See also ALLERGY, FOOD.)

dessert The last meal course. In the United States, dessert is likely to be a high-sugar, high-fat food: pastry-like cookies; cakes and pies; ice cream or other frozen dessert; custards or puddings; and gelatin desserts. Cheese, tarts, and custards are favorite desserts in Great Britain. In France, meals traditionally end with fruit, cheese, and a wine. In northern Europe cakes and tarts are often desserts. In Spain and Latin America, flan is traditional. Dessert may also include milk-based sweets with fruits. In India, sweet puddings and cakes flavored with honey, nuts, and rose water are typical dessert items. In many other cuisines, fresh fruit, tea, and coffee end the meal, without a sweet course. (See also DAIRY-FREE FROZEN DESSERTS.)

detoxification The chemical modification of foreign substances and waste products in order to help the body dispose of potentially harmful substances. Detoxification refers to treatment protocols designed to help the body rid itself of waste and toxic materials. The LIVER is a key actor in detoxification. Its battery of protective enzymes can oxidize and inactivate toxic compounds to increase their water-solubility so they can be excreted more readily. Liver enzymes add oxygen, break bonds, remove carbon atoms, and attach highly water-soluble materials such as amino acids and sugar derivatives to a wide range of compounds. Common examples of substances detoxified by the liver include ALCOHOL, oxidized to a derivative of acetic acid, AMMONIA, the toxic by-product of amino acid degradation, converted to nontoxic UREA, steroid HORMONES, and pollutants.

CYTOCHROME P450 refers to a major class of oxidizing enzymes of the liver, requiring IRON and RIBOFLAVIN. Cytochrome P450 enzymes can add oxygen atoms to otherwise very resistant compounds, including a variety of drugs and cyclic hydrocarbons.

A genetic defect in this cytochrome system, which occurs in about 20 million Americans, reduces their ability to break down drugs. Individuals with this defect are more likely to develop side effects when administered common prescription drugs such as painkillers at typical dosages.

Detoxification Procedures

A variety of treatments have been designed to help rid the body of toxins and environmental pollutants. The recommended approach entails a lifelong commitment to a healthful diet and regular physical exercise. With a substantial loss of body fat through supervised fasting or weight loss programs, there will be less fat available to accumulate fat-soluble contaminants like pesticides. In addition, drinking plenty of WATER helps the kidneys work efficiently to cleanse the blood and to excrete waste products. At least two quarts of water should be drunk daily. The diet should emphasize whole, minimally processed foods with fruits and vegetables and should supply adequate antioxidants including VITAMIN C, plus COPPER, MANGANESE, SELENIUM, and ZINC, needed by the body's detoxication enzymes to function optimally. Additional antioxidants, including vitamin E, may be prudent. Cabbage family vegetables (CRUCIFEROUS VEGETABLES) boost detoxifying enzyme levels. "Lipotropic" factors like CHOLINE, a nitrogen-containing compound used as a raw material for the phospholipid lecithin and for brain chemicals, and the essential sulfur-containing amino acid, METHIONINE, may help liver metabolism especially with fat-soluble materials. Milk thistle (*Silybum marianum*) and other botanical preparations have also been used to support liver metabolism.

Of course, limiting exposure to toxic agents is critically important. Gel-forming fibers like psyllium husk, guar gum, pectin, and oat bran can help bind ingested toxins and prevent their absorption. These can be combined with toxin-binding materials such as bentonite clay. The PESTICIDE burden can be reduced by eating organic produce and peeling waxed fruits and vegetables. Exposure to toxic chemicals, including drugs, should be minimized. Since many organic solvents are easily absorbed through the skin, direct contact with paint and solvents should be avoided. (See also ORGANIC FOODS.)

detoxification in recovery programs Supervised programs designed to assist in the recovery from a drug or an alcohol ADDICTION. Detoxification in this context involves abstaining from the addictive substance to allow the body to recover, while supplying support and counseling during critical phases. Withdrawal symptoms often initially accompany abstinence, including CONSTIPATION, FATIGUE, irritability, headache, joint ache, and perspiration. Severe symptoms may accompany withdrawal from ALCOHOL, tranquilizers, or sleeping pills and may require medical supervision.

After a detoxification program has been completed, exposure to even small amounts of the offending material may trigger a strong reaction.

In addition to abstinence, nutrition counseling is recommended. Eating nutritious meals with less fat, COFFEE, alcohol, white bread, pastry, and SUGAR forms a key part of the recovery process. Programs may recommend certain vitamins, amino acids, and ANTIOXIDANTS to diminish withdrawal symptoms and to boost the body's ability to dispose of toxic materials. (See also ALCOHOLISM; BEHAVIOR MODIFICATION.)

devil's claw (*Harpagophytum procumbens*) Native to southern Africa, this herbal painkiller is named for the miniature hooks that cover its fruit. For thousands of years, the Khoisan people of the Kalahari Desert have used devil's claw root in remedies to treat pain and complications of pregnancy and in topical ointments to heal sores, boils, and other skin problems. Since it was introduced to Europe in the early 1900s, its dried roots have been used to restore appetite, relieve heartburn, and reduce pain and inflammation.

Although devil's claw is odorless, it contains substances that make it taste bitter. It is a leafy perennial with branching roots and shoots whose secondary roots grow out of the main roots. The roots and tubers are used for medicinal purposes and contain iridoid glycosides that are believed to have strong anti-inflammatory effects. Harpagoside (one type of iridoid) is highly concentrated in devil's claw root and has been shown in some laboratory studies to have pain-relieving and anti-inflammatory properties.

The root is available either whole or ground, as well as in capsules, tablets, liquid extracts, and topical ointments. Teas (infusions) can be made from dried devil's claw root.

Devil's claw is considered to be nontoxic and relatively safe for most people, with virtually no side effects if taken orally at the recommended therapeutic dose for short periods of time. However, high doses can cause mild stomach problems in some individuals. It is not clear whether devil's claw becomes toxic if taken for long periods of time. Individuals with stomach ulcers, duodenal ulcers, or gallstones should not take devil's claw unless recommended by a health care provider. Devil's claw should not be used during pregnancy or breast-feeding.

Baghdikian, B., M. Lanhers, J. Fleurentin et al. "An Analytical Study of the Anti-Inflammatory and Analgesic Effects of *Harpagophytum procumbens* and *Harpagophytum zeyheri*," *Planta Med.* 63 (1997): 171–176.

Blumenthal, M., A. Goldberg, and J. Brinckmann. *Herbal Medicine: Expanded Commission E Monographs.* Newton, Mass.: Integrative Medicine Communications, 2000.

dextrin (maltodextrin) A sweetener containing a mixture of STARCH degradation products. Dextrin is obtained commercially by treating starch with enzymes, alkali, or acid. The source of starch is usually CORN, but POTATO and other starches are also used. Because starch is composed of GLUCOSE, dextrin yields glucose during digestion.

Dextrin also prevents sugar in candy from crystallizing and also serves as a thickening agent. Dextrin is used to encapsulate flavors used in powdered mixes. Dextrin holds water in foods and is used in baked goods, as well as gravies and sauces. It is incorporated into electrolyte-replacement sports drinks, where it serves as a readily used energy source.

dextrose A simple sugar also known as glucose that is used commercially as a sweetener. In foods, it occurs in FRUITS and HONEY. Dextrose contributes to the brown color of bread crusts and baked goods. Less sweet than sucrose, it is often used as a food additive when oversweetness is a problem, such as an additive in SOFT DRINKS to increase the flavor and make the beverage more appealing to the consumer. Dextrose is a refined carbohydrate and consequently adds only CALORIES and no other nutrients like vitamins and minerals, to food.

Glucose, whether ingested as a dextrose sweetener in processed food, or produced by starch digestion in the intestine, enters the blood very quickly and rapidly raises BLOOD SUGAR. Elevated blood sugar stimulates the pancreas to release INSULIN; in turn, this hormone causes tissues to absorb glucose, so that it can be burned for energy or converted to fat. (See also CARBOHYDRATE METABOLISM; GLYCEMIC INDEX.)

DHEA (dehydroxyepiandrosterone) A HORMONE made by the adrenal glands, testes, and ovaries. Like other steroid hormones, DHEA is fabricated from CHOLESTEROL and is released into the bloodstream where it is the most abundant of this hormone class. However, unlike the other steroid hormones, production of DHEA peaks between the ages of 25 and 30, and then declines with increasing age. While DHEA possesses complex, multiple roles in health and disease, its physiologic role is still not clear.

Research suggests that low blood levels of DHEA are linked to CARDIOVASCULAR DISEASE in men, perhaps by decreasing fat synthesis and the formation of LOW-DENSITY LIPOPROTEIN (LDL) cholesterol, the less desirable form of cholesterol. In addition, DHEA may reduce the risk of OSTEOPOROSIS and several forms of cancer. DHEA also can prevent the development of diabetes in mice with a predisposition to this disease. On the other hand, high DHEA levels in postmenopausal women can lead to increased abdominal fat, resistance to the blood-sugar lowering action of INSULIN and increased risk of cardiovascular disease.

DHEA supports a healthy immune response. Low DHEA blood levels increase the risk of infection. DHEA may be effective against autoimmune diseases such as RHEUMATOID ARTHRITIS and lupus. DHEA apparently increases the levels of a growth factor (insulin-like growth factor) that boosts cell metabolism and helps regulate immunity. In men, DHEA administration may activate T-cells, called natural killer cells, that combat viruses. Current research suggests that this powerful hormone plays a role in the aging process, and administering DHEA to older men and women can increase the sense of physical and mental well-being. However, this hormone does not prevent aging. (See also ADRENAL GLANDS; ENDOCRINE SYSTEM; IMMUNE SYSTEM.)

Zhang, Z. et al. "Prevention of Immune Dysfunction and Vitamin E Loss by Dehydroepiandrosterone and Melatonin Supplementation During Murine Retrovirus Infection," *Immunology* 96, no. 2 (February 1996): 291–297.

diabetes, gestational Persistently high BLOOD SUGAR that occurs in about 2 percent of pregnancies. In most cases, the mother's CARBOHYDRATE regulation generally returns to normal after birth. The American College of Obstetrics and Gynecology recommends that all pregnant women be screened for diabetes. Gestational diabetes seems to be caused when the hormones of pregnancy prevent INSULIN from acting normally. Like non-insulin dependent DIABETES MELLITUS, gestational diabetes is caused by reduced insulin sensitivity in muscle and other tissues. It increases the risk of difficult pregnancy, stillbirth, high birth weight, and birth defect. Women at risk include those with a family history of the disease or with high blood pressure; with previous difficult pregnancies; who are older than 30 to 35; or who are obese. (See also CARBOHYDRATE METABOLISM; GLUCOSE TOLERANCE; GLYCEMIC INDEX.)

diabetes insipidus A rare disease characterized by excessive urine production without glucose excretion. The resulting copious water loss creates an intense thirst (POLYDIPSIA). This condition is caused by the inadequate secretion of ANTIDIURETIC HORMONE from the PITUITARY GLAND, unlike DIABETES MELLITUS, which is caused by an imbalance in carbohydrate utilization. Diabetes insipidus can be associated with pituitary cancer, inflammation of the pituitary or hypothalamus, meningitis, and tuberculosis. Likewise, antidiuretic hormone production may be diminished after surgical or radiation damage to the pituitary gland, severe head injuries or unknown causes. (See also DEHYDRATION; ELECTROLYTES.)

diabetes mellitus A common disease characterized by excessive BLOOD SUGAR levels after a meal and by excessive production of urine containing an abnormal amount of GLUCOSE. When the body does not effectively absorb glucose from blood, blood sugar remains high for an abnormally long time. (In diabetes insipidus, altered kidney function leads to excessive urine production.)

Diabetes is one of the most common degenerative diseases in the United States, where it strikes one out of every 20 people. There is an epidemic of obesity and diabetes in the U.S., where it is increasing at the rate of 5 percent per year and is the third major killer in the United States. It is expected to affect 8.9 percent of the U.S. population by 2025. Significantly, half of those with diabetes are undiagnosed because the disease does not cause painful symptoms. Early symptoms include fatigue, numbness or cramping of legs, feet, or hands, and slowed wound healing. There are many complications of this disease, including DEHYDRATION (with increased thirst), ELECTROLYTE imbalance, muscle weakness, increased urinary tract infections, early ATHEROSCLEROSIS and high blood pressure, poor blood supply to arms and legs potentially leading to gangrene, eye problems and blindness, kidney disease, and shortened life span. A GLUCOSE TOLERANCE TEST would reveal abnormally high blood sugar levels if they remain elevated three to six hours after ingesting glucose. When blood sugar levels increase to about 180 mg/dl, the kidney passes glucose into the urine; extra water is drawn into the urine, resulting in frequent urination and excessive thirst.

In diabetes, two sorts of events may occur: Either microscopic cells of the pancreas produce too little INSULIN, the hormone needed by tissues to take up glucose, or the released insulin may be ineffective when tissues depending on it for the uptake of glucose become resistant to its normal action. During untreated, severe diabetes mellitus, the inability to use blood sugar creates a state resembling STARVATION. The body responds by degrading stored fat for energy, which can lead to excessive KETONE BODIES, acids from fat metabolism that produce acidic conditions (ACIDOSIS), mineral imbalance, and frequent urination.

Insulin-dependent Diabetes Mellitus (IDDM) (Type I, Juvenile Onset Diabetes)

IDDM is also known as Type I diabetes or juvenile onset diabetes. Patients with IDDM require insulin injections to lower blood sugar because the PANCREAS is damaged and cannot produce insulin. IDDM often begins suddenly and primarily affects children although it may begin in adulthood. IDDM appears to be an AUTOIMMUNE DISEASE in which malfunction of the immune system destroys insulin-producing cells. One of the earliest indications is the production of an antibody capable of attacking the insulin-producing cells. Viral infections such as (measles, mumps, flu, hepatitis), chemicals, or other agents, may trigger the immune system to backfire. There are no known means of preventing IDDM and there is no cure. However, researchers have identified some genetic markers for IDDM (Type 1) diabetes. Relatives of patients who have been diagnosed with this disease can now be tested to see if they, too, are at risk.

Non-insulin-dependent Diabetes Mellitus (NIDDM) (Type II, Adult Onset Diabetes)

NIDDM is also designated as "adult onset," or Type II diabetes. In general, patients do not depend on insulin injections; thus, NIDDM is a less severe form of the disease. NIDDM occurs five times more often than insulin-dependent diabetes. It progresses slowly and often is detected only in its later stages, when it primarily affects adults over the age of 40. Type II diabetes often affects the body's inability to use insulin efficiently. As an example, the number of insulin attachment sites on tissues diminishes with OBESITY, a condition to which NIDDM is frequently related. Inheritance can play a role; having relatives with diabetes increases the risk of developing NIDDM, possibly related to an inherited defect in sugar metabolism. Without treatment, patients gradually become increasingly resistant to insulin action, and they may reach a point at which they can no longer compensate for elevated blood sugar. However, individuals at risk for adult onset diabetes may reduce their risk by exercising and losing weight according to the Diabetes Prevention Program developed by the National Institutes of Health. Lifestyle and dietary changes can reduce the risk of developing type 2 diabetes by 58 percent. The program recommends losing 7 percent of body weight gradually over six months and exercising regularly, for example walking briskly for a total of 2 1/2 hours weekly. Exercise helps lower blood glucose levels by increasing glucose utilization and conversion to energy, both during and after exercise. Exercise also helps slow the development of cardiovascular disease. Women who regularly eat nuts and peanut butter have a reduced risk of type 2 diabetes. It is known that a diet that includes ample nuts can reduce the risk of heart disease, compared to a usual low fat diet.

Treatment

The treatment of diabetes focuses on stabilizing blood sugar at normal levels (60-160 mg/dl of blood), improving nutritional status, implementing a weight management strategy, and preventing secondary conditions including eye disorders, cardiovascular disease, kidney disease, nerve degeneration, reduced circulation, and infections. In IDDM, insulin must be administered and blood sugar and insulin must be balanced throughout the day, especially with carbohydrate meals. Excessive insulin administration can lead to severe HYPOGLYCEMIA.

General dietary guidelines include eating regular meals and snacks, minimizing consumption of sugar and sugary foods and sweets, minimizing high-fat foods, emphasizing whole or fresh or minimally processed foods, and exercising regularly. These steps can minimize a rapid increase in blood sugar, permit more effective regulation by insulin, and permit better utilization of fat.

Syndrome X is a constellation of signs and symptoms often related to NIDDM: obesity (especially "apple" or android obesity); elevated blood sugar, insulin (HYPERINSULINEMIA) and blood pressure; high LDL cholesterol; and low HDL cholesterol. A high carbohydrate diet contributes to the appearance of Syndrome X, which carries the risk of CARDIOVASCULAR DISEASE.

Recent discoveries shed light on mechanisms of weight control and diabetes. Defects in a gene ($beta_3$ adrenergic acceptor) that codes for the binding site for the NEUROTRANSMITTER norepinephrine, increase the risk of middle-age obesity and NIDDM. According to one model, fat tissue secretes LEPTIN, a protein that travels to the hypothalamus. There it could decrease production of neuropeptides that trigger appetite, and also activate sympathetic nerves that release norepinephrine. Normally this neurotransmitter directs fat cells to boost their metabolic rate to burn more fatty acids, but if their coupling site for norepinephrine is inefficient, fat calories may not be burned so easily. The question remains, does diabetes cause obesity or does obesity cause diabetes?

Several recommendations have been made to minimize the effects of type II diabetes: If overweight, weight loss and weight control are the primary means of prevention as well as treatment. If these strategies prove ineffective, oral hypoglycemics (blood-lowering drugs) may be prescribed. Often, patients who lose weight can reduce their need for medication.

Regular aerobic EXERCISE and fitness programs help the body burn glucose. Elevating the heart rate for at least 30 minutes three times weekly is recommended to burn glucose and increase the efficiency of insulin action.

While moderate amounts of SUCROSE (table sugar) in a simple meal may be tolerated by diabetics, excessive sucrose consumption can have undesirable effects on metabolism. Sucrose and fats containing table sugar must be substituted for other carbohydrate-rich foods, rather than adding them to a meal. SUGAR increases blood fat (TRIGLYCERIDES) and CHOLESTEROL levels in some people, and diabetics are prone to HEART DISEASE, which is linked to high lipid levels. Sugar-rich foods often contain extra fat and oils. Fructose has a lower glycemic response than sucrose; however, large amounts can raise LDL cholesterol and there is no clear advantage to using fructose.

Regarding fat consumption, a reasonable approach is to limit fat intake to no more than 25 percent to 30 percent of daily calories, with no more than a third coming from animal fat and hydrogenated vegetable oils. Increasing complex carbohydrate and increasing fiber from fruit and vegetables to 50 percent or more of daily calories, with reduced intake of refined carbohydrate, seems prudent. Weight loss diets need to be tailored carefully for the individual. A moderate reduction in daily calories (250–500) may be advised.

The American Diabetes Association recommends a balanced diet that follows the recommendations in the FOOD GUIDE PYRAMID. Regular exercise and well-balanced meals that are low in fat and sugar help diabetics manage their weight and keep blood glucose levels close to normal. Daily consumption of 20 to 35 grams of dietary fiber from a variety of plant foods is prudent. For example, an apple provides 3 to 5 grams of fiber and a slice of whole grain bread provides 1.5 to 2 grams of fiber.

Specific nutrients have been shown to help improve the body's ability to dispose of blood sugar, especially when deficiencies are present: vitamins including NIACIN, NIACINAMIDE, VITAMIN B_6, BIOTIN, VITAMIN C; and minerals such as CHROMIUM, VANADIUM, COPPER, MANGANESE, MAGNESIUM, and SELENIUM. Chromium supports the action of insulin and biotin supports glucose and fatty acid metabolism by the liver. Magnesium, vitamin B_6, zinc, and niacin have been found to improve the nutritional status of diabetics. Antioxidants, including vitamin E, vitamin C, and selenium, may help in preventing cataracts. Essential fatty acids containing GAMMA LINOLENIC ACID as supplied by borage, primrose or black currant seed oils may be correct imbalances in essential fatty acids. In addition, older women with type 2 diabetes may be able to reduce their risk of heart disease with supplemental soy products containing soy protein and isoflavones.

Sorbitol accumulation within cells is believed to be a major contributing factor in diabetic-related damage. This glucose derivative, once formed within cells, tends to disturb water balance and disrupt cell function. Sorbitol formation can be inhibited by vitamin C. In addition, vitamin C and other antioxidants slow the rate at which excess blood sugar attaches to proteins, a detrimental process that accelerates with elevated blood sugar levels. FLAVONOIDS work with vitamin C to enhance capillary strength and connective tissue integrity, which may be compromised in diabetics. Vitamin B_{12} can help prevent both neuropathy and retinopathy associated with diabetes. In older diabetic patients, digestive function may be compromised and digestive aids may be appropriate.

Gross, Jorge L. "Effect of a Chicken-Based Diet on Renal Function and Lipid Profile in Patients with Type 2 Diabetes: A Randomized Crossover Trial," *Diabetes Care* 25 (2002): 645–651.

Olefsky, J. M., and J. J. Nolan. "Insulin Resistance and Non-insulin-dependent Diabetes Mellitus: Cellular and Molecular Mechanisms," *American Journal of Clinical Nutrition* 61, supp. (1995): 980S–986S.

diarrhea A condition characterized by frequent, loose bowel movements. Diarrhea may be chronic, lasting for weeks or months, or it may occur abruptly and last a short time (acute diarrhea). Acute diarrhea is usually due to an intestinal viral disease, bacterial parasitic infection (dysentery), excessive FRUIT consumption, or a FOOD SENSITIVITY. Too much roughage or bulk in foods like fruit, bran, prunes, apples, and pears; psyllium products marketed as natural laxatives; chemical poisons; and certain medications like erythromycin and tetracycline may cause diarrhea.

Diarrhea involves different mechanisms:

- Osmotic diarrhea refers to excessive fluid retention in the intestines due to the increased concentration of water-soluble materials in the intestine. This can be caused by laxatives containing magnesium (milk of magnesia, epsom salts), carbohydrate malabsorption such as LACTOSE INTOLERANCE; excessive nonmetabolized sweeteners like SORBITOL; excessive VITAMIN C; and excessive consumption of legumes, like beans.
- Secretory diarrhea results from excessive secretion of ions into the intestine, which draws water into the stool. Laxative abuse, fat malabsorption syndromes, or infection by bacteria that produce toxins often trigger bouts of diarrhea.
- Inflammatory disease, such as COLITIS, CROHN'S DISEASE, bacterial infection, parasitic infection.

Reestablishment of normal intestinal bacteria may be important in treating diarrhea. Friendly bacteria like lacto-bacillus and BIFIDOBACTERIA limit the growth of disease-causing bacteria and have antifungal and antiviral activity. It is important to drink plenty of fluids during bouts of diarrhea to prevent DEHYDRATION. If diarrhea persists more than several days, or if it is accompanied by fever or weakness, a physician should be consulted for a detailed diagnosis and treatment plan. (See also ANTIBIOTICS; GIARDIASIS.)

diastolic blood pressure The lowest fluid pressure in arteries when the heart relaxes after its contraction (between heart beats). The normal range is 60 to 90 mm of mercury. Elevated diastolic pressure can result from constriction of arterioles (the smallest vessels carrying oxygenated blood to the capillaries) of the circulatory system, as during a response to stress.

Elevated diastolic pressure is a prime indicator of high blood pressure, one of the leading risk factors for CARDIOVASCULAR DISEASE. In adults, systolic pressure of 160 mm/Hg (the pressure during heart contraction) and a diastolic pressure of 95 mm/Hg (expressed as the ratio, 160/95) is considered to be high blood pressure. (See also BLOOD PRESSURE; CAFFEINE; SODIUM.)

diet The portions and types of foods and beverages consumed on a regular basis. A BALANCED DIET provides all nutrients at levels needed for growth and maintenance of health. A diet can also be a prescribed meal plan, specifying food consumption for a particular health condition or disease state. Four examples:

Bland Diet A traditional nutritional approach to the treatment of peptic ulcers. It is built around milk, soft-fiber foods, milk toast, poached eggs, creamed cereals, strained cream soups, white crackers, rennet milk pudding, custard and gelatin desserts, bananas, cooked vegetables as tolerated, fruit juice, cooked or canned fruit, potatoes, pasta, butter, or margarine. A bland diet omits foods that may cause distress: strongly flavored seasonings, olives, pickles, caffeinated beverages and COFFEE, fried pastries and rice, salad dressings, bran cereals, nuts, raw vegetables, most fresh fruits, and gas-forming foods like brussels sprouts, cabbage, cauliflower, and cucumber.

Clear-liquid Diet This contains foods that remain clear and liquid at room temperature. It is used to provide fluids and electrolytes and to prevent dehydration. This diet would contain BOUILLON, broth, carbonated beverages, coffee, filtered or strained fruit juices, gelatin desserts, and commercially prepared clear-liquid formulas.

Elemental Diet This diet contains nutrients in their simplest forms; for example, AMINO ACIDS may be included in the form of protein hydrolyzates rather than as proteins. An elemental diet is appropriate for those who cannot digest food adequately and therefore require simple nutrients.

Low-fat Diet When a group of American men with blocked arteries followed a diet providing no more than 10 percent of total CALORIES as fat, coupled with exercise, support groups, meditation, and counseling, their blocked arteries were cleared. They were able to keep off an average of 22 pounds from four to eight years afterward. It is not clear whether such a low-fat diet is generally appropriate for adults. Children and young adults into their early twenties continue to grow and have greater nutritional needs unlikely to be met with very low intake of fat. By eating mostly fruits, vegetables, and grains, and avoiding high-calorie food, people will often tend to lose weight. However, approximately 10 percent of Americans respond to a high-carbohydrate diet by increasing blood fat (triglyceride) levels, which can increase the risk of adult onset diabetes and possibly increase the risk of heart disease. (See also DIETING; ROTATION DIET.)

Downer, Nelda, and Janet Gregory. "Nationalizing Nutrition Education," *School, Foodservice & Nutrition* (June/July 1994): 88–93.

Woteki, Catherine E., and Paul R. Thomas eds. *Eat for Life*. Washington, D.C.: National Academy Press, 1992.

diet, high complex carbohydrate A high-fiber diet that typically emphasizes whole, fresh, and minimally processed foods to provide 60 percent or more calories as CARBOHYDRATE, mainly as COMPLEX CARBOHYDRATE; 10 percent to 15 percent as PROTEIN; and 30 percent or less as FAT. A high complex carbohydrate diet resembles a typical Asian meal. The fat comes from whole GRAINS, VEGETABLE OILS, lean MEAT and FISH, low-fat dairy products, and nuts and seeds; the protein comes from grains and lean meat, plus low-fat dairy products. Starchy foods like BEANS and lentils add protein and FIBER. Lentils also increase BLOOD SUGAR slowly, thus potentially increasing GLUCOSE TOLERANCE (the body's ability to dispose of blood sugar rapidly and effectively).

A high-fiber, high complex carbohydrate diet often helps improve the body's ability to manage blood sugar. Such a diet is associated with lower fasting blood sugar levels and lower insulin requirements. Dietary fiber slows the rate of DIGESTION by slowing the rate of food passing through the intestines, and water-soluble fiber seems to reduce the rate of glucose absorption.

High-fiber diets supplemented with fiber up to 50 g daily have been used to lower blood lipids and to lower blood cholesterol. On the other hand, high-fiber diets can raise blood lipids and/or blood sugar among diabetics, cause excessive insulin production and lower the desirable kind of blood CHOLESTEROL, HIGH-DENSITY LIPOPROTEIN (HDL).

Therefore, a high complex carbohydrate diet may not be advisable for some noninsulin-dependent diabetics and patients with high blood pressure. People who eat a high complex carbohydrate diet should monitor their blood fat and cholesterol. Other individuals may not tolerate a high-fiber diet because it can cause gas, cramping, and diarrhea. Obese diabetics should lose weight and exercise in addition to changing their diet. The combined strategy pays greater long-term dividends. (See also DIABETES MELLITUS; GLYCEMIC INDEX.)

Hirsch, J. "Role and Benefits of Carbohydrate in the Diet: Key Issues for Future Dietary Guidelines," *American Journal of Clinical Nutrition* 61, no. 4, supp. (1995): 996S–1,000S.

diet, low carbohydrate A diet providing inadequate CARBOHYDRATE with normal-to-high FAT and PROTEIN consumption. Many "eat all you want" diets specify high-fat and protein, with little carbohydrate (less than 100 g a day). Without enough carbohydrate in the diet, METABOLISM switches to a STARVATION mode, regardless of how much fat or protein is eaten. There is no evidence that this form of DIETING leads to permanent weight loss, and weight that is lost tends to be muscle rather than fat. Weight lost quickly represents water loss, accompanied by lost ELECTROLYTES.

The brain and nervous system require GLUCOSE (BLOOD SUGAR) for energy. When the diet does not provide enough carbohydrate, muscle protein breaks down to supply AMINO ACIDS. The liver converts them to glucose, which is released to raise blood sugar. Massive fat breakdown promotes the accumulation of KETONE BODIES in the blood, and disposal of these acids can cause DEHYDRATION and electrolyte imbalances. Side effects of low carbohydrate diets include nausea, low blood pressure, and fatigue. Fat may deposit in the liver because the normal fat-burning machinery is overwhelmed by extensive fat degradation. Children, pregnant women, and patients with a history of GOUT should not diet to lose weight without medical supervision. (See also DIETING; CRASH PROGRAMS; FAT METABOLISM; GLUCONEOGENESIS; KETOSIS.)

diet, very low-calorie Packaged, generally powdered formulations featuring low CARBOHYDRATE and CALORIES. VLC DIETS supply PROTEIN and carbohydrate to provide 300 to 600 calories a day, but without adequate protein and carbohydrate in the diet, the body will lose two ounces of muscle protein a day. VLC diet products available today represent improvements over earlier versions because they supply high-quality protein together with the required amounts of vitamins and minerals. These modifications help prevent the dangerous losses of heart muscle that sometimes accompany complete FASTING. Liquid or powdered formulations should meet the RECOMMENDED DIETARY ALLOWANCES (RDAs) for protein (AMINO ACIDS), VITAMINS, ELECTROLYTES, and TRACE MINERALS. Including a modest amount of carbohydrate in the formulation minimizes muscle breakdown and loss of lean body mass.

Many commercial weight management programs use VLC diets to get a client's weight loss program off to a fast start. However, their use is a severe strategy, to be followed for a short time only. VLC diets require supervision by qualified personnel, experienced in monitoring weight management. Optimally, supervision is coupled with behavior modification and nutrition education programs. VLC liquid protein diets are designed for obese adults who are at least 30 percent above their optimal body weight and for whom OBESITY creates a medical risk.

The drastic reduction in calories characteristic of very low calorie diets can damage heart muscle and can lead to HEART ATTACKS in susceptible individuals. Clinicians cannot predict who is most at risk. Furthermore, these diets induce DEHYDRATION and electrolyte imbalance. Side effects can be nausea, dry skin, and intolerance to cold. Drastic, short-term weight loss programs require routine monitoring by qualified professionals.

If the liquid protein formulation is to be used as a total weight loss diet, the label must warn that its use without medical supervision can lead to severe illness or death. If it is to be used to supplement a diet with more than 400 calories, the label must warn that the product cannot be used in weight loss diets supplying less than 400 calories a day.

VLC diets are not advised for infants, children, pregnant or nursing women, nor for patients with insulin-dependent diabetes or severe mental problems. (See also DIABETES MELLITUS; DIETING; CRASH PROGRAMS.)

Høie, L. H., and D. Bruusgaard. "Predictors of Long-Term Weight Reduction in Obese Patients After Initial Very Low-Calorie Diet," *Advances in Therapy* 16 (1999): 285–289.

dietary fiber See FIBER.

Dietary Guidelines for Americans Governmental recommendations to prevent disease and overnutrition, first published by the U.S. Department of Agriculture and the U.S. Department of Health and Human Services in 1980 and updated in 2000 (fifth edition).

As in earlier editions, the latest emphasizes balance, moderation, and variety and specifically encourages increased consumption of GRAINS, VEGETABLES, and FRUITS. For the first time the recommendations include a guide on how to keep food safe to eat, with particular emphasis on food preparation at home. The guidelines recommend:

Aiming for Fitness

This means choosing a lifestyle that combines sensible eating with regular physical activity. To be at their best, adults need to avoid gaining weight, and many need to lose weight. Being overweight or obese increases the risk for high blood pressure, high blood cholesterol, heart disease, stroke, diabetes, certain types of cancer, arthritis, and breathing problems. A healthy weight is key to a long, healthy life.

Daily Physical Activity

Being physically active and maintaining a healthy weight are both needed for good health, but they benefit health in different ways. Children, teens, adults, and the elderly all can improve their health and well-being and have fun by including moderate amounts of physical activity in their daily lives. Physical activity involves moving the body. A moderate physical activity is any that requires about as much energy as walking two miles in 30 minutes. Americans should aim to accumulate at least 30 minutes (adults) or 60 minutes (children) of moderate physical activity most days of the week, preferably daily.

Building a Healthy Base with Prudent Food Choices

Consumers should follow the FOOD GUIDE PYRAMID. Different foods contain different nutrients and other healthful substances; no single food can supply all the nutrients in the amounts needed. For example, ORANGES provide VITAMIN C and FOLATE but no VITAMIN B; CHEESE provides CALCIUM and vitamin B, but no vitamin C. People should choose the recommended number of daily servings from each of the five major food groups in the food guide pyramid. Dieters who avoid eating all foods from any one group should seek nutritional guidance to ensure they are getting the nutrients they need.

Consumers should choose a variety of grains daily, especially whole grains and a variety of fruits and vegetables.

Food Safety

It is also important to keep food safe from harmful BACTERIA, viruses, parasites, and chemical contaminants. Farmers, food producers, markets, food service establishments, and other food preparers have a role to keep food as safe as possible, but safe food handling also must be practiced at home. This means washing hands and preparation surfaces often with soap and water; separating raw, cooked, and ready-to-eat foods while shopping for, preparing, or storing food; cooking animal products to a safe temperature; chilling or refrigerating foods promptly; following food-handling instructions on labels; when serving keeping hot foods hot (140° F or above) and cold foods cold (40° F or below); and throwing away any food that may have been handled in an unsafe manner.

(See also DENTAL CARIES; DIETING; EXERCISE; FOOD; HEIGHT-WEIGHT TABLES; HYPERTENSION; TEETH.)

Nutrition and Your Health: Dietary Guidelines for Americans, Fifth Edition. Washington, D.C.: U.S. Departments of Agriculture and Health and Human Services, 2000.

Dietary Reference Intakes (DRI) The most recent set of dietary recommendations established by the Food and Nutrition Board of the Institute of Medicine. They update and expand the RECOMMENDED DIETARY ALLOWANCES—the benchmark of nutritional adequacy in the United States—that have been published by the National Academy of Sciences since 1941. The new DRIs will likely be used to update the REFERENCE DAILY INTAKE values, which were established by the U.S. FDA for use in nutrition labeling.

The DRIs are meant to shift nutritional focus from deficiency to lowering the risk of disease. They reflect the latest research on what levels of nutrients are best to combat diseases such as CANCER, OSTEOPOROSIS, and CORONARY ARTERY DISEASE. DRIs are not broken down by age group or sex; they are average values for the entire U.S. population. DRIs incorporate four nutrient-based dietary reference values:

- Estimated average requirement (EAR). The daily intake estimated to meet the nutrient requirements of people in a specific age or gender group.
- Recommended dietary allowance (RDA). The daily intake that meets the nutrient requirements of 97 percent to 98 percent of people in a specific age or gender group.
- Adequate intake (AI). When the EAR is not available to estimate an average requirement, this intake level is determined based on observing what amount of nutrients sustain health in a specific group of people.
- Tolerable upper intake level (UL). The daily nutrient intake that is unlikely to pose risks of adverse health effects to almost all healthy people of a specific age or gender.

dietetic foods Convenience foods processed especially for certain kinds of diets. Low-CHOLESTEROL, low-SODIUM, and low-CALORIE dietetic foods are typical. For a diabetic, several dietetic products may be helpful, including artificially sweetened SOFT DRINKS, ARTIFICIAL SWEETENERS, and sieved fruit packed in water, not syrup.

The following terms now have specific meanings:

"Low fat" means that the food contains no more than 3 g of fat per serving; or the food contains no more than 3 g of fat per 50 g of food (if the serving size is less than 30 g or 2 tablespoons).

"Low sodium" means that the food provides no more than 140 mg sodium per serving. If the serving size is 30 g or less, or no more than 2 tablespoons, the food will provide at most 140 mg of sodium per 50 g of food.

"Low cholesterol" means that the food provides less than 2 mg of cholesterol (and no more than 2 g of fat) per serving. If the serving size is 30 g or less, or no more than 2 tablespoons, the food provides at most 2 mg of cholesterol per 50 g of food.

In contrast with the above definitions, specifying foods as "dietetic" has no precise meaning because there are no standards to which food manufacturers must adhere for this designation. Dietetic foods may have reduced, although still appreciable, calories. (See also DIABETES MELLITUS; FOOD LABELING; FOOD PROCESSING.)

diet foods Processed foods marketed for individuals requiring low-CALORIE, reduced-calorie, or calorie-restricted diets according to FDA guidelines. These products often reduce calories by incorporating ARTIFICIAL SWEETENERS that provide little or no calories. (See also DIETETIC FOODS; DIETING.)

diet-induced obesity See YO-YO DIETING.

diet-induced thermogenesis Heat produced in the body as a result of digesting food and absorbing nutrients. Heat is normally produced as the body uses energy for any of its activities. In other words, thermogenesis is proportional to the total CALORIES used daily. The portion used for DIGESTION and assimilation accounts for 5 percent to 10 percent of total calories. Glandular secretions, synthesis and release of DIGESTIVE ENZYMES, uptake of nutrients by the intestine, and transport of fat and lipids in the blood account in part for this energy expenditure. The energy required to operate body functions while at rest (BASAL METABOLIC RATE) accounts for another 60 percent to 70 percent. The remainder represents energy needed for physical activity. (See also ENERGY; EXERCISE.)

Visser M. et al. "Resting Metabolic Rate and Diet-induced Thermogenesis in Young and Elderly Subjects: Relationship with Body Composition, Fat Distribution and Physical Activity Level," *American Journal of Clinical Nutrition* 61, no. 4 (1995): 772–778.

dieting Restricting food intake in order to control weight. Dieting is a major preoccupation in the United States where the term implies changing the physical appearance to fit society's image of beauty. This raises issues of high expectation, self-esteem, sacrifice, guilt, and denial of underlying emotional problems. At any given time, an estimated one out of every four Americans over the age of 18 is dieting to lose weight. Some studies show that as many as four out of five preadolescent girls believe being thin is attractive; girls as young as 8 years old are dieting. This attitude may explain in part the epidemic of BULIMIA NERVOSA and ANOREXIA NERVOSA in young women.

Women's metabolism generally seems to run slower than men's by an average of 50 calories daily, which means they burn fewer calories. In addition, women's bodies have higher levels of enzymes for storing FAT, and lower levels of enzymes for burning fat, than men do. Hypothetically, these differences in metabolism favor childbearing and fetal development.

Various methods are available to estimate an "appropriate" body weight based upon health standards, rather than an "ideal" body weight, which does not exist. Generally, it is healthier to be within 10 pounds of appropriate body weight than overweight. Recent evaluations support the premise that thinner individuals (down to 10 pounds below the average weight of their group in height and build) may live longer, provided they are healthy and do not smoke.

Individuals with health problems, pregnant and lactating women, and children should not undertake self-prescribed popular weight-loss diets. Heredity is another consideration; an estimated 25 percent of differences in body fat are due to genetic predisposition and family history.

Estimates of dieters' success rates (those who lose weight and maintain the new weight for at least a year) vary anywhere from 2 percent to 25 percent.

Research has provided clues as to why diets frequently fail: First, the dieter's eating habits: often did not change while undergoing the dieting program. Without changing eating patterns the weight lost in a dieting program returns as soon as the dieter resumes usual eating patterns.

Many obese people underreport the amount of food they consume. Careful analysis of caloric intake and fat deposition reveals that they may eat more that normal-weight people.

STARVATION or semistarvation is not a successful weight loss strategy. Drastically reducing food intake promotes a loss of five pounds a week, but it represents mainly water, not fat, loss, and the body regains the water immediately when the diet ends. Losing more than two pounds a week in an unsupervised diet, is not recommended because consuming fewer than 1,000 calories per day throws the body's physiology into a defensive mode for starvation. The BASAL METABOLIC RATE slows down to use fewer calories more efficiently. The body tends to keep the same amount of fat or to gain more weight later. Furthermore, starvation diets are too low in essential nutrients like vitamins and minerals, and chronic dieting can lead to serious health problems and malnutrition.

Often, dietary goals are unrealistic and set the person up for failure. People who keep weight off tend to do it for their own satisfaction, rather than for an external expectation or pressure.

In YO-YO DIETING (a cycle of on-again, off-again dieting) the body can adapt to periods of low calorie intake by increasing its energy efficiency, although the effect on metabolism is not firmly established. Some people find it easier to gain weight and harder to lose it, even without overeating. Negative psychological effects of yo-yo dieting include poor body image, problems with interpersonal relationships, and depression.

Some obese people cannot make permanent reductions in weight, even with severely restricted diets, without emotional repercussions. Some researchers have proposed that certain obese people have an altered metabolism. OBESITY may be locked into the number of an individual's fat cells, because children tend to follow the body build and fat cell distribution of their parents. Formerly obese individuals tend to store dietary fat as body fat rather than burning it. Recent research has demonstrated the presence of a hormone, LEPTIN, produced by fat cells that affects the appetite center in the brain to increase satiety and to curtail eating. In humans, obesity seems to be linked more frequently to the decreased sensitivity of the brain to leptin than to the inability to produce leptin. Nonetheless, it is unlikely that a single substance will treat obesity. Genes that are involved in weight control act together with diet and exercise, and probably no drug will substitute for either.

The lack of physical exercise is perhaps the most important factor in regaining lost fat. Exercise temporarily increases the body's metabolic rate even at rest, and it helps maintain lean body weight when dieting. It also seems to increase the sensitivity of the appetite control center, which tends to be blunted by a sedentary lifestyle.

Overweight people tend to prefer the taste of fattier food, and people who gain weight often eat high-fat foods like chips, fatty meats, fried food, CHEESE, and ice cream. Calories from fat are converted to body fat with a cost of 3 percent of calories. By comparison, 25 percent of calories from STARCH (GRAINS, LEGUMES, VEGETABLES, FRUIT) are burned in their conversion to fat.

To lose weight, experts recommend a variety of approaches. First, avoid yo-yo dieting or diet cycling, crash dieting, and reliance on diet beverages and ARTIFICIAL SWEETENERS. They are ineffective weight loss strategies. Artificial sweeteners do not help with weight control and they may actually promote weight gain, perhaps by creating a craving for sweets, or by creating a false sense of security in eating calorie-laden food.

Dieters should choose a well-balanced, low-calorie diet providing about 1,200 calories per day for women and about 1,600 calories per day for men for prudent weight loss. The diet should allow for a mixture of whole, fresh foods. A diet plan should be developed and followed after weight loss in order to subsequently maintain the current weight.

It's important to eat whole foods, instead of convenience meals in order to stock up on COMPLEX CARBOHYDRATES while cutting back on fat. Eating fruit instead of fruit juice and whole grains instead of white flour products provides more fiber. Chewing FIBER-rich foods puts a damper on hunger, and also helps fill the stomach, which leads to a feeling of satiation.

Dieters should eat less fat, which provides more than twice as many calories as carbohydrates, and enough PROTEIN (40 to 50 g per day) to help lose fat, not muscle. For example, dieters should eat 4 oz. of MEAT, FISH, or POULTRY and two glasses of skim MILK a day. Sweet and salty foods typical of many convenience and snack foods can stimulate HUNGER without satisfying it, and they may not satisfy hunger until excessive amounts have been eaten.

Refined sugars should be reduced, since they can increase hunger and promote weight gain. They boost the body's INSULIN level, which may be a hunger signal for the brain. Whole food snacks like unbuttered popcorn, apples, and bananas will not stimulate hunger. The fat in fatty foods such as doughnuts, ice cream, and pie is easier to convert to body fat than is complex carbohydrate.

Supplements can be used when needed. Many popular diet plans do not provide the RECOMMENDED DIETARY ALLOWANCE (RDAs) of VITAMINS and MINERALS, and supplements may be needed when the diet plan provides only 1,000 to 1,200 calories per day.

Breakfast should be the main meal of the day, instead of supper. Eating heavy meals at breakfast, followed by a medium lunch and a light supper, while consuming the usual amount of calories for the day, may help some overweight people to lose 5 to 10 pounds per month without restricting their calories. Eating only when hungry, and eating smaller meals, can be important dietary modifications.

Psychological support can be helpful. A support group and a qualified counselor can help define and support individual goals. BEHAVIOR MODIFICATION can help change deep-set patterns. Exposure to cues that trigger eating can be controlled. Hostile and anxious people have higher than usual blood cholesterol and greater risk of heart disease, perhaps related to their tendency to burn fat more slowly and make more cholesterol.

Thirty minutes of aerobic EXERCISE will burn 300 calories. With regular exercise, body fat can eventually be replaced with lean muscle, which burns calories at a higher rate. Because exercise increases the calories spent, calories are consumed rather than being stored as fat. Regular exercise helps maintain body weight at the end of the diet program because it counter-balances the body's adaptation to decreased food intake with lowered basal metabolic rate.

Dieting While Dining Away from Home

Eating out poses a challenge for anyone on a reduced-calorie diet. The following suggestions may help in maintaining a diet plan when eating out or eating while traveling.

- Exercising before eating out helps burn calories and takes the edge off HUNGER.
- A light snack if dinner will be late will help avoid nibbling high-calorie snacks such as CHEESE, dips, or cold cuts.
- Restaurants can be screened ahead of time to find those that offer low-calorie options.
- Fat and skin should be trimmed from POULTRY to reduce fat intake.
- ALCOHOL and soft drinks provide surplus calories. Mineral water, non-alcoholic BEER, or WINE are better choices. Drink more water to quench thirst.
- Dieters can share the order or order two appetizers or a soup and salad rather than ordering a full-course meal.
- Whole foods such as vegetables and legumes provide complex carbohydrates instead of fatty foods, which represent surplus calories.
- Baked, steamed, or poached foods are good choices, rather than fried or braised foods, which are cooked with fat or vegetable oil and supply surplus calories.
- BUTTER, sour cream, or salad dressings are essentially fat and should be avoided, together with rich, high-fat desserts for the same reasons.

(See also BODY MASS INDEX; DIETING; CRASH PROGRAMS; FAT METABOLISM; HEIGHT-WEIGHT TABLES.)

dieting, crash Drastically reducing CALORIES to lose weight rapidly, often by purging or using

APPETITE SUPPRESSANTS (AMPHETAMINES and DIURETICS). There is no evidence that crash DIETING leads to permanent weight loss, and it is also medically unsafe. Excessive weight loss (five pounds a week or more) represents water loss, not FAT loss, and the water returns when the diet ends. STARVATION diets do not provide adequate levels of essential nutrients like CARBOHYDRATE, PROTEIN, VITAMINS, and MINERALS. Without enough carbohydrate and protein, muscle protein can be lost at the rate of two ounces per day.

The body adjusts to starvation conditions by burning stored fat for ENERGY. In this process, it can overproduce KETONE BODIES, a readily transported form of fat calories. Excess ketone bodies acidify the blood (ACIDOSIS) and cause dehydration and ELECTROLYTE imbalance. Crash dieting can lead to YO-YO DIETING, a cycle of on-again, off-again dieting. The body may respond by storing fat, not losing it. Crash dieting for several days can also lead to critical losses of fluids and electrolytes.

Rather than crash dieting, patients should consider eating 1,500 calories a day to lose a maximum one to two pounds a week, and 2,000 calories a day to maintain weight. Adult females should consider eating 1,100 calories a day to lose 1 to 2 pounds a week, and eating 1,500 calories a day for stable weight. (See also BALANCED DIET; CONVENIENCE FOOD; KETOSIS; OBESITY.)

dietitian A health professional who provides dietary advice, plans and manages food preparation, and has successfully completed a course of study leading to professional certification. A dietetics educational program typically emphasizes nutrition; food science; food preparation; assessment and dietary management for common clinical situations, such as pregnancy; diabetes and weight control; and management training. Much of the dietitian's training occurs in clinic or institutional environments. Program variations may also emphasize mental health or other specialty areas.

College preparation to become a registered dietitian involves a four-year B.S. program, which qualifies graduates to take the certification examination administered by the American Dietetics Association. About half of the states require licensing. Applicants for licensing exams must be well prepared, with a degree in dietetics, food service management, nutrition, or the equivalent from an accredited institution. Alternatively, a master of science degree program that meets eligibility requirements for the certification exam can qualify an individual for state-approved certification.

diet margarine See MARGARINE.

diet pills A variety of drugs used to suppress HUNGER. AMPHETAMINES (Benzedrine, Dexedrine) are stimulants that have been prescribed for short-term weight loss (10 pounds or less). Newer drugs, such as mazindol phentermine, and diethylpropion, are safer than amphetamines. They mimic the effects of EPINEPHRINE (adrenaline) and block hunger signals in the brain so the patient will eat less food. Nonetheless, these drugs alone are not effective for large-scale weight loss because they do not lead to permanent changes, alter eating patterns, or deal with food-related emotional issues and exercising—essential ingredients of successful weight-loss programs. Because the use of these drugs does not lead to a permanent change in behavior, the lost weight often returns when medication ceases.

Amphetamine-type drugs gradually lose their effectiveness so that higher doses are required to get the original effect. Side effects of amphetamines include nervousness, irritability, insomnia, a false sense of well-being, dry mouth, and dizziness. Less common are blurred vision, vomiting, irregular heartbeat, HYPERTENSION, and impotence. An important consideration is that they are habit-forming. Furthermore, amphetamines are dangerous in combination with monoamine oxidase inhibitors or with other APPETITE SUPPRESSANTS because the combination can severely increase blood pressure. They should not be used by patients with kidney disease, glaucoma, heart problems, or a history of drug abuse or bouts of DEPRESSION.

Other diet pills incorporate DIURETICS, BULKING AGENTS, or thyroid hormone preparations. Diuretics are drugs that increase water excretion by the kidneys; therefore, they are used to control edema, water accumulation in the body, and they do not affect fat loss. Bulking agents add volume to food without calories. They contribute to a sense of feeling full (satiety); so theoretically less food is eaten. Thyroid hormones speed up metabolism; however, the fuel that is burned seems to be muscle protein rather than fat. Their use for weight control is controversial.

Two appetite suppressants, fenfluramine and dexfenfluramine, were taken off the market by the U.S. FDA in 1997 when it was discovered that thousands of patients who took these drugs developed potentially deadly primary pulmonary hypertension and heart valve abnormalities. Dexfenfluramine was shown to cause these injuries when taken alone, and fenfluramine was linked to valve problems in patients who combined it with the drug phentermine in a mixture popularly known as "fen-phen." Both fenfluramine and dexfenfluramine helped patients lose weight by increasing serotonin levels in the blood stream, which provided a sense of well-being and satiety. The problem, researchers discovered after the drugs were removed from the market, was that the drugs destroyed the body's ability to control the amount of serotonin circulating in the blood. Excessive amounts of serotonin can cause cell damage to cardiopulmonary structures.

In late 2000 the FDA issued a public health advisory warning patients about phenylpropanolamine hydrochloride (PPA). This drug is widely used in both over-the-counter and prescription-only nasal decongestants and for weight control in some over-the-counter drug products. The warning was issued after medical researchers published a study showing that phenylpropanolamine increases the risk of hemorrhagic stroke (bleeding into the brain or into tissue surrounding the brain) in women. Men may also be at risk. Since then the FDA has taken steps to remove PPA from all drug products. Many companies have reformulated their products to exclude PPA. No drug yet devised is completely safe and effective for treating OBESITY and for weight loss. (See also APPETITE SUPPRESSANTS; BEHAVIOR MODIFICATION; DIETING; MAO INHIBITORS; WEIGHT MANAGEMENT.)

Center for Drug Evaluation and Research, "Fen-Phen Safety Update Information." Available online. URL: http://www.fda.gov/cder/news/feninfo.htm. Updated March 27, 2001.

diet record A complete inventory of the kinds and amounts of all foods, beverages, and supplements consumed for one or more days in order to assess adequacy of nutrient intake. A DIET record (or diary) can be used to obtain an individualized estimate of daily calories. Typically, a record is kept for three days over a weekend, or for a week. The amounts of food are recorded in terms of the number of ounces, slices, cups, or tablespoons. For example, a piece of meat the size of a deck of cards is about two ounces. A NUTRITIONIST uses food composition tables compiled by the USDA to calculate the average daily consumption of essential nutrients, including vitamins, minerals, protein, carbohydrate, and fat. Sodium, CHOLESTEROL, SUGAR, and dietary FIBER can be calculated. Age, risk factors for disease, medical history, overall health and lifestyle, and dietary goals are other important parameters in evaluating the adequacy of a diet. (See also DIETING.)

digestibility A measure of nutrient uptake, based upon the difference between the amount eaten and the amount recovered in feces in healthy individuals. The index of digestibility, the "coefficient of digestibility," represents the percentage of a nutrient assumed to be absorbed. Typical values for PROTEIN, CARBOHYDRATE, and fat in the standard American diet are 92 percent, 97 percent, and 95 percent respectively, indicating efficient digestion of major, energy-producing nutrients under normal conditions. These are approximations because intestinal microflora ferment undigested nutrients.

digestion The breakdown of food to simple nutrients in the gastrointestinal tract. Food is a complex mixture of many nutrients, and during digestion it undergoes both physical and chemical changes to make these nutrients available to the body. In terms of physical changes, food is pulverized and mixed with SALIVA as a lubricant. STOMACH ACID produces further changes by denaturing (curdling) protein molecules. FAT, oils, and lipid-soluble materials are emulsified by detergent-like BILE salts. These physical changes make substances in foods more accessible to the action of digestive enzymes. Each of the major sources of energy—CARBOHYDRATE, FAT, and PROTEIN—undergoes HYDROLYSIS to release smaller molecules during digestion: PROTEINS yield AMINO ACIDS; fat and oils yield FATTY ACIDS and GLYCEROL; and STARCHES yield the single sugar GLUCOSE. Even table sugar (SUCROSE) must be broken down to its building blocks, glucose and FRUCTOSE. As food is digested, it is mixed, squeezed, and pushed down the GASTROINTESTINAL TRACT by the action of the muscle of the intestine alternately contracting and relaxing in a wave motion.

Many enzymes are necessary to digest food. The mouth initiates digestion. Saliva contains the enzyme AMYLASE, to begin starch digestion. The second site of digestion is the stomach. The stomach produces hydrochloric acid (stomach acid) to sterilize food as it is kneaded to a thick liquid. Protein digestion begins in the stomach with the enzyme PEPSIN, released by tiny gastric glands in the stomach wall and activated by stomach acid. The stomach also manufactures INTRINSIC FACTOR, a protein that binds VITAMIN B_{12} to facilitate absorption of this vitamin.

The SMALL INTESTINE completes digestion and absorbs most nutrients. In this process the pancreas plays a key role. Pancreatic juice enters at the beginning of the small intestine (DUODENUM), providing a battery of enzymes to break down fats, oils, starch, and protein, as well as minor food constituents like PHOSPHOLIPIDS, the building blocks of cell membranes. Secreted BICARBONATE neutralizes stomach acid. The intestine produces an activator of the protein-digesting enzymes. Bile released from the gallbladder emulsifies fat, prior to fat digestion by pancreatic LIPASES. In the last phase of digestion, the intestine produces a battery of enzymes that completely digest PEPTIDES (protein fragments), starch fragments (maltose, DEXTRINS), fat fragments (diglycerides), LACTOSE (milk sugar), and table sugar (sucrose). FIBER is not digested in the small intestine because the body does not manufacture enzymes capable of hydrolyzing this type of COMPLEX CARBOHYDRATE.

A family of hormones work together to regulate digestion. These hormones are produced in many different tissues and affect the gastrointestinal tract in different ways. The following are representative: GASTRINS from the lower region of the stomach stimulate the secretion of pepsin and hydrochloric acid (stomach acid) from gastric glands. Gastrins also stimulate the secretion of bile from the GALLBLADDER and of digestive enzymes from the pancreas. CHOLECYSTOKININ from the DUODENUM, the initial section of the small intestine, also stimulates bile release from the gallbladder and enzyme secretions by the pancreas. SECRETIN from the duodenum stimulates BICARBONATE secretion from the pancreas to neutralize stomach acid and pepsin release in the stomach. Gastric inhibitory protein from the small intestine blocks stomach acid secretion, while stimulating INSULIN production by the pancreas. Motilin from the intestine stimulates gastric and intestinal peristalsis (the rhythmic contraction and relaxation of muscles around the gastrointestinal tract), while enteroglucagon from the intestine blocks intestinal peristalsis. Vasoactive intestinal peptide from the intestine promotes digestive enzymes secretion by the pancreas and intestine, while inhibiting stomach motility.

Individual amino acids, simple sugars and fatty acids, together with vitamins and minerals freed by digestion, are efficiently absorbed by the villi, the fuzzy, rough surface of the small intestine. Most of these nutrients pass on directly to the bloodstream. Fatty acids are an exception. They must be reassembled into fat molecules (triglycerides); together with fat-soluble materials like cholesterol and fat soluble vitamins, they are packaged as CHYLOMICRONS (fat transport particles), then released into the lymph, which carries them to the bloodstream.

The COLON (large intestine) completes the digestive process. It absorbs WATER and minerals like CALCIUM and MAGNESIUM, and forms feces. It is the home of beneficial bacteria that supply VITAMIN K and BIOTIN and other nutrients while limiting the growth of undesirable microorganisms. Much of the fiber in ingested food is degraded by the gut microflora. They produce short-chain fatty acids, which nurture the colon.

Diarrhea, and intestinal disorders like CELIAC DISEASE and CROHN'S DISEASE, reduce intestinal absorption of nutrients. Intestinal inflammation due to FOOD SENSITIVITIES, medications, and infections can make the intestine porous, permitting foreign materials and toxic materials to penetrate the body.

The surfaces of the MOUTH, ESOPHAGUS, STOMACH, and INTESTINES possess important barriers to unwanted materials and pathogenic microorganisms. Cells lining these passageways secrete MUCUS, a slippery viscous material that tends to trap foreign materials. Mucus production especially in the intestine declines with STRESS. In addition to the physical barrier, the immune system is important. For example, cells beneath the intestinal lining secrete an ANTIBODY (secretory IgA) that can neutralize the huge load of foreign materials to which the intestine is subjected daily. Stress and inflammation can limit antibody production, thus setting the stage for infections and multiple food sensitivities. (See also DIGESTIVE ENZYMES; LEAKY GUT; PANCREAS; PERISTALSIS.)

digestive disorders See GASTROINTESTINAL DISORDERS.

digestive enzymes A collection of enzymes secreted by tissues that degrade foods and release nutrients. Four regions produce digestive enzymes: the mouth, the stomach, the PANCREAS, and the intestine.

AMYLASE (ptyalin) is a salivary enzyme that hydrolyzes STARCH to sugars.

GASTRIC JUICE from the stomach wall contains PEPSIN together with hydrochloric acid (STOMACH ACID). Pepsin initiates PROTEIN digestion and releases protein fragments. In the stomach, inactive pepsins (pepsinogens) released in gastric juice are rapidly activated by stomach acid.

The pancreas secretes many digestive enzymes into the intestine: Amylase completes starch DIGESTION initiated in the mouth. TRYPSIN, CHYMOTRYPSIN, and CARBOXYPEPTIDASES A and B represent a battery of proteolytic enzymes that digest proteins to amino acids. LIPASE hydrolyzes fats and oils to fatty acids. Phospholipase degrades PHOSPHOLIPIDS to free fatty acids. Deoxyribonuclease and ribonuclease break down DNA and RNA, respectively. An intestinal enzyme called enteropeptidase activates trypsin, which in turn activates other proteolytic enzymes. Therefore, the health of the small intestine is important in protein digestion.

The small intestine provides important enzymes that complete digestion, peptidases that degrade protein fragments called PEPTIDES to free amino acids and to very small peptides containing just two or three amino acids. All of these products of protein digestion are absorbed readily. Likewise, sugars assembled from smaller sugars (disaccharides) must be hydrolyzed to their constituents in order to be absorbed. LACTASE digests milk sugar (LACTOSE); MALTASE digests maltose; SUCRASE digests table sugar (SUCROSE); and small fragments (DEXTRINS) are digested to glucose by destrinase. Inadequate pancreatic enzyme levels lead to malabsorption of nutrients and eventually to malnutrition. Inadequate levels of digestive enzymes lead to maldigestion and malabsorption of nutrients. Cystic fibrosis and chronic inflammation of the pancreas (pancreatitis) can decrease pancreatic output of digestive enzymes. Low stomach acid production plays a role in disease processes: Normally, an acidic mixture of food paste leaves the stomach and stimulates pancreatic secretion, while an alkaline mixture does not, leading to maldigestion and malnutrition. Parasitic infections, bacterial infection, celiac disease, inflammatory bowel disease, and intestinal resection can diminish the absorptive surface of the small intestine, decrease sucrase and lactase production, and produce lactose or other carbohydrate intolerances. None of the digestive enzymes in humans possess the appropriate specificity to hydrolyze fiber like CELLULOSE or PECTIN, so they are fermented by colonic bacteria to varying degrees. (See also DIGESTIVE TRACT.)

digestive tract (digestive system, alimentary tract) The continuous cavity extending from the mouth to the rectum, together with accessory digestive organs devoted to food indigestion, DIGESTION, nutrient ABSORPTION, and waste elimination. These represent a huge task: During a lifetime, approximately 20 tons of food pass through the body.

The digestive tract consists of the mouth, esophagus, stomach, SMALL INTESTINE, and colon. Digestion begins in the mouth. Chewing (MASTICATION) breaks food into particles and mixes it with SALIVA. Saliva contains AMYLASE to begin STARCH digestion. It also provides MUCIN, which acts as a lubricant for swallowing. The ESOPHAGUS is the long tube that connects the mouth to the stomach. A muscular valve separates the esophagus from the stomach's acidic contents. Acid indigestion occurs when the valve stays open for a period of time, allowing stomach acid to back up into the esophagus.

The stomach is located on the left side of the body, below the diaphragm. It produces the enzymes PEPSIN to initiate protein digestion and hydrochloric acid (STOMACH ACID) to sterilize masticated food and to catalyze pepsin activation. The stomach also produces GASTRIN, a hormone that increases acid production, and INTRINSIC FACTOR, essential for VITAMIN B_{12} absorption in the small intestine. PERISTALSIS, wave-like contractions of muscles around the stomach and INTESTINE, moves chyme (a mixture of food paste and digestive fluids) through the stomach and intestine.

The intestine, a tube about 20 feet long, extends from the stomach to the rectum. The small intestine represents the upper three-fourths of the intestinal tract and begins at the pyloric valve, which regulates partially digested food leaving the stomach. The small intestine contains microscopic glands that produce enzymes to complete carbohydrate and protein digestion. Its enzymes also break down sugars like milk sugar, LACTOSE (with LACTASE), and table sugar (with SUCRASE) to simple sugars. It also digests small protein fragments (with aminopeptidases) to amino acids.

The small intestine consists of three regions. The first section, within a foot of the stomach, is called the DUODENUM, where BILE and pancreatic secretions flow into the intestine. Bile drains from the GALLBLADDER, after synthesis by the LIVER. The pancreatic enzymes are activated at this point. The JEJUNUM or middle region of the small intestine follows the duodenum. It is about 8 feet in length and ends with the ILEUM, which is about 12 feet long. The ileum joins the large intestine at a muscle-bound valve called the ileocecal valve.

Most nutrient absorption occurs in the small intestine. The highly folded surface is lined with fuzzy projections called VILLI, that create a velvet-like appearance of the intestinal wall. The number of villi, 10 to 40 per square millimeter, dramatically increases the surface area to maximize absorption. Furthermore, each absorptive cell possesses many microscopic, hairlike projections called MICROVILLI that further increase the surface area. Nutrients taken up by intestinal cells pass into capillaries and lymphatic vessels. Any undigested or unabsorbed material enters the colon.

The large intestine, or colon, represents the last 5 feet of the intestine. It is shaped like a hoop around the mass of the small intestine. The upward leg of the hoop represents the "ascending colon"; the top of the hoop represents the "transverse colon"; the downward leg represents the "descending colon." The sigmoid colon is the last short section before the rectum. No digestive enzymes are produced by the colon. It absorbs mainly water minerals like calcium and magnesium and short-chain fatty acids from the bacterial fermentation of undigested carbohydrate plus fiber, and it condenses undigestible wastes as feces. The colon houses several pounds of bacteria; most serve useful functions. In particular, they ferment fiber to produce short-chain fatty acids required by colon cells as fuel for normal growth. Colonic bacteria also produce vitamins and limit growth of disease-producing microorganisms. (See also CANCER; COLITIS; DIGESTIVE ENZYMES; MALABSORPTION.)

diglycerides A common type of FOOD ADDITIVE related to FAT and used to suspend fatty materials. Diglycerides prevent bread from going stale by blocking starch alterations; they also make bread soft. Diglycerides improve the stability of MARGARINE, and they improve the consistency of cake dough to make cakes fluffy. This additive also prevents the oil in peanut butter from separating. Diglycerides are common food additives, and Americans eat more than a half-pound of glyceride additives per person per year. Glyceride additives account for about 1 percent of the normal fat intake.

Diglycerides are composed of two FATTY ACIDS linked to glycerol, while fat and oils are TRIGLYCERIDES, containing three fatty acids bound to glycerol. Diglycerides are readily digested and are considered safe food additives. A variety of additives related to glycerides have been created by food technology. Ethoxylated monoglycerides and diglycerides are used as dough conditioners to improve the texture of baked foods. Sodium sulfacetate monoglycerides are used as an antispattering agent and as an emulsifier in margarine. Acetylated monoglyceride and diglycerides are waxy materials used in jelly beans and chocolate coatings. Glycerides are also coupled to LACTIC ACID, CITRIC ACID, and SUCCINIC ACID to form other emulsifiers.

dill (*Anethum graveolens;* false anise) An aromatic herb cultivated by ancient Mediterranean civilizations; the Romans regarded dill as a symbol of vitality. Dill leaves and seeds can season sour cream, fish dishes ranging from salmon to crayfish, as well as bean, cucumber, potato, and cabbage dishes. Bread and cheese may also be flavored with dill. Dill is also used in pickling.

dimethylpolysiloxane (methylsilicone, methylpolysilicone) An organic derivative of silicon. These silicon compounds are insoluble in water and chemically very stable. They find limited use in food manufacture compared to their widespread use in industry and in medicine. Dimethylpolysilicone prevents foaming during steps in the manufacture of refined sugar, GELATIN, chewing gum, and wine. Methylsilicone is added at one to 10 parts per million to VEGETABLE OILS to prevent foaming when these oils are used in cooking. Silicones are inert in the body and are classified as safe FOOD ADDITIVES, although dimethylpolysiloxane contains trace amounts of formaldehyde as a preservative. (See also EMULSIFIERS.)

dioctyl sodium sulfosuccinate (DSS) A FOOD ADDITIVE whose detergent-like properties improve the suspension of powders in water. Many powdered materials like starch, COCOA, and fatty acid derivatives tend to float on top of water. By coating these materials with DSS and similar detergent-like molecules, they more easily dissolve. DSS is used with thickening agents, powdered SOFT DRINK mixes, and cocoa milk beverages (to dissolve cocoa butter). DSS is also used as a detergent to clean fruit and vegetables, and in sugar manufacture. The U.S. FDA is considering adding DSS to a list of food additives that have a GENERALLY RECOGNIZED AS SAFE (GRAS) designation.

dioxin A widespread toxic pollutant. Dioxin refers to a family of chlorine-containing organic compounds that are industrial by-products; the most toxic member is TCDD. Dioxin now contaminates all populations in Western societies. Dioxin is a contaminant of commercial herbicides and the wood preservative pentachlorophenol, and it is created in wood stoves, in municipal incinerators, and wood pulp waste from pulp mills.

Trace amounts of dioxin have been found in people not directly exposed to dioxin. The average American carries five parts per trillion TCDD in fat tissue; and it is present in the BREAST MILK of nursing mothers. Despite this finding, experts of the U.S. EPA, the World Health Organization, and the La Leche League International advise that the advantages of BREAST-FEEDING outweigh potential disadvantages.

Dioxin can be found in MEAT, EGGS, POULTRY, and FISH. Fish likely to be contaminated include Great Lakes fish, walleye pike, and bass caught from polluted waters. It is found in root crops like carrots, potatoes, and onions grown in soil contaminated by spreading pulp mill sludge. Traces of dioxin contaminate paper and paper products like coffee filters, tampons, food packaging, milk cartons, teabags, and disposable diapers. Dioxin appears to migrate into microwaved meat from paper trays. Often the amounts of dioxin are extremely small, five to 13 parts per trillion. This is equivalent to adding one drop to the water carried by the tank cars of a 10-mile train. However, exposure to one part per billion is considered a potential hazard.

Dioxin's toxicity varies with the animal species. When digested by some species of animals such as rats and guinea pigs, TCDD is toxic to the fetus; it causes cleft palate and kidney abnormalities, damages the immune system in newborns, and disrupts the HORMONE system, causing feminization of male offspring. In some animal studies, dioxin causes CANCER in liver, thyroid, skin, and respiratory tract.

Human toxicity of dioxin is controversial. Although the EPA considers dioxin the most potent known animal carcinogen, until recently there was little evidence for specific toxic effects in humans other than serious ACNE. In 1991, German and U.S. studies indicated that at fairly high exposures, as experienced by chemical workers, dioxin is a human carcinogen. The possibility of long-term, subtle effects remains. A 1994 EPA review suggests that dioxin can lower immunity in humans.

To reduce exposure to dioxin: Drink filterless coffee. This reduces exposure due to bleached paper products. Consume organic produce or homegrown produce that has minimal contact with PESTICIDES. Peel or thoroughly wash fruit and vegetables in soapy water. Avoid freshwater fish caught from polluted waters. Eat less fatty portions of meat, and dairy products with high BUTTERFAT. Dioxin is a fat-soluble contaminant and accumulates in fat. (See also BIRTH DEFECTS; RISK DUE TO CHEMICALS IN FOOD AND WATER.)

dips High-fat spreads used as appetizers and snack foods. Commercial snack dips typically contain high levels of sodium and saturated fat (cream cheese, sour cream, hydrogenated vegetable oil, palm, and coconut oil). This is important because OBESITY remains a major health problem in the United·States, and fat is more easily stored as body fat than as carbohydrate. Saturated fat is considered a risk for ATHEROSCLEROSIS in susceptible people. Excessive dietary sodium can increase the risk of high blood pressure in sodium-sensitive people. Home-prepared dips based on low-fat yogurt or low-fat cottage cheese can cut the fat content by 90 percent. (See also DIETARY GUIDELINES FOR AMERICANS; PROCESSED FOOD.)

direct calorimetry A laboratory procedure to measure the number of CALORIES in a food. Food is burned completely in the presence of pure oxygen in a "bomb calorimeter," a sealed chamber immersed in water. Heat released is absorbed by the water. The increase in temperature is measured and converted to calories. A large calorie (kilocalorie) is defined as the amount of heat required to raise the temperature of 1 liter of water at 15° C by 1 degree. The amount of heat released when food is oxidized completely to carbon dioxide and water is the same whether the process occurs in the body or in the laboratory. The amount of heat released—the calories burned—can also be measured directly by immersing a subject in water in an insulated chamber. (See also ENERGY.)

disodium guanylate (GMP, guanosine monophosphate) A FLAVOR ENHANCER used commercially since 1940. GMP contains GUANINE, a nitrogen-containing bicyclic organic compound (base). GMP is found in high concentrations in several species of FISH and MUSHROOMS. GMP has little taste of its own; rather it accentuates natural food flavors. In particular, this FOOD ADDITIVE increases meat flavor without adding more expensive natural flavoring.

GMP appears in instant soups, chicken salad spreads, canned vegetables, and processed meat. GMP is degraded to the waste product URIC ACID and excreted. Individuals with GOUT (uric acid accumulation in joints) and with certain rare genetic diseases (related to PURINE metabolism) should not eat these foods. Otherwise, it is considered a safe food additive. (See also MONOSODIUM GLUTAMATE.)

disodium inosinate (IMP) A FLAVOR ENHANCER used commercially since 1960. Flavor enhancers accentuate food flavors without contributing their own taste. IMP occurs in a wide variety of FISH and animals where it contributes to the meat flavor of these foods. IMP is often used with DISODIUM GUANYLATE and MONOSODIUM GLUTAMATE (MSG), which act synergistically to produce a meaty flavor. By adding flavor enhancers, food manufacturers can use smaller amounts of expensive meat extracts in powdered soup mixes, ham and chicken salad spreads, sauces, and canned vegetables, which may contain IMP and disodium guanylate at levels ranging from 0.003 percent to 0.05 percent. Individuals with GOUT (uric acid accumulation in joints) and those who must avoid PURINES for genetic conditions should avoid this additive because the body converts it to uric acid. (See also FOOD ADDITIVES.)

distilled liquors Alcoholic spirits or liquors produced by distillation of products of FERMENTATION. Distillation concentrates ALCOHOL and characteristic essences of the material fermented. Thus, distillation of fermented sugarcane and juice, syrup, or molasses yields rum; fermented grain mashes yield whiskey; and rye whiskey comes from wheatmash. Rum and whiskey rely on fermentation of mashes by special strains of distiller's yeast (*Saccharomyces cerevisia ellipsoideus*), which produce high alcohol concentrations. Aging distilled liquors in charred oak barrels further modifies the composition. It is important to realize that the alcohol content of one shot (1.5 fluid oz.) of 80 proof gin, vodka, or rye whiskey contributes about 100 calories—and no other nutrients (EMPTY CALORIES). (See also DIETARY GUIDELINES FOR AMERICANS.)

distilled water See WATER.

diuresis The excretion of large amounts of urine. Normally the pituitary gland (neurohypophysis) produces the hormone ADH (ANTIDIURETIC HORMONE), which causes the kidney to remove water from urine and return it to the bloodstream, thus conserving body water. A deficiency of ADH causes DIABETES INSIPIDUS, characterized by excessive, dilute urine. This condition should not be confused with DIABETES MELLITUS, which is a disorder of insulin production and utilization and yields excessive urine with a high level of sugar (glucose) due to high blood sugar. The large quantities of unreabsorbed glucose hold water in kidney tubules, thus causing increased urine output.

Ingestion of certain drugs (DIURETICS), ALCOHOL, CAFFEINE, and large volumes of liquids increases urine output. In contrast, pain, stress, exercise, and anxiety increase ADH production and decrease urination, as do morphine, nicotine, and common medications (clofibrate, carbamazepine, and chlorpropamide). (See also ELECTROLYTES.)

diuretics Agents also known as water pills that increase urine production. Diuretics are prescribed to treat water retention and high blood pressure. These powerful drugs help the kidney lose sodium and water, so they increase the frequency of urination. Some of the safest and most effective are the thiazide diuretics. ALCOHOL and CAFFEINE also increase urine output, and thus are also classified as diuretics.

Thiazide diuretics should not be taken together with alcohol because the combination causes a dangerous drop in blood pressure which is potentially harmful to the heart. Thiazide-type diuretics can cause ELECTROLYTE imbalance, because they may increase the loss of POTASSIUM from the blood. Thiazides may also increase urinary excretion of MAGNESIUM, ZINC, RIBOFLAVIN, and CALCIUM. Triamterene can increase loss of SODIUM and lower blood levels of VITAMIN B_{12} and FOLIC ACID. Furosemide can increase losses of calcium and sodium, and lower serum levels of potassium.

Research studies link the use of diuretics to mild diabetes, increased blood CHOLESTEROL, and an increased risk of HEART ATTACK; and they should not be used as weight loss aids. The rapid weight loss they promote is water loss, not fat loss. (See also BULIMIA NERVOSA; DIETING; CRASH PROGRAMS.)

diverticulitis Inflammation of pouches or bulges (diverticula) in the COLON. Diverticulitis is a potentially serious condition when the contents of the colon are forced into pouches, leading to stagnation of fecal matter, infection, and inflammation. This disease does not, however, seem to lead to CANCER. Diverticulitis can be aggravated by FOOD SENSITIVITIES such as to MILK, WHEAT, and CORN. Symptoms include: cramps, alternating DIARRHEA and CONSTIPATION, gas, bloating, and indigestion.

Lifestyle changes may help prevent diverticulitis. Drinking plenty of WATER and eating enough FRUIT, vegetables, and whole grain foods can prevent complications by keeping the intestine toned and by keeping material flowing through the intestine at a normal rate. The diet should minimize SUGAR and refined CARBOHYDRATES. Increased FIBER intake up to 30 g daily may be helpful; however, a patient with acute diverticulitis, ulcerative COLITIS, or CROHN'S DISEASE should avoid fiber supplements because they may aggravate these conditions. Allergenic foods, foods causing gastrointestinal symptoms, and fruits with tiny seeds, such as STRAWBERRIES, RASPBERRIES, and TOMATOES, can irritate the colon. LAXATIVES and enemas can irritate the colon. Regular physical exercise may help some patients. (See also ALLERGY, FOOD; DIVERTICULOSIS; GASTROINTESTINAL DISORDERS.)

Angott, B. E. et al. "Overview and Treatment of Diverticular Disease," *Journal of the American Osteopathic Association* 101 (April 2001): S19–21.

diverticulosis A nondisease condition featuring diverticula (bulges) in the colon without symptoms. Hernias in the muscle wall of the intestine are very common later in life, and about two or three in 10 Americans develop this condition by the age of 60. The bulges are caused by straining to propel stools during constipation. A small fraction of individuals with diverticulosis develop inflamed bulges and pouches leading to cramps, alternating DIARRHEA and CONSTIPATION, gas, bloating, and indigestion. Measures to prevent constipation include increased FIBER (roughage) consumption and drinking plenty of water. This means eating more vegetables of all kinds, LEGUMES, FRUIT, and whole GRAINS. Safe, mild laxatives can also help avoid constipation. (See also DIVERTICULITIS.)

DNA (deoxyribonucleic acid) The chemical that contains the genetic information of the cell and thus controls heredity. Genes are informational units of DNA that determine the individual's structural and biochemical traits, which are passed from one generation to the next. DNA specifies the structure of all proteins in the body, as well as the mechanisms for duplication and repair of DNA. DNA synthesis require many nutrients, including ZINC, MAGNESIUM, and B vitamins like FOLIC ACID and VITAMIN B_{12}.

The structure of the DNA molecule is unique; human DNA is a meter long, yet it is tightly compressed into the cell's nucleus. DNA exists as compact clusters called chromosomes. DNA is classified as a polynucleotide, consisting of a sequence of four different kinds of cyclic compounds, resembling beads in a chain. The building blocks are called THYMINE and CYTOSINE, ADENINE and GUANINE. Their sequence defines (codes for) the sequence of amino acids in a protein.

Pairs of DNA chains twist about each other to form a double helix, resembling a double-railed spiral staircase with the steps composed of purine and pyrimidine extending inward. The sequences of bases in each DNA strand of the double helix are complementary to each other: a base of one DNA strand specifically pairs with its complementary base of the neighboring strand. The rule for complementary base pairing is simple: Adenine always pairs with thymine; guanine, with cytosine. DNA replication produces exact copies for new cells by using the parent DNA to serve as a template for synthesizing identical DNA chains.

Chemical agents in the environment as well as ionizing radiation can attack DNA, causing mutations, structural alterations in genes. The mutated DNA is passed on to successive generations. Changes in DNA structure alter the coding for specific amino acids, yielding mutant proteins with abnormal structures. Protein variants are common. For example, there are over 500 variants of HEMOGLOBIN in which a single amino acid is replaced by another. Most of these mutations are "silent" because the altered amino acid sequence does not impair biological activity. On the other hand, mutant proteins may be more or less inactive and can cause genetic diseases. Sickle-cell anemia, favism (sensitivity to broad beans), and familial HYPERCHOLESTEROLEMIA (inherited tendency for high blood CHOLESTEROL) illustrate the possible consequences of specific mutations. On the average, 10,000 DNA "hits" per cell are repaired daily. Consequently, mutations are infrequent events. As the organism ages, the DNA repair mechanisms become less effective. DNA damage accumulates in the cell nucleus as well as in the mitochondria, which contain a tiny chromosome. Cumulative DNA damage is believed to underlie the decline in immune function and the increased frequency of cancer associated with aging. (See also CARCINOGEN; GENE; GENETIC ENGINEERING; MUTAGEN; PROTEIN.)

Hartmann, Andreas et al. "Vitamin E Prevents Exercise-induced DNA Damage," *Mutation Research* 346, no. 4 (1995): 195–202.

docosahexaenoic acid (DHA) A large polyunsaturated FATTY ACID that is concentrated in cold-water oceanic FISH and their oils. DHA, together with its relative, EICOSAPENTAENOIC ACID (EPA), seems to lower the risk of coronary heart disease, possibly by reducing blood fat and CHOLESTEROL levels (when initial levels are high) by slowing the production of LOW-DENSITY LIPOPROTEIN (LDL), the less desirable form of cholesterol. Both acids reduce the synthesis of APOPROTEIN B, a key component of LDL.

DHA and EPA also reduce blood clot formation. EPA seems to block the formation of thromoxane A_2, a factor that causes blood platelets to stick together, by slowing its production, while DHA seems to alter cell membrane properties. DHA and EPA may also reduce inflammation associated with

AUTOIMMUNE DISEASE. DHA is necessary for normal development of the eye (retina) and the brain. Premature babies fed DHA-deficient formula have poorer vision six months after birth than similar infants fed DHA-supplemented formula. FISH OIL supplements help improve visual activity of DHA-deficient infants. DHA is a constituent of human milk, suggesting its importance in development. DHA levels are decreased in pregnant women with TOXEMIA and in the elderly.

DHA belongs to the omega-3 family of fatty acids derived from the ESSENTIAL FATTY ACID, alpha linolenic acid. It is a complex fatty acid with six double bonds and 22 carbon atoms. DHA and EPA can be synthesized to some extent by the liver from linonelic acid. However, the intake of this fatty acid may be low, and its conversion may be diminished by dietary factors such as an excess of the more common essential fatty acid, LINOLEIC ACID. Consequently, the consumption of fish oils and fish can be beneficial. (See also ESKIMO DIET.)

Cooper, Remi. *DHA: The Essential Omega-3 Fatty Acid.* Pleasant Grove, Utah: Woodland Publishing 1998.

dolomite A CALCIUM and MAGNESIUM mineral supplement that combines calcium and magnesium carbonates. Since dolomite is a mineral, its composition varies depending on the source. Because analyses indicate that dolomite may contain traces of LEAD, it is not recommended for children and pregnant women. (See also OSTEOPOROSIS.)

dong quai (*Angelica sinensis*) This herb has been used for more than a thousand years as a spice, tonic, and medicine in China, Korea, and Japan. Although there have been few definitive studies on dong quai, it is said to relieve constipation, increase red blood cell count, and ease menstrual cramps, irregular menstrual cycles, infrequent periods, premenstrual syndrome (PMS), and menopausal symptoms. In traditional Chinese medicine it is used for reproductive, circulatory, and respiratory conditions.

Dong quai grows in the mountainous regions of Asia, with smooth purplish stems and umbrella-shaped clusters of white flowers and winged fruits in July and August. The yellowish-brown thick-branched roots of the dong quai plant have a number of medicinal uses. After the plant reaches maturity in three years, the root is harvested and made into tablets and powders.

Dong quai contains compounds that may help reduce pain, dilate blood vessels, and stimulate and relax uterine muscles. Animal studies suggest that dong quai may be used to normalize heart rhythm, prevent atherosclerosis, protect the liver, promote urination and sleep, act as a mild laxative, and fight infection, but the scientific evidence in humans is weak. No substantiation exists for the claims made about dong quai.

Commercial dong quai preparations typically recommend doses of between 300 and 500 mg three times a day. This herb may be safe when used appropriately. Large amounts can cause skin sensitivity to the sun. Pregnant and breast-feeding women should not use this herb.

Seven different coumarin derivatives have been identified in dong quai, which act as vasodialators and antispasmodics. Others stimulate the central nervous system. Hypersensitivity to this herb may lead to excessive bleeding and occasional fever. The herb may also increase sensitivity to sunlight and interact with blood-thinning medications.

dopamine The parent compound of EPINEPHRINE (adrenalin), a key STRESS HORMONE and a brain chemical. In the ADRENAL GLANDS, dopamine is converted to the hormones norepinephrine and epinephrine. In the brain, dopamine serves as a NEUROTRANSMITTER, a chemical that relays nerve impulses.

PARKINSON'S DISEASE, an uncontrollable shaking of hands and arms, is caused by the degeneration of a part of the brain (substantia nigra) producing dopamine. Dopamine cannot penetrate the BLOOD-BRAIN BARRIER and therefore cannot serve as a therapeutic drug. However, its precursor, L-dopa, can enter the brain, and it has had some success in treatment of this disease.

double-acting baking powder See BAKING POWDER.

drug/nutrient interaction The ability of medications to interfere with the uptake or utilization of a nutrient. Interactions between foods and drugs are very common. Elderly persons are more susceptible to drug/nutrient interactions because they are more likely to be taking multiple medications; also, their bodies do not break down and inactivate drugs as effectively as younger people because their detoxifying enzymes are less active.

Drugs can affect nutrients themselves or they can increase the requirement for a nutrient by blocking its uptake or interfering with its normal function. The following are examples of drugs affecting specific nutrients.

- Pain relievers: ASPIRIN competes with FOLIC ACID for uptake by the intestine. Chronic aspirin users need more VITAMIN C. Excessive use promotes gastrointestinal bleeding and an increased IRON requirement.
- Antibiotics that are not absorbed (such as neomycin) can promote LACTOSE INTOLERANCE.
- The use of ANTACIDS based on aluminum hydroxide to decrease stomach acid can reduce CALCIUM phosphate, VITAMIN A, and VITAMIN D uptake.
- Anticonvulsive agents and sedatives like diphenylhydantoin, phenobarbital, and glutethimide increase vitamin D and VITAMIN K metabolism. They can create folic acid and VITAMIN B_{12} deficiencies as well.
- Resin-type CHOLESTEROL-LOWERING DRUGS (such as Questran) interfere with the absorption of fat-soluble VITAMINS.
- DIURETICS (to treat edema) such as chlorthiazide increase MAGNESIUM and POTASSIUM excretion.
- LAXATIVES. Mineral oil interferes with the uptake of fat-soluble vitamins like vitamins A, D, and E. Bulking agents and psyllium gum can interfere with RIBOFLAVIN absorption.
- Medication for Parkinson's disease. Levodopa increases the need for vitamin B_{12}, vitamin C, and VITAMIN B_6.
- Corticosteroids (cortisone, prednisone) have multiple effects. They increase urinary losses of ZINC, potassium, and vitamin C. They increase the need for vitamin B_6 and vitamin D and they can create blood sugar dysregulation.
- Hypotensive agents like hydralazine deplete vitamin B_6 stores.
- Oral contraceptives (conjugated estrogens, ethinyl estradiol) reduce bone loss and calcium excretion but deplete folic acid and vitamin B_6.
- Lithium (to treat bipolar disorder) reduces salt uptake. Conversely, a high sodium intake interferes with lithium.

Foods Can Also Interfere with Medications

- Milk and dairy products can bind some antibiotics like chloramphenicol used to treat infections and prevent their uptake. Patients should wait two hours after taking these drugs before eating dairy products.
- Patients should avoid liver, large amounts of cabbage, and dark-green leafy vegetables, including spinach, when taking anticoagulants, drugs used to thin blood and prevent blood clots. Their high vitamin K levels can promote blood clotting. Limit alcohol and caffeine consumption.
- Patients taking ANTIDEPRESSANTS (monoamine oxidase inhibitors) to treat depression and high blood pressure should avoid aged, sharp cheeses; chianti and red wine; pickled herring, yogurt, chicken liver, bananas, avocados, pastrami, pepperoni, salami, meat tenderizer, and yeast. They should also cut back on CHOCOLATE, cola beverages, and COFFEE. These products contain TYRAMINE, which can lead to severe high blood pressure in combination with the monoamine oxidase inhibitors.
- Patients taking thyroid medications (to increase thyroid function) should avoid BRUSSELS SPROUTS, SOYBEANS, turnips, and CABBAGE. An ingredient in these vegetables can counteract this medication.

(See also ALCOHOL; CYTOCHROME P450; DETOXICATION.)

dry milk See MILK.

dry weight The weight of a food after water has been removed. Water accounts for much of the weight of foods; the water content ranges from 40 percent to 90 percent. To standardize contents, ingredients or compositions are often expressed as a percentage of dry weight to provide a more accurate basis for comparison.

duck This member of the poultry family has been a food staple around the world for millennia. Its history as a domestic fowl can be traced back 4,000 years; the Chinese white-feathered Pekin duck dates to the Yuan dynasty, which lasted from 1279 to 1368 B.C.E. In America Native Americans and early colonists feasted on wild duck until fewer than a dozen Peking ducks were brought here from Asia in 1873, initiating domestic duck production.

In the United States duck is far less popular than chicken or turkey. The average American eats less than a pound of duck a year. This may be because there is less flesh on duck than on either chicken or turkey, and all duck meat is dark. Most of the duck sold in America (90 percent) is frozen.

Most of the duck in this country is raised on farms in the Midwest, although Long Island, New York, is still famous for its Peking duck farms. Ducks are fed corn and soybean meal that has been fortified with vitamins and minerals. The U.S. FDA prohibits use of hormones in domestic duck production, and antibiotics are rarely administered because few of these drugs have been approved for use in ducks.

Four varieties are popular. The Peking duck, the most popular variety in the United States, is typically between three and six pounds at slaughter. It has a mild flavor and larger bones than other varieties. The Muscovy, which originated in South America, is usually served in restaurants. It has a strong, gamy flavor and usually weighs between two and three pounds at slaughter. The mallard, which can be hunted in the wild or raised domestically, is about the size of a Cornish hen. It is called the meatiest of ducks because of its low fat content. The Moulard, a cross between the Muscovy and the Peking or another variety, is much larger than the other varieties and yields more meat, especially breast meat, which is dark and sweet.

Ducks can be roasted whole or cut up into pieces for sautéing. Roast duck is often accompanied by fruit-based (for example, ORANGE or CHERRY) sauces. Peking duck, a Chinese dish, is also popular but difficult to prepare at home because preparation includes blowing air into the skin to separate it from the meat and hanging the duck in an oven where air can constantly circulate around it.

Duck liver, or foie gras (French for "fat liver"), is considered a delicacy. It is produced by forcefeeding Moulard ducks for several days, causing their livers to grow to several times their normal size. Foie gras is often served as an appetizer called paté, which is very high in SATURATED FAT and CHOLESTEROL. One serving provides calories, 199; fat, 14 g; protein, 10 g; carbohydrate, 5 g; cholesterol, 291 mg; sodium, 146 mg.

Roasted skinless duck is a good source of IRON and PROTEIN and is low in FAT. Three ounces of skinless roasted duck breast yields calories, 119; protein, 23 g; fat, 2.1 g; cholesterol, 122 mg; iron, 3.8 mg; niacin, 8.9 mg.

dulse See SEAWEED.

duodenal ulcer An open sore or lesion in the wall of the duodenum, the first 12 inches of the small intestine. Duodenal ulcer is one of the two ulcerative disorders of the upper gastrointestinal tract. Duodenal ulcers occur four times more frequently in men than in women. The most common symptom is chronic pain below the stomach, usually occurring 45 to 60 minutes after meals and that can be relieved by ANTACIDS and by food. This condition may be aggravated by excessive exposure to stomach acid and pepsin, the digestive enzyme produced by the stomach. Patients with duodenal ulcers have twice the number of acid-secreting cells in their stomachs as individuals without ulcers. Other factors implicated in ulcer formation include food allergies, cigarette smoking, STRESS, aspirin and other nonsteroidal analgesics, ALCOHOL, and COFFEE.

An infection by the bacterium *Helicobacter pylori* is associated with more than 90 percent of cases of duodenal ulcer. Eradication of the bacterium in duodenal ulcers protects against relapses. Conventional treatment entails bismuth salts and antibiotics. Researchers have discovered that BROCCOLI and broccoli sprouts contain a chemical, SULFORAFANE, that kills *H. pylori* in mice. This bacteria has been linked to chronic stomach inflammation and stomach cancer. Similar studies on humans are ongoing.

Patients with ulcers in the digestive tract need medical attention, and complications such as perforation and hemorrhage present medical emergencies. A diet rich in whole foods that are high in

COMPLEX CARBOHYDRATES can promote tissue healing. VITAMIN A, VITAMIN E, and ZINC may be beneficial. Licorice has been reported to help with duodenal ulcers. (See also ALLERGY, FOOD; DIGESTION; GASTRIC ULCER; GASTROINTESTINAL DISORDERS.)

duodenum The first 12 inches of the small intestine. This region spans the upper region of the small intestine between the pylorus (the lower stomach opening) and the JEJUNUM (the middle section of the small intestine). It begins with the pyloric sphincter (valve) that regulates the flow of chyme, acidic food paste released by the stomach, into the stomach. BILE and pancreatic secretions flow into the intestine at this location through the common duct. The duodenum secretes an alkaline mucus to protect the intestinal wall from stomach acid and digestive enzymes. Chyme contains fat, partially digested protein, and hydrochloric acid and stimulates the small intestine to produce SECRETIN and CHOLECYSTOKININ, hormones that stimulate pancreatic secretions. In terms of disease states, the duodenum is often the site of ulcers. (See also DIGESTION; DIGESTIVE TRACT; DUODENAL ULCER; HELIOBACTER PYLORI.)

dysbiosis See INTESTINAL FLORA.

dyspepsia Indigestion or abdominal pain that occurs during a meal or shortly after eating. The symptoms include heartburn, nausea, belching, feeling stuffed, and flatulence. Many factors cause dyspepsia. It may be the result of a gastrointestinal disease such as FOOD POISONING, or it may be caused by nerve response to a disturbance in the abdominal cavity. Alternatively, food sensitivities, overeating, eating too quickly, eating under stress, and gulping air when swallowing are functional causes of dyspepsia. (See also ACID INDIGESTION; ANTACID; HIATUS HERNIA.)

dysphagia A difficulty in swallowing. Symptoms include food sticking in the throat, and coughing during swallowing. Dysphagia is associated with depression and anxiety. Food lodging in the lungs can promote respiratory infections. Possible causes of dysphagia include abnormalities in the structure of the mouth, throat, or esophagus as caused by a tumor; infection and inflammation (such as, tonsillitis); paralysis obstruction in the pharynx or esophagus, for example, following a stroke; diseases that affect nerves stimulating peristalsis, the wavelike contraction of the DIGESTIVE TRACT that propels food downward; and physical injury to the throat. (See also DEGLUTITION.)

E

eating disorders A class of diseases based on obsessive behavior related to eating: ANOREXIA NERVOSA, BULIMIA NERVOSA, and compulsive overeating. Eating disorders affect people from all socioeconomic classes, and ages range from 3 to 90. Although both men and women can develop eating disorders, predominantly women are affected.

Though factors vary among individuals, the cycle of eating disorders seems to be initiated by psychological injury, including physical and psychological abuse among family members, reduced self-esteem, oppression, social isolation, and nutritional insults, including faulty diet, abuse of drugs, alcohol, and medications, and food intolerance. The resulting behavioral changes and altered eating can lead to a cycle of altered diet, altered APPETITE, and hunger mechanisms worsened by nutritional imbalances, leading to further eating changes and compulsive behavior.

Anorexia nervosa, self-induced starvation out of an intense fear of becoming obese, was first described 100 years ago. It now occurs in an estimated 1 percent of American women. Although there is a genetic predisposition, social factors play key roles in determining the occurrence of anorexia nervosa. Symptoms include a markedly distorted body image and self-restricted dieting, leading to extreme weakness, muscle wasting, and loss of 25 percent of original body weight, and cessation of menstruation. Anorexia nervosa is potentially life-threatening.

Bulimia nervosa is characterized by recurring episodes of binge eating (rapid, excessive eating), followed by purging. Most bulimics are women. Bulimia was first described in the United States in 1980 and the incidence in America is increasing. It is characterized by frequent attempts to lose weight by severely restricted diets, followed by episodes of bingeing, followed by deliberate vomiting or abuse of diuretics or laxatives, to lose weight. Bulimics generally possess low self-esteem and fear an inability to stop eating. Frequent fluctuations in body weight are common.

The third category is compulsive overeating, which refers to episodes of excessive overeating or bingeing in secret. Compulsive overeating is accompanied by repeated attempts to lose weight and diet. The increased occurrence of compulsive overeating among American teenagers parallels their increased prevalence of OBESITY. Compulsive overeating can substitute for confronting life issues and dealing with emotions and their sources.

Hazards associated with eating disorders other than obesity include starvation, electrolyte and fluid imbalances, liver damage, kidney damage, stroke, cessation of menstruation, diabetes, internal bleeding, and ultimately death.

Eating disorders are complex conditions that profoundly affect health, and therapy entails multiple approaches including psychological counseling, support groups, nutrition counseling, and, in extreme cases, medical intervention. Strategies that focus on weight reduction or diet modification alone are of limited effectiveness in treating eating disorders because they fail to resolve underlying psychological issues. The most comprehensive treatment programs address emotional, social, physical, and spiritual components. Extended aftercare services as well as active participation in self-help groups support recovery.

Claude-Pierre, Peggy. *The Secret Language of Eating Disorders: The Revolutionary Approach to Understanding and Curing Anorexia and Bulimia.* New York: Random House, 1998.

eating patterns Trends in food consumption in the United States; patterns of eating behavior, reflecting food choices based on personal habits, taboos, customs, and family traditions. Food costs and food availability profoundly influence day-to-day food choices. Many personal values affect food choices: political conviction, such as conviction about the environment, or religious preferences (for example Catholic, Muslim, or Jewish); perceptions of social status; conditioning through advertising. Food purchases are often made according to health concerns, thus recent trends in eating fewer EGGS, less whole MILK, and less red MEAT are based in part upon consumers' concerns about CHOLESTEROL and clogged arteries.

The typical American diet, indeed the common pattern in industrialized nations, is low in fresh FRUIT and VEGETABLES and high in meat and processed food that is high in FAT, sodium, and sugar. Such a diet does not supply adequate FIBER, TRACE MINERALS, VITAMINS, and substances in plant foods whose antiaging and anticancer properties are still being discovered. Sweets and alcohol displace nutrient-rich foods, and lifestyle choices such as cigarette smoking and lack of EXERCISE alter nutrient needs.

Meal time has changed from eating at home with family to eating quick meals away from home. For many Americans, half of every dollar spent on food goes to outside meals. Generally, the odds of eating a less nutritious meal increase the more meals are eaten away from home. Often the choices rely on convenience foods and snack foods that contain high levels of fat, sugar, and sodium. Teenagers often obtain 20 percent of their food from such snacks, which has a long-term impact on their health.

The typical U.S. diet is imbalanced due to nutrient inadequacy and nutrient excess. The typical diet supplies too many CALORIES and too much FAT. Sweeteners in SOFT DRINKS, snacks, candy, ice cream, and pastry supply 25 percent of the calories. Each succeeding generation of Americans appears to get fatter. The typical diet supplies more fat than recommended to lower the risk of cancer and of heart disease. Paradoxically, women often have a problem in finding diets that will provide all the vitamins and minerals they need, while lowering their fat and calorie intake.

Results of Surveys

Surveys provide insight about what Americans are eating and how they make food choices. Recent polls to discover whether Americans are becoming more concerned about nutrition offer conflicting results. On the one hand, many Americans realize that diet is a factor in health risks. On the other hand, some results suggest that Americans have become less concerned about limiting high cholesterol food and obtaining adequate nutrients like vitamins. While heads of households have become more interested in many foods high in fiber and lower in fat and CHOLESTEROL, many also say that their health habits have not significantly changed. Sixty percent of American adults do not get enough physical activity and more than 25 percent are not active at all in their leisure time. Only about one-fourth of adults eat the recommended five or more servings of fruits and vegetables each day.

Recent data indicate that Americans are getting fatter; obesity has reached epidemic proportions. A 2000 survey by the U.S. Centers for Disease Control and Prevention (CDC) found that more than 45 million adults (about 60 percent of the adult population) are obese. The number of young people (age 6 to 17) who are considered overweight has more than doubled in the last two decades.

That the average American now weighs more than 20 years ago is perhaps related to the fact that food consumption has increased 20 pounds per person. The DIETARY GUIDELINES FOR AMERICANS recommend a diet that is low in saturated fat and cholesterol, yet more than half the adult population fails to meet the recommendations for saturated fat intake. The guidelines recommend no more than 30 percent of daily calories come from fat; the average adult gets 33 percent. Adults also consume too many foods high in sugar. Americans consume on average 20 teaspoons of sugar daily. Sodium consumption, too, exceeds recommended levels. The guidelines suggest limiting intake to no more than 2,400 mg a day. On average, men consume 4,000 mg and women consume 3,000 mg.

Eating healthier means changing one's lifestyle. A number of experts recommend gradual change and moderation, with ample information to enable people to make and support wise choices. A variety of food substitutions can be implemented in a stepwise fashion to achieve a gradual change to healthier alternatives. The following illustrates initial substitutions:

Food	Healthy Alternative	Healthier Alternative
whole milk	low-fat milk	nonfat milk
cottage cheese	low-fat cottage cheese	nonfat cottage cheese
sugar cereal	nonsugar cereal	whole-grain cereal, non-processed
fruit drink	orange juice	whole orange
soft drink with sugar, caffeine	diet soft drink	sparkling water or fruit juice
white bread	brown bread	100 percent whole-wheat bread
bologna	ham	turkey

(See also FAT, HIDDEN.)

Liebman, Bonnie. "The Changing American Diet," *Nutrition Action Healthletter,* 22:5 (1995): 9–10.

Physical Activity and Good Nutrition: Essential Elements to Prevent Chronic Diseases and Obesity. Atlanta, Ga.: Centers for Disease Control and Prevention, 2000.

Woteki, Catherine. "Consumption, Intake Patterns and Exposure," *Critical Reviews in Food Science and Nutrition,* 35:1,2 (1995): 143–147.

echinacea (*Echinacea angustifolia; E. purpurea*) A perennial herb that stimulates the body's immune system. Echinacea is native to North America, from Texas to the prairies of Canada. Native American tribes have long used this herb as an antiseptic and as an analgesic (pain reliever). The dried root is used most often. It contains echinacin, a polysaccharide (complex carbohydrate) that speeds wound healing and helps maintain connective tissue. Echinacea contains inulin, a polysaccharide composed of fructose that activates the "alternative" complements pathway, a system that increases defenses against viruses and bacteria, and speeds the migration of defensive white cells (such as neutrophils, monocytes, and lymphocytes) to injured or infected regions. Echinacea stimulates T-lymphocytes, which help direct immune defenses. It also stimulates the production of interferon (antiviral defense) and of lymphokines, chemicals of the immune system that stimulate natural killer cells and scavenger cells (macrophages). Echinacea is regarded as a safe herb.

eclampsia (toxemia of pregnancy) A serious medical condition that can accompany pregnancy. "Preeclampsia" is the early stage characterized by high blood pressure, headache, protein in urine, and swelling (EDEMA) of legs and feet. If untreated, the patient may develop true eclampsia.

Eclampsia develops in 0.5 percent of patients with preeclampsia. Convulsive seizures can occur between the 20th week of pregnancy and the first week after birth; eclampsia is usually fatal if untreated. In addition to the symptoms of preeclampsia, symptoms of eclampsia include severe headaches, dizziness, abnormal pain, nausea, convulsions, and possibly coma. The kidney, liver, brain, and placenta are affected. The causes of eclampsia are unknown. HYPERTENSION and kidney disease contribute to the problem. Treatment of eclampsia is medical. Salt restriction is not part of the treatment, and the use of DIURETICS may simply mask signs and symptoms.

Poor nourishment may predispose a woman to preeclampsia. Some studies indicate that poorly nourished women develop preeclampsia more often, but studies of calcium supplementation for preventing preeclampsia have had mixed results. A recent study showed that supplemental vitamin C and vitamin E may reduce preeclampsia in high-risk women, but the authors caution that it is too soon to recommend supplementation. Pregnant women should make sure their diet is adequate in food sources of these vitamins and take only the supplements prescribed by their prenatal care provider.

Anyaegbungm, A., and C. Edwards. "Hypertension in Pregnancy," *Journal of the National Medical Association* 86 (April 1994): 289–293.

Walsh, Scott W. "The Role of Fatty Acid Peroxidation and Antioxidant Status in Normal Pregnancy and in Pregnancy Complicated by Preeclampsia," *World Review of Nutrition and Diet* 76 (1994): 114–118.

eczema (atopic dermatitis) Persistent itchy and inflamed skin, often with scales, crusts, scabs, or small blisters. Eczema may be dry or there may be a discharge; the condition is not infectious. Allergies may be involved; many eczema patients test positive for allergies and they may exhibit hay fever symptoms. Emotional upset and stress can aggravate itching. Contact with chemical irritants can trigger eczema. Inheritance is a risk factor for eczema, and dietary factors are involved.

The Role of Diet

Often, eczema symptoms improve with an ELIMINATION DIET in which suspected allergy-producing foods are avoided, suggesting a linkage to food allergy in some cases. In infants, cow's MILK is the most common food allergy associated with eczema. ESSENTIAL FATTY ACIDS can help limit the inflammatory process. Omega-3 fatty acids are the essential fatty acids found in flaxseed oil and fish oils, while omega-6 fatty acids are found in EVENING PRIMROSE OIL and BORAGE oil. Vitamin C and FLAVONOIDS, plant substances that serve as ANTIOXIDANTS, appear to help control or limit inflammatory processes also. Vitamin A plays a key role in skin development and maintenance, and deficiencies should be corrected. Many eczema patients are ZINC deficient, and zinc supplementation may be helpful. This may be linked to the fact that low stomach acid is very common in patients with eczema, and low stomach acid contributes to mineral malabsorption, ultimately leading to eczema. Zinc is necessary to convert essential fatty acids to PROSTAGLANDINS, hormone-like substances that regulate inflammation, among other processes.

The diet of eczema sufferers should minimize convenience foods that supply high levels of fat, sugar, and other additives, while emphasizing whole foods, particularly fresh fruit and vegetables. Increasing consumption of polyunsaturated FAT (like SAFFLOWER oil) and FISH OIL may help decrease inflammation and boost the immune system. (See also ACNE; ALLERGY, FOOD; BREAST-FEEDING; LEUKOTRIENES.)

edema The swelling of any part of the body due to fluid accumulation. Allergies can cause edema when the allergic response releases HISTAMINE and other inflammatory agents that make capillaries porous so that fluid from BLOOD can then leak into surrounding tissue, causing puffy eyes and a swollen face, for example. Edema is also one of the symptoms of preeclampsia in pregnancy. Generalized edema can result from serious medical conditions such as HYPOTHYROIDISM, kidney failure, liver disease, and congestive heart failure.

Nutritionally-related causes of edema include excessive SODIUM, certain nutrient deficiencies, and food allergies. Excessive sodium can cause edema in about 20 percent of the American population who are sensitive to high salt intake. Edema is also associated with severe nutritional deficiency diseases such as BERIBERI (due to a deficiency of THIAMIN) and with protein MALNUTRITION.

Edema is often treated with DIURETICS (water pills), which increase urine production to remove water and salt from the body. The use of diuretics is considered potentially dangerous during pregnancy. Reduced salt intake can be helpful and low-sodium diets may be prescribed. (See also ALDOSTERONE; ECLAMPSIA; HYPERTENSION; KWASHIORKOR; SODIUM.)

edible portion The portion of food usually consumed. For example, husks, hulls, rinds, peels, seed, bones and gristle are usually excluded from weight measurements and nutrient compositions.

EDTA (ethylenediaminetetraacetic acid; disodium EDTA) A FOOD ADDITIVE used as an ANTIOXIDANT and a preservative to trap unwanted metal ion contaminants. As an antioxidant, EDTA blocks the formation of highly reactive forms of oxygen that attack fats and oils. Attack of food molecules by oxygen requires metal ions as catalysts. When metal ion contaminants are trapped by EDTA, they do not form free radicals. EDTA is often combined with butylated hydroxytoluene (BHT) and PROPYL GALLATE, which work together as antioxidants in processed foods.

EDTA is added to salad dressings, MARGARINE, MAYONNAISE, potatoes, peas, and vegetables. EDTA traps metal ions in canned SHELLFISH that would promote off-color and altered taste. In BEER it prevents excessive foaming and turbidity. SOFT DRINK producers use EDTA to stabilize ARTIFICIAL FOOD COLORS. Excessive EDTA would trap essential nutrients in the body, such as trace mineral nutrients and CALCIUM, and therefore typical usage is 0.01

percent in foods and beverages. The body absorbs only about 5 percent of an oral dose, and absorbed EDTA is excreted in the urine. EDTA is considered a safe additive. In medicine, EDTA is used to treat metal (LEAD) poisoning and as an alternative treatment in cardiovascular disease. (See also CHELATE.)

EFA See ESSENTIAL FATTY ACIDS.

egg As food, typically, the ovum of domestic fowl. Eggs are an inexpensive, nutrient-rich food that provides high-quality PROTEIN with all essential amino acids. Egg protein is often used as a reference protein in nutritional studies because it is readily digested and supplies a well balanced mixture of amino acids that are readily absorbed. A popular food, nonfertile chicken eggs are mass-produced, inexpensive, readily available, and easily prepared. Hens' eggs contain an inner fluid (the egg white) which contains half of the protein but no cholesterol; proteins protect the yolk from bacteria, such as AVIDIN, which tenaciously binds the B vitamin BIOTIN. Bacteria requiring this vitamin cannot grow in the egg white.

The yolk provides many nutrients such as minerals, vitamins, all of the CHOLESTEROL (213 mg), and 5 g of fat. The yellow color is due to the plant pigment xanthophyll (lutein). The egg yolk is also rich in LECITHIN, a phospholipid used to emulsify other lipids.

As food, eggs have limitations: Their CALCIUM content is low and they lack VITAMIN C. In recipes, egg yolks can often be substituted by using double the amount of egg white. Most commercial EGG SUBSTITUTES use egg whites only.

Eating more than a few eggs a week can raise blood cholesterol in sensitive people. On the other hand, moderate consumption seems safe for most healthy people. Perhaps as many as one-third of Americans are extremely sensitive to dietary cholesterol; their blood levels rise significantly when they eat cholesterol-rich foods. These individuals should limit their dietary cholesterol to no more than 300 mg per day. Particularly those with a family history of early heart disease or high cholesterol levels need to be watchful. More important than monitoring cholesterol in the diet is limiting fat consumption, especially consumption of SATURATED FAT. With a low-fat diet, egg cholesterol seems to have little impact on blood cholesterol levels.

Organic chicken eggs, farm fresh eggs, and mass-produced eggs contain the same amount of cholesterol, although mineral and vitamin content can vary according to the chicken feed. Efforts are being made to increase the content of ESSENTIAL FATTY ACIDS of eggs by varying the hens' diets.

Eggs can be contaminated by trace amounts of PESTICIDES from feed, so purchasing organic eggs might be desirable. Because raw or undercooked eggs can transmit food poisoning (SALMONELLA), raw cracked eggs should be discarded, and eggs should be cooked thoroughly. Eggs should be refrigerated to prevent bacterial contamination and age-related changes. One chicken egg (58 g) contains 79 calories; protein, 6.1 g; fat 5.6 g; cholesterol, 213 mg; calcium, 28 mg; iron, 1.04 mg; zinc, 0.61 mg; vitamin A, 78 retinol equivalents; thiamin, 0.04 mg; riboflavin, 0.15 mg; niacin, 0.03 mg. (See also BIOLOGICAL VALUE; ORGANIC FOODS.)

egg allergies A very common type of food allergy, usually due to a sensitivity to egg whites. Egg allergies may trigger symptoms quickly, including hives, asthma, watery eyes, swelling, and nausea shortly after the egg is consumed. Alternatively, a delayed sensitivity with symptoms such as headaches, DIARRHEA, or CONSTIPATION, can develop hours after the food is consumed. Because eggs are so common in processed foods, food labels of baked goods should be read carefully. (See also ALLERGY, FOOD; BIOLOGICAL VALUE; FOOD SENSITIVITY.)

eggplant (*Solanum melongena;* aubergine) A large, pear-shaped member of the NIGHTSHADE FAMILY that includes potatoes, tomatoes, and peppers. This vegetable probably originated in India and has been cultivated since antiquity. Eggplant is often dark purple with a glossy skin, but white, yellow, and striped varieties are also cultivated. It is a good source of FIBER and is an ingredient in many Middle Eastern dishes. Ratatouille, a dish based on eggplant, is part of southern French cuisine.

Unripened eggplant may contain the toxic alkaloid SOLANINE, which also occurs in green potatoes. Solanine can cause neurological symptoms and damage red blood cells.

One cup of cooked eggplant (160 g) contains 45 calories; protein, 1.3 g; carbohydrate, 10.6 g; fiber, 6 g; calcium, 10 mg; iron, 0.56 mg; potassium, 397 mg; vitamin A, 10 retinol equivalents; thiamin, 0.12 mg; riboflavin, 0.03 mg; niacin, 0.96 mg; vitamin C, 2 mg.

egg substitutes Cholesterol-free alternatives to eggs. By eliminating the yolk, food manufacturers have developed several cholesterol-free products. Egg substitutes usually contain egg white (egg albumin); a partially HYDROGENATED VEGETABLE OIL like CORN OIL; together with ARTIFICIAL FOOD COLORS, GUMS, EMULSIFIERS, and several VITAMINS and MINERALS found in a typical egg. Soy protein–based egg substitutes are also marketed.

eicosapentaenoic acid (EPA) A large, complex POLYUNSATURATED FATTY ACID found in FISH and fish oils. EPA belongs to the omega-3 family of polyunsaturates, derived from the ESSENTIAL FATTY ACID, ALPHA LINOLENIC ACID. EPA, with 20 carbons and five double bonds, is the parent compound for PROSTAGLANDINS (PGE_3 series) and thrombaxane A_3, hormone-like substances that help counterbalance inflammatory processes triggered by other prostaglandins (PGE_2 series) and other thromboxane A_2. The latter come from ARACHIDONIC ACID, an omega-6 polyunsaturate prevalent in meat. Therefore EPA and fish oil tend to balance some of the effects of a meat-heavy diet. Recent research has focused on the relationship between EPA and heart disease.

Population studies indicate that death due to heart disease is lower among those who consume an average of 30 g of fish daily, as compared with those who eat meat daily. Other studies have yielded mixed results. While the results are suggestive, it is not yet clear which of the constituents of fish oils are more important. EPA could reduce the risk of coronary heart disease by several mechanisms: EPA can inhibit clot formation indirectly. It blocks the formation of thromboxane A_2, a potent factor that causes platelets to clump. Clumping of these cellular fragments in the blood helps form blood clots within vessels. EPA is also converted to PGI_3, a prostaglandin that directly blocks platelet aggregation. EPA and related lipids seem to lower blood fat levels. They may lower serum cholesterol, if initial levels are elevated and diets are high in saturated fat, by depressing the formation of LOW-DENSITY LIPOPROTEIN (LDL), the undesirable form of cholesterol. EPA and its relatives may also block the early stages of atherosclerosis. The improvement of glucose utilization in diabetics who use fish oil supplement remains controversial.

Using fish oil as a supplemental source of EPA carries potential hazards. Depending on the source, it may contain industrial pollutants. Fish liver oil may contain high levels of VITAMIN A and vitamin D, which can be toxic in high doses, as well as pesticides and other contaminants. Guidelines regarding the optimal intake of EPA or of fish oil have not yet been established. (See also ESKIMO DIET; OMEGA-3 FATTY ACIDS.)

elastin A fibrous PROTEIN found in the lung, in large blood vessels and in the other elastic connective tissue such as ligaments. Elastin differs from other fibrous proteins like COLLAGEN in that it is capable of undergoing a two-way stretch, like a trampoline net. Synthesis of elastin requires copper, and an inherited inability to absorb copper (Menke's syndrome) causes defective arteries.

electrolyte replacement See SPORT DRINKS.

electrolytes Electrically charged atoms or molecules occurring in the blood and other body fluids and in solutions in general. Electrolytes control the distribution of water among the blood, cells, and tissues, and the spaces between them; thus, electrolytes help regulate blood volume and composition. The electrical charge of electrolytes enables them to function in the transmission of nerve impulses and in muscle contraction, including heart muscle. Electrolytes also help regulate ACID-base balance to maintain the pH of body fluids close to neutrality.

Electrolytes consist of positively charged ions (cations) and negatively charged ions (anions). The predominant cations are POTASSIUM, SODIUM, and MAGNESIUM, while the major anion is CHLORIDE. These electrolytes are not evenly distributed: Sodium and chloride are concentrated outside cells, while potassium and magnesium are concentrated in the cytoplasm (within cells).

Sodium, potassium, and chloride are nutrients. Low levels are excreted daily, and they must be regularly replaced through foods and beverages. The kidneys reabsorb these electrolytes and play an important role in regulating electrolyte balance. Electrolytes are secreted by the GASTROINTESTINAL TRACT in digestive juices and bile. For example, chloride is secreted by stomach glands as hydrochloric acid and pancreatic secretion, and the small intestine releases sodium and bicarbonate. However, much of sodium and chloride is reabsorbed and recycled.

The body malfunctions when electrolytes are lost—through vomiting, diarrhea, excessive urination caused by certain medications (diuretics) or uncontrolled diabetes, or through excessive perspiration. Too little sodium causes fatigue, muscle weakness, or even convulsions. Potent diuretics most frequently cause potassium losses because they rid the body of excess water. Diabetes, severe burns, and dietary deficiencies can also cause low potassium. Symptoms of potassium loss include a weak pulse, general weakness, and low blood pressure. Magnesium deficiency can be the result of diarrhea, chronic alcoholism, inflamed pancreas (pancreatitis), kidney disease, and inadequate diet. Chloride loss can occur with diarrhea and intestinal disease. Because chloride helps prevent excessive bicarbonate, which is alkaline, low chloride can cause the body to become excessively alkaline.

Mild losses of sodium and chloride are easily replaced by common beverages and processed foods. Potassium and magnesium are obtained from whole grains, green leafy vegetables, and fruits and juices. The loss of electrolytes and water can lead to life-threatening situations more rapidly than for losses of any other nutrient. With prolonged electrolyte imbalance, the brain, heart, and lungs do not function normally, and medical attention is required to replace fluids and electrolytes intravenously. (See also BULIMIA NERVOSA; DEHYDRATION; KETONE BODIES.)

electron transport chain A collection of ENZYMES responsible for the final stages of oxidation of FATTY ACIDS, CARBOHYDRATES, AMINO ACIDS, and other fuels in the presence of oxygen. The electron transport chain is part of the machinery of the MITOCHONDRIA, the cell's powerhouses. The oxidation-reduction enzymes are called CYTOCHROMES. Electrons pass sequentially from one cytochrome to the next like a bucket brigade. Nutrients like IRON and COENZYME Q are required for this process. In the last step, the enzyme cytochrome oxidase transfers electrons to molecular oxygen to yield water. Cyanide poisons cytochrome oxidase, accounting for the toxicity of this substance.

An essential feature of electron transfer between cytochromes is the simultaneous synthesis of ATP, which is the cell's energy currency. Chemical energy trapped in ATP meets almost all energy requirements of cells. (See also KREB'S CYCLE; OXIDATIVE PHOSPHORYLATION.)

elemental diet A DIET in which nutrients are present in their simplest, least combined forms. Free AMINO ACIDS and the simple sugar GLUCOSE are typical ingredients. Generally they contain no FIBER and very little FAT. Elemental diets require minimal digestive action in order to be absorbed and utilized by the body. Elemental diets are prescribed for INFLAMMATORY BOWEL DISEASE and other conditions in which the digestive and absorptive functions of the gastrointestinal tract are severely compromised: preparation for gastrointestinal surgery, treatment of burn victims, pancreatitis, and severe diarrhea. (See also DIGESTION; GASTROINTESTINAL DISORDERS.)

elimination diet/challenge test A simple way of detecting food allergies. During the initial phase of an elimination diet, all foods suspected of causing allergies are avoided for five to 14 days, to provide time for the IMMUNE SYSTEM to recover from the irritant. During the recovery phase, the diet is limited to "safe" foods and might include foods generally considered to be nonallergenic, such as lamb, rice, pears, and pure spring water or a chemically defined meal replacement that incorporates hydrolyzed protein such as rice protein.

When symptoms have diminished or disappeared, individual foods are added back to the diet, one at a time, for example, every two days. During this challenge period, the patient is instructed to record the recurrence of allergy symptoms when a questionable food is added back to the diet. This is a practical way to identify the offending food.

However, patients should not stay on an elimination diet for a long time because it is too restrictive, and patients on such a diet risk inadequate intake of vitamins and minerals. This method is also cumbersome when there are multiple food allergies and requires patience and persistence. For severe food allergy symptoms, medical supervision should be obtained before suspected foods are eaten. (See also ALLERGY, FOOD.)

ELISA (Enzyme-linked immuno-absorbent assays) These are sensitive analytical methods used in clinical diagnostic testing. These highly sensitive lab tests use manufactured ANTIBODIES (monoclonal antibodies), which bind with great specificity to a particular class of molecules, such as steroid HORMONES, tumor markers, viral antigens, parasitic antigens, and even other types of antibody molecules. The antibody used in the test is tagged with marker enzymes to permit measuring the degree of its binding. ELISA assays provide a previously unattainable window for assessing nutrient conditions and fundamental physiologic mechanisms, like circadian rhythm of hormone secretion, food allergies, and disease processes such as HIV-related (human immunodeficiency virus) conditions. (See also ALLERGY, FOOD.)

Emden–Meyerhoff pathway See GLYCOLYSIS.

emesis Vomiting of stomach contents, and possibly of intestinal contents in severe situations. Potential causes of emesis include food poisoning; chemical poisoning; viral infections; drug side effects; nervous conditions like brain injury, migraines, meningitis, seasickness; stimulation of the brain's vomiting center; gastric conditions such as cancer and peptic ulcers; and intestinal disorders like intestinal obstruction. Aggravating factors include excessive pain, sensitivity to certain foods, and toxic chemicals. Odors, shock, nervousness, anxiety, hysteria, morning sickness, coughing, and irritation of the pharynx can cause reflexive vomiting. Chronic vomiting can lead to ELECTROLYTE loss and tooth erosion due to gastric acid, DEHYDRATION and MALNUTRITION. (See also BULIMIA NERVOSA; EATING DISORDERS.)

emetic Any agent causing vomiting. Chemicals such as ipecac syrup, mustard, and zinc sulfate induce vomiting by local stimulation. Chemical emetics may be dangerous in pregnancy, GASTRIC ULCERS, CARDIOVASCULAR DISEASE, or hernia. Drinking large amounts of warm water can also induce vomiting. (See also BULIMIA NERVOSA; STOMACH ACID.)

empty calories Calories derived from burning food that provide excessive FAT, sugar, and/or white flour but contain far fewer key nutrients than those found in minimally processed foods. In particular, trace MINERALS, VITAMINS, PROTEIN, and FIBER are likely to be deficient. Foods supplying empty calories are said to have low NUTRIENT DENSITY. Alcoholic beverages, SOFT DRINKS, natural sweeteners like syrup and sugar, many manufactured foods, pastry, DESSERTS, CHIPS, and similar high-fat snacks lack the balance of nutrients found in whole foods and tend to crowd out more nutritious foods.

Most healthy people can tolerate an occasional splurge on junk food. However, problems arise when eating empty calorie foods becomes a habit. The more junk food a person eats, the more important it is for the remainder of the diet to supply important nutrients to make up for the deficiency. All too often, nutrient deficiencies such as folic acid, iron, calcium, even fiber occur. High-fat foods provide excessive calories, which favors weight gain. OBESITY is a growing problem for both American adults and children. Excessive fat and inadequate ANTIOXIDANT nutrients like VITAMIN C, VITAMIN E, and BETA-CAROTENE are linked to CARDIOVASCULAR DISEASE, AGING, and CANCER. (See also CONVENIENCE FOOD; DEGENERATIVE DISEASES; EATING PATTERNS; FAST FOOD; REFINED CARBOHYDRATES.)

emulsified vitamins Fat-soluble VITAMINS like vitamins A, D, and E that are processed as water-soluble emulsions. While not true solutions, emulsions consist of microscopic particles uniformly dispersed and stabilized so that oil and water do not separate. Like FAT, these vitamins are normally insoluble in water. Emulsified fat-soluble vitamins are absorbed directly by intestinal cells. Emulsification facilitates their uptake, an important consideration for individuals with MALABSORPTION. (See also VITAMIN A; VITAMIN D; VITAMIN E; VITAMIN K.)

emulsifiers (stabilizers, surfactants) A class of FOOD ADDITIVES widely used in manufactured foods to suspend oily materials in water. These chemicals, related to detergents, can suspend oils and lipids (water-insoluble materials) such as dyes in water as tiny droplets that do not coalesce or separate upon standing.

The most common commercial emulsifiers are DIGLYCERIDES, MONOGLYCERIDES, LECITHIN, POLYSORBATES, and sorbitan mono-stearate. Emulsifiers are used to keep bread from becoming stale; to stabilize fat in NONDAIRY CREAMERS for COFFEE; to keep cakes fluffy; to suspend flavors and food coloring in processed foods; and to stabilize ice cream. Egg lecithin is used to emulsify vegetable oils and vinegar to create MAYONNAISE. (See also CONVENIENCE FOOD.)

endive (*Cichorium endivia*) This bitter biennial or annual herb is a member of the aster family. It was used by ancient Egyptians and Romans and may have originated in India. Endive was adapted as food in France in the 14th century and is cultivated as a salad plant. Closely related to CHICORY, which it resembles, endive is a slightly bitter salad green. The leaves are finely divided and curly and are clustered in a loose head. To decrease their bitterness, the leaves are covered several weeks before harvest. It is an excellent source of BETA-CAROTENE. Nutrient content of 1 cup (50 g) is 28 calories; protein, 0.6 g; carbohydrate, 1.7 g; fiber, 0.46 g; calcium, 30 mg; 1.026 retinol equivalents; vitamin C, 3.2 mg; niacin, 0.49 mg; and small amounts of other nutrients.

endocrine system The collection of ductless glands that secrete HORMONES, chemical regulators of the body that travel to their target tissues via the bloodstream. As members of the body's system of checks and balances, ENDOCRINE glands respond to signals from the brain and to changes in chemicals in the blood, including BLOOD SUGAR, CALCIUM, and hormones.

The endocrine system consists of the ADRENAL GLANDS, PITUITARY (hypophysis), endocrine PANCREAS, THYROID, PARATHYROID, testes and ovaries, the pineal gland, and the thymus. The placenta also secretes hormones. Each endocrine gland produces a characteristic hormone, or set of hormones. Endocrine malfunctions create serious imbalances. Hyposecretion, in which inadequate levels of hormones are secreted, and hypersecretion, in which excessive amounts of hormones are secreted, cause many pathological conditions ranging from diabetes to excessive FATIGUE and CATABOLIC STATE.

The hypothalamus is the nerve tissue that links the brain with the pituitary gland. The hypothalamus indirectly controls many functions. It integrates and controls the autonomic nervous system, the grouping of nerves that regulates involuntary processes such as smooth muscle contractions (for example, the movement of food through the GASTROINTESTINAL TRACT and glandular secretions). In response to signals from the brain, and its own sensing mechanisms, the hypothalamus releases hormones that regulate the release of six hormones from the pituitary. The hypothalamus also forms two hormones, oxytocin and ANTIDIURETIC HORMONE (ADH), which travel to the posterior pituitary where they are released.

The functions of individual endocrine glands can be summarized as follows:

Pituitary Although it is only the size of a pea, the pituitary is considered the "master" endocrine gland because it regulates the activity of so many different glands throughout the body. ADH regulates SODIUM and WATER balance while oxytocin stimulates uterine contraction and the ejection of milk from mammary glands. The anterior pituitary makes "trophic hormones," hormones that activate other glands of the endocrine system. Trophic hormones include melanocyte-stimulating hormone (MSH) to regulate pigmented cells (melanocytes); PROLACTIN for milk secretion in women and for TESTOSTERONE production in males; interstitial cell stimulating hormone (ICSH), for testosterone production (men); luteinizing hormone (LH), for ovulation and progesterone production (women); follicle stimulating hormone (FSH), for development of ova and estrogen production (women) and sperm production in testes (men); thyroid stimulating hormone (TSH) for release of hormones from the thyroid gland; GROWTH HORMONE for tissue repair and maintenance; and ADRENOCORTICOTROPIC HORMONE (ACTH) for cortisol release from the adrenal cortex. The hypothalamus regulates the release of growth hormone, thyroid stimulating hormone, ACTH, FSH, and LH, and prolactin from the pituitary.

Adrenal Glands In response to ACTH, the adrenal glands produce the stress hormones EPINEPHRINE and NOREPINEPHRINE from the inner region of the adrenals to increase blood sugar, raise blood pressure, increase pulse rate, and similar effects that adapt the body to stress. The outer region of the adrenals produce steroids, like GLUCOCORTICOIDS, which raise blood sugar, increase the rate of breakdown of protein and fuels, and MINERALOCORTICOIDS, which conserve sodium and water.

Thyroid Gland Thyroid hormones regulate the rate of energy production of cells, the rates of tissue growth and development, and activity of the nervous system. Calcitonin lowers blood calcium levels.

Parathyroid Glands Parathyroid hormone raises calcium and phosphate ions and activates bone degradation.

Thymus Thymic hormones, thymosins, activate the immune system by promoting the proliferation of T cells, a major type of white blood cell.

Islets of Langerhans Clusters of endocrine cells scattered throughout the pancreas. The islets contain the alpha cells that produce GLUCAGON to increase blood glucose; and the beta cells that produce INSULIN to lower blood glucose.

Ovaries ESTROGENS (from the follicles) are female sex hormones that control the growth and development of female reproductive organs and secondary female characteristics and protein synthesis. They also produce PROGESTERONE (from the corpus luteum), which helps prepare the endometrium for implantation of a fertilized egg, and promotes milk production.

Gonads Produce testosterone in men. This hormone controls growth of male sex organs, body growth, secondary male characteristics, and sperm development.

Pineal Gland Produces melatonin, which has an inhibitory effect on ovaries. The pineal gland helps regulate circadian rhythms and may inhibit reproductive activities.

Placenta Serves as a temporary endocrine gland until birth. During pregnancy the placenta secretes chorionic gonadotropin, a hormone capable of stimulating the growth and function of the gonads, as well as estrogen and progesterone. (See also HOMEOSTASIS.)

endogenous carbohydrate Glucose that is synthesized in the body from noncarbohydrate compounds, excluding FATTY ACIDS, rather than obtained from the diet. The process, called GLUCONEOGENESIS, converts most AMINO ACIDS to glucose; thus, approximately 50 percent of dietary PROTEIN may be metabolized to glucose under normal (nonfasting) conditions. GLYCEROL from FAT breakdown yields glucose as does LACTIC ACID, PYRUVIC ACID, and such carboxylic acids of the KREB'S CYCLE as CITRIC ACID, SUCCINIC ACID, and OXALOACETIC ACID. (See also CARBOHYDRATE METABOLISM; FASTING.)

endoplasmic reticulum A membrane system found within the cytoplasm of many cell types. The endoplasmic reticulum functions in the synthesis, transport, and storage of a wide variety of exported products, such as DIGESTIVE ENZYMES. The endoplasmic reticulum of the LIVER also houses enzymes for cholesterol synthesis, for completion of long-chain FATTY ACIDS, and for powerful oxidizing enzymes (detoxifying enzymes) needed to modify toxic molecules and products of normal metabolism such as steroid hormones, to convert them to water-soluble materials that are more readily excreted. Long-term adaptation to repeated drug exposure produces a growth of "smooth" endoplasmic reticulum with increased levels of detoxifying enzymes in the liver. The portion of the endoplasmic reticulum devoted to protein synthesis machinery is called the "rough" endoplasmic reticulum. The cytoplasm of cells that manufacture huge amounts of protein, such as the PANCREAS and liver, is packed with rough endoplasmic reticulum to support their export of proteins. (See also CHOLESTEROL; CYTOCHROME P450; DETOXIFICATION.)

endorphins Brain chemicals involved in a wide variety of body processes, including pain control and emotions. Endorphins are produced by the body in response to pain, stress, and emotions, and they regulate the release of pituitary hormones, including growth hormone, ADRENOCORTICOTROPIC HORMONE (which triggers hormone release from the adrenal glands), and thyroid-stimulating hormone, among others. Endorphins also regulate cells of the immune system, white blood cells, antibody producing cells, and natural killer T-cells.

Endorphins are 50 to 100 times more potent than morphine as painkillers. Beta-endorphins may suppress pain by blocking the release of substance P, a neuropeptide that conducts pain-related nerve impulses to the central nervous system.

Endorphins bind to specific sites in the brain associated with pain perception and sedation. They also play a role in memory, learning, sexual drive, regulation of body temperature, and decreased blood pressure. Increased endorphin levels may be related to an increased sense of well-being or euphoria, much like the effects of morphine and other opiates. According to one hypothesis, individuals with chronic pain may have fewer brain endorphins than usual. EXERCISE may cause a natural "runner's high," a sense of euphoria and insensitivity to pain, when the brain is stimulated to form endorphins.

Endorphins may regulate APPETITE; and possibly certain foods like sweets may trigger the brain to produce endorphins, causing an "eater's high." Bulimics often binge on food, especially CARBOHYDRATE and sweets, and their CRAVING may represent the need to feel better by eating food that triggers endorphin production in the brain. Thus, a craving may be a form of "self-medication." Similarly, people with chemical dependencies may be deficient in certain neuropeptides and thus crave substances that stimulate endorphin production or opiate drugs, which substitute for them, because of their increased need for endorphin stimulation.

Enkephalins, brain compounds that block pain, were first discovered in 1975. Enkephalins are smaller than endorphins and contain only a few amino acids. Enkephalins are concentrated in the hypothalamus, parts of the limbic system of the brain, and in the spinal cord. They too are more potent painkillers than morphine. It is believed they inhibit pain pathways of the nervous system like endorphins. (See also ADDICTION; BULIMIA NERVOSA; NEUROTRANSMITTER.)

endosperm The starchy portion of kernels of CEREAL GRAINS that is concentrated in flour. During germination, the endosperm would normally supply the growing plant embryo with energy. In the production of flour, the milling of grains removes FIBER and GERM from kernels to yield a STARCH fraction that can be decolorized and bleached to yield white flour. (See also BREAD; WHEAT.)

energy The capacity to carry out work. In nutrition, energy is measured in large CALORIES (or kilocalories), defined as the amount of heat required to increase the temperature of 1 liter of water by 1° C–or in terms of kilojoules, a less common measure of energy used in medical literature.

There are two principal kinds of energy: potential energy (stored energy, such as chemical energy) and kinetic energy (motion). Energy takes many forms. Radiant energy is characterized by wave motion; heat and light are common examples. Chemical reactions involved in the breakdown of nutrients release some energy as heat, which cannot be used for cellular work. Electrical energy, based upon the flow of ions or electrons, is the form of energy essential for nerve impulses and for muscle cells.

The law of conservation of energy states that energy cannot be created or destroyed, only changed to other forms. This holds true for energy considerations of the body, where energy storage equals the difference between food consumed and energy output.

Energy is released when organic compounds are oxidized or broken down. On the other hand, the formation of bonds when biomolecules are assembled requires energy. Reactions involved in building processes (biosynthesis) require the input of energy supplied by the breakdown and oxidation of foods. Therefore, the body requires fuel to produce energy to drive all of the processes of growth, maintenance, and repair of the body.

The major fuels are FATS, CARBOHYDRATE, and, to a lesser extent, PROTEIN. Their oxidation yields a large amount of energy released as heat or trapped as chemical energy in the form of ATP, the energy currency of the cell. The end products of the complete oxidation of fuels are water and carbon dioxide. The process is quite efficient: Up to 40 percent of the energy released during glucose oxidation is trapped as chemical energy in the form of ATP. The amount of ATP present at any moment is very small; it is not a storage form of energy. Instead the body stores energy primarily as fats (triglycerides) in adipose tissue.

The total number of calories in a food can be determined in the laboratory by a process called direct calorimetry. In this procedure, a food is completely oxidized in a sealed chamber immersed in an insulated water tank. The heat released or the oxygen consumed are measured to obtain total calories. However, the calories in a food determined by direct calorimetry exceed the caloric yield in the body because not all food constituents are oxidized by the body to carbon dioxide and water. Tables of caloric values of foods are corrected for this discrepancy. Food energy values can be calculated using general energy conversion factors (4 calories per gram of protein or carbohydrate; 9 calories per gram of fat) and adding up the calories contributed by carbohydrate, fat, and protein. Most tables list physiologically available energy values based on specific energy conversions.

Energy Balance

Energy balance refers to the difference between calories consumed in food and the energy used for work and lost to the environment as heat and an increased state of disorder or randomness. The body requires a steady input of chemical energy to maintain all energy-requiring processes of the cell.

At "energy equilibrium," energy released from food consumed equals the work performed. There is no surplus, and body weight is stable. If the number of calories consumed exceeds energy needs, the excess energy is stored primarily as body fat and, therefore, weight increases.

Weight loss occurs when ingested food provides fewer calories than required to fuel the body, that is, when fuel expenditure exceeds intake. This fact is exploited by calorie-reduction diets, which are designed to assure that fuel intake is less than energy needs. The difference is made up by burning fat deposited in ADIPOSE TISSUE; muscle protein may also be broken down when calories are restricted. With gradual weight loss, the pounds lost represent the consumption of body fat.

The total number of calories in food consumed represents the energy intake. Energy expenditure consists of three categories. The resting energy expenditure (REE) is defined as the energy required to breathe, to pump blood, to keep the neurons of the brain active; in general, to maintain all body functions and normal temperature while at rest, awake, and at a typical room temperature. It represents the largest contribution to total energy requirements. REE accounts for approximately 60 percent of the energy output and reflects lean body mass. This accounts for the observed differences in REE between men and women, and between younger and older adults. In practice, the REE is easier to measure than the BASAL METABOLIC RATE (BMR), which is measured 12 hours after a meal, and soon after awakening in the morning. REE differs from BMR by only 10 percent, and for convenience REE is often used.

A second category of energy expenditure is a heat factor called the thermic effect of food (TEF), which represents the energy cost of digesting food and absorbing nutrients. This factor is small, approximately 5 percent to 10 percent of total energy expenditure.

Energy expended for physical activity represents the third category of energy output. This is the only component readily modified by lifestyle. Activity factors have been developed that correlate with different activity levels. The representative activity factor for resting (asleep) is 1.0; for very light work, 1.5; for light work, 2.5; for moderately heavy work, 5.0; and for heavy labor, basketball, football, soccer, and the like, 7.0.

The RDA (RECOMMENDED DIETARY ALLOWANCE) for energy takes into account differences among people based on their sex, body size, age, pregnancy, lactation, and activity level. For example, an average energy allowance for a healthy male between the ages of 25 and 50 and weighing 174 lb. is 2,900 calories per day. For females weighing 143 lb., the average energy allowance is 1,900 calories per day. (See also DIETING; EXERCISE; FASTING; WEIGHT MANAGEMENT.)

enrichment The addition of nutrients to foods as established by federal standards. In 1980 the U.S. FDA established guidelines for the addition of nutrients to food: decrease a nutritional deficiency for a given population; restore nutrients lost in processing; and improve the nutritional quality of food substitutes and imitations. Though enrichment is not required, the FDA has established standards for those enriched foods that include VITAMIN A, VITAMIN D, iodine, THIAMIN, RIBOFLAVIN, NIACIN, IRON, and calcium. The term FORTIFICATION is often used synonymously with enrichment, although fortification originally meant the addition of specific nutrients to foods, in excess of those usually found in those foods. These additions are usually in moderate amounts.

England and Canada have enrichment programs similar to that of the United States. Nutrients are commonly added to salt, milk, margarine, and CEREAL GRAIN products, including bleached flour and pasta, white rice, cornmeal, and bread and buns. FDA standards of enrichment include iodine in salt at a level of 7.6 mg per 100 g; vitamin D is added to milk at a level of 400 IU per quart; and vitamin A is added to margarine at a level of 15,000 IU per pound (the average vitamin A content of butter throughout the year). Bread may also be enriched by the addition of enriched flour, pure nutrients, or nutritional yeast with iron. Fortified beverages include vitamin A- and vitamin D-fortified milk; calcium- and vitamin B_{12}-fortified soy milk. Calcium is added to some orange juices and VITAMIN C is added to some synthetic beverages. (See also ERGOCALCIFEROL; FOOD ADDITIVES; FOOD FORTIFICATION.)

enteritis Inflammation of the intestine, particularly the layer of cells lining the intestine and also the underlying connective tissue. (See also INFLAMMATORY BOWEL DISEASE.)

enterohepatic circulation The absorption of nutrients and other materials by the INTESTINE, their transport to the LIVER and reutilization. A variety of substances released into the intestine can be reabsorbed by the intestine. Thus BILE salts released from the GALLBLADDER are absorbed by the small intestine, where they pass into the capillaries and then are transported to the liver via the portal vein. Bile salts can be taken up by the liver and released again in bile. Less than 1 percent of bile salts escapes this recycling process daily. This small loss nonetheless represents the major route by which CHOLESTEROL is altered and lost by the body. (See also FAT DIGESTION.)

enteropathy A general medical term referring to the broad class of intestinal disease. Typical examples are CROHN'S DISEASE, CELIAC DISEASE, INFLAMMATORY BOWEL DISEASE, and infectious DIARRHEA. Enteropathies can affect the small intestine, the colon or both portions of the intestine.

enteropeptidase An intestinal enzyme responsible for activating protein-degrading enzymes from the pancreas. The pancreas secretes enzymes that digest proteins as inactive precursors in order to prevent the pancreas from digesting itself. These inactive enzymes encounter enteropeptidase, which triggers the following cascade of events. Enteropeptidase activates trypsin, a powerful digestive enzyme. Trypsin in turn activates all other protein-digesting enzymes of the pancreas. Severe milk intolerance is linked to enteropeptidase deficiency, inadequate pancreatic enzymes, and, ultimately, to maldigestion. (See also DIGESTIVE ENZYMES.)

enterotoxin Bacterial products released or produced in the intestine that can cause illness. Certain bacterial species produce chemicals that cause food poisoning, including enterotoxin-producing strains of *ESCHERICHIA COLI* that can contaminate undercooked or raw meat. Staphyloccocal FOOD POISONING is caused by ingestion of bacterial toxins in contaminated food, usually in custards, milk products, and unrefrigerated meats, while *Shigella* species cause dysentery (very severe DIARRHEA) by releasing toxins at sites of infection. In contrast, the bacterium SALMONELLA causes food poisoning through rapid intestinal growth without the production of enterotoxins. (See also ACIDOPHILUS.)

environmental medicine A branch of medicine that focuses on the role of environmental factors in illness. Allergies or sensitivities to chemicals in food, water, and air, at home and at work, are relevant topics. Exposure to substances that cause symptoms can be physical or chemical, and usually symptoms are chronic and cyclic. Environmental ecologists believe that environmentally induced illness is the most common cause of chronic symptoms. Multiple organ systems are often involved. Treatment involves avoidance, control of air and water quality, and immunization therapy to control adverse responses and rotation diets. (See also CHEMICAL SENSITIVITY.)

enzymes A class of proteins that speed up (catalyze) the chemical reactions of cells. Enzymes are extremely important and dynamic proteins. The body carries out more than 100,000 different chemical reactions, and each of these requires a specific protein catalyst to speed up and control reactions. Because catalysts are not used up as they do their work, tiny amounts of enzymes can form a huge amount of products from substrates.

Enzymes play major roles in METABOLISM. They are required for DIGESTION, energy production, nerve function, muscle contraction, and regulation of blood pH. They help form all cell structures such as RNA and DNA—and much, much more. Chemical compounds that react in enzyme-catalyzed reactions are called substrates. A classic model is helpful to visualize how enzymes work: A key fits into a carefully constructed keyhole where chemical bonds are made or broken. The names of enzymes often use the suffix "-ase," for example, CATALASE, dehydrogenase, AMYLASE, and oxidase.

Like all PROTEINS, enzymes are long chains of amino acids (POLYPEPTIDES) composed of the 20 AMINO ACID building blocks. Each type of enzyme possesses a unique amino acid sequence, which is encoded in genes. The amino acid sequence determines both the structure and the function of a given enzyme. Mutations in genes are due to chemical modifications of DNA that lead to the production of proteins with altered amino acid sequences. Mutant proteins may not function as well as the unaltered protein; in the most severe cases, mutations can lead to completely nonfunctional enzymes and genetic diseases. PHENYLKETONURIA, an inherited inability to break down the amino acid phenylalanine, is an example.

The thousands of different enzyme reactions fall into just six categories. "Hydrolases" break chemical linkages in molecules by adding water (hydrolysis). Amylase (STARCH digestion), LIPASE (FAT digestion), and proteolytic enzymes like trypsin (protein digestion) are examples. "Transferases" move a group of atoms from one compound to another, for example, transaminases transfer amino ($-NH_2$) groups to carboxylic acids in order to form new amino acids. "Lyases" break bonds between carbon and carbon atoms, between carbon and nitrogen atoms (and carbon and oxygen atoms) of compounds without adding water molecules or oxygen. "Isomerases" catalyze rearrangements of atoms within molecules. Several reactions in glucose breakdown require isomerizations. "Ligases" utilize the energy of ATP to create new carbon compounds. Energy-requiring steps play key roles in the synthesis of fat from FATTY ACIDS, of proteins from amino acids, of complex carbohydrates from simple sugars. And finally, "oxidoreductases" carry out oxidation-reduction reactions. These enzymes are called "dehydrogenases" or "oxidases," for example, lactate dehydrogenase, which produces LACTIC ACID in the muscle during strenuous exertion.

Metabolic Pathways

Enzymes often participate in functional sequences of reactions called metabolic pathways. In metabolic pathways, the product of one enzyme becomes the substrate for the following enzyme, which modifies the intermediate product before passing it on to the next enzyme, much like a bucket brigade. A typical sequence can be illustrated as $A \rightarrow B \rightarrow C \rightarrow D$, in which enzyme 1 catalyzes the reaction $A \rightarrow B$; enzyme 2 catalyzes $B \rightarrow C$; enzyme 3 catalyzes $C \rightarrow D$; and so on.

Regulation

Enzyme pathways are often carefully regulated. The first enzyme committed to the pathway often controls a bottleneck step, limiting the flow of material through the pathway. Such rate-limiting enzymes can be activated to speed up the pathway or they can be inhibited, to slow it down. Thus, entire metabolic pathways can be turned on or off by regulating such key enzymes.

The body regulates enzymes in other ways as well. The amount of enzymes in tissues can be increased, for example, during adaptation to a carbohydrate-rich diet; fasting; embryonic and fetal development; pregnancy; and when taking drugs or medications. These changes are slow because they alter protein-forming machinery. Certain hormones are often enzyme inducers: Insulin induces biosynthetic enzymes associated with glycogen and fat formation for energy stores, while cortisol can increase levels of enzymes for fat degradation. Other hormones, such as the stress hormone EPINEPHRINE, can activate or inhibit enzymes quickly. The flow of molecules within cells can activate or block metabolic pathways quickly. In a common scenario a buildup of the products of a pathway can inhibit the first step of the pathway (FEEDBACK INHIBITION) to slow the flow of materials. As examples, ATP can shut down GLYCOLYSIS (glucose breakdown) and NADH (reduced NICOTINAMIDE ADENINE DINUCLEOTIDE) can shut down the KREB'S CYCLE, the central pathway in energy production of the cell's powerhouses (mitochondria).

Coenzymes and Cofactors

Many enzymes require nonprotein components to be active. TRACE MINERALS and the vitamins of the B COMPLEX assist in enzyme function. Trace mineral nutrients (like MAGNESIUM, MANGANESE, IRON, COPPER, ZINC, SELENIUM, and MOLYBDENUM) function as enzyme COFACTORS. For example, zinc helps DNA polymerase, the enzyme that makes DNA. Iron helps CYTOCHROMES, responsible for mitochondria production of ATP, with the transfer of electrons to oxygen to form water.

The body modifies vitamins of the B complex to form COENZYMES (enzyme helpers). An enzyme combined with its coenzyme is called a holoenzyme, while an APOENZYME lacks its coenzyme and consequently is completely inactive. NIACIN yields NAD (nicotinamide adenine dinucleotide), and RIBOFLAVIN forms FAD (FLAVIN ADENINE DINUCLEOTIDE) for oxidation reduction reactions, for example, in oxidizing fuels for energy. THIAMIN forms thiamin pyrophosphate, used in oxidation of carbohydrate. PANTOTHENIC ACID forms COENZYME A, used to carry fatty acids and acetic acid through reaction sequences. BIOTIN forms biocytin for reactions in which carbon dioxide is attached to compounds to form new acids, while FOLIC ACID forms tetrahydrofolate, used in shuttling single carbon atom fragments between molecules. VITAMIN B_6 forms pyridoxal phosphate for transferring nitrogen group, and VITAMIN B_{12} forms methylcobalamin used to regenerate the essential amino acid methionine, among others. As an example of the critical role that vitamins play in metabolism, consider that thiamin, riboflavin, pantothenic acid, and niacin are essential to burn fuels to produce ATP in the Kreb's cycle, the central energy pathway of mitochondria. A deficiency of any one of these vitamins impairs this pathway, and hence the ability of cells to produce energy.

Enzyme Inactivation (Loss of Enzyme Activity)

Enzymes are fragile and can be poisoned or destroyed by chemicals. Toxic HEAVY METALS like LEAD and MERCURY are poisons because they bind to enzymes. Enzymes are also sensitive to pH. If blood is too acidic (ACIDOSIS) or too basic (ALKALOSIS), enzymes may be inactivated. Heat, as used in cooking food and blanching vegetables, destroys enzymes. Soap destroys enzymes by causing the protein molecules to unfold and unwind. Oxidation and other chemical reactions can also irreversibly alter enzyme structure with loss of function.

Variability In Enzymes Among Individuals

Each person has somewhat different enzyme levels in body tissues. These slight but important differences in the enzyme makeup are the result of differences in heredity, age, sex, exercise pattern, diet history, state of health, lifestyle, exposure to environmental pollutants, medications, and drugs. The level of enzymes may increase as the body adapts to change. Thus drug-destroying enzymes of the liver will increase after prolonged drug exposure. (See also BIOCHEMICAL INDIVIDUALITY; CARBOHYDRATE METABOLISM; CARCINOGEN; FAT METABOLISM; TRACE MINERALS.)

EPA (Environmental Protection Agency) A federal agency established in 1971 to form and enforce laws to protect the environment and to control pollution. It is the largest independent regulatory agency of the federal government. The EPA administers clean water programs, clean air and solid waste disposal programs, and toxic waste clean-up; and conducts PESTICIDE research and programs to establish pesticide standards. The EPA establishes tolerance levels for toxic materials, pesticides, and even excessive noise. It also monitors radioactivity levels in the home and workplace. The EPA is responsible for setting limits based on lifetime exposure to toxic materials such as DIOXIN, LEAD, air pollutants, and pesticides found in FOOD, air, and WATER. It has outlawed a variety of pesticides and instigated reductions of sulfur dioxide and lead from automobile and industrial stack emissions. (See also FDA; USDA.)

ephedra (*Ephedra sinica*) An herb (also called ma huang) used in traditional Chinese medicine for more than 5,000 years primarily to treat asthma or bronchitis. Synthetic ephedrine compounds (such as pseudoephedrine) are widely used in over-the-counter cold remedies. Ephedra is also sold commercially as an energy booster, a weight-loss supplement, and an athletic performance enhancer. However, because of a number of reports of serious health problems and deaths linked to this herb, the U.S. government is studying ephedra and is expected to make a decision soon about whether to ban the herb. The ephedra industry, however, insists that its own scientific studies show the herb is completely safe. The federal government has cracked down on ephedra products sold illegally as an alternative to street drugs. But the law allows supplements that don't make illegal claims to be sold with little oversight.

Although some scientific evidence suggests that this herbal supplement may improve weight loss, the information overall regarding its effectiveness for weight loss, energy, and athletic performance has been controversial. Many ephedra-containing products sold for these purposes also contain caffeine, and the combination of the two increases the chance of side effects. Ephedra is banned by the U.S. Olympic Committee, the NFL, and the NCAA; the U.S. military has removed all ephedra products from its commissaries.

Ephedra (and its main active ingredient, ephedrine) can potentially stimulate the central nervous system, raising blood pressure and boosting heart rate to dangerous levels. Ephedra is also used to prepare illegal street drugs such as methamphetamine. In fact, ephedra has been the center of a major controversy between the herb industry and the U.S. Food and Drug Administration (FDA) since the 1990s.

Between 1997 and 1999 the FDA received 140 reports of adverse reactions associated with the use of ephedra and supplements containing ephedra alkaloids. Irregular heart rhythm with heart palpitations or extremely high blood pressure were among the most commonly reported adverse events; other problems reported included stroke, seizures, and death (10 fatalities have been reported in connection to the use of ephedra).

According to an analysis by the *New England Journal of Medicine,* dietary supplements for weight loss or increasing exercise capacity that contain ephedra and its related alkaloids have no apparent benefits and pose a serious health risk to some users. Users should also be careful with supplements containing norephedrine (another ephedra alkaloid, often called phenylpropanolamine), which can cause liver damage, bleeding, and stroke. The FDA issued a warning against norephedrine in November 2000 and requested that drug companies remove this product from the market.

In 2001 the national consumer research and advocacy organization Public Citizen Health Research Group petitioned the FDA to ban the production and sale of all dietary supplements containing ephedra and related compounds. The nutritional supplement industry, including the American Herbal Products Association (AHPA) and the Council for Responsible Nutrition (CRN), countered with their own proposal for much clearer labeling of the potential risks and appropriate dosing on ephedra-containing products. The AHPA and CRN claim that ephedra is generally safe if these warnings and precautionary measures are taken. For example, the CRN advocates that strict guidelines be established regarding a tolerable upper intake level (UL) for substances containing ephedra; their recommendation, based on scientific studies, is that no more than 90 mg per day of ephedra be taken in three divided doses for no longer than six months. The CRN states that use of amounts below this UL should avoid any dangerous adverse effects. Until more conclusive evidence becomes available, any supplements containing ephedra or its related compounds should be used only under the guidance and supervision of an appropriate health care professional.

Ephedra, a perennial evergreen that may grow up to four feet tall, grows on the tundra and the rocky and sandy slopes of Europe, Asia, and America. The plant has slender, cylindrical, yellow-green branches and underground runners and bears poisonous, fleshy red cones resembling berries. The young stems and branchlets are the parts used for medicinal preparations. It is available in dried and liquid preparations, but studies have found that there is wide variation in the amount of ephedra alkaloids present in supplements.

Ephedra can produce side effects such as irritability, restlessness, anxiety, insomnia, headaches, nausea, vomiting, and urinary problems in addition to its more serious side effects of high blood pressure, rapid or irregular heartbeat, stroke, seizures, addiction, and even death. Ephedra should be used only on a short-term basis because prolonged use may lead to addiction. The amount of time considered safe, however, is not clear; sources report anywhere from no longer than seven days to up to 12 consecutive weeks. It should be taken between meals without food. Pregnant and breast-feeding women should not use ephedra.

epidemiology The study of factors in populations that determine the frequency of diseases and their distribution in populations. Epidemiology requires the collection of data for groups of people to establish RISK factors and associations. "Retrospective" studies examine medical records to learn about past events. As an example, comparison of the occurrence of cancer in high-risk areas with low-risk areas where people rarely get a given type of cancer suggests that 80 percent to 90 percent of human cancer is preventable. One problem with linking diet to disease is that such studies usually depend on diet recall, that is, what people remember they ate, especially years ago when the initial events may have occurred. "Prospective" studies start with the selected group and follow a characteristic of that group for a period of time.

Several concepts are used in epidemiology. The "prevalence" of a disease or condition is like a "single snapshot" of a population; it answers the question of how many individuals are affected at a given moment. The "incidence" of a condition is a rate; it predicts the number of individuals who will be affected per unit of time, typically a month or a year.

Epidemiology demonstrated the link between cigarette smoking and increased risk of cancer, and the link between diets with ample fiber, fresh vegetables, and fruits and decreased risk of cancer. In addition to cancer, epidemiology has uncovered other associations between environment (diet) and disease. For example, diets high in FISH and marine lipids are linked to a decreased risk of heart attack. In the United States, diets high in SATURATED FAT are linked to an increased risk of CARDIOVASCULAR DISEASE; alcohol consumption increases the risk of FETAL ALCOHOL SYNDROME. Nonetheless, correlations between two variables alone cannot prove cause and effect because they deal with probabilities. Epidemiology can help calculate the probability, or odds, but it cannot predict events for a given individual. (See also FRAMINGHAM STUDY; RISK DUE TO CHEMICALS IN FOOD AND WATER.)

epinephrine (adrenaline) A HORMONE released by adrenal glands in response to STRESS. Epinephrine and a related hormone, norepinephrine, are synthesized from the amino acid TYROSINE by the inner portion of the adrenal gland. Epinephrine synthesis requires many nutrients in addition to tyrosine: COPPER, IRON, VITAMIN C, VITAMIN B_6, VITAMIN B_{12}, and METHIONINE.

The "flight or fight" response to physical stress or to situations perceived as threatening involves stimulation of the sympathetic division of the autonomic nervous system, the branch of the nervous system that controls involuntary responses. When epinephrine is released into the bloodstream in response to nerve stimulation, it constricts CAPILLARIES and reduces circulation in hands and feet, causing cold hands and feet. Epinephrine slows DIGESTION, increases heart rate, and relaxes bronchial smooth muscles to open air passageways and increase the oxygen supply to the lungs.

Epinephrine mobilizes the body's energy stores: It stimulates the release of FATTY ACIDS from ADI-

POSE TISSUE into the bloodstream, and it stimulates the release of GLUCOSE from liver GLYCOGEN to increase BLOOD SUGAR so they can be burned for quick energy. Epinephrine also triggers muscle glycogen breakdown to release glucose as an immediate fuel for muscle.

epithelial tissue (epithelium) The tissues lining the cavities and ducts of the body and all body surfaces. The epithelium forms the skin, the lining of the GASTROINTESTINAL TRACT and ducts of secretory tissues like the LIVER and PANCREAS, the urinary tract, the reproductive system, the respiratory tract and the blood vessels.

There are several fundamental types of epithelium. Simple squamous epithelium forms a single layer of flat cells, like a tiled floor, and lines the lungs, kidneys, heart, blood vessels, lymph vessels, and CAPILLARIES. Epithelial cells of the digestive tract (stomach, intestines, pancreas, liver, gallbladder) secrete digestive juices, a process controlled by long, columnar cells. Often they secrete complex polysaccharide, which forms MUCUS or a protective barrier. Epithelial cells of the gastrointestinal tract have a relatively short half-life. They constantly slough off, their protein is degraded and their amino acids are recycled in digestion.

Multilayered squamous epithelium functions as protection. A tough protective layer (keratinized tissue) form the outer layer of skin while softer, nonkeratinized tissues with moist surfaces are found in the mouth, tongue, ESOPHAGUS, and vagina. Glandular epithelium secretes products into ducts; these ducts include mammary glands, digestive glands like salivary glands, and the pancreas. Endocrine epithelium secretes hormones into blood. Examples are the pituitary gland, thyroid gland, ADRENAL GLANDS, ovaries and testes, and thymus gland. (See also DIGESTIVE TRACT; ENDOCRINE SYSTEM.)

ergocalciferol (calciferol, vitamin D_2) A common supplemental form of vitamin D. Ergocalciferol is readily manufactured from a plant lipid, ERGOSTEROL, by exposure to ultraviolet light. Ergocalciferol is the most common form of vitamin D used to fortify foods because it is readily available. Routine vitamin supplements containing more than 400 IU of vitamin D are not recommended because vitamin D can accumulate to toxic levels with excessive consumption; 1,800 IU of vitamin D (45 mcg) can cause symptoms in young children who are particularly susceptible. The levels of vitamin D in milk can vary widely and adults consuming several glasses of vitamin D–fortified milk daily may receive substantially higher levels of vitamin D. (See also HYPERVITAMINOSIS; RICKETS.)

ergogenic supplements Supplements that purportedly increase the potential for physical work by improving ENERGY production, or energy efficiency during EXERCISE. Ergogenic supplements are said to increase endurance and the capacity for exercise. However, in general, supplementation of specific nutrients above dietary allowances for healthy athletes does not improve athletic performance. So-called vitamin B_{15} or PANGAMIC ACID, mixtures of free AMINO ACIDS, ALCOHOL, bee pollen, GELATIN, HONEY, wheat germ oils, and inosine do not appear to consistently increase athletic performance.

Other substances have been periodically called "ergogenic." Tryptophan at large doses can increase growth hormone levels, but its effect in athletes has not been measured. In 1990 the U.S. FDA banned the sale of this amino acid supplement due to a toxic contamination. Aspartates, particularly potassium and magnesium aspartates, derived from the amino acid ASPARTIC ACID, have shown some positive effects in DOUBLE-BLIND, PLACEBO-controlled trials in which neither the investigator nor the subject knew who received aspartate and who received an inactive substance (placebo). Large doses of single amino acids can cause imbalances in susceptible individuals because the excess consumption of one can affect uptake of another.

CAFFEINE is a stimulant and may facilitate the use of fat stores for energy during exercise. (See also ARGININE; CARNITINE; OCTACOSANOL.)

Thein, L. A., J. M. Thein, and G. L. Landry. "Ergogenic Aids," *Physical Therapy* 75, no. 5 (1995): 426–429.

ergosterol A plant lipid found in yeasts and molds. This white, waxy substance is used commercially to synthesize vitamin D_2. Irradiated ergosterol or other forms of VITAMIN D are commercially added to MILK to ensure an adequate intake of this vitamin and to avoid vitamin D deficiency disease. (See also ERGOCALCIFEROL; FORTIFICATION; HYPERVITAMINOSIS.)

ergot A toxic substance produced by a fungus, *Claviceps purpurea,* which can infect rye and other grains. Ergot poisoning may occur from eating bread made from flour contaminated with this fungus, now a rare occurrence in developed nations. Historically, outbreaks of ergot poisoning were known as St. Anthony's Fire. Ingestion of ergot can cause tumors in experimental animals. (See also AFLATOXIN; FOOD POISONING; FOOD TOXINS; MOLD.)

erucic acid A monounsaturated fatty acid found in seed oils such as RAPESEED and MUSTARD seed, with 22 carbons. Research conducted in Canada and elsewhere in the 1960s demonstrated that consumption of large amounts of rapeseed oil by experimental animals resulted in impaired growth and pathological changes in heart muscle. Human toxicity was not reported; apparently, erucic acid can be broken down normally in humans. Nonetheless new varieties of rapeseed (*Canadian brassica*) were developed that contain little or no erucic acid. BORAGE oil contains a low level (1 percent to 3 percent) of erucic acid. (See also FATTY ACIDS; OLIVE OIL.)

eructation Belching. The noisy release of gas from the stomach. Drinking carbonated beverages, gulping food with excessive swallowing of air, and fermentation processes in the stomach can cause belching. (See also ACID INDIGESTION.)

erythema The redness of skin produced when CAPILLARIES close to the skin surface expand. Erythema is caused by inflammation, including allergies; reaction to food poisoning and to certain drugs; contact with toxic substances; and environmental factors such as heat, cold, and sunburn, as well as emotional upsets. (See also ALLERGY, FOOD.)

erythorbic acid (sodium erythorbate) A FOOD ADDITIVE used to protect processed foods against oxidation. Although it is a close relative of VITAMIN C, it is poorly absorbed. As an ANTIOXIDANT, erythorbic acid prevents undesirable changes in the color, aroma, and taste of processed foods.

Erythorbate and vitamin C are added to noncitrus fruits like apples, pears, and bananas, as well as vegetables such as eggplant, potatoes, and yams, to retard deterioration and browning reaction during processing.

Erythorbate is added to BEER after FERMENTATION to help prevent its darkening, turbidity, and taste deterioration. In cured meats such as SAUSAGE, HAM, and BACON, this antioxidant helps stabilize color and inhibit the formation of NITROSOAMINES, which are CARCINOGENS. (See also BHA; BHT; FREE RADICALS.)

erythrocytes See RED BLOOD CELLS.

erythropoiesis The formation of mature RED BLOOD CELLS (erythrocytes) from immature precursors ("stem" cells). Erythropoiesis is stimulated by the HORMONE erythropoietin, which is created by the kidneys when they are subjected to low oxygen levels. The kidneys respond by releasing a factor that converts a blood protein to erythropoietin. This hormone targets the bone marrow where immature precursor cells (erythroblasts) are induced to synthesize massive amounts of HEMOGLOBIN, the oxygen transport protein of red blood cells. Erythroblasts become reticulocytes, immature red blood cells released into the bloodstream where they mature into erythrocytes, full-fledged red blood cells, in one to two days. (See also ANEMIA; CIRCULATORY SYSTEM.)

Escherichia coli A rod-shaped bacterium that normally inhabits the colon (large intestine). *E. coli* is considered one of the friendly gut bacteria in fecal matter. By occupying an ecological niche, it can prevent potentially harmful organisms from growing. The presence of this bacterium in water and milk indicates fecal contamination. Normally nonpathogenic (nondisease-producing), *E. coli* can cause URINARY TRACT infections when it infects that tissue. Certain strains of *E. coli* are pathogens. A pathogenic strain causes at least 40 percent of traveler's DIARRHEA.

E. Coli 0157:H7

This strain of *E. coli* was discovered as a human pathogen in 1982. It damages the intestine and produces a toxic substance that can penetrate the body, damaging blood vessels and kidneys. It is the leading cause of bloody diarrhea in the United States. *E. coli* 0157:H7 also causes severe abdominal cramping. Infection by this strain of *E. coli* is the most common cause of hemolytic uremic syndrome, a serious disease that can cause kidney damage and death in children. The Centers for Disease Control and Prevention considered this to be the most serious public health problem relating to food-borne illness (1994). Estimates range from 200,000 cases per year; more states are requiring that cases of *E. coli* 0157:H7 be reported by doctors, so the picture will become clearer. Children under five are the most susceptible; infection can be spread by fecal contamination at day care centers or preschools.

Rare or uncooked meat, especially hamburger and ground beef, is a common source of *E. coli* 0157:H7 because fecal material often contaminates animal carcasses in meat packing plants. To be safe, meat must be cooked thoroughly until pinkness is gone and meat juices are clear. (See also ACIDOPHILUS; BIFIDOBACTERIA; FOOD POISONING.)

Mead, P., and P. M. Griffin. "*Escherichia Coli* 0157:H7," *Lancet* 352 (1998): 1,207–1,212.

Eskimo diet A "heart healthy" diet that includes coldwater ocean FISH, in addition to FAT and CHOLESTEROL from marine animals. This diet is rich in oils of coldwater fish; such oils contain high levels of omega-3 FATTY ACIDS. The rate of HEART ATTACK of Greenland Eskimos is only 10 percent that of U.S. adults. Omega-3 fatty acids lower blood CHOLESTEROL, reduce the tendency for blood to clot, and lower the risk of thrombosis. These factors, in turn, prevent cholesterol accumulation in arteries and therefore protect against heart disease. For Americans, eating fish regularly may help lower cholesterol only if fish is substituted for red MEAT, not added to a diet already high in SATURATED FAT. (See also DOCOSAHEXAENOIC ACID; EICOSAPENTAENOIC ACID; ESSENTIAL FATTY ACIDS; FISH OIL.)

esophagus The tube connecting the mouth and the upper end of the STOMACH. In the process of swallowing, chewed food is transported down the esophagus by the involuntary wavelike contraction and relaxation of smooth muscle walls (PERISTALSIS). The valve between the stomach and esophagus may not close properly (due to a reaction to food, or gulping air with food). When this occurs, stomach acid can back up into the esophagus, a condition called esophageal reflux, which causes ACID INDIGESTION or heartburn. (See also ANTACID; DIGESTIVE TRACT.)

essential amino acids Eight of the 20 AMINO ACIDS that are protein building blocks and must be supplied by the diet through the digestion of food proteins. The essential amino acids are the following: TRYPTOPHAN, PHENYLALANINE, METHIONINE, LYSINE, THREONINE, VALINE, ISOLEUCINE, and LEUCINE. Two other amino acids, HISTIDINE and ARGININE, are essential under special circumstances. Histidine supports growth in young children and arginine supports newborns and adults with damaged livers. When the diet does not provide adequate methionine, CYSTEINE becomes an essential amino acid because it is synthesized from methionine. These amino acids are therefore "conditionally essential" amino acids.

Because essential amino acids must be supplied in the diet on a daily basis, their levels in food are important to a balanced diet. The relative proportions of essential amino acids in a food protein determine whether it is "high-" or "low-"quality protein. Thus, a high-quality protein is one that supplies adequate levels of all essential amino acids to meet the body's requirements. POULTRY, FISH, and MEAT, together with milk products and EGGS, are the most common sources of high-quality protein in industrialized nations. Although there is no perfect protein, chicken eggs provide a mixture of essential amino acids in close-to-optimal amounts for healthy people and are the international standard by which other protein sources are measured. Plant protein is often relatively low in lysine, tryptophan, and methionine.

The following deficiencies are noted: corn (tryptophan and threonine); grain cereals (lysine); legumes (methionine); rice (tryptophan, threonine); soybean (methionine). Therefore, the limiting amino acids need to be complemented by mixing with plant protein sources. Combining rice protein and bean protein can satisfy the body's need for essential amino acids. Surplus essential amino acids from digestion as fuel are burned for ENERGY or are converted to FAT. (See also BIOLOGICAL VALUE; NET PROTEIN UTILIZATION; PROTEIN COMPLEMENTATION.)

essential fatty acids (EFA, vitamin F) Two fatty acids that cannot be synthesized by the body and must be provided by the diet. The essential fatty acids LINOLEIC ACID and ALPHA LINOLENIC ACID are polyunsaturated FATTY ACIDS, that is, they possess two or more double bonds and lack several hydrogen atoms found in saturated fatty acids. They differ in their location of double bonds, that is, bonds between carbon atoms that are deficient in hydrogen atoms. This small chemical difference has a huge nutritional impact. Linoleic acid contains 18 carbon atoms and belongs to the omega-6 family of fatty acids, in which the first double bond occurs at the sixth carbon atom of the molecular chain. Linoleic acid serves as the parent of a large polyunsaturated fatty acid, called ARACHIDONIC ACID. Arachidonic acid in turn forms PROSTAGLANDINS (PGE_2) and thromboxanes (TXA_2), hormone-like lipids that tend to promote blood clotting, induce pain and inflammation, and cause smooth muscle contraction. Another pathway converts arachidonic acid to LEUKOTRIENES, one of the most powerful inflammatory agents. Events triggering inflammation stimulate cells to synthesize prostaglandins (PGE_2) and thromboxanes (TXA_2). As a component of membrane lipids, linoleic acid helps maintain flexibility of cell membranes. Arachidonic acid is not a dietary essential unless a deficiency of linoleic acid exists.

The second essential fatty acid, alpha linolenic acid, is the major polyunsaturated fatty acid of plants. It contains 18 carbon atoms and three double bonds and belongs to the omega-3 family of fatty acids, in which the first double bond occurs at the third carbon of the fatty acid. Alpha linolenic acid is converted to a very long fatty acid, EICOSAPENTANEONIC ACID (EPA), which forms prostaglandins (PGE_3) and thromboxane (TXA_3) that counterbalance the effects of pro-inflammatory products derived from arachidonic acid by reducing the tendency to clot, reducing pain and inflammation. Dietary alpha linolenic acid will tend to inhibit arachidonic acid conversion to inflammatory agents, and thus further limit inflammation. Alpha linolenic acid occurs in high levels in BORAGE oil and flaxseed oil, while EPA occurs in high levels in fish and shellfish.

If the diet lacks adequate amounts of either linoleic or alpha linolenic acid, deficiency symptoms will develop that include scaly skin, hair loss, and slow wound healing. Omega-3 fatty acid deficiency leads to impaired brain and retinal development in experimental animals and possibly in premature births.

Polyunsaturated seed oils and fish oils supply the essential fatty acids in the typical U.S. diet. There is no RECOMMENDED DIETARY ALLOWANCE for linoleic acid or alpha linolenic acid. However, the amount of linoleic acid and related omega-6 fatty acids needed to prevent deficiency in adults is estimated to be 1 percent to 3 percent of calories, equivalent to approximately 6 g/day. Linoleic acid in typical American diets ranges from 5 percent to 10 percent of calories due to a high consumption of vegetable oils. It has been proposed that alpha linolenic acid represent 0.25 percent to 0.54 percent of daily calories for optimal health. Large amounts of polyunsaturated fatty acids may increase the requirement for antioxidants like VITAMIN E to prevent their chemical degradation. (See also DOCOSAHEXAENOIC ACID.)

essential nutrients Substances in FOODS that are indispensable for growth and maintenance and must be supplied by the diet. About 40 essential NUTRIENTS have been identified. For healthy adults, the essential nutrients include eight AMINO ACIDS, two ESSENTIAL FATTY ACIDS (LINOLEIC and ALPHA LINOLENIC ACIDS); VITAMINS (13 are so classified); MINERALS, including trace minerals and water. Foods must supply 15 minerals; none can be generated in the body. A certain minimal input of digestible CARBOHYDRATE is required to prevent excessive muscle protein and fat breakdown. Dietary FIBER maintains normal bowel function.

The amounts of these materials required for optimal health have not been specified.

A number of nutrients are best classified as conditionally essential, because under certain circumstances, the diet may not supply adequate amounts to meet the body's needs for growth, maintenance or repair and healing. The amino acids asparagine, histidine, methionine, and cysteine fall into this category. The need for nutrients such as TAURINE, a sulfur-containing compound derived from the sulfur amino acid cysteine, COENZYME Q_{10}, CHOLINE, and CARNITINE, a compound needed to degrade fatty acids, can increase during heart disease and other conditions. There is a growing awareness that vegetables and fruits supply a wide range of substances that support health beyond those traditionally recognized nutrients. These include complex aromatic compounds called FLAVONOIDS that affect liver detoxication, limit inflammation, strengthen capillary walls and serve as antioxidants. Dark green leafy and orange vegetables and fruits supply orange-yellow pigments called CAROTENOIDS that act as antioxidants and enhance the immune system. It may well be the case that such plant products are essential components of a balanced diet over a lifetime to prevent or retard chronic disease. (See also RECOMMENDED DIETARY ALLOWANCES.)

esterase An enzyme that breaks down esters. LIPASES are esterases that degrade fats and oils (TRIGLYCERIDES) to FATTY ACIDS and GLYCEROL during FAT DIGESTION and in LIPOLYSIS, the process of breaking down stored fat. Phospholipases digest PHOSPHOLIPIDS to fatty acids. An esterase plays a key role in the transmission of nerve impulses. Acetylcholine esterase breaks down the neurotransmitter ACETYLCHOLINE to its constituents, CHOLINE and ACETIC ACID. (See also DIGESTIVE ENZYMES.)

esters A class of organic compounds that includes fragrances, fruity flavors, FATS, oils, and WAXES. Esters contain two types of building blocks—ACIDS and ALCOHOLS. Esters that evaporate easily account for aromas and flavors of APPLES (methyl butanoate); oranges (octylacetate); pineapple (ethylbutanoate); and rum flavor (ethylformate). Artificial fruit flavors are primarily mixtures of low molecular weight esters.

Fats and OILS are triple esters containing the complex alcohol and long-chain FATTY ACIDS plus the triple alcohol, GLYCEROL, and are called TRIGLYCERIDES; they represent the most abundant LIPIDS. Digestion of fats and oils yields fatty acids that are readily absorbed.

Whether a triglyceride is a solid depends on its fatty acid composition. Triglycerides containing unsaturated fatty acids, such as OLEIC ACID and LINOLEIC ACID, are liquid at room temperature and are called oils. Corn oil, soybean oil, and wheat germ oil contain approximately 80 percent unsaturated oil and therefore these substances are liquids. On the other hand, triglycerides rich in saturated fatty acids, such as PALMITIC ACID and STEARIC ACID, are semisolid or solid at room temperature and are called fats. For example, beef fat (BEEF TALLOW) contains approximately 41.5 percent saturated fatty acids and is a waxy solid.

Naturally occurring waxes such as beeswax are esters containing a fatty acid combined with a large alcohol with a chain length from 16 to over 30 carbon atoms. Waxes are harder, more brittle, and less greasy than fats, and they are used in cosmetics, ointments, and time-release nutrient supplements, and are also used to coat produce in order to reduce moisture loss and to create a shiny appearance.

Other types of esters are important in cellular formation. Simple sugars like glucose must be esterified with phosphate before they can be used. Once phosphate is attached, sugars cannot leak out of the cell. Phosphate esters are also represented by a class of lipids called phospholipids, such as LECITHIN, which form cell membranes. Phosphate esters also link the building blocks of DNA and RNA. (See also CARBOHYDRATE METABOLISM; ESTERASE; FLAVORS; SUGAR.)

estrogen A class of steroid HORMONES that function as female sex hormones. Estrogens are formed by the follicles of ovaries. They serve many functions: They increase protein synthesis in targeted tissues; they are responsible for secondary female characteristics (such as the development of breasts and the deposition of fat); and they stimulate regeneration of epithelial tissue of the uterus. Estrogen levels increase in the postmenstrual phase of the menstrual cycle. Together with progesterone, estrogen prepares the endometrium for ovulation. Women's overall eating patterns are affected by the menstrual cycle, thus a decline in food consumption corresponds to a rise in estrogen levels at the time of ovulation.

Estrogen retards bone loss. When a woman goes through MENOPAUSE, her estrogen levels drop off sharply. Consequently, her bones may become brittle (OSTEOPOROSIS) and more prone to fracture. To decrease this risk many women in recent decades opted to undergo hormone replacement therapy (HRT), which involves taking the hormone drugs estrogen and progestin. Women who took the drugs were much less likely to suffer osteoporosis-related fractures.

However, in 2002 a study of hormone replacement therapy in 16,000 postmenopausal women was halted when researchers discovered that the hormone drugs caused a slight but significant increase in the risk of invasive breast cancer and also increased the risk of heart attack, stroke, and blood clots. Although researchers reported that the risk to any individual woman was small, they cautioned that the drugs' risks outweighed their benefits. After these results were announced, many women who had been on HRT stopped taking hormone medication. (See also CALCIUM; ENDOCRINE SYSTEM; TESTOSTERONE.)

Herrington, David M. et al. "Effects of Estrogen Replacement on the Progression of Coronary-Artery Atherosclerosis," *New England Journal of Medicine* 343 (August 24, 2000): 522–529.

Rossouw, Jack E. et al. "Risks and Benefits of Estrogen Plus Progestin in Healthy Postmenopausal Women," *Journal of the American Medical Association* 288, no. 3 (2002): 321–333.

ethanol (ethyl alcohol, grain alcohol) An ALCOHOL traditionally produced in the fermentation of carbohydrates and starches. Ethanol is present in fermented beverages and distilled liquors. Absolute alcohol contains 99 percent ethanol and 1 percent water. Ethanol is rapidly absorbed by the stomach and small intestine, and it is destroyed at a constant rate by the liver. Oxidation yields 7 calories per gram.

Ethanol is oxidized by ethanol oxidizing systems (EOS), an enzyme system that may be more active among heavy drinkers. Nonetheless, excessive alcohol can block the liver's ability to synthesize GLUCOSE, leading to low blood sugar (HYPOGLYCEMIA). Persistent overconsumption of ethanol can deplete the liver of vitamins and can lead to fatty liver and eventually to CIRRHOSIS.

Ethanol has several commercial uses; it is employed to extract herbal essences and is used in several patent medicines. Denatured alcohol is alcohol that has been rendered unfit for human consumption by the addition of a toxic substance; it is used commercially as a solvent. (See also ALCOHOLISM.)

ethylenediaminetetraacetic acid See EDTA.

ethyl formate A food additive used in artificial flavors including artificial LEMON and STRAWBERRY. Ethyl formate serves as a fungicide and as an agent to kill insect larvae in cereals and dried fruit.

etiology The cause of a disease or health condition. (See also EPIDEMIOLOGY.)

evaporated milk Concentrated milk, prepared from homogenized whole MILK through heating and evaporation. Each pint of evaporated milk is enriched with 400 IU of VITAMIN D. Upon dilution with water, evaporated milk provides the same food value and fat content as fresh milk. Evaporated skim milk is also available. Condensed milk is more concentrated than evaporated milk and is sweetened with sugar. (See also PASTEURIZATION.)

evening primrose oil The oil prepared from seeds of the evening primrose, which is used as a supplemental source of essential fatty acids. It contains 72 percent to 75 percent LINOLEIC ACID, an ESSENTIAL FATTY ACID; 9 percent GAMMA LINOLENIC ACID; and 9 percent OLEIC ACID, the nonessential fatty acid. The first metabolic conversion of linoleic acid to PROSTAGLANDINS, hormone-like fatty acid derivatives, is the transformation to gamma linolenic acid. This conversion is partially blocked by excessive saturated FATTY ACIDS, TRANS-FATTY ACIDS in processed vegetable oils, ALCOHOL, and zinc deficiency, and the process slows during diabetes and AGING. Dietary gamma linolenic acid can bypass this blocked step; furthermore it is metabolized to a type of prostaglandin (PGE_1) that inhibits the formation of pro-inflammatory prostaglandins, thus helping to reduce allergy symptoms and atopic ECZEMA in some cases. Both linoleic acid and gamma linolenic acid seem to have other diverse effects, including boosting the IMMUNE SYSTEM and reducing symptoms of premenstrual syndrome, lowering blood CHOLESTEROL, and slowing BLOOD CLOTTING. (See also ALLERGY, FOOD; ALPHA LINOLENIC ACID.)

exchange lists Food lists devised to help consumers plan nutritious, balanced meals. Exchange lists emphasize variety, freshness, fat, calorie control, and whole foods rather than processed foods. In the U.S. Exchange System, six groups categorize foods according to a similar content of CALORIES, CARBOHYDRATE, FAT, and PROTEIN: MILK; low-calorie VEGETABLES; FRUIT; grain products like BREAD and PASTA, plus starchy vegetables like lima beans and corn; a MEAT group including CHEESE and PEANUT butter; and fat, including oils.

This system simplifies the balancing of calories because each serving of a given food group has the same number of calories and the same amount of carbohydrates, protein, and fat, and interchanges within the group of foods are simplified. A further advantage is that fat content in foods is emphasized. For example, meats and cheeses are broken down into low-, medium-, and high-fat content foods. Meat items are given in terms of one-ounce portions, while a more typical portion size is three ounce or more. Exchange lists are available for diabetics, for those on weight-loss programs, and for individuals on salt-restricted, cholesterol-restricted, or fat-restricted diets. (See also BASIC FOOD GROUPS; DIABETES MELLITUS.)

excretion Processes by which the body eliminates waste products. Not only must the body take in nutrients, it must also rid itself of wastes. The body eliminates gaseous waste products (carbon dioxide, ACETONE) through the lungs, water-soluble wastes through the kidneys (urine), feces through the INTESTINE, and perspiration through the skin. Typical waste products include CARBON DIOXIDE and UREA, from the oxidation of foodstuffs, and also BILIRUBIN (from HEMOGLOBIN degradation) and URIC ACID (from DNA and RNA breakdown). The kidneys excrete urea, uric acid, creatinine, end products of HORMONE metabolism, in addition to processed drugs and ingested chemicals, for example, metal ions like ALUMINUM. Urea is the major nitrogen-containing waste product from protein degradation, while creatinine is a waste product of muscle. A variety of materials are absorbed but cannot be utilized by the body so they too are excreted in the urea. Several plant carbohydrates, sugar derivatives like mannitol, as well as the artificial sweeteners CYCLAMATE and SUCRULOSE are examples. Plant LIGNIN, a form of fiber that is neither digested nor absorbed by the COLON, is excreted in the feces.

Substances produced in the body in excessive amounts can be excreted in urine. Urinary excretion of KETONE BODIES during acute STARVATION, and GLUCOSE excretion during uncontrolled DIABETES MELLITUS, reflect excessively high blood levels of these substances. Overconsumption of substances such as water-soluble vitamins, VITAMIN C, and the B complex, beyond what the body can use or store, is also excreted. Alternatively, fat malabsorption or maldigestion can lead to the appearance of unusually large amounts of fat in feces. (See also ARTIFICIAL SWEETENER; CATABOLISM; DETOXICATION; FIBER.)

exercise Physical activity to maintain FITNESS or to strengthen the body. Regular aerobic physical exercise strengthens the oxygen delivery system (heart and lungs), increases endurance, and lowers the pulse rate, so the heart doesn't have to work as hard. Exercise assists in coping with emotional STRESS, and individuals who exercise are healthier and live longer than those who are sedentary. They maintain their body weight more easily. Active people tend to weigh less than sedentary people.

Moderate exercise, 30 minutes daily, promotes these beneficial effects: It increases, HIGH-DENSITY LIPOPROTEIN (HDL), the desirable form of cholesterol, insulin responsiveness to BLOOD SUGAR, bone strength, and antibody production. It lowers blood pressure and the risk of blood clots, CANCER, abdominal FAT, and cardiovascular disease. Sedentary people who start exercising might reduce their risk of dying from HEART DISEASE. Vigorous exercise strengthens the heart and blood vessels. Strenuous exercise (endurance events), however, can temporarily suppress the IMMUNE SYSTEM.

Regular exercise helps keep lost weight off after DIETING. Several factors are involved. Exercise increases muscle mass, and muscle burns calories more efficiently than fat tissue does. Examples of moderate exercises that burn 100 CALORIES include walking a mile, jogging a half-mile, swimming one-third of a mile, and cycling a quarter of a mile.

Calories are also burned more rapidly after exercising than not, although the duration and intensity of exercise needed to secure this benefit is an important question still being studied. If the individual is sedentary, moderate exercise seems to cause a 10 percent increase in basal metabolism for several hours. A moderately active individual may need to do aerobic exercise such as swimming, aerobic dancing, and jogging a total of six hours per week to increase the metabolic rate for several days afterward.

Exercise also seems to diminish the desire for fatty foods and increase the likelihood of eating CARBOHYDRATES, which contain fewer calories. Fat is a potential problem in the diet because the body more easily converts fat in food to body fat.

Carbohydrates are the best fuel during short, intense exercise such as sprinting, when muscles rely on GLUCOSE as fuel. During low to moderate intensity exercise, fat supplies about half the energy, while GLYCOGEN and blood SUGAR supply the rest. Fat is the major fuel during medium to intense exercise, when exercise lasts more than one to one and a half hours. Stored fat can supply as much as 70 percent of calorie needs for moderate exercise lasting four to six hours, especially when muscle glycogen stores are low. Afterward, PROTEIN supplies 5 percent to 15 percent of a person's energy needs.

APPETITE often stays the same with regular, moderate exercise (for example, 15 miles a week of jogging or walking). The appetite may increase to make up for the extra calories burned. Athletes burn more calories; while training for competition, the appetite of athletes increases because so many more calories are needed for strenuous physical activity.

Nutritional Needs During Exercise

Water Adequate water is essential for the body to use food and for the kidneys to dispose of waste. Perspiration controls body temperature. Drinking one to three cups of water or noncaffeinated beverage before exercise is recommended. Dehydration and overheating can be problems with prolonged exercise, especially during warm weather. Replacement of water losses may be needed before thirst is sensed, and adult athletes should drink 500 to 600 ml (16 to 20 oz.) of fluid during the two hours before exercise and up to 500 ml of fluid 10 to 15 minutes before an event.

Plain water or fruit juice is usually adequate; ELECTROLYTE replacement sports drinks are not necessary. During prolonged strenuous exercise, weakness due to low blood sugar can be remedied by drinking diluted carbohydrate beverages containing fruit sugar or glucose every 10 to 15 minutes, 150 to 250 ml (4 to 6 oz.). Fruit juices should be diluted to prevent delayed gastric emptying. Glucose-electrolyte sports drinks should contain between 6 percent to 10 percent carbohydrate for optimal uptake. Some contain maltodextran, short starch fragments that leave the stomach faster than plain sugar.

After an event, each pound of lost weight should be replaced with 500 ml (16 oz.) of fluid. Caffeinated and alcoholic beverages should be avoided. Alcohol and CAFFEINE act as diuretics, and dehydrate the body.

Protein The typical U.S. diet probably supplies up to twice as much protein as needed to maintain the body. However, it is important that the intake of calories be adequate. If calories are restricted, then protein needs will increase. For a sedentary adult, 0.8 g protein per kilogram of body weight per day is required to avoid deficiencies. Endurance athletes have increased protein requirements, estimated to be 1.5 g/kg/day. Athletes engaged in strength training may need as much as 2 g/kg/day. This protein requirement would be met by balanced diets providing 12 percent to 15 percent of their calories as protein. Loading up on protein powders or meat may promote calcium losses in female athletes. A high-protein diet tends to be high in SATURATED FAT, potentially harmful for the heart. A better approach is a diet with a mixture of carbohydrate, fat, and adequate protein.

Amino acids are a significant fuel source during endurance exercise, especially branched chain amino acids; and they have been used as supplements. However, single amino acids in large doses can cause amino acid imbalances, and the margins of safety are unknown. Large amounts of the amino acids ORNITHINE and ARGININE have been hypothesized to stimulate GROWTH HORMONE release and thus stimulate fat loss and protein buildup. However, reports on the anabolic effects of these amino acids remain inconclusive, and most available amino acid mixtures supply much lower doses of those amino acids than are found to be effective in some studies.

Carbohydrate During strenuous exercise (marathon running, for example), muscle glycogen becomes depleted; when this occurs, exhaustion sets in. For example, glycogen depletion can occur during exercise that requires near maximal bursts of effort (basketball, football, and soccer). Alternatively, glycogen depletion can occur gradually with repeated heavy workouts, in which glycogen breakdown exceeds its role of replacement. "Staleness" and FATIGUE can be due to overtraining and to inadequate carbohydrate consumption.

Complex Carbohydrate The typical American diet supplies only 46 percent carbohydrate, judged inadequate to meet increased energy needs of someone in training. Exercising for more than an hour per day increases the need for complex carbohydrates: whole GRAINS and CEREAL GRAINS, BREAD, VEGETABLES, LEGUMES, and FRUIT. Extra carbohydrate should supply 55 percent to 60 percent of calories. This means covering approximately two-thirds of a plate with carbohydrate foods at each meal. No more than 15 percent of calories should come from sugar. To prepare for strenuous exercise lasting more than an hour and a half by building up glycogen stores, a high carbohydrate diet (60 percent to 70 percent of daily calories) may be required for three days prior to the event together with a reduction in training. Carbohydrates eaten soon after strenuous exercise can refuel muscles with glycogen stores. Simple carbohydrates in juices and fruit will work best for the first few hours after a workout, followed by high complex carbohydrate meals.

Fat Fat is a significant source of energy during moderate exercise. Its utilization increases with duration. Although animal studies suggest that high-fat diets increase endurance, human studies have failed to reveal any advantage. There are many disadvantages to high-fat, low carbohydrate diets. They tend to raise blood cholesterol levels, which is linked to the increased risk of CARDIOVASCULAR DISEASE. They are hard to follow. High-fat diets increase the risk of OBESITY, because fat calories are more readily stored as body fat than carbohydrate. The National Research Council (U.S.) recommends that fats and oils should account for less than 30 percent of the calories for adults and saturated fat (animal fat, tropical vegetable oils) be limited to one-third of the total. Fatty foods should be avoided before exercise because they require three to four hours for digestion.

Supplements A BALANCED DIET supplying extra calories is adequate for increased needs due to exercise, although supplements can remedy nutrient deficiencies. Athletes on low-calorie diets to reduce body fat run the risk of malnutrition because they may not consume adequate VITAMIN E, VITAMIN D, or vitamins of the B COMPLEX like FOLIC ACID, CALCIUM, and IRON. Marginal VITAMIN C deficiency can impair performance. Iron intake for many women is marginal and exercising can worsen an iron deficiency, leading to ANEMIA.

There is no special set of recommended dietary allowances for vitamins and minerals for athletes. Some studies indicate an increased need for certain nutrients. Requirements for B complex and zinc may increase with exercise, and female gymnasts may be low in VITAMIN B_6, folic acid, calcium, iron, and zinc. Teenagers who are long-distance runners may be anemic because some blood is lost to the intestine through jarring. Eating mainly processed foods worsens the problem. POTASSIUM losses in perspiration are negligible, except under severe conditions, and are easily replaced by foods after a workout. Sodium replacement is also accomplished by the typical diet except for long, strenuous events and when the temperature is high or when additional electrolytes may be needed. However, salt pills can be dangerous because they can supply excessive SODIUM too rapidly. Sodium and electrolytes lost through sweating are easily made up with salt in food and by drinking diluted fruit juice. Recent studies indicate that vigorous physical exercise increases oxidative damage to the body due to the generation of free radicals and other reactive types of chemicals. The effects of moderate exercise are less clear. In any event, depletion of antioxidant defenses increases the body's vulnerability to oxidation, therefore, the consumption of sufficient antioxidants is important. Ample vitamin C, vitamin E, trace minerals such as zinc, copper, selenium, and manganese, and sulfur-containing amino acids are keys to maintaining antioxidant defenses. Whether people who exercise at moderate intensity need extra antioxidants is controversial. Endurance training has been shown to deplete vitamin E in subjects consuming a normal diet.

Clearly vitamin and mineral deficiencies will impair performance. Vitamin C, vitamin E, and B vitamins will not increase energy production or utilization by the body unless there is a deficiency. Vitamins and mineral supplements cannot be used to "patch up" a faulty diet—one based on fatty, fried, or convenience foods.

Meals Before Competition A light meal (300 to 800 calories) two to four hours before running may be recommended. The meal should be served in a comfortable setting; it should be easily digested and low in fat and protein. Eating during the hour before competition and consuming excessive sugar before exercise could stimulate insulin production, possibly leading to lower blood sugar (HYPOGLYCEMIA) during the event and hindering performance. Symptoms of hypoglycemia include feeling light-headed and shaky, blurred vision, and fatigue. Foods and beverages with simple sugar sweeteners such as SOFT DRINKS, candy, and fruit juices, should be avoided within an hour of exercising.

(See also CARBOHYDRATE METABOLISM; FAT METABOLISM; GLYCOGEN LOADING.)

Clarkson, Pricilla M. "Antioxidants and Physical Performance," *Critical Reviews in Food Science and Nutrition* 35, nos. 1, 2 (1995): 131–141.

Katzel, Leslie I. et al. "Effects of Weight Loss vs Aerobic Exercise Training on Risk Factors for Coronary Disease in Healthy, Obese, Middle-aged and Older Men—A Randomized Controlled Trial," *Journal of the American Medical Association* 274, no. 24 (December 27, 1995): 1,915–1,921.

exotic fruits and vegetables The public demand for these foods has increased dramatically in recent years. As many people have tried to adopt more healthy eating habits, they have begun eating more fruits and vegetables. Americans also have become more aware of other cuisines because of the growing diversity of the American population, together with increased business and leisure travel to countries such as Korea, Vietnam, and India.

Many of these exotic foods are imported, but some domestic producers are beginning to locally grow varieties. A few of the more prevalent exotic fruits and vegetables appearing in American supermarkets include:

Bok Choy Also called Chinese mustard, this member of the CRUCIFEROUS VEGETABLES family has long white stalks with oblong or oval dark green leaves. Bok choy is similar to celery in flavor but is less stringy and can be substituted for that vegetable in any dish. It is high in vitamins C and A.

Chayote Also known as the "vegetable pear" because of its shape, this relative of summer squash tastes similar to zucchini but has a slightly tangy flavor. It is a good source of vitamin C.

Chinese Cabbage Also called napa cabbage, this member of the cruciferous family has long, pale-green, crinkly leaves. It has a delicate cabbage flavor and is a good source of vitamins A and C.

Cilantro Also known as Chinese parsley, this herb has a uniquely pungent flavor that is used often in Hispanic cooking. The seeds are a spice called coriander.

Enoki Mushrooms These small-capped, fragile white mushrooms with long stems are often used in Japanese cooking. They are crunchy, have a mild sweet flavor, and can be used to flavor cooked foods (often soups) or served raw in salads.

Jicama Also called the Mexican potato, this member of the legume family has radish-shaped roots that usually weigh between two and five pounds when sold for consumption. The tuber flesh is crisp and sweet when eaten raw. When cooked it resembles the potato. One cup, raw, offers 45 percent of the RECOMMENDED DAILY ALLOWANCE (RDA) of vitamin C and 4 percent of the RDA of iron.

Kohlrabi A member of the turnip family with a stem that is usually white and purple and can be eaten like a turnip, but is juicier and has a milder, sweeter flavor. The dark green leaves that grow from the stem are cooked like KALE or COLLARD greens. They are rich in vitamin C.

Mango A popular fruit around the world, mangoes are grown domestically in Florida. The sweet, juicy fruit can best be compared to a tangy peach. The mango has a large, flat pit. To serve, the fruit should be sliced lengthwise close to the pit. Then each half should be scored in a cross-hatch pattern before folding the edges back until the center pops up. Mangoes are a good source of vitamins A and C.

Papaya These tropical fruits vary in size but are most often sold in sizes that range between one and three pounds. Papaya has a light-green rubbery skin that gives slightly to pressure when the fruit is ripe. The flesh is juicy, sweet, and has a delicate flavor. The center cavity contains several small black seeds; these are edible but are usually scooped out before serving. Papaya is an excellent source of vitamin C.

Shiitake Mushroom A large medium-brown mushroom with firm flesh and a meaty flavor. It can be eaten raw but is more often served grilled or sautéed.

Star Fruit Grown domestically in Florida, this pale-green fruit is shaped like a football, with deeply scored ridges. When sliced cross-wise, the fruit resembles a five-pointed star. Its flavor is a cross between plum, pineapple, and lemon. It is a good source of vitamin C.

extracellular fluid Fluid that lies outside of the cells of the body. The human body is 60 percent WATER, by weight. Water is indispensable because it forms a major constituent of every tissue and every cell and is the medium for nearly all functions and chemical transformations. Water in the body distributes itself in two general compartments. Water within cells is considered INTRACELLULAR FLUID, which represents 60 percent of the body's water content. Extracellular fluid includes fluids between cells and tissues and in the circulatory systems. Less than 20 percent occurs in blood and lymph systems. (See also BODY FLUIDS; CYTOPLASM; DEHYDRATION.)

F

FAD See FLAVIN ADENINE DINUCLEOTIDE.

fad diets Drastic weight-reduction programs. Fad diets are potentially dangerous because they employ one or more of the following flawed strategies:

Severely Restricting Calories

With less than 1,000 CALORIES a day the body adapts to semistarvation by burning its fat and muscle, regardless of whether or not a little PROTEIN or CARBOHYDRATE is consumed. This adaptation raises the possibility of excessive water loss and excessive buildup of acidic products of fat metabolism (KETOSIS). Water loss disrupts fluid and ELECTROLYTE balance, which can harm the heart. The harmful aspects of severe caloric restriction are worsened by the use of laxatives, DIURETICS, or induced vomiting, which can cause electrolyte imbalance and flush water out of the body. The resulting weight loss represents water loss, not fat loss.

Consuming No Carbohydrates

Without dietary carbohydrate, the body switches into a CATABOLIC STATE in which stored fat is oxidized and KETONE BODIES (metabolic acids) accumulate, a situation called ketosis. As excessive ketone bodies are excreted in the urine, extensive water losses promote DEHYDRATION, while the loss of sodium causes electrolyte imbalance. The brain requires GLUCOSE for ENERGY, and when carbohydrate is not supplied by the diet, BLOOD SUGAR must be synthesized from AMINO ACIDS, derived from muscle protein breakdown.

Eating Just One Kind of Food for a Long Time

Unless the diet supplies adequate amounts of protein and carbohydrate, body chemistry switches over to fat and muscle breakdown. No single food or supplement supplies all the required nutrients in the appropriate ratios needed to maintain health.

Using Appetite Suppressants

This class of compounds includes benzocaine, BULKING AGENTS, and PHENYLPROPANOLAMINE, a commonly used APPETITE SUPPRESSANT in diet pills. Benzocaine numbs the taste buds without bringing about a long-term change in eating behavior, while phenylpropanolamine causes only a temporary appetite reduction and may raise blood pressure. (See also AMPHETAMINES; ATKINS DIET; DIET, LOW CARBOHYDRATE; DIET, VERY LOW CALORIE; DIETING: CRASH PROGRAMS; FASTING; GLUCONEOGENESIS.)

familial hypercholesterolemia An inherited tendency to have high CHOLESTEROL levels, which greatly increases the risk of coronary heart disease. About 1 in 500 people carry a defective gene causing a two- to threefold increase in serum cholesterol from birth. Individuals who possess the defective gene in both sets of chromosomes are much more severely affected. Their cholesterol may be five to six times normal, and they may have heart attacks by the age of 20 due to clogged arteries (ATHEROSCLEROSIS). Therefore, a family history of premature coronary heart disease greatly increases a person's risk.

One form of hypercholesterolemia is characterized by the inability of tissues to remove LOW-DENSITY LIPOPROTEIN cholesterol (LDL) from circulation. LDL transports cholesterol to the various tissues of the body where it must bind to specific docking sites on cell surfaces. As a result, LDL cannot be effectively taken up by cells. Recent investigations have revealed that this condition is often the result of mutations of the gene for the LDL receptor.

Patients with familial hypercholesterolemia are likely to be placed on low-cholesterol diets and to be given medications in order to lower their cholesterol levels. (See also CHOLESTEROL-LOWERING DRUGS; HYPERLIPOPROTEINEMIA.)

FAO See FOOD AND AGRICULTURAL ORGANIZATION.

fast food Meals that are mass-produced and often sold by franchised restaurant chains. Typical offerings include fried CHICKEN, chicken nuggets, pizzas, fried FISH, roast BEEF, HOT DOGS, HAMBURGERS, FRENCH FRIES, nachos, tacos, chili, pasta salads, and doughnuts. There are more than 215,000 fast-food restaurants in the United States, where it is often possible to order a meal and eat it within 10 to 15 minutes.

Nearly one out of every four Americans eats fast food every day, and more than half of the money spent on meals away from home goes for fast food. The immense popularity of fast foods rests on convenience, dependable quality, and moderate expense. Two-income households have less time for home chores, including cooking, and they have more money to spend. Busy schedules for each member of the family place a premium on time spent in planning, preparing, and eating a meal. Fast food is also appealing to travelers and commuters. The fast-food industry has expanded overseas sales as well as branching out into hospitals, airports, colleges, and airline in-flight meal service.

Fast-food chains have responded to nutrition awareness of consumers, so that many now offer salad bars, low-fat roast beef, low-calorie salad dressing, corn on the cob, and baked potatoes. Several chains reduced the CALORIES and FAT in their hamburgers. It is now often possible to obtain a "heart healthy" meal with less salt, less SATURATED FAT, and more vegetables and fresh fruit than before. Several restaurant chains provide nutritional information about calories, fat, and SODIUM content, as well as additives such as SULFITES, MONOSODIUM GLUTAMATE (MSG), and LACTOSE. Nutritional information has not yet found its way to labels on fast-food products, however.

With prudent selection from a fast-food menu, most healthy people can eat fast foods occasionally without compromising their health. The health costs of relying on fast foods, however, are high.

Overnutrition Many fast-food items contain excessive fat (especially saturated fat), SUGAR, salt, and calories. Fast food supplies 20 percent of the fat in American diets and much of it is saturated. A single meal can easily supply all the calories and sodium needed for an entire day.

Although fish, chicken, and POTATOES alone are relatively low-calorie foods, they become high-fat, high-calorie foods when dipped in batter and fried. In addition, chicken skin, which is essentially fat, is added to chicken nuggets. If the fat used in cooking is BEEF TALLOW, fried foods—regardless of their source—are also high in CHOLESTEROL and in saturated fat, believed to promote clogged arteries. Several fast-food chains have switched to soybean oil or to saturated vegetable oils to avoid the potential problems and negative image of animal fat. Pasta salads are usually high in fat because of added dressings, cheese, or processed meat toppings. A typical 3/4-cup serving can provide fat equal to the amount in a fast-food cheeseburger (nearly four teaspoons).

Undernutrition Many menu options that are high in sugar and fat calories are often low in critical nutrients. These include FIBER, vitamins (like VITAMIN A, VITAMIN C, VITAMIN E, and FOLIC ACID), and minerals (like chromium, manganese, magnesium, ZINC, and IRON). There is a growing appreciation of the importance of the nonnutrient constituents in plant foods called phytochemicals, which seem to protect against chronic diseases associated with aging, such as cancer. Between 10 percent and 20 percent of the U.S. population consumes the minimum recommended five servings of fruits and vegetables daily.

Poor Digestion Eating a meal in 10 minutes may not provide enough time for adequate digestion. Adequate chewing is a signal to start the digestive juices flowing, and minimal chewing means less efficient breakdown and assimilation.

To cut down on fat while still enjoying fast foods:

1. Eat less fried food.
2. Peel off the batter coating of fried fish or chicken, which retains the fat.

3. Select the salad bar but cut back on salad dressing, pasta salad, bacon bits, and potato salad. These contain extra fat. Add flavor with low-fat COTTAGE CHEESE, pepper, spices, or KETCHUP.
4. Substitute a baked potato for french fries, which retain much of the fat and oil they were fried in.
5. Omit sour cream, CHEESE, and BUTTER (all high in saturated fat) on salads and baked dishes.
6. Select roast beef instead of hamburger. A lean roast beef sandwich plus a salad without heavy dressing or a seafood salad provides a balanced meal.
7. Eat less butterfat. Croissants, sweet rolls, milk shakes, and ice cream are all sources of saturated fat.

(See also ADVERTISING; ATHEROSCLEROSIS; BALANCED DIET; CONVENIENCE FOOD; EATING PATTERNS; FAT; MALNUTRITION; OBESITY.)

Schlosser, Eric. *Fast Food Nation*. Boston: Houghton Mifflin, 2001.

fasting Choosing not to eat. Fasting for a day with adequate water is generally safe for healthy adults. Children are more susceptible to problems associated with fasting because their energy reserves of GLYCOGEN and FAT are smaller; prolonged fasting causes major metabolic changes that can eventually be harmful.

On the first day of fasting, carbohydrate stored in the liver (glycogen) is broken down to supply blood GLUCOSE. During the first week, body fat begins to be broken down to meet the energy requirements of the body. Muscle protein breakdown yields AMINO ACIDS, which the liver converts to BLOOD SUGAR (GLUCONEOGENESIS) to fuel the brain. With prolonged fasting, the body's metabolic rate slows in order to conserve energy and fuels are used more efficiently. With excessive fat breakdown, KETONE BODIES (water-soluble acids derived from fatty acids) can accumulate in the blood. They acidify the blood and cause excessive urination, which, in turn, causes DEHYDRATION and loss of ELECTROLYTES. Severe imbalance of ions in the blood can lead to heart failure.

Three commonly stated reasons for fasting include:

- Weight loss. Fasting is not a recommended weight loss strategy. Fasting causes considerable weight loss initially (up to 5 pounds per week), but this represents extensive water loss, not fat loss. Such lost weight will be regained rapidly upon return to the usual DIET. Studies show that during fasts, muscle is lost, as well as fat, and lost muscle may be rapidly replaced by fat at the end of the fast.
- Detoxification (a procedure for the removal of toxins). As body fat is consumed, materials trapped or stored in fatty tissue may be released. Weakened cells in tissues are selectively destroyed by the immune system. The buildup of toxic materials released into the bloodstream can create an additional metabolic burden and oxidative stress for the liver, which is responsible for disposing of toxic materials.
- An altered state of consciousness. During fasting, individuals sometimes experience a greater clarity of mind, and fasting has traditionally accompanied forms of meditation.

Precautions regarding fasting:

1. No one should fast more than a day or so without medical supervision.
2. Pregnant or lactating women, children, adolescents whose bodies are growing, and diabetics should not fast.
3. It is important to drink plenty of liquids; the production of metabolic wastes continues at a high rate during fasting. A juice fast is safer than drinking water alone because the carbohydrate, vitamins, and electrolytes of fruit juices help maintain body functions more adequately, and the carbohydrate they contain is needed to fuel the brain.
4. To end a fast, patients should resume eating food with several small meals rather than with one large one. Fatty foods should be added back slowly because fat is harder to digest than carbohydrates and protein.
5. During fasting, the production of ketone bodies in the urine can be monitored by using a "dip stick" available at drug stores. The presence of ketone bodies in urine indicates a state of KETOSIS, excessive fat breakdown.

(See also ACIDOSIS; DIET, VERY LOW CALORIE; DIETING: CRASH PROGRAMS.)

fasting blood sugar The blood glucose level that is maintained between meals. Normally, BLOOD SUGAR is maintained at a concentration between 60 and 100 mg per deciliter. An elevated fasting blood sugar level can indicate a diabetic or prediabetic condition. Adequate blood sugar is maintained by the liver, which breaks down GLYCOGEN, a starch-like carbohydrate synthesized from glucose after a meal. Maintenance of blood sugar is controlled by hormones. GLUCAGON and GLUCOCORTICOIDS help raise blood sugar levels by directing the liver to synthesize glucose from AMINO ACIDS released from muscle and INSULIN stimulates glucose uptake after a meal. (See also GLUCONEOGENESIS; GLUCOSE TOLERANCE TEST.)

fat (triglyceride, triacylglycerol) An oily nutrient that is the most concentrated form of ENERGY, supplying 9 calories per gram, more than twice as much energy as in CARBOHYDRATE or protein. Fat is one of the most abundant nutrients in foods, and it is a major fuel for the body. Dietary fat supplies about 36 percent of total calories in the standard American diet. Fat serves two other functions: It carries flavors in foods and helps fat-rich foods create a feeling of satiety (feeling full) by slowing the rate of stomach emptying.

Fat is classified as a LIPID because it dissolves in organic solvents like hexane rather than in water. Although often considered a "fat," cholesterol is a very different compound, although they are both insoluble in water and thus are both lipids. Fat functions as an energy reserve; it is usually broken down to carbon dioxide to supply energy, while cholesterol is converted only to steroid hormones and BILE salts. From a dietary perspective, a low-cholesterol diet also lowers saturated fat intake because both fat and cholesterol occur in meat.

Fats and oils contain three FATTY ACIDS bonded to GLYCEROL (glycerin) like streamers hung from a flagpole. During digestion, fat is broken down by the enzyme pancreatic lipase and is released into the intestine. Fat can also be broken down in the test tube by a process called saponification in which fats and oils react with alkali to produce soaps.

Fats are classified as saturated or unsaturated, according to their fatty acid compositions. Saturated fat is solid at room temperature; examples are LARD and HYDROGENATED VEGETABLE OIL (VEGETABLE SHORTENING). Saturated fat contains relatively high levels of saturated fatty acids (40 percent for lard, to 50 percent for BEEF TALLOW, to 62 percent for butterfat). If a fat contains less than one-third saturated fatty acids, it is considered unsaturated.

Oils contain more unsaturated fatty acids, or they contain smaller than usual saturated fatty acids (medium-chain fatty acids). Examples of the oils with higher amounts of unsaturates are vegetable oils (corn, safflower, soybean, sunflower, olive oils) and FISH OIL. Examples of saturated-fat oils are PALM OIL and palm kernel oil. Several unsaturated oils contain relatively high levels of unsaturated fatty acids (89 percent for sunflower oil, 91 percent for safflower oil, 86 percent for olive oil and 87 percent for corn oil).

Fat calories in food are not the same as carbohydrate calories because the body converts dietary fat to body fat much more efficiently than it converts carbohydrate to fat. That is, 23 percent of the calories in starches and sugars are consumed in converting them to fat, while only 3 percent of the calories in dietary fat are expended in converting it to stored fat.

Many authorities recommend fat intake of less than 30 calories daily. As an example, for a woman eating 1,600 calories daily, the limit for fat would be 44 g (3 tablespoons). For a man eating 2,400 calories per day, the limit would be 67 g of fat. To help visualize this, five tablespoons of any vegetable oil or three-quarters of a stick of butter equals 70 g of fat. (See also DIETING; DIET RECORD; FAT, TISSUE; OBESITY.)

fat, hidden The invisible FAT in foods. Visible fat is readily identified and measured, in such foods as butter, margarine, lard, and cooking oils. The U.S. Department of Agriculture's Center for Nutrition Policy and Promotion estimated that Americans lowered the percent of caloric intake from total fat between 1965 (45 percent of calories) to 1995 (34 percent of calories). However, that decrease in percent of calories from fat is a result of increased total caloric intake, not decreased fat consumption. In fact, the average daily fat consumption in grams increased from 1990 to 1995 by an overall average of 15 percent. In 1990 the average for adult men was 89 g, and in 1995 it was 101 g. For women the average in 1990 was 64 g, and in 1995 it was 65 g. Despite documented cutbacks on obvious fat sources like fatty red meat, butter, and whole milk, the average consumption of fat in prepared foods and other high-fat foods significantly increased.

Fats and oils are found in most cheeses and spreads; in salad dressing; corn, potato, and wheat CHIPS; cookies, muffins, pastries, and CRACKERS; fried FISH and fried CHICKEN; FRENCH FRIES; GRANOLA; and whipped cream substitute. Nondairy coffee whitener often has more SATURATED FAT than butter because it contains coconut oil. HAMBURGER legally can contain up to 30 percent fat. CHEESE and dairy products are high-fat foods. Hidden fat can supply 60 percent to 75 percent of their calories; BEEF and PORK have much more fat than chicken or fish. However, when fish and chicken are breaded and deep-fat fried, their calorie content increases dramatically due to hidden fat. Processed meats such as HOT DOGS, SAUSAGE, BOLOGNA, and luncheon meats are generally extremely fatty.

Food labels can help sort out high-fat foods. The U.S. FDA has instituted wide-ranging changes in food labels, including listing the number of fat calories. Governmental dietary guidelines recommend that fat calories not exceed 30 percent of the total calories.

Claims such as "98 percent fat-free" on a food label have been misleading, and such claims are not permitted under the revision of food labels. "Fat free" means the food contains less than 0.5 g fat per serving. "Low fat" means the food contains 3 g or less per serving, while "reduced fat" or "less fat" indicate the food contains at least 25 percent less fat per serving than the reference food. (See also CONVENIENCE FOOD; EMPTY CALORIES.)

fat and chronic disease There is a general consensus that excessive fat consumption is a contributing factor in OBESITY, CANCER, and HEART DISEASE. The prevailing medical opinion is that Americans eat too many fatty foods. Excessive fat consumption has been singled out as the number one dietary problem in the United States; average fat consumption is 130 pounds a year per person, which includes animal fat, VEGETABLE OIL, SHORTENING, MARGARINE, and partially HYDROGENATED VEGETABLE OILS. This consumption is about twice as much fat and oil as is considered healthy by some experts. The DIETARY GUIDELINES FOR AMERICANS (U.S.) recommend cutting back on fat by at least 25 percent, so that total fat accounts for no more than 30 percent of daily calories for adults.

Fat contributes to obesity in part because it is easier to gain weight from eating excess fat than it is from eating excess CARBOHYDRATE. The body's metabolism is not efficient in converting sugar to fat; about a quarter of the calories in sugar are lost in the conversion. On the other hand, only 3 percent of the calories in consumed fat is expended in converting dietary fat to body fat. A high-fat diet promotes water loss and electrolyte imbalance and may increase uric acid levels and increase the risk of gout. It also increases the risk of kidney dysfunction.

Cancer

A high-fat intake is one of the strongest risk factors for CANCER, after cigarette smoking. For example, lung cancer risk increases with diets high in saturated fat. High-fat diets decrease the ability of the IMMUNE SYSTEM to destroy cancer cells, and eating less animal fat and vegetable oil lowers the risk of colon, prostate, and, possibly, breast cancer.

Overconsumption of fat increases the risk of heart disease in American populations. A diet with too much animal fat tends to raise blood CHOLESTEROL. On the other hand, polyunsaturated vegetable oils help lower blood cholesterol levels, believed to decrease the risk of heart disease. FISH and FISH OIL also seem to protect against heart disease. A special ingredient of fish oil, OMEGA-3 FATTY ACIDS, balances the immune system, and decreases inflammation. Fish and fish oils slow down blood clotting, lower serum fat, and perhaps cholesterol levels, and may reduce the risk of heart attacks. People who are generally angry or anxious have higher cholesterol levels; they degrade fat more slowly than others. Consequently, slow fat breakdown may be one of the risk factors in heart attacks.

A very-low-fat diet, with 10 percent of calories from fat, was incorporated into a program to reduce the risks in people with heart disease. The program included exercise, stress reduction, counseling, and support groups. Men who changed their lifestyle managed to reverse clogged arteries and to keep off lost weight for four to eight years.

Recommendations to Reduce Fat Calories

- Eating less fat by eating fewer servings and smaller portions. Being realistic about expectations rather than totally eliminating favorite fatty foods. Dairy products like BUTTER and sour cream and plant-derived fat, like COCONUT OIL, palm and PALM kernel oil, shortening, margarine, and CHOCOLATE, are sources of saturated fat. Vegetable oils such as SAFFLOWER oil, CORN OIL, SOYBEAN oil, and mayonnaise represent unsaturated fat. Substituting low-calorie margarine and low-calorie mayonnaise. Using spices, vinegar, or lemon juice rather than oily salad dressing.
- Reducing consumption of fat in MEAT by trimming off visible fat or by using only lean meat ("select" or good quality beef). Eating fewer hot dogs, hamburgers, and sausage. Draining fat after browning meat. Removing skin from chicken and turkey. Broiling, baking, poaching, or steaming food rather than eating fried foods.
- Chilling soups and discarding coagulated fat. Cooking vegetables in water and herbs instead of sauteing them in butter. Eating tuna packed in water, not oil. Baking fish with lemon juice instead of butter.
- Avoid pastry and rich desserts like ice cream.
- Using skim milk, nonfat yogurt, and lowfat cottage cheese rather than products derived from whole milk. Avoiding adding sour cream and cheese toppings to baked potatoes.

(See also ATHEROSCLEROSIS; BODY MASS INDEX; DIETING; EATING PATTERNS.)

fat digestion The breakdown of fat to its building blocks: FATTY ACIDS and the polyalcohol GLYCEROL. Fat DIGESTION is primarily an intestinal process requiring LIPASES, fat-splitting enzymes secreted by the pancreas. The pancreatic protein colipase assists in this process.

After digestion, fat follows a complex route through the body. BILE released from the gallbladder provides bile salts needed to absorb fatty acids into the intestine, where they are reassembled into fat, then packaged as CHYLOMICRONS, a lipid-protein complex that transports dietary fat first through the lymphatic system, then through the bloodstream.

Fat in chylomicrons is degraded by a special lipase in capillaries to fatty acids, which are absorbed by muscle to be oxidized for energy and by adipose tissue to be stored as fat.

In contrast to usual dietary fats and oils, a fat containing medium-chain fatty acids (MEDIUM-CHAIN TRIGLYCERIDES) is used therapeutically with compromised digestion and maldigestion syndromes, because it passes directly into the bloodstream without chylomicron formation and is delivered to the liver, where it can be used immediately. (See also DIGESTIVE ENZYMES; DIGESTIVE TRACT.)

fat fold test (skin fold test) A convenient method of estimating body FAT. This test relies on a measurement of the width of a fold of skin on the back of the upper arm or other part of the body. Skin fold measurements, together with measurements of waist and hip circumference, have been used to estimate bone growth and changes in muscle mass during weight loss or weight gain. A caliper that applies a fixed pressure is used to measure skin fold thickness. A fat fold of more than an inch wide reflects OBESITY. The fat at the back of the arm or from the upper back is roughly proportional to total body fat. When fat is gained, or lost, the fat fold increases and decreases proportionately. The test requires an experienced assessor for reliable results.

The distribution of fat is important in considering the risk of CARDIOVASCULAR DISEASE because abdominal fat, not hip fat, is correlated with an increased risk. Abdominal fat seems to be more easily metabolized by the liver and converted to LOW-DENSITY LIPOPROTEIN (LDL), the undesirable form of CHOLESTEROL. (See also BODY MASS INDEX; HEIGHT/WEIGHT TABLES; LEAN BODY MASS.)

fatigue Feelings of persistent tiredness and lethargy, unrelieved by rest. This is a multifaceted condition and may be the result of MALNUTRITION, fluctuations in BLOOD SUGAR levels, and allergic reactions. Glandular imbalances, depression, cancer, infections, autoimmune diseases, diabetes, heart disease, AIDS, parasites, chronic pain, drugs, and liver disease can also cause fatigue. Deficiencies of most VITAMINS, MINERALS, CARBOHYDRATE, and PROTEIN promote fatigue as do conditions that affect the delivery of oxygen to tissues. These include ANEMIA, emphysema, and other respiratory problems. Fatigue is also a symptom of HYPOTHYROIDISM, which lowers basal metabolism and contributes to the sluggishness of many functions, including muscular activity. The overproduction of CORTISOL, a steroid hormone produced by the ADRENAL GLANDS, can be the result of adaptation to chronic stress and can cause fatigue. Inadequate cortisol production contributes to low blood sugar (HYPOGLYCEMIA), which leads to fatigue. (See also CHRONIC FATIGUE; STRESS.)

fat metabolism (post-digestion) Reactions in the body encompassing the synthesis of FATTY ACIDS and FAT, as well as fat degradation and fatty acid oxidation. Fat stored in the body (ADIPOSE TISSUE) is constantly synthesized and constantly broken down. When the number of calories consumed exceeds the energy needs of the body, the surplus fuel is converted to fat for energy storage. Consumption of an excess of ALCOHOL, CARBOHYDRATE, PROTEIN, or fat can therefore lead to weight gain. Alternatively, when fewer calories are consumed than needed for extended periods, stored fat is gradually depleted as it is needed for energy production.

Fat (Triglyceride) Synthesis

Fat synthesis occurs after a high-carbohydrate meal. Fat is made mainly in the liver and fat cells (adipose tissue) in response to the hormone INSULIN, but not in muscle. The liver and adipose tissue convert GLUCOSE, the simple sugar with six carbon atoms, into acetic acid, which contains only two carbon atoms and represents the raw material for fat synthesis.

In the next phase, eight molecules of activated acetic acid are chained together to create a long saturated fatty acid with 16 carbon atoms known as PALMITIC ACID. The enzyme system that performs this complex conversion is called fatty acid synthetase. The B vitamins BIOTIN and NIACIN are required to synthesize fatty acids. In the final step of fat synthesis, three fatty acids are attached to GLYCEROL, a three-carbon fragment of glucose, to form a fat molecule known as a triglyceride.

Palmitic acid can be lengthened to produce STEARIC ACID, a common saturated fatty acid containing 18 carbon atoms. The body can also make simple monounsaturated fatty acids such as OLEIC ACID, which is deficient in two hydrogen atoms and possesses one double bond from saturated fatty acids.

To summarize, neither palmitic acid, nor stearic acid, nor oleic acid are dietary essentials. On the other hand, the body cannot create most fatty acids with multiple double bonds, such as the ESSENTIAL FATTY ACIDS, LINOLEIC ACID, and ALPHA LINOLENIC ACID.

Fat synthesized by the liver is transported in the bloodstream as a water-soluble carrier particle called VERY-LOW-DENSITY LIPOPROTEIN (VDL), which delivers newly formed fat molecules to fat cells where it can be stored.

Fat Degradation

When too few calories are consumed to meet the body's energy needs, the body breaks down stored fat, its primary stored fuel. The hormone EPINEPHRINE activates an enzyme in fat cells called LIPASE, which cleaves stored fat molecules to free fatty acids; these enter the bloodstream and are carried to tissues.

Tissues rapidly absorb circulating fatty acids, which last only a few minutes before being absorbed. Muscle cells oxidize this fuel to produce ATP to meet their energy needs. In contrast, glucose is the major fuel for the brain, because fatty acids do not cross the BLOOD-BRAIN BARRIER.

To be oxidized, fatty acids are first transported into MITOCHONDRIA, the cell's energy-producing factory, using a carrier molecule called CARNITINE. Carnitine may be an essential nutrient for elderly people and patients with heart disease. In mitochondria, fatty acids are completely burned to carbon dioxide for energy by the KREB'S CYCLE, the central energy-producing mechanism of mitochondria. Fatty acid oxidation requires enzyme helpers from three B vitamins: PANTOTHENIC ACID, niacin, and RIBOFLAVIN. Mitochondria trap energy as ATP. The amount of ATP from the oxidation of fatty acids is more than double the amount from glucose oxidation. This reflects for the fact that fat provides more than twice as many calories per gram as carbohydrates. (See also ELECTRON TRANSPORT CHAIN; METABOLISM; RESPIRATION, CELLULAR.)

fat replacer See FAT SUBSTITUTE.

fat substitute A FOOD ADDITIVE that partially replaces FATS and oils in processed foods. Fat substitutes are classified as protein-, carbohydrate-, or lipid-based. Their presence tricks the mouth into sensing flaky, tender baked goods or creamy foods without the presence of fat and its associated calories. Carbohydrate- and protein-based fat substitutes break down at high temperature and cannot be cooked.

Among carbohydrate fat replacers are the following:

- DEXTRINS and maltodextrins. These STARCH fragments prepared from WHEAT, TAPIOCA, POTATO, CORN, or OAT flour, are used in salad dressing, puddings, frozen desserts, dairy products, margarine, spreads, and fillings.
- Modified food starch. Chemically treated starch is prepared from corn, potato, wheat, rice, or tapioca and used in processed meat, salad dressing, frosting, and frozen desserts.
- Microcrystalline CELLULOSE. This highly purified form of cellulose is prepared from wood pulp and ground into tiny particles. It is used in dairy products, sauces, and frozen desserts.
- GUMS. Plant gums, including xantham gum, guar gum, locust bean gum, and carrageenan, are used in reduced calorie and fat-free salad dressing and processed meats.
- Fruit fiber. Fiber from apples, figs and prunes is used in baked goods.

Fat substitutes can also be classified in terms of their digestibility. Digestible fat substitutes yield calories, while nondigested fat substitutes do not. An example of a digestible fat substitute is SIMPLESSE, approved in 1990 by the U.S. FDA as the first synthetic fat substitute for the U.S. market. This product is derived from EGG white and milk PROTEIN by a process of blending and heating. Simplesse is digested and used by the body as protein. Simplesse cannot be used in cooking because frying or baking causes it to lose its creamy consistency. It may appear more frequently in products like frozen desserts, MAYONNAISE, salad dressing, and cheese spreads.

SUCROSE POLYESTER (Olestra) is an example of an indigestible fat substitute that does not yield calories. Its structure resembles fat, except that it has a molecule of sugar at its core instead of glycerol and has eight attached fatty acids instead of three. It has a new structure that cannot be digested and has been the center of controversy. Despite considerable controversy, sucrose polyester has been approved by the FDA as a food additive. Long-term animal studies suggest that it might cause liver problems and could interfere with the absorption of fat-soluble vitamins; other studies indicate it is safe. It is being marketed with supplemental fat soluble vitamins, in potato chips and snack foods. However, the FDA has received more than 18,000 adverse reaction reports related to olestra—more than the FDA has received for all other food additives in history combined. Products containing olestra are required to carry a label warning that it may cause abdominal cramping and diarrhea. As a result of these reports, in 2000 Health Canada rejected olestra for use as a food additive in Canada.

Oatrim is made from oat flour and contains soluble fiber. It was developed by the USDA in 1993 and is being used in cheeses, ground beef, cookies, and muffins. Other products are being developed. Oatrim supplies 1 calorie per gram, in contrast with fat, which supplies 9 calories per gram. Like any other high-fiber food, it can cause gas and bloating.

Modification of the structure of the fat molecule has yielded another family of digestible fat replacers. These products employ short-chain fatty acids, like acetic acid and propionic acid, which provide fewer calories than the usual fatty acids found in fats. These modified triglycerides provide 5 calories per gram.

Whether fat substitutes will help people eat less fat is unknown. By analogy to ARTIFICIAL SWEETENERS, fat substitutes may contribute to a false sense of security, leading consumers to eat additional amounts of high-calorie foods. Artificial sweeteners do not help people change their diets significantly. Even if Simplesse were incorporated into all foods for which FDA approval was sought, it would reduce fat intake by at most 14 percent, assuming no further change in the diet. Many low-fat foods contain sugar, while sugar-free foods may contain fat. The reason is that it is difficult to take both sugar and fat out of a food and have it taste good. In the final analysis, no fat substitute or other food additive can replace wise food choices and regular exercise for weight control.

fat, tissue Fat found in ADIPOSE TISSUE, which is the only tissue specialized to store fat, the major fuel of the body. Body fat also insulates the body against changes in cold and serves as a shock absorber for sensitive organs like the kidneys. Stored fat comes from two different sources. It can be made from carbohydrate or ethanol or even from an excess protein, carbohydrate meal, or it can come from excessive dietary fat.

Body fat accumulates during early childhood and adolescence, when the number of fat cells increases. At other times, fat is deposited in preexisting fat cells when caloric intake exceeds calories spent. For example, METABOLISM slows and people tend to EXERCISE less, while continuing to eat high-calorie food as they get older. This accounts for the weight gain often seen at middle age.

Body fat can be burned up when the diet does not provide adequate calories. In response to stress, ADRENAL GLANDS secrete EPINEPHRINE, which signals fat cells to break down their stored fat to fatty acids, which are released into the bloodstream, absorbed by muscle, and oxidized for energy production. Women have greater levels of enzymes for storing fat and lesser amounts of enzymes to degrade fat than men do. This may help to partially explain why some women have greater difficulty in dieting and maintaining body weight than men do. Chronically hostile and anxious people may burn fat more slowly than less upset and more emotionally balanced people who do not suppress anger.

A person's optimal amount of body fat depends on many factors, including inheritance, body build, sex, and age. Women's average body fat is about 20 percent to 25 percent of their body weight, while men's weight is typically 15 percent to 20 percent fat. Women usually have more fat than men because fat is important in pregnancy and lactation. Athletes who train vigorously (like marathon runners) have less fat. Fat may be 7 percent of a male athlete's body weight and 10 percent of a female athlete's weight. The distribution of excessive body fat is linked to HEART DISEASE. Fat around the middle (abdominal obesity) is a greater risk for heart disease than fat accumulated around hips and thighs (the "pear" profile).

(See also CELLULITE; FAT DIGESTION; FAT METABOLISM; LIPOSUCTION; SET POINT; STRESS.)

fatty acids A class of organic acids (CARBOXYLIC ACIDS) containing short, medium, or long chains of carbon atoms. Fatty acids are the major constituent of fat and represent the major energy source of the body. When oxidized for fuel, fatty acids yield 9 calories per gram, more than twice as much energy as from sugar.

Short-Chain Fatty Acids

Short-chain fatty acids contain two, three, and four carbon atoms; they are, respectively, ACETIC ACID, PROPIONIC ACID, and BUTYRIC ACID. These acids are products of microbial digestion of fiber in the gut and are a significant energy source, especially for intestinal epithelial cells. The oxidation of protein, fat, and carbohydrate for energy production yields acetic acid, attached to a carrier called COENZYME A, which plays a central role in energy production.

Medium-Chain Fatty Acids

Medium-chain fatty acids are saturated fatty acids containing five to 12 carbon atoms. An example is CAPRYLIC ACID, with eight carbons. Medium-chain fatty acids are commonly bound to GLYCEROL to form medium-chain triglycerides. Commercially, medium-chain triglycerides are prepared primarily from coconut and palm oils. They have long been used in intravenous formulations for patients who do not absorb fat efficiently. Medium-chain triglycerides are digested by pancreatic lipase to free acids in the intestine and are transported in the blood and rapidly absorbed by tissues for energy production. Medium-chain fatty acids do not require special transport mechanisms, unlike usual fats.

Long-Chain Fatty Acids

Long-chain fatty acids are common building blocks of fats and oils and therefore are the major fat components in a typical diet. Long-chain fatty acids may be either saturated or unsaturated. Saturated fatty acids are filled up with hydrogen atoms; PALMITIC ACID (16 carbon atoms) and STEARIC ACID (18 carbon atoms) are the most abundant saturated fatty acids in the body.

Unsaturated fatty acids lack pairs of hydrogen atoms and contain one or more double bonds, and this difference sets them apart from saturated fatty acids. Those with a single double bond (monounsaturates) are represented by palmitoleic acid (16 carbon atoms) and OLEIC ACID (18 carbon atoms), which is the most common. Polyunsaturates contain two or more double bonds. Because the typical unsaturated fatty acids possess a bent shape, they do not pack together easily to form solids at room temperature and therefore tend to be liquids. Fats high in unsaturated fatty acids are oils. Saturated fatty acids lack built-in kinks and they tend to stack together in parallel, like cords of wood, and they solidify easily. Therefore, fat containing mainly saturated fatty acids is solid at room temperature.

Two types of polyunsaturated fatty acids must be supplied in the diet because the body cannot fabricate them: LINOLEIC ACID and ALPHA LINOLENIC ACID. Certain details like the position of the double bonds are important distinctions for these fatty acids because the body is very selective in how they are used.

Both linoeic acid and alpha linolenic acid possess 18 carbon atoms: The former possesses two double bonds, while the latter possesses three double bonds. Linoleic acid belongs to the omega-6 family of polyunsaturates, with double bonds beginning at the sixth carbon atom from the end of the fatty acid; while alpha linolenic acid belongs to the omega-3 class, with double bonds beginning at the third carbon atom from the end of the fatty acid. Omega-3 fatty acids and omega-6 fatty acids cannot be converted one to another. In general, the ESSENTIAL FATTY ACIDS can be converted to more complex fatty acids and hormone-like substances such as PROSTAGLANDINS, compounds that can stimulate or inhibit many physiologic processes, and LEUKOTRIENES, very powerful inflammatory agents.

Omega-6 Fatty Acids

The smallest member of the omega-6 family is linoleic acid, an essential fatty acid. Linoleic acid is converted to more complex omega-6 fatty acids, including GAMMA-LINOLENIC ACID, which can give rise to the PGE_1 series of prostaglandins that help counterbalance inflammatory processes and return the body to normal. The conversion to gamma-linolenic acid is hampered in cases of zinc deficiency, ALCOHOLISM, or diabetes. Human milk contains a high level of gamma-linolenic acid, suggesting an important role in growth and development.

Linoleic acid is also converted to the largest member of the omega-6 family, ARACHIDONIC ACID, which yields the PGE_2 series of prostaglandins, the 2 series of thromboxanes (TXA_2) and leukotrienes that increase physiological responses to stress. The PGE_2 prostaglandins increase inflammation, especially involving joints and skin; produce pain and fever; increase blood pressure; and induce blood clotting.

Deficiency symptoms of linoleic acid include DEPRESSION, irritability, rough skin, ECZEMA, ACNE, psoriasis, dandruff, hair loss, slow wound healing, ANEMIA, blurred vision, and lowered immunity. Deficiencies have been linked to an increased risk of multiple sclerosis, HYPERTENSION, some forms of CANCER, and HEART DISEASE.

Dietary omega-6 fatty acids have long been known to reduce serum CHOLESTEROL and thus may lower the risk of ATHEROSCLEROSIS. Chronic low intake correlates with an increased risk of heart attack among Americans. The general conclusion is that a modest increase in dietary omega-6 fatty acids can help protect against cardiovascular disease. Consequently, dietary strategies to lower cholesterol have often specified lowering the intake of saturated fatty acids while increasing the intake of omega-6 unsaturated fatty acids. Although such diets can lower LOW-DENSITY LIPOPROTEIN (LDL), the undesirable form of cholesterol, they also lower HIGH-DENSITY LIPOPROTEIN (HDL), which protects against coronary heart disease.

In the United States, linoleic intake ranges from 5 percent to 10 percent of calories. The U.S. National Research Council recommends a maximum 10 percent of calories as omega-6 fatty acids. Common sources of linoleic acid include vegetable oils like SOYBEAN oil, sunflower, and SAFFLOWER

(safflower oil is the richest source). A tablespoon of polyunsaturated vegetable oil daily meets the daily requirement. EVENING PRIMROSE OIL and BLACKCURRANT OIL are common supplemental sources of gamma linolenic acid.

All polyunsaturated fatty acids are susceptible to oxidation. Oxidized fatty acids contain lipid peroxides, which can generate free radicals, can damage cells, and can cause cancer. Therefore, increased consumption of polyunsaturates increases the need for VITAMIN E as an ANTIOXIDANT.

Omega-3 Fatty Acids

The smallest member of the omega-3 fatty acids is alpha linolenic acid, an essential fatty acid that is the building block for all other longer chain omega-3 fatty acids. It occurs in certain plants, pumpkin seeds, and walnuts. FLAXSEED OIL and FISH OIL are used as supplemental sources. This fatty acid also occurs in phytoplankton, which are consumed by coldwater ocean fish. They convert alpha linolenic acid to larger members of the omega-3 family, EICOSAPENTAENOIC ACID (EPA), 20 carbon atoms, 5 double bonds (20:5), and DOCOSAHEXAENOIC ACID (DHA), 22 carbon atoms, 6 double bonds (22:6), which are found in highest concentrations in fish and fish oil.

A growing body of evidence indicates that a diet enriched in omega-3 fatty acids conveys significant health and mental health benefits, though this area is controversial. They may decrease inflammation common to degenerative diseases like rheumatoid arthritis. At the molecular level, the body converts omega-3 fatty acids to families of regulatory substances including prostaglandin (PGI_3), thromboxane (TXA_3), and leukotrienes, which counterbalance products of omega-6 fatty acids that promote platelet aggregation, blood clotting, and inflammation. EPA is a source of prostacyclin PGI_3, a substance that decreases blood platelet clumping, an important step in blood clot formation (thrombogenesis). In addition, omega-3 fatty acids can block the formation of substances that trigger inflammation.

Fish and fish oils that are enriched in EPA and DHA seem to lower the risk of heart attack by lowering blood cholesterol, if the initial levels are high. They generally lower the level of blood fat and VERY LOW-DENSITY LIPOPROTEIN (VLDL), which transports fat in the blood. The mechanism seems to involve blocking the synthesis of VLDL and LDL, the undesirable forms of serum cholesterol.

A deficiency of the omega-3 fatty acids is associated with retarded growth, retarded retinal development in infants, and abnormal brain development in experimental animals. Furthermore, anyone whose diet relies on highly processed foods might be deficient in omega-3 fatty acids. The omega-3 fatty acids in general, and alpha linolenic acid specifically, are deficient in the standard American diet. There is little or none in fast foods, including fried fish, fried chicken, or hamburgers. Processing removes or destroys omega-3 fatty acids because they are susceptible to rancidity and shorten the shelf life of processed foods. Furthermore, the high levels of omega-6 fatty acids in conventional American diets, which emphasize meat, block the production of EPA from alpha linolenic acid.

Optimal levels of alpha linolenic acid in the diet are unknown, although recommended daily intakes range from 1 percent to 2.5 percent of daily calories. The recommendation of the American Heart Association is to eat several servings of fish weekly. The optimal ratio of omega-6 to omega-3 fatty acids is not known. In the traditional Japanese diet, the ratio is 4:1; in the American diet, the ratio is more like 10:1 and may be too high. With increased consumption of polyunsaturated fatty acids, there is an increased need for fat-soluble antioxidants like VITAMIN E.

Fish oil and flaxseed oil are very susceptible to rancidity and are often packaged with vitamin E as an antioxidant. To minimize their oxidation, fish oil supplements as well as any unsaturated oils should be refrigerated in capped containers. Flax oil and other highly unsaturated oil should not be used for cooking because they are too easily oxidized when heated.

fatty liver A deposition of FAT in LIVER tissue. Normally, lipids are transported out of the liver. With a massive breakdown of fat during STARVATION, DIABETES MELLITUS, crash DIETING, and chronic ALCOHOLISM, the fat tissue releases free fatty acids into the bloodstream. They enter liver cells and are converted back to triglycerides, leading to lipid deposits in the liver. Decreased fatty acid oxidation by the liver during alcoholism further adds to fat accumulation in the liver.

Chemical poisons such as carbon tetrachloride, alcoholism, and protein malnutrition, slow the liver's ability to export fat and increase fat accumulation. Over time, accumulated fatty deposits impair liver function. Eventually, if liver cells die and are replaced by scar tissue leading to irreversible damage, the result is liver scarring. (See also CIRRHOSIS; FAT METABOLISM.)

favism A condition that causes the rupture of red blood cells. Favism occurs in genetically susceptible individuals when they eat seeds or inhale pollen of *Vicia faba,* the BROAD BEAN (fava bean). The disease occurs in Mediterranean and Middle Eastern countries and in western China. Children are more susceptible to favism than adults.

The acute stage associated with fever, abdominal pain, headache, ANEMIA (and in severe cases, coma) lasts 24 to 48 hours and symptoms usually diminish. Favism is linked to a deficiency of an enzyme that supports the antioxidant system required to maintain the structure in red blood cell membranes (glucose-6-phosphate dehydrogenase). Enzyme deficiencies make red blood cells more susceptible to damage by external agents. (See also FOOD SENSITIVITY.)

FDA (U.S. Food and Drug Administration) A federal agency founded in 1972 that is responsible for enforcing the Federal Food, Drug, and Cosmetic Act, together with its amendments, the Fair Packaging and Labeling Act, and sections of the Public Health Service Act. The FDA inspects, tests, approves, and sets standards for most foods, including imported foods, drugs, and cosmetic products like lipstick, perfume, shampoo, deodorant, and toothpaste. Similarly, the FDA approves and monitors medical devices such as thermometers, sunlamps, artificial body parts, and drug testing kits. The FDA approves and monitors prescription drugs, as well as labels for over-the-counter drugs. The FDA assures the efficiency and long-term effects of drugs such as heart medications, vaccines, over-the-counter medications, AIDS drugs, CANCER drugs, breast implants, and drugs that treat baldness and skin conditions. (MEAT, POULTRY, and EGGS are regulated by the U.S. Department of Agriculture (USDA).)

The FDA is responsible for verifying the contents of drugs, foods, and supplements. With regard to foods, the FDA regulates food handling to assure sanitary, safe foods, free of harmful chemical contaminants and spoilage. Low levels of additives and pesticide residues that may cause cancer are permitted, provided the risks are negligible, according to the Food Quality Protection Act of 1996, which supersedes the DELANEY CLAUSE of the amended Food, Drug, and Cosmetic Act. The FDA monitors pesticide residues in foods, including illegal drug use in livestock and chemicals released from food packaging. If pesticide or chemical residues are too high, the FDA can order a crop destroyed. The FDA monitors more than 2,800 FOOD ADDITIVES currently approved for foods. It regulates new food additives and reviews additives already in use. The FDA also regulates interstate food shipment.

The FDA is concerned with new food products and nutritional claims. It also sets and maintains standards for safe and adequate food labeling. In 1990, Congress passed the Nutrition Labeling and Education Act, which gave the FDA the responsibility of creating a national FOOD LABELING standard. The FDA issued its proposals in 1991; they became law in 1993. (See also FOOD LABELING.)

FD&C-approved food colors Synthetic color additives approved for food and beverages. The abbreviation stands for Food, Drug, and Cosmetics to designate intended use. Ninety percent of all dyes are synthetic and employ FD&C designations such as "FD&C No. 1," "FD&C No. 2" and so on. (See also ARTIFICIAL FOOD COLORS; FOOD ADDITIVES.)

fed state Refers to changes in energy production and physiologic processes in response to a meal. The fed state favors the synthesis of protein, fat, and glycogen, a chain of GLUCOSE molecules that serves as an energy storage mechanism. In contrast, fat degradation, fatty acid oxidation, and glycogen breakdown are blocked after a meal.

A complex series of events unfolds at the end of a meal. After eating carbohydrate, digestion produces glucose, which is absorbed by the small intestine into the bloodstream. BLOOD SUGAR rises more or less rapidly, then gradually declines to the fasting level maintained between meals. The hormone INSULIN dominates the body's response to an increased blood sugar. This hormone is released by the pancreas in response to elevated blood sugar and promotes glucose uptake by most tissues, thus lowering blood sugar levels. Muscle converts surplus glucose to glycogen, the liver forms glycogen and fat, and adipose tissue forms fat. In addition, insulin stimulates muscle to take up circulating amino acids, particularly BRANCHED CHAIN AMINO ACIDS (LEUCINE, ISOLEUCINE, and VALINE) for protein synthesis.

After eating a fatty meat, digested fat is absorbed by the intestine and packaged as CHYLOMICRONS, water-soluble fat carriers that distribute fat to tissues via the bloodstream. The short-term rise in serum fat level after a meal is termed "postprandial hyperlipidemia." Dietary fatty acids released from fat in chylomicrons are taken up by many tissues and burned for energy. Adipose tissue also absorbs and reincorporates fatty acids into fat for storage. (See also ANABOLISM; CATABOLIC STATE.)

feedback inhibition A common control mechanism in the regulation of biochemical reactions of the body and/or a mechanism for maintaining processes within normal limits (HOMEOSTASIS). Feedback inhibition can refer to a way of regulating a system of enzymes that operate to create a final product (metabolic pathways) or it can refer to hormonal regulation. In a metabolic pathway, very often the first unique step is catalyzed by a "bottleneck" enzyme, which regulates the rate at which material flows through the pathway.

In feedback inhibition of a metabolic pathway, the buildup of the final product of that pathway shuts down the bottleneck or regulating enzyme. When the product is consumed, inhibition is released and more product can be synthesized by the pathway. This type of regulation is quite common. As an example, HEME, the iron pigment of hemoglobin in red blood cells, is an end product of a system of enzymes devoted to its synthesis. If levels of heme build up due to overproduction or a slowdown in consumption, heme inhibits the key enzyme regulating heme synthesis. As another example, an excess of ATP, the cell's energy currency, blocks GLYCOLYSIS, the pathway that degrades GLUCOSE to produce energy.

Feedback is a common occurrence in the regulation of endocrine glands that secrete certain hormones that stimulate other glands to release hormones. As an example, the anterior pituitary secretes thyroid-stimulating hormone (TSH), which in turn stimulates THYROXINE (thyroid hormone) production by the thyroid gland. When the blood levels of thyroxine build up to an optimum level, the anterior pituitary senses this level and stops secreting TSH. Consequently, the thyroid stops producing excess thyroxine and the blood level falls. (See also CATABOLISM; ENDOCRINE SYSTEM.)

Feingold diet A diet based on the studies of Benjamin Feingold, M.D., a pediatric allergist who in 1973 proposed treating HYPERACTIVITY and learning disorders with diet modifications instead of medications. He evolved a diet that eliminates foods containing synthetic colors and flavors, as well as the antioxidant preservatives BHA and BHT. It also eliminates foods, beverages, and medications containing salicylates, which are compounds related to ASPIRIN. Naturally occurring salicylates are found in ALMONDS, APPLES, APRICOTS, berries, CLOVES, COFFEE, NECTARINES, ORANGES, PEACHES, PLUMS, TANGERINES, TEAS, TOMATOES, and oil of wintergreen.

The Feingold diet is a controversial plan. Parents who use it successfully for hyperactive children stoutly defend it, although a panel of experts of the U.S. National Institutes of Health concluded there aren't enough clinical studies to grant official approval. While the Feingold diet has been effective in some cases, it is very restrictive for children. Eating away from home while maintaining this diet is difficult; common foods like luncheon meats, sweets, and even nonfood items like toothpaste, are artificially colored and flavored. As with any diet modification program, there must be a supportive home environment for a permanent dietary change to occur in children. (See also ARTIFICIAL FLAVORS; ARTIFICIAL FOOD COLORS; FOOD ADDITIVES.)

Stubberfield T. G., and T. S. Parry. "Utilization of Alternative Therapies in Attention Deficit Hyperactivity Disorder," *Journal of Pediatrics and Child Health* 35 (1999): 450–453.

fennel (*Foeniculum vulgare*) An aromatic vegetable belonging to the parsley family that is native to Mediterranean regions. Common fennel is a perennial with characteristic bright-green feathery leaves and stalks resembling celery. Its flavor is similar to anise, though less pronounced. Fennel leaves and bulbs are used for seasonings, soups, stews, and salads, wile fennel seed is a spice in cooking, candy, and certain liqueurs. Fennel oil extracted from seeds is used in perfumes, soaps, and several medications.

fen-phen See DIET PILLS.

fermentation The microbial degradation of CARBOHYDRATE, particularly simple SUGARS. Characteristics of the fermentation depend upon the nature of the carbohydrate, the type of microorganism, and conditions such as degree of acidity and the amount of available oxygen. BACTERIA, MOLDS, and YEASTS commonly carry out fermentations by degrading sugars without the direct participation of air or oxygen (anaerobically).

Alcoholic Fermentation Under anaerobic conditions, specific strains of yeast ferment sugar (GLUCOSE) to alcohol in the preparation of alcoholic beverages. In WINE making, yeast ferments the sugar in GRAPE juices. Alcohol can be prepared by the fermentation of other FRUIT juice. Ale and BEER are the product of fermentation of sugar from starch in malted grains. In this case, partly sprouted grains produce enzymes that release sugars from starch. In VINEGAR manufacture (acetic acid fermentation), the alcohol in wine and beer is further oxidized by microbial fermentation to ACETIC ACID.

Lactic Acid Fermentation Lactic acid-producing bacteria (lactobacillus strains) ferment LACTOSE in MILK to sour milk. In cheese production, the enzyme RENNET is used to clot milk, and the resulting curdled milk protein is fermented with bacteria or mold strains to ripen cheese. YOGURT is milk that has been boiled and then inoculated with lactic acid-producing bacteria.

The many other fermented foods include the dough in leavened baked goods containing yeast enzymes; SAUSAGE; fermented vegetables such as SAUERKRAUT, BORSCH, and kimchi. Far Eastern fermented foods are prepared from SOYBEANS, RICE, LEGUMES, and FISH. Other types of fermentations produce critic acid from glucose (citric acid fermentation) and oxalic acid from glucose (oxalic fermentation).

COLON bacteria ferment undigested carbohydrates in dried beans, lactose (due to LACTOSE INTOLERANCE), and FIBER. Excessive fermentation can cause FLATULENCE or DIARRHEA. Normally, much of dietary fiber is fermented anaerobically to produce short-chain fatty acids: ACETIC ACID, PROPIONIC ACID, and BUTYRIC ACID. These fatty acids are absorbed and are the preferred fuel of cells lining the colon. (See also ACIDOPHILUS.)

ferritin An iron storage PROTEIN in tissues that represents the major form of stored iron in the body. Ferritin accounts for 20 percent of the total iron in adults. Ferritin functions both in iron absorption and iron recycling. APOFERRITIN, the protein portion of ferritin, is formed by intestinal mucosa, LIVER, spleen, and bone marrow. These tissues combine apoferritin with inorganic iron (ferric phosphate and ferric hydroxide) obtained from iron carried in the blood by the serum protein TRANSFERRIN. Iron released from ferritin can be transported to other tissues via the bloodstream.

During early stages of iron deficiency, a decreased serum ferritin level is the first sign of decreased iron stores. On the other hand, many conditions elevate serum ferritin: inflammation, cancer, infections, and liver disease. Iron overload disease, HEMOCHROMATOSIS, a potentially damaging condition, is associated with iron buildup in tissues. (See also ANEMIA.)

ferrous gluconate Iron salt of gluconic acid, an acidic derivative of glucose. Ferrous gluconate is used to darken OLIVES to a uniform black color. As a nutritional supplement, it is a readily absorbable form of ferrous IRON. (See also CHELATE; VITAMIN.)

fetal alcohol syndrome (FAS) A congenital condition in children whose mothers drank ALCOHOL during their pregnancy. One in 300 to 500 babies are born with FAS. It is characterized by mental retardation; facial deformities, particularly of the upper lip and eyelids; hyperactivity; low birth weight; and heart problems. Some children may be permanently brain damaged, and the average IQ of adults with fetal alcohol syndrome is 68. While the dosage of alcohol that can damage the fetus is unclear, even moderate alcohol consumption during pregnancy can affect the newborn, and the American College of Obstetricians and Gynecologists recommends abstaining from alcohol completely during pregnancy.

FAS can have long-term effects as well. Mental deficiencies and emotional problems make it difficult for adults with FAS to adapt to normal living, and there is an increased need for society to prevent the dysfunction, chronic mental illness, and homelessness so frequently observed in older patients with this disorder. (See also BIRTH DEFECTS.)

fiber Undigested plant residues that represent the outer coating or plant wall material of VEGETABLES, GRAINS, seeds and FRUITS. Fiber is considered essential to maintain a healthy digestive tract. A low-fiber diet has been associated with CONSTIPATION, colon CANCER, spastic colon, HIATUS HERNIA, varicose veins, hemorrhoids, HEART DISEASE, HYPERTENSION, GALLSTONES, diabetes, OBESITY, COLITIS, and CROHN'S DISEASE.

Fiber can help curb appetite because the stomach feels full. Fiber-rich foods require longer chewing, which stimulates digestive juices and helps digestion. Fiber displaces fat calories and slows fat digestion and absorption by binding bile salts and, therefore, it may help control OBESITY.

Fiber also helps fight heart disease. In a study of more than 40,000 U.S. middle-aged men, researchers have found that heart attacks were 41 percent less common among men who consumed at least 28 g fiber daily compared with men who ate less than 13 g daily as typical of the usual U.S. diet. It is estimated that fiber-deprived men reduced their risk of heart attack by 20 percent to 44 percent for each 10 g of additional fiber, without lowering their fat intake. The largest reduction was among men who ate wheat bran, which represents mainly insoluble fiber.

Recent studies have confirmed that a high-fiber diet does not reduce risk of colon cancer because it seems to have no effect on the growth of precancerous colon polyps. In one study researchers at the National Cancer Institute (NCI) put one group of people on a high-fiber diet and told another group to simply eat what they usually eat. All the participants had had at least one precancerous polyp removed from their colon in the six months before the study. Four years later the researchers found that the risk of developing another polyp was the same in both groups.

In the other study researchers at the Arizona Cancer Center asked one group of people to eat half an ounce of wheat fiber daily and gave another group a tenth of an ounce. Again, three years later the risk of developing a precancerous polyp was the same in both groups. Bacterial degradation of dietary fiber releases organic acids, such as butyrate and acetate, which promote a healthy colon. A high intake of whole grains, vegetables and fruits, and derived fiber seems to reduce the risk of cancers of the upper digestive tract and ovarian cancer. In women, increased fiber intake is associated with a reduced risk of cardiovascular disease and heart attacks, according to 2002 research.

It is estimated that Americans consume only one-third to one-half the optimal amount of fiber daily. The National Cancer Institute recommends doubling or tripling fiber intake from 12 g to 20 to 35 g per day. At this level, there is minimal interference with nutrient ABSORPTION, while assuring normal maintenance of intestinal function. However, there is as yet no formal RECOMMENDED DIETARY ALLOWANCE for fiber because the exact amount required for health has not been established.

"Dietary fiber" refers to the fiber content in plant foods that resists digestion by enzymes of the GASTROINTESTINAL TRACT, and dietary fiber is the usual designation for fiber content in foods. Lab methods for measuring dietary fiber are more gentle than those for crude fiber, which measure only material that resists strong acid treatment. Values for dietary fiber can be up to four times higher than for crude fiber contents.

Food labels are required to list the amount of dietary fiber as a percentage of daily value, based upon the needs of a 2,000 calories per day diet.

Listing the amount of soluble and insoluble fiber is voluntary.

Major Types of Fiber

Fiber consists of a mixture of very different nonstarch complex carbohydrate and noncarbohydrate materials. The major classes of dietary fiber are cellulose, HEMICELLULOSES, PECTIN, mucilage, GUMS, algal materials, and LIGNIN.

- Cellulose is a linear chain of glucose units.
- Hemicelluloses are highly branched structures found in plant cell walls. They are a diverse group with varying sugar compositions, including the simple sugars MANNOSE, GLUCOSE, GALACTOSE, xylose, arabinose, and an acid derived from glucose called glucouronic acid. Some hemicelluloses are water-soluble.
- Pectins function as a glue that holds plant tissues together, and they contain an acidic sugar derived from galactose, galacturonic acid, in the primary chains, with side chains or branches containing less common sugars: arabinose, fucose, and xylose.
- Gums are plant secretions and contain acidic sugars.
- Algal polysaccharides are products of edible seaweed.
- Lignin is a noncarbohydrate insoluble material and a principal structural material of wood.

Insoluble Fiber

It is convenient to break down fibers according to whether they are insoluble or water-soluble. Insoluble fiber includes CELLULOSE and lignin. This type of fiber swells in water, increases stool weight and stool frequency, and helps prevent constipation, colonic inflammation (DIVERTICULITIS) and hemorrhoids, by softening stools and speeding up the movement of waste through the intestine. Cellulose is not digested, although colon bacteria break down 40 percent to 80 percent of cellulose. Lignin is not degraded and passes through the digestive tract unchanged. Lignin softens stools, increases regularity and may lower blood cholesterol.

Bran is the most common source of insoluble fiber, derived from the outer husk of kernels of WHEAT and other CEREAL GRAINS. It contains cellulose and other cell wall materials and slows the rise in blood sugar after a meal. Bran can protect against heart disease in middle-aged men; oatmeal is also effective, though more may need to be consumed to get the same effect as wheat bran.

Soluble Fiber

This type of plant fiber swells in water and forms glue-like gels. Soluble fiber is made up of noncellulose carbohydrates, including pectins, gums, algal polysaccharides and some types of hemicellulose. Soluble fiber has important physiologic effects. It becomes viscous, thus softening stools and slowing the rate of stomach emptying. Soluble fiber also slows starch digestion and glucose uptake, in turn lowering the amount of insulin needed to process blood glucose after a meal, and it may help diabetics. Eating oat BRAN (2 oz.) regularly each day may effectively lower blood sugar levels. Despite the popularity of oat bran as a source of water-soluble fiber, it provides both water-soluble and insoluble fibers.

The water-soluble fibers are completely degraded by intestinal microorganisms to SHORT-CHAIN FATTY ACIDS, which are used as fuels to help maintain the intestinal lining.

Soluble fiber also seems to lower blood CHOLESTEROL. Regular consumption of oat bran and legumes may lower blood cholesterol. Fiber binds bile salts in the intestine, which could reduce their resorption, thus forcing the LIVER to remove more cholesterol from the blood to make more bile. Pectin, guar gum, and locust bean gum have been reported as effective in this regard. Because it believes that long-term health benefits are not yet proven, the U.S. FDA does not permit health claims linking fiber consumption with the prevention of either heart disease or certain types of cancer.

Good sources of fiber include dried BEANS, LENTILS, lima beans, pinto beans, SWEET POTATOES, BROCCOLI, BRUSSELS SPROUTS, SPINACH, ALMONDS, CORN, wheat, oat bran, and fruit (blackberries, pears, apples). In general, the less processed a food is, the more fiber it has. Therefore, eating whole, minimally processed foods assures a mixture of soluble fiber and insoluble fiber; both kinds are needed for health.

Sources of insoluble fiber include skins of vegetables and fruits, whole grains (not white flour), high-fiber cereals, dried beans, broccoli, and bulgur wheat. Bran is a common and inexpensive source of insoluble fiber. Cold bran cereals have more insoluble fiber than hot cereals. Bran is lost in preparing white flour and it is not replenished by ENRICHMENT.

Good sources of soluble fiber are fruits, cooked dried beans, CHICKPEAS, BARLEY, LENTILS, navy beans, vegetables such as SQUASH and CARROTS, plus barley, oat, and rice bran. GUAR GUM, GLUCOMANNAN, and pectin are common soluble fiber supplements. Fructo oligo saccharides are also considered to be a form of fiber.

When increasing fiber consumption, the recommendation is to begin gradually because excessive fiber intake causes bloating, gas, cramps, nausea, and DIARRHEA. A month may be required to adapt to a high-fiber diet. Initial steps can be eating whole fruit instead of juices; popcorn instead of potato chips; whole WHEAT instead of white BREAD; and a baked potato with its skin instead of mashed potatoes. Patients should consult a physician when planning to take fiber supplements if they have a serious digestive disease, or if they plan a daily consumption over 35 g of fiber. Following the FOOD GUIDE PYRAMID, which specifies eating six to 11 servings of grain-based foods and two to four servings of fruits and three to five servings of vegetables daily, will satisfy the recommended fiber intake.

Fiber Supplements

Supplements are a popular way of increasing dietary fiber intake, although the National Cancer Institute recommends increasing fiber intake through whole, fiber-rich foods. Fiber supplements often contain bran, guar gum, pectin, or PSYLLIUM. Since they swell in water and help create a feeling of being full, fiber supplements have been used in weight-reduction programs to control APPETITE. It is not clear that they help with permanent weight loss, however. Fiber from psyllium seeds is the primary ingredient of several popular brands of nonchemical LAXATIVES.

Patients with serious intestinal disorders such as DIVERTICULITIS, ulcerative colitis, or Crohn's disease should avoid taking fiber supplements without medical supervision. Patients should consult a physician before consuming more than 35 g of fiber supplements a day; high levels of fiber can block the uptake of IRON, CALCIUM, ZINC, COPPER, and other minerals and cause calcium losses. Patients should also avoid fiber supplements that contain APPETITE SUPPRESSANTS like phenylpropanolamine, which can cause side effects.

DIETARY FIBER CONTENT OF SELECTED FOODS

	dietary fiber	grams
cereals		
wheat bran	(1 oz.)	8.4
shredded wheat	(" ")	2.6
oat meal	(" ")	0.5
grains		
wheat germ	(3 tbsp.)	3.9
barley	(1/2 cup)	3.0
corn	(" ")	2.9–3.9
whole wheat bread	(slice)	1.5–2
white enriched bread	(slice)	0.5
oat bran	(1/3 cup)	4.0
vegetables		
brussels sprouts	(1/2 cup)	2.3
cauliflower	(")	1.1
chickpeas	(")	8.0
kidney beans	(")	8.0
lettuce	(")	0.3
potato	(")	2.5
sweet potato	(")	4.0
fruit		
apple	(1)	2.8
orange	(1)	3.0
prune	(1)	1.0
raspberries	(1/2 cup)	4.6
strawberries	(1/2 cup)	1.7
banana	(1)	2.2
figs (dried)	(3)	4.6

Ornish, D. et al. "High Fiber Diet and Colorectal Adenomas," *New England Journal of Medicine* 343 (September 7, 2001): 736–738.

fibrin An insoluble, fibrous protein that forms a gel-like blood clot to seal openings in blood vessel walls. Fibrin is produced from its precursor in the blood, fibrinogen, by the enzyme THROMBIN, one of a series of coagulation factors that are protein-degrading enzymes. BLOOD CLOTTING is a VITAMIN K-dependent process because the vitamin is required in the processing of thrombin. Therefore, a vitamin K deficiency can increase the tendency to bleed (hemorrhage). Individuals with disorders that prevent fat absorption may experience uncontrolled bleeding because vitamin K uptake is inadequate to produce enough thrombin. Calcium is also required for thrombin activation. In the final step of the clotting pathway, thrombin produces fibrin, a fibrous protein that forms insoluble clumps at a site of injury. Cell fragments called blood platelets embed themselves in the fibrin clot to complete the blood clotting process. Once a clot is formed, it plugs the ruptured area of the vessel, preventing hemorrhaging. Fibrin threads gradually retract because platelets pull on them. This helps close the hole in the vessel by pulling the edges of the wound closer together.

fibrocystic disease See BREAST CYSTS.

fibromyalgia syndrome A condition characterized by widespread aching pain with tenderness on both sides of the body. The prevalence of fibromyalgia is about 4 percent for adults after the age of 60, and it occurs more frequently in women than in men.

Common complaints include persistent pain in the neck, shoulders, low back, and hips; morning stiffness; fatigue; and fitful sleep patterns. There may also be numbness in hands and feet, headaches and intolerance to heat or cold. At a cellular level, energy production may be sub-par.

Patients with fibromyalgia syndrome may have food allergies and sensitivities to toxins and chemicals in the environment. One common denominator is LEAKY GUT, in which inflammation makes the intestine more permeable to materials that should normally be excluded, such as incompletely digested food proteins and bacterial breakdown products. A leaky gut can result from the destruction of beneficial intestinal bacteria during prolonged use of antibiotics or nonsteroidal anti-inflammatory agents. Patients with fibromyalgia may be helped by avoiding materials to which they are sensitive, for example, household chemicals (such as cleansers) and food allergens. Supplementation with nutrients that support antioxidant defenses and energy production—including minerals (ZINC, SELENIUM, MAGNESIUM, MANGANESE), and enzyme helpers (COENZYME Q, VITAMIN C, and the B complex vitamins)—may help. Patients may also benefit from an individualized plan that includes exercise, physical therapy and manipulation, and dietary options to meet all of their nutritional needs. (See also FATIGUE; STRESS.)

fibrous proteins Highly elongated, water-insoluble PROTEIN that helps protect and support the body. Fibrous proteins form static, insoluble rigid rods (hair) or sheets (skin, connective tissue), which are stabilized by crosslinks between protein segments. In contrast, proteins such as ENZYMES and ANTIBODIES are dynamic: They attach to other molecules for biological function and, generally, they are globular in shape and water-soluble. Extended arrays of fibrous proteins form the structure of skin, tendon, bone, and connective tissue, while KERATIN is the protein of hair and outer layers of the skin. COLLAGEN is the primary fibrous protein of connective tissue, and MYOSIN forms fibers that cause muscle contraction. Two other fibrous proteins are worth mentioning. FIBRIN forms blood clots, while ELASTIN forms ligaments and the valves of large blood vessels.

The insolubility and high degree of cross-linking of fibrous proteins in connective tissue limits their digestion in meat. COOKING softens myosin fibers in muscle and gelatinizes collagen, making meat more digestible.

fig (*Ficus carica*) The pear-shaped fruit of the fig tree. The fig is native to southwestern Asia; approximately 700 varieties are now cultivated throughout the Mediterranean area. California is the source of most domestic figs. Red, purple, white, and green figs are the basic types. Figs possess a tough skin and a soft pulp. Because the fresh fruit has a short life span, 90 percent of household figs are either dried or canned. Dried figs are a rich source of sugar, dietary fiber, and minerals. The Calimyrna, Black Mission, and Brown Turkey are the most popular dried figs. Figs are among the sweetest of all fruits. Food value for 10 dried figs (187 g) is 477 calories; protein, 5.7 g; carbohydrate, 122 g; fiber, 24 g; calcium, 269 mg; iron, 4.2 mg; magnesium, 11 mg; potassium, 1,331 mg; zinc, 0.94 mg. Figs contain moderate amounts of B vitamins; thiamin, 0.13 mg; riboflavin, 0.13 mg; niacin, 1.3 mg.

fight or flight response The physiologic response to real or perceived STRESS. Stress may be physical (exposure to disease-producing organisms and to toxic agents, or injury) or psychological (fear or joy associated with a crisis). There are three phases of adaptation to stress; each is regulated by the adrenal glands.

The body initially responds to stress with an "alarm" that mobilizes the body for immediate physical activity—to confront or flee from a threatening situation. The brain perceives the threat and activates the ADRENAL GLANDS to secrete norepinephrine and EPINEPHRINE (adrenaline). These hormones, released by the adrenal medulla, stimulate energy production and promote a state of alertness, increase the heart rate to pump more blood to the brain and muscles, and increase blood pressure. Blood is channeled to muscles and brain and away from the skin and the organs, except the lungs and the heart. Epinephrine and norepinephrine increase the rate of breathing to supply more oxygen to the heart, skeletal muscles, and the brain. The hormones promote BLOOD CLOTTING, increase BLOOD SUGAR rapidly, and mobilize stored fat to increase free FATTY ACID levels in blood. The release of digestive juices drops and PERISTALSIS slows to severely restrict digestive processes, and perspiration increases.

In the second phase of adaptation to stress, the resistance reaction allows a more sustained adaptation to a stressor to enable the body to carry out strenuous work, cope with emotional upsets and ward off infection. In response to ACTH (adrenocorticotropin) from the pituitary gland, the adrenal cortex produces steroid hormones to adapt the body to long-term stress. Glucocorticoids like CORTISOL stimulate catabolic (degradative) processes and favor the breakdown of muscle protein to amino acids, which are converted by the liver to blood sugar. Glucocorticoids stimulate fat breakdown as well.

Continued high cortisol output contributes to fatigue. High cortisol also suppresses the immune system and antibody production, thus increasing the risk of infection, and alters bone metabolism. Normally, cortisol output follows a circadian rhythm: Levels are highest in the morning, dropping to a plateau between noon and 4 to 5 P.M. and reaching a nadir at midnight. This pattern can be disrupted in chronic stress.

To manage stress, EXERCISE, relaxation techniques, and nutritional support are preeminently important. Regular exercise leads to an increased ability to deal with stress and also reduces the risk of stress-related conditions such as heart disease and depression. Relaxation through prayer, yoga, meditation, or biofeedback reverses the physiologic effects of the fight or flight response. Nutrients that are required to support adrenal function include VITAMIN C, the B complex VITAMINS, especially VITAMIN B_6 and PANTOTHENIC ACID, and zinc and magnesium. POTASSIUM losses reduce adrenal function, therefore potassium levels need to be maintained. (See also CATABOLISM; GENERAL ADAPTATION SYNDROME.)

firming agents Food additives that maintain firmness and crispness of vegetables and fruits when canned or pickled. CALCIUM and ALUMINUM compounds are added to pickles and maraschino cherries, as well as to canned peas, tomatoes, potatoes, and apples. Examples of firming agents include aluminum sulfate, calcium lactate, and calcium chloride. (See also FOOD ADDITIVES.)

fish An aquatic cold-blooded vertebrate used as a food source since prehistoric times. Edible bony fish fall into two categories: saltwater fish and freshwater fish. Important saltwater fish include COD, FLOUNDER, HALIBUT, HADDOCK, HERRING, MACKEREL, SALMON, sole, swordfish, sea bass, and TUNA; freshwater fish include BASS, CATFISH, pike, sturgeon, PERCH, and TROUT. Fish contribute high-quality protein to the diet and supply MAGNESIUM, COPPER, ZINC, IODINE, and B vitamins, together with modest amounts of IRON and CALCIUM. Fish can replace red meat in a healthy diet because it does not contain high levels of saturated fat.

Coldwater ocean fish and their oils contain high levels of essential fatty acids, polyunsaturated FATTY ACIDS derived from the omega-3 family. These fatty acids are believed to lower serum fat and cholesterol levels, to lower the risk of blood clots and of CARDIOVASCULAR DISEASE. Fish and FISH OIL also seem to reduce inflammation associated with chronic disease. Oily fish and fish liver oils contain significant amounts of VITAMIN A and VITAMIN D.

A variety of studies have demonstrated the benefits of fish on health. The Multiple Risk Factor Intervention Trial involving 13,000 U.S. men showed that the risk of dying from heart attack was 40 percent less for those eating the most fish. Dutch studies have shown that men eating fish several times weekly were less likely to die of heart attack or stroke. The Physician' Health Study did not observe a connection between fish and heart attacks.

Besides replacing saturated fat meals with unsaturated fat, the addition of fish to the diet may reduce platelet stickiness, making these cell fragments less likely to form clots; may lower high blood fats (triglycerides) that may indirectly promote cholesterol-clogged arteries; and may help stabilize heart muscle and prevent deadly, abnormal heart rhythms during heart attacks.

On the other hand, fish oil impairs blood clotting, possibly increasing the risk of stroke due to bleeding into the brain (hemorrhagic stroke).

The optimal amount of fish in the diet is unknown, although eating average servings (4 oz.) of fish instead of red meat several times a week seems to offer protection against heart attacks. Health benefits seem to increase when total dietary fat, especially saturated fat, consumption decreases, and more polyunsaturated fats are consumed. Shark, SHELLFISH, rainbow trout, and striped bass are fair to good sources of omega-3. To preserve the essential oils in fish, it should be poached, steamed, or baked at medium temperatures. Fast-food fish contain almost no omega-3 fatty acids.

Fresh frozen seafood has generally a better flavor and texture than canned or frozen fish because it is frozen within four hours after being caught. Fresh fish sold in supermarkets may be 10 days old by the time it is purchased by the consumer. Fresh fish has almost no odor; if fish smells after cooking, it should be discarded. Fresh fish should be refrigerated and eaten soon after purchase. Frozen fish should be stored no more than a month. Freshly caught game fish should be cleaned as soon as possible to eliminate major bacterial contamination.

Seafood Safety Issues

Only a small percentage of the fish and seafood consumed in the United States is currently inspected, and the adequacy of SEAFOOD INSPECTION programs has been questioned. Seafood safety is a prominent issue because fish spoil more rapidly than most other foods and may be contaminated by hard-to-degrade pollutants because they are at the top of the aquatic FOOD CHAIN. In addition, to meet increased consumer demand, fish and shellfish are being harvested closer to shore, where pollution levels are higher.

Fish that scavenge food from sediment lake beds and the sea floor may be likely to contain industrial contaminants deposited in sediments. Great Lakes fish, freshwater fish grown in polluted water, and certain predatory species like swordfish, tuna and walleye pike, and fatty fish, are more likely to contain fat-soluble pollutants like pesticides, PBBs, PCBs, and mercury. These could harm a fetus and increase the risk of cancer. Tuna can accumulate mercury and swordfish and lake whitefish tend to be high in mercury or PCBs. Sole and flounder may contain less pollutants, and fish harvested from relatively clean areas like the Northern Pacific may be even less contaminated. The general recommendation is to eat a variety of fish several times weekly.

Raw fish can contain worms (*Aniskis simplex* and *Pseudoterranova decipiens*) that are destroyed by adequate cooking or freezing. However, partial cooking and short-term microwave cooking may not kill worms or their eggs. Sushi is a raw fish dish from Japan whose growing popularity in the United States raises questions about the safety of eating raw fish. In the United States, fish has traditionally been smoked or cooked before eating, but salting, smoking, or marinating may not kill all parasites.

Symptoms of parasitic infections include vomiting, diarrhea, and stomach cramps. Parasitic diseases are difficult to diagnose. Diagnosis usually relies on analysis of stool or blood. (See also BREAST-FEEDING; OMEGA-3 FATTY ACIDS; PARASITES IN FOOD AND WATER.)

fish oil Supplements containing lipids from cold-water fish. These fish accumulate large, highly unsaturated fatty acids—EICOSAPENTAENOIC ACID (EPA) and DOCOSAHEXAENOIC ACID (DHA)—belonging to the omega-3 family of essential fatty acids. In fact, fish and fish oils are the major concentrated source of these polyunsaturated fatty acids, which form a class of HORMONE-like substances (PROSTAGLANDINS and thromboxanes) of the omega-3 series that reduce pain and inflammation and counterbalance inflammatory processes in the body and help restore equilibrium in the body after stress and injury. (In contrast, red meat supplies ARACHADONIC ACID, which generates pro-inflammatory prostaglandins and thromboxane.) Eating fish seems to lower the risk of cholesterol-clogged arteries, and fish oils may do the same. Population studies suggest that the more ocean fish consumed, the lower the risk of HEART DISEASE, even when consumption of CHOLESTEROL is high, as is the case for Greenland Eskimos. Eating oily fish several times per week provides about 0.5 g of omega-3 long-chain fatty acids. Modest amounts of fish oil can reduce levels of blood fats known as VERY-LOW-DENSITY LIPOPROTEIN (VLDL), which transports fat in the bloodstream in healthy people as well as type II diabetics. It may also reduce LOW-DENSITY-LIPOPROTEIN (LDL, the less desirable form of serum cholesterol) in normal people (if the diet is high in saturated fat). The issue is by no means clear-cut because fish oils sometimes raise rather than lower LDL levels in people with high blood fat levels.

Fish oil is a complex mixture of lipids, and the relative importance of each constituent in lowering the risk of heart disease is not known. In some studies, beneficial effects reported for people with high fish intake could be due to other dietary modifications. Negative results with fish and fish oils are sometimes explained by the fact that olive oil, used as a control, itself may lower the risk of heart disease and is not a neutral substance.

Other possible effects of fish oils are wide ranging. Together with ASPIRIN and anticoagulants, fish oil capsules help preserve the effects of coronary artery widening. Fish oil in foods can reduce the risk of dying from coronary heart disease, acute heart attack, and stroke. A recent Italian study suggests that fish oil lipids can dramatically reduce the risk of sudden death and death overall in people who have had heart attacks. More than 11,000 heart attack survivors were divided into four groups: one was given a gram of n-3 polyunsaturated fatty acids a day, one received 300 mg of vitamin E a day, the third group took both, and the last took a placebo. Those participants who received the fatty acid supplements had fewer sudden deaths than those who did not. Fish oils have potent anticlotting effects: They inhibit the production of a blood protein called fibrinogen, which triggers clot formation when activated. High fibrinogen levels are a risk factor for heart diseases. Fish oils also reduce the stickiness of platelets, small cell fragments in the blood that promote blood clotting. Fish oils also seem to block the action of a substance called thromboxane TXA_2, which promotes blood clot formation. In addition, EPA generates the prostaglandin PGI_3, which inhibits clumping of blood platelets and reduces the risk of blood clots.

Fish and fish oils reduce inflammation and may lessen symptoms of AUTOIMMUNE DISEASES like rheumatoid ARTHRITIS, lupus erythematosus, and other diseases related to an abnormal response of the immune system, such as psoriasis and multiple sclerosis. Eating fish regularly reduces the risk of chronic bronchitis and emphysema among cigarette smokers. In terms of inflammation, fish oils and omega-3 fatty acids appear to block the production of LEUKOTRIENES and other potent inflammatory agents like prostaglandin PGE_2.

Fish oils may help prevent fatal changes in heart rhythm (ventricular fibrillation) following a heart attack. Fish oils from supplements or fish also can reduce high levels of triglycerides by between 20 percent and 60 percent, and fish oils reduce prostate cancer risk. Very large doses many have a modest effect on high blood pressure. Fish oil-fortified formula seems to help visual development of premature infants. Standard infant formula does not include fish oil or the long-chain OMEGA-3 FATTY ACID, docosahexaenoic acid, which normally accounts for a third of the fatty acids in the retina and the gray matter of the brain. The system for fabricating this fatty acid is ineffective in infants, and DHA can be considered a "conditionally" essential nutrient for preterm babies.

Basic question about fish oil supplements remain unanswered. It is not known how much fish oil to take, why it needs to be taken, who should take it, or how long it should be taken. For these reasons, the American Heart Association does not recommend fish oil for treatment of heart disease nor does the U.S. FDA permit health claims to be made regarding fish oil and disease.

There are several precautions to be taken in using fish oil supplements. Those with high blood fat (TRIGLYCERIDES) or high blood cholesterol levels should not self-medicate; consultation with an expert on heart disease is warranted. Diabetics need to be aware that larger doses of fish oil can increase blood sugar and therefore blood sugar should be carefully monitored when using these supplements. Asthmatics who cannot tolerate aspirin can experience more frequent asthma attacks after taking fish oil supplements. Some fish oils (including COD LIVER OIL) contain significant amounts of cholesterol. Fatty fish can be contaminated with industrial chemicals like MERCURY, PCB, PBB, and PESTICIDES. Cod liver oil is a very concentrated form of VITAMIN A and VITAMIN D. It is easy to overdose with these vitamins because they are stored by the body. Large amounts of fish oils increase bleeding tendencies and they may decrease the ability of white cells to fight infections. Excessive fish oil increases the need for vitamin E. (See also BREAST-FEEDING; DDT; ESKIMO DIET.)

Harris, W. S., and W. L. Isley. "Clinical trial evidence for the cardioprotective effects of omega-3 fatty acids." *Curr. Atheorscler. Rep.* 316 (November 2001): iii.

fish protein concentrate (FPC) An inexpensive protein FOOD ADDITIVE. The flesh of less desirable commercial fish is minced, defatted, and dehydrated to produce the powdered protein concentrate. It is added to bread, cookies, and tortillas to increase their PROTEIN quality. When 5 percent to 10 percent FPC is added to wheat flour or corn flour that is low in several ESSENTIAL AMINO ACIDS, the protein quality matches that of milk, which is high quality. (See also NET PROTEIN UTILIZATION; TEXTURIZED VEGETABLE PROTEIN.)

fitness The physiologic adaptation to physical exertion. Fitness implies increased muscular endurance or the ability of muscles to sustain repeated contractions, which correlates with strength. Regular, sustained EXERCISE significantly increases the body's ability to use and store ENERGY efficiently. At maximal exertion, skeletal muscles increase their overall metabolic rate by over tenfold. Conditioning increases the ability of muscles to oxidize FAT because muscle cells produce more of the fat-metabolizing machinery, MITOCHONDRIA, to meet the increased demand for energy due to increased work. As a result, muscles burn fat more rapidly even between periods of exercise, which assists in weight control. Conditioned muscles will burn fat longer before beginning to use muscle carbohydrate stores (glycogen), thus contributing to endurance.

Regular physical exertion increases the capacity of the lungs and heart to deliver oxygen. Well conditioned individuals typically have a lower heart rate than sedentary people, which means the heart does not need to work as hard during physical exertion. Regular aerobic exercise lowers LOW-DENSITY LIPOPROTEIN (LDL), the less desirable form of cholesterol, and increases HIGH-DENSITY LIPOPROTEIN (HDL), the desirable form, thus decreasing risks associated with CARDIOVASCULAR DISEASE. Exercise has also been found to help in recovery from heart attacks. Even moderate exercise stimulates the immune system. (See also FAT METABOLISM.)

5-hydroxytryptophan (5-HTP) An amino acid produced by the body from the essential (not produced by the body) amino acid tryptophan. It can then be converted to SEROTONIN, a chemical that in the brain functions as a NEUROTRANSMITTER, increasing feelings of well-being and reducing pain and appetite.

It is sold in the United States as a DIETARY SUPPLEMENT and promoted as a treatment for depression, obesity, insomnia, and pain associated with fibromyalgia. Some studies confirm that because of its serotonin enhancing, 5-HTP shows promise as a treatment for these conditions. However, because it is sold as a dietary supplement rather than a drug, its safety and efficacy have not been tested by any governmental agency.

In 1989 the U.S. Food and Drug Administration (FDA) temporarily removed all tryptophan supplements from the market after reports that the dietary supplement L-tryptophan was contaminated with a substance that caused a potentially fatal disorder called eosinophilic myalgia syndrome. Such contaminants may be present in 5-HTP preparations. Side effects that have been reported by patients taking the supplement include nausea and heartburn. It may also interact negatively with medications, especially those used to treat depression, Parkinson's disease, pain, and insomnia.

Cangiano, C. et al. "Effects of Oral 5-hydroxy-tryptophan on Energy Intake and Macronutrient Selection in Non-insulin Dependent Diabetic Patients," *Interna-*

tional Journal of Obesity and Related Metabolic Disorders 22 (1998): 648–654.

flatulence The production of gas in the stomach and INTESTINES. Excessive flatus gas in the digestive tract is responsible for bloating and gas pains after eating. Normally, the intestine produces gases from COLON BACTERIA, fermenting undigested SUGARS, CARBOHYDRATES, and FIBER. Products of fermentation are carbon dioxide, methane, hydrogen, and volatile sulfur and nitrogen-containing compounds from protein degradation, which have an unpleasant odor (skatole, putrescine, and others). Little research has been carried out on the causes of gas, or on its remedy. Individuals differ in their tolerance to foods, and tolerance can change daily. Possible causes of gas and bloating include:

Swallowed Air When chewing gum or gulping food, excessive air may be swallowed.

Lactose Intolerance Individuals with the inability to digest milk sugar should avoid MILK and milk products such as ice cream. When undigested, LACTOSE can be fermented by colonic bacteria. Alternatively, LACTASE, an enzyme that degrades lactose to simpler sugars GLUCOSE and GALACTOSE, can be used in digesting milk sugar. Preparations of lactase are commercially available as tablets or drops.

Flatulence-causing Foods Foods likely to cause gas include APPLES, BEANS, BAGELS, BRAN, BROCCOLI, BRUSSELS SPROUTS, CABBAGE, CAULIFLOWER, CITRUS FRUIT, ONIONS, RAISINS, GRAINS like WHEAT and OATS, CARROTS, prunes, and APRICOTS. These foods contain fiber and other undigested carbohydrate that can be broken down by bacteria. Less of a problem are BREAD, pastries, radishes, EGGPLANT, BANANAS, CELERY, lettuce, POTATOES, and CORN. It is best to modify the diet to avoid those foods that provoke a reaction. To remove the bulk of flatulence-producing sugars in beans (stachyose and raffinose), they should be soaked four to eight hours in hot water, and cooked in fresh water.

Carbonated Beverages These can worsen a gas problem because of released carbon dioxide in the beverages that one drinks.

Fatty Foods Fat slows down gas moving through the digestive tract and should be limited.

Stress Prolonged STRESS can alter gastrointestinal function.

(See also ACID INDIGESTION.)

flavin adenine dinucleotide (FAD) A type of enzyme helper (COENZYME) formed from RIBOFLAVIN (VITAMIN B_2). FAD functions as an electron carrier in key oxidation-reduction reactions in energy production by mitochondria, the cellular powerhouse. Specifically, FAD assists enzymes in the KREB'S CYCLE, the central energy-yielding pathway ultimately responsible for oxidizing fat, carbohydrate, and protein breakdown to carbon dioxide; and in the oxidation of fatty acids. In addition, FAD helps to detoxify potentially harmful molecules like cigarette smoke and pesticides.

Flavin Adenine Mononucleotide (FMN)

FMN is a type of coenzyme formed of riboflavin that serves a more limited oxidation-reduction role than FAD. FMN assists enzymes participating in the oxidation of certain AMINO ACIDS and in the ELECTRON TRANSPORT CHAIN, the bucket brigade sequence of enzymes that ultimately consumes oxygen and produces ATP in mitochondria when fat and carbohydrate are oxidized. (See also CARBOHYDRATE METABOLISM; CATABOLISM; GLYCOLYSIS.)

flavonoids (bioflavonoids) A large family of widely distributed plant substances, formerly designated as vitamin F. However, flavonoids are not classified as essential nutrients, nor do they have a vitamin status. These compounds are often pigments and occur in high concentrations in all fruits, especially CITRUS FRUITS; purple berries and apples; as well as in VEGETABLES, including onions; tea; and whole grains. They are responsible for astringency of certain fruits and tea.

Flavonoids include flavones (such as QUERCETIN), ISOFLAVONES (from soybeans), FLAVANONES (such as naringen and HESPERIDIN and RUTIN from citrus), ANTHOCYANINS (blue, purple, and red plant pigments) and flavononols (including catechins, ellagic acid and TANNINS). Typical examples of major flavonoids and common sources are listed in the accompanying table.

Research before World War II demonstrated that vitamin C taken with flavonoids (called "vitamin F" at that time) strengthens capillaries, and in the 1950s flavonoids were frequently prescribed for bleeding. Subsequently the U.S. FDA ruled that they were ineffective despite medical experience to the contrary. Flavonoids have been used as supportive treatment for menstrual bleeding, bruising, frostbite, and cold sores.

Flavonoids can also strengthen the blood-brain barrier to increase protection of the nervous system against foreign substances and they help reduce damage due to inflammation, thereby reducing allergy symptoms and allowing tissues to normalize. They accomplish this in the following ways: Flavonoids strengthen and repair connective tissue by stimulating the synthesis of COLLAGEN, the fibrous protein of the connective tissue that holds cells together and by inhibiting collagen breakdown. Furthermore, these plant materials slow the infiltration of neutrophils, immune cells that can cause damage, into an inflamed area. Flavonoids also stabilize defensive cells in tissues (mast cells), making them less likely to release substances such as histamine, protein-degrading enzymes and LEUKOTRIENES that initiate inflammation. Flavonoids can even block the production of proinflammatory PROSTAGLANDINS as well as leukotrienes and they act as ANTIOXIDANTS to prevent FREE RADICAL damage and lipid oxidation that triggers inflammation. Free radicals are highly reactive molecules that tear electrons away from neighboring molecules to make up for their own deficiency.

Populations studies indicate that consumption of flavonoids from tea, onions, and apples by northern European men can decrease the risk of heart attack, and the consumption of black tea is associated with a lower risk of STROKE. Two properties may account for these effects. Flavonoids make small blood cells called platelets less sticky, thus they can reduce the risk of dangerous blood clots. Flavonoids also act as antioxidants, possibly preventing the oxidation of LDL-cholesterol, believed to be an initiating event in atherosclerosis. Other studies suggest that certain flavonoids such as concord grapes, block cancers (anticarcinogenic activity). They can activate or inhibit various DETOXICATION enzymes in the liver, thus they may prevent the activation of carcinogens.

The amounts of key flavonoids in foods and beverages have been determined and dietary intakes can be computed. How much of a given flavonoid needs to be consumed to achieve a protective effect is uncertain, although a diet that provides 25 to 50 mg of key flavonoids offers a degree of protection against heart disease. How flavonoids are processed in the intestine by gut bacteria, how they are absorbed and how they are assimilated remain largely unknown factors. Very likely, combinations of flavonoids together with other factors in foods will be most beneficial. The long-term effects of purified flavonoids on health have not been fully investigated. It should be pointed out that certain

FLAVONOIDS THAT MAY BENEFIT HEALTH

Flavonoid	Typical Sources	Possible Beneficial Effects
Anthocyanin	Blueberries, blackberries, raspberries, grapes, eggplants, red cabbage, wine	Antioxidants. May dilate blood vessels.
Ellagic acid	Strawberries, grapes, apples, cranberries, blackberries, walnuts	Antioxidant. May block damage of DNA from carcinogenics.
Catechin	Green tea, black tea	Antioxidant. May stimulate detoxication enzymes and protects liver. Strengthens capillaries. Blocks inflammation. May inhibit tumor formation.
Tannin	Green tea, black tea	Antioxidant. May stimulate detoxication enzymes and strengthen capillaries. Blocks inflammation. May inhibit tumor formation.
Kaempferol	Strawberries, leeks, kale, broccoli, radishes, endives, red beets	Antioxidant. May stimulate detoxication enzymes and strengthen capillaries. Blocks inflammation. May inhibit tumor formation.
Quercetin	Green tea, onions, kale, red cabbage, green beans, tomatoes, lettuce, strawberries, sweet cherries, grapes	Antioxidant. May stimulate detoxication enzymes and strengthen capillaries. Blocks inflammation. May inhibit tumor formation.

flavonoids can actually increase oxidation (prooxidant effects) and that high levels could inhibit the thyroid gland. (See also BILBERRY; GRAPE SEED EXTRACT; PYCNOGENOL; PHYTOCHEMICALS.)

Manthey, J. A. "Biological Properties of Flavonoids Pertaining to Inflammation," *Microcirculation* 7 (2000): S29–S34.

flavor enhancers FOOD ADDITIVES used to increase the effect of certain flavors. Enhancers themselves contribute little flavor to a food. First used in fish and meat dishes, they now intensify desired flavors and mask unwanted ones in beverages, processed fruit and vegetables, and baked goods like breads and cakes. Flavor enhancers work to enhance each other; therefore, mixtures are usually used. MONOSODIUM GLUTAMATE (MSG), DISODIUM GUANYLATE and DISODIUM INOSINATE are common examples. (See also HYDROLYZED VEGETABLE PROTEIN.)

flavors (flavorings) One of the largest groups of FOOD ADDITIVES. About two-thirds of all additives are flavors or FLAVOR ENHANCERS. Flavors stimulate the sense of taste and/or smell. Except for sweet, bitter, salty, and sour taste sensations, flavors are the result of odor perception. In spite of their wide usage, only tiny amounts of flavorings are consumed yearly (about an ounce per person) in the United States. Therefore, the U.S. FDA has less stringent regulations for them than for other food additives. Despite the small quantity consumed individually each year, food manufacturers use flavors extensively in manufactured foods because they can either replace natural flavors lost in processing, or they can replace expensive natural flavors with less expensive ingredients.

Most natural flavorings are either extracted or derived from plant products. SPICES, HERBS, YEAST, FRUIT, and leaves, buds, and roots of certain plants are used to provide natural flavors. Examples of natural flavors are allspice, bitter ALMOND, ANISE, balm, BASIL, caraway, cardamom, cinnamon, celery seed, chervil, citron, CLOVES, coriander, CRESS, CUMIN, DILL, FENNEL, fenugreek, GINGER, LEMON, LICORICE, MARJORAM, mint, MUSTARD, NUTMEG, OREGANO, PAPRIKA, PARSLEY, ROSEMARY, SAGE, savory, tarragon, thyme, TURMERIC, VANILLA, and wintergreen.

Artificial Flavors

Artificial flavors are manufactured; their chemical structure may be the same as those flavors that occur naturally. For example: Artificial vanilla contains vanillin, the same compound as from vanilla beans. Artificial flavors may be new flavors or they may be new compounds that create familiar flavors. They have several advantages: Synthetic flavors can withstand processing; they cost less than natural flavors; they are readily available; and they are consistent in quality. Flavors are often very complex mixtures of ingredients, whether naturally occurring or created from synthetics, and food technologists have gone to great lengths to assure that the blend of synthetic flavors will meet with consumer acceptance. A wide variety of synthetic flavors are used in processed foods. Artificial flavors (like artificial cherry, raspberry, strawberry, watermelon, and vanilla) can cover up the absence of more expensive ingredients in manufactured foods like mixes and SOFT DRINKS.

There are hundreds of flavoring compounds. These examples illustrate their versatility:

- allyl butyrate: pineapple odor, apple taste;
- allyl cinnamate: berry flavors, grape and peach;
- bornyl acetate: minty flavor;
- cinnamaldehyde: cinnamon, cola blends;
- cyclohexyl propionate: banana, rum;
- 2-ethyl butyraldehyde: chocolate, cocoa;
- hexyl hexanoate: strawberry, vegetable flavors;
- 5-hydroxy-4-octanone: butter, cheese, nuts;
- lactic acid: dairy flavors;
- d-limonene: citrus flavor;
- menthol: mint flavor, toothpaste;
- myrcene: citrus imitation, fruit blends;
- nonanoic acid: coconut;
- nonyl isovalerate: fried fatty food aroma and flavor;
- phenethyl isovalerate: apple, pineapple, pear, peach mixtures;
- 4-phenyl-2-butanol: melon flavors;
- 2-thienyl mercaptan: coffee-roasted flavors;
- valeraldehyde: chocolate, coffee, nut flavors;
- vanillin: vanilla, chocolate;
- zingerone: spice, root beer, raspberry.

(See also FAST FOOD; PROCESSED FOOD.)

flaxseed oil A rich source of ALPHA LINOLENIC ACID, one of two ESSENTIAL FATTY ACIDS. Flaxseed oil contains 57 percent alpha linolenic acid, 16 percent LINOLEIC ACID (the second essential fatty acid) and 18 percent oleic acid, a nonessential fatty acid. Essential fatty acids are polyunsaturated FATTY ACIDS, that is, they lack pairs of hydrogen atoms and are sensitive to oxidation. They cannot be manufactured by the body and therefore must be supplied by foods or supplements. Alpha linolenic acid belongs to the omega-3 family of fatty acids. This family is converted to certain PROSTAGLANDINS, HORMONE-like lipids that normalize key processes of the body. For example, the omega-3 fatty acids help balance the immune system, decrease inflammation, decrease blood pressure, and decrease the tendency to form blood clots. The typical diet supplies twice as much omega-6 oils as needed while supplying little omega-3 fatty acids. Most of the plant oils Americans consume—CORN OIL, peanut oil, SAFFLOWER oil, and sunflower oil, to name a few—are omega-6 oils. A deficiency of omega-3 fatty acids is associated with several health problems. Omega-3 oils may improve conditions associated with heart disease, diabetes, inflammatory conditions such as allergies, and rheumatoid ARTHRITIS.

There are several advantages to obtaining omega-3 fatty acids from plant sources. Flaxseed oil has none of the cholesterol, VITAMIN A or VITAMIN D that occur in fish liver oils and can accumulate in the body. Fish oil may be contaminated with pesticides and industrial chemicals, depending on where the fish lived. However, there is no clear evidence to indicate how much flaxseed oil is optimal.

Flaxseed oil is very easily oxidized and should never be used as cooking oil. To avoid rancidity, this oil needs to be refrigerated and protected from light and oxygen. BETA-CAROTENE and VITAMIN E are often added to flaxseed oil as ANTIOXIDANTS.

flora, intestinal Bacteria that normally inhabit the intestinal tract. More bacteria live in the human intestinal tract than there are cells in the body. By far, most live in the large intestine (COLON). Lactic acid-producing bacteria, *LACTOBACILLUS ACIDOPHILUS* and *L. bifidus,* are important examples of "good" bacteria. Optimally, the relationship between intestinal bacteria and the host is symbiotic: Beneficial bacteria produce VITAMIN K, BIOTIN, and other nutrients, which are absorbed. They provide the intestinal lining with a substantial part of its energy. Intestinal microorganisms promote localized acidic, anaerobic environments that inhibit the growth of potential disease-producing (pathogenic) organisms. Lactic acid–producing bacteria *L. acidophilus* and *L. bifidus* are important in this regard. Beneficial gut bacteria can also produce antimicrobial substances that limit the growth of pathogenic organisms and stimulate the IMMUNE SYSTEM.

The composition of colonic bacteria varies with the composition of the diet, the transit time (the speed with which food passes through the GASTROINTESTINAL TRACT), and use of antibiotics. A low-fiber diet contributes less carbohydrate for bacterial fermentation. Products of fermentation include short-chain FATTY ACIDS that are primary fuels for cells lining the colon. A short transit time limits the ability of acid-producing bacteria to create an acidic environment to inhibit growth of potential pathogenic organisms. Broad-spectrum antibiotics destroy beneficial bacteria as well as pathogenic bacteria. This alteration of the intestinal environment can permit opportunistic organisms such as yeast to proliferate, causing disease. (See also ACIDOPHILUS; BIFIDOBACTERIA; *CANDIDA ALBICANS*.)

flounder A large family of saltwater FISH that includes gray sole, lemon sole, and winter flounder. Flounder are bottom-feeding fish (they feed off the ocean floor). Their flat bodies, with eyes on top of the head, are adaptations to this mode of feeding. This important food fish is lean and delicate. A 3-oz. (8.5 g) serving of baked flounder provides 80 calories and: protein, 17 g; fat, 1 g. It contains moderate amounts of iron, 1 mg; cholesterol, 75 mg; calcium, 34 mg; niacin, 2.9 mg; riboflavin, 0.1 mg; and small amounts of other vitamins. (See also SEAFOOD INSPECTION.)

flour Finely ground powder generally prepared from cereal GRAIN, although flours are also prepared from legumes, vegetables, and fish. Flour is the primary ingredient in baked goods. It provides starch (complex CARBOHYDRATES) and varying amounts of protein and other nutrients. In cooking, flour thickens soups, gravies, and batters (mixtures of flour, water, and oil) and are used in sautéing and frying foods. Flour is prepared by milling (grinding with steel rollers and sieving) grains to separate the larger starchy layer (ENDOSPERM) of the kernel from its hard outer layer (BRAN) and the oil-rich germ. In whole-grain flours, bran and endosperm are added back at this point. Wheat flour is further purified by removing oil to prevent rancidity, bleaching to remove a yellow endosperm color, and then aging by chemical treatment to produce white flour for baking.

In 1998 the U.S. FDA began requiring all enriched grain products, including flour, to be fortified with folic acid at the rate of 140 mcg per 100 g of grain. This action was taken based on studies that showed that only about 25 percent of women of childbearing age regularly consumed enough folic acid. Women who consume at least 400 mcg daily have a significantly lower risk of bearing children with neural tube defects such as spina bifida.

Twenty-two nutrients are more or less removed or destroyed at most of these preparation steps: trace minerals (ZINC, MANGANESE, MAGNESIUM); vitamins (VITAMIN B_6, folic acid, riboflavin, thiamin, niacin); ESSENTIAL FATTY ACIDS; VITAMIN E; both soluble and insoluble FIBER, and even proteins to an extent. Most states require that white flour be enriched with thiamin, riboflavin, and niacin, plus iron to partially compensate for the loss of nutrients. Minerals, like zinc and manganese; vitamins, like vitamin B_6, and fiber are not added back, however.

Wheat flour is favored throughout the world because it forms elastic doughs that contribute a light texture to baked goods with yeast or other leavening agents. Wheat flour contains GLUTENS, a family of proteins (GLIADEN and glutein) that gives dough its elasticity. Aging partially oxidizes the protein and creates a flour that yields an even more elastic dough for baking. "Hard" wheat contains more protein than "soft" wheat. Most flours are blends. All-purpose flour has a higher percentage of soft wheat, while bread flour has a higher protein content. Biscuit flours are produced from soft wheat, as are cake flours.

Whole wheat flour, milled from the entire wheat kernel, contains many of the nutrients of all whole grain. Consequently, whole wheat BREAD is generally more nutritious than white bread. Because it contains oils, whole wheat flour can become stale unless it is refrigerated. It does not create a fine pastry flour; often a 50/50 mixture of whole wheat to white flour is appropriate for baking.

"All-purpose" flours are used for baking bread or pastries and in thickening. All-purpose flour is enriched and may be bleached or unbleached, and some contain more protein than others. Flour with 11 g or more of protein per cup will yield more tender yeast breads. Bran and cracked wheat flour, as well as oat flour, are all-purpose flours that contain wheat flour plus another grain. Pastry flour is not as coarse as all-purpose flour nor as finely milled as cake flour; it is suitable for pastry doughs. Bread flour is milled from hard wheat and has more protein, making a stronger dough. Self-raising flours also contain chemical leavening agents and salt; they are suitable for quick breads, cakes, and cookies. SEMOLINA, made from durum wheat, is a granular flour, suited for pizza dough because of its high protein content.

Other flours are available at health food stores and supermarkets, including arrowroot, RYE, BUCKWHEAT, soy, CORNMEAL, OAT, TAPIOCA, POTATO, and AMARANTH flours. Amaranth and buckwheat flour are alternatives for those with grain allergies; they belong to plant families unrelated to the grass family, of which wheat is a member. (See also BAKING POWDER; BAKING SODA; ENRICHMENT.)

Wharton, B., and I. Booth. "Fortification of Flour with Folic Acid," *British Medical Journal* 323 (2001): 1,198–1,199.

flour substitute (imitation flour) A FOOD ADDITIVE used as a flour filler to reduce calories and to increase the FIBER content of bread and baked goods. A flour substitute consists of CELLULOSE that has been highly purified from wood, corn husks, and other plant materials. Although purified, finely ground cellulose can be classified as a form of insoluble fiber, it probably doesn't reduce the risk of CONSTIPATION or high blood cholesterol as well as the cellulose in whole foods. LEGUMES, GRAINS, fruits, and vegetables can also provide additional fiber for bread. (See also IMITATION FOOD.)

fluid balance Regulation of WATER distribution in the body. Water is the most prevalent compound in the body, accounting for approximately 60 percent of body weight. Body water exists within cells (cellular water), in tissues (between cells), in body cavities and in the circulation (blood and lymph). The water content in each of these compartments is carefully regulated to assure normal function of all systems. Water diffuses freely through cell membranes and capillary walls. Excessive water distends cells, altering their membrane properties; inadequate water interferes with metabolism, which relies on a watery environment for normal function.

Water distribution is regulated by serum PROTEINS, highly charged proteins that normally do not cross the membranes of cells and capillary walls, and by ELECTROLYTES, ions whose transport across membranes is carefully regulated. Water follows the distribution of these ions, and they work together to maintain appropriate osmotic pressure. The kidneys filter 180 liters of fluid daily while producing about 2 liters of urine a day. Therefore, a liter of fluid must be ingested to make up for this loss. Kidney malfunction can alter the fluid composition of the body, which is under hormonal control. For example, ALDOSTERONE from the adrenal glands regulates SODIUM levels in the blood by directing the kidneys to take up sodium from urine. Since water follows the movement of sodium, aldosterone regulates water retention by the kidneys as well. Excessive water loss, through DEHYDRATION, DIARRHEA, bleeding, and vomiting, upsets water and electrolyte balance. (See also EXTRACELLULAR FLUID.)

fluoridated water WATER treated with controlled amounts of sodium fluoride. About half of the municipal water supplies in the United States are fluoridated, and today half of the children in the United States between the ages of five and 17 have no cavities. The reduction in cavities in people drinking fluoridated water has been consistently observed, although this effect is not as large as earlier believed. The increased use of fluoride dental treatment, of fluoride mouth washes and toothpaste, as well as consumption of fluoridated water, could explain the reduction in dental caries in recent years. The reduction could also be due to a complex array of factors including diet changes, oral hygiene, and, perhaps, increased immunity.

Fluoridation remains a controversial issue. Those opposed to fluoridation often view it as a personal rights issue, in which exposure to a potentially toxic agent is a health risk about which they should have a choice. The American Academy of Pediatrics, the U.S. Public Health Service, and the American Dental Association traditionally support fluoridation of water as an effective way of reducing tooth decay. They recommend fluoride supplements for children, if drinking water does not contain fluoride. They feel there are no harmful effects at the optimal level of 1 mg of fluoride per liter of water.

The Centers for Disease Control and Prevention (CDC) has listed water fluoridation as among the 10 greatest public health milestones of the 20th century, crediting it with dramatic reductions in tooth decay. The CDC recommends adding small amounts of fluoride to drinking water, about one part per million, and requiring bottled water to list fluoride content.

A committee of the National Research Council concluded that at the presently allowed level in drinking water, fluoride does not increase the odds of cancer, bone disease, or kidney failure. On the other hand, high levels can adversely affect the nervous system, a possible link to learning problems. Some tooth pitting and discoloration are possible at somewhat higher levels. With a high intake, fluoride can alter BONE structure. Evidence indicates that patients with kidney disease have an increased RISK of bone abnormalities due to fluoridation. (See also CALCIUM; FLUOROSIS; TEETH.)

fluoride An essential TRACE MINERAL required to build strong bones and teeth. Fluoride is the ionized form of the element fluorine. The estimated safe and adequate daily dietary intake of fluoride for adults is 1.5 to 4 mg. Most research regarding fluoride has focused on the relationship of fluoride to preventing tooth decay because fluoride hardens tooth enamel. Fluoride is absorbed by gums and incorporated into the structure of developing teeth as a fluoride-containing mineral, fluorapatite. This mineral strengthens the enamel and dentine, making them more resistant to bacterial decay. Traces of fluoride also occur in soft tissues but its role there is unclear.

Adult intake of fluoride in the United States from various sources may reach 0.5 to 1.0 mg daily. Seafood and tea are especially good sources of fluoride. Low levels are present in many foods and in drinking water. Two fluoride-containing compounds, stannous fluoride and sodium fluorophosphate, are common ingredients of toothpaste and mouth rinse. Most toothpastes contain one milligram of fluoride per gram of paste, and a fluoride overdose is possible if it is swallowed.

Side effects of chronic fluoride overdose include stomach ulcers, stress-induced bone fractures, and swollen joints. Questionable evidence for fluoride being a carcinogen in rats was found by the Natural Toxicology Program in 1990. The connection between fluoride and cancer in humans is still unclear, but a 1999 CDC report found no evidence supporting claims that water fluoridation increased the risk of cancer, Down syndrome, heart disease, osteoporosis and bone fracture, acquired immunodeficiency syndrome, low intelligence, Alzheimer's disease, or allergic reactions. Several studies indicate that fluoride can increase the risk of osteoporosis. Four separate studies noted an increased risk of hip fractures in people over 65 who had been drinking fluoridated water. (See also FLUORIDATED WATER; TEETH.)

Centers for Disease Control and Prevention. "Achievements in Public Health, 1900–1999: Fluroidation of Drinking Water to Prevent Dental Caries," *Morbidity and Mortality Weekly Report* 41 (October 22, 1999): 933–940.

fluorosis A disease resulting from excessive FLUORIDE consumption, which can lead to the mottling of tooth enamel during tooth development. The ingestion of fluoride at levels 100 times the optimal level may lead to fluoride toxicity, characterized by bone overgrowth, brittle bones, and stiff joints. Excessive fluoride in drinking water can cause fluorosis. However, fluorosis does not occur in communities where fluoride is added to drinking water because the level is raised to only 1 mg/liter. (See also TEETH.)

folacin See FOLIC ACID.

folic acid (folacin, folate) A water-soluble vitamin and a member of the B COMPLEX family that is essential for cell division (especially in RED BLOOD CELLS and the immune system), for growth and for reproduction. The Reference Daily Intake (RDI) for folic acid is 400 mcg for adults while the RDA (RECOMMENDED DIETARY ALLOWANCE) is 200 mcg for men and 180 mcg for women (who are not pregnant or lactating).

Folic acid deficiency is one of the most common vitamin deficiencies worldwide. In 1998 the U.S. FDA began requiring all enriched grain products, including cereals, breads, pasta, and rice to be fortified with folic acid at the rate of 140 mcg per 100 g of grain. This action was taken based on studies that showed that only about 25 percent of women of childbearing age in the United States regularly consumed enough folic acid. Women who consume at least 400 mcg daily have a significantly lower risk of bearing children with neural tube defects, such as spina bifida. In 2001 the U.S. Centers for Disease Control and Prevention reported that the number of children born with these defects had dropped by 19 percent since the enrichment program began. Specific groups more likely to be folate deficient include: alcoholics; women taking oral contraceptives or who are pregnant; people who rely on convenience foods; and elderly people. A variety of drugs interfere with folic acid uptake and utilization: oral contraceptives, GLUCOCORTICOIDS, barbiturates, ANTACIDS, ASPIRIN, dilantin for epilepsy, and some anticancer drugs.

Deficiency symptoms include fatigue, sore tongue, mental disturbances, megaloblastic anemia, digestive disturbances, and growth problems. Mild folate deficiency that does not cause anemia has been linked to NEURAL TUBE DEFECTS (SPINA BIFIDA), TOXEMIA of pregnancy, some types of CANCER (lung, esophagus, breast, colon), and cervical dysplasia, a precancerous state. Researchers have found that the risk of heart attack and heart disease is greater with low folic acid consumption. The link seems to be HOMOCYSTEINE, a by-product of the amino acid METHIONINE. High homocysteine levels in blood increases the risk of atherosclerosis, leading to heart attacks and strokes. Homocysteine accumulates with suboptimal folic acid intake and homocysteine possibly injures blood vessels. Most people's level of homocysteine drops with supplemental folic acid, at least 400 mcg daily. There is yet no clinical study demonstrating that lowering homocysteine levels protects against heart disease.

In the body, folate forms an important enzyme helper (COENZYME) called tetrahydrofolate. This coenzyme transfers single-carbon fragments from amino acid breakdown to create building blocks (PURINES and THYMINE) of DNA and RNA. Inadequate supply of these building blocks reduces the rate of DNA synthesis, hence of cell replication. Tetrahydrofolate also plays an important role in recycling METHIONINE, an essential AMINO ACID, from homocysteine. Methionine is required to synthesize CHOLINE (employed in neurotransmitter synthesis to help carry signals between nerve cells) and EPINEPHRINE (a hormone synthesized by adrenal glands to help adapt the body to stress).

Sources of folic acid include dark green leafy vegetables, BEANS (legumes), BROCCOLI, SPINACH, citrus fruits, breakfast cereals, nuts, LIVER, SALMON, and whole GRAINS. Cooking and food processing destroy this fragile vitamin.

Doses of folic acid in the range of 5 to 10 mg per day may reduce the risk of some kinds of cancer, especially colorectal cancer. Experiments in mice indicate that insufficient levels of folic acid can increase the risk of ALZHEIMER'S DISEASE. These findings complement other studies linking elevated levels of HOMOCYSTEINE with Alzheimer's disease, because folic acid reduces homocysteine levels. In combination with vitamin B_{12} and vitamin B_5, folic acid can lower homocysteine levels and decrease the risk of arterial closure after coronary angioplasty. Folic acid is also used to treat anemia and to prevent atherosclerosis, coronary heart disease, cervical dysplasia, and malabsorption syndromes.

Folate supplements are not considered to be toxic at the usual therapeutic doses. Huge doses (10 to 20 g per day) may induce convulsions in epileptics. Folate supplementation may mask a VITAMIN B_{12} deficiency, common in older Americans, and this can lead to nerve damage. Consequently, folate and vitamin B_{12} are administered together when used therapeutically. (See also BIRTH DEFECTS; ECLAMPSIA.)

Morrison, H. J., D. Schaubel, M. Desmeules, and D. T. Wigler. "Serum Folate and Risk of Fatal Coronary Heart Disease," *Journal of the American Medical Association*, 275 (June 26, 1996): 1,893–1,896.

food Edible substances that provide nourishment for growth and maintenance of health. Foods are mixtures of NUTRIENTS—broadly classified as MINERALS, VITAMINS, CARBOHYDRATES, PROTEINS, FATS, and OILS—and WATER. FIBER is essential for a healthy intestinal tract.

Foods are neither "good" nor "bad." To evaluate the appropriateness of a particular food for an individual, it is important to know its nutrient content; the quantity being consumed and the frequency of consumption; the overall DIET and the effects of lifestyle on the diet; the health and nutritional status as well as the age. Genetic susceptibility to CANCER, HEART DISEASE, HYPERTENSION, and diabetes need to be taken into account. Specific foods can either reduce or increase the risk of disease. A given food may be undesirable for those with FOOD SENSITIVITIES, food allergies, or inherited conditions such as PHENYLKETONURIA (an inherited inability to process acid phenylalanine). Most healthy people can tolerate splurging occasionally on cookies, CHOCOLATE, or ice cream. However, moderation and a variety of fresh, whole (minimally processed) foods are hallmarks of a BALANCED DIET.

The question of whether foods and specific nutrients can prevent or minimize the effects of degenerative diseases cannot be answered in detail; this area is being researched vigorously. Clearly, a reliance on highly PROCESSED FOODS can lead to health problems because such a diet does not provide adequate nutrition. On the one hand, such a diet may supply inadequate vitamins and minerals, while on the other, some nutrients are provided in excess—typically, salt, SUGAR, SATURATED FAT, and TROPICAL OILS, together with HYDROGENATED VEGETABLE OIL. These additives can pose problems in susceptible individuals. Consequently, a "junk food" diet with a surplus of calories and minimal trace nutrients is not recommended. (See also CHOLESTEROL; DEGENERATIVE DISEASE; DIETARY GUIDELINES FOR AMERICANS; SODIUM.)

food additives Substances intentionally added to food products. Food additives are used for a variety of reasons: to make food look more appealing to consumers; to maintain freshness; to make food safer or more nutritious; or to ease food manufacture or processing. Unintentional (incidental) food additives are inadvertently present in foods. They have no planned function in food, but become incorporated during processing, packaging, or storing. There are nearly 3,000 intentional additives.

Many are derived directly from foods, like LECITHIN, a lipid related to fat. Certain additives are needed to prevent spoilage and to maintain freshness of foods that must be distributed to consumers far from the point of manufacture or origin. Paradoxically, scientists' ability to detect food additives in foods, whether intentional or incidental, exceeds their ability to interpret the results in terms of human health.

The Federal Food, Drug and Cosmetic Act (1938) is the basic food law; it gives the U.S. FDA the responsibility for the safety of foods. Three amendments strengthened this act in 1954. The Miller Pesticide Act provided for establishing safe tolerances for pesticides in raw agricultural products. The Food Additives Amendment of 1958 required premarketing clearance by the FDA for food additives. It includes the DELANEY CLAUSE, which made it illegal to add cancer-causing chemicals to foods. The Color Additive Amendment (1960) regulated the certification of food colors. The FDA legally classified substances added to food into four categories: food additives, GENERALLY RECOGNIZED AS SAFE (GRAS) substances, prior sanctioned items, and food colors. Hundreds of food additives were classified as GRAS in 1958, based on common experience and apparent safety record. These include SUGAR, salt, SPICES, VITAMINS, MINERALS, milk, and egg protein. The GRAS list is periodically updated as new safety data are available. Thus CYCLAMATE, SULFITES, several food colors and SACCHARIN were removed when their safety was found wanting. Prior sanctioned additives are those agreed on before 1958. NITRITE used as a preservative for processed meat is an example. That a food is prior-sanctioned or that it is on the GRAS list does not assure safety; it must be evaluated in light of more current knowledge and more advanced technology.

Excluding salt, sweeteners, and sugar, the average yearly U.S. consumption of food additives like flavors, preservatives, and colors is 5 to 10 pounds per person. Food additives are used extensively by the food industry to help create a huge variety of processed foods. These manufactured foods tend to have a high level of fat and oil, salt, sugar, preservatives, and artificial coloring, and lower levels of several important nutrients.

Common functions of food additives:

1. ANTICAKING AGENTS are added to powdered or crystalline products to prevent lumping, e.g., silicon dioxide, CORNSTARCH, calcium silicate.
2. Antimicrobial agents preserve foods by preventing growth of bacteria, molds, and yeasts, e.g., CALCIUM PROPIONATE, sodium benzoate.
3. ANTIOXIDANTS retard deterioration or rancidity and discoloration due to oxidation, e.g., VITAMIN C (ascorbic acid), VITAMIN E, BHA, BHT, propyl gallate.
4. Curing and pickling agents provide characteristic flavors and increase shelf life, e.g., sodium NITRATE, sodium nitrite.
5. Emulsifiers establish a uniform dispersion, e.g., lecithin, carrageenan.
6. Enzymes can improve food processing, e.g., glucose oxidase, MEAT TENDERIZERS.
7. FLAVOR ENHANCERS increase original taste without imparting their own flavors, e.g., DISODIUM GUANYLATE, DISODIUM INOSINATE, HYDROLYZED VEGETABLE PROTEIN.
8. Flavorings impart a taste or aroma to food, e.g., SODIUM chloride, SUCROSE, and many artificial flavoring agents.
9. Flour treatment agents are bleaching and maturing agents added to flour, e.g., BENZOYL PEROXIDE, AZODICARBONAMIDE.
10. Food colors or color adjuncts are used to enhance a color or impart a color to a food, e.g., canthoxanthin, caramel, FD&C colors (Blue No. 1, Red No. 3, Yellow No. 5, and others), grape skin extract. Certain chemicals can stabilize or fix a food color.
11. HUMECTANTS absorb water and help keep foods moist, e.g., invert sugar, DEXTROSE, glycerin (GLYCEROL).
12. LEAVENING AGENTS produce CARBON DIOXIDE in baked goods, e.g., sodium BICARBONATE, yeast.
13. ARTIFICIAL SWEETENERS have less than 2 percent of the caloric value of sucrose (table sugar) when used at the same level of sweetness. They include saccharin and ASPARTAME.
14. Nutrient additives like IRON, THIAMIN, and RIBOFLAVIN enrich white flour and partially replace some of the nutrients lost in preparing

bleached flour. Iodide (the chemical form of iodine) is used to fortify salt.

15. Nutritive sweeteners include sucrose, dextrose, CORN SYRUP, and high FRUCTOSE CORN SYRUP.
16. Many pH control agents change or maintain the acidity or alkalinity of a food. These include ACIDS, BASES, and BUFFERS like dihydrogen phosphate, ACETIC ACID, phosphoric acid, and citric acid.
17. Processing aids include clarifying agents, clouding agents, and crystallization inhibitors. Filter aids are used to clarify BEER, for example.
18. Propellants are used to expel a product. Carbon dioxide and other gases have replaced chlorofluorocarbons in foams and aerosols.
19. Sequestrants combine with metal ions to form complexes. This action improves product stability, e.g., CITRIC ACID, ethylenediaminetetraacetic acid (EDTA).
20. Thickeners produce viscous solutions while stabilizers form stable suspensions (emulsions). They impart "body" to foods or beverages, e.g., CAROB BEAN GUM, AGAR, and alginates, as found in salad dressing, whipped cream, cheese, pudding, and frozen desserts.
21. Surface finishes increase palatability, preserve gloss and inhibit food discoloration, e.g., polishes, waxes, and glazes.
22. Texturizers alter the appearance and "mouth feel" of food; e.g., PECTINS, GUM GHATTI, and GUM ARABIC.

Safety

The most questionable additives are artificial food colors because they may cause cancer and/or allergic reactions and their use is strictly cosmetic. Consumer advocates claim they could be eliminated without altering the nutritional value of the food. Other food additives are potentially harmful; for example, sodium nitrite, a preservative, can be converted to a class of compounds (in the stomach and intestine) that cause cancer. Saccharin, an artificial sweetener, also causes cancer in lab animals. Its use has been continued through congressional action, though saccharin-containing food must bear a warning label.

Nutritive sweeteners like sugar (sucrose) and salt are by far the most common food additives. Sweeteners represent EMPTY CALORIES because they do not supply minerals, vitamins, protein, or fiber. Americans eat 28 billion pounds of sweeteners each year; the yearly per capita consumption is 130 to 150 pounds. There is consensus that excessive sugar consumption contributes to tooth decay and to obesity, now considered a leading disease in the U.S. Salt (sodium) is often added to processed foods because they lack flavor. The yearly U.S. consumption of salt per person is 10 to 15 pounds. A high-sodium diet contributes to high blood pressure in some people, who have an increased risk of dying from heart disease. There is no easy way to identify those who are sensitive to sodium ahead of time. (See also CHELATE; DIETARY GUIDELINES FOR AMERICANS; EATING PATTERNS; FAST FOOD; HYPERTENSION; NITROSOAMINES; PROCESSED FOOD.)

food advertising See ADVERTISING.

food allergy See ALLERGY, FOOD.

Food and Agricultural Organization (FAO) A branch of the United Nations that has long been concerned with worldwide nutrition and health. It presents a world forum for dealing with international problems concerning food, agriculture, and fisheries, and helps developing nations with agriculture and food production. As examples of its nutrition-related activities, the FAO has published standards for nutrient intakes, similar to the RECOMMENDED DIETARY ALLOWANCES of the United States. The FAO sets world standards for key nutrients such as PROTEIN and has published tables based on egg protein as the standard for evaluating the compositions of ESSENTIAL AMINO ACIDS of food proteins. The FAO has also developed regulations and standards for PESTICIDES, an important function because pesticide use is increasing worldwide and is not monitored carefully on a global basis. (See also EPA; HUNGER; PROTEIN QUALITY.)

Food and Drug Administration, U.S. See FDA.

food and the nervous system The relationship among food, behavior and emotions. Research over the last two decades has brought a deepened understanding of brain chemistry, together with a renewed interest in the effects of diet on behavior and mental well-being.

One focus is on NEUROTRANSMITTERS, chemicals that carry signals between individual nerve cells. The synthesis of at least five neurotransmitters may be affected by the brain concentrations of certain raw materials. Significantly, diet can influence concentrations of these raw materials. Most research on food and neurotransmitters has focused on SEROTONIN, which normally induces relaxation, increased tolerance to pain and decreased carbohydrate consumption. It has been proposed that serotonin may inhibit eating behavior because some bulimics (binge-purge eaters) are deficient in serotonin. The brain converts the amino acid TRYPTOPHAN to serotonin, and a high-carbohydrate meal may lead to increased TRYPTOPHAN levels in the brain, increased brain serotonin, and sleepiness. On the other hand, a high-protein meal may promote mental alertness temporarily because after protein digestion, relatively more of the amino acid TYROSINE is taken up by the brain. This may lead to a rise in norepinephrine, a neurotransmitter responsible for maintaining a state of alertness. These effects do not seem to extend beyond a single meal, however. The body generally controls total caloric intake rather precisely, but not protein and carbohydrate intake, which can vary considerably from meal to meal.

A second category of brain chemicals implicated in food and behavior is neuropeptides and peptide hormones. These are composed of chains of amino acids (polypeptides), though they are much smaller than proteins. Neuropeptides, such as endorphins and enkephalins, are synthesized by nerves, while peptide hormones regulating food intake are produced in several different tissues, including fat cells; the stomach, and the small intestine. Current research focuses on a complex array of factors that stimulate or inhibit appetite and food consumption. Neuropeptides and hormones participate in a complex gut-brain communication system to regulate food intake.

As examples, insulin can block the production of galanin in the brain, a neuropeptide that stimulates fat intake in the hypothalamus. Other factors that stimulate appetite include the hormone ghrelin, produced by the gastrointestinal tract and neuropeptide Y, which acts as a transmitter. Neuropeptides believed to inhibit eating include:

- CHOLECYSTOKININ A polypeptide hormone that suppresses appetite for fat and carbohydrate.
- Cyclo His-Pro (histidyl-proline diketopiperazine) This small molecule is derived from just two amino acids: HISTIDINE and PROLINE. It is released into the bloodstream after a meal and may be present for up to 12 hours afterward.
- Neuropeptide Y stimulates APPETITE for carbohydrate within minutes after it appears in the brain of experimental animals. The effect lasts for 24 hours. Levels increase between meals and decrease after eating. The hormone ghrelin, produced by the small intestine and stomach, acts as a powerful appetite stimulant. Blood levels of ghrelin increase in dieters and generally just before meals.

Substances that decrease appetite include neurotransmitters such as serotonin and norepinephrine, and several peptide hormones, including corticotropin-releasing hormone from the hypothalamus and peptide YY3-36 (PYY) produced by the small intestine. Intestinal release of cholecystokinin in response to ingested fat and protein stimulate nerve endings in the gut to reduce food intake. Leptin, produced by fat cells, regulates the hypothalamus to inhibit food consumption while increasing fat metabolism. When PYY is released into the bloodstream, this hormone travels to the hypothalamus, where it turns off neurons that stimulate hunger. These appetite-regulating hormones, their receptors, and mimics are the focus of current research to control obesity.

Food choices are based on many factors other than HUNGER, including state of physical and emotional health, cultural beliefs, food preferences, and economic status, among others. While socioeconomic factors affect which foods are chosen, biochemical mechanisms, including sugar consumption, nutrient deficiencies, exposure to toxic materials, and food sensitivities, help regulate the kinds of foods selected, the time of eating, and the amount of food consumed.

Sugar and Mood This is a controversial area. A variety of clinical studies suggest that sugar does not generally cause changes in mood or hyperactivity. Other studies and considerable anecdotal evidence suggest that in susceptible people, excessive sugar consumption can alter BLOOD SUGAR levels, change brain function and cause mood swings. Blood sugar may temporarily drop several hours after eating. Thus, a heavy lunch tends to exaggerate the afternoon slump, possibly because large meals apparently increase blood flow to the gut, away from the brain. A drop in blood sugar (HYPOGLYCEMIA) can cause irritability, depression, FATIGUE, and moodiness because the brain is exquisitely dependent on blood sugar to meet most of its energy needs.

Nutrient Deficiencies It is well established that vitamin and mineral deficiencies can have long-term effects on mood. Severe, chronic deficiencies of VITAMIN B_6, VITAMIN B_{12}, VITAMIN C, FOLIC ACID, and NIACIN can cause symptoms resembling SENILITY, DEPRESSION, and schizophrenia. However, these are complex illnesses that probably have multiple causes. To the extent that nutritional deficiencies contribute to mental disturbances, supplementing with vitamins can sometimes help alleviate symptoms. Experts stop short of claiming that vitamin supplements can cure mental illness. Indirect evidence links oxidative damage from free radicals to a decline in brain function with aging and with certain degenerative diseases of the nervous system. The implication is that antioxidants are essential for healthy brain function. In experimental animals, deficiencies in the above nutrients, as well as in IRON, COPPER, and ZINC, impair neurotransmitter synthesis. It is not clear to what extent subclinical deficiencies affect the brain and behavior. Some lines of research suggest that abnormal levels of copper and other minerals may predispose males to violent behavior.

Toxic Metals Exposure to HEAVY METALS can have many effects on the nervous system and behavior. As examples, too much CADMIUM can partially block the uptake of the essential trace mineral zinc. LEAD pollution lowers intelligence and scholastic performance, especially in younger children.

Food Sensitivities Traditionally, food sensitivities and allergies have not been considered important influences of behavior. However, evidence is accumulating that indicates food allergies can trigger mood swings, anxiety, and fatigue in susceptible individuals when the allergic attack focuses on the nervous system. Sensitivities to whole milk and other foods have been implicated in schizophrenia, depression, and aggressive behavior in some instances. (See also ALLERGY, FOOD; APPETITE; BULIMIA NERVOSA; FEINGOLD DIET; HUNGER.)

White, J. W., and M. Wolraich. "Effect of Sugar on Behavior and Mental Performance," *American Journal of Clinical Nutrition* 62, supp. (1995): 242S–249S.

Rosenthal, N. E. et al. "Psychobiological Effects of Carbohydrate- and Protein-Rich Meals in Patients with Seasonal Affective Disorder and Normal Controls," *Biological Psychiatry* 25 (1998): 1,029–1,040.

food banks Organizations that provide donated free food. Since the 1970s, many grassroots organizations have been established in the United States to help combat hunger in communities. Food can be donated by private citizens, large food distributors like supermarkets, and the U.S. Department of Agriculture (USDA). Surplus commodities like RICE, BUTTER, FLOUR, HONEY, CORNMEAL, and MILK have been provided free by the USDA, as specified by the Temporary Emergency Food Program of 1983. A food bank may be administered by a larger agency, offering a variety of services ranging from clothing assistance to pre-employment training. Eligibility requirements vary depending on the particular agency or organization. Typically, individuals and families needing assistance can obtain a sack of groceries several times a week.

food-borne arthritis Chronic joint inflammation and degeneration resulting from food poisoning due to the bacterium SALMONELLA (salmonellosis), one of the fastest growing food-borne illnesses. Salmonellosis can cause ARTHRITIS as a long-term side effect, as well as other chronic illnesses. In both the United States and Canada cases of salmonellosis have steadily increased since the 1970s. Salmonella bacteria cause an estimated 4 million cases of salmonellosis in the United States each year, and one in 10,000 of these people will develop reactive arthritis, a condition called Reiter's syndrome. (See also AUTOIMMUNE DISEASES; EGG; FOOD POISONING.)

food chain The linkage of the feeding habits of animals to each other and to the plants they consume. As the ultimate consumer of foods, humans are at the top of the food chain. Livestock, which live on grain and grasses, are slaughtered for human consumption. Carnivorous food fish, like tuna, live on small fish that, in turn, live on plankton.

The food-chain concept has several important ramifications: The higher up the food chain, the less efficiently a species uses the energy in food. According to the "10 percent rule," animals at each rung on the ecological ladder use approximately 10 percent of the energy trapped by life forms in a lower rung. In other words, cattle use about 10 percent of the energy trapped in GRAIN, and humans utilize only 10 percent of the energy trapped in BEEF. Thus, 3,000 calories of energy (gas, oil, cultivating, planting, harvesting, fertilizer, and PESTICIDES) are required to produce one pound of sweet corn, which contains the equivalent of 375 calories. A cow has to eat approximately 80 pounds of corn (representing 29,500 calories) to produce 5 ounces of beef, which then contributes 375 calories in a meal. By eating foods lower down on the food chain, people can conserve energy and resources like water because less of each is needed to produce plant foods. In terms of energy conservation and global awareness, a greater reliance on plant food will decrease the demands on the world's resources of water and fuel.

A second ramification of the food chain is that materials not effectively degraded by microorganisms in the environment tend to accumulate in plants and small organisms and therefore in the animals that eat them. In this way, pollutants can be passed up the food chain, to be concentrated in the species highest on the food chain, whether bird, carnivorous fish, or mammal, which are therefore the most susceptible to the toxic effects of accumulated pollutants. Falcons and hawks have been most damaged by DDT in their food supply. Ocean fish like swordfish and tuna are often contaminated with MERCURY, while walleye pike, a freshwater species, is contaminated with many industrial wastes. Scavengers like crabs and catfish are more likely to be contaminated when they consume foods that are laden with pollutants. Humans are especially vulnerable because of the consumption of many other species likely to possess high concentrations of fat-soluble waste chemicals that are poorly degraded and poorly excreted. As one consequence, nearly all Americans carry traces of CADMIUM, LEAD, and mercury, as well as pesticides, DIOXIN, PBB, PCB, and other chemicals in their tissues without having been directly exposed to these pollutants. (See also CHLORINATED HYDROCARBONS; HEAVY METALS.)

food coloring, natural Food colors are derived from plants, insects, and, historically, even minerals. Plant colorings approved by the U.S. FDA include ANNATTO, BETA-CAROTENE, PAPRIKA, SAFFRON, and TURMERIC. Their colors range from yellow to red. Caramel and roasted cottonseed flour create brown colors. Powdered algae, yellow corn oil, and tagetes (Aztec marigold) are added to chicken feed to yellow chicken skin and augment the color of egg yolk. Fruit JUICES and vegetable juices can be used to color foods. As examples, grape extract can be used to create purple-red foods, dehydrated beets contribute a dark red, while carrot oil and a related plant pigment CANTHAXANTHINE create orange-colored foods. Insect pigments appear rarely. Carmine comprises 10 percent of the extract of cochineal insects; about 2,000 pounds are used annually in the United States.

Certain inorganic compounds are approved by the U.S. FDA as coloring agents. Ferrous gluconate develops a black color in ripe OLIVES, and titanium oxide can be used up to 1 percent in foods as a whitener. Sodium NITRITE contributes pink color to processed meats like HOT DOGS and HAM and processed meat products, but it is considered a preservative.

Only about 5 percent of food coloring currently being used is derived from natural products. The rest represents artificial dyes, synthesized from petroleum products. Careful studies (lasting more than a year) have not been carried out on most of these plant-derived coloring agents. While there is no evidence so far that they are in any way harmful, the question of their long-term safety remains unanswered. (See also ARTIFICIAL FOOD COLORS; FOOD ADDITIVES.)

food combination Eating certain foods in combinations based on the belief that PROTEIN-rich foods should not be eaten with fruits, vegetables, or starchy foods. There is little evidence to support the contention that protein DIGESTION and CARBOHYDRATE digestion would interfere with each other. In the first place, most foods are mixtures of protein and carbohydrates, and normally the body is well suited to efficiently digesting both nutrients simultaneously. Both pancreatic AMYLASE and pancreatic proteolytic enzymes are secreted simultaneously. Carbohydrate consumed within four hours of protein can enhance protein breakdown and can provide raw materials for nonessential AMINO ACIDS that can help increase protein synthesis. In this respect, adequate supplies of dietary fuels, carbohydrates and FAT lower the dietary requirement for protein; consequently, amino acids from food protein are retained more effectively to be utilized in building new protein. For people with multiple food allergies or with maldigestion problems, there may be a benefit to following such guidelines.

food complementation Eating a variety of VEGETABLES, GRAINS, and LEGUMES in order to supply the body with the appropriate amounts of amino acids that it cannot make (essential amino acids). Individual plant foods are often deficient in one or more essential amino acid. When eating a variety of plant foods it is unnecessary to determine the amino acid composition or the grams of protein in each type of food, nor is it necessary to eat a mixture of protein sources with each meal. Simply eating generous portions of a variety of foods that represent each of the vegetables, legumes, and grains families each day assures an adequate supply of essential amino acids. (See also BIOLOGICAL VALUE; COMPLETE PROTEIN; VEGETARIAN.)

food composition data Tables prepared by the U.S. Department of Agriculture (USDA) defining the nutrient compositions of many foods. These tables describe the caloric content, the content of PROTEIN, CARBOHYDRATE, FIBER, and FAT together with the content of VITAMINS, MINERALS, and CHOLESTEROL. Typically, CALCIUM, IRON, MAGNESIUM, PHOSPHOROUS, POTASSIUM, SODIUM, and ZINC are included. These tables usually omit certain trace nutrients such as IODINE, COPPER, SELENIUM, and chromium.

Among water-soluble vitamins, THIAMIN, RIBOFLAVIN, NIACIN, VITAMIN B_6, FOLIC ACID, and VITAMIN C and one fat-soluble vitamin, vitamin A, are routinely listed. Other fat-soluble vitamins (VITAMIN D, VITAMIN K, and VITAMIN E) and certain water-soluble vitamins (VITAMIN B_{12}, BIOTIN, and PANTOTHENIC ACID) are omitted. The tables indicate the portion size, whether the food has been trimmed (edible portion) or whether the food is fresh or raw.

Many factors influence the reported nutrient values: mineral content in the soil in which the food was grown, method of processing, method of storage, genetic characteristics of the harvested plant, time of year the food was harvested, methods used for nutrient analysis, different moisture contents of the food, methods of cooking, and the like. Therefore, the nutrient data are close approximations, rather than exact values. (See also DIET RECORD.)

Food, Drug and Cosmetic Act (U.S.) The basic food law that gives the Food and Drug Administration (FDA) the responsibility for the safety of foods. The first Food and Drug Act (1906) was designed to prevent the use of toxic preservatives and dyes in foods and to regulate the safety of patent medicines. In 1927, the Food, Drug and Insecticide Administration was formed, which later became the Food and Drug Administration. In 1938 the Federal Food, Drug and Cosmetic Act broadened the scope of the 1906 act by including coverage of medical devices and cosmetics, and requirements for assuring the safety and efficacy of new drugs; by setting tolerances for unavoidable toxic materials in food; by setting standards of identification for certain foods; by authorizing food manufacturing and processing factory inspections and providing for court injunctions with regard to seizures and possession.

Three amendments strengthened this act. The Miller Pesticide Act (1954) provides for establishing safe tolerances for pesticides in raw agricultural products. The Food Additives Amendment (1958) requires premarketing clearance by the FDA for food additives; it includes the DELANEY CLAUSE, which made it illegal to add CANCER-causing chemicals to foods. The Color Additive Amendment (1960) regulates the certification of food colors. In 1958, the term "food additive" was legally defined to exclude

PESTICIDES, food colors, new animal drugs, and substances listed on the GENERALLY RECOGNIZED AS SAFE (GRAS) list. (See also CARCINOGEN; USDA.)

food fortification The addition of nutrients to foods without the intention of replacing nutrients lost in preparation. The added nutrient may or may not have been present in the original food. If normally present in the food, the amount of the nutrient added could be well above the amount found naturally. Often, the term *fortification* is used synonymously with *enrichment,* that is, addition of a nutrient to levels at or near the original food before processing. General criteria for a nutrient to be used in fortification are as follows:

> The consumption of the nutrient in question should be low in the diets of a significant number of people. The food to be fortified should be frequently consumed. The nutrient should be readily absorbed and it should not become inactive during processing and storage. It should not interfere with the nutrient qualities of the food. There should be no toxicity of the nutrient associated when an excess of the food is eaten. And the nutrient should not contribute to a nutritional imbalance.

Many new products are being fortified, including fruit juices (with calcium and vitamin C and other antioxidants), peanut butter (with vitamins and minerals), nonfat yogurt (with vitamins, minerals and lactic acid-producing bacteria), and a wide range of herbal products and beverages. Processed foods and synthetic beverages may be fortified and, at the same time, still be deficient in other nutrients. Enriched white bread contains added IRON, niacin, riboflavin, and thiamin, but lacks the VITAMIN B_6, MANGANESE, and FIBER found in the original food, for example. Whole, minimally processed foods are more nutritious options.

To improve health and minimize the risk of nutrient deficiencies, salt is generally fortified with IODINE (sodium iodide) at a level of 76 mcg iodine per g and MILK is fortified with VITAMIN A (50 IU per cup) and VITAMIN D (80 IU per cup). CALCIUM is now added to several juices and beverages. Iron is added to FLOUR and GRAIN products; otherwise, grains are poor sources of iron. Enriched white bread contains 0.7 mg iron per slice (25 g); enriched cornmeal, 1.1 mg per 25 g meal; enriched breakfast cereals, 4 to 11 mg per 25 g (1 cup). The U.S. FDA has mandated that folic acid be added to bread and grain products such as pasta, grits, breakfast cereals and rolls. All U.S. wheat, rice, and corn are fortified at a rate of 140 mcg per 100 g of grain. Iron is now added to so many products there is a concern that excessive dietary iron over the years might promote iron accumulation disease (HEMOCHROMATOSIS) in susceptible people, especially men. (See also ENRICHMENT; SODIUM.)

food grading A process used to classify foods according to standard criteria. Usually, sensory qualities are used, including flavor, texture, and appearance or color. A higher grade does not imply a higher nutritional content. As an example, maple syrup can be graded Fancy, Grade A, or Grade B. Grade B is the darkest and most strongly flavored. Graded food meets standards set by the U.S. Department of Agriculture (USDA) for MEAT and POULTRY products, while the National Marine Fisheries Service grades FISH and fish produce similarly. USDA grades are not based on nutritional content. MILK and milk products generally carry a "Grade A" label, based on FDA recommended sanitary standards for milk production and processing. This grade does not refer to nutrient content, though the FDA requires specific levels of VITAMIN A and VITAMIN D for certain milk products.

food guide pyramid A food guide plan released in 1991 by the USDA. It is designed to replace the "Basic Four Food Groups," in use since 1956. The pyramid attempts to demonstrate graphically the relative importance of food groups as layers on a pyramid. Minimal daily servings are given. At the bottom of the pyramid are GRAINS, including BREAD, CEREAL, RICE, and PASTA (9 to 11 servings). The next layer up consists of VEGETABLES (3 to 5 servings) and FRUITS (2 to 4 servings). By depicting produce and grains as the dietary foundation, the federal government is moving away from viewing MEAT as the dietary foundation, as it was in the old four food groups. The larger areas also stress foods that have less fat. Recommended consumption of fruits and vegetables is therefore a minimum of 5 servings daily. In 1993 less than 10 percent to 20 per-

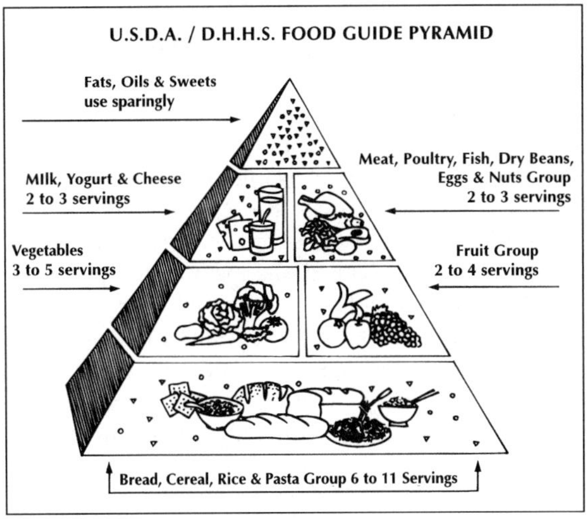

cent of the U.S. population ate this much. The third layer up consists of dairy products: MILK, YOGURT, and CHEESE (2 to 3 servings for men and 3 to 4 servings for women) and red meat, POULTRY, and FISH. Included is another group of high-protein foods: dry BEANS, EGGS, and NUTS (2 to 3 servings). The peak of the pyramid, covering the smallest area, indicates food items to be used sparingly: FAT, oils, sweets, ALCOHOL, BUTTER, MARGARINE, CANDY, cookies, cakes, and SOFT DRINKS.

The old Basic Four guide considered only PROTEIN, CALCIUM, THIAMIN, NIACIN, RIBOFLAVIN, VITAMIN A, and VITAMIN C as "leader NUTRIENTS." The belief was that when people consumed enough of these nutrients, the consumption of more than 40 other nutrients would also be adequate. As early as 1974, it was shown that DIETS based on the Basic Four were low in many key trace nutrients. The importance of fiber in the diet was not acknowledged in the Basic Four, nor was that guide designed to prevent overnutrition. A high-fat, low-fiber diet is linked to increased risk of HEART DISEASE and may be linked to the most common cancers unrelated to smoking: prostate, breast, and colon.

Vegetarians should note that a food pyramid for vegetarians emphasizes fresh fruits and vegetables as well as whole grain breads and cereals. Nuts and seeds, legumes, low-fat dairy products, fortified soy substitutes, and limited eggs are the recommended protein sources. Consumption of a good food source of ascorbic acid with meals will further enhance absorption of available iron. Those whose nutrient needs are especially high due to growth, pregnancy, lactation, or recovery from illness can generally meet their nutrient requirements on well planned vegetarian diets containing dairy products.

Vegan or veganlike diets that exclude animal products can be healthy as long as they include adequate amounts of vitamin D, trace minerals such as zinc and iron, and vitamin B_{12}. If, however, intake of these nutrients is not sufficient to meet the recommended daily allowance, supplements may be necessary.

There are several caveats attached to the food guide pyramid. The USDA's first edition poster depicted PEAS and LENTILS together with high-fat foods like meats. Although they provide protein, LEGUMES are low-fat foods that are rich in fiber and should not be classified as fats, nor should they be restricted because of fat content. The serving size is not clear; potato represents two servings, while a slice of bread counts as a single serving.

The food guide pyramid is based on the 1990 DIETARY GUIDELINES FOR AMERICANS, which recommends decreasing fat consumption to less than 30 percent of daily calories. Many nutritionists recommend that less than 25 percent of food calories should be derived from fats and oils. It may well be that no more than 20 percent of total calories should come from fat for maximum protection from chronic disease. Furthermore, non-animal sources of calcium can provide extra calcium, and they may be more beneficial than high-fat dairy products. (See also GLYCEMIC INDEX.)

Achterberg, C., E. McDonnell, and R. Bagby. "How to put the Food Guide Pyramid into practice," *Journal of the American Dietetic Association,* 94, no. 9 (September 1994): 1,030–1,035.

food handling and public health Foods that are extensively handled and are not thoroughly reheated before serving represent possible health hazards. Most items in kitchens are not sterile, and manipulation of food will contribute to the risk of food contamination. For example, handlers of raw MEAT and animal products may be asymptomatic carriers of bacteria and viruses that can cause disease. Staphyloccal infections can be spread easily because they occur frequently in the nose and skin. Many disease-producing microorganisms are transmitted by fecal contamination; HEPATITIS A outbreaks in restaurants have been traced to poor personal hygiene of employees. Food handlers with gastric enteritis caused by salmonellosis can spread this disease because of the increased risk of fecal organism contamination with DIARRHEA. Careful attention to personal cleanliness, the use of disposable gloves, separate work areas and personnel to handle raw and cooked foods, rigorous cleaning schedules and disinfectant procedures can minimize microbial contamination. (See also FOOD POISONING.)

food interactions See DRUG/NUTRIENT INTERACTION.

food intolerance Physiologic reactions to foods that can be the result of toxins, metabolic diseases, or enzyme deficiencies. There are two broad categories of food intolerances: those based on a response of the IMMUNE SYSTEM and those independent of the immune system. In the former situation, food-derived molecules can trigger an allergic reaction and activate the immune system. Food allergens can be absorbed by the intestine if it is inflamed and if the protective mucosal barrier is inadequate. True food allergy attacks can be immediate (immediate onset food allergy) or delayed (delayed onset food allergy), with symptoms occurring hours after exposure to the provoking substance.

Food intolerances not regulated by the immune system include the following types of situations. Avoidance of the provoking substance(s) is important in recovery from this form of food intolerance.

- Reactions to FOOD ADDITIVES, such as ARTIFICIAL FOOD COLORS (e.g., FD&C yellow No. 5), MONOSODIUM GLUTAMATE (MSG), and SULFITES.
- Reactions based on natural substances that behave as drugs. Some substances affect blood vessels (vasoactive amines) and mimic hormones. Examples are tryptamine and TYRAMINE (in aged cheese and cured meats); phenylethylamine (in CHOCOLATE); HISTAMINE and amines (in red WINE, oranges, plums, pineapples, and tomatoes). Other active substances are methylxanthines such as CAFFEINE (in COFFEE, TEA, colas, chocolate, and COCOA). These can cause headache, palpitations, anxiety, or vomiting.
- Reactions based on a metabolic imbalance or a metabolic defect (enzyme deficiency) or altered body chemistry. LACTOSE INTOLERANCE due to a deficiency of LACTASE, the enzyme responsible for digesting milk sugar, is the most common of this type. PHENYLKETONURIA is an example of an inherited metabolic disease based upon an intolerance of PHENYLALANINE due to a deficiency of an enzyme required to degrade this amino acid. Sugar sensitivity or HYPOGLYCEMIA are metabolically based conditions that may reflect hormonal imbalances.
- Reactions classified as FOOD POISONING. Bacterial toxins (BOTULISM) and mold toxins (AFLATOXIN) are possible causes. (See also ALLERGY, FOOD; ALLERGY, IMMEDIATE; ELIMINATION DIET; ENTEROTOXIN.)

food irradiation Sterilization of food using radiation. The intent of food irradiation is to extend the shelf life of a food and to kill potentially dangerous microorganisms and insects. Another advantage is that irradiation can also delay ripening and inhibit sprouting of POTATOES and WHEAT. Food irradiation in the United States is currently approved for SPICES, WHEAT, fresh FRUIT like strawberries, fresh vegetables including POTATOES, PORK, fresh poultry and frozen, uncooked poultry, meat, medical supplies, and some drugs. Irradiation of chickens is permitted in order to kill salmonella bacteria, which can cause food poisoning. Irradiated foods are required to be labeled as such; the warning symbol is a floral emblem. Prepared foods do not need to be labeled, though they may have been irradiated. Presently, no law requires labeling fast foods.

Proponents argue that irradiation could replace post-harvest PESTICIDES on fruit and vegetables and reduce the threat of salmonella food poisoning in CHICKEN. However, irradiation is turning out to be more expensive and sometimes less effective than predicted. The only foods being irradiated worldwide are GRAINS (eastern Europe) and potatoes (Japan). Irradiated food does not become radioactive, though it may be exposed to radioactive elements. The irradiation process breaks up molecules in pests as well as in the food itself, and VITAMIN C and VITAMIN E plus THIAMIN are thus destroyed. The high doses of radiation required to kill pests create new substances (called radiolytic products) from the production of molecular fragments (free radicals). The radiolytic products are potential CARCINOGENS, and critics of irradiation argue that not enough testing has been done to establish long-term safety of irradiated food.

The presently permitted irradiation dose does not completely sterilize grains and nuts, thus leaving them susceptible to potentially dangerous molds when stored for extended periods. Opponents of food irradiation contend that the salmonella problems should be corrected through more sanitary processing in slaughterhouses and meat-packing facilities. On the other hand, food irradiation is endorsed by the World Health Organization, the American Dietetic Association, and the U.S. National Academy of Sciences, which believe the production of harmful chemicals is negligible. (See also FOOD PROCESSING.)

Olson, D. G. "Irradiation of Food," *Food Technology* 52 (1998): 56–62.

food labeling Consumer information required by the U.S. FDA and the FOOD SAFETY AND INSPECTION SERVICES for about 90 percent of processed foods. Nutrition labeling and nutrient lists are required of most foods regulated by the FDA, excluding restaurant foods and foods served for immediate consumption on airplanes, in hospitals and by food service vendors; deli and bakery goods prepared on-site; foods sold in bulk and not for resale; foods produced by small businesses; medical foods, such as those designed for specific patient needs; plain coffee and tea; and products for export. Foods in small packages (less than 12 sq. in., such as a candy bar 1-in. thick, 2 in. wide and 6 in. long) need not have nutrition information unless a nutritional claim is made. Labeling for meat and poultry products is regulated by the U.S. Department of Agriculture (USDA).

The new food label in place as of 1994 features an improved nutrition panel called "Nutrition Facts." Serving sizes are more consistent than before and are stated in household and metric units, based on the amount customarily eaten at a given time. Reference amounts are broken down into 139 categories regulated by the FDA and 23 meat and poultry categories (regulated by the USDA). For example, cookies have a reference amount of 30 g; for breads it is 50 g. The top of the food label provides the number of servings per container and the total number of calories, as well as the calories derived from FAT. One of the most useful features is a listing of how much sodium, fat, CHOLESTEROL, fiber, sugar, and other nutrients as a percentage of the daily allotment is in a serving.

Food labeling

Nutrition Facts	Amount/serving	% DV*	Amount/serving	% DV*
Serv. Size 1/3 cup (56gf)	Total Fat 1g	2%	Total Carb. 0g	0%
Servings about 3	Sat Fat 0g	0%	Fiber 0g	Ê0%
Calories 80	Cholest. 10mg	3%	Sugars 0g	
Fat Cal. 10	Sodium 200mg	8%	Protein 17g	
*Percent Daily Values (DV) are based on a 2,000 calorie diet.	Vitamin A 0%•Vitamin C 0%•Calcium 0%•Iron 6%			

Nutrition Facts

Serving size 1 can (360mL)

Amount Per Serving	
Calories 140	
	%Daily Value*
Total Fat 0g	0%
Sodium 20mg	1%
Total Carbohydrate 36g	12%
Sugars 36 g	
Protein 0g	0%

*Percent Daily Values are based on a 2,000 calorie diet.

The new mandatory components (underlined) are listed below in the order in which they must appear, together with certain permitted voluntary components.

- <u>total calories</u>
- <u>calories from fat</u>
- calories from saturated fat
- <u>total fat</u>
- saturated fat
- polyunsaturated fat
- monounsaturated fat
- <u>cholesterol</u>
- <u>sodium</u>
- potassium

- total carbohydrate
- dietary fiber
- soluble fiber
- insoluble fiber
- sugars
- sugar alcohol (for example, the sugar substitutes xylitol, mannitol, and sorbitol)
- other carbohydrate (the difference between total carbohydrate and the sum of dietary fiber, sugars, and sugar alcohol, if declared)
- protein
- vitamin A
- percent vitamin A represented by beta-carotene
- vitamin C
- calcium
- iron
- other essential vitamins and minerals may be listed.

If a claim is made about any of the optional components as to health benefits, or if a food is fortified or enriched with them, nutrition information for these components is required.

Amounts in grams are listed both in terms of grams (or milligrams) and as a percent of the Daily Value (DV), based on the amounts supplied by a typical daily diet supplying 2,000 calories. Certain variations of the format are mandatory. For example, to prevent parents from restricting fat intake for young children, the labels for foods for children under two years of age cannot list information on fat or calorie content. (Rules for labeling infant formulas are covered under a separate act, the Infant Formula Act of 1980.) Food labels for children under four such as infant formulas and baby foods cannot list Daily Values or percentages for calories, fat, protein, and carbohydrate because they have not been determined for such young children, although Daily Values for vitamins and minerals is permissible.

Packaged foods must list the common (generic) name of the product such as spaghetti or chicken soup; the name and address of the manufacturer, distributor or packer, and net contents. Standards of identity (standard recipes long in use and approved by the FDA) exist for 300 or so staples like catsup, mayonnaise, ice cream, peanut butter, salt, sweeteners, and preservatives, and their contents need not be listed.

Sometimes, the daily values are maximum levels; the daily value for fat is 65 grams or less. Other values are minimums; the daily value for carbohydrates is equal to 300 g or more.

Three categories of claims can be used on foods and dietary supplement labels:

- Health claims. These describe a relationship between a food substance and a disease or health-related condition.
- Structure/function claims for supplements. These may claim a benefit related to a nutrient deficiency disease (like vitamin C and scurvy). However, the claim must also state how widespread the disease is in the United States. Structure/function claims can also describe how a nutrient or dietary ingredient affects a structure or function in humans. For example, "Calcium builds strong bones." They can also describe how a nutrient or dietary ingredient acts to maintain a structure or function. For example, "Fiber maintains bowel regularity." Alternatively, they may simply say the nutrient provides general well-being.
- Nutrient content claims. These describe the level of a nutrient or dietary substance in the product, such as "good source," "high," or "free."

The responsibility for ensuring the validity of these claims rests with the manufacturer, the FDA, or, in the case of advertising, the Federal Trade Commission.

Terminology

Certain terms on food labels presently have no legal meaning: "natural," "dietetic," "health food." Other terms are now defined by the FDA and the USDA:

1. High: High indicates a benefit to the consumer by providing more than 20 percent of the amount of a given nutrient recommended for daily eating (daily value), as in "high protein."
2. Good Source: This term indicates a given food is beneficial in providing 10 percent to 19 percent of the amount of the daily value per serving.
3. Light: A food labeled light contains one-third fewer calories than a comparable food. When

used otherwise, light must specify its reference to look, taste, or smell, as in "light in color."

4. More: Indicates that a food has at least 10 percent more of the nutrient than a comparable food.
5. Fresh: Raw food. Refers to food that has never been frozen, processed, or preserved.
6. Lean: Per 100 g lean, cooked meat or poultry contains less than 10 g of fat (less than 4 g of saturated fat) and less than 95 mg of cholesterol.
7. Extra Lean: Extra-lean cooked meat or poultry contains less than 5 g of fat (and less than 2 g of saturated fat) and less than 95 mg of cholesterol per 100 g.
8. Imitation: Both the FDA and the USDA require that a product be labeled "imitation" if it contains an ingredient making it nutritionally inferior to the product with the traditional ingredient. Taking pizza as an example, the FDA requires that if the product uses less than 100 percent real cheese, it must be labeled imitation.

The following illustrate definitions for "free," "reduced," "low," and "less" as they pertain to sugar, calories, fat, cholesterol, sodium, and fiber—as provided by the FDA Consumer Special Report, "Focus on Food Labeling" (May 1993).

Sugar

- "Sugar free": less than 0.5 g per serving.
- "No added sugar," "Without added sugar," "No sugar added":

1. No sugars added during processing or packing, including ingredients that contain sugars (for example, fruit juices, apple sauce or dried fruit).
2. Processing does not increase the sugar content above the amount naturally present in the ingredients. (A functionally insignificant increase in sugars is acceptable from processes used for purposes other than increasing sugar content.)
3. The food that it resembles and for which it substitutes normally contains added sugars.

- "Reduced sugar": at least 25 percent less sugar per serving than reference food.

Calories

- "Calorie free": fewer than 5 calories per serving.
- "Low calorie": 40 calories or less per serving or, if the serving is 30 g or less or 2 tablespoons or less, per 50 g of the food.
- "Reduced calories" or "Fewer calories": at least 25 percent fewer calories per serving than reference food.

Fat

- "Fat free": less than 0.5 g of fat per serving.
- "Saturated fat free": less than 0.5 g per serving and the level of trans-fatty acids does not exceed 1 percent of total fat.
- "Low fat": 3 g or less per serving, or if the serving is 30 g, or less or 2 tablespoons or less, per 50 g of the food.
- "Low saturated fat": 1 g or less per serving and not more than 15 percent of calories from saturated fatty acids.
- "Reduced fat" or "Less fat": at least 25 percent less per serving than reference food.
- "Reduced saturated fat" or "Less saturated fat": at least 25 percent less per serving than reference food.

Cholesterol

- "Cholesterol free": less than 2 mg of cholesterol and 2 g or less of saturated fat per serving.
- "Low cholesterol": 20 mg or less and 2 g or less of saturated fat per serving or, if the serving is 30 g or less or 2 tablespoons or less, per 50 g of the food.
- "Reduced cholesterol" or less cholesterol: at least 25 percent less and 2 g or less of saturated fat per serving than reference food.

Sodium

- "Sodium free": less than 5 mg per serving.
- "Low sodium": 140 mg or less per serving or, if the serving is 30 g or less or 2 tablespoons or less, per 50 g of the food.
- "Very low sodium": 35 mg or less per serving or, if the serving is 30 g or less or 2 tablespoons or less, per 50 g of the food.
- "Reduced sodium" or "Less sodium": at least 25 percent less per serving than reference food.

Fiber

- "High fiber": 5 g or more per serving. (Foods making high-fiber claims must meet the definition for low-fat, or the level of total fat must appear next to the high-fiber claim.)

- "Good source of fiber": 2.5 g to 4.9 g per serving.
- "More fiber" or "Added fiber": at least 2.5 g more per serving than reference food.

The number of grams of fat and of saturated fat are listed. The phrase "partially hydrogenated" can designate any vegetable oil that is from 5 percent to 60 percent saturated. Unfortunately, few foods indicate the percentage of total calories derived from fat. This is vital information in terms of nutritionists' recommendations that fat contribute a maximum of 30 percent of calories, and that saturated fat contribute no more than 10 percent of calories.

Tips for Reading a Food Label

If the first ingredient listed on the label is VEGETABLE OIL or SUGAR, the food is very high in calories. If the food label contains several alternative names for refined sugar—DEXTROSE, FRUCTOSE, high FRUCTOSE CORN SYRUP, SUCROSE, malt sugar, maltose, HONEY—it is a high-sugar food. The phrase "made with pure vegetable oil" may mask the fact that the food is made with COCONUT OIL or PALM OILS, vegetable oils that are more saturated than BUTTER and lard. SATURATED FAT is a suspected cause of HEART DISEASE. To minimize intake of a given potential problem ingredient, a rule of thumb is to avoid any product listing that particular ingredient among the first five additives.

Food containers and wrappers often provide other types of information that do not deal with nutrient content, such as FOOD GRADING, product dating, and universal bar codes.

Product Dating Four kinds of dating are used for perishable foods and milk and dairy products. "Pack date" refers to the day the food was manufactured, processed, or packaged. "Pull" or "sell date" is the last date on which the product should be sold, assuming proper storage and handling. MILK, YOGURT, ice cream, and cold cuts are examples of food with pull dates. "Expiration dates" define the last date the food should be eaten; infant formulas display "use by" dates. A "freshness date" resembles an expiration date, but baked goods can still be used after the freshness date. While safe and wholesome, the food beyond the freshness date might not taste as good as the fresh product. Generally, product dating is not regulated by the FDA.

Universal Product Code (UPC) A bar code, a block of parallel lines of various widths, with numbers, that appears on most food labels. Each code designation is unique to a given product. Stores equipped with computerized checkout can read these codes and automatically record sales. Together with a computerized system, UPC functions as an automatic inventory system to follow the rate of sales and reordering data. The universal product code is not regulated by the FDA. (See also FOOD ADDITIVES; FOOD GRADING; PESTICIDES.)

Food and Drug Administration. "Claims That Can Be Made for Conventional Foods and Dietary Supplements," Washington, D.C. (2001).

Kurtzweil, Paula. "Answers to Consumer Questions about the Food Label," *FDA Consumer* 29, no. 5 (June 1995): 6–9.

food poisoning Diseases caused by microorganisms that are transmitted through food. Estimates of food-borne gastroenteritis (irritation of the stomach and intestines often accompanied by vomiting and diarrhea) range from 33 million to 81 million annually, depending on the estimates of unreported cases. Bacteria, viruses, fungi, worms, and protozoa are major causes of food-borne disease throughout the world. Disease-producing organisms are usually transmitted by the oral-fecal route, generally through contamination of food and water. Most food poisoning in the United States is caused by bacteria, which can produce toxins rather than cause infections. Food inherently contains bacteria unless sterilized, but bacteria can also be introduced from external factors, such as soil, dust, poor sanitary habits, inadequate hygiene, household pets, and insects.

Microbial contamination causes problems in foods that are not cooked long enough or are handled improperly after cooking. Heating food destroys most viruses and bacteria; however, bacteria can rapidly multiply in food left at room temperature or kept warm. Refrigeration slows bacterial growth, while freezing prevents it. If food is left unattended for a long enough time, certain bacteria will produce very toxic substances that may not be destroyed by heating (or freezing).

The following are prominent examples of possible microbial contamination of food:

Salmonellosis The bacterium SALMONELLA can contaminate raw or undercooked beef or poultry and foods coming into contact with them or their juices, as well as raw or undercooked eggs. Since salmonella is spread by fecal contamination, inadequate hygiene by food handlers increases the risk. Symptoms (nausea, vomiting, cramps, chills) usually begin within 12 to 48 hours. Salmonellosis can be fatal to children, elderly persons and those with low immunity.

Shigellosis The bacterium *Shigella* can contaminate foods handled by an infected person with poor hygiene, or foods undercooked or stored at room temperature. Symptoms (nausea, bloody stools) appear in one to seven days. Shigellosis can be serious in elderly people, infants, and those with lowered immunity.

Infectious Hepatitis (Type A) The hepatitis virus type A can contaminate food handled by infected food handlers and shellfish contaminated by raw sewage. Symptoms (jaundice, liver damage) appear in 15 to 50 days. This disease can be fatal.

Escherichia Coli 0157:H7 Can cause hemmorhagic colitis and hemolytic uremic syndrome. This strain of *E. coli* is linked to contaminated raw or undercooked meat and to contaminated beverages. Symptoms include bloody diarrhea, severe abdominal cramping, and kidney damage. The disease can cause permanent kidney damage and death in young children.

Staphylococcal Food Poisoning The bacterium *Staphyloccus* contaminates food that has been handled under unsanitary conditions and by infected food handlers, especially those with skin infections. It may be present in foods like potato or tuna salad. Symptoms (nausea, diarrhea, abdominal cramping, vomiting) can begin in one to eight hours.

Parahemolytic Food Poisoning Species of the bacterium *Vibrio* may contaminate fish and shellfish exposed to raw sewage. Symptoms (abdominal pain, diarrhea, headache, chills, bloody stools) can begin in 15 to 24 hours.

Viral Gastroenteritis Intestinal viruses (rotaviruses, enteroviruses, Norwalk virus, parvovirus) can contaminate foods processed by infected food handlers. These viruses also occur in shellfish contaminated by raw sewage. Symptoms (vomiting, nausea, diarrhea) occur in 12 to 48 hours.

Campylobacteriosis The bacterium *Campylobacter* can contaminate meat and poultry and by fecal exposure in packing plants. Typical sources are undercooked or raw beef, poultry, shellfish, and untreated water. Symptoms (fever, diarrhea, bloody stools, cramps) can begin within two to five days.

Perfringens Food Poisoning The bacterium *Clostridium perfringens* can contaminate foods that are slowly cooled or held at room temperature too long. Typically, these are meat and poultry dishes that are covered or wrapped with limited exposure to air. Symptoms (diarrhea, abdominal pain, nausea, vomiting) are usually mild and begin in eight to 24 hours.

Botulism The bacterium *Clostridium botulinum* can contaminate improperly cooked low-acid foods, like green beans or corn, that are home cooked. It also can grow in potatoes covered with butter or oil and left at room temperature for too long a period. This bacterium produces an extremely powerful nerve toxin that causes double vision, difficult breathing, and in extreme cases, death. Symptoms begin within eight to 36 hours.

Worms Parasites that are found in fish (causing clonorchiasis, opisthochiasis) and pork (causing TRICHINOSIS, cysticercosis, balantidiasis), among others.

Seafood Poisoning SCROMBOID poisoning is an example of fish poisoning; shellfish poisoning can be the result of red tide contamination.

Suggestions for Preventing Food Poisoning

1. Wash hands with soap before preparing food. Use a fresh dish towel. Many food-borne illnesses are due to fecal contamination.
2. Assume that all raw meat, fish, and poultry are contaminated. Do not mix raw meat (especially HAMBURGER, PORK, and roast beef) with fresh vegetables. Do not use the same cutting board, sponges, or utensils for raw meat and fresh vegetables. Do not use the same utensils or even the same kitchen sponge for both raw meat and cooked meat. This can reintroduce bacteria into the cooked meat.
3. Cook food thoroughly. Meat should not be pink and juice should run gray. Freeze or refrigerate leftovers, particularly any food that is wrapped or coated with breading. Refrigerator temperature

should be kept below 40° F. Do not leave food at room temperature for more than one hour.

4. Thaw meat or poultry in the refrigerator, microwave, or in cold running water rather than at room temperature.
5. Do not stuff a turkey ahead of roasting time and then refrigerate it. This could allow time for disease-producing bacteria to multiply. Stuff the bird and cook it immediately.
6. Marinate meat and poultry in the refrigerator rather than at room temperature.

Schardt, David, and Stephen Schmidt. "Keeping Food Safe," *Nutrition Action Healthletter* 22, no. 3 (April 1995): 4–7.

food preservation Strategies to preserve food and prevent spoilage. Common methods include DEHYDRATION, ANTIOXIDANTS, PRESERVATIVES, FERMENTATION, refrigeration, freezing, and heat processing.

Dehydration This is an ancient method of food preservation. The removal of water from foods deprives microorganisms of an environment suitable for their growth. Heat is used to dehydrate fruit, herbs, milk, meat, and fish. To better maintain nutrients, foods may be freeze-dried. In this process, water is removed by evaporation from foods that have been rapidly frozen and maintained at low temperature and low pressure. Restricted exposure to air helps to prevent oxidation of sensitive nutrients in dehydrated foods. Therefore dehydrated foods are sealed against air and moisture.

Antioxidants To control oxidation, a wide variety of substances can be added to foods. ANTIOXIDANTS prevent the reaction of oxygen with sensitive materials in foods. Thus, they reduce rancidity and increase product shelf life. Butylated hydroxytoluene (BHT), butylated hydroxyanisole (BHA) and VITAMIN C (ascorbic acid) delay browning and preserve color and freshness of foods.

Preservatives Compounds such as CALCIUM PROPIONATE, SODIUM BENZOATE, sodium NITRATE, SODIUM chloride, and SULFITES retard microbial growth in many processed foods.

Fermentation Fermented foods are generally more stable than unfermented ones. Mold and bacteria can produce LACTIC ACID, ethanol or other substances that inhibit microbial degradation. CHEESE, YOGURT, kefir, and BUTTERMILK are more stable than fresh milk.

Pickling Pickling involves the addition of vinegar, salt and spices to vegetables (like cucumbers), fish (pickled herring), or meat.

Refrigeration Freezing and refrigeration slow the reaction of food constituents with oxygen and with enzymes in foods themselves. Lowered temperatures also retard microbial proliferation and prevent spoilage.

Cooking Heat processing destroys microorganisms and can destroy endogenous ENZYMES that would alter food quality. BLANCHING destroys surface microorganisms and inactivates enzymes that could change their color, flavor, or nutritive value. PASTEURIZATION inactivates a portion of the microorganisms present in MILK and delays spoiling. Sterilization requires heating foods at 100° C to 120° C in order to destroy bacterial spores. Heat will cause the loss of certain nutrients like FOLIC ACID and vitamin C, depending on the temperature and duration of heating.

food processing Methods used to preserve and to prepare agricultural and livestock products as foods. Historically, food processors have emphasized safety, convenience, and acceptability, and there is a growing awareness of nutritive value as a major quality. "Minimally processed" foods are treated by routine kitchen procedures only, including slicing, mixing, chilling, freezing, drying, grinding, mincing, and cooking procedures such as boiling, braising, or baking.

Industrial preservation methods include refrigerating, freezing or chilling, drying, fermentation as in pickling, adding chemical preservatives as in salting or curing, and more recent innovations such as freeze-drying. Food technology also incorporates procedures such as blanching (short-term heating), extracting, fractionating (separating into fractions), and extruding (pushing through a small hole).

Advantages of Food Processing

Food processing helps prevent food from spoiling and packaging reduces losses from insects and rodents during storage. Food preservation prevents food from deteriorating quickly and seems essential in order to provide an adequate food supply throughout the year in all regions of America.

Some processing procedures improve food safety: Adding preservatives and antioxidants to foods and pasteurizing beverages are examples. Canned goods must be heated rigorously to destroy all microorganisms, though this destroys some vitamins. Sometimes processing destroys antinutrient factors. As an example, heating soybeans and other beans destroys a trypsin inhibitor, a protein that blocks the action of a digestive enzyme. Processed foods may require less meal preparation time, an important consideration for anyone attempting to save time and effort.

CONVENIENCE FOODS are either partially or completely prepared before sale. They need not be low in nutrients if made primarily from basic ingredients. On the other hand, some convenience foods do not equate with home-prepared foods. Certain prepared dinners have been found to be low in THIAMIN, VITAMIN B_6, and VITAMIN E. Reheated frozen TV dinners tend to be low in folic acid. The concern among nutritionists is that American children may associate salty, sweet, and high-fat foods with good taste and good diet.

Fabricated foods are either imitations or completely new food forms. TEXTURIZED VEGETABLE PROTEIN, fish protein (powder), modified STARCH, corn sweeteners, sodium CASEIN (milk protein), COCONUT OIL, and PALM OIL are combined in a myriad of innovative ways to create foods ranging from nondairy creamer, nondairy imitation cheese, imitation whipped cream, imitation pecans, breakfast bars, and a host of sweets and synthetic drinks. Some fabricated foods are designated "food analogs" designed to imitate a natural food. Meat analogs are made from extruded soy protein or other texturized vegetable protein. In animal feeding experiments, engineered foods, which by chemical analysis seem nutritionally equivalent to conventional foods, may be inferior in some cases.

When a food is made to resemble a familiar or conventional food, the U.S. FDA requires that it be labeled "imitation" unless the food is nutritionally equivalent to the original in all respects except fat and caloric content. If the fabricated food contains as much vitamins, minerals, and protein as the food it resembles, the food can be given a new descriptive name, although it need not contain real foods such as apples, blueberries, or lemon. The term "formulated food" usually applies to food that is designed for a specific need; INFANT FORMULAS are a well-known example. Such products find use in hospitals for total or supplemental feedings, such as liquid diet formulations.

Disadvantages of Food Processing

Most controversy has centered on highly refined or highly processed foods. Although some food processing methods improve nutritional quality, loss of some nutrients frequently occurs during processing. The degree and type of processing influences the extent of losses. Compare a baked potato with a fabricated potato chip, which has been cooked, mashed, dehydrated, rehydrated, mixed with additives, shaped, and fried. The final product is a popular snack food low in nutrient density and high in fat and salt. Additives are commonplace in highly processed foods. Salt is usually used for added flavor, far in excess of the amount used in home cooking. Because consumers become accustomed to the taste of highly salted commercially prepared foods, they may come to view home cooking as bland.

Added sugar sweetens foods, making them more appealing to consumer's sweet tooths, and increases the ease of processing in some instances. The sugar content of commercially processed foods can be needlessly high. Popular dry BREAKFAST CEREALS can be 50 percent sugar; even canned fruit may be packed in syrup. Furthermore, a product can be high in refined sugar although the word "sugar" does not appear on the food label. Thus DEXTROSE, maltodextrins, CORN SYRUP, corn syrup solids, high FRUCTOSE CORN SYRUP, HONEY, corn sweeteners, and MOLASSES on a food label all indicate that refined sugar has been added to the food. Fat is added to create pleasant textures and taste in cookies, crisp snack foods like CHIPS and CRACKERS, muffins, and even granola. The added fat is likely to be saturated or hydrogenated for stability and extended shelf life. (See also FOOD ADDITIVES; FOOD LABELING.)

Food Safety and Inspection Service (FSIS) A regulatory arm of the U.S. Department of Agriculture (USDA), its mission is to protect the public by ensuring that meat, poultry, and egg products are safe, wholesome, and accurately labeled. Under the authority of the Federal Meat Inspection Act, the Poultry Products Inspection Act, and the Egg Products Inspection Act, the FSIS regulates the inspection of all meat, poultry, and egg products sold in interstate commerce and reinspects imports to ensure their safety. Annually, the FSIS conducts reviews of inspection systems in foreign countries that can import meat and poultry products to the United States to ensure they are as stringent as are those in the United States. The agency is also responsible for setting requirements for meat and poultry labels. Following reports of foodborne health hazards and diseases, the FSIS works with the Centers for Disease Control and Prevention in conducting epidemiological investigations.

food sensitivity Any negative physiologic reaction to a food. Food sensitivity is the broadest category of responses to foods and includes both physiological and psychological causes.

Food sensitivities include two broad categories: food intolerances, which do not involve the immune system, and food allergies, which reflect reactions of the immune system.

Food sensitivities can cause a variety of symptoms such as abdominal pain and alternating diarrhea and constipation resembling IRRITABLE BOWEL SYNDROME. Typical examples include sensitivity to MOLDS or to certain added chemicals in foods; the inability to digest foods; psychological disorders relating to food (such as bulimia and anorexia nervosa); and conditioned responses to food.

Food Sensitivity

The following are considered common food sensitivities:

Lactose Intolerance The most common food intolerance is due to the inability to digest milk sugar (lactose). Although infants and young children produce the enzyme needed to degrade lactose, production declines in many adults, so that mild sugar in dairy products and processed foods can overwhelm the digestive tract. Colonic fermentation produces gas and diarrhea in many Asians, African Americans, and people of Mediterranean heritage.

MSG (Monosodium Glutamate) Sensitivity (MSG Related Syndrome) Some people react to large amounts of this flavor enhancer added to prepared foods in Chinese and Italian restaurant cooking. MSG-related syndrome ("Chinese restaurant syndrome") may involve a burning sensation and chest pain. MSG is a component of hydrolyzed vegetable protein, also used as a flavor enhancer.

Sensitivity to Red Wine Susceptible people can get headaches after drinking red wine. The cause is not clear; possibly tannins, complex pigments from grape skins, may trigger a reaction.

Sensitivities to Artificial Food Coloring and Preservatives People who are sensitive to FD&C Yellow #5 food coloring are often sensitive to aspirin. Some parents report that reducing these substances in the diet relieves symptoms associated with hyperactivity. Sulfites can trigger reactions in susceptible people. Sulfites are found in certain preserved foods like sauerkraut and dried fruit and wine.

The diagnosis of food sensitivities is the first step. There are several time-honored strategies to pinpoint cause and effect, including a complete medical history and food or diet diaries. A challenge test involves introducing a suspected food after avoiding it for several weeks and noting any subsequent reactions. Optimally, neither the patient nor the health care provider knows the identity of the challenge substance.

Food Allergy

Food allergies may cause a rapid response such as asthma, hay fever, swelling, and hives or they may cause delayed symptoms, like headache, diarrhea and fatigue. Some food allergies can be life-threatening when the food causes severe shock (anaphylactic shock). The most common foods that produce immediate reactions include eggs, milk, wheat, soybeans, seafood, nuts, and peanuts (a legume, not a true nut). Delayed hypersensitivity is very common and does not lead to anaphylaxis. A variety of laboratory tests are designed to assess specific antibody levels to specific substances in foods. (See also ALLERGY, FOOD; ANOREXIA.)

Brostoff, Jonathan, and Linda Gamlin. *Food Allergies and Food Intolerance: The Complete Guide to Their Identification and Treatment.* Rochester, Vt.: Healing Arts Press (2000).

food spoilage The decay or decomposition of food due to microbial metabolism. BACTERIA and MOLDS are always present on foods exposed to air. In an appropriate environment, with suitable temperature and moisture, they will begin to break down constituents in food. Refrigeration slows the process because microbial metabolism is based on chemical reactions that slow at lower temperatures. However, several species of yeasts and molds that can spoil food grow slowly at refrigerator temperatures, and will eventually decompose even refrigerated foods. Unlike bacterial contamination in foods, moldy food (like moldy bread and cheese) is visible. Organisms that cause FOOD POISONING generally cannot grow in the refrigerator; Campylobacter (CAMPYLOBACTERIOSIS) is one important exception.

Spoiled or rotten food is usually obvious because it tastes and smells bad. On the other hand, organisms that cause food poisoning cannot be spotted so easily. Besides microbial attack, food can also be destroyed by insects, endogenous enzymes, spontaneous chemical reactions (such as reaction with oxygen), burning during excessive cooking, and physical changes brought about by freezing, heating, and handling. (See also BOTULISM; SALMONELLA.)

Food Stamp Program A federal program (Food Stamp Act of 1977 and Food Stamp Act of 1964) designed to maintain health and to raise the level of nutrition of low-income people by enabling them to buy nutritious food in greater variety. Administered by the U.S. Department of Agriculture (USDA) in cooperation with county and state welfare agencies, the program is designed to increase a household's purchasing power. Food stamps are currently given free to families who are certified, as by Aid to Families with Dependent Children.

Specific regulations frequently change; however, in general, eligibility criteria specify limits for monthly net income and financial resources. U.S. citizens and some resident aliens may qualify. The Welfare Reform Act of 1996 closed the program to many legal immigrants, although Congress later restored benefits to many minor and elderly immigrants as well as other groups. The Welfare Reform Act also placed time limits on benefits for unemployed, able-bodied, childless adults. Their net value depends on the size and resources of the household. In 2000 the average monthly benefit was $73 per person and $173 per household. Stamps are used like money for buying food (except pet food); beverages (except alcoholic beverages); and seeds and plants for growing food. The maximum allotment of stamps is equivalent to the U.S. Department of Agriculture's Thrifty Food Plan. This plan was developed by the Agricultural Research Service to provide adequate quantities of most nutrients, but not all, as a guide to making healthful food choices.

Consumer freedom of food choice means that consumers may purchase foods with low nutrient value. Thus, effectiveness of the program is restricted by the degree of nutrition education, which may be limited. Funding remains a continuing problem. In 2000 7.3 million households and 17.2 million individuals participated in the program. (See also DIETARY GUIDELINES FOR AMERICANS.)

food toxins Substances in foods that adversely affect health. Toxins can be classified as CARCINOGENS, pharmacologic agents and agents that block nutrient function.

Carcinogens are natural cancer-causing agents that may occur in the following:

- moldy grains and nuts (AFLATOXIN)
- barbecued meat (BENZOPYRENES)
- CABBAGE (thiourea)
- certain herbs (ALKALOIDS)
- certain vegetables and processed meat products (NITRATE and NITRITES, which are converted to NITROSOAMINES)
- fermentation products (ethyl carbamate) in pickled herring and sauerkraut.

Pharmacologic agents in foods affect organ function and/or cellular metabolism. They include:

- CHEESES: TYRAMINE affects the nervous system.
- nuts and pits: ALMOND, APPLE, APRICOT, cherry, peach, pear, and plum. These products contain cyanogenetic GLYCOSIDES, which release cyanide and block cellular respiration.
- mussels and CLAMS: After ingesting the dinoflagellate responsible for red tides, contaminated mussels and clams can cause muscle weakness and paralysis.
- cheeses, preserved meat, and preserved fish: These products may contain nitrosoamines, which cause cancer and liver damage.
- legumes: These vegetables contain a family of proteins called hemagglutinins, which can rup-

ture red blood cells and damage intestinal mucosa in susceptible people and slow growth. Cooking inactivates hemagglutinin.

- brassica family (including cabbage, KALE, BRUSSELS SPROUTS, CAULIFLOWER, BROCCOLI, TURNIPS, and RUTABAGA): contain glucosinolates, which produce the inorganic ion thiocyanate. Thiocyanate can cause hyperplasia of the thyroid gland, GOITER, because it blocks iodine assimilation, required for thyroid hormone formation.
- certain fish: A variety of fish toxins can poison the nervous system.
- RHUBARB: An acid in rhubarb called OXALIC ACID binds CALCIUM; in excess, oxalic acid can contribute to kidney stones.
- fungi: A variety of mycotoxins can damage the liver and affect the nervous system.

Certain materials or enzymes in foods interfere with nutrient assimilation or function, but are often inactivated by heating and cooking:

- beans and soybeans: Thorough cooking destroys a protein called trypsin inhibitor, which blocks protein digestion; hemagglutinin, which retards growth; and lipoxidase, an enzyme that destroys VITAMIN A.
- cottonseed oil: This oil contains sterculic acid, a fatty acid that interferes with reproduction in experimental animals when consumed in large amounts.
- fish and clams: Raw seafood contains varying amounts of thiaminase, an enzyme that breaks down the B vitamin THIAMIN.)
- milk: Milk contains LACTOSE (milk sugar), which can create diarrhea in individuals who cannot digest this carbohydrate.
- cereal grains: These contain varying amounts of PHYTIC ACID, a phosphate-containing acid that binds calcium and IRON.
- vegetables and fruit: Fresh produce contains variable amounts of an enzyme called ascorbic acid oxidase that destroys VITAMIN C when exposed to air.
- raw eggs: Raw egg white contains ovamucoid, a protein that blocks protein digestion, and AVIDIN, a protein that binds BIOTIN and blocks its absorption. (See also FOOD POISONING.)

food trends See EATING PATTERNS.

food wrap Film plastic wrap and shrink wrapping are used to wrap and package food. Plastic food wrap contains plasticizers that have caused tumors in mice. While their effect in humans are unknown, it is not advisable to wrap plastic around food that is to be cooked. Plasticizers are absorbed by fatty and oily foods, even with refrigeration. Thus fatty foods like cheese should be stored in containers rather than wrapped in plastic sheeting.

Components that leach out of packaging into foods are known as indirect additives. Moist foods, especially those containing ALCOHOL, fat, or acids, favor migration of organic compounds into a food. The U.S. FDA monitors packaging that comes into contact with food, and manufacturers are required to obtain FDA approval for all materials used in food packaging. Migration of package components usually is not a problem if the food is dry. (See also MICROWAVE COOKING.)

formula See INFANT FORMULA.

fortification See FOOD FORTIFICATION.

four food groups See BASIC FOOD GROUPS.

frame size An assessment of a person's bone size and musculature. Bone mass correlates with muscle mass, and larger-boned people generally have larger muscles. The breadth of the elbow bones is used as an index of frame sizes for insurance-derived HEIGHT-WEIGHT TABLES. These in turn are used to estimate an optimal body weight. The weight tables also employ heights based on one-inch heels and weights based on fully clothed people. (See also DIETING; OBESITY.)

Framingham Study An early U.S. study of factors associated with HEART DISEASE. This population study was designed to estimate risk factors in the development of heart disease by studying 5,000 men and women aged 32 to 60, living in Framingham, Massachusetts between 1949 and 1969. Subjects enrolled in this study initially did not have signs of coronary heart disease. They were examined every two years for signs and symptoms of CARDIOVASCULAR DISEASE. The risk of heart disease was found to increase with the following:

- smoking: All other factors being equal, the risk of heart disease for smokers was 1.5 times higher than for nonsmokers.
- obesity: Individuals 20 percent or more heavier than "optimal" body weight had three times the risk of death due to heart attack.
- male gender: Other factors being equal, 45-year-old men were found to be three times more likely to develop heart disease as women.
- physical inactivity: Active persons had one-third to one-half the risk of heart attack or angina as sedentary individuals.
- elevated blood pressure. People with readings (systolic blood pressure) of 180 or higher were about twice as likely to have heart disease as those who had a systolic pressure of 120, other factors being the same.
- high blood sugar levels: Glucose intolerance (blood sugar level of 120 or greater, or passing sugar in the urine) was associated with a greater risk of heart disease. Thus the risk of angina or sudden death for obese diabetics was 2.5 times as great as for obese nondiabetics.
- Elevated CHOLESTEROL levels: This alone accounted for a modest increase in risk of heart disease; but when associated with other risk factors, high cholesterol increased the risk. (See also AGING; DIETARY GUIDELINES FOR AMERICANS.)

frankfurter A sausage made of BEEF, PORK, turkey, or VEAL, or a combination of these. The meat, together with seasonings and nitrates, is placed in casings, then smoked, steamed, and finally chilled. Frankfurters are a high-FAT, high-SODIUM food, and most of the fat is saturated. A beef and pork frankfurter provides 145 calories; protein, 5.1 g; carbohydrate, 1.1 g; fat, 13.1 g; iron, 0.52 mg; sodium 504 mg; zinc, 0.83 mg; niacin, 1.2 mg. It contains 23 mg of cholesterol. For comparison, a turkey frankfurter provides 102 calories: protein, 6.4 g; carbohydrate, 0.7 g; fat, 8.3 g; iron, 0.77 mg; sodium, 550 mg; zinc, 1.0 mg; niacin, 1.77 mg; and cholesterol, 44 mg. (See also CONVENIENCE FOOD; DIETARY GUIDELINES FOR AMERICANS; HOT DOG.)

free radicals Highly damaging molecules or ions that often contain oxygen. Free radicals possess a single electron; unlike stable molecules with pairs of electrons, these renegades attack harmless molecules of the cell by removing an electron to make up for their own electron deficiency. Once they have been produced, free radicals can multiply via chain reactions, making them even more dangerous to the cell.

Free radicals likely to be encountered in the body include superoxide, NITRIC OXIDE, hydroxyl radicals, and lipid radicals (lipid peroxyl radicals). Certain activated forms of oxygen, including singlet oxygen, lipid peroxides, and HYDROGEN PEROXIDE, can generate free radicals, though they are not radicals themselves.

Numerous health conditions are possibly linked to free radical damage, including CANCER, ATHEROSCLEROSIS, high blood pressure, ALZHEIMER'S DISEASE and SENILITY, weakened IMMUNE SYSTEM, CATARACTS, lung disease, ARTHRITIS, emphysema, Parkinson's disease, and AGING. Free radicals damage cells by attacking vulnerable sites, the most important being DNA ENZYMES, and lipids and proteins that make up cell membranes.

Sources of Free Radicals

Exposure to free radicals is unavoidable because the body uses oxygen to derive energy from burning fuel molecules. For example, as mitochondria, the cell's powerhouses, consume oxygen, they produce highly unstable forms of oxygen, including superoxide and hydroxyl radicals, when functioning under par. In addition, hydrogen peroxide, which can break down to form free radicals, is a normal byproduct of many types of cells containing peroxisomes, small bodies within cells that can degrade fatty acids and other substances.

Free radicals are also generated by defensive cells. Phagocytes, cells that engulf foreign invaders, destroy bacteria and virus-infected cells by bursts of toxic chemicals, including superoxide, NITRIC OXIDE (another radical), and hydrogen peroxide. Chronic infection and the ensuing inflammation can create prolonged oxidative stress on the body. Nitric oxide also functions in the body as a nerve chemical (neurotransmitter) and regulatory molecule.

Detoxifying enzymes like CYTOCHROME P450 in the liver, which is responsible for inactivating pollutants and toxic compounds, can yield byproducts that form free radicals. It is ironic that in making some molecules more easily excreted, the body's defense system can create more dangerous substances.

People who are prone to iron storage disease (HEMOCHROMATOSIS) or who consume excessive iron may increase their risk of free radical damage because reduced iron atoms can spontaneously react with oxygen to produce free radicals.

Environmental factors play a key role in free radical damage. Besides being produced by normal physiologic processes, free radicals are generated by ultraviolet light and ionizing radiation such as X rays, radon, and gamma rays. Some environmental pollutants like ozone and nitrogen oxides react within the body to form free radicals.

Consequences of Free Radical Attack

In view of the prevalence of free radicals, it is not surprising that cells experience free radical damage frequently. An estimated 10,000 damaging attacks are made on a cell's genes daily, although nearly all of this damage is normally repaired by enzymes. However, free radicals can damage and inactivate repair enzymes over time. Cumulative damage to repair enzymes can slow the DNA repair so that DNA damage increases with age, as does the risk of mutations and cancer. Besides DNA and protein, lipids can be targets. Free radical attack on polyunsaturated FATTY ACIDS yields oxidized lipids (lipid peroxides) that can break down to free radicals and toxic fragments.

Materials outside of cells can also be injured by free radicals. LOW-DENSITY LIPOPROTEIN (LDL), which transports CHOLESTEROL to tissues via the bloodstream, is another free radical target. Oxidized LDL is implicated in the development of plaque formation in arteries (atherosclerosis). According to the free radical theory of aging, the body possesses a powerful collection of antioxidant defenses; however, some free radicals inevitably escape and are able to attack cells. Over time, the body's defensive mechanisms reach the point at which cellular repair can no longer keep up with oxidative damage and damaged proteins, lipids, and DNA accumulate. Ultimately, a point is reached at which cells are impaired and consequently organ function declines. Eventually, the body's ability to ward off cancer and to maintain itself is compromised.

Antioxidants

Antioxidants are substances that can block the oxidation of target molecules in the cell. Antioxidants can either quench free radicals ("chain breakers") or they can block the initiation of free radical attack ("preventive inhibitors"). Chain breakers include VITAMIN E and VITAMIN C. Preventive inhibitors include defensive enzymes, such as CATALASE, SUPEROXIDE DISMUTASE, and GLUTATHIONE PEROXIDASE. Trace mineral nutrients function as antioxidants when they function as cofactors of enzymes. COPPER, MANGANESE, and ZINC are cofactors for the enzyme superoxide dismutase, which inactivates superoxide. SELENIUM is a cofactor for glutathione peroxidase, an enzyme that converts peroxides to safe intermediates, while catalase degrades hydrogen peroxide to water and oxygen.

Glutathione, the sulfur-containing antioxidant of the cytoplasm and beta-carotene quench active forms of oxygen or bind metal catalysts that could otherwise produce free radicals. These antioxidants complement each other: Vitamin C is a powerful, water soluble antioxidant, while beta-carotene and vitamin E are fat-soluble free radical traps. The increased consumption of polyunsaturated vegetable oils increases the requirement for vitamin E. Plant substances called FLAVONOIDS also can act as powerful antioxidants. The long-term health benefits of eating adequate fruits and vegetables is due in part to these important substances.

Much previous research indicates that the consumption of ample amounts of fruits and vegetables helps prevent disease. These foods contain multiple antioxidants including hundreds of carotenoids in addition to beta-carotene. Combinations of free radical quenchers as found in foods, rather than a single antioxidant, will best prevent free radical damage in the body. Investigators hypothesize that boosting protection against free radical damage by dietary antioxidants may help people live longer. For example, vitamin E or vitamin E with carotenoids seem to help prevent cancer or heart disease.

Thomas, M. J. "The Role of Free Radicals and Antioxidants: How Do We Know That They Are Working?"

Critical Reviews in Food Science and Nutrition 35, nos. 1, 2 (1995): 21–39.

french fries A high-fat, common FAST-FOOD menu item. To make french fries, potatoes are usually sliced into strips and fried. Fast-food french fries are precooked at the factory, then refried immediately before serving. Some fast-food restaurants use vegetable oil to avoid cholesterol, rather than lard or beef tallow for frying. However, the hydrogenated vegetable oil that is commonly used is more saturated then untreated oils, and contains modified fats called *trans* fats. As a result, french fries may contain as much artery-clogging fat as potatoes fried in beef tallow. Nonetheless, fried potatoes absorb FAT: French fries provide about 50 percent of their calories as fat. Any food providing more than 30 percent of its calories as fat can be considered a fatty food. In 2002 Swedish research revealed that some fried carbohydrate-rich foods such as french fries and potato chips contain a likely cancer-causing substance called ACRYLAMIDE. Experts around the world agreed more research was needed before dietary changes could be recommended because it was still too early to evaluate the real risk to people. Scientists at Stockholm University had published research indicating that acrylamide, already known as a probable cancer-causing agent, was formed in very high concentrations when carbohydrate-rich foods such as rice, potatoes, and cereals were fried or baked. The researchers estimated acrylamide could be responsible for several hundred of the 45,000 cancer cases in Sweden each year based on experiments in which rats were fed fried food.

The U.S. Environmental Protection Agency classifies acrylamide, a colorless, crystalline solid, as a "medium hazard probable human carcinogen." Scientists still do not know whether the formation of acrylamide is linked to the temperature at which the food is cooked, but the level of acrylamide produced during food preparation was reported in the Swedish studies to increase with the temperature at which the food is cooked.

The Swedish National Food Administration (NFA) stressed that current knowledge does not allow for a balanced analysis of risks and benefits of staple foods containing acrylamide. As a result, the Swedish NFA can currently issue only general advice regarding the risk management of acrylamide to the food industry and consumers. A plain baked potato (202 g) contains 220 calories; plus fat, 0.2 g; vitamin C, 26 mg; and sodium, 16 mg. An equivalent amount of french fries (200 g cooked in vegetable oil) provides almost three times as many calories: 632 calories; fat, 33.2 g; sodium, 432 mg; and vitamin C, 20 mg (See also ACRYLAMIDE; CONVENIENCE FOOD; FRIED FOOD.)

freshness Product freshness refers to the degree of chemical change in a food due to breakdown by enzymes and chemical processes within the food itself. Oxidation, change in color and texture or flavor of a food, and loss of nutrients like VITAMIN C are possible consequences. In contrast, spoilage represents the action of MOLDS, fungi, YEASTS, and BACTERIA growing on the food. (See also FOOD ADDITIVES; FOOD SPOILAGE.)

fried food Food that has been cooked in fat or oil. Fried foods are both high-FAT and high-CALORIE because of the absorption of cooking fat or oils. Foods cooked with a batter or breading also absorb high levels of fat. This is a concern for two reasons: Excessive fat is linked to an increased risk of clogged arteries (atherosclerosis) and cancer, and a surplus of calories is a major contributor to OBESITY in the United States. Dietary fat is one of the largest contributors to obesity and to cancer (after cigarette smoking). According to the DIETARY GUIDELINES FOR AMERICANS, fat should account for no more than 30 percent of daily calories.

POLYUNSATURATED VEGETABLE OILS like safflower, corn, sunflower, and soybean oil are often used in frying. High temperatures convert these oils to potentially harmful products. Their oxidation products (peroxides and epoxides) yield free radicals and reactive compounds called aldehydes that can damage the LIVER, slow growth and cause chromosomal damage in lab animals. There is less of an oxidation problem in cooking with fresh oil at medium temperatures. However, there is no guarantee that the fried food eaten in restaurants has not been overheated.

It is generally recommended that consumption of fried foods be reduced. Many more healthful options exist, including baked or broiled foods. (See also CHICKEN; CONVENIENCE FOOD, DIETING; EATING PATTERNS; FAST FOOD.)

frozen desserts, fat-free Frozen desserts made without milk FAT or cream. Several fat-free options are now available that contain no cream and no CHOLESTEROL. Frozen nonfat yogurts, sorbets, sherbets, and fruit bars fall into this category. They may contain FRUCTOSE or polydextrose (derived from cornstarch) as sweeteners, cellulose gel and gums as thickeners, nonfat milk or whey, and flavors. Calories range from 50 to 90 per half-cup serving and there may be only 1 g of fat. Such desserts are more healthful than standard ice cream, which contains 150 calories and 8 g of fat. Fat substitutes are now being marketed in frozen desserts.

Nonbutterfat frozen desserts can be useful in lowering daily fat intake. The DIETARY GUIDELINES FOR AMERICANS recommends reducing daily fat consumption to less than 30 percent of total calories. Cholesterol intake should be reduced to the equivalent of no more than four egg yolks per week. Nonetheless, low-fat, low-cholesterol desserts should not take the place of whole foods like grains, vegetables, and fruits. In terms of weight control, there is no substitute for exercise and good eating habits. (See also DAIRY-FREE FROZEN DESSERTS; OBESITY.)

frozen entrees CONVENIENCE FOODS that often provide excessive CALORIES, FAT, and SODIUM. Gourmet and "lite" varieties are increasingly being marketed. To reduce the consumption of fat, food additives and calories from frozen entrees, consumers should:

- read labels: "Light, low fat" designations on food labels are best. As a guideline, less than 10 g of fat per meal should be eaten. If the CALCIUM, VITAMIN, and FIBER contents are low, the food is probably processed and contains more fat. Consumers should eat fewer foods in which fat contributes more than 30 percent of the calories; this is the limit recommended in DIETARY GUIDELINES FOR AMERICANS for overall fat consumption.
- avoid SULFITE. This preservative is often added to seafood entrees, sauerkraut, and other canned vegetables and dried fruit. Sulfite can cause strong reactions in sensitive people.
- avoid MONOSODIUM GLUTAMATE (MSG) and its cousin, HYDROLYZED VEGETABLE PROTEIN: These flavor enhancers can cause reactions in sensitive people, including migraines and mood swings.
- be aware that SURIMI is artificial shellfish: If the food label lists pollack and other fish, ARTIFICIAL FOOD COLORS, and other food additives, surimi and not real shellfish is being offered.
- Americans consume two to five times more salt than needed. The maximum level is 3,000 mg per day. A single frozen dinner may easily supply this much. (See also MSG RELATED SYNDROME; OBESITY.)

fructogligosaccharides (FOS) See PROBIOTICS.

fructose A simple sugar found in HONEY and FRUIT, especially dried fruit. Fructose is three times sweeter than table sugar (SUCROSE). Typically, fructose accounts for 10 percent of the daily CALORIES for the U.S. population; much of it comes from sucrose, which is half fructose. As a refined CARBOHYDRATE, fructose is increasingly used as a FOOD ADDITIVE. In the form of high FRUCTOSE CORN SYRUP, processed from cornstarch, it is added to almost all soft drinks in place of table sugar, and consumption has increased 250 percent over the last 15 years.

Fructose has been recommended as a sweetener for diabetics because it is converted to BLOOD SUGAR more slowly. Consequently, there is less need for insulin, the hormone that increases blood glucose uptake by tissues. However, if DIABETES isn't controlled, even fructose can eventually lead to excessively high blood sugar in susceptible people.

It is estimated that a fructose intake twice the average consumption can increase blood fat (TRIGLYCERIDES), blood CHOLESTEROL, and URIC ACID in 10 percent to 15 percent of adults with elevated blood fat (triglycerides) and insulin levels. Diets high in fructose and low in copper and magnesium also increase blood lipids and increase the risk of heart disease. There is a risk of CATARACTS and kidney stones in susceptible individuals with long-term high consumption of fructose. High consumption of any kind of sugar depletes the body of CHROMIUM, required with insulin to stimulate cells to absorb and metabolize blood sugar. In individuals with elevated blood insulin and blood sugar, as in a prediabetic condition, excessive fructose consumption can aggravate a chromium deficiency. (See also GLYCEMIC INDEX; NATURAL SWEETENERS.)

fructose corn syrup A major food additive that often replaces table sugar (SUCROSE). It is prepared from CORN SYRUP, which consists mainly of GLUCOSE. Fructose corn syrup contains 40 percent to 90 percent FRUCTOSE; because it is sweeter than table sugar, less needs to be added to achieve the equivalent level of sweetness.

While table sugar consumption has declined in recent years, high fructose and fructose corn syrup consumption has more than made up the difference. Thus the total sweetener consumption rose from 118 pounds per person in 1975 to the current annual consumption of about 150 pounds. This is equivalent to eating a cup of sugar daily. On average, SOFT DRINKS represent 65 percent of fructose corn syrup consumption. It is used in cranberry juice and sauces, fruit sherbet and ice cream, jellies and jams, catsup, MAYONNAISE, spaghetti sauce, sweet pickles, cookies, syrup, bread, peanut butter, and wine coolers.

There is a risk of cataracts and kidney stones with long-term use of fructose in susceptible individuals. Large amounts of dietary fructose can increase blood lipids and may increase the risk of HEART DISEASE. (See also DIETARY GUIDELINES FOR AMERICANS; EATING PATTERNS; FOOD ADDITIVES; NATURAL SWEETENERS; TEETH.)

fruit The pulpy tissue associated with seeds. In botany, the ovary of a plant; according to this definition, EGGPLANT, CUCUMBERS, and PUMPKINS are fruits. However, the USDA prefers to define a fruit as a plant food if it is usually eaten as a DESSERT or as a snack between meals, or accompanies breakfast, rather than being a main course of a meal.

Fruits are often classified into the following groups:

- Aggregate fruits consist of many tiny seed-bearing fruits combined in one mass and developed from many ovaries. Strawberries, BLACKBERRIES, and RASPBERRIES are examples.
- Berries are fruits from a single ovary but they may contain more than one seed. GRAPES and persimmons belong to this group. According to this classification, BANANA is a berry that has lost the ability to form seeds.
- Drupes are fruits that contain a single seed fruit that develops entirely from a single ovary. CHERRY and PEACH are examples.
- Hesperidium refers to CITRUS FRUITS; they contain a many-seeded, multisectioned fruit enclosed by a tough skin. LEMONS and ORANGES are typical.
- In multiple fruits, ovaries and receptacles derived from a common base become the fruit. PINEAPPLE and FIGS belong to this category.
- False berries are represented by BLUEBERRIES and CRANBERRIES. These fruits are the result of a fusion of an ovary and a receptacle.
- Pomes are represented by APPLES and PEARS. This many-seeded fruit results from the fusion of an ovary and receptacle.

Worldwide, the leading fruit crops are grapes, bananas, and plantains (varieties used before ripening), citrus fruits (oranges, tangerines, lemons, limes, grapefruit, and pomelos), followed by apples, melons, and mangoes. In the United States, citrus fruits, grapes, and apples are the leading fruit crops. Citrus fruit production is limited primarily to California, Texas, and Florida. Because of domestication, many fruit-bearing plants have been altered so extensively that they cannot be grown without human propagation. Fruit production has increased steadily this century because of increased popularity in most countries and the expansion of food processing, which allows fruits to be eaten year-round. In recent years much of the increased consumption in the United States has been in processed fruit, rather than fresh fruit.

Fruits are generally rich sources of VITAMIN C, POTASSIUM, soluble and insoluble FIBER, FLAVONOIDS (plant antioxidants), and simple SUGAR. The most common sugars in fruits are GLUCOSE and FRUCTOSE: The sugar content varies from 6 percent to 20 percent. Bananas and figs are among the highest in sugar content. The net caloric content is also a function of processing, because canned fruit is often packed in syrup, which adds extra calories.

Fruit Juice

Common beverages are prepared from fruits such as oranges, grapes, apples, or more exotic fruits like guavas or papayas. Fresh fruit juices are excellent sources of vitamin C and potassium. Their caloric content is derived almost exclusively from simple sugars. The vitamin C content may have been depleted in the processing of commercially available juices.

The amount of fruit juice actually put into a juice drink varies, and the U.S. FDA does not require manufacturers to specify how diluted a juice drink is. If the product label specifies "juice" only, the product contains pure fruit juice. If the label says anything else, for example, juice drink, juice cocktail, juice blend, or fruit punch, the product is diluted juice. Cranberry "cocktail" is less than one-third cranberry juice. In 1994, federal regulators estimated that 10 percent of all fruit juice sold in the United States had been adulterated, most often by adding sugar or orange by-products. Young children drink large quantities of fruit juices, such as apple juice, and this may displace higher calorie, more nutrient-rich foods in their diet, causing malnutrition, diarrhea, and tooth decay.

Dried Fruit

Most commonly, apples, APRICOTS, DATES, figs, NECTARINES, peaches, PLUMS, prunes, and seedless grapes are commercially dried in the United States. When the water content of a fruit is reduced to about 24 percent from about 90 percent, spoilage is reduced. Sulfuring or sulfiting agents, which are used as preservatives in the drying process, can destroy thiamin. Dried fruit is a rich source of fructose, glucose, fiber, iron, and potassium. Raw or stewed dried fruit can help with bowel regularity. (See also BALANCED DIET; DEHYDRATION; EXERCISE; PECTIN.)

fruitarian A VEGETARIAN whose diet relies primarily on fruits. (See also LACTO-OVO-VEGETARIAN.)

fruit leather A snack food prepared from fruit pulp and dried as a thin sheet. Fruit leathers are not as nutritious as fresh fruit because they contain lower amounts of vitamins. However, they have less fat and less added sugar than candy. Fruit leathers often contain added sweeteners. (See also CANDY; SULFITES.)

fruit sugar See FRUCTOSE.

fumaric acid An additive used to provide tartness in foods and beverages. Fumaric acid finds use in gelatin desserts, puddings, pie fillings, candy, and powdered soft drinks. It is also used as an acidic ingredient in LEAVENING AGENTS (agents used to make dough rise). Fumaric acid is recognized as a safe additive. It is an intermediate of the KREB'S CYCLE, the central energy-producing pathway of metabolism, hence is readily broken down. (See also FOOD ADDITIVES.)

fumigants Gaseous PESTICIDES. A typical example of a fumigant is methyl bromide, a post-harvest fumigant used to control insects in stored GRAINS, nuts, fruits, and vegetables. Methyl bromide is also used for macadamia nuts, BROAD (fava) BEANS, SWEET POTATOES and other root crops, kiwi fruit, cereal, FLOUR, spices, LENTILS, and leafy vegetables. Direct exposure to this chemical by workers causes toxicity.

functional foods Foods or food ingredients that have been modified so that they provide health benefits above and beyond the levels they traditionally contain. The food can benefit physical performance, overall health and mental well-being in addition to its ability to supply given nutrients.

A functional food can be part of a daily diet, and it can enhance specific body functions, such as enhancing the IMMUNE SYSTEM in the prevention of disease, or it can aid in the recovery of a disease. Examples include protein-enriched sports drinks with collagen, soft drinks with fiber and iron, calcium-rich beverages, tea fortified with calcium, bread with soluble fiber, cereals with bran, iron-fortified candy, candy with fructooligosaccharides, sausage with fiber, and milk and yogurt with lactobacillus species and bifidobacteria. The judicious use of such foods in the diet could provide a more individualized program tailored to meet specific needs. (See also BIOCHEMICAL INDIVIDUALITY; GENETIC ENGINEERING.)

fungicides PESTICIDES used to prevent MOLDS from developing in produce during shipping and storage. Most fungicides have been shown to cause cancer in experimental animals. A typical example is CAPTAN, used on FRUITS such as APPLES, PEACHES, and STRAWBERRIES, and on VEGETABLES such as CORN, GARLIC, CABBAGE, LETTUCE, CARROTS, BEETS, PEAS, BEANS, KALE, and SPINACH. Captan is sometimes used in packing boxes for post-harvest treatment. Captan has been found in oils and shortening because it is fat-soluble. This fungicide can cause CANCER in experimental animals and is toxic to fish, birds, and bees. Chlorothalonil (Bravo), a fungicide used on vegetables, including beans, TOMATOES, ONIONS, BROCCOLI, cabbage, CUCUMBER, lettuce, and on fruit, including watermelon and CANTALOUPE, causes tumors in rats and mice. A family of fungicides called EBDs (Maneb, Mancozeb, and Metiran) is now permitted by the EPA on 43 crops including apples, corn, tomatoes, potatoes, cucumbers and onions because it is now believed to cause only a minor cancer risk (one additional cancer patient per million people over a lifetime). (See also CARCINOGENS; DELANEY CLAUSE.)

fungus A member of a broad division of plants lacking the green photosynthetic pigment chlorophyll. MOLDS, YEASTS, and MUSHROOMS belong to this plant family. Fungi degrade dead organic materials or living tissue for nutrients.

Edible mushrooms and molds used in the maturation of CHEESE are useful fungi, and yeasts are used in FERMENTATION for WINE and BEER. Several antibiotics are fungal products.

As pathogens, fungi can cause ringworm, athlete's foot, and thrush. Several species of fungi produce toxic agents (mycotoxins). (See also AFLATOXIN; ASPERGILLUS; *CANDIDA ALBICANS*.)

furcelleran A natural GUM obtained from seaweed. Furcelleran resembles CARRAGEENAN, also obtained from a seaweed. It is used occasionally as a FOOD ADDITIVE to thicken processed foods and to help puddings gel. Its long-term safety has not been carefully examined.

G

galactose A simple SUGAR found in the diet in milk sugar (lactose). Galactose is a six-carbon sugar, as is the more common GLUCOSE (BLOOD SUGAR). Unlike glucose, however, it does not occur by itself in foods. DIGESTION of lactose by the intestinal enzyme LACTASE yields equal amounts of galactose and glucose. Before galactose can be used by the body for energy, it must first be transformed into glucose by the LIVER. Certain people have a genetic susceptibility to galactose accumulation. (See also CARBOHYDRATE METABOLISM; GALACTOSEMIA.)

galactosemia A rare genetic disease due to an inability to degrade the sugar GALACTOSE normally. The most common defect is the inability to convert galactose to GLUCOSE, an essential preliminary step for galactose to be used for energy production. Because galactose cannot be extensively degraded when the path to glucose is blocked, it accumulates in the blood of galactosemic patients. This leads to severe mental retardation unless special galactose-free (milk-free) diets are administered shortly after birth. The prevalence of galactosemia is about one in 50,000. (See also CARBOHYDRATE METABOLISM.)

gallbladder A dark green organ that concentrates and stores BILE from the LIVER. Bile is a mixture of powerful emulsifiers needed to digest and absorb FAT and oils and fat-soluble vitamins. When the INTESTINE detects food and fat released by the stomach, the intestine releases the hormone CHOLECYSTOKININ into the bloodstream, which causes the gallbladder to release bile into the DUODENUM, the upper section of the small intestine. (See also DIGESTIVE TRACT.)

gallstones Gravel-like deposits in the gallbladder in which BILE is stored; the gallbladder releases bile during meals to aid fat digestion and absorption.

Many people consuming Western diets develop gallstones, although the causes of gallstones are unknown. Risk factors include high-FAT, low-FIBER diets, female gender, obesity, aging, CROHN'S DISEASE, cystic fibrosis, and alcoholic cirrhosis of the liver.

The more refined and processed the foods in the diet, the greater the risk of developing gallstones. High-fiber diets may increase bile flow, thus preventing stone formation. For example, pre-1950s northern Canadian Inuit populations consuming a traditional diet had no record of gallstones. As a Western diet became more popular, the incidence of gallbladder disease increased dramatically.

Food allergies are also a contributing factor, especially allergies to egg, pork, and onion. Hypochlorhydria (low stomach acid) may underlie maldigestion and food allergies, thus contributing to symptoms such as abdominal pain, bloating, and gas.

The composition of gallstones ranges from almost pure CHOLESTEROL to mixtures of bile salts, cholesterol, calcium carbonate, and BILE PIGMENT (bilirubin). In the United States, most stones are of the mixed variety. Frequently, stones are small enough to pass through the duct leading to the intestine. Other stones often remain in the gallbladder without causing discomfort. When large stones become lodged in the common bile duct, this triggers a painful gallbladder attack called choledocholithiasis.

It is clear that materials normally dissolved in bile create stones, and that stone formation begins with bile saturation. Bile contains cholesterol emulsified by bile salts and LECITHIN for digestion. Cholesterol will precipitate when there is a decrease in bile acids, water, or lecithin content in bile. For example, less bile salt is made as one ages, making cholesterol more insoluble.

gamma globulins A family of specialized proteins (antibodies) that are the first line of defense against foreign invaders such as BACTERIA and viruses in the bloodstream. Unlike most serum proteins that are made by the LIVER, gamma globulins are products of B cells and related plasma cells of the IMMUNE SYSTEM. Most antibodies in the blood belong to the IgG class. Together with circulating white blood cells, they constitute "humoral immunity." Gamma globulin shots temporarily boost immunity for protection against diseases such as HEPATITIS. (See also ALLERGEN; ALLERGY, FOOD; ANTIBODIES.)

gamma hydroxybutyric acid A compound that has been promoted by some body builders as a muscle-enhancing agent. It occurs naturally in the central nervous system, and it has been used as a general anesthetic and hypnotic or tranquilizing substance. However, gamma hydroxybutyric acid has caused comas and convulsions in susceptible individuals, and the U.S. FDA has warned consumers against its use because of possible serious adverse side effects.

gamma linolenic acid (GLA) A polyunsaturated FATTY ACID found in seed oils such as borage, evening primrose, and blackcurrant. GLA is the raw material for a family of PROSTAGLANDINS, HORMONE-like lipids that regulate many physiologic processes. GLA forms the PGE_1 class of prostaglandins that counterbalance the effects of other prostaglandins (PGE_2) by decreasing inflammation, expanding blood vessels (vasodilation), lowering blood pressure and reducing the tendency to form blood clots. This may be the basis for the observation that GLA may help reduce pain associated with rheumatoid arthritis.

GLA is derived from LINOLEIC ACID, the ESSENTIAL FATTY ACID, and belongs to the omega-6 family of fatty acids. GLA possesses 18 carbons. Its three double bonds are located at different points along the chain. The structure of GLA differs from ALPHA LINOLENIC ACID, an omega-3 essential fatty acid. Therefore GLA and alpha linolenic acid are not interchangeable and serve different functions in the body.

Specific nutrients NIACIN, VITAMIN B_6, VITAMIN C, and ZINC participate in the formation of PGE_1. The ability to produce GLA from linoleic acid seems to diminish with age, diabetes, high ALCOHOL consumption and high blood CHOLESTEROL. Therefore, supplementation may be helpful in certain situations. GLA is one of the polyunsaturated fatty acids of BREAST MILK, suggestive of its importance in development and growth.

gamma-oryzanol (ferulate; ferulic acid) A plant extract derived from rice bran oil. It is also found in other grains and in some fruits, vegetable, and herbs. Gamma-oryzanol has been used in Japan for decades as a treatment for anxiety, digestive disorders, menopause, and elevated cholesterol, LDL cholesterol, and triglyceride levels. Some studies done in Japan support use of gamma-oryzanol for these conditions. However, the results are questionable because either the subjects studied were laboratory animals or the number of humans studied was too small to produce conclusive evidence of efficacy.

In the United States gamma-oryzanol is available as a dietary supplement. It has gained popularity among some athletes and bodybuilders who believe it can increase muscle mass and enhance strength and endurance. However, a study of male weightlifters who took supplements for nine weeks showed that gamma-oryzanol had no effect on exercise performance. Other studies indicated the substance retards production of growth hormones.

Gamma-oryzanol may have a positive effect on the body's production of endorphins, chemicals that produce a feeling of well-being. Although this claim has not been proven, many athletes claim taking supplements can reduce fatigue and pain associated with hard physical training.

Because gamma-oryzanol is sold as a dietary supplement and not a drug, its safety and efficacy have not been tested by any government agency. Because there is inadequate safety information, pregnant and breast-feeding women should not use this product.

Fry, A. C. "The Effects of Gamma-Oryzanol Supplementation During Resistance Exercise Training," *International Journal of Sport Nutrition* 7 (1997): 318–329.

garbanzo bean See CHICKPEA.

garlic (*Allium sativum*) This bulbous plant is closely related to ONIONS, leeks, and chives. The ancestor of modern garlic grows in Central Asia, and garlic has been cultivated for at least 5,000 years. The underground compound bulb is made up of cloves or sections. Garlic is strongly scented and strongly flavored, and has many culinary applications. Most of the garlic produced in the United States comes from California. Much of the commercially grown garlic is processed to garlic powder.

The healing power of garlic has been recognized by Chinese folk traditions dating back thousands of years. Research has shown that garlic can lower blood CHOLESTEROL, especially the undesirable fraction of serum cholesterol LOW-DENSITY LIPOPROTEIN (LDL) and serum fat in animals and humans. Garlic also can significantly lower high blood pressure. Eating half a clove of garlic a day may lower blood cholesterol by 9 percent. Garlic reduces the tendency to form blood clots, although the conjecture that garlic decreases the risk of CARDIOVASCULAR DISEASE has been challenged. The suggestion has also been made that eating garlic and onions (not supplements) on a regular basis may lower the risk of stomach CANCER because materials isolated from garlic inhibit cancer production in experimental animals. Garlic can prevent dietary nitrites, used as a preservative in processed meat, from forming nitrosoamines, which can cause cancer, or can block their action. Garlic boosts the IMMUNE SYSTEM by increasing natural killer cells and phagocytic activity of white cells, and this may explain its anticancer activity.

Garlic contains 0.4 percent volatile oil containing a variety of unusual organo-sulfur compounds, believed to be responsible for most of the pharmacologic and antimicrobial actions. "Allylsulfides" increase the production of so-called phase 2 liver detoxification enzymes (glutathione transferases) that increase the water solubility of cancer-causing compounds and toxins, speeding their excretion. Diallylsulfide may protect against lung cancer and stomach cancer. Other compounds in garlic seem to limit tumor cell growth. However, garlic yields different active ingredients depending on the way it is prepared. Garlic juice possesses antibacterial activity, antifungal activity, and antiviral activity. Allicin causes the pungent odor of raw garlic and seems to be partly responsible for antimicrobial activity.

Garlic has been reported to lower blood pressure in experimental animals and in humans and to inhibit blood platelet clumping, a necessary step in clot formation in vessels. Garlic reduces inflammation by blocking the formation of agents that induce it, including PROSTAGLANDINS, thromboxanes, and LEUKOTRIENES. Steam distillation of garlic juice produces a sulfur product called ajoene, which inhibits a prostaglandin, PGE_2, which induces pain. Garlic sauteed in oil produces still other sulfur compounds, vinyldithiins, which are bronchial relaxers (they open air passageways in the lungs).

Garlic supplements have yielded mixed results. Although odoriferous, fresh garlic seems to be generally more effective than garlic powders and oils. Certain products carefully prepared from freeze-dried garlic appear to be effective. Garlic usually does not cause side effects, but in sensitive people garlic can cause allergic symptoms. Gastrointestinal upsets can be diminished by mixing crushed fresh garlic in oil and mixing this with food.

Researchers have found garlic supplements can interfere with the beneficial effects of a type of medication to treat HIV/AIDS. Investigators from the National Institutes of Health (NIH) found that garlic supplements sharply reduced blood levels of the anti-HIV drug saquinavir.

Piscatelli, S. C. et al. "The Effects of Garlic Supplements on the Pharmacokinetics of Saquinavir," *Clinical Infectious Diseases* 34 (January 15, 2001): 234–238.

gas See FLATULENCE.

gastric acid See STOMACH ACID.

gastric juice Secretions from glands lining the stomach. Up to 700 ml of gastric juice are secreted daily. Different types of secretory cells produce gastric juice. "Chief cells" produce pepsinogen, the inactive form of the stomach's protein-digesting enzyme, PEPSIN. "Parietal cells" produce hydrochloric acid (STOMACH ACID). This very strong acid creates a pH of 1.2 to 3.0, equivalent to 10 to 50 ml of dilute hydrochloric acid. The acid unfolds food PROTEINS, making them more accessible to attack by digestive enzymes. To further aid digestion, acid activates pepsin to initiate protein DIGESTION. The strong acid also helps sterilize ingested food and destroy bacterial toxins.

Gastric juice contains a LIPASE or fat-degrading enzyme that, when secreted, can liberate BUTYRIC ACID from BUTTER-FAT; as well as INTRINSIC FACTOR, a protein that binds VITAMIN B_{12} and aids VITAMIN B_{12} absorption by the small intestine. Chloride in gastric juice is efficiently absorbed by the intestine and is recycled. (See also ACHLORHYDRIA.)

gastric ulcer An open sore (also known as peptic ulcer) in the lining of the stomach. There are two major forms of ulcers: duodenal ulcer in the upper region of the small intestine, and gastric or stomach ulcer.

Gastric ulcers are somewhat less common. Most patients with gastric ulcers report abdominal discomfort about an hour after a meal, or during the night. Acid secretion is normal or reduced, rather than excessive. Eating or using ANTACIDS relieves the pain.

There are several causes of gastric ulcer. ASPIRIN, phenylbutazone, indomethacin, and other nonsteroidal anti-inflammatory agents can cause stomach bleeding and ulcer formation. ALCOHOL, smoking, and COFFEE (whether decaffeinated or not) decrease tissue resistance and may play a causative role. ACHLORHYDRIA (the absence of stomach acid) is associated with gastric ulcers. Heredity is a factor. The bacterium *HELICOBACTER PYLORI* (*H. pylori*) is associated with chronic gastric inflammation and ulcers. Infection increases the risk of stomach cancer. High levels of antibodies against *H. pylori* can often be detected in the blood of gastric ulcer patients, and long-term eradication of *H. pylori* often clears up stomach ulcers and inflammation and prevents ulcer recurrence. Researchers have discovered that BROCCOLI and broccoli sprouts contain a chemical, SULFORAFANE, that kills *H. pylori* in mice. Similar studies on humans are ongoing. Ulcer patients have a tendency to suppress emotions. Whether stress is involved in the development of ulcers is controversial.

Conventional medical treatment involves the use of drugs that block stomach acid secretion (cimetidine, ranitidine) or agents that coat ulcers and bowel. Cimetidine (Tagamet) is the second most commonly prescribed drug in the United States. Food sensitivities are implicated in experimental and clinical studies of gastric ulcer, and ELIMINATION DIETS have been used in preventing recurrent ulcers. Calcium carbonate antacids should not be used for gastric ulcer because they trigger excessive stomach acid secretion later (rebound effect). In botanical medicine, a licorice extract called deglycyrrhizinated has been used as an anti-ulcer agent, shown to be as effective as cimetidine and ranitidine. Eradication of *H. pylori* requires treatment with antibiotics and bismuth compounds. (See also ACID INDIGESTION.)

Sepulveda, A. R., and L. G. Coelho. "Helicobacter pylori and gastric malignancies." *Helicobacter.* 7 Suppl. 1 (2002): 37–42.

gastrin A hormone formed by pyloric glands in the lower region of the stomach. In response to food, gastrin is released into the bloodstream where it stimulates the secretion of stomach acid by specific cells in the stomach lining called parietal cells. Gastrin also stimulates intestinal peristalsis. (See also DIGESTION.)

gastritis Any inflammation of the stomach lining. Gastritis may be accompanied by nausea and vomiting, or by a sense of fullness after eating a small meal. Gastritis is one of the most common stomach ailments and it increases the risk of stomach cancer.

A variety of causes have been implicated, including excessive consumption of ALCOHOL, rich food, COFFEE, tea, and other irritating foods. Among the most common causes of gastritis is ASPIRIN, which may cause stomach bleeding. Other drugs can cause acute symptoms: sulfonamide, certain antibiotics, and quinine. Viral and bacterial infections may be involved. Pernicious ANEMIA (due to

VITAMIN B_{12} deficiency), gastric ulcer and polyps, diabetes and adrenal insufficiency often accompany chronic gastritis.

Symptoms, which are intermittent and variable, include loss of appetite, mild nausea, a feeling of fullness or abdominal pain, recurrent heartburn or pain in the upper abdominal region, and vomiting.

Eliminating the offending irritant and avoiding alcohol, caffeine, smoking, and foods that provoke a response may help reduce pain. Symptoms may be relieved by medications (such as cimetidine) that coat the lesions or reduce acid production. Deglycyrrhizinoted licorice has been used to help heal peptic ulcers.

Recurrent, chronic gastritis can indicate an underlying problem. For example, food allergies can cause gastric inflammation and other gastrointestinal symptoms. The bacterium *HELICOBACTER PYLORI* is frequently associated with chronic stomach inflammation. Elimination of infection by antibiotics and bismuth compound treatments can eliminate recurrent episodes. (See also ACID INDIGESTION.)

Fay, M., M. B. Fennerty, J. Emerson, and M. Larez. "Dietary habits and the risk of stomach cancer: a comparison study of patients with and without intestinal metaplasia," *Gastroenterology and Nursing* 16, no. 4 (1994): 158–162.

gastroenteritis An inflammation of the stomach and large and small intestines. It is most often caused by viruses like rotaviruses and adenoviruses, but it can also be caused by bacteria or parasites in food and water. Bacterial causes include SALMONELLA and *ESCHERICHIA COLI* 0157. It can be easily passed on to others in bodily fluid. It can also be a reaction to LACTOSE INTOLERANCE.

Symptoms include vomiting, diarrhea, stomach cramps, headaches, and fever. ANTIBIOTICS can help if the cause is bacterial. There are as many as 90 million cases of gastroenteritis each year in the United States.

gastroenterology A specialized branch of medicine focusing on the structure, function, and pathology of the STOMACH, INTESTINES, ESOPHAGUS, and related organs like the LIVER and PANCREAS. (See also GASTROINTESTINAL DISORDERS.)

gastrointestinal Concerning the stomach and intestines. (See also DIGESTION.)

gastrointestinal disorders A wide variety of conditions affecting the gastrointestinal tract, including food sensitivities; structural defects; infections by VIRUSES and BACTERIA (such as *Helicobacter pylori* and *Escherichia coli*) and by organisms causing food poisoning; parasites such as giardia; fungal pathogens such as YEAST; STRESS; and glandular imbalances, such as low stomach acid. Diet is directly related to problems due to nutritional deficiencies, food allergies, food sensitivities, and low fiber intake. LACTOSE INTOLERANCE is an example of a common food sensitivity.

In the United States, overall rates of gastrointestinal illness range from 1.5 to 1.9 illnesses per person per year. Diarrheal illnesses are second only to CARDIOVASCULAR DISEASE as a cause of death worldwide, and they are the leading cause of childhood death. The following is a listing of important gastrointestinal disorders:

- GASTRITIS: Characterized by gastric pain due to a generalized inflammation of the stomach lining.
- GASTRIC ULCERS and DUODENAL ULCERS: Open sores in the stomach or intestinal wall. The pitting may be severe enough to cause internal bleeding.
- GASTROENTERITIS: An illness that can cause diarrhea, stomach cramps, vomiting, nausea, fever, and headache.
- Chronic constipation.
- Chronic DIARRHEA.
- COLITIS: Inflammation and/or ulcer of the colon and rectum.
- ILEITIS: An inflammation and ulceration of the small intestine that causes alternating diarrhea and constipation, occasionally with vomiting.
- LIVER CIRRHOSIS: Scarring of the liver.
- HEPATITIS: Inflammation of the liver, often due to viral infection.
- Stomach cancer.
- Hiatus hernia: The bulging of the stomach through the diaphragm.
- MALABSORPTION: Maldigestion and infection by bacteria and parasites.
- MALDIGESTION: This can lead to secondary nutrient deficiency states. Inadequate pancreatic

enzymes, low stomach acid (hypochlorhydria), and carbohydrate intolerance (such as lactose intolerance) may be involved.

- DIVERTICULITIS.
- Hemorrhoids.

(See also CELIAC DISEASE; FLATULENCE; INFLAMMATORY BOWEL DISEASE; LACTOSE INTOLERANCE; SPRUE.)

Chang, L. et al. "Perceptual Responses in Patients with Mild Inflammatory and Functional Bowel Disease," *Gut* 47 (2000): 497–505.

gastrointestinal tract That part of the DIGESTIVE TRACT represented by the stomach and the intestines and their ancillary glands, including the liver and pancreas. (See also DIGESTION.)

gastroplasty A surgical procedure that reduces the functional size of the stomach by stapling a portion (sealing off). This is a drastic weight-reduction strategy used for severely obese individuals. Weight loss ensues because the capacity for food intake is reduced. (See also DIETING; OBESITY.)

gastrostomy A surgical procedure introducing a passageway from the STOMACH cavity through the abdominal wall (fistula). When the ESOPHAGUS is closed off, for example due to tumors, or when swallowing reflexes are inhibited, as in some stroke patients, food may be introduced into the stomach through such an opening. (See also DIGESTION.)

gavage Liquid feeding that occurs with a tube through the nasal passage to the ESOPHAGUS and the STOMACH (nasal gavage). Gavage also refers to feeding via a stomach tube (gastrogavage).

gelatin A processed form of animal PROTEIN that dissolves when mixed with hot water and gels upon cooling. Gelatin absorbs 5 to 10 times its weight as water. It is commercially prepared by the breakdown of connective tissue protein, especially COLLAGEN, from the bones of slaughtered animals. Gelatin is a low-quality protein because it is deficient in many essential AMINO ACIDS, including TRYPTOPHAN and METHIONINE.

Gelatin is used as a culinary thickening and stabilizing agent. It is used with flavorings in desserts and pudding mixes, and in candy, jellies, and ice cream. Commercial gelatin desserts usually contain high levels of SODIUM, SUCROSE, and artificial coloring to make them look and taste like fruit desserts. Despite popular opinion, gelatin neither strengthens nails nor helps cure ulcers. (See also BIOLOGICAL VALUE.)

gemfibrozil A cholesterol-lowering drug that has been shown to raise HIGH-DENSITY LIPOPROTEIN (HDL), the desirable CHOLESTEROL. (See also CHOLESTEROL-LOWERING DRUGS.)

gene A unit of heredity that defines a trait or characteristic. A gene represents a region of DNA that codes for the sequence of AMINO ACIDS of a specific protein. Consequently DNA is said to be the "blueprint" of the cell's proteins. The cell nucleus contains a set of chromosomes with many thousands of genes.

MUTAGENS are agents that alter genes by attacking the DNA molecule, changing the genetic structure and causing mutations. Once a mutation has occurred, it is passed from one generation to the next. Mutagens are a diverse group of agents: Certain endogenous chemicals in plants, as well as pollutants, certain PESTICIDES and some synthetic FOOD ADDITIVES, even ultraviolet light, can cause mutations. This is a major concern because most mutagens are cancer-causing agents (CARCINOGENS).

In the nucleus of a human cell, chromosomes occur in pairs. Each member of a pair of genes is called an allele, which may be dominant or recessive. In a simple scenario, one or both genes of a pair of alleles may be dominant; therefore the trait or characteristic determined by the gene is expressed. A recessive trait (autosomal recessive gene) will not be expressed if it is paired with a dominant gene, though it will nonetheless be carried along through inheritance. Individuals who carry the recessive trait possess one normal gene and one modified gene and are classified as heterozygotes (hybrids). A gene coding for a defective protein would be expressed when two recessive genes are inherited (homozygotes), leading to the occurrence of certain rare genetic diseases at birth.

Several genetic diseases are based upon altered metabolism due to mutant enzymes. About 5 percent of cases with highly elevated blood cholesterol are due to genetic alterations in proteins responsible for cholesterol metabolism or transport. Typical examples are PHENYLKETONURIA, which reflects a defect in the metabolism of the amino acid PHENYLALANINE, and GALACTOSEMIA, the result of a defect in the metabolism of the SUGAR GALACTOSE. The severe effects of PKU can be avoided by strict dietary measures initiated soon after birth to avoid ingesting excessive amounts of phenylalanine. Early detection is the best strategy. Individuals who carry a recessive gene and a normal gene usually do not experience the genetic disease. For example, about one person in 100 carries the trait for phenyketonuria while those with PKU possess a pair of abnormal genes—a much rarer occurrence (one out of 10,000 births).

Genetic polymorphism refers to the multiple genetic variants for a given protein, such as HEMOGLOBIN, the oxygen carrier protein of red blood cells. Most of the protein variants function more or less normally and do not directly cause disease. On the other hand, it is the slight differences in proteins reflecting differences in genetic makeup that account for individual traits among people. As a consequence, there will be slightly different nutrient requirements for optimal health among different persons. Their levels of liver detoxication enzymes will also vary. This variation partially explains why different individuals vary in their susceptibility to toxins, medications, anesthetics, and even cigarette smoke. (See also BIOCHEMICAL INDIVIDUALITY; GENETIC ENGINEERING.)

generally recognized as safe (GRAS) Substances added to foods that are judged as safe because of their long history of usage without apparent harmful effects. Because of public concern for the safety of an increasing number of new food additives, in 1958 the Food Additive Amendment was appended to the federal Food, Drug and Cosmetic Act requiring *pre*-market approval of all food additives. Developers must demonstrate "reasonable certainty of no harm" of a new food additive. Otherwise, foods containing the additive may be considered adulterated under the original act. The amendment, however, contains an important exception: If an additive is "generally regarded as safe" (GRAS), then the additive is *exempt* from formal premarket safety review. The intent of this exception was to prevent common food additives such as salt and pepper from having to undergo unnecessary safety testing. The determination of GRAS status is not a formal process, and the developer may presume an additive to be GRAS, only to be contradicted later by the FDA. The 1958 law regulating food additives exempted about 700 apparently safe chemicals and materials, which were approved by the U.S. FDA as food additives without further study. Subsequently developed food additives have had to meet requirements for premarket clearance in the FDA.

The GRAS "grandfather" clause is controversial because the safety of some have been questioned. As a result, the FDA has reevaluated the GRAS listings and banned or restricted some substances on the basis of new data indicating potential health problems.

The process by which an additive is cleared for use is complex. The responsibility for proving a substance belongs on the list is borne by the manufacturer, who must first prove to the FDA that the proposed additive is effective and that the additive can be detected and measured in the final product.

The next step requires the manufacturer to study the effects of the substance on animals who ingest large amounts of the additive to make sure that the substance does not cause cancer, birth defects, or other injury. If the additive meets these requirements, the FDA validates the research and then schedules a public hearing to discuss expert testimony for and against the substance. A ruling is then issued by the FDA. Once the substance is approved for the GRAS list, the FDA determines in what amounts and for what purposes the substance may be used. (See also FOOD, DRUG AND COSMETIC ACT.)

genetically modified foods The chemical modification of genes of plants, animals, and microorganisms. Typically, additional genetic messages are removed from one organism and inserted into chromosomes of another type to create the ability to synthesize new proteins in the recipient. For example, a genetically engineered BOVINE GROWTH HORMONE being sold in the United States can boost milk production in cows by 10 percent. Genetic engineering also may improve the protein quality of plant foods and feed for livestock. A renewed interest in the disease-prevention and the health-enhancing properties of foods has sparked other efforts to improve these characteristics in foods; for example, breeding carrots with increased levels of the antioxidant BETA-CAROTENE.

Technology is producing plants resistant to insects to viral diseases and to HERBICIDES. Some of the first experiments with genetically engineered crops have yielded tomato plants that produce animal antibodies against viral infections, conferring disease resistance. Alternatively, infection-resistant genes from other plant species have been inserted into tomatoes, making them resistant to bacterial infection. Planting crops that have herbicide-tolerant genes may help farmers control weeds in crops that would otherwise be damaged. One method is to insert an altered gene for a specific plant enzyme normally targeted or inactivated by a given herbicide. The change can make the enzyme insensitive to the herbicide. Another approach is to insert a gene for a new enzyme that detoxifies the herbicide. For example, a gene from petunia protects soybean plants from herbicides; and bacterial gene inserted into corn protects it against the European corn borer.

Genetic alteration may yield crops that can grow in cooler or warmer, wetter or drier climates. Plants may someday produce drugs such as vaccines and human hormones. Genes from other species can be incorporated in plants to develop products that are more nutritious or are sweeter; have a better flavor or more color for consumer appeal; and/or have a longer shelf life.

Viruses affect many crops, ranging from wheat, corn and POTATOES to TOMATOES and CITRUS FRUIT. By inserting a gene coding for a protein of an attacking virus into a susceptible plant species, the recipient plants tolerate tobacco, alfalfa, and cucumber mosaic viruses as well as potato viruses. Virus-resistant potatoes and tomatoes have been field-tested.

A number of concerns have been expressed by food scientists, consumer groups, and policymakers about genetic engineering. There is concern that plant geneticists may engineer crops to improve processing and yield at the expense of good nutrition. Cosmetic changes could be developed that might mask unripe or overripe foods.

Safety is another concern. Genetically engineered plants could make higher levels of known toxic substances. Viral genes that can increase a plant's resistance to a pest could produce altered plant viruses that may harm plants.

Transferring genes could cause allergies. For example, genes from a peanut plant inserted into another plant could make the new variety able to trigger reactions in those with peanut allergies. The FDA does not require special labeling for genetically engineered foods, except to potential allergens. Another possibility is the production of plant toxins in genetically engineered food.

One type of genetically modified corn became the subject of a class-action consumer lawsuit in the late 1990s. Starlink corn seed, developed by Aventis, contained the insecticidal protein Cry9C. Corn containing this protein was protected from attack by corn boring insects. Starlink corn was registered and annually renewed for domestic animal feed and nonfood industrial use in the United States in 1998, 1999, and 2000. In mid-2000 fragments of Starlink corn began appearing in the food supply, specifically taco shells. Dozens of people claimed they became ill after eating food containing Starlink corn. By the end of 2000 Aventis had withdrawn its registration for Starlink corn.

Three federal agencies regulate genetically engineered products in the United States. The Department of Agriculture (USDA) must first approve field tests of transgenic (genetically engineered) plants. The Environmental Protection Agency (EPA) establishes the tolerance levels of all synthetic pesticides in such food crops. The FDA evaluates all genetically engineered plant foods to determine whether the new genetic trait constitutes a FOOD ADDITIVE or other major plant alteration. The FDA does not require special labeling or review unless alteration of a food changes its nutritional value or produces possible toxins or allergens. (See also DNA; FUNCTIONAL FOODS; GREEN REVOLUTION.)

geophagia The consumption of inedible materials such as clay, dirt, and chalk. Famine has been associated with earth and clay eating, but clay eating is not limited to hardship. Clay is consumed around the world in spices, condiments, or relishes. The hypothesis that clay eating is a response to deficiencies of minerals like IRON or CALCIUM has not been supported by hard evidence, possibly because the minerals in clay may be readily absorbed. Another proposal is that clay eating is a detoxifying strategy allowing people to make wider use of plants as food. In certain cultures, pregnant women have traditionally eaten clay to settle their stomach. A common over-the-counter remedy for diarrhea is kaolinate, a major mineral in clay.

germ The nutrient-rich embryo of seeds or kernels. This area is vitamin-rich and contains VITAMIN E plus THIAMIN, RIBOFLAVIN, NIACIN, and plant oils. Wheat germ is removed during the milling and refining process to obtain white flour. (See also BRAN, WHEAT; ENDOSPERM; GRAIN; WHEAT.)

gestational diabetes See DIABETES, GESTATIONAL.

ghee See BUTTER, CLARIFIED.

giardiasis An intestinal infection caused by the protozoan parasite *Giardia lamblia.* This disease usually is associated with contaminated drinking WATER that may look clean. Water chlorination may not destroy giardia cysts, therefore water treatment may not remove this parasite. In the United States, giardiasis is the most frequent cause of waterborne diarrhea, and an estimated 2 percent to 5 percent of adults are infected. The numbers are higher for children; in some counties of the western United States, the percentage of infected adults may be as high as 13 percent. It can be transmitted by fecal contamination, and thus by infected food handlers. Children at day care centers, and individuals with low stomach acid and compromised IMMUNE SYSTEMS, are more likely to acquire giardia.

Symptoms include DIARRHEA, stomachache, FLATULENCE, ANOREXIA, nausea, and vomiting. Giardiasis promotes atrophy of the surface of the small intestine, which can result in LACTOSE INTOLERANCE and MALABSORPTION. However, chronic giardiasis may cause only mild symptoms and people without symptoms are reservoirs of this parasite. In order to minimize the risk of infection, campers are advised to boil water for 10 minutes, or use water purification tablets or a portable water filtration unit. (See also GASTROINTESTINAL DISORDERS; MICROVILLI.)

ginger (*Zingiber officinale*) A spice originating in the East Indies, now cultivated in many tropical areas including Jamaica, and regions of Nigeria, India, and Japan. Ginger is a yellow or reddish-brown underground stem called a rhizome and belongs to a family of reedlike perennials. Several hundred varieties of ginger exist. The characteristic peppery taste of ginger is produced by a compound called gingerin. When harvested at the appropriate time, it is not fibrous, nor does it have a bitter aftertaste. Ginger is used fresh or dried, powdered or crystallized, in pickling spices, ginger bread, cakes, puddings, stews and curry bases. Ginger, boiled and preserved in syrup, is known as Canton ginger and is used in desserts.

Dried ginger has been used in folk medicine to treat complaints of the digestive tract, such as gas and bloating, nausea and vomiting, diarrhea and stomach cramps. Ginger also has a long history in treating rheumatism and reducing inflammation; clinical studies suggest it can help ease knee pain in osteoarthritis.

gingivitis Inflammation of gums (gingiva), a chronic DEGENERATIVE DISEASE. Gingivitis affects 70 percent of Americans over the age of 65. Inflammation can lead to bleeding gums, recession of gums, destruction of the bony tooth matrix, and, eventually, to tooth loss. Gingivitis is associated with vitamin deficiencies and metal poisoning and can be caused by pathogenic organisms associated with dental plaque accumulation. Ill-fitting appliances and dentures can also cause gingivitis. Flossing and prophylactic cleaning by a dental hygienist are the best approaches to prevention. (See also FLUORIDE.)

ginkgo (*Ginkgo biloba*) An ancient species of deciduous tree whose leaves have long been used in Asian medicine. Ginkgo is native to China, and extracts of ginkgo leaves have been used to support heart, brain, and lung function for nearly 5,000 years. Ginkgo leaf extracts are standardized in terms of their active components. The leaves contain substances called ginkgolides and bilobalide, complex organic compounds that help fight disease. Ginkgo also contain FLAVONOIDS that function as ANTIOXIDANTS, which limit damage due to reactive forms of oxygen and can help reduce inflammation. Furthermore, ginkgo extracts can help maintain normal blood flow in arteries, veins, and capillaries and maintain circulation.

Ginkgo leaf extracts can increase and normalize blood flow by relaxing blood vessel walls. They can also improve blood flow to the brain, thereby improving brain function. Ginkgo extracts inhibit the action of a substance called platelet activating factor, which triggers inflammation through the production of oxidized lipids and the migration of attacking white blood cells. They therefore protect areas such as the lungs and intestine against inflammation and tissue damage. Clinical studies suggest that ginkgo leaf extracts can stabilize, slow the progression, and sometimes improve certain aspects of Alzheimer's disease or mixed dementia. They may also improve cognitive function in older adults with mild to moderate age-dependent memory deficits. Lower doses of 120 mg/day were as effective as 600 mg/day. Pain-free walking may improve in patients with intermittent claudication. Ginkgo may also benefit some patients with PMS, or those with age-related macular degeneration. In addition ginkgo leaf extract has been used to prevent altitude sickness.

Side effects are rare and may include headaches and stomach upsets. Crude ginkgo preparations, but not the widely used leaf extracts, can cause severe allergies. Safety data on ginkgo extract is insufficient regarding its use by pregnant or lactating women. (See also SENILITY.)

ginseng (*Panax ginseng;* Chinese ginseng, Korean ginseng) A medicinal herb native to northern China and Korea. Ginseng is widely cultivated in Korea, China, and Japan. It is available as white ginseng, from the dried root, or as red ginseng, which has been steamed. (Siberian ginseng, *Eleuthrococcus senticosus,* is a distant relative to the more popular Panax ginseng. Its properties are similar to *Panax ginseng.* Most research on Siberian ginseng has been conducted in Russia and the former Soviet Union.) Ginseng is a famous herb of Chinese medicine, long used to restore "yang" energy, specifically to support normal healing processes during infections, to overcome fatigue, and to counter elevated blood pressure and high blood lipids (fat and cholesterol). Ginseng can stimulate the IMMUNE SYSTEM, especially natural killer cells and scavenger immune cells (macrophages) in the liver, spleen, and lymph nodes, and antibody-producing cells. In experimental animals, ginseng has prevented viral infection. However, excessive amounts of ginseng can inhibit the immune response during serious infections. Ginseng may lower the risk of some types of CANCER in experimental animals. Ginseng can also lower elevated BLOOD SUGAR levels and high blood pressure.

Human studies performed in the former Soviet Union support ginseng's role in increasing stamina. Animal studies indicate that it can improve metabolism of the central nervous system and nerves controlling muscles, and spare GLYCOGEN, the glucose reserve, in exercising muscle. A class of plant compounds called saponins appears to be the active ingredient. In terms of adapting to stress, ginseng saponins (ginsenosides) stimulate the adrenal glands by promoting the release of adrenocorticotropin (ACTH) and ENDORPHINS, the brain's own opiates, from the PITUITARY GLAND. The adrenals are responsible for adapting the body to stress by producing hormones such as epinephrine (adrenaline) and cortisol.

Ginseng can affect the body in many ways, and long-term consumption of excessive amounts may have negative consequences. It may depress the central nervous system, and cause vaginal bleeding and breast pain in postmenopausal women. Long-term use can lead to "ginseng abuse syndrome," with possible high blood pressure, DIARRHEA, skin eruptions, loss of sleep, edema, nervousness, feminization of males, and masculinization of females. One of the problems with ginseng is the wide variation in quality of commercially available products, which range from chewing gum and teas to capsules. Preparations standardized for content of an active ingredient (ginsenoside) and prudent application of ginseng are recommended. Safety data for *Panax ginseng* are inadequate for use by pregnant or lactating women.

GI tract See DIGESTIVE TRACT.

gland An organ or cell group specialized to secrete products used elsewhere in the body. Simple glands consist of a few cells, while compound glands possess clusters around a lumen or cavity and their secretions leave by a common duct.

Endocrine glands produce HORMONES, and are ductless glands whose secretions directly enter the blood or lymph. Pancreatic islets, the PITUITARY, THYROID, THYMUS, and ADRENAL GLANDS are endocrine glands. Major endocrine glands are located in the ovaries, testes, duodenum (upper portion of the small intestine), and stomach.

Exocrine glands export their secretions to other regions via ducts. The exocrine pancreas secretes digestive enzymes, and the LIVER secretes BILE for digestion in the intestine through a duct leading to the small intestine. Mucous glands produce protective materials to coat the surface of the digestive tract and other cavities. Gastric glands in the lining of the stomach secrete GASTRIC JUICE for digestion. The parotoid and salivary glands produce SALIVA. Sudoriferous glands in the skin produce perspiration. (See also ENDOCRINE SYSTEM; PANCREAS.)

gliaden A protein found in wheat, rye, and other grains. Together with glutenin, the other major type of GLUTEN protein, gliaden is responsible for the stickiness of dough. The high gluten content of wheat FLOUR creates an elastic, versatile dough for baking. Gliaden contains unusually large amounts of nonessential amino acids, GLUTAMINE and PROLINE. On the other hand, wheat protein and gliaden are low in the essential AMINO ACIDS.

globulins A group of PROTEINS that are insoluble in pure water but are soluble in salt solutions at neutral pH. An important globulin is serum ALBUMIN, which represents 55 percent of total soluble protein of blood. Serum albumin helps maintain the osmotic pressure of vessels and appropriate concentration of ELECTROLYTES in blood because it does not cross vessel walls.

Alpha, beta, and gamma globulins of blood have different net electrical charges, permitting their separation by an electric field. Alpha globulins include HIGH-DENSITY LIPOPROTEIN (HDL), the lipoprotein that scavenges CHOLESTEROL; ceruloplasmin for COPPER transport; and VERY LOW-DENSITY LIPOPROTEINS (VLDL), which transport fat synthesized by the liver. Beta globulins include TRANSFERRIN, which transports IRON; LOW-DENSITY LIPOPROTEINS (LDL), which transport cholesterol from the liver to other tissues; and fibrinogen, responsible for blood clotting. The liver also produces inactive enzymes like prothrombin that, when activated, promote clot formation. GAMMA GLOBULINS are circulating ANTIBODIES.

Other globulins occur in plants; edestin (WHEAT); phaseolin (BEANS); legumin (beans, peas); tuberin (POTATO); amadin (ALMONDS); and arachin (peanuts).

glomerular filtration The first step in the process of urine production. Nephrons, microscopic filtration units of the kidney, permit some substances to pass into the kidney while excluding others. They are composed of a knot of vessels and a microscopic tube called a glomerulus. The filtration rate into the glomerulus is high; for the normal adult the kidneys filter about 48 gallons (180 liters) of fluid per day. Many compounds pass through the pores in the capillary walls, but serum ALBUMIN and most proteins are normally not filtered.

As filtrate passes downstream, tubules allow selective reabsorption of ions like SODIUM and BICARBONATE and small molecules like GLUCOSE, AMINO ACIDS, and water. As sodium is transported back into the blood from the tubules, it draws water along with it; therefore most of the water is reabsorbed (taken back up into the bloodstream). Passage of the remaining water is regulated by a pituitary hormone, triggered when the brain (hypothalamus) senses an increase in osmotic pressure (lower water concentration). The tubules also help regulate the pH of the blood. When concentrations of KETONE BODIES, acids produced during severe caloric restriction, or of glucose, produced in uncontrollable diabetes, exceed a point at which they are no longer efficiently reabsorbed, they are also excreted in the urine, causing increased urine production and possible dehydration. (See also ALDOSTERONE; ANGIOTENSIN; ANTIDIURETIC HORMONE.)

glossitis Tongue inflammation. Acute glossitis is a painful condition in which the tongue is irregularly fissured and ulcerated. Inflammation of the tongue is accompanied by a loss of the rough surface (filliform papillaes) or "bald tongue." The pain associated with glossitis can make eating difficult. Glossitis may be associated with nutritional ANEMIAS and nontropical SPRUE (a digestive disorder characterized by malabsorption of fat and other nutrients, together with deficiencies of NIACIN, RIBOFLAVIN, and VITAMIN B_{12}). (See also AVITAMINOSIS; MALNUTRITION.)

glucagon A HORMONE that increases the levels of BLOOD SUGAR (glucose). Glucagon is produced by alpha cells of the endocrine pancreas and is released into the bloodstream when blood sugar drops. Glucagon has the opposite effect of INSULIN, which is released after a meal to lower blood glucose. Both are constructed of AMINO ACIDS.

To increase blood sugar levels, glucagon stimulates GLYCOGEN breakdown and glucose release by the liver. Glycogen is the glucose polymer for temporary storage. Glucagon also stimulates the liver to convert amino acids to GLUCOSE (a process called GLUCONEOGENESIS). (See also CARBOHYDRATE METABOLISM; ENDOCRINE SYSTEM; EPINEPHRINE.)

glucocorticoid A hormone produced by the adrenal glands, responsible for maintaining BLOOD SUGAR, limiting inflammation, and suppressing the immune response. The principle glucocorticoid is CORTISOL (hydrocortisone). Like other steroid hormones, it is synthesized from cholesterol. Extreme STRESS can lead to an overproduction of glucocorticoids, which places the body in a "catabolic state," with increased muscle breakdown, decreased antibody production, and increased susceptibility to infection and fatigue. Inadequate glucocorticoid production can lead to HYPOGLYCEMIA (low blood sugar) as well as excessive fatigue. (See also ADRENAL GLANDS; ADRENOCORTICOTROPIC HORMONE; HYPOTHALAMUS.)

glucomannan A form of water-soluble FIBER obtained from Konjac tubers, which originated in Japan. Glucomannan readily absorbs water and swells to form a gel. The increased bulk contributes to a feeling of satiety, and glucomannan has been used as an APPETITE SUPPRESSANT. Like pectin, glucomannan has an effect of lowing cholesterol levels. Glucomannan tablets can lodge in the throat if not predissolved in water. (See also BULKING AGENTS.)

gluconeogenesis The enzymic system responsible for producing GLUCOSE from noncarbohydrate sources. Gluconeogenesis occurs primarily in the LIVER in response to lowered BLOOD SUGAR. The liver stores surplus glucose as GLYCOGEN, long chains of glucose units, after feeding. Between meals glucose is released from glycogen stores. However, gluconeogenesis becomes important in maintaining blood sugar levels with prolonged fasting. During severe dietary restriction (caloric or carbohydrate restriction) muscle protein is substantially degraded to provide amino acids that the liver readily transforms to glucose. The liver also manufactures glucose from a variety of noncarbohydrate molecules, including from lactic acid during strenuous exercise; from glycerol during fat breakdown; and from PYRUVIC ACID, CITRIC ACID, and other intermediates of the KREB'S CYCLE, the central energy-producing pathway of the cell. Gluconeogenesis is lowered in individuals who abuse alcohol or who are susceptible to HYPOGLYCEMIA. (See also CARBOHYDRATE METABOLISM; CORTISOL; GLUCAGON.)

gluconic acid An ACID derived from glucose and a naturally occurring ingredient in food. Several forms of gluconic acid are also used as FOOD ADDITIVES. Sodium gluconate is used in nonalcoholic beverages and in processed fruit juices to bind (chelate) metal ions that promote spoilage. A derivative of gluconic acid called FERROUS GLUCONATE is used to blacken olives. Another widely used derivative, called gluconolactone, is used in cake mixes, CHEESES, powdered SOFT DRINKS, gelatin desserts, processed fruits and vegetables, imitation dairy products, and certain cured meats. (See also CHELATE.)

glucosamine (D-glucosamine) A building block of cartilage. Glucosamine is a raw material for GLYCOSAMINOGLYCANS, structural materials needed for healthy joints. It is also a component of mucins, slippery materials that are part of mucous secretions, and cell coat materials. Glucosamine is normally synthesized from glucose (blood sugar). Apparently, the ability to synthesize and maintain cartilage declines with age. Glucosamine is selectively absorbed and supplementation has been reported to relieve joint pain in OSTEOATHRITIS by exerting a protective effect on joint tissue and in supporting cartilage repair.

The typical forms of glucosamine found in supplements are glucosamine sulfate and glucosamine hydrochloride. Studies of the effectiveness of glucosamine sulfate in relieving the pain of osteoarthritis have lasted up to three years. It may be as effective as common nonsteroidal anti-inflammatory drugs but is better tolerated.

So far, it has not been established whether alterations in blood lipids or insulin are clinically relevant. Individuals who are susceptible to diabetes, high blood pressure, or high cholesterol should use glucosamine with caution. Because glucosamine is derived from shellfish, this may be a concern for those with shellfish allergies. (See also CHONDROITIN.)

glucose A simple sugar that is one of the most important CARBOHYDRATES in plant and animal metabolism. As an hexose (six-carbon sugar), glucose has a formula of $C_6H_{12}O_6$. Photosynthesis converts carbon dioxide and water to glucose, which is stored in leaves, stems, fruits, roots, pods, and seeds, as glucose, as other sugars or as STARCH, composed of long chains of glucose units. DIGESTION converts starch back to glucose.

Glucose occurs naturally in food. It is a major ingredient of HONEY and SUCROSE (table sugar) and consists of half-glucose and half-fructose, while milk sugar (lactose) contains half-glucose and half-GALACTOSE. Free glucose occurs in fruit (grape sugar). Glucose is a common food additive, listed as DEXTROSE. Glucose from any of these sources is absorbed easily by the small intestine, raising blood glucose levels rapidly.

Glucose is the most important carbohydrate in the body. As BLOOD SUGAR, it is key, supplying about 20 percent of normal energy needs. Simple sugars such as FRUCTOSE and galactose must first be converted to glucose by the liver to be used for energy. Like all carbohydrate nutrients, glucose yields four calories per gram. Glucose is the major fuel of the brain because it readily crosses the BLOOD-BRAIN BARRIER. The brain accounts for only 3 percent of total body weight, yet this organ consumes 20 percent of the glucose in the blood.

The speed at which different sources of starch are digested affects the rate at which glucose is absorbed and blood sugar rises. Slower digestion results in a slower rise in blood sugar and a decreased need for insulin. The rate at which blood sugar rises after a carbohydrate-rich meal depends on the source and type of carbohydrate, how it has been processed, how it is used after digestion, and whether fat has slowed gastric emptying. Generally, the less processed the starchy food, the slower starch conversion to glucose, the slower the increase in blood sugar, hence less insulin will be required. (See also CARBOHYDRATE METABOLISM; GLYCEMIC INDEX.)

glucose metabolism Chemical processes by which the body uses the simple sugar GLUCOSE—the most important carbohydrate fuel of the body. It is oxidized by all tissues including RED BLOOD CELLS for ENERGY.

Glucose Degradation

GLYCOLYSIS is the first pathway of carbohydrate utilization, yielding ATP, the energy currency of the cell. Glycolysis converts glucose to a simple three-carbon acid called PYRUVIC ACID. The process is anaerobic: Oxygen does not participate in the reactions. Mitochondria, the "power houses" of the cell, oxidize pyruvic acid to ACETIC ACID, as an activated form called acetyl coenzyme A. Acetyl CoA in turn enters the KREB'S CYCLE, the central energy-yielding pathway, to be oxidized to CARBON DIOXIDE. The complete glucose oxidation traps 40 percent of the chemical energy in glucose as ATP, a remarkably efficient process.

Glucose is also oxidized anaerobically by the PENTOSE phosphate pathway to ATP and five carbon sugars (pentoses), required for DNA and RNA formation. This pathway also provides NADPH (reduced NICOTINAMIDE ADENINE DINUCLEOTIDE phosphate), the reducing agent for all biosynthetic reduction reactions such as occur in FAT and CHOLESTEROL synthesis. Glucose is the raw material for fat and cholesterol. Surplus glucose yields surplus acetyl coenzyme A, which is converted to saturated FATTY ACIDS and fats by the liver and by adipose (fat) tissue (LIPOGENESIS).

Glycogen Formation

Surplus glucose in stored as GLYCOGEN, long chains of glucose units, in the LIVER and muscle. The liver release glucose from glycogen into the bloodstream when the blood glucose level drops between meals or in the early stages of fasting in response to hormone signals from the pancreas and adrenal glands. Muscle glycogen supplies muscle cells with glucose for quick energy during strenuous EXERCISE. Muscle glycogen cannot be released from muscle cells as glucose. During vigorous physical activity muscles produce LACTIC ACID as the end product of glycolysis, rather than pyruvic acid, the usual product of glycolysis (see above). Lactic acid accumulation partially accounts for the FATIGUE and cramping associated with vigorous exertion. Lactic acid migrates out of muscle cells into the blood, which transports it to the liver for resynthesis as glucose and eventual storage as glycogen.

Regulation of Blood Sugar

Blood sugar is carefully regulated by homeostatic mechanisms (physiologic processes that tend to keep the body functioning on an even keel). The range is normally maintained between 60 and 100 mg glucose per deciliter of blood by several different hormones. The body must deal with two possible situations: elevated blood sugar and low blood sugar. The hormone INSULIN is released into the bloodstream in response to elevated blood glucose levels after a high-carbohydrate meal. Insulin lowers elevated blood sugar by promoting glucose uptake by tissues and stimulating glycogen, fat, and protein synthesis. Abnormally high blood glucose (HYPERGLYCEMIA) is a characteristic of diabetes, a severe disease if left untreated.

Abnormally low blood glucose is called HYPOGLYCEMIA. This condition can profoundly affect the nervous system because of its dependency on glucose for energy. GLUCAGON, CORTISOL, and other hormones counterbalance insulin by raising blood glucose levels. Glucagon promotes glycogen breakdown in the liver. Cortisol promoters the conversion of amino acids, released from muscle protein degradation, to glucose by a pathway called GLUCONEOGENESIS. In time of need, glucose can also be synthesized from lactic acid, pyruvic acid, products of glycolysis, as well as acidic intermediates of the KREB'S CYCLE, such as CITRIC ACID.

Low-carbohydrate diets are the basis of many fad weight-loss programs. When the diet does not supply enough carbohydrate to maintain blood sugar levels, the body switches over to a starvation mode in order to supply blood glucose. The body adapts to inadequate carbohydrate/calorie intake by breaking down muscle protein into amino acids, to be converted to glucose to supply the brain with energy, as well as by breaking down body fat for more general energy needs. (See also DIET, LOW CARBOHYDRATE; DIET, VERY LOW CALORIE; EXERCISE; GLYCEMIC INDEX.)

glucose oxidase An enzyme used to degrade GLUCOSE. A product of MOLD culture, glucose oxidase is used by the food industry to destroy glucose in egg white and whole egg products. Glucose removal facilitates product drying and helps prevent product deterioration. Glucose oxidase helps extend the shelf life of canned SOFT DRINKS and is also used to remove traces of oxygen in packaged foods including dehydrated products, mayonnaise, and canned foods. This step minimizes changes in color and flavor during storage. (See also FOOD ADDITIVES.)

glucose tolerance The efficiency with which the body can take up and dispose of glucose, thus lowering elevated blood GLUCOSE. Blood sugar levels higher than normal (HYPERGLYCEMIA) are classified as impaired glucose tolerance. DIABETES MELLITUS is the most common cause of chronically high blood glucose levels. The hormone INSULIN stimulates glucose uptake by tissues; diabetics may produce inadequate insulin, or insulin that is produced may not be able to work effectively at the target tissues. Glucose tolerance can decrease with age, due to decreased tissue responsiveness to insulin. The increased proportion of body fat present in some older people also decreases insulin sensitivity.

glucose tolerance factor An agent that assists the action of INSULIN in lowering BLOOD SUGAR (GLUCOSE). Together with glucose tolerance factor, insulin promotes the cellular uptake of glucose and of amino acids and the increased synthesis of fat and protein. Glucose tolerance factor apparently enhances the effects of insulin; it is inactive unless insulin is present. Glucose tolerance factor may be released into the blood, perhaps by the liver, whenever there is a marked increase in blood glucose or insulin.

Glucose tolerance factor contains the trace mineral nutrient CHROMIUM combined with NIACIN (vitamin B_3) and several amino acids. The factor has been isolated from liver and yeast; one of the best dietary sources of the factor is BREWER'S YEAST. (See also CARBOHYDRATE METABOLISM.)

glucose tolerance test A diagnostic procedure that measures how effectively a person clears a large dose of glucose from the bloodstream. Typically, the patient consumes 100 g of glucose in water before breakfast (after fasting overnight). BLOOD SUGAR levels are subsequently measured at intervals for several hours. In a normal response, the blood sugar level rises sharply during the first hour after ingesting glucose, then returns to the resting or fasting level within three hours as INSULIN in released. If the blood sugar level remains elevated, diabetes or a prediabetic condition may be indicated. HYPOGLYCEMIA may be indicated if the blood sugar dips below normal and only slowly returns to the resting level while the patient experiences typical symptoms such as shakiness, sweating, and weakness.

The glucose tolerance test may cause significant discomfort in susceptible people. Hypoglycemic individuals can experience blackouts, sleepiness, or irritability as their blood sugar plummets. A three-hour test may not be long enough to assess glucose tolerance; five or six hours may be more appropriate. It has been suggested that a more realistic test is a "food tolerance" test, designed to see how the body responds to sugar released by DIGESTION of foods. A diagnosis is strengthened by a simultaneous insulin tolerance test that measures the blood levels of insulin after the glucose challenge. Candidates for a glucose tolerance test include those at risk for diabetes through inheritance, and pregnant women. (See also CARBOHYDRATE METABOLISM; DIABETES MELLITUS.)

glucostat A hypothetical mechanism in the brain by which BLOOD SUGAR levels help regulate APPETITE. According to this proposal, a drop in blood glucose affects the HYPOTHALAMUS, the region of the brain that regulates involuntary activities and integrates response to stress. The hypothalamus responds by activating neural pathways to arouse eating behavior. This seminal concept formed the basis for much of the essential research on brain function and glucose utilization. Evidence continues to accumulate that the hypothalamus contributes to regulating feeding behavior. The fat cell hormone LEPTIN may affect the region of the hypothalamus that regulates satiety. (See also CRAVING; OBESITY.)

glucosuria The excretion of abnormal amounts of glucose in the urine. Glucosuria often indicates elevated BLOOD GLUCOSE (HYPERGLYCEMIA) caused by DIABETES MELLITUS. Healthy people secrete little glucose in the urine because glucose is rapidly reabsorbed (salvaged) from the filtered fluid by the KIDNEY. However, when blood glucose concentrations reach 300 mg/100 ml, the kidneys' transport maximum absorption rate is exceeded, and glucose is secreted in the urine. Excretion of glucose requires additional water, and DEHYDRATION is a likely consequence due to frequent urination. (See also GLOMERULAR FILTRATION.)

glutamic acid (Glu; glutamate) One of the 20 AMINO ACIDS that are the building blocks of PROTEIN. Glutamic acid is an acidic, nonessential amino acid because the body easily manufactures it as needed from alpha ketoglutaric acid, a common intermediate produced by amino acid degradation and by the KREB'S CYCLE, the pathway central to carbohydrate metabolism. When glutamic acid is neutralized it is called "glutamate." The body converts glutamic acid to GLUTAMINE, another nonessential amino acid. Glutamine formation is a key in the disposal of ammonia for the brain because it crosses the BLOOD-BRAIN BARRIER and transports the nitrogen from ammonia to other tissues for eventual disposal as UREA, a nontoxic end product.

Glutamic acid functions as a NEUROTRANSMITTER, a chemical employed in transmitting signals between nerve cells, and is concentrated in the brain. During a STROKE, glutamic acid is released from cells damaged by the loss of oxygen. It has been proposed that in large amounts, glutamic acid can damage nerve cells; thus a stroke may be related to glutamate-induced damage. Glutamic acid is related to brain function in another way: It is the parent of the inhibitory neurotransmitter gamma aminobutyric acid.

Glutamic acid also appears in supplements and FOOD ADDITIVES. Glutamic acid hydrochloride is a supplement used to increase gastric acidity and to counterbalance a deficiency of hydrochloric acid (STOMACH ACID). MONOSODIUM GLUTAMATE (MSG) is a combination of glutamic acid and sodium. MSG is used as a FLAVOR ENHANCER in prepared and CONVENIENCE FOODS. In susceptible people, excessive MSG in food can cause MSG Related Syndrome, including a tingling or burning sensation, heart palpitations, anxiety, urination, thirst, or stomachache. Other food enhancers incorporating glutamate are potassium glutamate and HYDROLYZED VEGETABLE PROTEIN. (See also ACHLORHYDRIA; FOOD LABELING.)

glutamine (Gln, L-glutamine) One of the 20 AMINO ACIDS that serve as raw materials for PROTEINS. The body manufactures this amino acid from GLUTAMIC ACID, therefore, it is not classified as an essential amino acid. The brain and muscle synthesize glutamine to dispose of AMMONIA, a toxic metabolic by-product.

Glutamine is released into the bloodstream and transported to the intestine, where it is a preferred fuel. There it is broken down to glutamic acid and ammonia. Ammonia travels directly via the portal vein to the liver, which incorporates it into urea, the end product of nitrogen metabolism. Urea is then released into the bloodstream and excreted by the kidneys.

Though glutamine is normally the most prevalent amino acid in blood, it may be limited in cases of severe trauma such as recovery from surgery or severe burns, and glutamine supplements may be recommended. Glutamine supplements have been used in drug detoxification centers to help minimize the symptoms of drug and alcohol withdrawal. Glutamine may help maintain the integrity of the small intestine. (See also ALCOHOLISM; AMINO ACID METABOLISM.)

Teran, J. C., K. D. Mullen, and A. J. McCullough. "Glutamine—A Conditionally Essential Amino Acid in Cirrhosis?" *American Journal of Clinical Nutrition* 62 (1995): 897–900.

glutathione The principal sulfur-reducing agent of the cell and a primary ANTIOXIDANT. Glutathione contains three amino acids, including the sulfur amino acid CYSTEINE. Glutathione helps maintain the structure of red blood cell membranes and other cellular proteins and it helps maintain the cytoplasm in a reduced state. Low levels of reduced glutamine are associated with oxidative stress (AGING, toxic exposure, AIDS). As an antioxidant, glutathione assists an enzyme (glutathione peroxidase) that inactivates hydrogen peroxide and oxidized lipids (lipid peroxides), and prevents them from liberating damaging, highly reactive agents. It can also quench free radicals directly.

Glutathione plays an additional, protective role in the liver, where it combines with toxic materials and waste products to permit more efficient excretion. Glutathione also functions as a carrier in the transport of the sulfur-containing amino acids, cysteine and METHIONINE, into cells, and it assists the synthesis of LEUKOTRIENES, extremely potent inflammatory agents. (See also CARBOHYDRATE METABOLISM; DETOXICATION; FREE RADICALS.)

glutathione peroxidase A widely distributed ENZYME that functions as an ANTIOXIDANT. Glutathione peroxidase inactives oxidized lipids (lipid peroxides) and HYDROGEN PEROXIDE, which spontaneously break down to FREE RADICALS, highly reactive chemical species that can damage cells. This enzyme converts hydrogen peroxide to oxygen and water and converts peroxides of polyunsaturated FATTY ACIDS to nontoxic, fatty acids. Glutathione peroxidase requires the trace mineral nutrient SELENIUM as a cofactor. For this reason, selenium is acknowledged as an antioxidant nutrient. (See also BETA-CAROTENE; CATALASE; VITAMIN C; VITAMIN E.)

gluten The major PROTEIN fraction of wheat FLOUR. Gluten consists of an equal mixture of two fractions, GLIADEN and glutenin. When moistened, these proteins yield an elastic dough that is easily shaped. The unique rising qualities of WHEAT flour dough are due to its ability to trap carbon dioxide bubbles released by LEAVENING AGENTS. Baking coagulates gluten so that baked goods maintain their shape without crumbling. Hard wheat contains more gluten than soft varieties. The proteins, hordenin from BARLEY, and oryenin from RICE, resemble glutenin.

Gluten-Free Diet

Only the gliaden portion of gluten has been demonstrated to cause severe malabsorption (CELIAC DISEASE) in sensitive people. Although similar proteins occur in other grains including RYE, barley, TRITICALE, and OATS, wheat contains by far the largest percentage of gluten; corn and rice contain little gluten-type protein. Individuals with celiac disease need to avoid gluten-containing products, a difficult task because wheat flour is added to a huge variety of foods. Rice, potato, legumes like soybeans and lima beans, or foods classified as grains but belonging to different plant families such as AMARANTH and QUINOA yield flour that can substitute for wheat in many dishes and baked goods. (See also BREAD.)

gluten-sensitive enteropathy See CELIAC DISEASE.

glycemic index A measure of how rapidly a food or nutrient raises the BLOOD SUGAR level relative to ingestion of a sample of pure sugar, GLUCOSE. Foods with a high glycemic index increase blood sugar almost as rapidly as eating glucose alone. Not all starchy foods are digested and assimilated with equal ease. Those with a low glycemic index are digested slowly and cause a slower rise in blood sugar. Factors influencing the rate of carbohydrate digestion include the type of food and methods of storage, processing, and cooking. Furthermore, the presence of one food can affect digestion of another.

Before the development of the glycemic index in 1981, scientists assumed that the human body absorbed and digested simple sugars quickly, producing rapid increases in blood sugar level. This was the basis of the advice to avoid sugar, a warning recently relaxed by the American Diabetes Association and others. Now scientists know that simple sugars don't make blood sugar rise any faster than do some complex carbohydrates (although simple sugars are empty calories and still should be minimized for that reason).

Scientists have so far measured the glycemic indexes of about 750 high-carbohydrate foods. Many of the glycemic index results have been surprises. For example, baked potatoes have a glycemic index considerably higher than that of table sugar. The key is to eat less of those foods with a high glycemic index and more of those foods with a low index.

The index is especially useful to people with diabetes who want to plan their diets to minimize the incidence of high blood sugar, or spikes, because it measures how fast the carbohydrate of a particular food is converted to glucose and enters the bloodstream. The lower the number, the slower the action.

When the body digests food more slowly, or converts the food to blood sugar more slowly, less INSULIN is needed to compensate for the increase in blood sugar. For example, FRUCTOSE is slowly converted to glucose by the liver; consequently this refined sugar has a low glycemic index. Foods with a low glycemic index include whole, unprocessed foods like LEGUMES, BEANS, cracked WHEAT, BRAN cereals, and bulgur wheat. These foods contain FIBER and minimally processed starch. Foods with a high (less desirable) glycemic index include table sugar and sugar-rich foods, white BREAD, rice puffs, corn flakes, rye crisps, corn CHIPS, some vegetables, and instant POTATOES. These foods raise blood sugar almost as rapidly as sugar alone because food processing partially breaks down their starch.

However, the utility of the glycemic index in meal planning for diabetics is limited. For example, ice cream, a food with a high content of FAT and SUCROSE (table sugar), has a low glycemic index because fat slows stomach emptying and lowers the rate of entry of sugar into the intestine. This does not mean a diabetic should overindulge in ice cream, because an excess of fatty foods is potentially hazardous to health.

The glycemic index is about the quality of the carbohydrates, not the quantity. Obviously, quantity matters, but the measurement of the glycemic index of a food is not related to portion size. It remains the same whether a person eats 10 g or 1,000 g. This is because to make a fair comparison, tests of the glycemic indexes of food usually use 50 g of available carbohydrate in each food. This means that a person can eat twice as many carbohydrates in a food that has a glycemic index of 50 than in one that has a glycemic index of 100 and have the same blood glucose response. (See also CARDIOVASCULAR DISEASE; DIABETES MELLITUS; DIETARY GUIDELINES FOR AMERICANS.)

Wolever, Thomas, and Janette B. Miller. "Sugars and Blood Glucose Control," *American Journal of Clinical Nutrition* 62, supplement, (July 1995): 212S–221S.

glycerol (glycerin) A syrupy, clear, odorless liquid with a sweet taste; used as a FOOD ADDITIVE. Glycerol maintains moisture in foods and helps dissolve flavors in prepared foods like MARSHMALLOWS, CANDY, fudge, and baked goods. It is used in amounts ranging from 0.5 percent to 10 percent. Glycerol is classified as a generally recognized as safe (GRAS) food additive by the U.S. FDA.

As a NUTRIENT, glycerol occurs in chemical combination with FATTY ACIDS in lipids, fat, and oils (triglycerides). Glycerol contains three oxygen groups that link up with fatty acids. Glycerol itself is derived from GLUCOSE metabolism and can be converted back to glucose by the liver. (See also CARBOHYDRATE METABOLISM; FAT METABOLISM; GLYCOLYSIS.)

glycine (Gly) The smallest of the 20 AMINO ACIDS that form PROTEIN. Glycine is the only common amino acid that is symmetrical, and therefore no mirror image (D, L) forms. The body coverts the amino acid SERINE to glycine; consequently it is not a dietary essential amino acid.

Glycine plays a pivotal role in biosynthesis: Glycine is a building block of HEME, the iron-binding center (porphyrins) of HEMOGLOBIN of RED BLOOD CELLS and oxidation-reduction enzymes (CYTOCHROMES) of the MITOCHONDRIA. It is also a building block of creatine, which is used to replenish ATP in skeletal muscle. Glycine helps form PURINES, nitrogen-containing cyclic compounds that form half the bases of DNA and RNA. The LIVER combines glycine with chemicals to inactivate them and render them water-soluble for excretion. (See also AMINO ACID METABOLISM; DETOXIFICATION; FOLACIN.)

glycocholic acid An acid in BILE that is important in emulsifying FAT for DIGESTION and absorption. It is synthesized from the amino acid GLYCINE and cholic acid, itself a bile component formed by the oxidation of CHOLESTEROL by the liver. As a FOOD ADDITIVE, glycocholic acid serves as an EMULSIFIER to suspend water-insoluble materials. (See also FAT DIGESTION.)

glycogen A storage CARBOHYDRATE in animal tissues. Glycogen resembles STARCH, which is the storage form of GLUCOSE in plants. Both are large molecular weight chains composed of glucose building blocks. Unlike starch, glycogen has a very highly branched structure. Because of its high degree of branching, glycogen binds 3 to 5 g of water per gram of glycogen. A normal adult weighing 150 pounds (68 kg) possesses approximately 800 g of glycogen, found predominantly in skeletal muscle and in the LIVER. Muscle accounts for approximately two-thirds of the glycogen in the body.

Liver Glycogen Metabolism

The liver helps regulate BLOOD SUGAR through the synthesis and degradation of glycogen. After a carbohydrate meal, the liver absorbs glucose from the blood and incorporates it into glycogen in response to the pancreatic hormone INSULIN. With low blood glucose, EPINEPHRINE (adrenaline) from the adrenal glands and GLUCAGON from the pancreas signal glycogen breakdown. The liver, alone, can disengage glucose from cellular reactions and release it into the bloodstream.

Muscle Glycogen Metabolism

Insulin, released in response to elevated blood sugar levels, stimulates glucose uptake by skeletal muscle, where it is deposited as glycogen. Muscle glycogen does not form blood sugar. To provide quick energy, epinephrine (adrenaline) activates the enzyme responsible for breaking down muscle glycogen to glucose, which directly enters GLYCOLYSIS for rapid oxidation and conversion to energy.

During vigorous physical EXERCISE, muscle cells oxidize a portion of the glucose to LACTIC ACID, which can promote muscle cramping and muscle fatigue. Lactic acid eventually escapes from muscle cells into the bloodstream, where it enters the liver and is converted back to blood glucose. During recovery from strenuous exercise, muscles take up blood glucose to restore depleted glycogen. The recovery period may last a day or two.

Glycogen in food is not a significant source of carbohydrate. Meat and fish normally contain very little glycogen because their tissues rapidly break down glycogen during slaughter or capture. Oysters, mussels, scallops, and clams contain a little glycogen when eaten. (See also CARBOHYDRATE LOADING; CARBOHYDRATE METABOLISM; GLYCOGENOLYSIS.)

glycogen loading See CARBOHYDRATE LOADING.

glycogenolysis The breakdown of glycogen in the LIVER and muscle to glucose. EPINEPHRINE, a hormone of the adrenal glands, signals glycogenolysis in muscle for quick energy and, to a lesser extent, in the liver in response to stress, while GLUCAGON from the endocrine PANCREAS triggers glycogenolysis in the liver to compensate for low blood sugar.

Glycogenolysis is carried out by a specific ENZYME called glycogen phosphorylase, which senses change in blood glucose for the liver. Thus, high blood glucose levels rapidly inactivate the enzyme, because the need for glycogen degradation to supply glucose vanishes. (See also CARBOHYDRATE LOADING; CARBOHYDRATE METABOLISM; GLUCOSE TOLERANCE; GLYCOLYSIS.)

glycolysis The degradation of GLUCOSE to small, organic acids, such as PYRUVIC ACID or LACTIC ACID, to produce ENERGY without the participation of oxygen (anaerobically). Glycolysis is a primary energy-yielding pathway of carbohydrate metabolism: Ten different kinds of ENZYMES work together, like an assembly line in a factory, to cleave and oxidize glucose in order to produce energy as ATP. To completely release all of the energy locked in the original glucose molecule, pyruvic acid is further oxidized with oxygen-requiring enzymes to CARBON DIOXIDE, yielding more ATP than released simply from glycolysis.

Glycolysis is regulated by enzyme-feedback mechanisms and by HORMONES. In the liver, it is increased by INSULIN, a major biosynthetic hormone, and it is inhibited by GLUCAGON, a hormone signaling the liver to increase blood glucose, rather than consuming it. This pathway is inhibited when ATP or CITRIC ACID accumulates in the cell, indicating a saturation of another energy-yielding pathway (the KREB'S CYCLE).

RED BLOOD CELLS and other cells without the mitochondria cannot use oxygen to oxidize fuels and rely strictly on anaerobic glycolysis to produce ATP and lactic acid. Muscles use gycolysis to metabolize glucose for energy, and during vigorous EXERCISE, glucose can be anaerobically converted to lactic acid to provide extra ATP when muscle cells receive limited oxygen to burn fuels. During FERMENTATION to prepare WINE and BEER, yeast utilize anaerobic glycolysis to convert glucose to ethanol (alcohol). (See also BLOOD SUGAR; CATABOLISM; FEEDBACK INHIBITION; GLUCONEOGENESIS; GLYCOGEN.)

glycoproteins PROTEINS containing CARBOHYDRATE segments. Glycoproteins represent many classes of proteins including certain ENZYMES, ANTIBODIES, HORMONES, and membrane components likely to be involved in cell recognition (for example, that determine blood type) and slippery proteins called mucins. Sugars such as GALACTOSE, MANNOSE, and nitrogen derivatives of GLUCOSE and galactose are building blocks as well as acidic sugars. Proteins with very large carbohydrate chains

(GLYCOSAMINOGLYCANS) form connective tissue like cartilage while mucins form mucus to protect moist surfaces of tissues. (See also HEPARIN.)

glycosaminoglycans (mucopolysaccharides) Large carbohydrate chains that support connective tissues such as skin, tendons, cartilage, ligaments, and BONE. Glycosaminoglycans also support the structure of ears, auditory tubes, and heart valves. Glycosaminoglycans such as chondroitin sulfate are jelly-like substances that help lubricate surfaces of joints and provide resiliency, so that joints resist compression. Other glycosaminoglycans help maintain fluid compartments. For example, hyaluronic acid occurs in the fluid of the eye and joint spaces, while heparin serves as an anticoagulant in veins and arteries. Mucus, secreted to lubricate and protect moist surfaces of the body, is also composed of glycosaminoglycans.

Cells produce glycosaminoglycans from simple sugars or compounds derived from them. For example, amino sugars—GLUCOSAMINE and galactosamine—and the sugar acid, glucuronic acid, come from GLUCOSE (blood sugar). These building blocks are assembled into long chains. SULFUR in the form of sulfate may be attached, and the completed glycosaminoglycans are released into the surrounding (extracellular) space. The synthesis of healthy connective tissue and its repair depend on adequate supplies of glycosaminoglycan building blocks, including the amino acids GLUTAMINE, METHIONINE, and CYSTEINE. Vitamins, such as VITAMIN C, NIACIN, and PANTOTHENIC ACID and the trace minerals MANGANESE, COPPER, IRON, and ZINC function as enzyme helpers in the process. It is important to note that pain killers, such as nonsteroidal antiinflammatory drugs, are often taken to relieve joint pain, although they can interfere with the rebuilding process and slow recovery from joint injury. (See also COLLAGEN; CHONDROITIN POLYSACCHARIDES.)

Boeve, E. R. et al. "Glycosaminoglycans and Other Sulphated Polysaccharides in Calculogenesis of Urinary Stones," *World Journal of Urology* 12, no. 1 (1994): 43–48.

glycoside A compound composed of a simple SUGAR bound to another sugar or other substance. Thus, LACTOSE (milk sugar) is a glycoside of GALACTOSE and GLUCOSE. Plant glycosides contain sugars attached to a variety of other compounds besides sugars. Cyanogenic glycosides found in seeds of apricots and apples yield toxic cyanide upon decomposition. Digitalis (digitoxin) is a glycoside that is a heart stimulant. FLAVONOIDS are a group of plant substances that generally exist bound to sugars and serve as ANTIOXIDANTS and in other useful functions. (See also HESPERIDIN.)

glycyrrhizin (glycyrrhizic acid) A principal flavor of LICORICE. One of the sweetest natural substances, glycyrrhizin is 50 to 100 times sweeter than SUCROSE. Ammoniated glycyrrhizin is prepared from licorice root extracts and used as a FOOD ADDITIVE. It is used in beverages (root beer), candy, chewing gum, and baked goods.

Glycyrrhizin possesses powerful physiologic effects. Excessive ingestion of licorice (several ounces of licorice daily for extended periods) may result in lowered blood potassium levels, lowered aldosterone levels with sodium and water retention, HYPERTENSION, fatigue, and, in extreme cases, heart failure.

Licorice root has long been used in Chinese medicine in the treatment of lung infections and digestive disorders. Glycyrrhizin has antiviral activity, and in Western medicine it has been used to treat peptic ulcers and Addison's disease. Its anti-inflammatory effects may be the result of an inhibition of the formation of pro-inflammatory PROSTAGLANDINS, derivatives of essential fatty acids. Because licorice can exhibit estrogenic and steroid properties and can stimulate uterine contractions, pregnant women should avoid licorice.

goat's milk A MILK sometimes used as a substitute for cow's milk that contains more VITAMIN A and fat than cow's milk, but contains the same amounts of LACTOSE (milk sugar). Goat's milk is low in FOLIC ACID and VITAMIN B_{12}. Although it lacks CASEIN, the major cow's milk protein, goat's milk may cause milk sensitivity, and there is often a crossover allergy between goat's milk and cow's milk. Two-thirds of the children allergic to cow's milk cannot tolerate either goat's milk or cow's milk. (See also ALLERGY, FOOD.)

goiter An enlargement of the THYROID GLAND often due to IODINE deficiency, which represents an attempt by the body to compensate for a shortage of the iodine required for synthesizing thyroxine, the thyroid hormone that contains iodine. An iodine deficiency decreases thyroxine production, and lowered thyroxine production leads to increased production of thyroid-stimulating hormone by the pituitary, which stimulates further growth of the thyroid. Excessive consumption of raw soybeans, thiocyanate-containing drugs used to treat high blood pressure, and even excessive iodine can produce goiters.

The first European use of iodine compounds to treat goiter occurred in 1816; however, the ancient Chinese recommended treating goiter with seaweed and burnt sponge, now known to contain large amounts of iodine. They also administered dried animal thyroid glands. Until the early 1920s, goiters were common in the southern United States where the soil contains little iodine. Iodine in the form of sodium iodide was added to SALT in the 1920s. With this addition, goiters disappeared in the United States. People living in certain regions of the world still suffer from iodine deficiency, and goiter is likely to be found inland, where the availability of seafoods is limited, and in areas where the topsoil has negligible iodine, such as the plains of Africa, Asia, and South America. (See also FOOD TOXINS; GOITROGENS.)

goitrogens Plant compounds that can cause thyroid hormone deficiency and GOITER formation. This class of compounds liberates thiocyanate, which can block IODINE uptake and use. CABBAGE, RUTABAGA, TURNIP, KALE, CAULIFLOWER, BROCCOLI, RADISH, and KOHLRABI contain low levels of goitrogens. In most cases, cooking inactivates goitrogens. Realistically, goitrogens are a potential problem only if rutabagas and turnips are used as a staple and if the diet is iodine-deficient, an unlikely situation in the United States. A dietary excess of calcium and fluorine enhances the effects of goitrogens. (See also FOOD TOXINS; THYROID GLAND.)

goldenseal (*Hydrastis canadensis*) A medicinal plant of North America with a long history of Native American use. Goldenseal is now cultivated in the Pacific Northwest. Goldenseal together with barberry (*Berberis vulgaris*) and Oregon grape (*Mahonia aquifolium*) produce alkaloids called berberine, berberastine, canadine, and hydrastine, which stimulate the IMMUNE SYSTEM and act as antibiotics. Goldenseal has been used to treat inflammatory conditions such as digestive disorders, ulcers, COLITIS, and infections of the digestive tract like traveler's diarrhea, as well as infections of the lungs, throat, sinuses, and urinary tract. Goldenseal can also lower fever.

The dried root and underground stem are used as supplements; alternatively, purified berberine can be used. Berberine attacks a wide variety of disease-producing organisms, including parasites, bacteria, yeast, and fungi. In addition, it prevents such pathogens from binding to tissues, thus preventing adherence to the host, a first step in the infectious process. Berberine also activates macrophages, cells of the immune system that scavenge bacteria, viruses, and tumor cells. It also helps support the spleen, an organ that filters and cleans the blood. Berberine-containing plants are not recommended during pregnancy, and consumption of large amounts can block the utilization of B complex vitamins. Goldenseal is probably unsafe for newborns, and pregnant or breast-feeding women.

gooseberry (*Ribes grossularia*) The tart fruit of a prickly shrub, closely related to the currant. Gooseberries grow singly, rather than in clusters. They are usually small, although varieties can be an inch in diameter. They turn amber when they ripen. Gooseberries are native to both Europe and America. European cultivation probably began in the 10th century. Commercial production began in the 1800s. Gooseberry production in the United States was restricted in the early 1900s when it was discovered that gooseberries were a carrier of a pine blister rust that had caused extensive damage to pine forests by the turn of the century. In the United States, gooseberries are grown in Michigan, Oregon, and Washington. Different varieties can be either red, white, green, or yellow. Raw, 100 g provides 39 calories; carbohydrate, 1.7 g; 1.9 g of fiber; and vitamin C, 33 mg.

Gotu kola ***(Centella asiatica)*** A medicinal herb native to China, India, Indonesia, and the South Pacific, including Australia. Since prehistoric times, Gotu kola has been used for healing wounds and skin conditions. Tradition relates that it promotes longevity. The plant contains triterpenes—including asiaticoside—substances which seem to promote growth of connective tissue and skin. Extracts contain a mixture of substances that are responsible for its multiple effects, ranging from improving mental function to correct varicose veins. Although extracts are generally well tolerated, repeated application of isolated asiatoside has been reported to cause skin cancer. Pregnant women should not use this herb.

gout A painful joint inflammation, especially of the hands and feet (specifically the big toe of men). Gout may affect the kidneys and the heart as well. Gout is fairly common in America: It occurs in three people per thousand and is 20 times more common in men than in women. This disease is due to abnormal deposits of URIC ACID, the normal end product of PURINE degradation that occurs in the blood and is excreted in the urine. Purines are nitrogen-containing, cyclic compounds that are building blocks of DNA and RNA. Uric acid is borderline soluble at typical blood pH.

The causes of gout are unknown, though OBESITY, inheritance, and chronic lead poisoning can contribute to the risk. Elevated uric acid in the blood (hyperuricemia) is associated with gout in susceptible people. Uric acid can accumulate for several reasons. In "primary" gout, uric acid accumulation is the result of certain inherited enzyme deficiencies. In these cases, specific enzyme defects can cause excessive purine breakdown or overproduction of purines. In "secondary" gout, uric buildup is associated with cancer, hemolytic ANEMIA, and certain toxic drugs and kidney disease. In the latter situation, the excretion of uric acid is reduced, allowing a buildup to occur. Certain drugs also affect kidney performance and can cause gout: thiazide DIURETICS, salicylates like ASPIRIN, probenecid, and ethanibutol.

A high-protein diet and purine-rich foods like caviar, organ meats, YEAST, poultry, and ANCHOVIES can contribute to the risk of gout in susceptible people. The accumulation of LACTIC ACID, ALCOHOLISM, toxemia of pregnancy, and excessive KETONE BODIES (acidic products of fat metabolism during uncontrolled diabetes) can lead to excessive blood acidity, which can promote uric acid precipitation.

Treatment of gout may involve controlling weight in obese people, avoiding alcohol and reducing consumption of purine-rich foods. Other dietary measures include a liberal intake of liquids (2 quarts of fluid daily) to avoid kidney stones; low-fat, low-protein intake; and increased complex carbohydrate consumption. FISH OIL supplementation has been used to reduce joint inflammation. CHERRIES are claimed to relieve symptoms of gout. Gout can be treated with medications to lower uric acid blood levels, and low doses of the drug colchicine may reduce deposition of uric acid crystals in joints.

Flieger, Ken. "Getting to Know Gout," *FDA Consumer* 29, no. 2 (March 1995): 19–22.

graded foods Eggs, milk, milk products, and meat are graded according to palatability, size, color, texture, appearance, and maturity by the U.S. Department of Agriculture (USDA). Food packers and processors pay for the grading service. In contrast, food inspection is mandatory for food involved in interstate commerce. Food grading is voluntary and has nothing to do with food safety. (See also FOOD, DRUG AND COSMETIC ACT; FDA.)

grain Cereal grains are members of the grass family. They include WHEAT, MILLET, OATS, RICE, RYE, SORGHUM, TRITICALE, and CORN. The development of ancient civilizations relied upon the cultivation of grain, which allowed for more effective food production from the land. Wheat and barley farming began as early as 7,000 B.C. Dried grains store well, and their cultivation spread rapidly in Asia, Africa, and Europe. In the New World, corn spread from Mexico into other regions of North America. Much of modern grain production is devoted to livestock feed for meat production.

Cereal grains account for about 40 percent of the world crop production. Americans eat about 150 pounds of grains per person a year. However, in the early 1900s the average person ate twice as much, 300 pounds a year. This decline correlates with increased consumption of SUGAR and FAT. Grains are dietary STAPLES throughout the world due to their high content of COMPLEX CARBOHYDRATE (STARCH and FIBER), their PROTEIN and the ease of cultivation. Grains generally lack VITAMIN C, VITAMIN D, VITAMIN B_{12}, and VITAMIN A. Yellow corn contains small amounts of BETA-CAROTENE, the precursor of vitamin A. Grains are low in calcium, and their protein is generally low in the essential AMINO ACIDS such as LYSINE. In modern times, cereal grain products and FLOUR have been FORTIFIED/enriched with amino acids, vitamins, and minerals to increase their nutritional value.

In 1998 the U.S. FDA began requiring all enriched grain products, including cereals, breads, pasta, and rice to be fortified with folic acid at the rate of 140 mcg per 100 g of grain. This action was taken based on studies that showed that only about 25 percent of women of childbearing age in the United States regularly consumed enough folic acid. Women who consume at least 400 mcg daily have a significantly lower risk of bearing children with neural tube defects, such as spina bifida.

Cereal technology involves modifying starch through malting or sprouting. Seeds are germinated to activate enzymes that partially degrade starch to sugar. This strategy is used in brewing, baking, and the production of distilled alcoholic beverages. Milling refers to grinding and crushing (rolling) grains to remove fibrous hulls and to produce meal or flour for baking. Products from cereal grains include BREAD and other baked goods, BREAKFAST CEREAL, FLOUR, infant cereal, and popular snack foods like CHIPS and CRACKERS.

Grain substitutes are important alternatives, particularly for those with wheat and GLUTEN sensitivities. AMARANTH, BUCKWHEAT, and QUINOA are not related to grains, so cross allergies with wheat are less likely (See also BRAN; ENRICHMENT.)

grain alcohol See ALCOHOL.

granola A dry, whole grain BREAKFAST CEREAL and snack food. There are many variations of granola. Typically, commercial varieties contain rolled OATS, HONEY, nuts, and dried fruit like DATES. Often, COCONUT OIL and PALM OIL are added to make the mixture tastier. These granolas are often high in fat and sugar and may provide more CALORIES than other breakfast cereals.

granulated sugar See TABLE SUGAR.

grape (*Vitus*) A pulpy, smooth-skinned berry, growing in clusters on vines. The grape was domesticated before 5,000 B.C. and is one of the oldest cultivated fruits. The three basic types of grapes are European, North American, and hybrids. Seeded and seedless varieties are available. North American grapes are hardy, disease-resistant varieties, including *Vitis abrusca* (Catawba, Concord, Delaware, and Niagara are common varieties). Hybrids were developed mainly for wine production. Some are adapted for table use, including Thompson seedless and Tokay/Emperor. Other varieties include Black Beauty, Calmeria (Lady fingers), Cardinal, Champagne (source of dried currants), Flame Seedless, Italia Muscat, Perlette Seedless, Red Globe, and Ribier. Raisins are several varieties of sun-dried grapes. European grapes (*Vitus vinifera*) account for about 95 percent of grapes grown worldwide and represent the common table grape and are used in the production of famous wines. Worldwide grape production is around 67 million metric tons, 60 percent of which is produced by Europe. The United States accounts for about 7 percent of the world's production. California produces over 95 percent of U.S. grapes, mostly the European varieties. American grape varieties are grown primarily in New York, with Pennsylvania, Michigan, Kansas, Virginia, and Washington also contributing.

Grapes are traditionally used in wine making because their high sugar (GLUCOSE) and low acid content make them ideal for fermentation. The best wine-making grapes contain 18 percent to 24 percent sugar and 0.5 percent to 1.5 percent acidic substances. The acidity decreases and sweetness increases with ripening. Grapes provide low to moderate amounts of vitamins and minerals, but some varieties provide substantial VITAMIN C and FIBER. Red and purple grapes contain anthocyanin, a form of FLAVONOID that functions as an antioxidant. Food value of 10 seedless grapes (50 g): calories, 35; protein, 0.3 g; carbohydrate, 8.9 g; fiber, 1.0 g; potassium, 105 mg; vitamin C, 5.4 mg; thiamin 0.05 mg; riboflavin, 0.03 mg; niacin, 0.15 mg.

grapefruit (*Citrus paradisi*) A large yellow-skinned member of the citrus family. A grapefruit can weigh between 2 and 12 pounds, with a diameter ranging from 3 to 6 inches. The yellowish white or pink pulp is juicy and characteristically bitter.

Grapefruit originated in Barbados in the 18th century. Later mutations yielded the Thompson seedless pink variety (1913) and Ruby seedless red variety (1929). The U.S. produces 50 percent of the world's grapefruit crop. Florida leads in domestic grapefruit production, providing 80 percent of the U.S. crop. More than half of the domestic crop is processed as grapefruit juice, juice concentrate, and canned grapefruit sections. One of the most popular eating varieties is the Marsh Seedless, which yields pink and red grapefruits (Pink Seedless and Ruby Red Seedless). Star Ruby is a newer red variety. Red and pink grapefruit owe their color to small amounts of BETA-CAROTENE, enough to supply 5 percent to 12 percent of the RDA of VITAMIN A. Grapefruit is an excellent source of FLAVONOID, a plant material that serves as an antioxidant and anti-inflammatory agent. The flavonoid that contributes most of the bitter taste of grapefruit is called naringin. Grapefruit also provides pectin, a form of soluble FIBER that can lower cholesterol levels in blood, in addition to potassium, and VITAMIN C. Grapefruit juice provides vitamin C but not, of course, the fiber of the whole fruit. Food value for half a fruit with peel: calories, 37; protein, 0.8 g; carbohydrate, 9.9 g; fiber, 1.5 g; vitamin C, 47 mg; potassium, 175 mg; thiamin, 0.04 mg; riboflavin, 0.02 mg; niacin, 0.32 mg. One cup of grapefruit juice, sweetened, canned, provides 115 calories; protein, 1.4 g; carbohydrate, 28 g; potassium, 405 mg; vitamin C, 67 mg; thiamin, 0.1 mg; riboflavin, 0.06 mg; niacin, 0.8 mg. (See also CITRUS FRUIT.)

grape juice One of the sweetest juices. Grape juice is made from crushed grapes. A purple-colored juice indicates that it was prepared from grapes with purple skins, usually Concord grapes. Usually, grape juice provides no VITAMIN C unless it has been added by the manufacturer. Because of its high sugar content, an 8-oz. glass of grape juice provides 128 to 155 calories, higher than orange juice. If the label specifies "grape juice" it must contain 100 percent juice. Any other wording such as "drink" or "punch" indicates that the product contains little grape juice and is a mixture of sugar (corn syrup) and water. Researchers have discovered that the flavonoids in purple grape juice, like those in wine, can prevent the oxidation of LOW-DENSITY LIPOPROTEIN (LDL) cholesterol, the so-called bad cholesterol that leads to formation of plaque in arteries. Participants who drank purple grape juice daily for 14 days had noticeably improved blood flow and lower cholesterol rates. Purple grape juice has also been shown to prevent blood from clotting, thereby reducing the risk of stroke. One cup of grape juice, bottled, provides 155 calories; protein, 1.4 g; carbohydrate, 38 g; fiber, 1.26 g; potassium, 160 mg; thiamin, 0.05 mg; riboflavin, 0.03 mg; niacin, 0.15 mg.

grapeseed oil An oil extracted from seeds after grapes have been pressed to prepare wine or grape juice. Grapeseed oil is sometimes marketed as an alternative to olive oil. In individuals with elevated serum CHOLESTEROL on low-fat diets, this oil may raise the level of HIGH-DENSITY LIPOPROTEIN (HDL), the desirable form of cholesterol, without affecting overall cholesterol levels. A variety of materials in foods, such as soluble FIBER in OAT bran and PSYLLIUM, can lower LOW-DENSITY LIPOPROTEIN (LDL) cholesterol, but few foods have been shown to raise HDL levels. Moderate ALCOHOL consumption and some cholesterol-lowering drugs have been shown to raise HDL. (See also ATHEROSCLEROSIS; DIETARY GUIDELINES FOR AMERICANS.)

grape sugar See GLUCOSE.

GRAS See GENERALLY RECOGNIZED AS SAFE.

green number 3 See ARTIFICIAL FOOD COLORS.

Green Revolution A period between the late 1960s and early 1970s when high-yield cereal grains and synthetic fertilizers were exported to developing nations with the aim of increasing crop production. Advances in farming technology in the 1960s offered the potential of doubling or even tripling grain production in certain regions in developing countries. This technology, in conjunction with international agricultural research centers that produced new varieties of WHEAT, CORN, and RICE, could dramatically improve production per acre of cultivated land. Many special varieties of cereal grains required extra water, fertilizer, and PESTICIDES to obtain maximum yields.

By the 1970s, petrochemical pesticides and fertilizers and widespread irrigation in developing nations permitted massive crop cultivation and high productivity. It is estimated that the Green Revolution was responsible for an extra 50 million tons of grain annually.

More recent advances pose the prospect of a second Green Revolution, and biotechnology is capable of producing new plant strains with desirable qualities. However, the question remains whether technology alone will eradicate HUNGER in the world. The Green Revolution did not address the questions of high birth rates and population growth, illiteracy, disenfranchised small farmers, poverty, inadequate food distribution, civil strife, or the increased resistance of insects to pesticides. Malnutrition often occurred as cereal grains displaced legumes in the food supply in some developing countries. In addition to advances in agricultural technology, political and economical solutions are also needed to overcome world hunger.

In a shift of emphasis, 13 international agricultural research centers, working under the Consultative Group on International Agricultural Research, embarked upon a plan to broaden their focus (1990). They emphasize management of natural resources, including forestry, fisheries, irrigation management, and farming systems research (See also GENETIC ENGINEERING.)

grits Coarsely ground cereal grain, from which the outer layer (BRAN) and nutrient-rich germ have been removed. Grits are more finely ground than groats, although both have had their hulls removed. Grits from CORN are known as hominy grits. Grits are also prepared from BUCKWHEAT, RYE, OATS, and RICE.

In contrast, groats represent larger fragments of hulled grains. Groats can be prepared from buckwheat, oats, BARLEY, WHEAT, and corn. Cracked wheat refers to either a wheat groats or grits. Buckwheat groats, also known as KASHA, are commonly used.

ground beef See HAMBURGER.

growth hormone (GH, somatotropin) A hormone that primarily stimulates growth and maturation of tissues, rather than controlling the developmental processes. When growth hormone is administered to elderly men, their short-term and long-term memory improves, their body fat diminishes, and their lean body mass (muscle) increases. Growth hormone is the only hormone produced by the anterior pituitary that does not affect other hormone-secreting glands. It increases protein synthesis, as well as fat and carbohydrate utilization, and it increases amino acid uptake in muscles. Growth hormone enhances bone synthesis and the formation of red blood cells.

Growth hormone release follows a circadian rhythm: Blood levels peak during sleep and decline during the day. EXERCISE increases growth hormone production. It is regulated by "growth hormone release inhibiting factor" and "growth hormone releasing factor" from the HYPOTHALAMUS, the part of the brain that regulates the PITUITARY GLAND, the master gland of the ENDOCRINE SYSTEM (hormone secreting glands). (See also AGING; ANABOLISM; BOVINE GROWTH HORMONE.)

growth promoters See ANIMAL DRUGS IN MEAT.

GTF See GLUCOSE TOLERANCE FACTOR.

guanine A nitrogen-containing base that is a building block of DNA and RNA. Guanine in one DNA chain pairs with ADENINE in a second (complementary) DNA strand. This specificity between strands of DNA helps direct the replication of DNA and the formation of RNA, which directs protein synthesis. Guanine also forms guanosine triphosphate, GTP, a high-energy compound like ATP, required as an energy source for protein synthesis, activating internal enzymes when regulatory molecules like hormones bind to the outer cell surface, and other processes.

Guanine is not a dietary essential, because it is readily synthesized in the body from three amino acids (ASPARTIC ACID, GLYCINE, and GLUTAMINE) together with derivatives of the coenzyme of FOLIC ACID (tetrahydrofolate). It is also salvaged and reused by the body. Guanine occurs in all plant and animal foods, especially organ meats like liver and glandular tissues, and also in seeds. It is degraded by the body to URIC ACID and excreted. (See also DISODIUM GUANYLATE; GOUT; PURINE.)

guar gum A vegetable GUM used as a thickening agent, Guar gum is obtained from the guar plant, *Composia teragonolobus,* grown in India and the United States. Guar gum is a form of soluble FIBER and contains long chains composed of the sugars MANNOSE and GALACTOSE. Guar gum dissolves in cold water, readily forms gels and is one of the most widely used gum stabilizers in foods. It is used commercially to thicken beverages, ICE CREAM, gravies, salad dressing, doughs and batters, snack foods, and even pet foods, and it provides resiliency to dough, batters, and artificial whipped cream. Guar gum is considered a safe FOOD ADDITIVE.

Guar gum gel may help lower blood cholesterol. It has been used as an appetite suppressant; because it swells in water, it has also been used as a BULKING AGENT to promote the sensation of being full. It does not help prevent constipation because it slows movement of material through the gastrointestinal tract. Unlike bran, guar gum is broken down in the gut by microorganisms.

guava (*Psidium guajava*) A round, yellow to white, aromatic fruit that is a native of the Caribbean. Guavas are cultivated in tropical regions and in California and Florida. Guavas range in size from that of a cherry to that of an apple. The pulp is generally white, although some varieties produce a crimson pulp. The fruit is used in fruit salads and fruit juices, in jam, jelly, and pie fillings, and as a condiment for meat dishes. Guavas are an excellent source of soluble FIBER (pectin), which can help lower blood cholesterol, and of VITAMIN C. The nutrient content per 3.5 oz. (100 g) serving is 60 calories; protein, 0.77 g; carbohydrate, 14.5 g; fat, 0.57 g; vitamin A, 285 retinol equivalents; vitamin C, 234 mg; niacin, 1.12 mg; thiamin, 0.051 mg; riboflavin, 0.046 mg.

guidelines See DIETARY GUIDELINES FOR AMERICANS.

guggul (gum guggulu) A yellowish resin produce by the mukul myrrh (*Commiphora mukul*) tree, which grows throughout India, where it has been used medicinally since ancient times to treat a variety of conditions, including arthritis, obesity, skin disorders, and high cholesterol. Preliminary studies indicate guggul may be effective in treating ATHEROSCLEROSIS by lowering blood levels of triglycerides and "bad" LOW-DENSITY LIPOPROTEIN (LDL) and VERY LOW-DENSITY LIPOPROTEIN (VLDL) cholesterol while raising "good" HIGH-DENSITY LIPOPROTEIN (HDL) cholesterol levels in people with high blood lipid levels. It has been approved for that use in India. However, because these studies were limited in scope the results are unreliable. Other small studies indicate guggul may help to treat acne.

Guggul is available in the United States as a dietary supplement. Consequently, its safety and efficacy as a cholesterol- and triglyceride-lowering substance have not been tested or proven by any government agency. Some studies indicate it can stimulate the thyroid, so it may counter the effects of some thyroid medications. Other reported side effects include headache, nausea, and skin rashes. Guggul is probably unsafe for pregnant women. Safety data for breast-feeding women are inadequate.

gum A form of fiber used as a FOOD ADDITIVE. Gums form gels and are used by manufacturers to thicken and stabilize many foods, including ice cream, whipping cream, dough, gravies, salad dressing, and snack foods. Gums are also used to change food textures and to increase the moisture-holding capacity in canned meats. Several gums have been used as bulking agents to avoid constipation. Because they swell in water and increase the feeling of satiety, some have also been used as APPETITE SUPPRESSANTS. Gums consist of long chains of sugar units, such as glucose, galactose, and sugar acids, linked together, thus representing a form of COMPLEX CARBOHYDRATE. Some gums contain repeating units of multiple sugars.

Natural gums occur in microorganisms and in plant cell walls. Gums are often secreted by plants to heal wounds in the bark. Gums from tree extracts include arabic, ghatti, karaya, larch, and tragacanth. Certain gums occur in seeds, including guar, locust bean, psyllium, and quince. AGAR, algin, CARRAGEENAN, and FURCELLERAN represent gums isolated from species of SEAWEED. Microbial fermentation produces XANTHAN GUM, while beta-glucan is derived from OATS and BARLEY. Synthetic gums are made of chemically modified CELLULOSE, microcrystalline cellulose, carboxymethylcellulose, and modified starches, such as carboxymethyl starch and hydroxyethyl starch. Chemically modified versions of ALGINATES, PECTIN, locust bean gum, and GUAR GUM are also employed as thickeners.

Gums are classified as water-soluble FIBER, and they exert several important physiologic effects:

- increased glucose tolerance: Soluble fibers such as guar gum and pectin reduce the rate at which glucose is absorbed by the intestine when mixed with foods, and they have been used in the diets of diabetics to decrease blood glucose levels after a meal. Guar gum reduces blood glucose levels and insulin responses to an oral glucose load.
- slowed lipid absorption: Soluble fiber and gums slow fat digestion.
- lowered cholesterol: Guar gum, GUM ARABIC, oat gum, and pectin lower blood cholesterol levels. Since gums bind BILE salts, synthesized from cholesterol, it has been proposed that they reduce the reabsorption, and thus reutilization, of cholesterol and bile acids by the liver. According to this theory, cholesterol would be diverted to bile salt synthesis and excretion away from the blood. Gums may therefore indirectly increase the ability of the liver to remove cholesterol from the blood.
- colonic fermentation: Gums are degraded by intestinal bacteria to simple sugars that are fermented to short-chain, saturated fatty acids (ACETIC ACID, PROPIONIC ACID, BUTYRIC ACID). These supply substantial fuel for the colonic mucosal cells and the body. (See also GUM GHATTI.)

gum arabic A soluble GUM obtained from the acacia tree in Sudan. Gum arabic is a form of complex carbohydrate containing GALACTOSE and acidic derivatives of GLUCOSE, among other sugars. Gum arabic is used to stabilize buttered syrup and dry mixes (such as pancake mixes and powdered drinks), ice cream, and the foam in BEER. It is used to prevent granulation of candy and helps dissolve oils like flavors in SOFT DRINKS. Like other natural gums, it is not digested but is fermented by COLON BACTERIA. Occasionally, gum arabic causes an allergic reaction, but gum arabic is considered a safe FOOD ADDITIVE although few tests to establish long-term safety have been performed.

gum disease See GINGIVITIS.

gum ghatti A vegetable GUM produced by a tree found in India (anogeissus). It is a form of complex carbohydrate containing xylose, GALACTOSE, MANNOSE, and an acid derivative of GLUCOSE. Relatively small amounts are imported for use in salad dressing and butter-flavored syrups (See also FIBER; FOOD ADDITIVES.)

H

haddock (*Melanogrammus aeglefinus*) A lean saltwater FISH related to COD. Haddock is an important food fish; its white flesh has a pleasant, somewhat bland taste that can be prepared in any recipe for cod or FLOUNDER. Smoked haddock is called finnan haddie. Haddock is an excellent source of high-quality PROTEIN; raw, 3.5 oz. (100 g) provides 79 calories; protein, 18.3 g; fat, 0.66 g; calcium, 23 mg; cholesterol, 60 mg; niacin, 3 mg; thiamin, 0.04 mg; riboflavin, 0.06 mg.

hair analysis A convenient, reasonably inexpensive preliminary screening tool for detecting mineral imbalances. Because minerals accumulate in hair as it grows, hair analysis can be used to screen for accumulated toxic metals, including MERCURY, ALUMINUM, COPPER, LEAD, and CADMIUM. Hair analysis also has been used to assess body levels of trace minerals (iron, copper, manganese, zinc) and to compare minerals in populations living in different regions with differing degrees of pollution and soil depletion of minerals. These hair samples are easily obtainable, and analytical methods (atomic absorption spectrometry, X-ray fluorescence spectrometry, among others) are sufficiently sensitive to permit accurate analysis of small samples.

However, hair analysis is a controversial test. Some laboratories do not provide reproducible results, and hair is easily contaminated with shampoo, conditioners, dyes, and air pollutants. Moreover, findings can be overinterpreted. For example, hair levels of some MINERALS such as SODIUM and POTASSIUM do not correlate with body levels. (See also HEAVY METALS.)

halibut (*Hippoglossus*) A flat saltwater FISH found in all oceans that is one of the most important food fishes. Resembling a huge FLOUNDER, the lean flesh is firm with a pleasant flavor and texture. Halibut liver oil is an excellent source of VITAMIN A and VITAMIN D and is a primary commercial source of these vitamins. Food value of 3.5 oz. (100 g) raw has: calories, 100; protein, 19.0 g; fat, 1.1 g; calcium, 13 mg; cholesterol, 50 mg; niacin, 8.3 mg.

ham The rear leg of a hog. Ham is a red MEAT containing 34 percent of total CALORIES derived from saturated FAT that provides high-quality PROTEIN together with many VITAMINS and MINERALS. The glistening greenish sheen on the surface of sliced ham is a sign of oxidation, not necessarily spoilage.

To minimize SODIUM intake, patients should reduce consumption of all cured pork products, including ham. Roasted ham contains per 3 oz. (85 g): calories, 207; protein, 18.3 g; fat, 14.2 g; cholesterol, 53 mg; iron, 0.74 mg; sodium, 1,009 mg; zinc, 1.97 mg; thiamin, 0.51 mg; niacin 3.8 mg; riboflavin, 0.21 mg. For comparison lean, roasted ham contains per 3 oz.: calories, 133; protein, 21.3 g; fat, 4.7 g; and sodium, 1,128 mg. Canned ham contains per 3 oz.: calories, 140; protein, 17.8 g; fat, 7.2 g; sodium, 908 mg. (See also DIETARY GUIDELINES FOR AMERICANS; FAT, HIDDEN; FATTY ACIDS.)

hamburger Ground BEEF to which beef fat (beef tallow) can be added to bring the fat content up to 30 percent by weight. Hamburger is the most commonly eaten MEAT in the United States, representing a major contributor of total fat and saturated fat to the average diet. The average fat in lean ground beef is 21 percent, while extra-lean hamburger contains 15 percent fat. When fat is drained after cooking, both regular hamburger and extra-lean have about the same cooked weight. Hamburger can be prepared from fresh or frozen beef. Fat, water extenders or binders cannot legally be added. Only 12 states presently require that the fat content of ground beef be listed on food labels. Hamburger and ground beef need to be cooked thoroughly to destroy possible disease-producing strains of the bacterium *E. coli,* a leading cause of food poisoning in the United States.

There is no fixed definition of ground beef; however, if ground beef is designated on the label as being derived from a particular cut of meat, then the product must consist of beef derived entirely from the cut so identified.

Ground round roast or top round steak are lower fat alternatives to hamburger. These cuts of meat contain only 6 percent fat, representing 29 percent of the total calories. Food value of lean hamburger, per 3 oz. (85 g) broiled is: calories, 230; protein, 21 g; fat, 16 g; cholesterol, 74 mg; calcium, 9 mg; iron, 1.8 mg; zinc, 3.74 mg; riboflavin, 0.18 mg; niacin, 4.41 mg; thiamin, 0.04 mg; B_6, 0.39 mg. For "regular" hamburger, the value per 3 oz. (85 g) broiled is: calories, 245; protein, 20 g; fat 17.8 g; cholesterol, 76 mg. (See also ANTIBIOTICS; CHOLESTEROL.)

hard cider See CIDER.

hardening of the arteries See ARTERIOSCLEROSIS.

hard water See WATER.

hawthorn (*Crataegus oxyacantha*) A spiny tree or hedge native to Europe whose berries have medicinal properties. Folk traditions describe the use of berries and flowers as beneficial supplements for INFLAMMATION ranging from ARTHRITIS to sore throats; for vascular conditions such as angina, high blood pressure, and clogged arteries. Substances in hawthorn extracts inhibit constriction of blood vessels and strengthen arterial walls, potentially protecting against plaque deposits.

Hawthorn berries and blossoms contain FLAVONOIDS, particularly anthocyanins and proanthocyanins, colored pigments of berries including blueberries, cherries, and grapes. These flavonoid compounds stabilize collagen, the primary structural protein of connective tissue, as well as of tendons, cartilage, and ligaments. They act as antioxidants, prevent FREE RADICAL damage, and prevent the release and synthesis of substances that promote inflammation, such as prostaglandins, histamines, and leukotrienes. Hawthorn is unsafe for pregnant women; data for breast-feeding women are inadequate.

Hazard Analysis and Critical Control Points (HACCP) A food safety program initially adopted by the U.S. FDA in 2001 for seafood and juice; eventually, the agency plans to expand it to the entire U.S. food supply. Based on a similar program developed for astronauts in the 1970s, HACCP focuses on preventing hazards that could cause food-borne illnesses by applying science-based controls, from raw material to finished product.

The FDA describes the seven principles of HACCP as follows:

- **Analyze hazards.** Potential hazards associated with a food and measures to control those hazards are identified. The hazard could be biological, such as a microbe; chemical, such as a toxin; or physical, such as ground glass or metal fragments.
- **Identify critical control points.** These are points in a food's production, from its raw state through processing and shipping to consumption by the consumer, at which the potential hazard can be controlled or eliminated. Examples are cooking, cooling, packaging, and metal detection.
- **Establish preventive measures with critical limits for each control point.** For a cooked food, for example, this might include setting the minimum cooking temperature and time required to ensure the elimination of any harmful microbes.
- **Establish procedures to monitor the critical control points.** Such procedures might include determining how and by whom cooking time and temperature should be monitored.
- **Establish corrective actions to be taken when monitoring shows that a critical limit has not been met.** This might entail, for example, reprocessing or disposing of food if the minimum cooking temperature were not met.
- **Establish procedures to verify that the system is working properly.** This might involve, for example, testing time-and-tempera-

ture recording devices to verify that a cooking unit is working properly.

- **Establish effective record-keeping to document the HACCP system.** This would include records of hazards and their control methods, the monitoring of safety requirements, and action taken to correct potential problems. Each of these principles must be backed by sound scientific knowledge: for example, published microbiological studies on time and temperature factors for controlling food-borne pathogens.

This new food safety program was adopted by the FDA as a way to meet the challenges of increasing numbers of food pathogens, including *ESCHERICHIA COLI* 0157:H7 and SALMONELLA.

hazelnut (filbert, cobnut) A sweet, grape-sized nut of a deciduous shrub or small tree that is related to the birch. The hazelnut is one of the world's largest nut crops; it is commercially grown in the United States, Spain, Turkey, and Italy. A native of Europe and Asia Minor, it grows well in regions with mild, moist winters and cool summers. "Divining rods" made from the wood of the tree were believed to have the power to seek out treasure or pockets of valuable minerals. Chopped or ground hazelnuts are often used as flavorings in desserts and sweet snacks. The brown whole nuts are often included in holiday mixes at Christmas. A quarter cup serving provides: calories, 180; fat 16 g; fiber, 4 g; protein, 5 g.

HCl See STOMACH ACID.

HDL See HIGH-DENSITY LIPOPROTEIN.

head cheese A cold cut prepared from the MEAT of a calf and pig heads, (including cheeks, snouts, lips) together with brains, hearts, tongues, and feet. The cooked meat, stripped from bones, is ground, seasoned, and then pressed to create a single jellied mass. (See also BEEF; FOOD PROCESSING; HAM.)

heart attack A condition (also known as myocardial infarction) resulting from a blocked coronary artery, an artery feeding the heart. When oxygen supplied to the heart muscle is compromised, the tissue may be irreparably damaged.

Symptoms include prolonged pressure or painful tightness at the center of the chest, possibly spreading to the left arm and shoulder and to the neck and jaw. There may also be nausea and vomiting, shortness of breath, and sweating.

The odds of heart attack increase with well-established risk factors: a family history of heart disease; high blood pressure; obesity; diabetes; increasing age; cigarette smoking; low folic acid; a high intake of saturated fat; a sedentary lifestyle; and repressed anger/anxiety. A healthful diet, regular exercise, stress management, social and emotional support, maintaining a desirable body weight, avoiding smoking, and a semi-vegetarian diet with reduced fat are recommended.

Blood clots are one of the dangers of clogged arteries. When clots lodge in arteries feeding the heart, they block blood flow. The heart requires a constant supply of nutrients and oxygen from the blood, and being deprived of oxygen even briefly will damage the heart muscle.

It is critically important to secure immediate medical care for a heart attack by dialing 911. Many heart attack patients die before they get to the hospital, and delays in summoning help can be fatal. (See also ATHEROSCLEROSIS; BLOOD CLOTTING; CHOLESTEROL; CORONARY ARTERY DISEASE; HOMOCYSTEINE; STROKE.)

Morrison H. I. et al. "Serum Folate and Risk of Fatal Coronary Heart Disease," *Journal of the American Medical Association* 275, no. 24 (June 26, 1996): 1,893–1,896.

U.S. Department of Health, Education and Welfare, *How Doctors Diagnose Heart Disease.* Washington, D.C.: DHEW Publication No. (NIH) 78–753.

heartburn See ACID INDIGESTION.

heart disease See ATHEROSCLEROSIS; CARDIOVASCULAR DISEASE; CORONARY ARTERY DISEASE; HEART ATTACK; STROKE.

heart-healthy diet See CHOLESTEROL; DIETARY GUIDELINES FOR AMERICANS.

heat inactivation The loss of biological activity of a substance, such as an ENZYME, when heated to sufficiently high temperatures. In the case of enzymes, heat alters structures critical for catalysts. COOKING at high temperatures destroys vitamins such as VITAMIN C, FOLIC ACID, and THIAMIN. Through oxidation or other chemical changes, polyunsaturated FATTY ACIDS and even CHOLESTEROL become oxidized when heated at sufficiently high temperature in the presence of air. The essential AMINO ACID, LYSINE, is partially destroyed when grain protein and carbohydrate are heated together. Several processed BREAKFAST CEREALS contain less lysine than that present in flour because they have been baked.

heavy metals Industrial chemicals of LEAD, MERCURY, CADMIUM, CHROMIUM, NICKEL, antimony, and ARSENIC. These chemicals are general enzyme poisons, and the toxic effects of these industrial wastes is well established. As an example, lead exposure causes ANEMIA by blocking a key step in the synthesis of HEMOGLOBIN, required for the formation of RED BLOOD CELLS.

As a general rule, the greater the exposure to a toxic metal, the greater the risk of poisoning. Widespread pollution has created chronic low-level exposure in many regions of the United States, thus increasing the risk of heavy metal poisoning. Therefore, minimizing heavy metal exposure in air, food, and WATER can lead to dramatic, long-term health benefits.

Nutrients like sulfur-containing amino acids, selenium, and VITAMIN C seem to have the ability to counteract heavy metals in the body, while diets low in CALCIUM, IRON, or ZINC increase lead uptake. The body has several defense mechanisms against toxic exposure. One of these is metallothionens, proteins rich in the sulfur amino acid CYSTEINE that bind heavy metals and speed their removal. Metallothionen synthesis is triggered by exposure to heavy metal ions. The following are specific examples of common toxic metals:

Arsenic, which occurs in PESTICIDES, smog and cigarette smoke, is believed to interfere with neurological development, and high doses increase the risk of some types of cancer. Cadmium may cause high blood pressure and heart abnormalities, bronchitis, lung fibrosis, and emphysema. Small amounts are common in consumer items ranging from cigarettes and pesticides to food. Drinking water may be contaminated with cadmium because soft water dissolves the cadmium in galvanized pipes.

Lead exposure leads to distractibility, DIARRHEA, irritability, and lethargy. More serious consequences are smaller fetal brain size, increased BIRTH DEFECTS, decreased IQ, anemia, CHRONIC FATIGUE, aching limbs, kidney disease, and sometimes coma. Though the U.S. EPA banned leaded paints and has required lowered lead levels in gasoline, Americans still are exposed to lead through drinking water, glazed ceramic dinnerware, old paint, and decades of environmental pollution.

Selenium is a water and soil contaminant in some regions of the United States. In trace amounts, the appropriate chemical form of selenium is an essential nutrient. However, the margin of safety of selenium is small, and ingesting only five times the level deemed safe and adequate can cause toxic side effects. (See also BREAST-FEEDING.)

height/weight tables Standards of weight and height by age used to assess an appropriate body weight for normal people. Several different tables have been developed. The Metropolitan Life Insurance Company assembled the best-known height/weight table, based upon the heights and weights of policy holders. It was later realized that weight depends on body build; therefore, values for an "IDEAL BODY WEIGHT" were adjusted by including different values for "small," "medium," and "large" body sizes. Since ideal body weight implies making a judgment and is subjective, a more liberal version of these tables was published in 1983, based on data obtained from 1959 to 1983. The 1983 revision came up with a "desirable body weight" that is 10 percent greater than that on the older table. This revision suggests that a woman of average frame and average height (5 feet 4 inches) wearing 3 pounds of clothing and wearing one-inch heels would weigh 126 to 138 pounds. For an average man (5 feet 9 inches tall, wearing five pounds of clothing), the range is 148 to 160 pounds.

Several limitations of life insurance tables restrict their usefulness. Their weights are based on values that were simply reported, not measured. Insurance policy holders for whom the data were collected do not represent the whole U.S. population. High blood pressure, smoking, and diabetes—factors that can affect general health and body weight—are not considered. There is no firm definition of "frame size." Thus, tables of this kind represent a subjective evaluation. The tables would suggest that a wide range of weights (30 to 40 pounds) poses no risk, in contradiction to common experience. Newer information indicates that excess FAT, not weight, is critical. Furthermore, it is important to establish how the fat is distributed in order to assess risks. (See also BODY MASS INDEX; OBESITY.)

***Helicobacter pylori* (*Campylobacter pylori*)** A spiral-shaped bacterium that can infect the stomach and cause GASTRIC ULCERS, duodenal ulcers and symptomatic, atrophic GASTRITIS (stomach inflammation), and a higher risk for stomach cancer. Almost 90 percent of patients with the most common type of stomach CANCER, intestinal-type gastric adenocarcinoma, are infected with *H. pylori.* While stomach acid kills many bacteria, *H. pylori* burrows deep into the mucus layer to the underlying mucosal cell surface, where it is protected from stomach acid. Half of all Americans over the age of 50, and 75 percent of subjects older than 65 have antibodies against *H. pylori,* suggesting a wide prevalence of infection. While many adults exhibit evidence of antibodies to this bacterium, it is not clear why only a small percentage develop duodenal ulcers. On the other hand, irradiation of *H. pylori* with bismuth compounds combined with several antibiotics decreases the risk of ulcer relapse and yields a significant improvement in ulcers and stomach inflammation. Researchers have discovered that BROCCOLI and broccoli sprouts contain a chemical, SULFORAFANE, that kills *H. pylori* in mice. Similar studies on humans are ongoing. (See also GASTROINTESTINAL DISORDERS.)

hematocrit A clinical lab test used to assess the health of red blood cells. The hematocrit represents the volume of packed red blood cells, expressed as the percentage of total blood volume. For men, the average hematocrit is 47 percent with a range of 40 percent to 54 percent and for women, the average is 42 percent with a range of 37 percent to 47 percent. Children's hematocrit varies depending on the age. Serious fluid loss without cell loss, as in DEHYDRATION, raises the hematocrit, while blood loss or ANEMIA lowers the hematocrit. (See also HEMOGLOBIN.)

heme An IRON-containing red pigment found in red blood cells. HEMOGLOBIN, the oxygen transport protein of blood, requires heme to bind molecular oxygen reversibly. Heme also functions as a helper group of CYTOCHROMES, enzymes responsible for transporting electrons in energy-generating reactions of MITOCHONDRIA.

Heme is synthesized in the bone marrow by the parents of red blood cells (reticulo-endothelial cells). Iron is bound within a complex ring structure, synthesized from small building blocks: GLYCINE, the simplest AMINO ACID, and SUCCINIC ACID, produced from fat and carbohydrate breakdown. Heme synthesis requires VITAMIN B_6, and LEAD inhibits the process. Therefore vitamin B_6 deficiency and lead poisoning cause ANEMIA. When the spleen removes wornout red blood cells it converts heme to the BILE PIGMENT, bilirubin, and recycles the released iron.

Much of the iron in meat, fish, and poultry occurs as heme, which is readily absorbed by the intestine. Absorption of this heme iron is not diminished by PHYTIC ACID, a metal binder occurring in certain plant materials, nor is it increased by VITAMIN C. In contrast, most of the iron in vegetables is not bound to heme and is less readily absorbed. The efficiency of nonheme iron absorption from plant sources is only 10 percent to 20 percent that of heme iron. Vitamin C increases the uptake of iron from nonheme sources. Some forms of FIBER bind minerals and lower intestinal absorption of nonheme iron.

hemicellulose A form of dietary FIBER, plant material resistant to digestive enzymes. Hemicellulose helps form plant cell walls. Annual plants contain 15 percent to 30 percent hemicellulose by dry weight in their cell walls, while wood contains 20 percent to 25 percent hemicellulose. Dietary sources of hemicellulose include FRUIT, vegetables, LEGUMES, cereal, BRAN, whole-grain flours, nuts, and seeds. Dietary hemicelluloses absorb water, provide bulk, and soften stools. They are broken down by intestinal bacteria. Excessive amounts of hemicelluloses may interfere with mineral absorption.

Hemicellulose is structurally distinct from water-soluble fibers such as gums and pectin and insoluble fiber like CELLULOSE. Hemicellulose contains long chains of repeating sugar units. Pentosans are chains of PENTOSES, five-carbon sugars like xylose and arabinose. Pentosans form the largest group and occur in CEREAL GRAINS. Galactosans, chains of the simple sugar GALACTOSE, form a second group. Acidic hemicelluloses also occur in food.

hemochromatosis A rare condition caused by excessive IRON deposits in tissues, including the LIVER, PANCREAS, and skin. Symptoms include liver enlargement, weakness, moderate weight loss, bronzed skin, diabetes, and, eventually, heart failure. Hemochromatosis is 10 times more frequent in men than in women.

Abnormal iron metabolism can be caused by a genetic defect (primary hemochromatosis) characterized by increased accumulation of iron in tissues. The inherited trait for iron storage disease is relatively common among whites, affecting perhaps as many as one person in two hundred. This suggests that the tendency to accumulate dietary iron is a more general problem in the U.S. than generally recognized. Alternatively, excessive iron consumption can lead to abnormally high iron storage (secondary hemochromatosis). This can occur with chronic iron supplementation in men, because they do not usually lose iron, and in alcoholics, because several alcoholic beverages contain iron. (See also FERRITIN.)

hemoglobin The oxygen transport protein of blood and the predominant protein in red blood cells. Hemoglobin is a complex PROTEIN; it contains a total of four individual amino acid chains called globins. Adult hemoglobin contains two alpha globin chains and two beta globin chains. Hemoglobin also contains the iron-containing pigment HEME, which is required to bind oxygen. Heme imparts a red color to hemoglobin and to red blood cells.

Hemoglobin is a dynamic molecule and changes its shape and oxygen-carrying characteristics to help regulate oxygen delivery and blood pH. It binds oxygen when the oxygen concentration is high in blood exposed to air in the lungs. Next, arteries carry oxygen-rich red blood cells from the lungs to capillaries, where hemoglobin responds by releasing more of its bound oxygen (the Bohr effect). The released oxygen then diffuses into cells to enable them to continue the oxidation of fuel molecules. During this process of shedding oxygen molecules hemoglobin binds carbon dioxide and hydrogen ions and returns them to the lungs via the veins. In the lungs hemoglobin picks up more oxygen and simultaneously releases carbon dioxide and hydrogen ions.

An adult normally produces 6.25 g of hemoglobin daily. The hemoglobin blood content of women is 12 to 16 g per 100 ml of blood, and of men, 14 to 18 g. ANEMIA is a deficiency of normal red blood cells. Deficiencies of IRON, VITAMIN A, VITAMIN B_6, VITAMIN B_{12}, VITAMIN D, VITAMIN E, and FOLIC ACID may cause anemia.

Over 400 mutant hemoglobins are known. Most do not alter normal physiological function of hemoglobin. However, certain mutations lead to abnormal hemoglobins that malfunction and produce fragile red blood cells and, consequently, anemia, including sickle cell anemia and thalassemias. Alteration of a single amino acid in a chain of 146 amino acids causes sickle cell anemia.

Environmental factors can decrease hemoglobin function. Carbon monoxide poisons hemoglobin, and cigarette smokers' blood contains much more carbon monoxide than that of nonsmokers. Furthermore, babies born to smoking women are smaller than average because they receive less oxygen during fetal development. (See also ERYTHROPOIESIS; HEMATOCRIT.)

Davie, Sarah J. et al. "Effect of Vitamin C on Glycosylation of Proteins," *Diabetes* 41 (1992): 167–173.

hemolytic anemia A deficiency of red blood cells caused by their rapid destruction and characterized by chronic fatigue. Typically, hemoglobin breakdown products accumulate, leading to JAUNDICE, the accumulation of yellow pigment in the skin and in the whites of the eyes. Rapid turnover of red blood cells may be caused by genetic diseases that lead to the production of abnormal HEMOGLOBIN, as in sickle cell ANEMIA and thalassemias. Defects in red blood cell enzymes can also cause hemolytic anemia. A deficiency of one such enzyme, glucose-

6-phosphate dehydrogenase that helps maintain adequate levels of GLUTATHIONE, a cellular ANTIOXIDANT, is the most common of these defects. Acquired hemolytic anemia can be caused by exposure to potentially damaging chemicals, including certain drugs (antimalarials, pimaquine, and Atrabine). (See also IRON.)

hemolytic-uremic syndrome See *ESCHERICHIA COLI.*

hemosiderosis A condition associated with excessive iron deposition, particularly in the LIVER and spleen. Hemosiderin is the insoluble iron complex formed in the liver with iron accumulation. Hemosiderosis can be caused by:

1. excessive red blood breakdown associated with chronic infection, malaria, hemolytic anemias, PERNICIOUS ANEMIA, or multiple blood transfusions;
2. excessive uptake of dietary iron;
3. impaired utilization of iron.

Under severe conditions, with extreme accumulation of iron, the resulting disease is called HEMOCHROMATOSIS. This condition in turn causes liver damage and pancreatic damage, which can lead to DIABETES.

heparin A carbohydrate that is a naturally occurring anticoagulant (prevents blood from clotting). Heparin is produced by mast cells (cells that also contain inflammatory agents like histamine) in connective tissue, the liver and certain white blood cells. Heparin prevents the formation of FIBRIN clots. (Fibrin is the insoluble protein produced when blood clotting is triggered.) In capillaries, heparin also activates the lipoprotein LIPASE, the enzyme that releases FATTY ACIDS from CHYLOMICRONS and VERY LOW-DENSITY LIPOPROTEINS, particles that transport fat in the blood. (See also FAT METABOLISM; GLYCOSAMINOGLYCANS.)

hepatic Refers to the LIVER.

hepatitis Chronic inflammation of the LIVER. Symptoms include JAUNDICE, liver enlargement, fever, and gastrointestinal disturbances. Hepatitis can cause a loss of APPETITE, headache, and a change in taste sensation. It can interfere with DIGESTION, leading to MALNUTRITION. Hepatitis can be caused by drugs, poisons, and viruses.

Infectious hepatitis refers to a family of viral diseases spread orally. Hepatitis A is caused by the hepatitis A virus usually transmitted orally through fecal contamination of food utensils, due to poor hygiene by food workers who have been infected with the virus. Fecal contamination can also spread through drinking WATER. Eating shellfish contaminated by raw sewage is a common cause of infectious hepatitis. The long incubation period, three to six weeks, makes it difficult to associate hepatitis with a specific food. GAMMA GLOBULIN may prevent the disease, provided the shots are administered soon after exposure. Travelers to countries typified by poor sanitation may be advised to receive gamma globulin shots, which will offer protection for up to three or four months. Hepatitis E is an enteric (small intestinal) form of hepatitis that has been associated with waterborne outbreaks of hepatitis in developing countries. Other forms of hepatitis (such as hepatitis B and hepatitis C) are spread through blood. (See also FOOD POISONING.)

Fried, M. W. "Therapy of Chronic Viral Hepatitis," *Medical Clinics of North America* 80, no. 5 (September 1996): 957–972.

herbal medicine (botanical medicine) The branch of medicine that emphasizes the therapeutic properties of plants. Ancient medical traditions from India (ayurvedic medicine) and China (oriental medicine) and others emphasize the health benefits of specific plants and plant products, and medicinal plants provided the foundation of the modern pharmaceutical industry. Recent environmental awareness of the diversity of species in threatened tropical rain forests has rekindled research in the pharmacological effects of indigenous plants. Although natural products, they offer the advantage of containing multiple active principles that possess a variety of often complementary properties. Often, the active ingredients of herbs correct an underlying problem rather than simply treating a symptom. Most herbal preparations are considered foods by the U.S. FDA and they cannot be labeled with health claims.

Quality control is an issue with herbal preparations. Their potency is affected by the plant's age at the time of harvest, the season of harvest, the type of soil used for cultivation, the climate, and the methods of storage and preparation. Producers often measure the amounts of active ingredients in a given herbal preparation or extract and then adjust the strength to a standard level to assure a reproducible activity.

The appropriate amount consumed is a second concern; an amount that is safe for an adult may not be safe for a child. Some herbs are appropriate for short-term use, and not for long periods.

A third concern is safety. According to the U.S. FDA, extracts of the following plants are potentially dangerous: arnica, belladonna (deadly nightshade), Culcana, blood root, Scotch broom, buckeye nuts, heliotrope, hemlock, henbane, jalop root, jimsonweed, lily of the valley, lobelia, mandrake, mistletoe, morning glory, periwinkle, St.-John's-wort, spindle bean, tonka bean, snakeroot, and wormwood (once used to flavor absinthe, a liqueur).

Often foods themselves provide substances that promote health. Beyond the nutrients they contain, ONIONS, GARLIC, CHILI PEPPERS, LICORICE, TURMERIC, CRANBERRY, GINGER, DANDELION, BLUEBERRIES, and cherries contain a variety of substances that fight infection, reduce the risk of cancer, stimulate the nervous system or reduce inflammation. (See also ALFALFA; CHAMOMILE; COMFREY; GINSENG; GOLDENSEAL; HAWTHORN; PEPPERMINT; SARSAPARILLA; STRAWBERRY.)

Wehrbach, M. R., and M. T. Murray. *Botanical Influences on Illness*. Tarzana, Calif.: Third Line Press, 1994.

herbicides A diverse family of chemicals used to kill weeds during cultivation of crops. Many herbicides are suspected of causing CANCER or BIRTH DEFECTS. The health risks of herbicides are greatest for those with chronic exposure, such as farm workers and professional applicators. The following herbicides are examples currently in use:

- Alachlor is a widely used herbicide and is among the most dangerous.
- Atrazine accounts for about 10 percent of PESTICIDE sales in the United States and was restricted by 1991. This herbicide has been found to widely contaminate underground water supplies in the United States.
- Dinoseb was subject to an emergency ban by the EPA in 1986 because of a possible link to birth defects, skin rashes, cancer, and sterility in experimental animals. Because a substitute was not developed, the EPA permitted the continued use of Dinoseb on LENTILS, PEAS, CHICKPEAS, green beans, and RASPBERRIES.
- Linuron is a common herbicide used on SOYBEANS, carrots, celery, asparagus, corn, potatoes, and wheat. It is associated with tumors in experimental animals. Linuron frequently contaminates water supplies,
- Paraquat is used to treat fields before planting or before harvest. It is used extensively in soybean agriculture and in orchards. Paraquat cannot be washed off produce, and direct exposure to this chemical is hazardous. Inhalation of its mist causes lung inflammation and repeated exposure can lead to kidney and lung damage. It is also toxic to fish.
- 2,4-D is widely used by home owners and home gardeners to kill dandelions. It is the toxic agent in over 1,500 pesticide products. Exposure is greatest for children and animals who play in treated areas. Farmers use 2,4-D on CORN, WHEATS, and hay. A National Cancer Institute study linked this weed killer with cancer of lymphoid tissue in experimental animals. (See also DIOXIN; PESTICIDES.)

herbs The leaves, shoots, stems, and seeds of many widely distributed plants. In contrast, SPICES are prepared from the FRUIT, bark, or pepper corns from tropical plants. Culinary herbs have appealing aromatic or savory characteristics and make food tasty and flavorful. In addition many herbs affect physiological processes, which is the basis for their medicinal properties. In some cases, research has provided deeper insights into the active ingredients.

Culinary herbs that exhibit physiologic effects include:

- ANISE and CARAWAY may relieve gas and stomach cramps. Caraway contains carvacrol, a compound that eases muscle spasms.
- Carrot seed may relax smooth muscles, relieve stomach cramps, and lower blood pressure.

- Celery seed contains phthalides, chemicals that are sedatives. Celery seed has antibiotic activity. Celery juice may lower blood pressure.
- CHERVIL contains the mild carcinogen estragole, which is also found in basil and tarragon.
- Coriander (cilantro) may lower BLOOD SUGAR and increase GLUCOSE TOLERANCE. Coriander lowers blood fat. According to folklore, it curbs bad breath.
- Dill oil reduces cramps, lowers blood pressure, and slows heartbeat in experimental animals. Dill water reduces colic, according to folklore.
- FENNEL contains sulfur compounds that relieve cramps. According to folklore, it helps with colic and upset stomach.
- LOVAGE seeds, leaf, and root can be steeped in boiling water to prepare a tea, used in folk medicine to reduce water retention and ease joint pain. Lovage increases urination and water loss in experimental animals.
- PARSLEY lowers blood pressure and stimulates uterine contractions in experimental animals. Parsley acts as a mild LAXATIVE and also freshens the breath. Parsley oil contains apiol and myristicin, which induce menstruation. Parsley oil can induce miscarriages and should not be administered during pregnancy.

Herbs of the mint family that exhibit physiologic effects:

- BASIL relieves FLATULENCE and gastrointestinal discomfort.
- Lemon balm is an ANTIOXIDANT. Animal studies suggest the oil relieves inflammation.
- MARJORAM may relax smooth muscles and relieve stomach cramps. According to folklore, marjoram tea eases cramps and upset stomach.
- OREGANO can function as an antiseptic. Its oil contains carvacrol, which possesses broad antimicrobial properties. It relieves upset stomach and is a smooth muscle relaxant. According to folklore, chewing oregano reduces toothache pain.
- ROSEMARY and SAGE contain strong antioxidants. Like CLOVES, oregano, and GINGER, they have long been used to preserve food. Sage is used commercially to preserve salad oil and potato chips. According to folklore, rosemary aids memory and induces sleep.
- THYME contains thymol, an antiseptic. Thyme is used as a mouth wash. Oil of thyme causes dangerous side effects, however.

hermetically sealed Refers to food containers that do not permit entry of either microorganisms or air. For example, bottled or canned foods are hermetically sealed. (See also FOOD PROCESSING.)

herring (*Clupea harengus*) A small, saltwater FISH related to the shad and SARDINE. Silvery and streamlined, the herring reaches a length of 10 in. at maturity. A freshwater variety is known as cisco. Herring is an important food fish that is also processed for animal feed. Intensive fishing practices worldwide have placed this fish in jeopardy.

Herring is an oily fish, and most of the fat is unsaturated. It is available frozen, pickled, or smoked. Herring roe is used to prepare CAVIAR. Pickled herring, 3 oz. (85 g), provides calories, 190; protein, 17.3 g; fat, 12.8 g; cholesterol, 66 mg; calcium, 31 mg; iron, 1.2 mg; sodium, 1.38 mg; zinc, 0.85 mg; vitamin A equivalents, 20; niacin, 2 mg; thiamin, 0.04 mg; riboflavin, 0.18 mg.

hesperidin A substance found in rinds of ORANGES and lemons and in the peels of ripe fruit. A mature orange contains about a gram of hesperidin. Citrus FLAVONOIDS are commercially extracted from the pulp remaining after juicing oranges and lemons. Hesperidin is believed to strengthen capillary walls in conjunction with VITAMIN C. Like most flavonoids, it is also an ANTIOXIDANT and limits oxidative damage. (See also CITRUS FRUIT.)

heterocrine Refers to tissues that secrete different types of materials. The PANCREAS is a notable example; it combines an endocrine function (secretion of hormones INSULIN and GLUCAGON directly into the blood) and an exocrine function (secretion of digestive enzymes into the intestine). (See also ENDOCRINE SYSTEM.)

heterocyclic amines (HCAs) A family of cancer-causing agents that occur in cooked MEAT. HCAs tend to form inside meat with longer cooking times and higher temperatures of barbecuing. They cannot be scraped off and once eaten they can become activated to attack DNA of cells, a possible first step in cancer development. HCAs can also inflame the heart.

There are several ways to minimize the risk of HCAs. Precooking hamburger for a short time before barbecuing seems to eliminate some of the compounds that can form HCAs. On the other hand, green and black tea contain tannins, bitter substances in brewed tea, that can block the ability of HCAs to damage DNA. Garlic and onions behave similarly. The green plant pigment chlorophyll can also block the damaging effects of HCAs. Supplementing with the bifidobacteria can protect the COLON against HCAs. (See also CARCINOGEN.)

hexose A large class of simple sugars composed of six carbon atoms that can serve as an energy source. FRUCTOSE and GLUCOSE are the two most important hexoses in the diet. As BLOOD SUGAR, glucose is the most important CARBOHYDRATE fuel in the body. Hexoses also function as building blocks for more complex sugars and for important large molecular weight carbohydrates. Thus, fructose is linked to glucose in table sugar, and LACTOSE contains two hexoses, GALACTOSE and glucose. Polymerized MANNOSE is found in glucomannan, a form of fiber. STARCH, GLYCOGEN, and CELLULOSE are polysaccharides made from glucose. (See also NATURAL SWEETENERS.)

hiatus hernia (hiatal hernia) The protrusion or bulging of the STOMACH through the esophageal opening (hiatus) of the diaphragm into the chest. Aging or damage of supportive tissue can lead to hiatus hernia and DIVERTICULOSIS, which is the bulging of the large intestine. For Americans, there is a 50 percent chance of having a hiatus hernia after the age of 40. Symptoms resemble DYSPEPSIA, including a burning pain under the breastbone and heartburn in which stomach contents regurgitate into the ESOPHAGUS, causing inflammation. Inability to breathe deeply and frequent belching are also experienced. Symptoms are most noticeable after a large meal, when straining or when stooping.

Hiatus hernia is often a recurrent condition. Several steps can be taken to minimize its effects. Consumers should:

- Practice good posture to allow less crowding of organs in abdominal area.
- Eat light meals that are less likely to force the stomach through the diaphragm.
- Eat in a peaceful environment.
- Receive physical manipulation by a skilled therapist or bouncing on one's heels to move the stomach down into place.
- Avoid swallowing air; this inflates the stomach.
- Take licorice extract.

hidden fat See FAT.

high blood pressure See HYPERTENSION.

high-calorie foods See FAT, HIDDEN.

high complex carbohydrate diet See DIET, HIGH COMPLEX CARBOHYDRATE.

high-density lipoprotein (HDL) A type of lipid-protein complex or particle in the blood that scavenges CHOLESTEROL from peripheral tissues and transports it to the LIVER for disposal. HDL's function is opposite that of LOW-DENSITY LIPOPROTEIN (LDL), which transports cholesterol to tissues. HDL can transfer cholesterol to another lipid carrier, VERY LOW-DENSITY LIPOPROTEIN (VLDL), prior to its conversion to LDL.

Because HDL possesses the highest protein content, which is more dense than lipid, HDL is the densest of the various circulating lipoproteins. HDL precursor is synthesized by the liver. HDL_3 is an intermediate form, to which lipids and proteins are added from other lipoproteins in the circulation. The mature, spherical HDL is called HDL_2. Generally speaking, the higher the HDL level, the lower the risk of ATHEROSCLEROSIS. Women have a lower risk of heart disease than men and their HDL levels are higher. Evidence suggests that HDL_3 is inversely linked to the risk of coronary heart disease more strongly than HDL_2.

HDL contains proteins that determine its role. For example, Apoprotein D catalyzes cholesterol transfer between HDL and LDL, and Apoprotein CII is transferred to VLDL and CHYLOMICRONS, enabling these lipoproteins to interact in capillaries

evaporate and will dissipate with time. Adding an acidic ingredient like vinegar or mayonnaise blocks enzyme action and decreases the flavor. Horseradish can be served with fatty meats, cocktail sauces, cold cuts, and FISH. Horseradish contains low levels of GOITROGENS. High levels of these agents block IODINE uptake by the thyroid gland, needed to produce thyroid hormone. However, usual consumption of such vegetables and condiments is not deemed harmful, and they add variety and nutritional value to many dishes. (See also SPICE.)

hospital-induced malnutrition Malnutrition occurs during hospitalization after patients have been fed inadequate diets for several weeks. A study reported in the 1970s suggested that 30 percent to 50 percent of hospitalized people left the hospital in worse nutritional condition than when they arrived as patients. Hospitals generally have improved their menus since then, although hospitalization still does not guarantee optimal nutrition. A 1996 study of 57 hospitals found that only four routinely offered patients menus that met all federal dietary guidelines: Fewer than 20 percent kept cholesterol below 300 mg/day, while half kept salt intake below 6 g/day and dietary fiber at more than 20 g/day. (See also DIETARY GUIDELINES FOR AMERICANS; MALNUTRITION.)

hot dog A heavily processed meat product resembling a sausage in shape. Though viewed as a PROTEIN source, a typical hot dog contains only about 5 g of protein, the same as an average hot dog bun. Red meat hot dogs are a high-fat food: FAT accounts for 80 percent of the CALORIES. This is true even when the label indicates hot dogs are "80 percent fat free." The USDA permits the designation of "80 percent fat free" to indicate any hot dog containing less than the standard 30 percent fat by weight, provided the standard is also listed on the food label. This term refers to fat content by weight and provides no indication of fat calories.

"Lean" hot dogs may contain 20 percent fat, rather than the usual 30 percent. Because half of the weight of the hot dog is WATER, the percentage of calories from fat is 71 percent higher than 20 percent. Often, CHICKEN and turkey hot dogs contain 8 to 9 g of fat, as much as red meat hot dogs; they are not low-fat foods. TOFU hot dogs are meat-free and contain 30 percent less fat than regular hot dogs and no CHOLESTEROL.

Manufacturers add nitrates and NITRITES to hot dogs and other cured meat foods to prevent the growth of disease-producing bacteria, to add flavor, and to enhance their color.

These preservatives from nitrosoamines in the digestive tract, which may pose a cancer risk. (See also DIETARY GUIDELINES FOR AMERICANS; FAT, HIDDEN; FOOD LABELING.)

humectant A FOOD ADDITIVE used to maintain moisture, texture, and freshness in prepared foods. Humectants attract water in air and tend to retain water. CORN SYRUP, GLYCEROL, glycerol monostearate, propylene glycol, and SORBITOL are common examples of humectants. They are used to keep candies, shredded COCONUT, and MARSHMALLOWS from drying out. They are generally considered as safe food additives.

hunger A compelling need to eat caused by food deprivation. Hunger is often accompanied by a painful feeling and weakness and is unpleasant. Energy stores are mobilized with hunger. In contrast, APPETITE is usually associated with pleasure during food consumption. Rhythmic contractions (PERISTALSIS) of an empty stomach are responsible for hunger pangs; these become more frequent the longer a meal is delayed. To a limited extent, stomach contractions are regulated by blood sugar levels and by distension of the stomach when filled. Hunger is regulated primarily by several brain centers, including the hypothalamus, via a "feeding center" and a "satiety center." Normally the hypothalamus functions as an integration center for a variety of signals; possibly brain centers sense a decline in blood sugar levels, for example. Other hypotheses involve the production in the brain of neuropeptides. Some are identical with gut peptides, where they stimulate or inhibit eating. Cholecystokinin, formed in the gut and in the brain, inhibits eating. Long-term control of body weight relies upon mechanisms that are currently being defined. LEPTIN, a protein produced by body fat, signals the brain to stop producing signals that stimulate feeding. Leptin could curtail production of specific brain peptides and it could block norepinephrine and related neurotransmitters that trigger hunger and increase basal metabolism. Overall, eating patterns reflect internal regulatory mechanisms; psychological influences such as stress and mood; environmental factors like climate; and diseases such as mental illness, BULIMIA NERVOSA, and ANOREXIA NERVOSA. (See also OBESITY.)

hunger, world HUNGER continues to be an international issue. An estimated 1.1 billion people in the world are malnourished. Hunger is common among developing nations as well as among subpopulations of developed nations. Pregnant women and children are the most vulnerable to MALNUTRITION. In developing countries of Asia and Africa, BREAST-FEEDING assures adequate nutrition until about six months of age. Subsequently, hunger takes a greater toll. Practices such as relying on formula feeding rather than breast-feeding are detrimental when the formula is diluted or cannot be prepared with sterile water or refrigeration. Failure of children to grow at a normal rate indicates chronic, severe problems. Malnourished infants who survive chronic hunger bear the emotional and physical burden, with mental retardation as a possible consequence. Indirect consequences of marginal nutrition include infectious diseases, diarrhea, and parasitic diseases such as malaria. Protein-calorie malnutrition due to severe food restriction is the most prevalent form among children.

Maternal nutrition is often marginal where hunger is endemic, and women in developing countries often bear the brunt of hunger within a family. The mother often feeds her family first and subsists on what is left. These women also often provide physical labor required to obtain food for families, even during pregnancies.

Poverty and hunger are linked by lack of education, poor health, little political voice, inadequate food distribution, and lack of technical information—enforced by those possessing education and political and military power, who control resources and rely on cash crops, and who hold a monopoly on technology. Overpopulation is another pressing concern worldwide. The world is now populated by more than 6 billion people. In another century, it is projected to be 12 billion. However, poverty links hunger and overpopulation.

World food production can provide all people with ample calories, according to the United Nations' FOOD AND AGRICULTURAL ORGANIZATION. Generally, when there has been economic growth and equal distribution of resources among most groups in a population, population growth rates have declined. Land reform in which more people have an input in food production also seems essential. The GREEN REVOLUTION of the 1960s failed to achieve its goal of making countries self-sufficient in food production because it generally ignored local culture, traditional agriculture, and economic factors such as dependency on imported chemical fertilizers. Food distribution is a critical factor. The problem of unequal distribution of resources is compounded by the fact that in most countries governments dictate daily life. In addition, at least 20 percent of total food produced yearly is wasted by spoilage and pests, contributing to food shortages.

Multinational corporations involved in exporting plantation crops and a preoccupation with profitability may indirectly contribute to hunger when cultivated land is used for luxury and export crops, rather than for traditional staples, despite starvation and local severe malnutrition. Thus, regions of Africa are net exporters of COFFEE, COCOA, PEANUTS, and cattle, as well as beans and barley, despite having the greatest incidence of severe malnutrition among children.

The 1980 Presidential Commission on World Hunger concluded that nations have the capability of remedying global hunger and that the global demand for food requires political and technical solutions to the above problems, that assistance programs need to focus on self-reliance, and that developing countries need to develop effective food production and distribution systems and to emphasize education. (See also INFANT FORMULA.)

Center on Hunger, Poverty and Nutrition Policy, Tufts University School of Medicine. *Statement on the Link Between Nutrition and Cognitive Development in Children.* 1994.

hunger suppressants See APPETITE SUPPRESSANTS.

huperzine A A purified ALKALOID derived from a rare Chinese herb, used in traditional Chinese medicine to treat fever. In limited studies huperzine A has exhibited anticholinesterase activity and improved memory and cognitive function in patients with dementia. It is being investigated as a possible treatment for or preventive of ALZHEIMER'S DISEASE. There is inadequate safety data for pregnant or breast-feeding women.

Skolnick, A. A. "Old Chinese Herbal Medicine Used for Fever Yields Possible New Alzheimer Disease Therapy," *JAMA* 277, no. 10 (March 1997): 776.

HVP See HYDROLYZED VEGETABLE PROTEIN.

hydrochloric acid See DIGESTION.

hydrocortisone See CORTISOL.

hydrogenated vegetable oil Vegetable oil that has been modified by the addition of hydrogen. Hydrogenation is an industrial process that adds hydrogen atoms to double bonds of oils, polyunsaturated FATTY ACIDS. Hydrogenation creates a more saturated FAT (filled up with hydrogen atoms) and thus hardens or solidifies vegetable oils. Most commercially available polyunsaturated oils (CORN OIL, SOYBEAN OIL, SAFFLOWER oil, SUNFLOWER oil, and COTTONSEED OIL) are partially hydrogenated to retard rancidity, to increase shelf-life, and to make them thicker and more spreadable.

The degree of hydrogenation varies with the type of product. Solid fats like stick MARGARINE and vegetable SHORTENING are the most hydrogenated. Vegetable shortening is highly hydrogenated vegetable oil, the equivalent to LARD, although less saturated than BEEF TALLOW. Tub margarine is made of partially hydrogenated oils and is 20 percent saturated. However, it is much less saturated than BUTTER, which is 66 percent saturated. Partially hydrogenated vegetable oils are somewhat more saturated than untreated oils. For example, soybean oil is initially 15 percent saturated and ends up 20 percent saturated after partial hydrogenation.

During hydrogenation some of the polyunsaturated fatty acid content is converted to monounsaturates with a single double bond instead of multiple double bonds. Also during hydrogenation, a fraction of the polyunsaturated fatty acids are converted to TRANS-FATTY ACIDS, in which some of the existing double bonds straighten. Trans-fatty acids raise cholesterol levels and are associated with an increase in the risk of heart attack. Whether the risk is greater than with saturated fats is unknown. Hydrogenated vegetable oil supplies 80 percent of the trans-fatty acids Americans ingest. The long-range health effects of these industrial by-products are unknown.

Partially hydrogenated vegetable oils, including soybean, cottonseed, corn, and rapeseed oils, are commonly added to increase the flavor and taste of processed foods. Foods with partially hydrogenated or hydrogenated vegetable oils include foods such as most kinds of CHIPS (potato chips, corn chips, and the like), CRACKERS, rye crisps, margarines, shortening, frozen pizzas, salad dressing, low-cholesterol MAYONNAISE, and even FROZEN ENTREES. Food labels presently list fat content and often use the term PARTIALLY HYDROGENATED OIL without further explanation, which provides little detailed information. Nonetheless, added oil indicates added calories. The general recommendation is to cut back on all fats and oils to lower the risk of cancer and heart disease. Eating an excess of saturated fat, whether it is animal fat or hydrogenated vegetable oil, increases the risk of CARDIOVASCULAR DISEASE. (See also CONVENIENCE FOOD; DIETARY GUIDELINES FOR AMERICANS; PROCESSED FOOD.)

hydrogen peroxide A powerful oxidizer. Solutions of hydrogen peroxide are colorless and have a biting taste. They are used as a bleaching agent, and as a bactericide and a disinfectant for the mouth, nose, and throat. Hydrogen peroxide can spontaneously break down into FREE RADICALS, a highly reactive chemical species.

Hydrogen peroxide also is a product of METABOLISM, especially in the LIVER. It is generated in organelles called PEROXISOMES. Additionally, scavenger white blood cells (phagocytic leukocytes) produce a burst of highly reactive forms of oxygen, including hydrogen peroxide, to destroy engulfed microorganisms. The body's antioxidant system generates hydrogen peroxide. SUPEROXIDE DISMUTASE is an enzyme that degrades a free radical called superoxide to hydrogen peroxide. Hydrogen peroxide is decomposed very rapidly by glutathione peroxidase and CATALASE, other ANTIOXIDANT enzymes.

hydrolysis An important type of chemical reaction that forms the basis of DIGESTION. During hydrolysis, a bond between atoms of a compound is split by incorporating a water molecule, giving rise to the name hydrolysis (hydro = water, lysis = splitting). Hydrolysis creates two smaller molecules (fragments). Digestive enzymes catalyze (speed up) the hydrolysis of food molecules.

LIPASES are enzymes that hydrolyze (break down) FATS and OILS to produce GLYCEROL and FATTY ACIDS. Proteolytic enzymes (PROTEASES) like TRYPSIN and PEPSIN catalyze the degradation of proteins to amino acids. AMYLASE, a pancreatic enzyme, hydrolyzes STARCH to maltose, a sugar containing two glucose units. Intestinal enzymes help complete carbohydrate digestion. Thus MALTASE digests maltose to glucose and LACTASE digests LACTOSE (milk sugar) to glucose and GALACTOSE. (See also CARBOHYDRATE; CARBOHYDRATE METABOLISM; DIGESTIVE TRACT.)

hydrolyzed vegetable protein (HVP) An additive in PROCESSED FOODS used to enhance the flavor of meat dishes like beef stew, instant soups, sauces and gravy mixes. HVP is no longer added to BABY FOODS. It is prepared by breaking down PROTEIN of SOYBEANS, PEANUTS, WHEAT, or CORN into AMINO ACIDS and small fragments. On a food label, HVP can legally be called a "natural flavor" with no further description, though often it contains up to 20 percent MSG (MONOSODIUM GLUTAMATE) and is a hidden source of this FLAVOR ENHANCER. (See also ARTIFICIAL FLAVORS; FOOD LABELING.)

hydrophilic Refers to the ability of certain compounds to attract WATER molecules. Ions (electrolytes) like those of SODIUM, POTASSIUM, and CHLORIDE are hydrophilic, as are water-soluble organic compounds such as sugars, simple acids (lactic ACID, VITAMIN C, acetic acid), B VITAMINS (niacin, biotin, riboflavin, thiamin), and AMINO ACIDS. Large molecules can also be hydrophilic, and thus dissolve in water solutions. Many proteins found in blood and the cytoplasm fall into this category. Certain insoluble substances like cellulose, while water-insoluble attract water molecules and form "wettable" surfaces. The surfaces of cells contain carbohydrate structures and phospholipids that attract water and permit the cell to survive in an aqueous medium. Foreign materials that enter the body through water, food, and air or are ingested directly like medication may accumulate unless they are chemically modified to make them more water-soluble so they can be secreted. Particularly the liver is well stocked with a large group of "detoxifying" enzymes that increase the hydrophilic properties of these substances. (See also BUFFER; EMULSIFIERS; MICELLE.)

hydrophobic Refers to the ability of certain compounds to be attracted to organic solvents such as hexane and oils in FAT and to repel water. Hydrophobic substances include lipids, a diverse family of water-insoluble substances like fats, oils, and CHOLESTEROL. When transported in blood, which is primarily water, these hydrophobic substances are enclosed by a layer of proteins and phospholipids as microscopic droplets (micelles) that are water-soluble. These particles are called LIPOPROTEINS and include LOW-DENSITY LIPOPROTEIN (LDL) cholesterol (so-called bad cholesterol) and HIGH-DENSITY LIPOPROTEIN (HDL) cholesterol (a desirable form of cholesterol). Agents such as BILE acids act like detergents to suspend fats and oils as MICELLES in water-based digestive juices. Bile acids and bile salts, as well as phospholipids, possess a hydrophobic end and a hydrophilic (water-attracting) end. They form a ball-shaped shell, in which the attracting portions of the molecules face outward to interact with water, while their hydrophobic regions point inward, embedded in the oily droplet they surround.

Certain amino acids possess hydrophobic regions (side chains): PHENYLALANINE; METHIONINE, TRYPTOPHAN, ALANINE, LEUCINE, ISOLEUCINE, and VALINE. When they are building blocks of functional proteins like ENZYMES, serum proteins and antibodies, the hydrophobic amino acids are buried within the interior of the protein molecule away from the surrounding water molecules rather than on the exterior. In contrast, insoluble proteins of skin and hair (keratins) repel water because their hydrophobic amino acids are exposed. (See also EMULSIFIERS; VITAMIN.)

hydroxybutyric acid See BETA HYDROXYBUTYRIC ACID.

hydroxycitric acid (HCA) A compound prepared from the Malabar tamarind (*Garcinia cambogia*), a fruit native to Southeast Asia where it is often used as a condiment in curry dishes. HCA is similar to citric acid in its chemical structure.

Preliminary animal studies indicated HCA could be helpful as a weight-reduction aid. However, more recent and reliable studies in human subjects showed no significant weight loss in patients who took supplements of HCA for 12 weeks.

HCA is available in the United States as a dietary supplement. Consequently, its safety and efficacy as a weight-loss aid have not been tested by any government agency. Safety data for pregnant and breast-feeding women are inadequate.

Heymsfield, Steven et al. "*Garcinia cambogia* (Hydroxycitric Acid) as a Potential Antiobesity Agent: A Randomized Controlled Trial," *JAMA* 280, no. 18 (November 11, 1998): 1,596–1,600.

hydroxyproline An oxidized form of amino acid PROLINE that is a feature of COLLAGEN, the structural protein of connective tissue. Hydroxyproline is not classified as a dietary essential amino acid, nor is it used to assemble proteins because it is formed from proline after a protein chain is synthesized. Hydroxyproline in collagen stabilizes its fibrous structure. Hydroxyproline is synthesized by the enzyme, proline oxidase, which requires VITAMIN C. Chronic vitamin C deficiency therefore prevents connective tissue maturation, resulting in capillary fragility, susceptibility to bruising and bleeding gums, and joint pain. (See also SCURVY.)

hyperacidity See HYPOCHLORHYDRIA.

hyperalimentation Orally administered liquid diets providing high levels of one or more nutrients. In medicine, intravenous hyperalimentation refers to the administration of a solution containing all essential nutrients, including AMINO ACIDS (3.5 percent), GLUCOSE (25 percent), VITAMINS and ELECTROLYTES (ionic substances) required to sustain life. Three liters daily supplies 3,000 CALORIES and 105 g of amino acids. It is usually infused into a major vein leading into the heart (superior vena cava) via a catheter, so that highly concentrated solutions are quickly diluted in the blood. This procedure is usually used in cases of severe illness, including PANCREATITIS, CANCER, severe MALNUTRITION, gastrointestinal blockage, trauma, and other medical conditions.

hypercalcemia An excess of CALCIUM in the blood. Regulatory mechanisms involving calcitonin, a HORMONE from the thyroid gland that lowers blood calcium; parathyroid hormone from the PARATHYROID GLANDS that raises blood calcium; and VITAMIN D help maintain blood calcium levels within very narrow limits, regardless of diet. Hypercalcemia therefore is most often caused by a hormonal abnormality. Possible causes include CANCER, overproduction of calcitonin by the parathyroid glands or excessive ingestion of vitamin D. Symptoms associated with hypercalcemia include vomiting, loss of appetite, and possibly kidney stones. (See also ENDOCRINE SYSTEM.)

hyperchlorhydria (hyperacidity) The excess in secretion of hydrochloric acid in the stomach. In the absence of food, hyperchlorhydria causes a burning sensation after meals. Excessive acid production is associated with strong emotional responses and HUNGER pains, and it may aggravate DUODENAL ULCERS. Emotional disturbances and food sensitivities can cause excessive production of STOMACH ACID. Hormonal imbalance may relate to an increased sensitivity of parietal cells (acid-secreting cells of the stomach) to the hormone GASTRIN, which stimulates acid production; to hyper-secretion of gastrin after meals; or to a decreased ability to inhibit gastrin release when the acidity of GASTRIC JUICE contents drops.

Pain associated with hyperchlorhydria can be relieved by ANTACIDS. However, the use of calcium carbonate antacids is associated with a rebound in gastric juice (stomach acid) production. (See also DIGESTION.)

hypercholesterolemia High blood CHOLESTEROL. This condition affects an estimated 25 percent of Americans. This is a concern because elevated cholesterol is a risk factor for ATHEROSCLEROSIS and HEART DISEASE.

Opinion varies regarding the level of cholesterol that is considered abnormal. Some guidelines consider that moderate risk of heart disease exists when the cholesterol value is higher than 200 mg/deciliter for people between the ages of 20 and 29 years; or greater than 220 for those between 30 and 39 years; or greater than 240 for those 40 or older. Cholesterol levels that are 20 points greater for any age bracket put the individual into the high risk category (high hypercholesterolemia). In other words, the high risk threshold is 220 for 20 to 29 year olds; 240 for 30 to 39 year olds; and 260 for those 40 or older.

Causes of hypercholesterolemia include long-term unhealthy dietary and lifestyle choices, diabetes, kidney disease, high blood pressure, and inheritance. Familial hypercholesterolemia (Type IIA HYPERLIPOPROTEINEMIA) refers to an inherited tendency toward high cholesterol values (excessive LOW-DENSITY LIPOPROTEIN, LDL, the less desirable form of cholesterol). Elevated blood cholesterol due to inheritance accounts for only 5 percent of cases. In this disease, the body's mechanism for the removing of LDL from blood can be defective, allowing cholesterol to accumulate in the blood, where it is more likely to clog arteries.

Individuals with hypercholesterolemia may be advised to lower their FAT intake, especially saturated fat, to less than 10 percent of fat calories; to restrict cholesterol intake to less than 200 mg daily; to reduce their weight (if overweight); and to stop smoking. Eating a variety of foods, emphasizing whole grains, vegetables, lean meat, fish, and poultry helps to lower cholesterol. Eating less fatty red meat and less processed food that contains COCONUT OIL and PALM OIL also helps lower fat consumption. Drug therapy may be recommended when the cholesterol is very high, when the cholesterol value doesn't drop with diet therapy and other lifestyle changes, and when the risk of cardiovascular disease is high for other reasons, such as heredity. (See also CHOLESTEROL-LOWERING DRUGS.)

hyperglycemia **(HYPERINSULINISM)** Elevated BLOOD SUGAR (GLUCOSE). Normally, blood sugar rises within 30 to 60 minutes after eating starchy foods, then returns to a baseline level within three to five hours as starch is digested to glucose and is absorbed. If the blood sugar level remains elevated, a prediabetic or a diabetic condition may be indicated. In this case, the PANCREAS may not synthesize enough INSULIN or the cellular mechanisms responding to insulin may be defective. Sustained high blood-sugar levels promote the bonding of glucose to proteins, including HEMOGLOBIN. The resulting proteins do not function normally. Their gradual accumulation may contribute to altered organ deterioration associated with uncontrolled diabetes mellitus. (See also CARBOHYDRATE; CARBOHYDRATE METABOLISM; DIABETES MELLITUS; GLUCOSE TOLERANCE; HYPOGLYCEMIA.)

hyperinsulinism Excessive secretion of INSULIN by the endocrine (hormone-secreting) PANCREAS. Sustained high blood insulin levels can produce unusually low BLOOD SUGAR (HYPOGLYCEMIA). Extreme hyperinsulinism represents a glandular imbalance. On the other hand, a short-term, transient insulin excess may occur when blood glucose rises in response to ingesting a large amount of SUGAR or NATURAL SWEETENERS, causing a subsequent drop in blood sugar. This situation represents an overcompensation by the pancreas called "postprandial" hypoglycemia (low blood sugar after eating). Chronic hyperinsulinism, that is, resistance to the action of insulin for years, is linked to a constellation of signs and symptoms related to noninsulin-dependent DIABETES MELLITUS, such as OBESITY, increased blood pressure, elevated blood sugar, blood triglycerides and LOW-DENSITY LIPOPROTEIN (LDL) cholesterol, with decreased HIGH-DENSITY LIPOPROTEIN (HDL) cholesterol (SYNDROME X). Chronic stress and elevated adrenal hormone, especially CORTISOL, are also associated with syndrome X. Furthermore, insulin resistance may turn out to be almost as serious a risk factor for CORONARY HEART DISEASE as such well-known factors as cigarette smoking and high blood pressure. (See also ENDOCRINE SYSTEM; HORMONE.)

hyperkalemia Excessive levels of POTASSIUM in the blood. Normally, potassium is concentrated inside cells, where it helps maintain fluid volume.

During nerve transmission and muscle contraction, potassium moves out of cells and SODIUM moves in as these ions briefly trade places across the cell membrane. Excessive potassium in the blood causes a serious sodium-potassium imbalance that interferes with muscle contraction and the transmission of nerve impulses. The heart dilates and gradually becomes weaker. Overdosing with potassium supplements or using excessive amounts of SALT SUBSTITUTES can significantly raise blood potassium levels. Hyperkalemia is a serious complication of kidney failure, shock, and severe DEHYDRATION. (See also ELECTROLYTES; MINERALS.)

hyperlipemia Excessive lipids in the blood. The accumulated lipids may be cholesterol, fat (triglycerides), or both. (See also HYPERLIPOPROTEINEMIA; HYPERTRIGLYCERIDEMIA.)

hyperlipoproteinemia (hyperlipidemia) Excessive level of lipid-protein complexes in the blood. LIPOPROTEINS transport CHOLESTEROL and FAT (also known as TRIGLYCERIDES) through the bloodstream. Although these lipids are insoluble in blood, which is mainly water, they become soluble when emulsified, as when bound to certain proteins called apolipoproteins and phospholipid. The levels of lipoproteins are influenced by diet, hormonal balance, age, weight, stress, and illness. Severely elevated blood lipids may be due to heredity. High levels of cholesterol and fat in the blood warrant medical attention. The American Heart Association recommends a gradual reduction of total fat, saturated fat, and cholesterol as a dietary approach to treating hyperlipoproteinemia. It recommends restriction of total fat intake to less than 30 percent total calories; restriction of saturated fat consumption to less than 10 percent of fat calories and restriction of cholesterol to less than 300 mg daily. Weight reduction is also advised, and medication under a doctor's supervision may be appropriate. In a Step 2 program, cholesterol consumption would not exceed 200 mg daily and saturated fat would represent no more than 7 percent of total daily calories. Consumption of fish and fish oil can significantly reduce blood triglyceride levels when elevated (hypertriglyceridemia).

There are four major lipoproteins of the blood:

- VLDL (VERY-LOW-DENSITY LIPOPROTEINS): carries fat synthesized by the liver to tissues.
- CHYLOMICRONS: transport fat from digested food to tissues, first through the lymphatic system, then through the bloodstream.
- LDL (LOW-DENSITY LIPOPROTEINS): transports cholesterol from the liver to tissues.
- HDL (HIGH-DENSITY LIPOPROTEINS): carries cholesterol from tissue back to the liver for disposal.

In one of the most widely used classification systems, hyperlipoproteinemias are categorized according to the types of lipoprotein that accumulate:

Type I is characterized by elevated chylomicrons (triglycerides plus cholesterol). This rare inherited condition is often caused by a deficiency of lipoprotein lipase, the enzyme in capillaries that releases fatty acids from chylomicrons so they can be taken up by cells. Type I usually appears in childhood.

Type IIa is a common inherited disease, characterized by elevated LDL and cholesterol. In severe cases it leads to early ATHEROSCLEROSIS and premature death. Milder forms are not obviously due to family history. Secondary forms of Type IIa may be due to excessive dietary cholesterol, liver disease, or hypothyroidism.

Type IIb is characterized by elevated LDL, VLDL, cholesterol, and triglycerides. Often this is a rare inherited condition; milder forms may be sporadic. Type IIb is usually not detected until adulthood.

Type III (relatively uncommon compared to the other types) is characterized by elevated VLDL (which contains cholesterol plus triglycerides), due to an abnormal composition of VLDL. Type III is frequently an inherited condition, usually detected in adulthood.

Type IV is a common disease, characterized by elevated VLDL and triglycerides with normal or elevated cholesterol due to an elevated production of normal VLDL. It is probably an inherited condition. Often half of the patients' close adult relatives will also have Type IV.

Type IV is worsened by obesity and alcohol consumption and often appears after the age of 20. Secondary causes include diabetes, pregnancy, ALCOHOLISM, and kidney disease.

Type V (uncommon) is characterized by both elevated chylomicrons and elevated VLDL (triglycerides plus cholesterol), thus representing a "mixed" type hyperlipidemia. When inherited, more than half of a patient's close relatives have Type IV or Type V hyperlipoproteinemia. Clinically, Type V resembles Type I. (Elevated chylomicrons and VLDL may also result from alcoholism, kidney disease, or diabetes.)

(See also CHOLESTEROL-LOWERING DRUGS; FAT METABOLISM; HYPERCHOLESTEROLEMIA.)

hyperplasia The overproduction of tissue mass without the formation of a tumor. Often, a gland or organ responds to increased demand, excessive use or nutrient deficiency by increasing tissue mass. GOITER is an overgrowth of the thyroid gland responding to chronic IODINE deficiency. (See also GROWTH HORMONE.)

hypertension The medical term for high blood pressure. Up to 50 million American adults have abnormally high pressure. Millions more have increased risk because their blood pressure is on the high side of normal. Added together, as many as 75 percent of Americans over the age of 35 may face dangerously high blood pressures in their lifetimes. This is a major public health concern because, typically, there are no obvious symptoms for 15 to 20 years, until STROKE, HEART ATTACK, kidney failure, and/or blindness strike. Even after reducing hypertension to normal, the risk of illness and death is greater than in people without a history of hypertension.

Blood pressure is a measure of fluid pressure against vessel walls. Optimal blood pressure is considered to be 110/70, while a normal acceptable blood pressure is below 120/80. The first number is the "systolic" pressure due to heart pumping, measured in millimeters of mercury. The second number represents the "diastolic" pressure between beats, when the heart rests. Although there are no precisely defined rules regarding abnormal blood pressure, as a general guideline, consistent systolic pressures of 150 to 160 or consistent diastolic readings of 99 or above signal hypertension that requires medical treatment and need to be controlled. The risk of CARDIOVASCULAR DISEASE and kidney disease increases when either systolic or diastolic pressures are consistently high, and the odds increase further when both numbers are high.

Blood pressure values representing mild hypertension vary with age. For young adults, 140/90 is considered borderline high, but it may be considered high normal for those over 60. Mild forms of hypertension do not have to be treated with drugs, because diet modification and lifestyle changes can usually control mild forms of hypertension. A diastolic pressure of 85 to 89 represents borderline hypertension.

Diastolic hypertension is caused by the restriction of small arteries (arterioles) flowing into the capillary bed. Systolic pressure rises temporarily after stress, physical exercise, eating, and drinking; thus, there is no single cause for this condition. Hypertension is more common in men than in women and is more common among African Americans than whites. The risk increases with age, and after the age of 50 it is more common in women. Hypertension also runs in families. Having parents or siblings with hypertension increases the risk. Other causes relate to hormone imbalance, abnormal capillary structure of nervous system–directed constriction of blood vessels. ARTERIOSCLEROSIS causes hypertension in elderly persons. Hypertension can also result from chronic kidney disease, as well as from LEAD and CADMIUM exposure.

The role of diet and environment is illustrated by the observation that blood pressure has increased with age only in industrialized nations. Prevention focuses on education in the following big areas. Several recommendations pertain to diet.

Patients should consume adequate CALCIUM, ZINC, and MAGNESIUM. Deficiencies of these minerals increase the risk of hypertension. Studies suggest that hypertensive individuals consume less calcium than people with normal blood pressure, and calcium supplementation seems to help with mild to moderate hypertension. Low cellular magnesium levels correlate with increased blood pressure (hypertensives) and adequate magnesium intake is essential for cardiovascular health. However, there is no guarantee that calcium supplementation will lower blood pressure. Taking calcium supplements daily can lessen hypertension in a majority of patients, while it can worsen hypertension in a minority.

Increasing dietary FIBER consumption with whole GRAINS, FRUIT, and VEGETABLES. A high-fiber, high complex carbohydrate diet may prevent many forms of cardiovascular disease.

Reducing intake of saturated and total fat. Consuming low-fat dairy products can help achieve this goal. A low-fat diet may lower blood pressure. In particular, vegetable oils rich in essential fatty acids, including LINOLEIC ACID, can decrease hypertension.

Reducing SODIUM (salt) consumption while increasing POTASSIUM from fresh fruit and vegetables. Low potassium intake is linked to hypertension. Americans consume much more salt and other sources of sodium than necessary for body functions. In a survey of 32 countries, people with normal weight but high sodium intake were up to seven times more likely to have high blood pressure than those whose weights were low and whose sodium intake was low. About one-third of hypertensives are sensitive to sodium. In these people, excessive consumption of salt (sodium chloride) together with inadequate dietary potassium seems to induce hypertension. Lowering sodium consumption can often decrease blood pressure in people with normal blood pressure, as well as those with hypertension.

Reducing ALCOHOL consumption. Drinking increases blood pressure due to increased EPINEPHRINE production by ADRENAL GLANDS. More than one or two drinks daily increases the odds for many diseases. An estimated 5 percent to 7 percent of hypertensive cases can be accounted for by excessive drinking.

Other Lifestyle Changes are Important

- If overweight, losing weight and maintaining normal body weight. OBESITY increases blood pressure, and those who are overweight face odds that are two to six times greater than people with normal weight. Surplus body weight accounts for 20 percent to 30 percent of hypertensive cases.
- Exercising regularly. The exercise and weight management programs need to be tailored to the individual. Aerobic exercise is one of the most effective ways to normalize blood pressure. People who exercise regularly do not generally experience an age-related increase in blood pressure. Daily exercise is most effective; low-intensity (walking) to moderate-intensity (jogging) exercise seems to be as effective in lowering blood pressure as high-intensity exercise (running).
- Reducing stress. Anxiety and the suppression of anger increase the risk of hypertension in middle-aged men and in teenagers. Many techniques, including biofeedback, yoga, meditation, and self-hypnosis, are effective.
- Treating DIABETES and high blood cholesterol for cardiovascular health. Elevated blood sugar increases the odds of hypertension in middle-aged women, and diabetes increases the risk of vascular disease generally.
- Stopping smoking. Smoking is a contributing factor in hypertension, independent of all other factors. There are many reasons for stopping smoking, including decreasing the risk of cancer, heart attack, and stroke.
- Avoiding common DIET PILLS. PHENYLPROPANOLAMINE can raise blood pressure.

In assessing hypertension, a number of risk factors need to be evaluated. Lifestyle changes and weight reduction may be the first therapeutic strategy, rather than medication. There is an increased emphasis on nondrug therapy because of potentially harmful drug side effects. (See also HEART DISEASE.)

Liebman, Bonnie. "One Nation, Under Pressure," *Nutrition Action Healthletter* 22, no. 6 (July/August 1995): 1, 6–9.

hyperthyroidism Overactivity of the THYROID GLAND leads to profound systemic changes, due to overproduction of thyroxine, the major thyroid HORMONE. This hormone increases the BASAL METABOLIC RATE, the rate at which energy is consumed to maintain body functions at rest. Symptoms include hyperactivity, weakness and, in extreme cases, weight loss, heat intolerance, excessive sweating, increased heart rate, and sexual dysfunction. (See also ENDOCRINE SYSTEM; HYPOTHYROIDISM.)

hypertriglyceridemia Chronically elevated blood FAT, also called TRIGLYCERIDES.

A normal serum triglyceride value after an overnight fast is around 100 mg per deciliter. Values greater than 500 increase the risk of CARDIOVASCULAR DISEASE, HEART ATTACK, and PANCREATITIS. If elevated LOW-DENSITY LIPOPROTEIN (LDL, the undesirable form of cholesterol) accompanies elevated triglycerides, the risk of heart disease doubles. Hypertriglyceridemia is often an inherited disorder. Obesity, consumption of excessive alcohol, use of oral contraceptives, estrogens, thiazide DIURETICS, or beta blockers also increases the odds of this condition. Excessive VITAMIN A, CAFFEINE and alcohol consumption and low CHROMIUM intake aggravate this condition. Fatty or sugary foods raise blood fat levels only temporarily after a meal.

Treatment calls for reduction of dietary fat, especially SATURATED FAT, and increased dietary COMPLEX CARBOHYDRATES together with weight reduction. Fish oil also can reduce blood triglycerides. Diabetics on high-fiber, high complex carbohydrate diets need to monitor their serum triglyceride levels, which can rise with such diets. (See also DIET; FAT METABOLISM; FIBER; HYPERLIPOPROTEINEMIA.)

U.S. Department of Health and Human Services. *Treatment of Hypertriglyceridemia,* Washington, D.C.: National Institutes of Health Consensus Development Conference Summary, 4:8.

hyperuricemia Excessive URIC ACID levels in the blood. Although most people with high uric acid in the blood have no symptoms, this increases the risk factor for GOUT, a painful inflammation of joints due to deposits of uric acid. Elevated uric acid can result from inherited alterations in metabolism, such as the overproduction of the precursors of PURINES, building blocks of DNA, the genetic material, and of RNA, which directs protein synthesis. Factors favoring the precipitation of uric acid include excessive ALCOHOL consumption; accumulation of KETONE BODIES, acids produced during uncontrolled diabetes; and occasionally the use of DIURETICS (water pills). A low purine diet restricts consumption of purine-rich food like ANCHOVIES, SARDINES, and organ meats. (See also ARTHRITIS.)

hypervitaminosis Toxicity due to an excessive intake of VITAMINS, especially overdosing with fat-soluble vitamins. Fat-soluble vitamins are not readily excreted and thus accumulate in fatty tissue. In contrast, the water-soluble vitamins are excreted by the kidney and, with the exception of VITAMIN B_{12}, are not stored.

Chronic high levels of VITAMIN A (e.g., 25,000 retinol equivalents or more per day) are linked to birth defects. Recent studies indicate that even 10,000 IU or 3,000 retinol equivalents per day are linked to an increased risk of birth defects. The consumption of 50,000 retinol equivalents for several months can cause toxic symptoms in adults such as headache, fatigue, nausea, hair loss, and blurred vision. Liver damage is possible. Symptoms disappear when vitamin A intake is restricted. VITAMIN D excess (25,000 to 250,000 IU daily for several months) can cause kidney stones, kidney failure, and heart irregularities. Excessive VITAMIN K can also be toxic. Symptoms include liver damage and JAUNDICE. VITAMIN E appears to be the safest of the fat-soluble vitamins.

Rothman, K. J. et al. "Teratogenicity of High Vitamin A Intake," *New England Journal of Medicine* 333, no. 21 (November 23, 1995): 169–173.

hypoalbuminemia An abnormally low level of serum ALBUMIN in the blood. Serum albumin represents 55 percent of the soluble protein of blood and as such it helps maintain the proper water concentration between blood and tissues. When less serum protein is synthesized, fluid tends to accumulate in tissues (EDEMA). Severe protein deficiency (starvation) causes the liver to decrease production of all serum proteins. The result is more readily observed with serum albumin. Thus, a starving child may appear fat because of the severe edema. (See also EMACIATION; MALNUTRITION.)

hypocalcemia Abnormally low blood CALCIUM. Circulating calcium concentration is maintained within a very narrow range, in spite of fluctuation in dietary calcium. This condition most frequently represents a kidney abnormality or glandular disturbance, especially a deficiency of the parathyroid hormone, parathormone, the hormone responsible for raising blood calcium levels. (See also GLOMERULAR FILTRATION; PARATHYROID GLANDS; VITAMIN D.)

hypochlorhydria Inadequate production of hydrochloric acid (STOMACH ACID). Although some free acid is present in gastric juice, it is inadequate to digest PROTEIN efficiently. Because there is inadequate acid to sterilize stomach contents, lowered stomach acid increases susceptibility to chronic infection by pathogenic bacteria, yeast, and parasites and increases the likelihood of other gastrointestinal imbalances, including inflammation, maldigestion, and nutrient MALABSORPTION. Diabetes, chronic GASTRITIS, FOOD SENSITIVITIES, and SPRUE (severe intestinal malabsorption) can lower stomach acid production. Cimetidine, Tagamet, and Zantac are medications that severely reduce gastric juice secretion. (See also ACHLORHYDRIA; ANTACIDS.)

hypoglycemia Chronic low BLOOD SUGAR that occurs during fasting (between meals). Symptoms are persistent and include headache, FATIGUE, lethargy, confusion, and, in extreme cases, amnesia and unconsciousness. Hormonal imbalances, such as HYPOTHYROIDISM, low cortisol production, drug side effects, and tumors can cause chronic fasting hypoglycemia. Individuals with disorders of the metabolism of glycogen (the storage form of carbohydrate) are also prone to fasting hypoglycemia. Underlying causes need to be treated to ameliorate this condition. (See also HYPOGLYCEMIA, POSTPRANDIAL.)

hypoglycemia, postprandial A marked decline in BLOOD SUGAR within two to five hours after a meal, typically to less than 60 mg of glucose per deciliter. Postprandial hypoglycemia may be an early signal of non-insulin-dependent DIABETES in middle-aged individuals. Normally, blood sugar is maintained between 70 and 110 mg per deciliter in order to supply the brain with glucose, its primary energy source. After eating a carbohydrate meal, the PANCREAS may overreact by releasing too much INSULIN, causing blood sugar to plummet below normal, baseline levels. Other mechanisms more slowly respond to raise blood sugar levels. The adrenal gland secretes EPINEPHRINE and GLUCOCORTICOIDS; the pancreas secretes GLUCAGON and the pituitary produces GROWTH HORMONE to increase blood sugar levels.

Hypoglycemia typically causes the midmorning and midafternoon slumps. Any of the following may be observed during hypoglycemic episodes: sweating, anxiety, intense heartbeat, trembling, craving for food, hunger pangs, feeling lightheaded, inability to concentrate. However, the symptoms are transient. The feelings and perceptions of a patient undergoing a test to measure blood sugar levels after eating carbohydrate need to be monitored. Note that some symptoms resembling postprandial hypoglycemia occur with several serious disorders not involving hypoglycemia, and medical expertise is recommended to rule them out.

A variety of factors affect the level of blood sugar after a meal, including:

- Glucose uptake: The nutrient composition of the meal can prevent a precipitous drop in blood sugar due to an insulin overshoot. Certain types of carbohydrate (unrefined complex carbohydrates) are digested more slowly to glucose than others. Fat and fiber slow the rate of carbohydrate digestion and sugar absorption.
- High blood insulin: Secretion by the pancreas may be excessive. This is more likely to occur in response to a sudden, high rise in blood sugar. Alternatively, excessive insulin medication can cause high insulin levels. In either case, excessive insulin promotes a dramatic decline in blood sugar.
- Altered carbohydrate metabolism: A key to maintaining blood sugar levels between meals is the ability of the liver to synthesize glucose (GLUCONEOGENESIS) and to liberate glucose from stores (GLYCOGEN).

Frequent causes of postprandial hypoglycemia include:

- ALCOHOLISM: Consuming alcohol while eating may cause hypoglycemia if too much insulin is released and if glucose formation is blocked after drinking. A more serious situation can develop if liver glycogen stores are minimal, as occurs during chronic alcoholism. In this case, three to 10 drinks can prevent the liver from manufacturing enough blood glucose to fuel the brain, and a crisis can occur between six and 36 hours after drinking, sometimes leading to unconsciousness and death. Alcohol-induced hypoglycemia is particularly treacherous because symptoms resemble intoxication and glucose may not be administered in time to prevent unconsciousness.
- Chronic, severe stress and adrenal exhaustion: The adrenal glands may not produce enough CORTISOL to promote protein breakdown and

thus supply inadequate AMINO ACIDS for gluconeogenesis. This condition can also be the result of chronic starvation, and disease with fever.

- Dietary factors: Excessive consumption of refined carbohydrate and natural sweeteners can cause erratic blood sugar due to a rapid rise in blood sugar followed by overcompensation by the pancreas, liberating excessive insulin.
- Starvation: Too little carbohydrate is consumed to maintain normal blood sugar.
- Carbohydrate maldigestion: This can lead to inadequate carbohydrate assimilation, even when carbohydrate intake is normal.
- Liver disease: This can diminish the ability to produce glucose from amino acids and other noncarbohydrate building blocks of glucose.
- Strenuous exercise: can temporarily deplete blood sugar.

Treatment of postprandial hypoglycemia often involves eating small, frequent meals, high in PROTEIN (20 percent of total calories) and COMPLEX CARBOHYDRATES (35 percent to 45 percent of calories) to maintain a slow, steady liberation and uptake of glucose.

It is also important to avoid SUGAR, refined sweeteners (CORN SYRUP, high FRUCTOSE CORN SYRUP, DEXTROSE, FRUCTOSE) and sweets to minimize sudden increases in blood sugar levels and over-reaction by the pancreas, and to consume fewer CONVENIENCE FOODS and high-calorie foods that generally have a high sugar and highly refined carbohydrate content. Hypoglycemics should also avoid COFFEE and alcohol, which can accentuate the symptoms of hypoglycemia. Reducing stress with meditation or yoga can normalize endocrine function. Many individuals can manage stress effectively if they eat properly and exercise. Finally, it is important to control FOOD SENSITIVITIES, which may accentuate blood sugar variations.

hypokalemia Low blood POTASSIUM. Typically this accompanies severe DIARRHEA because potassium in secretions is lost. Hypokalemia can occur during treatment for diabetes (ketoacidosis) involving the accumulation of ketone bodies, acidic products of fat metabolism. In addition, certain DIURETICS cause excessive potassium excretion. Symptoms of hypokalemia include muscle weakness and muscle cramps. (See also HYPERKALEMIA.)

hypothalamic-pituitary-adrenal axis (HPA axis) A pivotal integration of the nervous system and the endocrine system. The HPA axis integrates fundamental physiological and metabolic processes, including circadian (daily) rhythms. The hypothalamus monitors the autonomic nervous system. The autonomic nervous system regulates visceral activities such as dilation of blood vessels, blood pressure and rate of heartbeat, movement of the gastrointestinal tract, and most glandular secretions (sweat glands, salivary glands, gastric and intestinal glands, and the pancreas). Most changes occur involuntarily and automatically. The sympathetic division stimulates activity of an organ, whereas the parasympathetic division decreases activity.

The hypothalamus in turn regulates the pituitary, the master hormone-secreting gland. In particular the pituitary regulates ENDOCRINE glands such as the adrenal cortex, which is triggered to release CORTISOL into the bloodstream. In turn, cortisol regulates many metabolic processes including protein breakdown, fat turnover, and blood sugar formation. Subsequently, elevated blood cortisol binds to receptors in the HYPOTHALAMUS and the PITUITARY, which limits further adrenal stimulation. Such finely timed feedback loops assure precise integration of these regulatory processes. (See also HOMEOSTASIS.)

hypothalamus An array of nerve cells and fibers, located near the upper region of the brain stem, that regulate body temperature, water and ELECTROLYTE balance, blood pressure, reproduction, APPETITE, and possibly body weight and HUNGER. The hypothalamus is classified as a neuroendocrine gland because it is made up of nerves and at the same time it produces HORMONES. The hypothalamus processes emotions like embarrassment, anger and fright, and at the same time it integrates the autonomic nervous system, responsible for regulating many involuntary functions like heartbeat, blood pressure, peristalsis (contraction of smooth muscles of the DIGESTIVE TRACT), and the secretion of most glands, including sweat glands, glands producing digestive juices (salivary glands, pancreas, stomach, and intestinal glands), and even a portion of the

ADRENAL GLAND (adrenal medulla), which releases the stress hormone EPINEPHRINE (adrenaline).

The hypothalamus produces two hormones, transported to and secreted by the posterior lobe of the pituitary: ANTIDIURETIC HORMONE (ADH), which accelerates reabsorption of WATER into blood from the urine in kidney tubules, and OXYTOCIN, which stimulates contractions of the uterus at the termination of pregnancy and stimulates milk release. The hypothalamus regulates the PITUITARY GLAND, the master gland of the ENDOCRINE SYSTEM, by means of a battery of hormones.

Thyrotropin-releasing hormone directs the pituitary gland to release thyroid stimulating hormone. Corticotropin-releasing factor directs the pituitary to release ACTH, which activates the adrenal glands. The hypothalamus also secretes growth hormone releasing hormone, and growth hormone inhibiting hormone (somatostatin), which regulate pituitary secretion of growth hormone; luteinizing hormone releasing hormone, which directs the pituitary to release luteinizing hormone to help regulate the menstrual cycle; and prolactin releasing hormone, which directs the pituitary to release prolactin, a hormone that helps control breast development and milk formation during pregnancy. Finally, the hypothalamus produces follicle stimulating-hormone releasing hormone which directs the pituitary to release follicle stimulating hormone to help regulate the menstrual cycle.

Body fat signals the hypothalamus to stop feeling hungry by secreting a protein called LEPTIN into the bloodstream. Leptin is believed to direct the brain to curtail eating by shutting down production of hunger signals. Hunger, craving, and satiety are complex phenomena involving the integration of a vast amount of information by the brain and central nervous system. The hypothalamus plays a central role in this integration. (See also HOMEOSTASIS; HYPOTHALAMIC-PITUITARY-ADRENAL AXIS.)

Chrousos, J. S. "The Hypothalamic-pituitary-adrenal Axis and Immune-mediated Inflammation," *New England Journal of Medicine* 332, no. 20 (May 18, 1995): 1,351–1,362.

hypothyroidism The condition resulting from inadequate production of thyroid HORMONES, which, together with THYROXINE and triiodothyronine, help regulate metabolism throughout the body. Any decrease in the production or utilization of those hormones would affect major processes such as energy production.

FATIGUE and low body temperatures may indicate the THYROID GLAND is not working with maximum efficiency, and thyroid hormone production may be low. In some cases, the pituitary gland may produce inadequate thyroid stimulating hormone (TSH) Clinical laboratory tests frequently measure levels of thyroid hormones as well as TSH and thyroid releasing hormone (TRH). Severe adult hypothyroidism is called myxedema and is characterized by a puffy, bloated face with dry, rough skin and hair loss.

The thyroid gland helps regulate the body's temperature and metabolic rate; hypothyroidism can lower the BASAL METABOLIC RATE by 35 percent to 40 percent, which in turn causes reduced muscle tone, depression, sluggishness, low body temperature, and excessive fatigue. In children, hypothyroidism can delay growth and mental development. In women, there may be heavy menstrual bleeding. The efficiency of using protein, carbohydrate, and fat as fuels declines, and blood CHOLESTEROL and FAT levels generally increase, increasing the risk of CARDIOVASCULAR DISEASE. During aging hypothyroidism becomes more and more common, especially in women (10 percent of all women over age 50 show signs of a failing thyroid).

Mild hypothyroidism is common in the Great Lakes region, possibly due to low iodine content in midwestern soils. Other conditions can cause fatigue, including low adrenal steroid hormones, infection, ALLERGY, and MALNUTRITION. There have been reports of childbirth correcting mild hypothyroidism. Chronic hypothyroidism warrants medical attention. Clinical laboratory tests can measure serum thyroid hormone levels (T_3 and T_4), as well as thyroid stimulating hormone from the pituitary, to help uncover underlying imbalances. (See also CHRONIC FATIGUE; CORTISOL; ENDOCRINE SYSTEM; HYPOGLYCEMIA.)

Singer, Peter A. et al. "Treatment Guidelines for Patients with Hyperthyroidism and Hypothyroidism," *Journal of the American Medical Association* 273, no. 10 (1995): 808–812.

I

iatrogenic malnutrition See HOSPITAL-INDUCED MALNUTRITION.

IBD See INFLAMMATORY BOWEL DISEASE.

IBS See IRRITABLE BOWEL SYNDROME.

iceberg lettuce See LETTUCE.

ice cream A frozen DESSERT containing flavored, sweetened frozen cream and MILK products, and SUGAR. Frozen desserts based on EGGS, cream, and milk were apparently invented in the 1600s, although frozen blends of fruits were served in ancient China, where salt mixtures were used to lower the temperature below freezing. Americans eat an average of 15 quarts a year per person.

Ice cream is a high-CALORIE, high-FAT, and high-sugar food. Unless it is homemade, ice cream will usually contain artificial coloring, flavorings, and stabilizers such as LOCUST BEAN GUM, GUAR GUM, CARRAGEENAN, GELATIN, and alginic acid or cellulose derivatives. Federal law requires that ice cream contain at least 10 percent fat (BUTTERFAT), and most regular ice creams provide 10 percent to 12 percent butterfat. Super-premium vanilla ice cream contains 16 percent to 20 percent butterfat. In contrast, ice milk contains 2 percent to 7 percent fat, while sherbet contains 1 percent to 2 percent fat. Ice cream usually contains sugar or other sweeteners and emulsifiers like POLYSORBATES and MONOGLYCERIDES stabilize ice cream during processing.

Nondairy frozen desserts resembling ice cream have no legally defined butterfat content, and although they are low-fat options, sometimes these desserts have more total calories per serving than traditional ice cream due to their high sweetener content.

One cup of rich vanilla-flavored ice cream with about 16 percent fat provides: 349 calories; protein, 4.1 g; carbohydrate, 32 g; fat 23.7 g; cholesterol, 88 mg; calcium 151 mg; vitamin A, 219 retinol equivalents; thiamin, 0.04 mg; riboflavin, 0.28 mg; niacin, 0.12 mg.

One cup of regular vanilla ice cream with about 11 percent fat provides: 269 calories; protein, 4.8 g; carbohydrate, 31.7 g; fat, 14.3 g; cholesterol, 59 mg; calcium, 176 mg; vitamin A, 133 retinol equivalents; and similar amounts of thiamin, riboflavin, and niacin to those found in rich vanilla ice cream.

One cup of vanilla-flavored ice milk with about 4 percent fat provides: 184 calories; protein, 5.2 g; carbohydrate, 29 g; fat, 5.6 g; cholesterol, 18 mg; calcium, 176 mg; vitamin A, 52 retinol equivalents; and similar amounts of other vitamins. (See also DAIRY-FREE FROZEN DESSERTS; DIETARY GUIDELINES FOR AMERICANS.)

ideal body weight An outmoded standard for body weight that originated from data collected by U.S. life insurance companies from their policy holders who lived the longest. Ideal body weight was listed as the average weight for a given age, height, body, or "frame" size. From these data grew the classic definition for OBESITY as a weight 20 percent greater than the ideal body weight. Part of the problem with this standard of ideal body weight lies in the nature of HEIGHT-WEIGHT TABLES. Weight charts and tables do not take into account individual variations in body structure (muscles and bone mass); consequently, there is no standard for measuring small, medium, or large body frames.

There is no single ideal body weight for a group of people because every person has an individual, desirable weight. Selecting a realistic body weight as a goal has proven to be far more useful than striving for a rigidly defined standard. A realistic body weight is one that can be readily maintained without intermittent DIETING.

A measure of body FAT is more useful than total body weight because body weight may not correlate with the amount of fat on a lean person. Furthermore, ideal body weight provides no indication of fat distribution. Some fat deposits are riskier for heart disease than others. Methods of accurately measuring body fat at clinics include buoyancy testing with underwater weighing (requiring a special tank) and SKIN FOLD thickness measured by skin calipers or by skin resistance measurements.

Suggestions for estimating an optimal body weight include: For males, take 106 pounds for the first 5 ft. of height, then add six pounds for each additional inch of height. For females, take 100 pounds for the first 5 ft., then add five pounds for each additional inch. (See also BODY MASS INDEX; FAT-FOLD TEST.)

idiopathic A medical term that is applied to a disease or condition arising spontaneously from an unknown cause. Idiopathic GOUT and high blood pressure are examples.

ileitis See CROHN'S DISEASE.

ileum The last three-fifths of the small INTESTINE that joins the large intestine (COLON). The length of the ileum varies among individuals, ranging from 15 to 30 ft. in adult men. The ileum absorbs FAT, fat-soluble vitamins, CALCIUM, MAGNESIUM, VITAMIN B_{12}, and AMINO ACIDS. BILE salts, which act as the detergents in bile required for fat DIGESTION, are also absorbed in the ileum and are recycled by the liver to released once again in bile.

Flow of material between the ileum and colon is regulated by the ileocecal valve. (See also ENTEROHEPATIC CIRCULATION.)

illness Ill health or disease; the opposite of wellness. Illness reflects imbalanced body functions and can thus be regarded as a change away from the healthy state, in which all systems function within normal limits (HOMEOSTASIS).

An illness may be localized, in which a limited region of the body is affected, or it may be systemic, in which several parts of the body or the whole body are affected. Pain is often associated with illness, although pain is not equivalent to disease. Pain generally indicates that an imbalance exists in the body. The imbalance could reflect an unhealthy lifestyle, such as dietary excess or deficiency, or it could be associated with infection and inflammation.

Most illnesses are self-limiting, meaning that the body generally can cure itself when given the opportunity. It is now clear that the body's systems work together to maintain health. Particularly important are the IMMUNE SYSTEM, the NERVOUS SYSTEM, and the ENDOCRINE SYSTEM (hormone-producing system). An imbalanced immune system affects the brain, and the brain alters immunity and hormone production. Hormones in turn affect nerve function. As an example, perceived STRESS can trigger a FIGHT OR FLIGHT RESPONSE by the brain. The stress response is modified by hormones, and sustained, elevated adrenal hormones due to prolonged stress affect the immune system and decrease the immune response to foreign invaders.

Whether or not an individual becomes ill depends on a complex interplay of many factors, broadly categorized according to medical history and environmental influences. Family history reflects patterns of inheritance, over which one has no control. Genetic predisposition thus increases the risk of many chronic, degenerative diseases of AGING, such as OSTEOPOROSIS, heart disease and STROKE, high blood pressure, and DIABETES. Health history can have a profound effect on susceptibility to illness. Thus, prior injury, deficiency, or illness can set the stage for a subsequent illness. For example, arthritis can begin at the site of a former injury, and prolonged treatment with a broad-spectrum antibiotic can destroy beneficial gut bacteria and promote a yeast infection. Prior drug treatment can alter the body's ability to destroy alcohol, and pretreatment with alcohol can alter the body's ability to degrade many drugs. In terms of public health, immunization against polio, flu, or tetanus reduces the risk of these diseases. At the beginning of the 20th century, niacin deficiency caused widespread pellagra and associated mental illness in the South. The enrichment of bread and grain products with the B vitamin NIACIN in the 1920s essentially eliminated pellagra as a public health issue in the United States.

Due to differences in inheritance and environment, toxic exposure, nutritional status, and medical history, each person is biochemically unique. Thus, individuals vary in their ability to protect themselves against damaging effects of FREE RADICALS, and to detoxify potentially dangerous chemicals that they eat or drink or breathe at home or in the workplace.

Although neither a family history nor a medical history can be altered, lifestyle choices can profoundly impact susceptibility to illness. The most frequently cited RISK factors for illness and premature death include the use of tobacco and alcohol, accidental injury, unwanted pregnancy, drug abuse, and inadequate nutrition. The growing awareness that prevention is the most cost-effective and permanent solution to many health issues has lead many physicians to work with their patients as partners in health to empower them in making healthful choices for themselves and their families.

This approach could possibly decrease American deaths before the age of 65 by two-thirds, even without further breakthroughs in medicine and nutrition.

Prevention and Personal Responsibility

The health-conscious individual can focus on four essential steps in maintaining health and preventing illness: positive attitude, a healthy diet, regular exercise and minimizing toxic exposures. Humanistic psychology emphasizes the importance of a positive mental attitude in preventing illness and maintaining health. The immune system and the repair mechanisms of tissues are well designed to ward off infection, to cure disease and to repair injury. DEPRESSION seems to diminish this capacity. For example, depression causes a drop in the production of interleukin, proteins that help regulate the immune response and help activate cancer-killing lymphocytes. Clinical statistics in the United States suggest psychological stress can harm the heart, increasing the risk of rehospitalization among patients with cardiac problems. Group therapy, meditation, and other practices may improve cardiovascular health in patients with clogged arteries by modifying their response to psychological stress.

Susceptibility to disease reflects nutritional status; the nutritional environment affects the expression of inherited traits. Either overnutrition or UNDERNUTRITION can set the stage for chronic illness. Excessive fat consumption increases the risk of cancer and obesity, while inadequate amounts of most nutrients eventually lower the body's defense against disease, including cancer. On the other hand, a healthy diet provides optimal amounts of all nutrients to assure health, while avoiding detrimental food constituents.

Probably the best strategies to avoid chronic illness associated with aging are regular physical exercise coupled with wise food choices. A sedentary lifestyle is linked to an estimated 250,000 deaths annually in the United States. Exercise decreases the risk of heart disease, stroke, high blood pressure (hypertension), adult onset diabetes, osteoporosis (thin bone disease), and colon and breast cancer.

Minimizing exposure to potentially damaging agents such as solvents, pollutants, and cigarette smoke is also important. The amount, type, and length of exposure to a toxic material at home or in the workplace affects health. Only recently have studies been undertaken to determine additive, long-term effects on health of continued low level-exposure to pesticides and industrial pollutants in food and water and air. (See also ANTIOXIDANT; BIOCHEMICAL INDIVIDUALITY; DEGENERATIVE DISEASES; DETOXIFICATION.)

imitation fat See FAT SUBSTITUTE; OLESTRA; SIMPLESSE.

imitation flour See FLOUR SUBSTITUTE.

imitation food A processed food that is nutritionally inferior to the real food. The designation "nutritionally inferior" on a food label means that the food contains 10 percent less of one or more nutrients than the food for which it substitutes. The food industry has devoted considerable financial resources toward producing imitation food, most often substitutes for MEAT, FISH, dairy products, and FRUIT. For example, SURIMI is imitation seafood. Compared to real foods, imitation foods often have a longer shelf life and may be tastier. Food additives are carefully selected for this purpose. Imitation foods are often less expensive than the real foods, but are generally less nutritious than the foods they replace because processing destroys or removes important nutrients. Relatively few nutrients are added back.

Current regulations specify that food labels must list ingredients in descending order according to weight, meaning that the first ingredient listed is the most predominant. If the first item listed on the food label is one of the following, the food is likely to be fabricated or highly processed: any natural sweetener such as corn sweetener, high FRUCTOSE CORN SYRUP, HONEY, DEXTROSE, SUCROSE, or corn syrup solids; TEXTURIZED VEGETABLE PROTEIN; and sodium caseinate. The presence of artificial food colors, MSG (MONOSODIUM GLUTAMATE), COCONUT OIL, palm or palm kernel oil, and PRESERVATIVES also indicates that the food is imitation or highly processed. (See also CONVENIENCE FOOD; FOOD ADDITIVES; FOOD LABELING.)

immune system An elaborate, finely tuned defense system to destroy and counter the effects of viruses, bacteria, yeasts, and foreign substances that operate within tissues and cells and in the bloodstream. The immune system recognizes "self" from "nonself," substances not part of the body. Another feature of the immune system is memory. It can remember previous invaders and mount a rapid response to them when they reappear. When the immune system is healthy, it destroys foreign elements without causing symptoms, but an imbalanced immune system can set the stage for disease. Foreign substances and microorganisms may not be recognized or destroyed, resulting in chronic infection or even CANCER and AIDS. An imbalanced immune system can attack the body's own tissues, creating AUTOIMMUNE DISEASES, or it can over-respond to common substances, creating allergies, such as food allergies.

Organization of the Immune System

The two branches of the immune system are "cellular immunity" and "humoral immunity." The first depends on the active participation of different types of cells. Cellular immunity includes macrophages, cells that engulf foreign invaders. These scavengers are amoebalike cells that surround and digest foreign particles, viruses, and bacteria. Macrophages live in tissues like the spleen (splenocytes), the LIVER (Kupffer cells), the lymph (wandering macrophages), the spinal cord, the brain (microglia), and connective tissue.

Lymphocytes are an important type of white blood cell. T cells are highly specialized lymphocytes that attack viruses, tumors, and transplanted cells and regulate the immune system. T cells are processed by the THYMUS GLAND. They work with B cells, which produce defensive proteins called ANTIBODIES. In a typical scenario, macrophages first engulf foreign materials called ANTIGENS and transform fragments of the antigens for display on their cell surfaces. Certain T "helper" cells, acting as "generals," "read" these antigens, and in turn stimulate the production of specialized T "killer" cells, foot soldiers that destroy abnormal cells or foreign materials. The gut is the largest immune organ, which is called the Gut-associated lymphoid tissue (GALT). GALT produces more antibodies than any other tissue in the body.

The different types of immune cells communicate with each other via protein messengers called LYMPHOKINES. For example, macrophages produce a lymphokine called interleukin-1 to activate T helper cells, which in turn produce interleukin-2, to stimulate the production of the killer T cells. Helper T cells also produce gamma INTERFERON, which activates killer T cells.

Mast cells are a type of T cell that lives in tissues and fights local infection. When they contact foreign materials and cells, mast cells destroy them. Mast cells also release special chemicals like HISTAMINE, as well as certain lymphokines that trigger inflammation marked by swelling (EDEMA), redness, itching, sneezing, and runny nose. Lymphokines also trigger phagocytes (macrophages) to destroy foreigners and dispose of signal proteins once they have done their work.

Humoral immunity pertains to blood and lymph. It relies on cells that release defensive PROTEINS called complement and antibodies into the bloodstream to fight infection. Antibodies (gamma globulins) are Y-shaped proteins designed to target a particular antigen, by which a substance is recognized as being foreign. An antibody can neutralize the enemy either by binding to it or by targeting it for attack by other cells and chemicals. After antibodies bind foreign cells, complement ruptures them. Complement also triggers localized inflammatory reactions, leading to common symptoms of pain, redness, and swelling, as well as to an increased concentration of defensive cells at the point of injury or infection.

B cells, which originate in bone marrow, are a type of lymphocyte that yield plasma cells, specialized to produce antibodies when exposed to foreign invaders. B cell proliferation, maturation, and antibody production are stimulated by T helper infected cells. Another type of T cell, called T suppressor cells, gear down the immune system by turning off B cell production. Thus T suppressor cells limit allergic attacks and auto-immune reactions.

Immunity

Immunity is a hallmark of the immune system. The recovery from an infection renders the individual immune to subsequent attack by the particular disease-causing agent. Immunity to chicken pox is a common example. The underlying mechanism relies on memory T and memory B cells in the bloodstream, which signal a red alert for a quick attack the next time a conquered virus invades again. These memory cells multiply rapidly when they again encounter any antigen they remember.

Nutrients that May Benefit the Immune System

The immune system requires a rich array of nutrients, including protein, FATTY ACIDS, VITAMINS, and MINERALS, for normal function. A JUNK FOOD diet can lead to overnutrition (too many calories and fat) and malnutrition (too little trace minerals and vitamins) that weaken the immune system. Malnourished individuals lacking adequate protein or calories are prone to disease. Low-level deficiencies of many nutrients seem to lower the effectiveness of the immune system. Supplements can boost immunity, especially in elderly people. It seems clear that a wise approach to support the immune system nutritionally includes a varied diet—reducing fat to less than 30 percent of daily calories and emphasizing whole foods, FRUITS, and VEGETABLES, especially those rich in VITAMIN C, BETA-CAROTENE, and other carotenoids. Supplementing the diet with 100 percent of the RDA, (RECOMMENDED DIETARY ALLOWANCE) of B vitamins and trace minerals for insurance may also be prudent when a diet is compromised by junk food or when the diet provides fewer than 1,600 calories.

ANTIOXIDANT nutrients such as vitamin C, VITAMIN E, SELENIUM, COPPER, MANGANESE, and beta-carotene may enhance immune responses by lowering the burden of FREE RADICALS, thus protecting immune cells against the cumulative oxidation and free radical attack due to the release of powerful oxidizing agents as superoxide, hydrogen peroxide, and hydroxyl radicals.

Vitamin C deficiency lowers the immune response in animal models. Adequate vitamin C increases T and B cell production and helps attacking cells migrate to sites of infection while making viruses and bacteria more sensitive to destruction. Furthermore, vitamin C acts as an antioxidant, and it protects cells against reactive chemicals produced by mast cells used to destroy foreigners.

Vitamin E enhances both humoral and cell-mediated immunity, while vitamin E deficiency contributes to reduce T cells, killer cells, and macrophage function. Vitamin E supplementation boosts the immune system in elderly men and women consuming a typical diet, suggesting that older people require more vitamin E than specified by the adult Recommended Dietary Allowance to assure a fully functional immune system.

Selenium is a cofactor for an important antioxidant enzyme, glutathione peroxidase, which neutralizes lipid peroxide that could damage the immune cells. Selenium works with vitamin E to stimulate the immune response to infection in experimental animals. Together they may help protect against cancer. Selenium increases T helper cells and increases antibody production in experimental animals. However, excessive selenium depresses the immune system.

Other specific nutrients support the function of the immune system:

FOLIC ACID is required for immunity and lymphocyte production. Folic acid is often deficient in the American diet.

IRON is required to produce T and B cells. Iron deficiency is associated with increased incidence of common infection among children.

MAGNESIUM is needed by the complement system to activate phagocytes. It is also required for antibody production. Americans typically do not consume enough magnesium.

PANTOTHENIC ACID and VITAMIN B_6 help keep the lymphatic system and thymus gland healthy.

VITAMIN A and beta-carotene help maintain thymus gland function during stress. Overproduction of cortisol, a stress-induced hormone from the adrenal glands, tends to shrink the thymus gland, which is critical for fully functioning T cells. Beta-carotene is the precursor of vitamin A. Limited studies suggest that beta-carotene may also stimulate helper T cells. Studies of children in developing nations indicate that there is a direct relationship between vitamin A deficiency and decreased resistance to infection. On the other hand, excessive vitamin A can decrease immune system function.

Vitamin B_6 plays an important role in maintaining optimal immunity, including antibody production and phagocytic activity. Vitamin B_6 deficiency impairs the immune system in a number of ways. It lowers cell-directed immune responses, described earlier, and leads to decreased thymus function. Vitamin B_6 deficiency during gestation in experimental animals impairs immune functioning even in first and second generation offspring.

ZINC helps maintain lymph glands and the thymus gland, thereby helping to fight chronic infection. Zinc is required for many important enzymes, and it is not surprising that zinc deficiency decreases T cell and B cell function and macrophage activity. However, too much zinc can depress immunity. Zinc, in combination with other trace minerals including copper, iron, and manganese, appears to improve B and T cell function in older people.

Copper deficiency is associated with an increased risk of infection. Copper deficiency diminishes the effectiveness of the humoral system in lab animals. Copper is an essential component of SUPEROXIDE DISMUTASE, an antioxidant system, and CYTOCHROME C oxidase, an enzyme system required for energy production.

Immunity, Stress, and Exercise

Physical or emotional stress can alter hormonal output and immune response. A high level of stress increases the risk of illness and injury in the following year and shortens the life span.

Emotional well-being is supported by proper diet and regular physical EXERCISE. Moderately intense exercise increases the production of ENDORPHINS, the brain's own opiates, which can bolster parts of the immune system. Studies indicate that interleukin-1 and interferon, which help the body respond to infection or injury, increase after moderate exercise. Moderate exercise also increases killer cell activity.

Strenuous aerobic exercise may decrease efficiency of the immune system and temporarily increase susceptibility to illness by increasing the production of adrenal stress hormones. Among the hormones produced is cortisol, which limits inflammation by blocking the immune system. With continued stress, production of protective antibodies (such as secreted IgA, the antibody that protects the intestine and other body cavities against invasion by foreign substances). Chronic stress also decreases killer cell activity, increasing a person's susceptibility to disease. (See also AGING; B COMPLEX; ENDOCRINE SYSTEM; MALNUTRITION; NERVOUS SYSTEM; PSYCHONEUROIMMUNOLOGY.)

Chandra, R. K. "Nutrition and the Immune System from Birth to Old Age," *European Journal of Clinical Nutrition* 56, supp. 3 (August 2002): 573–576.

inborn errors of metabolism Abnormal gene products can cause metabolic imbalances, resulting in disease. Generally the inherited defect leads to the inadequate formation of an enzyme. Occasionally, inadequate formation of a COENZYME (enzyme helper) limits enzyme function or the protein-based signalling system that regulates a given enzyme's function. Most genetic defects are classified as autosomal recessive, meaning that they are not sex-linked. Full expression of the imbalance can occur only when both chromosomes contain the defective gene coding for a given enzyme and normal genes coding for that enzyme are absent. Examples of genetic diseases related to nutrients include familial HYPERCHOLESTEROLEMIA (high blood CHOLESTEROL), sickle cell anemia, GALACTOSEMIA, and PHENYLKETONURIA. PKU is an inherited inability to metabolize the essential AMINO ACID, PHENYLALANINE. PKU responds to nutritional intervention. During infancy and childhood PKU patients receive carefully balanced diets that provide only enough phenylalanine to support growth. Labels for foods containing the artificial sweetener ASPARTAME must warn phenylketonurics because of its phenylalanine content. (See also DNA; FOOD LABELING; MUTATION.)

Brusilow, S. W., and N. E. Maestri. "Urea Cycle Disorders: Diagnosis, Pathophysiology and Therapy," *Advances in Pediatrics* 43 (1996): 127–170.

indigestion See GASTROINTESTINAL DISORDERS.

individuality See BIOCHEMICAL INDIVIDUALITY.

induction The increased production of an ENZYME in response to external stimuli. Enzymes function as biological catalysts of cellular chemical reactions. The body can adapt to a limited extent to changes in the diet and to environmental influences by altering the levels of enzymes in a given tissue. For example, a high-carbohydrate diet leads to increased production of AMYLASE, the starch-digesting enzyme of the pancreas. Starvation decreases levels of digestive enzymes and enzymes responsible for fat and glycogen synthesis but induces enzymes required for fat and carbohydrate degradation. Enzymes that synthesize BLOOD SUGAR (glucose) from amino acids are also induced by starvation.

Excessive alcohol consumption induces liver alcohol oxidizing systems so that alcohol will be cleared from the blood more efficiently. Similarly, many medications induce liver enzymes responsible for drug degradation. Certain cellular enzyme levels increase in response to hormones and to growth promoters. Examples include the hormones ESTROGEN (female sex hormone), CORTISOL (adrenal hormone regulating energy metabolism and degradation), and GROWTH HORMONE (a pituitary hormone involved both in growth and maintenance of tissues, especially muscles). INSULIN provides the broad impetus for increased enzyme production in many tissues. Insulin from the PANCREAS is perhaps the most general anabolic hormone; that is, it promotes enzymes leading to the accumulation of protein, fat and carbohydrates. (See also DETOXIFICATION.)

infant formula A manufactured food designed to nurture the infant during the first year of life, until weaning. Commercial infant formulas are either nonfat cow's MILK-based or soybean-based. Common formulas are available in powdered form, as concentrates, or as ready-to-feed liquid with no prior preparation. No formula exactly reproduces human milk; on the other hand, formulas can provide adequate nutrition for babies.

In the late 1970s, production of chloride-deficient formulas caused delayed speech, slowed growth, and poor muscle control in babies who had consumed the products. Partially in response to this disaster, Congress passed the Infant Formula Act of 1980, which mandates the U.S. FDA to see that this synthetic food meets nutrient standards based upon the American Academy of Pediatrics' recommendations to assure infant growth and development.

In 1982, the FDA adapted quality-control procedures to monitor the production of this food. As a result, infant formulas are nutritionally similar though not identical to BREAST MILK in total protein, total fat, calcium-to-phosphorus ratio, energy content (calories/100 ml), content of the essential fatty acid linoleic acid, and electrolytes (sodium, potassium, chloride).

There are advantages to infant formulas. There is no limit to the supply, and a mother has greater freedom to care for other children or to return to work. Other family members can participate in feeding sessions, developing the warmth of that association. The mother of a formula-fed infant can offer the same closeness and stimulation as the BREAST-FEEDING mother.

In 1998 an estimated 29 percent of women in the United States were breast-feeding their infants 6 months after leaving the hospital. Several weeks of breast-feeding assures that the mother's antibodies will be present in the infant.

Cow's milk formula resembles its source in terms of type of milk protein, total fat, and calcium to phosphorus ratio. It has been adjusted so that the total protein content, carbohydrate, fat, major minerals, linoleic acid, and vitamins are similar to breast milk. The La Leche League International does not recommend substituting formula or breast milk with cow's milk until the baby is a year old or older (eating the equivalent of three baby food jars of solid food per day). Unprocessed cow's milk is not a suitable food for infants for many reasons.

Cow's milk contains three times as much protein as human milk, and this protein is more difficult for babies to digest. Manufacturers either presoften or predigest this protein, or they add whey to adjust the protein ratio. Butterfat is also poorly digested by infants; therefore it is replaced by vegetable oils. Because the higher concentration of phosphate and other dissolved minerals in cow's milk increases the burden on immature kidneys, minerals are adjusted to resemble breast milk. Lactose or corn syrup solids are used to adjust the carbohydrate content. Bovine milk protein contains much more of the essential amino acid phenylalanine than human milk protein. This situation could affect infants who cannot tolerate high phenylalanine for genetic reasons (see PHENYLKETONURIA).

Cow's milk in infant formulas sometimes triggers an ALLERGY, especially if there is a family history of allergies. Cow's milk-based formula as a supplement to breast-feeding is less of a problem when the baby is six months or older.

For infants who are sensitive to cow's milk, liquid formulas containing soy protein fortified with the essential amino acid methionine and with soybean oil are available. A variety of formulas are prepared from coconut oil and corn oil, but these oils contain very little alpha linolenic acid, an essential fatty acid. Human milk contains substantial amounts of a large fatty acid called DOCOSAHEXAENOIC ACID (DHA). DHA, which is necessary for normal brain and eye development, is not added to formula. There is a consensus that formula should at least contain linolenic acid, the precursor of DHA, which the infant's body may convert to DHA.

A wide variety of infant formulas is available to meet special needs. Infants with lactose intolerance can drink formulas in which lactose is replaced by other carbohydrates. Formulas can be adapted to adjust protein ratio, linoleic acid content, or to lower sodium content. Special formulas are available for preterm babies.

Ready-to-use formula, as well as powdered formula, sometimes contains ALUMINUM. This is not a problem for babies with normal kidneys; however, premature babies may tolerate it poorly. CARRAGEENAN-containing formula should not be given to premature infants. This SEAWEED product is used to stabilize fat by forming gels in milk.

In the past, the infant formula industry employed questionable marketing practices in developing countries, which led to a 1977 consumer boycott against the Swiss-based Nestlé company. For example, they dressed staff in hospital garb while introducing infant formula to new mothers, and used misleading ads. In 1979, Nestlé, which accounted for 50 percent of formula sales to the developing world, and the U.S. government formally agreed to voluntary guidelines that banned marketing abuses in developing nations.

In 1981, the United Nations World Health Organization voted overwhelmingly to approve an international code of conduct to restrict advertising and marketing of baby formula, which can lead to infant malnutrition and death when improperly used. Although not binding, the new guidelines apply to infant formula promotion in industrialized nations as well as developing nations. Proper use of infant formula is often impossible in poorer areas of the world, where the water used to mix the formula is often contaminated. (See also BABY FOOD.)

Ryan, A. S. "The Resurgence of Breast-feeding in the United States," *Pediatrics* 99, no. 4 (1997): e12.

Scariati, Paula D. "Risk of Diarrhea Related to Iron Content of Infant Formula: Lack of Evidence to Support the Use of Low-Iron Formula as a Supplement for Breast-fed Infants," *Pediatrics* 99, no. 3 (1997): e2.

inflammation A defensive response by the body to irritation, injury, or infection usually characterized by heat, redness, swelling, and pain at the injury site. This response is triggered by physical agents, chemical agents, or disease-producing organisms. Swelling is due to increased blood vessel leakage of fluids, and redness is due to the increase in diameter of blood vessels, (especially capillaries) so that they carry more blood. With increased vessel leakage, substances normally retained in blood such as water, antibodies, phagocytic cells, and clot-forming components, migrate into tissues at the site of injury.

Cellular Materials that Promote Inflammation

HISTAMINE, kinins, PROSTAGLANDINS, LEUKOTRIENES, and complement contribute to inflammation. Histamine, derived from the amino acid HISTIDINE, is released from white cells (basophils), mast cells, and other cells when injured. Kinins are proteins that induce vasodilation, increase vessel leakiness, attract phagocytic cells, and cause pain. Prostaglandins are hormone-like materials that function in the immediate area where they are produced. They play many roles, including intensifying pain and promoting fever, which helps combat infections. Leukotrienes are extremely powerful inflammatory agents. Complement is a group of blood proteins that stimulate histamine release, destroy bacteria, and promote phagocytosis (engulfing other cells and fragments). Pain can result from injured nerves or from irritation by released microbial products. Inflammation generates free radicals, which are highly damaging chemical fragments. Chronic inflammation therefore can produce cellular damage and oxidative stress, leading to an unbalanced immune response. Many chronic degenerative diseases involve inflammation and oxidative damage. Examples include rheumatoid arthritis, atherosclerosis, as well as side effects resulting from radiation and chemotherapy during cancer treatment.

Nonsteroidal anti-inflammatory drugs (NSAIDS) are often used to combat inflammation. These drugs, which are often nonprescription items, can themselves cause damage to the stomach or intestinal lining; in some instances they may harm the liver when used in excess. (See also ASPIRIN; IMMUNE SYSTEM.)

inflammatory bowel disease (IBD) A chronic inflammation of the intestinal wall involving painful swelling and open sores. Eventually, the intestinal wall becomes scarred, which narrows the intestinal opening. IBD affects 1 million to 2 million Americans. It differs from CELIAC DISEASE, a grain (especially wheat) intolerance, and from IRRITABLE BOWEL SYNDROME (spastic colon), a much more common, less serious condition involving muscle contractions, rather than chronic inflammation. Two distinct disorders are classified as inflammatory bowel disease: CROHN'S DISEASE and ulcerative COLITIS. Crack-like ulcers and abnormal granular growths in the intestine often accompany Crohn's disease, while ulcerative colitis occurs only in the large intestine and involves inflammation and ulceration.

IBD symptoms include persistent (sometimes bloody) DIARRHEA, flatulence, cramps, low-grade fever, and weight loss, as well as problems such as ARTHRITIS and inflamed eyes or skin. Children may be affected by retarded growth and retarded sexual development. IBD increases the risk of colon CANCER.

IBD is reported mainly in developed countries, where it is most common between the ages of 12 and 40. The causes of IBD are unknown. It does not seem to be caused by stress. One theory is that IBD is an AUTOIMMUNE DISEASE in which the person's own immune system attacks the intestine. Clearly, immune imbalances seem to play a part. Another view is that bacteria, viruses, or toxic chemicals initiate IBD. Food sensitivity has also been implicated in some cases.

Conventional medical treatment involves drugs and/or surgery. Drugs reduce inflammation and can lead to a remission. However, steroids have side effects like high blood pressure, diabetes, and thinning of bones. Typical treatment recommendations include:

- Eating a well-balanced diet that provides adequate nutrients to maintain and repair the intestinal tract. It is important to correct any nutrient deficiencies caused by the disease (especially iron, folate, and calcium).
- Eating several small meals throughout the day. This may be more effective for good digestion and assimilation than eating three big meals.
- Avoiding irritating foods that could increase inflammation. These differ from person to person, though seeds, nuts and corn, lactose and dairy products, fried or greasy foods, and coffee are often the culprits.
- Getting enough exercise and managing stress. Severe stress suppresses the immune system and encourages inflammation.
- Seeking expert medical advice. The National Foundation for Ileitis and Colitis provides important information to patients and their families.

Gross, V. et al. "Free Radicals in Inflammatory Bowel Diseases—Pathophysiology and Therapeutic Implications," *Hepato-Gastroenterology* 41 (1994): 320–327.

inhibition Restricting the activity of a cellular or physiologic process. Several different mechanisms are involved in inhibition.

Hormones Hormones may serve as inhibiting agents because they can inhibit the release of other hormones. Thus, the ovaries produce inhibin (a hormone that inhibits the secretion of the ovarian hormones), follicle stimulating hormone, and lutenizing hormone, at the end of the menstrual cycle. Elevated CORTISOL from the adrenal glands inhibits the release of ADRENOCORTICOTROPIN (ACTH) from the PITUITARY GLAND. ACTH stimulates the release of cortisol.

Enzymes Enzymes are protein catalysts that lose activity when blocked by inhibitors. Competitive enzyme inhibitors are compounds that mimic the chemical that the enzyme usually alters.

Enzyme poisons like toxic heavy metals—LEAD, MERCURY, and CADMIUM—can bind to enzymes without competing with substances and can permanently inactivate enzymes.

Certain key regulatory enzymes may be reversibly inhibited by the accumulation of key products of metabolism. One example is the feedback inhibition of a METABOLIC PATHWAY, a sequence of functionally linked enzymes. In this type of inhibition, a surplus of the final product of the pathway can inhibit the pathway. For example, the buildup of ATP, the energy currency of the cell, can inhibit enzyme systems like GLYCOLYSIS that generate ATP. Such feedback mechanisms help the cell avoid wasteful overproduction of products. (See also ENDOCRINE SYSTEM; INDUCTION.)

inosine One of the basic compounds composing cells and a precursor to adenosine, an important energy molecule and building block of DNA and RNA. Although some European scientists believed it could have energy-boosting effects, controlled studies concluded that inosine does not improve athletic performance. Athletes often take between 5,000 and 6,000 mg of inosine a day, but research does not support the use of this supplement in any amount.

However, some animal research studies have suggested it may be helpful in the treatment of stroke and other central nervous system disorders. Inosine occurs in organ meats and brewer's yeast and can be taken as a supplement. Although there are no reports of side effects, any inosine that is not used by the body is converted to uric acid, which could be a problem for people at high risk for gout. Safety data are inadequate for pregnant and breastfeeding women.

Starling, R. D., T. A. Trappe, K. R. Short et al. "Effect of Inosine Supplementation on Aerobic and Anaerobic Cycling Performance," *Medicine and Science in Sports and Exercise* 28 (1996): 1,193–1,198.

inositol (myoinositol) An essential building block of cell membrane LIPIDS. Chemically, inositol is a cyclic ALCOHOL with six hydroxyl groups, one per carbon atom. Inositol is a constituent of phosphatidylinositol, a component of inner-cell membranes. Derivatives of inositol function as HORMONE relay signals in cells. Diverse hormones such as VASOPRESSIN (from the pituitary gland), EPINEPHRINE (from the adrenal gland) and releasing factors from the HYPOTHALAMUS stimulate the release of inositol triphosphate from phosphatidylinositol.

Animal studies show that inositol may protect against ATHEROSCLEROSIS and against hair loss. Inositol is also supposed to help reverse nerve damage caused by diabetes in animals. Oral supplementation in human diabetics has not verified this result. Diabetics should consult their health care providers before taking inositol supplements. Inositol has a low toxicity.

Nutritionists have not yet established the optimum amount of inositol in the diet. It is widely distributed in food and is also manufactured in the body. Sources include CITRUS FRUIT (except lemons), CANTALOUPE, whole grain bread, cooked beans, green beans, and nuts. Inositol occurs in grains such as PHYTIC ACID, in which six phosphate groups are attached to the inositol molecule. Phytic acid can bind minerals and limit their uptake. Safety data are inadequate for pregnant and breastfeeding women. (See also VITAMIN.)

Shamsuddin, Abulkalaman M. "Inositol Phosphates Have Novel Anti-Cancer Function," *Journal of Nutrition* 125, supp. 3 (1995): 725S–732S.

insulin A protein HORMONE, secreted by beta cells in the PANCREAS, that stimulates the uptake of BLOOD SUGAR by many tissues. Insulin counteracts the effects of GLUCAGON, the pancreatic hormone responsible for raising blood sugar. Insulin is used therapeutically to treat DIABETES MELLITUS and is either purified from pork or beef pancreas or is genetically engineered of human origin. Insulin is produced by small cell clusters in the pancreas called the islets of Langerhans. Insulin itself is hormonally regulated. An increase in blood sugar levels stimulates insulin release. PANCREOZYMIN, an intestinal hormone, also stimulates insulin release. The trace mineral CHROMIUM, which appears in the form of GLUCOSE TOLERANCE FACTOR, is required for optimal insulin activity.

Insulin exerts a profound effect on glucose HOMEOSTASIS. Once glucose is absorbed it can be oxidized for energy production or it can be converted to triglycerides (fat). More generally, this hormone favors the formation of GLYCOGEN, LIPIDS, and PROTEIN. Muscle and fat cells require insulin to absorb surplus glucose from the blood after a meal. On the other hand, the brain utilizes blood glucose independently of insulin. In ADIPOSE TISSUE, insulin activates fat synthesis from glucose, while in MUSCLE, insulin promotes the storage of glucose as glycogen, the polymer that functions as the storage form of glucose. Insulin also promotes amino acid uptake and increased muscle protein synthesis. In the liver, insulin stimulates the formation of triglycerides and glycogen from glucose while blocking glucose formation and glycogen breakdown.

Excessive insulin can lead to low blood sugar (HYPOGLYCEMIA). In postprandial HYPOGLYCEMIA, blood sugar drops after eating carbohydrates. One reason for this is that the pancreas overreacts to the sudden rush of glucose by releasing excessive insulin. The subsequent drop in blood sugar may cause fatigue, irritability, and other symptoms.

The mechanism of insulin action is still not completely understood, although the hormone was discovered over 70 years ago. Insulin increases glucose transport into cells, activates or inactivates certain enzymes responsible for glucose metabolism and storage, and changes the level of protein synthesis at the gene level. Initially, insulin binds to specific binding sites called hormone receptors on the cell surfaces of target tissues. Binding causes the release of one or more intracellular messengers that lead to altered metabolism. The nature of the signal mechanism is under active investigation. Insulin may activate certain enzymes called protein kinases, regulatory enzymes that in turn modulate enzymes required for energy utilization. One outcome is the activation of enzymes for glycogen synthesis.

Insulin Resistance

A low response to insulin is called insulin resistance, which typically elevates blood sugar levels. Up to 25 percent of nonobese Americans are estimated to have an inherited inefficient response to insulin. European and American research implicates insulin resistance and elevated blood sugar in the development of some forms of CORONARY ARTERY DISEASE. The mechanism by which insulin resistance might cause heart disease remains unknown.

The most extreme case of insulin resistance is diabetes. Most diabetic patients exhibit a degree of insulin resistance. In non-insulin-dependent diabetes (Type II diabetes), there is a loss of insulin sensitivity and a decline in the maximal response elicited by insulin. According to one scenario the problem may reflect the inability to use insulin effectively because of too few insulin binding sites on target cells. Thus, insulin resistance can be caused by defective insulin receptors or other defective proteins, and it can provoke a decline in insulin production.

Secondary factors that can affect insulin resistance in target cells include: STRESS, fever, FASTING and STARVATION, as well as liver CIRRHOSIS, KETOSIS, OBESITY, puberty, high blood sugar, and AGING. Also, the excessive production of hormones like CORTISOL, glucagon, EPINEPHRINE, and GROWTH HORMONE can induce insulin resistance. With obesity there is a loss of insulin sensitivity by peripheral tissues, also due to a decrease in relative amounts of hormone receptors. (See also AMINO ACID METABOLISM; CARBOHYDRATE METABOLISM; DIABETES MELLITUS; ENDOCRINE SYSTEM.)

Gerstin, H. C., and Salim Yusuf. "Dysglycaemia and Risk of Cardiovascular Disease," *Lancet* 347 (April 1996): 949–950.

insulin-dependent diabetes See DIABETES MELLITUS.

interferon A family of proteins secreted by virus-infected cells that function as the body's first line of defense against a wide variety of viruses. Three basic types of interferon have been identified: White blood cells secrete leukocyte interferon; connective tissue cells produce fibroblast interferon;

and immune system cells produce lymphocyte interferon. Most interferons can block viral proliferation in infected cells by binding to adjacent cells, converting them to a virus-resistant state. Lymphocyte interferon also modulates the immune system on T cells, a class of immune cells derived from the THYMUS GLAND. The interferon also acts as a growth factor and stimulates T cell proliferation, also stimulating the killing action of certain T cells. Consequently, interferon has been used on a limited basis as an anticancer agent. Interferon differs from ANTIBODIES, which are proteins synthesized by specialized cells of the IMMUNE SYSTEM to combat a specific foreigner. Antibodies can attack bacteria as well as viruses in the bloodstream but do not fortify cells against viral attack.

international unit (IU) A standardized amount of physiologically active material such as a HORMONE, an ENZYME, or a VITAMIN. International units are based on measurements of biological effects, such as increased growth rate in experimental animals.

The weight of active material represented by an international unit varies with the specific material. For example, fat-soluble vitamins are sometimes listed on supplement labels in terms of IU. The REFERENCE DAILY INTAKE (RDI) for VITAMIN D is 400 IU, equivalent to 10 mcg, based on experiments with rats and chicks, while the RDI for VITAMIN E (alpha-tocopherol) is 30 IU, equivalent to 20 mg. For VITAMIN A (retinol), the RDI is 5,000 IU, representing 1,500 retinol equivalents or 1,500 mcg. (See also RECOMMENDED DIETARY ALLOWANCES.)

interstitial fluid Fluid that bathes cells and tissues; it buffers cells against extreme pH, delivers oxygen and nutrients to cells, removes wastes and serves as an avenue for defensive cells of the immune system.

Interstitial fluid contains white BLOOD cells (LEUKOCYTES) that also enter tissue fluid from the bloodstream by squeezing through capillary walls and migrating to the site of infection and inflammation. Interstitial fluid, together with blood and lymph, help maintain the internal environment within normal limits. When interstitial fluid flows through lymphatic vessels, it is called LYMPH.

Cell-free constituents of blood and fluid normally penetrate capillaries. Whole blood does not penetrate vessel walls unless they are injured. These materials include water, ions like SODIUM and CHLORIDE, GLUCOSE, and other nutrients, as well as small proteins. PLATELETS, small cell fragments that promote clotting, together with serum proteins, blood, and RED BLOOD CELLS, are retained within vessels and do not appear in the interstitial fluid. (See also BUFFER; ELECTROLYTES; HOMEOSTASIS.)

intestinal flora Microorganisms (chiefly bacteria) that normally occupy the the latter part of the small intestine and extensively colonize the COLON. Intestinal bacteria are more numerous than all of the cells of the body. Bacteria living in the intestine weigh several pounds and represent one-third of the dry fecal weight. An estimated 400 different bacterial species inhabit the digestive tract, and the concentration in the colon far exceeds the level in the small intestine. Twenty species comprise 75 percent of the total number of bacterial colonies, and anaerobic (oxygen-sensitive) bacteria greatly outnumber aerobic bacteria. Many types of gut bacteria have established a symbiotic relationship through evolution. Most are anaerobic and thrive without oxygen, while others can live under both aerobic and anaerobic conditions.

Bacteria implant in the infant's intestine shortly after birth. *Bifidobacterium infantis* is promoted by BREAST-FEEDING. Later in life, a full complement of bacteria is normally in place. Different bacteria favor different regions of the intestine. *Bifidobacterium bifidum* is a major component of the large intestine in adults, while *LACTOBACILLUS ACIDOPHILUS* inhabits both the small and large intestine. *Streptococcus faecalis* and *Escherichia coli* are normal inhabitants of the intestine. However, if *E. coli* spreads to the urinary tract, it can cause bladder infections. Virulent species of *E. coli* produce enterotoxins that cause diarrhea.

Beneficial Effects of Gut Flora

The normal gut flora degrade toxins and foreign compounds. They break down food constituents such as fiber and undigested starch into short-chain fatty acids like ACETIC ACID, PROPIONIC ACID, and BUTYRIC ACID, which serve as major fuels. Butyrate is a preferred energy source for cells lining the colon. Intestinal bacteria enhance bowel function, such as PERISTALSIS, increasing the time required for material to pass through the digestive system. Intestinal bacteria also provide B vitamins like biotin and fat-soluble VITAMIN K. By occupying an important biological niche, beneficial bacteria control the spread of undesirable microorganisms. They produce factors that limit growth of potential pathogens and create an acidic, anaerobic environment that also limits the growth of undesirable species. Some strains of normal gut bacteria produce substances that suppress potential pathogens. YEASTS are generally present in very low number, if at all, because they are held in check by beneficial bacteria like the acid-producing varieties.

Imbalanced Gut Flora

An unhealthy gastrointestinal tract can alter gut flora. Thus, imbalanced intestinal flora can be caused by low stomach acid, diarrhea or constipation, or by malnutrition. Broad-spectrum antibiotics can wipe out entire populations of beneficial bacteria. When stomach acid is low, food is not sterilized; surviving microorganisms can proliferate in the warm, moist, and nutrient-rich intestine, thus setting the stage for intestinal disease due to yeast, parasites, and pathogenic bacteria. Low stomach acid also increases the probability of maldigestion.

Altered gut flora can in turn cause intestinal damage, maldigestion, and MALABSORPTION. Incompletely digested foods can provide unusual substrates for gut bacteria, which they can convert to harmful substances. For example, a high meat diet induces certain bacteria to break down amino acids to amines and phenols, compounds that can damage intestinal cells.

Endotoxins (poisonous materials released by bacterial overgrowth) also can inflame the gut. This increases intestinal permeability or leakiness, permitting further toxin uptake. Alternatively, bacterial enzymes can break down BILE salts and estrogens, altering LIVER regulation of these materials. Maldigestion can occur when intestinal inflammation causes decreased production of intestinal digestive enzymes. For example, atrophy of the intestinal lining accompanies infestation by giardia, a common intestinal parasite. Likewise, poor absorption of nutrients will occur under these conditions.

Gut flora can be normalized by taking lactobacillus and bifidobacteria supplements, as well as supplementing other beneficial bacteria, by drinking plenty of clean water, by eating fewer refined foods and less fat and meat, and by eating more whole (minimally processed) foods and more fiber from vegetables and fruits. Nutrients that support the immune system and stress reduction also help balance gut microorganisms. (See also CANCER; HYPOCHLORHYDRIA.)

Roberfroid, M. B. et al. "Colonic Microflora: Nutrition and Health," *Nutrition Reviews* 53, no. 5 (1995): 127–130.

intestine The long tube connecting the stomach and anus that is divided into two segments, each with different functions.

Small Intestine

The small intestine leads to the large intestine (colon). Narrower and longer than the colon, the small intestine is the major site of digestion and uptake of nutrients, including CARBOHYDRATE, AMINO ACIDS, FATTY ACIDS, WATER, MINERALS, and VITAMINS released by stomach and intestinal secretions.

The small intestine begins at the valve regulating the opening of the stomach (pyloric sphincter) and coils its way through the abdominal cavity before joining the large intestine. The average diameter of the small intestine is 1 inch and the length is about 20 feet in an adult.

The surface of the small intestine looks like a wrinkled shag rug, which increases the efficiency of nutrient absorption. The highly convoluted surface is coated with fuzzy, microscopic projections called VILLI. There are 10 to 40 villi per square millimeter. Cells lining the small intestine possess microscopic, hairlike projections called MICROVILLI, which further increase the surface area so that the total surface area of the inner surface of the small intestine is about the size of a tennis court. The small intestine secretes important digestive enzymes that complete the process of DIGESTION. They include LACTASE, MALTASE, and SUCRASE, which break down carbohydrate to simple sugars together with enzymes capable of digesting protein fragments to amino acids. Once nutrients like sugars, vitamins, minerals, and amino acids are absorbed by cells lining the intestine, they pass into CAPILLARIES and enter the bloodstream or pass into the LYMPHATIC SYSTEM if they are fat soluble.

Because of its huge surface area and daily exposure to many foreign materials and microorganisms, the intestinal tract is subject to disease. The intestine protects itself against the onslaught of bacteria, bacterial cell wall fragments, and products of bacterial metabolism, and against food antigens by several mechanisms. The lining secretes MUCUS, a thick viscous fluid that creates a physical barrier, and lysozyme, an enzyme that attacks certain bacteria. The intestine also secretes a major ANTIBODY called secretory IgA. This antibody binds to specific organisms and keeps them from attacking the mucosal cells, often a prerequisite for infection. It also binds specific antigens like food proteins and prevents their penetration. Stress can lower secretory IgA production, increasing the likelihood of intestinal imbalance and infection.

Colon (Large Intestine)

The large intestine is about one-quarter of the length of the small intestine and averages 2.5 inches (6.5 cm) in diameter. The opening between the terminal portion of the small intestine (ILEUM) and the large intestine is regulated by the ileocecal valve. Digestive enzymes are not secreted in the colon, which is the site of the last stage of food breakdown. Colonic bacteria degrade much of the undigested material received from the small intestine (CHYME). FIBER and undigested carbohydrates are metabolized to CARBON DIOXIDE, hydrogen, methane, and simple saturated acids like ACETIC ACID and BUTYRIC ACID, which are absorbed and used as fuels. Colonic bacteria also degrade certain amino acids to compounds responsible for fecal odor. BILE PIGMENT (bilirubin) is converted to brown pigments. B vitamins and VITAMIN K synthesized by bacterial action are absorbed in the large intestine, as are SODIUM, CHLORIDE, and other minerals. The large intestine also absorbs water from fecal material, creating a formed stool.

Different types of bacteria occupy different regions of the intestine. *Bifidobacterium bifidium* is a major component of the large intestine in adults, while *LACTOBACILLUS ACIDOPHILUS* favors the small intestine. Strains of *ESCHERICHIA COLI* are normal inhabitants of the intestine. Yeasts are generally in very low numbers, if present at all. However, reduction in beneficial bacterial populations can permit yeast and other potential pathogens to proliferate. INFLAMMATORY BOWEL DISEASE, DIARRHEA, IRRITABLE BOWEL SYNDROME, CONSTIPATION, ILEITIS, LEAKY GUT syndrome, several types of FOOD POISONING, and parasitic diseases like giardia are a few of the more common intestinal disorders. (See also ACIDOPHILUS; BIFIDUS FACTOR; *CANDIDA ALBICANS*; DIGESTIVE DISORDERS; DIGESTIVE TRACT.)

intoxication See ALCOHOL.

intracellular fluid The total amount of WATER contained within cells that accounts for twice as much water as outside of cells and represents nearly 40 percent of the total body weight.

EXTRACELLULAR FLUID refers to water excluded from cells. Because water readily diffuses across cell membranes, the intracellular and the extracellular compartments are linked. Consequently, massive water losses will draw water out of cells and eventually alter cell function. Physiologic processes ranging from regulation of body temperature, waste removal, and kidney function to the function of the central nervous system and distribution of oxygen and nutrients, rely upon water balance. (See also CYTOPLASM; DEHYDRATION; ELECTROLYTES.)

intrinsic factor A protein produced by the stomach lining and required for intestinal absorption of VITAMIN B_{12}. Gastric PARIETAL CELLS normally secrete intrinsic factor during digestion. Intrinsic factor binds tightly vitamin B_{12} released from food during intestinal digestion. The resulting B_{12}-intrinsic factor complex is selectively absorbed by the epithelial cells lining the ILEUM, the latter portion of the small intestine. If the stomach does not secrete enough STOMACH ACID (a condition called HYPOCHLORHYDRIA), it probably does not make enough intrinsic factor either. With too little intrinsic factor, vitamin B_{12} cannot be assimilated by the body, leading to a chronic deficiency. This causes PERNICIOUS ANEMIA, as well as neurological symptoms. Vitamin B_{12} is required for DNA synthesis and cell proliferation. Restricted vitamin B_{12} uptake due to a lack of intrinsic factor leads to ANEMIA because the BONE marrow cannot produce adequate red blood cells without adequate vitamin B_{12}. The linkage between vitamin B_{12} deficiency and neurological damage is poorly understood.

Abnormal intrinsic factor production is genetically linked; susceptibility runs in families. Vitamin B_{12} injections, and possibly oral supplementation of massive amounts of vitamin B_{12} (1,000 mcg or more per day), may permit adequate vitamin B_{12} assimilation when intrinsic factor and stomach acid production are low. Because FOLIC ACID also supports cell proliferation similar to vitamin B_{12}, folic acid is usually administered with vitamin B_{12}. (See also ACHLORHYDRIA; AGING; SENILITY.)

inulin A POLYSACCHARIDE that is composed primarily of the simple sugar FRUCTOSE. Inulin plays a minor role in the diet; it is found in only a few foods, including ARTICHOKES, ONIONS, and GARLIC. Fresh foods contain higher levels of inulin than stored foods because most of the inulin might be broken down to fructose during storage. Inulin is poorly digested, but once it is absorbed it is filtered by the glomerulus, the KIDNEY structure that removes materials from the blood during urine formation. Since inulin is excreted in urine by the kidney, its rate of appearance in urine is a measure of GLOMERULAR FILTRATION rate, the rate at which the kidney can remove soluble materials from blood.

invert sugar A mixture of GLUCOSE and FRUCTOSE, the two simple sugars that make up table sugar (SUCROSE). Sucrose hydrolysis by acid or by the enzyme invertase yields a 50/50 mixture of these two sugars that is both sweeter and more soluble than table sugar. Invert sugar is an additive in the manufacture of candy because it prevents the sugar in candy from crystallizing. Like all sugar sweeteners, it contributes only calories to the diet. (See also FOOD ADDITIVES; NATURAL SWEETENERS.)

iodine (iodide) An essential trace mineral nutrient required to produce thyroid hormones. The element iodine occurs in food and in the body as the ionized or chemical form called iodide. The THYROID GLAND combines iodide with the AMINO ACID, TYROSINE, to produce thyroxine and triiodothyronine. These hormones control the body's idling speed (BASAL METABOLIC RATE) and support normal growth and development.

Symptoms of iodine deficiency include sluggishness (HYPOTHYROIDISM), weight gain, and, in extreme cases, an enlarged thyroid gland (GOITER). During pregnancy, iodine deficiency can cause severe mental retardation (cretinism) in children. Before salt was iodized in the 1920s, goiters were common in areas of the United States, especially the South, with iodine-deficient soils. Though rare, goiter sometimes occurs in women and children in certain areas of California, Texas and the South, and in Manitoba and Saskatchewan, Canada. Goiter is still common in parts of Africa. Certain substances called GOITROGENS in vegetables like CASSAVA and rutabagas block iodine uptake and may contribute to the occurrence of goiter when excessive amounts of these foods are consumed.

Sources of iodide include SEAWEED; shellfish like shrimp, clams, and oysters; marine fish; and iodized salt. Iodine occurs in food in other chemical forms besides iodide. SODIUM iodate, a commercial dough oxidizer, occurs in some commercially baked goods. Milk and milk products may contain traces of free iodine, used as a disinfectant for milk cows and in milk production.

The typical diet supplies more than twice the U.S. REFERENCE DAILY INTAKE (RDI) of 50 mcg. Consuming 2 mg per day is generally considered safe for healthy adults. BREAST-MILK contains iodine to provide for the infant's requirements, and lactating women require extra iodide in their diets. An additional 50 mcg of iodine per day is recommended. Iodine as supersaturated potassium iodide has been used clinically in the treatment of asthma, slow lymphatic drainage, sebaceous cysts, and fibrocystic breast disease, and to promote desirable balance of estrogens. Iodine, as a water purifier, possesses antiviral and antibacterial activity. Excessive amounts of iodide can cause iodine-induced goiter. Other side effects include rash and allergies.

Iodized Salt

In the United States, sodium iodide has been added to table salt (sodium chloride) since 1924 to create "iodized salt." With 76 mcg of iodine per gram of salt, this ENRICHMENT was responsible for the virtual disappearance of goiter in the United States. Small amounts of additives stabilize iodine in iodized salt and prevent caking: They include GLUCOSE, sodium thiocyanate, sodium aluminum silicate, or sodium BICARBONATE. SEA SALT is not a good source of iodine. Although sea water is rich in iodide, it is lost during purification. Note that sea salt and iodized salt contribute the same amount of sodium as standard table salt. (See also FORTIFICATION; HYPERTENSION; TRACE MINERALS.)

iron A versatile trace mineral nutrient that performs essential functions in the body. The presence of iron is responsible for the red color of BLOOD. Red blood cells contain vast amounts of HEMOGLOBIN, the red oxygen transport protein of blood. Hemoglobin is red because it contains HEME, the red, iron-rich pigment that actually binds oxygen and transports it to tissues. Iron deficiency leads to a low level of red blood cells (ANEMIA).

Muscles contain a red, iron-containing protein called myoglobin, which stores oxygen for muscle contraction. The body contains a total of 3 to 5 g of iron. Hemoglobin represents 65 percent of this iron; about 30 percent occurs as FERRITIN, the iron storage complex found in the LIVER, spleen, and BONE marrow.

Iron plays many roles. It is required to oxidize fuels to produce energy needed to maintain tissue functioning. Iron functions in CYTOCHROMES and other mitochondrial enzymes that burn CARBOHYDRATE and FAT to form ATP, the cell's chemical energy currency. In this context, it is noteworthy that iron promotes the formation of CARNITINE, a compound required to transport fatty acids into mitochondria to be burned.

Connective Tissue This is the matrix that holds cells and tissues together. Iron-containing enzymes are involved in the formation of structural proteins COLLAGEN and ELASTIN, required to form connective tissue.

Defensive Cells The bacteria-killing white blood cells (neutrophils) depend upon iron to help generate highly reactive forms of oxygen that function as bacteriocides. Inadequate iron reduces the effectiveness of the immune system. The production of T-lymphocytes and red blood cells requires rapid DNA synthesis. An iron-dependent enzyme synthesizes DEOXYRIBOSE, the carbohydrate building block of DNA. Iron deficiency slows DNA synthesis.

Nervous System Iron is required in the synthesis of neurotransmitters, DOPAMINE, SEROTONIN, and norepinephrine. Neurotransmitters are chemicals that help conduct impulses between nerve cells.

Liver Glucose (BLOOD SUGAR) formation from amino acids requires iron. CYTOCHROME P450 is an iron-dependent enzyme system that helps the liver destroy toxic chemicals and waste products.

Antioxidant Enzyme Iron assists the action of CATALASE, a ubiquitous enzyme that degrades HYDROGEN PEROXIDE to water and oxygen. Hydrogen peroxide is a by-product of cellular reactions and it is a powerful oxidizing agent unless inactivated.

Iron Deficiency

Iron deficiency is one of the most common nutritional problems worldwide; about 1 billion people are to some extent iron deficient. Half the world's inner city and rural poor may not be getting enough iron. Iron deficiency is the major nutritional deficiency among children, notably 1 to 2 year olds and older children from low-income households. This is a concern in developing nations where the diet is inadequate and parasitic diseases such as schistosomiasis and malaria are common. As many as 60 percent of the U.S. population may not get enough iron. Teenagers who rely on a junk food diet, dieters and pregnant or lactating women, individuals with liver disorders or blood loss, and low-income elderly persons may develop iron deficiency. An estimated 10 percent to 20 percent of women of childbearing age in the United States, Japan, and England may be anemic due to poor eating habits and blood loss through menstruation. Inadequate iron absorption among the elderly, due to use of antacids and low stomach acidity, frequently causes iron deficiency.

Mild iron deficiency, due to diminished iron storage without full-blown symptoms of iron deficiency, occurs long before anemia develops. Symptoms include FATIGUE, decreased alertness and learning and memory problems in children, muscle weakness, susceptibility to chronic infections and frequent colds, low stomach acid and poor digestion, slow growth, dizziness, and rapid heartbeat. Iron deficiency impairs work capacity and endurance.

Anemia represents the final stage of chronic, severe iron deficiency. Depleted iron reserves cause excessive fatigue due to inadequate oxygen delivery to tissues. Iron supplementation will cure anemia due to iron deficiency, but it will not cure pernicious anemia, which is due to VITAMIN B_{12} deficiency, nor will iron cure anemias based on other nutritional deficiencies such as vitamin B_6.

A variety of laboratory tests are used to evaluate iron deficiency. The most sensitive clinical test for mild iron deficiency measures serum ferritin. Serum ferritin may decline to 12 mcg/liter without visible symptoms. With serious iron deficiencies, the level of the iron-transport protein in the blood, transferrin, is elevated, but it contains less iron than usual (less than 16 percent saturation). With severe deficiency hemoglobin levels decline and small red blood cells appear, a condition called microcytic anemia, and the packed volume of red blood cells, the HEMATOCRIT, declines.

Sources of Iron

Animals are the best food sources of iron because the iron in flesh (heme) is highly absorbable. These include MEAT, especially liver, POULTRY, and FISH, as well as iron-fortified flour, egg yolk, BREAD, and cereals. Iron uptake is increased by cooking acidic foods in an iron skillet. Red wines often contain iron. Nonheme iron, as found in vegetables and iron-fortified foods, is often poorly absorbed. Nonheme iron also occurs in meat. Only 1.4 percent of the iron in spinach and of the iron in soybeans is absorbed because it is tightly bound to plant materials that resist the action of digestive enzymes. Absorption is increased by the addition of VITAMIN C and small amounts of animal protein. Iron uptake in blocked by substances in grains called PHYTIC ACID, by the TANNINS in tea, ANTACIDS, ASPIRIN, the fiber in wheat BRAN, as well as excessive use of zinc supplements. The iron content in typical foods (milligrams per 100 g) is as follows: almonds, 4.7; dried beans, 2.4–2.7; beef, 3.0; blackstrap molasses, 16.1; bread, 2.2–2.4; milk chocolate, 1.0; caviar, 11.8; chicken, 1.3–1.8; eggs, 2.3; liver, 8.8–14.2; oyster, 8.1; peanut butter, 2.0; popcorn, 2.1; pork, 2.6; sardines, 2.9; shrimp, 2.0; tofu, 1.9. Organically complexed iron, for example with CITRIC ACID, SUCCINIC ACID, or with vitamin C, is well absorbed. Oxidized iron (ferric, Fe^{3+}) is not as well absorbed as reduced iron (ferrous, Fe^{2+}).

Requirements

The body hoards iron and efficiently recycles it; only small amounts (1.0 mg per day for adults) are excreted. The RECOMMENDED DIETARY ALLOWANCE (RDA) for pre-menopausal women (15 mg/day) is higher than for men (10 mg/day) to compensate for blood losses. The upper tolerable limit is 45 mg. per day.

The RDA for iron varies with age, and the RDA during pregnancy and lactation is greater. The recommended daily intake during pregnancy is 60 mg per day. Iron supplements are required to achieve this level and are usually prescribed for pregnant women in the United States. Treatment of iron deficiency anemia calls for increased dietary iron, under professional guidance. A chronic iron deficiency may set the stage for excessive menstrual blood loss, thus causing a vicious cycle. Iron supplementation can remedy this situation. Iron supplements should be taken at a different time than vitamin E because iron rapidly oxidizes vitamin E. Iron supplements often contain chelated iron, that is, iron bound to organic compounds in order to facilitate absorption. Examples include iron gluconate and iron aspartate.

Safety

Iron supplements may cause stomachache, diarrhea, constipation, and dark stools, although iron complexed with protein may cause fewer side effects.

Iron overload can occur with inherited iron storage disease (HEMOCHROMATOSIS). Men who are susceptible to hemochromatosis and who take high iron supplements for long periods may develop iron overload; they should probably avoid iron supplements.

Iron supplements should probably be avoided by healthy, nondeficient people for additional reasons: Excessive iron suppresses the immune system. High blood levels of iron are associated with increased risk of FREE RADICAL damage and cancer. Stored iron (ferritin) can be a risk factor for coronary diseases. U.S. men with high blood concentrations of ferritin (more than 200 mcg per liter) are more likely to suffer heart attacks as men with lower ferritin values. It is postulated that too much iron can promote the formation of highly reactive forms of oxygen (free radicals) that can attack LOW-

DENSITY LIPOPROTEIN (LDL), a particularly dangerous type of CHOLESTEROL. Oxidized LDL is more likely to stick to arterial walls and trigger fatty plaque buildup, which can clog arteries. Scientists also speculate that free radicals themselves damage arterial walls and heart muscle tissue. Patients should not exceed 18 mg of iron per day unless advised to do so by a physician. Iron is the most common cause of pediatric poisoning deaths.

Several thousand children are poisoned each year by iron supplements. As few as six iron supplement tablets can kill a child. (See also CATABOLISM; ERYTHROPOIESIS; GLUCONEOGENESIS; MITOCHONDRIA; TRACE MINERALS.)

irradiated food See FOOD IRRADIATION.

irritable bowel syndrome (IBS) A common intestinal disorder characterized by spasms of the COLON or large intestine, with alternating CONSTIPATION and DIARRHEA and heartburn, cramps, and gas. Through the years IBS has been called by many names—colitis, mucous colitis, spastic colon, spastic bowel, and functional bowel disease. Most of these terms are inaccurate. Colitis, for instance, means inflammation of the large intestine (colon). IBS, however, does not cause inflammation and should not be confused with another disorder, ulcerative colitis.

The cause of IBS is not known, and as yet there is no cure. Although IBS can sometimes be simply a mild annoyance, for some people it can be disabling, keeping them from social events, a job, or travel. Most people with IBS, however, are able to control their symptoms through medications prescribed by their physicians, diet, and stress management. In this situation, food does not move normally through the intestine, and cramps result. Excessive STOMACH ACID is a secondary problem.

IBS accounts for half of all gastrointestinal problems among Americans, and it is more common than HEPATITIS or ulcerative COLITIS. Women are the most susceptible to IBS. The disease often begins between the ages of 20 and 40.

Symptoms may resemble CROHN'S DISEASE, peptic ulcer, or gynecological problems. LACTOSE INTOLERANCE can mimic symptoms of IBS, as can reaction to excessive fructose or sorbitol used as sweeteners. Reactions to CORN, WHEAT, CITRUS FRUIT, TEA, and COFFEE have been implicated in IBS. Recent research suggests that the IMMUNE SYSTEM overreacts, imbalancing the control of inflammation. Gut microflora may also be imbalanced; parasitic or bacterial infection can adversely affect the health of the intestine and cause symptoms resembling IBS.

The most likely conditions to aggravate IBS are diet and emotional stress. Eating causes contractions of the colon, which normally causes an urge to have a bowel movement within 30 to 60 minutes after a meal. In people with IBS the urge may come sooner, with cramps and diarrhea. The strength of the response is often related to the number of calories in a meal and especially the amount of fat in a meal. Fat in any form (animal or vegetable) is a strong stimulus of colonic contractions. Many foods contain fat, especially meats of all kinds, whole milk, cream, cheese, butter, vegetable oil, margarine, shortening, avocados, and whipped toppings.

Extra FIBER may be beneficial in the treatment of constipation; food sources include whole GRAINS, whole fruits, PEARS, berries, PEAS, prunes, and BRUSSELS SPROUTS. PSYLLIUM seed powder, various fiber supplements, and fiber cookies are other options. For many people, eating a proper diet can help. High-fiber diets keep the colon mildly distended, which may help to prevent spasms from developing. Some forms of fiber also keep water in the stools, thereby preventing hard stools that are difficult to pass. Doctors usually recommend eating just enough fiber to produce soft, easily-passed, and painless bowel movements. Although high-fiber diets may cause gas and bloating, within a few weeks these symptoms often go away as the body adjusts to the diet. However, a health care provider should be consulted before beginning a high fiber diet in the presence of digestive disease. Large meals can cause cramping and diarrhea in people with IBS. Symptoms may be eased by eating smaller meals more often or just eating smaller portions, especially if meals are low in fat and high in carbohydrates such as pasta, rice, whole-grain breads and cereals, fruits, and vegetables. Stress also stimulates colonic spasm in people with IBS; stress reduction and relaxation training and counseling help relieve IBS symptoms in some people. However, doctors are quick to note that this does not mean IBS is the result of a personality disorder. IBS is at least partly a disorder of colon motility. Patients should avoid coffee and fatty, gas-provoking, and irritating foods. Stress reduction and gut-directed hypnotherapy can help in some cases. (See also ALLERGY; CAFFEINE; DIGESTION; DIGESTIVE DISORDERS; DIGESTIVE TRACT; INFLAMMATORY BOWEL DISEASE.)

irritable colon See IRRITABLE BOWEL SYNDROME.

ischemia The reduction of oxygen supply to the heart so that cardiac muscle cells are weakened. Ischemia is often caused by the narrowing of arteries such as in ATHEROSCLEROSIS or by blood clot formation. Angina pectoris or chest pain is due to ischemia of the heart muscle. (See also CARDIOVASCULAR DISEASE; CHOLESTEROL; HEART ATTACK.)

isoflavone A class of nonnutrient plant substances with potential anticancer effects. Isoflavones occur in relatively high concentrations in soy products and in varying amounts in several hundred other plants. The content varies with the variety, time of harvest, and geographic location. Isoflavones belong to the general class of FLAVONOIDS; they possess complex ring structures with oxygen atoms attached. Genistein and daidzein are two examples of isoflavones. Their general shape resembles the steroid hormone estrogen, a major female hormone. It is possible that isoflavones block estrogen from binding to targets, a needed step in hormone-dependent cancers like cancers of the breast, ovary, and endometrium. They could also stimulate the production of an estrogen-binding protein in the blood, or they could block liver enzymes that activate compounds to become cancer-causing agents (carcinogens). Vegetarians whose diets are enriched in soy products and tofu have a lower risk of cancer.

Clarkson, T. B. et al. "Estrogenic Soybean Isoflavones and Chronic Disease," *Trends in Endocrinology and Metabolism* 6, no. 1 (1995): 11–16.

isoleucine (Ile, L-isolucine) A dietary essential AMINO ACID. Isoleucine is classified as a nonpolar (water-repelling) amino acid. It possessed a side chain resembling a lipid and does not attract water molecules. The side chain of isoleucine is branched, and like LEUCINE and VALINE, the other BRANCHED CHAIN AMINO ACIDS, it cannot be assembled by the body. These amino acids are largely degraded in the MUSCLE, rather than by the LIVER. Infants require an estimated 70 mg per kilogram of body weight daily, children (2 to 12 years) about 30 mg per kilogram daily, while adults require 10 mg per kilogram daily. These figures reflect the high growth rates of children. The total amount of high-quality PROTEIN needed daily to support growth and maintenance increases from about 13 g per day for infants to 46 to 63 g per day for adults due to their increased body weight. (See also AMINO ACID METABOLISM; BIOLOGICAL VALUE.)

isothiocyanate A family of sulfur-containing plant substances with potential anticancer effects. Isothiocyanates and related thiocyanates occur in high levels in vegetables of the cabbage family (CRUCIFEROUS VEGETABLES). Isothiocyanates seem to block the reactions of cancer-causing agents at sensitive sites within the cell, and they also seem to suppress the expression of cancer after cancer has been initiated. Animal studies indicate that isothiocyanates can inhibit dangerous chemical changes to DNA in the cancer-generating stages. Possibly these substances increase liver production of protective "phase II" enzymes. These detoxication enzymes attach innocent molecules to potentially harmful compounds to help flush them out of the body (glutathione transferase is an example).

Zhang, Yuesheng, and Paul Talalay. "Anticarcinogenic Activities of Organic Isothiocyanates: Chemistry and Mechanism," *Cancer Research* 54, supp. (April 1, 1994): 1,976S–1,981S.

IU See INTERNATIONAL UNIT.

J

jam A preservative prepared from boiled SUGAR syrup and crushed or pureed FRUIT. Jams need a single cooking step. Fruits like ripe APPLES, QUINCES, currants, CRANBERRIES, GOOSEBERRIES, and PLUMS contain PECTIN, a complex carbohydrate that will gel upon cooling. Low-pectin fruit like BLUEBERRIES, APRICOTS, CHERRIES, BLACKBERRIES, GRAPES, and PINEAPPLE or stalks of RHUBARB have to be mixed with pectin—or pectin-containing fruits—to obtain a thicker consistency. Jam flavor reflects the amount of sugar used in syrup. The less sugar, the more pronounced the fruity flavor. Jam, like jelly, is a high-calorie, refined CARBOHYDRATE food: A quart of jam typically contains 2 to 2.5 cups of sugar. (See also NATURAL SWEETENER.)

jaundice A yellowing of skin, mucous membranes, and whites of the eyes due to the buildup of BILE PIGMENT (bilirubin) in the body. Jaundice itself is not a disease, but indicates an underlying problem.

Three conditions promote jaundice (bilirubin accumulation). Prehepatic jaundice reflects the excessive breakdown of red blood cells. Bilirubin is produced during the degradation of the red pigment of the oxygen-carrying protein HEMOGLOBIN during disposal of aged red blood cells. Bilirubin travels to the LIVER, where it is processed for excretion. In prehepatic jaundice the rate of bilirubin production exceeds the liver's ability to process incoming bilirubin, for example in hemolytic ANEMIA.

Hepatic jaundice reflects abnormal liver function. HEPATITIS, liver CIRRHOSIS, and certain liver diseases imbalance liver metabolism and decrease the liver's ability to process bilirubin.

Extrahepatic jaundice occurs when interference with BILE release from the GALLBLADDER forces bilirubin to back into the liver. Bile duct obstructions commonly include GALLSTONES. (See also DIGESTION; HEME.)

jejunum The middle segment of the small intestine. The jejunum is about 8 feet long and lies between the DUODENUM (the first 10 inches) and the ILEUM, the last 12 feet of small intestine. Like other regions of the small intestine, the jejunum possesses a large surface area due to its highly wrinkled surface. It is covered by numerous hair-like protrusions called VILLI. Furthermore, each villus cell surface is covered with microscopic projections called MICROVILLI. These physiologic features dramatically increase the absorptive area and aid nutrient absorption and assimilation. (See also DIGESTION; DIGESTIVE TRACT.)

jelly A sweet, thickened spread composed of boiled FRUIT juice. Jellies are used on toast and in biscuits and pastry. Commercial jelly contains at least 55 percent fruit. Home-prepared jellies can contain as much as 60 percent sugar. Jelly is therefore a source of refined CARBOHYDRATE and a high-calorie food with few nutrients other than sugar. Jelly requires two cooking steps. In the first, JUICE is extracted from the fruit and filtered. The clear juice is then cooked with sugar until a gel forms. Often juices are extracted by pressure cooking. However, high temperatures destroy PECTIN, a form of fiber required for gel formation. Pectin is added back in this case. (See also EMPTY CALORIES; NATURAL SWEETENER.)

joule The international scientific standard unit for ENERGY measurement used for all branches of science. Recommended by the International Organization for Standardization, the joule was adopted by the U.S. Bureau of Standards in 1964. One joule is equal to 4.184 calories and is a measure of mechanical energy while the calorie is based on heat (thermal energy). Nutrition references still use KILOCALORIES as a measure of energy in foods. For example, caloric values (in kilocalories) of foods are published by the USDA; they can be converted to kilojoules (thousands of joules, abbreviated kJ.) by multiplying the listed calories by 4.184.

juice The liquid extract of FRUITS and VEGETABLES. Juices typically contain only small amounts of FIBER and pulp, which are removed by filtration. Juices can be freshly prepared, concentrated, frozen, canned, or bottled. Juices contain sugars, soluble minerals, and vitamins that can be released when plant tissues are crushed or pulverized. Plant leaves yield green, chlorophyll-rich juices.

Preparing juices at home with juicers is popular in the United States. On the other hand, consumers spend more than $9 billion on prepared fruit juices and fruit drinks annually. These preparations are subject to food labeling regulations. The U.S. FDA does not require manufacturers to specify the amount of fruit juice used in a given juice. Manufacturers must list ingredients in order of predominance, but not by percentages. Listing percentages of ingredients would indicate the actual ratios of the more expensive juices such as kiwi, strawberry, or peach. If the product label specifies "juice" only, then the product contains only pure fruit juice. Any other designation indicates a diluted juice. Apple juice and white grape juice are among the least expensive juices to produce and are frequently used in mixtures. Proposals by the FDA would require manufacturers to reveal how much juice is actually in "juice cocktail" or "juice drink."

A juicer/juice extractor is a popular mechanical device that extracts juices from vegetables and fruits. Juicers pulverize the vegetable or fruit by rotary blades. The pulp, seeds, and skin are separated from the juice by centrifugal filtration. In contrast, blenders combine pulp and juice.

Fresh juices provide a convenient way of increasing consumption of vegetables and fruits while cutting back on SOFT DRINKS as part of a healthful diet that includes lower fat, more whole grains, vegetables, and fresh fruit. Eating whole fruits and vegetables can provide essential nutrients and lower the risk of cancer and help reduce the risk of diseases associated with deficiencies and aging. However, no juice is a panacea. Juicing removes most fiber and pulp, which retain significant amounts of vitamins, minerals, and perhaps as yet unknown materials that promote health. Fiber may have beneficial effects, including lowering the risk of colon cancer. There are few studies on the stability of vitamins in juices or on the efficacy of vitamins in the extracts.

Fresh juices served immediately are better than those stored because oxidation begins to change the color, flavor, and nutritional quality after the juice is made. Juice combinations of vegetables may begin to separate soon after they are made. The juice is only as good as the produce used; therefore, using organically grown produce and cleaning produce before juicing make sense when whole produce is to be juiced. Ginger and mint can improve the flavor of many juice mixtures. (See also AGING; BALANCED DIET.)

junk food A highly processed FOOD. Compared to unprocessed foods, junk foods generally contain less nutritive value beyond their caloric content due to added sugar, refined starch, fat or oils. Junk food therefore represents a major source of "empty calories" in the typical American diet. Junk food is often based on refined grains, such as white flour. Obvious examples include CHIPS, CRACKERS, doughnuts, cookies, packaged sweet snacks, and sugar-laden BREAKFAST CEREALS. Gelatin desserts, soft ice cream, candy and soft drinks fit into this category as well. One-third of the average American's diet is junk food, according to a recent study.

Potential Problems with Junk Food Diets

Individual foods are neither "good" nor "bad." Whether a food is appropriate depends on how much and how often it is eaten, as well as on the health and nutritional status of the individual consuming it. Reliance on junk food is often a direct cause of nutrient-deficient diets in the United States. Food manufacturing removes many nutrients; consequently, junk foods contain less FIBER;

less trace minerals such as ZINC, MANGANESE, SELENIUM, CALCIUM, CHROMIUM, COPPER, and IRON; and less vitamins like VITAMIN A, VITAMIN B_6, VITAMIN C, and FOLIC ACID than usually found in unprocessed or minimally processed foods. Simultaneously, food manufacturing adds many materials not present in the original whole food, including: salt, SUGAR, SATURATED FAT and OIL, synthetic preservatives like BHA and BHT, artificial colorings, and flavors. To partially correct for nutrient losses in processing, FLOUR and grain products (such as processed breakfast cereals) are enriched with NIACIN, THIAMIN, and RIBOFLAVIN to bring them up to the levels found in whole grain. However, enrichment replaces few of the vitamins and trace minerals, and none of the fiber lost during food manufacture.

Overnutrition is a second consequence of diets relying on junk foods. Junk food is a major source of surplus calories and saturated fat in the typical U.S. diet, and a high fat intake is directly tied to a higher risk of CANCER and coronary heart disease. Excessive junk food is a major cause of OBESITY, a critical health problem in the United States. Saturated fats—such as HYDROGENATED VEGETABLE OIL, COCONUT OIL or palm kernel oil, LARD, and BUTTER—generally increase CHOLESTEROL levels, perhaps setting the stage for clogged arteries. Characteristically, junk food contains large amounts of refined sweeteners such as high FRUCTOSE CORN SYRUP, DEXTROSE, maltose malt sugar, corn sweetener and HONEY, as well as SUCROSE.

On any given day 46 million Americans eat FAST FOOD, which now shapes many children's eating habits. Studies suggest that children between the ages of six and 11 are more likely to eat cookies than fruit for snacks. Children between one and five are just as likely to drink powdered and carbonated soft drinks as they are to drink orange juice. (See also CONVENIENCE FOOD; FOOD PROCESSING.)

Kant, Ashima. "Consumption of Energy-Dense, Nutrient-Poor Foods by Adult Americans; Nutritional and Health Implications. The Third National Health and Nutrition Examination Survey, 1988–1994," *American Journal of Clinical Nutrition* 72 (2000): 929–936.

juvenile diabetes See DIABETES MELLITUS.

K

kabob Chunks of seasoned meat grilled or roasted on skewers. The name comes from the Turkish *sis kebab,* meaning "skewered, roasted meat." Traditionally, marinated mutton or lamb is skewered with pork fat or mutton fat. American variations of ingredients include veal, meatballs, and vegetables like onions, peppers, mushrooms, and tomatoes. (See also BARBECUED MEAT.)

kale (*Brassica oleracea acephala*) A dark green, leafy vegetable of the cabbage family that is closely related to the European wild CABBAGE. There are many different leaf forms of kale, from curly to plain, and colors range from bluish-green to red-brown and purple. Kale withstands the stress of cold weather and severe frosts, and gardens can provide fresh greens into autumn.

Kale holds its texture when cooked, making it a useful ingredient in soups, meat loafs, stews, and the like. Eaten raw, it can be used in mixed salads. Kale can be blanched, steamed, sauteed, or microwaved. Like other leafy greens, kale contains high levels of BETA-CAROTENE (provitamin A). One cup, cooked (130 g), provides: 42 calories; protein, 3.5 g; carbohydrate, 7.3 g; fiber, 3.7 g; calcium, 94 mg; potassium, 296 mg; vitamin A, 962 retinol equivalents; thiamin, 0.07 mg; riboflavin, 0.009 mg; niacin, 0.70 mg; vitamin C, 53 mg. (See also CHARD; SPINACH.)

karaya gum A FOOD ADDITIVE that serves as a thickening agent and is not absorbed by the INTESTINE. Karaya GUM, obtained exclusively from the sterculia tree in India, prevents fats and oils from separating in whipped products and salad dressing and in the meat juices in sausages. It also improves the texture of ice cream and has been used as a LAXATIVE. Karaya gum is unique in that it expands to up to 100 times its dry volume when wet.

Some individuals are allergic to karaya gum, but it is presumably safer than other thickening agents since little of it is absorbed. However, long-term safety studies have not been performed. The question of whether this gum binds nutrients and prevents their absorption has not been resolved. (See also BULKING AGENTS.)

kasha Roasted BUCKWHEAT; a coarse or finely ground, hulled GRAIN that can be cooked like RICE. The roasting process conveys a nutlike flavor. Buckwheat is not a grass, therefore it is not related to the cereal grains. Individuals who are allergic to GLUTEN can often tolerate buckwheat. In the United States, buckwheat is most commonly eaten as an ingredient in pancakes. Kasha is also an eastern European dish. Russian kasha refers to small buckwheat pancakes. Polish kasha is a sweet pudding prepared either with BARLEY or with SEMOLINA.

kava (*Piper methysticum,* kawa) A plant native to South Pacific islands, where the root of the plant is often ground into the fine paste and used in a traditional ceremonial beverage. It has been sold in the United States as an herbal supplement to ease generalized anxiety, sleeplessness, and anxiety during menopause. In 2002 the U.S. FDA issued a consumer advisory warning that kava-containing products had been associated with liver-related injuries, including hepatitis, cirrhosis, and liver failure in patients taking normal doses for as little as 1 to 3 months. It is therefore not recommended; kava is banned in Switzerland and Germany is considering a ban.

kefir Fermented milk. A traditional beverage of the Middle East and southern Russia. Originally, kefir was prepared from camel's MILK; now cow's milk is fermented instead of camel's milk. The fermentation process produces LACTIC ACID, which gives kefir its tangy flavor. Fermentation also produces a low level of ALCOHOL (generally about 1 percent). One cup provides 150 calories; protein, 9.3 g; carbohydrate, 8.8 g; fat, 4.5 g; calcium, 350 mg; potassium, 205 mg; vitamin A, 155 mg; thiamin, 0.45 mg; riboflavin, 0.44 mg; niacin, 0.30 mg. (See also YOGURT.)

kelp See SEAWEED.

keratin A PROTEIN that is the major constituent of skin, hair, nails, and the protein matrix of tooth enamel. Keratin is a highly insoluble protein, classified as a structural protein. Its role in protecting the body is passive only. Alpha keratin occurs in mammals and consists of highly coiled protein chains that form insoluble fibers. This protein contains high levels of the sulfur-containing AMINO ACID, CYSTEINE. The cysteine sulfur atoms of adjacent keratin chains cross-link with each other, making keratin resistant to stretching and contributing to water insolubility and strength of hair. For this reason, keratin also resists digestion. Keratin in skin is softer than in hair and nails because it has less sulfur content, and therefore less cross-linking. Toxic HEAVY METALS bind to keratin in hair, and mineral analysis of hair samples can reveal the accumulation of toxic elements like LEAD, CADMIUM, or MERCURY. (See also HAIR ANALYSIS.)

ketchup (catsup) In North America, a thick tomato sauce used to flavor MEAT, FISH, HAMBURGERS, FRENCH FRIES, and HOT DOGS. Ketchup is made of tomato puree, SALT, VINEGAR, and a variety of spices, Typical ketchup contains 25 percent SUGAR and represents one of the hidden sources of this sweetener, though it is not considered sweet. One tablespoon (17 g) contains 18 calories; protein, 0.3 g; carbohydrate, 4.3 g; sodium, 156 mg; and trace levels of vitamins. (See also CONDIMENT; FOOD PROCESSING.)

keto acid A class of weak ACIDS with a carbon atom skeleton. The keto acids are more highly oxidized acids than FATTY ACIDS and appear as intermediates in metabolic pathways of the body, which oxidize fatty acids and CARBOHYDRATES for energy production. Keto acids contain a keto group, an oxidized carbon atom found in a class of organic compounds called ketones.

Typical keto acids of cellular METABOLISM include: PYRUVIC ACID (three carbon atoms), produced from the single sugar GLUCOSE by GLYCOLYSIS, the major pathway of glucose degradation. Alpha ketoglutaric acid (five carbon atoms) and OXALOACETIC ACID (four carbon atoms) are intermediates of the KREB'S CYCLE, the central energy-producing pathway of the cell. Oxaloacetic acid is important for several reasons. It is both the starting point and the end point of the KREB'S CYCLE. Furthermore, oxaloacetic acid can be converted to glucose for BLOOD SUGAR.

Keto acids are produced in the degradation of certain AMINO ACIDS by removal of their amino groups (nitrogen-containing groups). Thus, the amino acid ALANINE yields pyruvic acid; ASPARTIC ACID yields oxaloacetic acid; and GLUTAMIC ACID yields alpha ketoglutaric acid. The process is reversible so that an addition of an amino group to pyruvic acid forms alanine; to oxaloacetic acid, forms aspartic acid; an addition to alpha ketoglutaric acid forms glutamic acid. Because these amino acids are readily synthesized by the body from common keto acids, they are not essential to the diet. (See also AMINO ACID METABOLISM; CARBOHYDRATE METABOLISM; GLUCONEOGENESIS.)

ketogenic Refers to compounds converted to KETONE BODIES, a kind of metabolic acid, during their chemical breakdown for energy production. Ketogenic compounds include free FATTY ACIDS and the amino acid LEUCINE. Most amino acids are both ketogenic and "glycogenic"; that is, their complex structures are broken down into both ketone bodies and the sugar GLUCOSE. Excessive accumulation of ketone bodies may acidify the body, leading to imbalances. (See also ACIDOSIS; AMINO ACID METABOLISM.)

ketone bodies The water-soluble products of excessive fat breakdown. Ketone bodies represent ACETOACETIC ACID, BETA HYDROXYBUTYRIC ACID, and ACETONE, which are synthesized by the liver. They accumulate in the blood during prolonged fasting, STARVATION, crash DIETING, and ALCOHOLISM. Each of these conditions promotes high rates of fat degradation. Fatty acids cannot be completely oxidized for energy under these conditions and are instead converted to ketone bodies. The accumulation of ketone bodies in the blood and their excretion in the urine indicates a potentially hazardous metabolic imbalance. (See also ACIDOSIS; FAT METABOLISM; KETOSIS.)

ketosis The accumulation of KETONE BODIES in the blood due to incomplete oxidation of FATTY ACIDS. Excessive fat breakdown can occur during uncontrolled diabetes, ALCOHOLISM, crash DIETING, and with high-fat, low-carbohydrate diets. Prolonged high levels of ketone bodies (ACETOACETIC ACID and BETA HYDROXYBUTYRIC ACID), can acidify the blood (ACIDOSIS). Furthermore, ketone body excretion in the urine can lead to excessive water loss (starvation diuresis). DEHYDRATION is potentially hazardous. Ketosis causes disturbances in ELECTROLYTES (dissolved minerals like SODIUM, POTASSIUM, and CHLORIDE) in body fluids. Imbalanced electrolytes can alter heart function and nervous system responses. Severe ketosis can cause coma and, ultimately, death.

kidneys Organs that regulate the amounts of key ingredients in blood, including WATER, the pH (acidity) and the levels of minerals (ELECTROLYTES), and in excreted waste products. By regulating water excretion in urine, kidneys also regulate BLOOD PRESSURE. There are two kidneys, located close to the backbone at the back of the abdomen. Each is about 4 in. (10 cm) long and each contains approximately one million filtering units called NEPHRONS, resembling small tubes. The nephrons filter a huge amount of fluid; about 425 gallons (1,930 liters) per day for adults. However, only a very small fraction, (2 liters) is excreted as urine, because most of the water, and most of the other useful blood constituents, are reabsorbed and recycled.

Nephrons are supplied with blood from the kidney artery, and a small cluster or "tuft" of capillaries (glomerulus) feeds each nephron. The glomerulus acts as a filter under pressure. The filtrate, the fluid emerging from the glomerulus, contains small molecules like water, salts (dissolved minerals, SODIUM, POTASSIUM, CHLORIDE), GLUCOSE, UREA (the end product of protein degradation), and creatinine (the waste product of muscle metabolism). Larger particles like proteins and cells are retained in the blood by the glomerulus.

The filtrate passes through the convoluted tubules of the nephron, where most of the sodium chloride is reabsorbed into the blood. The tubules help regulate the sodium content and the pH of the blood by exchanging electrolytes like AMMONIA, potassium, and chloride. The final product is urine.

Glucose at normal blood concentrations is completely reabsorbed by the kidneys into the blood. In DIABETES MELLITUS the blood sugar concentration may be so high that more glucose appears in the filtrate than can be reabsorbed, and thus it passes into the urine (glucosuria). Because water follows the glucose, frequent urination accompanies glucose in the urine and may cause DEHYDRATION. Certain metabolic acids called KETONE BODIES may accumulate in the bloodstream with ALCOHOLISM, untreated diabetes, crash DIETING, and other situations. Once their levels exceed the kidney threshold, ketone bodies are excreted in the urine. This, too, can cause dehydration and electrolyte imbalances that further compromise the patient's health.

Urine represents the concentrated waste; 99 percent of the water has been reabsorbed by the time urine reaches the ureters, which are tubes that drain into the bladder. The kidneys regulate water balance. If there is too much fluid in the body, the kidneys excrete more water as urine. When there is too little fluid, they retain more water and urine becomes more concentrated. Environmental temperature also affects kidney function because sweating increases water losses, prompting the kidneys to retain more water. Kidneys add potassium and hydrogen ions, ammonia, and bicarbonate to the filtrate to control blood pH.

HORMONES regulate kidney function. Water retention can be regulated by a pituitary hormone, ANTIDIURETIC HORMONE (ADH). Release of this hormone is stimulated when the brain (HYPOTHALAMUS) detects a low blood-water concentration. ADH increases water loss from cells, allowing more water to pass back into the blood. ALDOSTERONE, a hormone from the adrenal glands, regulates sodium excretion. If the sodium level drops, for example from sweating or DIARRHEA, aldosterone levels increase, salt reabsorption from the filtrate increases, and water is retained.

The kidneys also process hormones. VITAMIN D is activated by the kidneys; they convert calcidiol (25-hydroxyvitamin D) to the hormone calcitriol (1,25 dihydroxyvitamin D). They also produce erythropoietin, a hormone that stimulates BONE marrow to produce RED BLOOD CELLS, and renin, a hormone that controls blood pressure. (See also BLADDER INFECTIONS; GLOMERULAR FILTRATION; KIDNEY STONES.)

kidney stones Mineralized particles occurring in the kidney and upper urinary tract. Most kidney stones contain CALCIUM as carbonate, phosphate, or oxalate. In the United States, they are quite common and more prevalent than stone formation in the gallbladder. An estimated 10 percent of men and 15 percent of women over 30 years of age will eventually develop kidney stones.

A kidney stone is formed when the concentration of mineral salts in urine increases to the point of saturation, at which time the mineral will spontaneously crystallize. DEHYDRATION and increased calcium in urine favor stone formation. High urinary calcium can reflect a high intake of VITAMIN D, too much ALUMINUM or MILK, overactive THYROID (hyperthyroidism), lengthy immobilization, or kidney disease. Calcium oxalate stones are more likely with vitamin B_6 deficiency; with high consumption of foods like SPINACH rich in the organic acid OXALIC ACID; intestinal disease (particularly of the ileum); fatty stools; and abnormal metabolism of certain organic acids.

Possible Causes

Certain metabolic diseases, such as parathyroid malfunction and certain diseases of the bone, can cause kidney stones. MILK ALKALI SYNDROME is associated with an increased risk. Many toxic metals, especially CADMIUM, increase the risk of stone formation. In addition, several dietary factors are often linked. Inadequate water intake prompts the formation of insoluble salts. Inadequate VITAMIN K could promote stone formation because the vitamin assists in the synthesis of a protein that inhibits stone formation. INSULIN insensitivity and OBESITY increase the risk of stone formation. Certain foods contain high oxalic acid levels; therefore, reduced intake of COCOA, tea, spinach, chard beet leaves, RHUBARB, and PARSLEY decreases the risk. Consuming more FIBER-rich foods, like fruit and vegetables, is likely to decrease the risk of kidney stones. VITAMIN B_6 deficiency is also linked to oxalate-stone formation. URIC ACID occasionally forms stones, a process favored by the excessive consumption of nucleic acid-rich foods like yeast and organ meats, and by certain anticancer drugs.

The prevention of kidney stones relies on dietary changes:

- Drinking plenty of water. Adequate water is needed to keep salts dissolved.
- Avoiding sugar, refined carbohydrate, and excessive animal protein, salt, and caffeine. These tend to increase the level of calcium in urine.
- Avoiding cola soft drinks. These contain phosphate, which promotes stone formation.
- Avoiding over-consumption of aluminum containing antacids.
- Minimizing alcohol consumption. High alcohol consumption favors dehydration.
- Emphasizing magnesium-rich foods. Magnesium deficiency is linked to kidney stone formation, so eating foods with a high magnesium content—barley, wheat bran and other whole grains, avocados, bananas and lima beans—or supplements can reduce the risk.
- Citric acid keeps calcium solubilized, and citric acid supplementation has been used to reduce the incidence of kidney stones.

(See also GALLSTONES.)

Burtis, William J. et al. "Dietary Hypercalciuria in Patients with Calcium Oxalate Kidney Stones," *American Journal of Clinical Nutrition* 60, no. 3 (September 1994): 424–429.

kilocalorie A measure of ENERGY content frequently used in nutrition. The term CALORIE is frequently used synonymously with kilocalorie although strictly speaking it should be capitalized (Calorie). The prefix "kilo" means 1,000. Thus, one kilocalorie (abbreviated kC.) is the amount of heat required to increase the temperature of 1,000 g(1 l) of water by 1° C (from 15.5° C to 16.5° C), while a calorie (small c.) refers to heating 1 g of water by 1° C. The caloric content of foods and daily energy requirements are given in kilocalories. A small calorie is one-thousandth of a kilocalorie. However, the international standard for energy content is based on the JOULE; 1 kilocalorie equals 4.18 kilojoules.

kiwi fruit ***(Actinidia chinensis)*** An egg-sized fruit that originated in China and is now cultivated in New Zealand, France, Israel, and California. Kiwi fruit has a thin, brown, hairy skin. The fruit is pale green with a tangy taste and is eaten raw, used in fruit salads and tarts or as a garnish with meat and fish. Each raw fruit (46 g, peeled) provides 46 calories; protein, 0.8 g; carbohydrate, 11.3 g; fiber, 1.16 g; calcium, 15 mg; potassium, 80 mg; vitamin C, 31 mg; thiamin, 0.02 mg; riboflavin, 0.01 mg; niacin, 0.06 mg.

kohlrabi ***(Brassica oleracea, var. caulorapo)*** A stem vegetable of the CABBAGE family. Its bulbous stalk (resembling a turnip) distinguishes its appearance from other members of the cabbage family. Kohlrabi was popular in the Middle Ages in central and eastern Europe. Currently, kohlrabi is grown in California. Kohlrabi is a source of VITAMIN C, CALCIUM, and IRON. Small stems are more tender than the more mature vegetable. It is cooked like a turnip or celery root. Cooked, sliced kohlrabi (1 cup, 165 g) provides 48 calories; protein, 3 g; carbohydrate, 11.4 g; fiber, 2.3 g; calcium, 50 mg; iron, 0.66 mg; potassium, 561 mg; vitamin C, 89 mg; thiamin, 0.07 mg; riboflavin, 0.03 mg; niacin, 0.64 mg. (See also CELERIAC.)

kombu See SEAWEED.

konjac ***(Amorphophallus konjac)*** A tuber cultivated in the Far East that is a traditional ingredient in Japanese cooking. The tuber is processed to yield a light-colored flour. Konjac has been used to make noodles (shiritaki noodles) and heat-stable gels such as mitsumame, a fruit dessert. The flour is used in food processing as a thickener for soups, sauces, and desserts. Konjac flour provides a form of FIBER, a complex carbohydrate called GLUCOMANNAN that forms viscous solutions in water. When added to processed foods, konjac helps other plant-based thickeners like CARRAGEENAN, XANTHAN GUM, and CORNSTARCH work more efficiently. (See also FOOD ADDITIVES; PASTA; THICKENING AGENTS.)

kosher Foods permitted by Jewish law. Jewish dietary laws, known as kashruth, define the fitness and appropriateness of foods. Acceptable and unacceptable foods fall into three food groups: *Milchig* refers to dairy products and MILK; *fleishig* refers to MEAT, fowl, and products derived from them; and *pareve* refers to foods that can be eaten with either milk or meat. These neutral foods are FRUITS, VEGETABLES, GRAINS, FISH, and EGGS. Acceptable fish have fins and scales; SHELLFISH are excluded. Domestic fowl are permitted, as are animals with a split hoof that chew cud, a group that includes cattle, goats, sheep, and deer. Pigs (pork) are not acceptable. CONVENIENCE FOOD is not kosher unless certified by rabbinical authority, signified by the name and insignia on the package. BREAD must be baked by observant Jews under rabbinical supervision. Bread is normally a pareve food.

All meat and fowl must be killed according to prescribed methods. Kosher slaughter involves the use of a sharp knife to quickly sever the carotid arteries, jugular bone, and windpipe of a live animal by a trained slaughterer (*schochet*). Kosher slaughter of poultry must also be done by hand. Some Jews follow a stricter interpretation of rules concerning acceptability. *Glatt* kosher meat means the organs, especially the lungs of kosher-killed animals, have been inspected for blemishes or defects. Glatt kosher meat and must be soaked and salted within 72 hours of slaughter.

GRAPE JUICE and WINE, traditionally used in religious ceremonies, must be prepared by observant Jews. To be kosher, grape juice must be properly separated and heated. If grape-flavored sodas with real fruit juice are not prepared in this way, the soda is not kosher. The Union of Orthodox Jewish Congregations of America has published guidelines regarding the kosher status of food and beverage ingredients.

Jews who keep kosher may not eat insects. This poses a problem for fresh produce, especially green, leafy vegetables, which may require inspection. Aphids are a common problem, and fresh produce from health food stores and roadside outlets requires inspection.

The Passover holiday has additional kosher requirements extending over an eight-day period. Many products, kosher for the rest of the year, are not kosher for Passover. Leavened grain and related materials are avoided to commemorate the departure of the Jews from Egypt. Legumes, corn, rice, and mustard are not eaten during Passover by Jews of European ancestry.

To separate meat and dairy, the kosher kitchen employs two sets of pots, pans, dishes, utensils, and table linen to be used separately for dairy and meat. Pareve foods can be prepared and eaten with either set. The utensils are washed and stored separately. Currently, an estimated 500,000 families in the United States and perhaps 50,000 families in Canada abide by kosher dietary laws. Some non-Jewish groups, such as Seventh Day Adventists and Muslims, sometimes purchase specific kosher foods to meet their religious needs, and some consumers consider the kosher seal an indicator of quality. (See also EATING PATTERNS.)

Kreb's cycle (citric acid cycle, tricarboxylic acid cycle) A branch of metabolism consisting of a coordinated sequence of enzymes that operate in a cyclic fashion to oxidize the major fuels of the body to produce ENERGY. The Kreb's cycle is a major METABOLIC PATHWAY and produces approximately 90 percent of the body's energy production by oxidizing FATTY ACIDS, AMINO ACIDS, and CARBOHYDRATES to carbon dioxide. The Kreb's cycle occurs in MITOCHONDRIA, particles in the cell's cytoplasm that function as cellular powerhouses.

Prior to entering the Kreb's cycle, fuel molecules are broken down to ACETIC ACID, a two-carbon molecule that is attached to a carrier molecule called COENZYME A. The product, ACETYL COENZYME, feeds into the Kreb's cycle. The acetic acid unit (two carbon atoms) combines with a simple acid with four carbon atoms, OXALOACETIC ACID, to create CITRIC ACID (six carbon atoms), the first true product of the Kreb's cycle. Subsequent oxidations release carbon dioxide and regenerated oxaloacetic acid, which can again react with incoming acetyl COA to continue the cycle.

Certain B complex VITAMINS support energy production from food in part because they assist the Kreb's cycle. They include NIACIN, RIBOFLAVIN, PANTOTHENIC ACID, and THIAMIN. B vitamins must first be converted to a COENZYME or enzyme helper to catalyze chemical reactions performed by the cycle. Thus, coenzyme A is the coenzyme form of pantothenic acid.

The Kreb's cycle is coupled with other pathways supporting energy production by mitochondria, the cell's powerhouses. Coenzymes of niacin and riboflavin, as well as COENZYME Q, carry electrons from the oxidations of the Kreb's cycle to the terminal ELECTRON TRANSPORT CHAIN, which reduces OXYGEN to form WATER and simultaneously forms ATP, the cell's energy currency. When the Kreb's cycle slows down, this slowdown inhibits glucose oxidation, allowing it to be shunted to storage mechanisms by the liver. (See also CARBOHYDRATE METABOLISM; FAT METABOLISM.)

Barron, John T., Stephen I. Kopp, and June Tow. "Fatty Acid, Tricarboxylic Acid Cycle Metabolites and Energy Metabolism in Vascular Smooth Muscle," *American Journal of Physiology* 267 (August 1994): Part 2, H764–H769.

kudzu (*Pueraria lobata*) A fibrous root vegetable, native to subtropical Asia; kudzu is used as a source of complex carbohydrate. It is chopped into cubes and cooked with soups in order to thicken them, and is available in Asian food markets. The food value, in 100 g (raw) is: calories, 120; protein, 2.1 g; carbohydrate, 27.8 g; fiber, 0.7 g; and essentially no fat. (See also STARCH.)

kumquat (*Fortunella spp.*) A small CITRUS FRUIT, with a sweet rind and a sour pulp. Kumquats are about the size of a quail's egg and have a thin, orange-red skin that is eaten with the fruit. Kumquats originated in China and are now cultivated in Australia, the Far East, Florida, and California. Kumquats can be eaten raw with skins, in jam and in baked goods like cakes. Nutrient content of one fruit (raw, 20 g) provides 12 calories; protein, 0.17 g; carbohydrate, 3.1 g; fiber, 0.7 g; vitamin C, 7.1 mg; thiamin, 0.02 mg; riboflavin, 0.02 mg.

kwashiorkor A severe malnutrition disease caused by a chronic protein-deficient diet. Kwashiorkor is the classic protein deficiency disease in which caloric intake may be adequate, but consumption of too little PROTEIN causes serious MALNUTRITION. Protein and ENERGY are required for growth and maintenance of the body. People consuming too little food to supply either will degrade their own body protein and fat. Thus, protein malnutrition and energy malnutrition overlap. Symptoms include EDEMA, apathy, decreased resistance to disease, delayed development, depigmented hair, and scaly skin. Symptoms in children include bloated belly, DIARRHEA, fatty liver, and ANEMIA.

Kwashiorkor is more common in developing tropical and subtropical nations. In low socioeconomic regions of Africa, the Near East, Asia, and Central and South America, the disease often begins with the birth of a second child. The weaned, first-born child must then rely on cereals, often a protein-deficient diet within the community. This does not supply enough amino acids to maintain a child, nor to support growth. It can be prevented by diets providing adequate protein and energy to meet the child's growth requirements. (See also BALANCED DIET; HUNGER, WORLD; STARVATION.)

L

label See FOOD LABELING.

labile Refers to the chemical alteration of molecules, often leading to the loss of biological function. Cells are composed of a huge array of molecules ranging from ultra-stable, very simple minerals like SODIUM chloride to complex molecules assembled from carbon atoms (organic compounds). Very large molecules (macromolecules) such as PROTEINS, and nucleic acids like DNA and RNA, are among the most complex organic molecules in the body. Macromolecules are hundreds to many thousands of times larger than simple sugar molecules. Such huge molecules tend to be fragile: They are easily altered with heat, cooking, or by acidic or alkaline conditions.

Certain nutrients are labile as well: Dissolved VITAMIN C is readily oxidized by air, while excessive cooking destroys the B complex vitamins THIAMIN and FOLIC ACID. Baking dough at high temperatures can destroy the essential amino acid LYSINE in wheat protein. Polyunsaturated FATTY ACIDS, major constituents of fats and oils, are readily oxidized when exposed to air, light, and heat; fat RANCIDITY (decomposition) is the culmination of this process. Internal processes can destroy biomolecules as well. Certain hormone-like derivatives of ESSENTIAL FATTY ACIDS, PROSTAGLANDINS, and LEUKOTRIENES are exceedingly labile and break down in a matter of seconds. The chemical currency of the cells, ATP, survives only minutes in cells before being broken down (hydrolyzed). (See also FREE RADICALS.)

lactalbumin The major protein of whey, which is the soluble protein fraction remaining after MILK has curdled. Untreated cow's milk contains 20 percent lactalbumin and 80 percent CASEIN. Lactalbumin occurs in two forms, alpha-lactalbumin and beta-lactalbumin. Alpha-lactalbumin is a constituent of lactose synthetase, the enzyme that synthesizes LACTOSE (milk sugar). In a milk allergy, the immune system recognizes as foreign a milk protein such as lactalbumin. It will mount an allergic response when exposed to this food constituent. (See also ALLERGY, FOOD; ANTIGEN.)

lactase The intestinal enzyme that digests LACTOSE (milk sugar). Lactase breaks down lactose to its simple sugar building blocks, GLUCOSE and FRUCTOSE. This is an essential step in digestion because lactose itself cannot be absorbed by the intestine into the bloodstream, while glucose and fructose are readily absorbed. No other digestive enzyme can perform this task.

Intestinal lactase levels are high during infancy and early childhood, until the age of five to six. Whether lactase activity persists into adulthood is genetically determined. In most populations of the world, lactase activity and the ability to digest milk drop dramatically after weaning ("primary lactase deficiency"). In contrast, northern and western Europeans and their descendants often maintain high lactase levels throughout adulthood. Secondary lactase deficiency can occur as a result of intestinal disease. For example, infection by an intestinal parasite giardia (GIARDIASIS) correlates with and often causes gut inflammation and lactase deficiency. (See also FOOD SENSITIVITY; LACTOSE INTOLERANCE.)

lactase deficiency See LACTOSE INTOLERANCE.

lactic acid (lactate) A common acidic food additive. Lactic acid is used as an acidifier in CHEESE, carbonated fruit, beverages, frozen desserts, and green olives. It prevents discoloration of fruit and vegetables. Calcium lactate, the calcium salt of lactic acid, is used in condensed milk and powdered milk. Certain bacteria like lactobacillus degrade carbohydrate to lactic acid. Commercial lactic acid is produced by fermenting CORNSTARCH, MOLASSES, potato starch, or whey. Lactic acid bacteria ferment milk sugar (LACTOSE) in the formation of cottage cheese, YOGURT, and sour milk. Fermentation in SAUERKRAUT and related food processing yields lactic acid, which acts as a preservative. Lactic acid is naturally produced in the body by glycolysis, the enzyme system in the body that degrades the simple sugar GLUCOSE to provide energy without the participation of oxygen. Lactic acid is produced by muscles during strenuous exercise, when oxygen availability is limited. Lactic acid buildup is partially responsible for muscle cramps and FATIGUE related to vigorous EXERCISE. Lactic acid migrates out of muscle cells into the bloodstream. It is carried to the liver, where it changes back to glucose. The liver releases glucose to be returned to muscles and again broken down to lactic acid.

Venema, G. et al. *Lactic Acid Bacteria: Genetics, Metabolism and Applications.* New York: Kluwer Academic Publishers, 1996.

Lactobacillus acidophilus A beneficial, acid-producing bacterium that is normally found in the healthy intestine. *Lactobacillus* species, which tend to occupy the lower portion of the gut, are considered "friendly bacteria" because they produce nutrients like vitamins (BIOTIN, VITAMIN K) and short-chain fatty acids, especially BUTYRIC ACID, used as fuels by the intestinal lining. These bacteria help combat disease-causing microorganisms; they produce factors that inhibit the growth of undesirable organisms and, by filling an ecological niche, they prevent them from proliferating. Many potential pathogens do not thrive in an acidic, anaerobic environment that is created by beneficial bacteria. Extensive exposure to "broad-spectrum" antibiotics like penicillin and tetracycline destroys beneficial intestinal bacteria as well as the disease-producing bacteria, leaving the intestine prone to overgrowth by yeast and other species. In clinical trials strains of other lactic acid bacteria (*Lactobacillus rhamnosus*) have been used in children with diarrhea from rotavirus infection to reduce symptoms of diarrhea in malnourished children, and to prevent diarrhea associated with antibiotic use in children. (See also ACIDOPHILUS; *CANDIDA ALBICANS;* INTESTINAL FLORA.)

lactoferrin An IRON-binding protein in BREAST MILK. Lactoferrin helps block the growth of potentially pathogenic bacteria that require IRON for growth in the infant's intestine. Lactoferrin secretion varies among healthy women for unknown reasons. (See also LACTALBUMIN.)

lacto-ovo-vegetarian A person who eats no red MEAT, FISH, or fowl. The diet consists of FRUIT, GRAINS, VEGETABLES, seeds, nuts, MILK, and EGGS. (See also VEGETARIAN.)

lactose (milk sugar) The major carbohydrate of MILK. This sugar is a primary energy source for infants. It also improves intestinal absorption of CALCIUM and other minerals. Because the human INTESTINE does not absorb lactose, it must be digested to be used. Lactose digestion occurs in the intestine of infants, growing children, and some adults. The enzyme LACTASE breaks down lactose to its simple sugar constituents GALACTOSE and GLUCOSE, which are easily absorbed into the bloodstream by the intestine. Glucose is used directly; galactose is converted to glucose by the liver. A deficiency of lactase in adults leads to LACTOSE INTOLERANCE (lactose maldigestion).

Lactose is a very common, safe FOOD ADDITIVE. It enhances flavors and helps in the browning of baked goods such as BREAD, waffles, biscuits, and brownies. Lactose may also be found in frozen VEGETABLES, soups, salad dressing, cereals, breakfast drinks, sauces, hot chocolate, gravies, sherbet, processed meat, and cake mixes. Lactose is also used to manufacture pills because it makes firm tablets when compressed. It is included in 20 percent of prescription pills and 5 percent of nonprescription pills.

lactose intolerance An adverse reaction to MILK and dairy products due to the inability to digest milk sugar (lactose). Lactose is the primary carbohydrate in cow and human milk. Lactose intolerance is the result of a deficiency of lactase, the intestinal enzyme responsible for lactose digestion. Lactose intolerance represents a FOOD SENSITIVITY, not a food ALLERGY, and the IMMUNE SYSTEM is not involved.

Lactase is normally produced until early childhood. In adults, production of this enzyme is genetically controlled. Large populations are deficient in lactase. In the United States, lactose intolerance occurs in 79 percent of Native Americans, 75 percent of African Americans, 51 percent of Hispanics, and 21 percent of whites. In Asia, Africa, and Latin America, the prevalence ranges from 15 percent to 100 percent of the population. A secondary lactase enzyme deficiency, parasitic infections like giardiasis intestinal damage from prolonged use of nonsteroidal antiinflammatory drugs can also lead to lactose intolerance.

When undigested lactose reaches the COLON, it is fermented by bacteria to produce acids and gases: methane, hydrogen, and carbon dioxide. In excess, these fermentation products can cause symptoms such as abdominal bloating, DIARRHEA, and stomach cramps. Lactose intolerance covers a range of sensitivities. Some individuals who maldigest lactose may be able to consume a small amount of lactose, such as a cup of milk (8 g of lactose), without symptoms. The type of dairy product also determines symptoms. YOGURT containing viable cultures of bacteria used in its preparation, such as *Lactobacillus bulgaricus,* contains less lactose and may be tolerated. Aged cheese also contains less lactose, and it may not cause symptoms, especially if aged for six months or more. Cheese manufacture discards most of the lactose as whey; aging of cheeses converts the remaining lactose to LACTIC ACID. Enzyme-treated milk can help reduce symptoms. Commercially prepared lactase drops can be added to milk to lower the lactose content by 70 percent after 24 hours in the refrigerator. Alternatively, lactase tablets can be ingested before eating dairy foods to lower lactose burden.

Lactose intolerance can be confirmed by medical diagnosis. The test involves ingesting 50 g of lactose in water (for fasting adults). After ingestion, the extent to which lactose is digested can be measured indirectly by assessing an increase in the level of blood glucose, or by measuring hydrogen produced by intestinal fermentation by breath testing.

Aranda-Michel, Jaime. *Living Well with Lactose Intolerance.* New York: Avon, 1999.

laetrile A compound that has been used as an anticancer treatment in humans worldwide but that has not been approved by the U.S. Food and Drug Administration (FDA) as a treatment for cancer in the United States. Although the drug is manufactured and distributed as a cancer treatment in Mexico, variations in commercial preparations of laetrile have been documented, with incorrect product labels and samples contaminated with bacteria and other substances.

Because of several court cases in the 1970s that challenged the FDA's role in determining which drugs should be available to cancer patients, laetrile was legalized in more than 20 states. In 1980 the U.S. Supreme Court overturned decisions by the lower courts, reaffirming the FDA's position that drugs must be proven both safe and effective before permitting widespread use in humans.

The term *laetrile* is an acronym (laevorotatory and mandelonitrile) used to describe a purified form of the chemical amygdalin, which is a plant compound that contains sugar and produces cyanide. Amygdalin is found in the pits of many fruits and raw nuts and in other plants such as lima beans, clover, and sorghum. Cyanide is believed to be the active cancer-killing ingredient in laetrile.

Although the names *laetrile, Laetrile,* and *amygdalin* are often used interchangeably, they are not the same product. The chemical makeup of Laetrile, which was patented in the United States, is different from the laetrile and amygdalin produced in Mexico. The patented Laetrile is a semisynthetic form of amygdalin, while the laetrile and amygdalin manufactured in Mexico is made from crushed apricot pits.

Amygdalin was first isolated in 1830 and was first used as an anticancer agent in Russia as early as 1845. However, it was not used as a chemotherapy drug in the United States as a treatment for cancer until the 1920s. Work with the compound was discontinued when scientists decided that the early pill form of amygdalin was too toxic. In the 1950s a reportedly nontoxic semisynthetic form of amygdalin was developed and patented in the United States as Laetrile. Laetrile gained popularity in the 1970s as an anticancer agent and as part of a special treatment program involving a special diet, high-dose vitamin supplements, and pancreatic enzymes (proteins that help digest food). By 1978 more than 70,000 people in the United States had reportedly been treated with Laetrile.

Despite numerous studies of laetrile in the lab and with animals, there has been little evidence that it is effective against cancer. In 1978 the National Cancer Institute (NCI) requested case reports from practitioners who believed their patients had benefited from treatment with laetrile. Of the 93 cases submitted the NCI considered 67 complete enough to be evaluated. An expert panel concluded that two of the 67 had complete responses and that the tumors in four people grew smaller.

Based on these six cases, the NCI sponsored clinical studies with laetrile in the late 1970s and early 1980s. Results were negative, and the NCI concluded that no further investigation of laetrile was necessary. No controlled clinical trials of laetrile have been conducted.

Side Effects

The side effects associated with laetrile are similar to the symptoms of cyanide poisoning, including nausea, vomiting, headache, dizziness, bluish discoloration of the skin, liver damage, very low blood pressure, droopy upper eyelids, walking problems, fever, confusion, coma, and death. The side effects worsen if the patient simultaneously eats raw almonds, crushed fruit pit, certain types of fruits and vegetables including celery, peaches, bean sprouts, and carrots or takes high doses of vitamin C. The side effects of laetrile also appear to depend on the method of administration; taking laetrile by mouth results in more severe side effects than when it is given by injection.

lamb The flesh of a young sheep. It is considered a red MEAT. In practice, lambs or yearlings fall into the lamb category, while mutton refers to adult sheep. Mutton is much darker muscle meat than lamb meat and has a stronger flavor. While mutton is eaten in other parts of the world, lamb is preferred in North America because of its juiciness, tenderness, and flavor. The fat is highly saturated, like beef tallow. Lamb accounts for only about 1 percent of the total meat production in the United States, and Americans generally eat less than two pounds per person per year on average. Lamb chops (cooked, 2.2 oz, 63 g) provide 220 calories; protein, 20 g; fat 15 g; cholesterol, 7.7 mg; calcium, 16 mg; iron, 1.5 mg; thiamin, 0.04 mg; riboflavin, 0.16 mg; niacin, 4.4 mg. (See also PORK.)

lamina propria The layer of connective tissue lying beneath the lining of the gastrointestinal tract. This layer surrounds the DIGESTIVE TRACT and contains lymph vessels and lymph nodes, masses of lymphatic tissue, and blood vessels. Blood and lymph vessels transport absorbed nutrients to other parts of the body. The lamina propria protects the body against disease because it releases an ANTIBODY called secretory IgA to help neutralize the huge load of foreign materials to which the digestive tract is subjected with each meal. Secretory IgA binds potentially pathogenic organisms to prevent them from attaching to the mucosal lining; it also binds food proteins and other foreign materials and limits their penetration into the body. (See also ANTIGEN; INTESTINE.)

La Pacho (*Tabebuia avellanedae*) Also known as *pau d'Arco* or *taheebo*. This is a tree from South America that produces bark with medicinal properties. La Pacho has a long history of folk use in treating infections.

The tree produces a complex mixture of quinones, which are compounds with complex, oxygen-containing ring structures, including lapachol.

Extracts possess strong antimicrobial activity. They are effective against the yeast *CANDIDA ALBICANS*, staphylococcus, and other disease-producing bacteria, as well as against certain parasitic infections. Extracts of La Pacho bark have been used to reduce inflammation and vaginitis. A beverage is prepared by boiling the whole bark in water. In South America, La Pacho is used to treat certain forms of cancer and infections. Although isolated ingredients in high amounts may produce anemia and increase blood clotting in animals after long-term usage. La Pacho is possibly unsafe with typical oral doses. Safety evaluations have not been performed using typical doses, however, toxicity has occurred with higher doses.

lard FAT released from cooking and processing of PORK. One of the highest grades of lard is kettle-rendered lard, prepared from fat trimmings. Refined lard is bleached and purified and has a mild flavor. Commercial lard contains added hydrogenated fat to increase its melting point to make it firmer. The antioxidants—BHA, BHT, VITAMIN E, and PROPYLGALLATE—retard RANCIDITY. Lard is considered a saturated fat.

Like all fat, lard provides nine calories per gram. Lard consumption in the United States has steadily declined since 1950 from a yearly per capita consumption of 13 pounds to less than two pounds. Lard is used commercially in processed foods such as baked beans, chili, baked goods like muffins, and refried beans. VEGETABLE SHORTENING has largely replaced home use. Shortening is prepared from hydrogenated COTTONSEED OIL, PEANUT oil, SOYBEAN oil or COCONUT OIL, and mixtures of vegetable oils and animal fat. (See also BEEF TALLOW; HYDROGENATED VEGETABLE OIL.)

lasagna A PASTA or dried wheat dough cut in wide ribbons. The flat ribbons are usually cooked with alternating layers of minced meat topped with tomato sauce and cheese. Green lasagna is flavored with SPINACH, and pink lasagna is flavored with tomatoes. Typical of pasta, hard glutinous wheat is used to make flour for lasagna. To prepare this form of pasta, paste made from moistened flour is shaped by pressing it through extruders; then it is dried. (See also MACARONI; STARCH.)

lathrogen A toxic substance found in certain members of the pea family that can cause lathyrism, a condition characterized by muscular weakness and spastic paralysis of the legs. CHICKPEAS, the flat podded vetch (*Lathyrus cicera*) and the Spanish vetchling (*L. clymenum*) possess an amino acid (beta N-oxayl.L-alpha beta diaminopropionic acid) that is toxic to nerve cells. Outbreaks of lathyrism have occurred in certain regions of North Africa and Asia after poor wheat crops and famine when seeds of the Lathyrus family were harvested for food. (See also FOOD SENSITIVITY.)

lauric acid A saturated FATTY ACID occurring in MEDIUM-CHAIN TRIGLYCERIDES, a readily absorbable and easily metabolized oil. Lauric acid occurs in small amounts in BUTTER, COCONUT OIL, PALM OIL, and several other vegetable oils. Because it contains 12 carbon atoms, it is classified as a medium-chain fatty acid. The more common long-chain saturated fatty acids in the body possess 16 carbons (PALMITIC ACID) or 18 carbons (STERIC ACID). All of these fatty acids are "saturated," that is, they are filled up with hydrogen atoms. (See also FAT; SHORT-CHAIN FATTY ACIDS; TRIGLYCERIDES.)

laxative A material or drug that induces bowel movements to relieve CONSTIPATION. Laxatives can be classified as BULKING AGENTS, which increase the water content of the stool; as agents that increase bowel contraction; and as lubricating agents.

Bulking agents are the safest laxatives. BRAN, and other vegetable-based natural FIBERS, such as flaxseed, and fiber-rich foods will soften the stool by absorbing water and encouraging rapid transit through the digestive tract. Bulking agents can interfere with absorption of some vitamins and medications (aspirin, digitalis, antibiotics, anticoagulants) and should be taken between doses of medications.

Certain medications increase water content by drawing water into the intestine, thus softening the stool. MAGNESIUM salts, Epsom salts and milk of magnesia all have this effect. Lubricants include mineral oil and glycerin suppositories. The prolonged use of mineral oil blocks the uptake of minerals (ZINC, CALCIUM, and POTASSIUM) and of VITAMINS A, D, E, and K, and excessive use can promote OSTEOMALACIA, a soft bone disease. In general, laxatives should not be used extensively without medical supervision because they can mask root causes of persistent constipation such as colon cancer, kidney disease, underactive thyroid gland, mental depression, improper diet, or lack of exercise. (See also PSYLLIUM.)

LDL See LOW-DENSITY LIPOPROTEIN.

lead A toxic HEAVY METAL and widespread industrial pollutant. People today have a thousand times more lead in their bones than did their prehistoric forebears. By 1980, almost one-third of urban Americans had seriously high levels of lead in their blood. This led the EPA to ban leaded gasoline and leaded paints; subsequently, the percentage of Americans with high lead levels has fallen to 2 percent of the population. However, lead poisoning remains an epidemic for children. According to the Centers for Disease Control and Prevention, nearly one in 20 American children suffer from lead poisoning, and lead affects more than 1 million children under age six. Pregnant women, young children and elderly people are most sensitive to lead. Chronic lead exposure among children remains a concern because the average amount detected is enough to cause subtle lead poisoning. The United States Public Health Service estimates between 3 and 4 million children under the age of five may suffer delayed development due to lead toxicity, and some children one to three years old who are exposed to lead may suffer permanent damage (lowered IQ). About 1.5 million schoolchildren have high enough lead levels in their blood to cause serious health problems.

Symptoms of subacute lead poisoning include distractibility, diarrhea, irritability, and lethargy. More serious consequences are smaller fetal brain size, increased birth defects, hearing difficulties, impaired memory, and decreased IQ. These may lead to an individual being stigmatized as a slow learner or underachiever. Children should have less than 10 micrograms per deciliter (10 μg/dl) of blood lead concentration. Lead hinders children's growth. Lead may affect the pituitary gland, or it may inhibit factors guiding bone growth. Growth hormone and insulin-like growth factor production diminish with lead exposure, as does another pituitary hormone, thyroid stimulating hormone. Adults run an increased risk of high blood pressure and decreased male fertility with lead exposure.

Symptoms of acute lead poisoning include severe ANEMIA, hair loss, CHRONIC FATIGUE, pallor, headache, CONSTIPATION, aching limbs, kidney disease, high blood pressure, nerve damage (hearing loss and mental retardation), GOUT, and sometimes coma. Diets low in CALCIUM, IRON, and ZINC increase lead absorption, while increased calcium absorption blocks lead uptake.

Sources of Lead Contamination

Glazed Ceramics Glazed dinnerware can be deadly because the pigments often contain lead. Poorly glazed pottery or pottery fired at low temperatures is often a problem with homemade or tourist goods, because the lead soaks out of this pottery into acidic foods like fruit juices and tomatoes.

Canned Milk or Canned Seafood Containers Soldered seals can contribute high lead levels to the contents.

Bone Meal This is not a recommended calcium supplement because animal bones often contain high levels of lead.

Dust from Remodeling of Older Homes Pre-1950 houses in the United States usually incorporated lead-based paint. Pregnant women must avoid paint dust during remodeling.

Wine Bottle Stoppers Wine bottles sealed with lead foil can leach lead into the stopper, thus contaminating the contents.

Drinking Water Lead leaches out of soldered joints and any lead plumbing. Recent checks show that many building water coolers contaminate water with lead because of soldered joints and lead alloys in fixtures. The EPA estimates that one out of every five people ingests excessive lead from home drinking water due to soldered joints of copper pipes and leaded water pipes in houses 80 years or more old. To minimize the risk, consumers should run the water five minutes before drinking. Charcoal filters don't remove lead from drinking water. (See also INHIBITION.)

Markowitz, M. "Lead Poisoning," *Pediatrics in Review* 21, no. 10 (2000): 327–335.

leaky gut A condition characterized by the increased intestinal uptake of potentially harmful materials. Leaky gut is caused by conditions that create intestinal inflammation, including excessive alcohol; the prolonged use of certain medications, especially non-steroidal antiinflammatory drugs or broad-spectrum antibiotics; chronic intestinal infections due to viruses, parasites, yeast, or bacteria; maldigestion; or nutritional deficiencies, such as IRON deficiency in children. Bacterial toxins (endotoxins) and ingested toxic materials can also injure the intestine, rendering it more porous. Leaky gut is associated with compromised immunity and with INFLAMMATORY BOWEL DISEASE, such as Crohn's disease.

Depletion of beneficial bacteria and growth of potentially dangerous bacteria (a situation termed dysbiosis) increase the likelihood of leaky gut. FIBROMYALGIA and CHRONIC FATIGUE are linked to leaky gut as well. Note that the intestine can become so damaged in certain disease states that nutrient uptake slows down and maldigestion of protein and carbohydrate and MALNUTRITION can occur. For example, CELIAC DISEASE (severe wheat protein sensitivity) is associated with decreased gut permeability.

As a result of increased intestinal uptake, partially digested food proteins can be absorbed, which promotes multiple food allergies. Damaging toxins may also find their way into the body. These materials may overburden the liver so that its ability to dispose of toxic materials may be compromised. The influx of foreign substances may also overtax the immune system, creating a long-term drain on the body's reserves. Circulating immune complexes, aggregates of antibodies and toxic materials, can lodge at different locations and can trigger autoimmune reactions, in which the body's defenses attack tissues; RHEUMATOID ARTHRITIS and lupus are possible outcomes.

Treatment involves eliminating the underlying condition, whether it is an infectious agent, alcohol, or medication overuse. Improving the diet to avoid excessive amounts of food with low nutrient content, such as highly processed, fatty convenience foods, is an important consideration. Specific nutrients become important with a leaky gut. Antioxidants help curb inflammation; BETA-CAROTENE, VITAMIN C, FOLIC ACID, VITAMIN A, VITAMIN E, and trace minerals such as ZINC are special keys to intestinal health. These nutrients also boost the immune system and the intestinal immune cells to ward off attack. Other nutrients specifically promote intestinal health, including fiber and the amino acid glutamine. STRESS is known to lower immunity, including decreased production of the major antibody of the intestine, secretory lgA. Correcting imbalanced gut flora (dysbosis) with lactobacillus and bifidobacteria species and fructose-containing fiber may help normalize gut function. Therefore, stress reduction and exercise may be beneficial. (See also ACIDOPHILUS; FATIGUE.)

Zoli, G. et al. "Effect of Oral Glutamine on Intestinal Permeability and Nutritional Status in Crohn's Disease," *Gastroenterology* 108 (1995): A766.

lean body mass A term used to indicate fat-free weight, representing primarily MUSCLE weight. The concept of lean body mass is important in terms of the effectiveness of weight loss and weight management programs. Optimally, weight loss programs that incorporate exercise and gradual weight loss (no more than one to two pounds per week) facilitate fat loss while minimizing potentially damaging losses of muscle protein. On the other hand, severe caloric restriction and crash DIETING programs will cause loss of both fat and muscle. Often the lean body mass lost with such programs is replaced by fat when previous diet and lifestyle are resumed at the end of a weight loss program. (See also OBESITY.)

lean meat See MEAT.

leavening agents Materials added to dough that make it rise before baking. The most common examples of leavening agents are BAKING SODA (sodium bicarbonate), BAKING POWDER, and BAKER'S YEAST. All of these agents generate carbon dioxide, which is trapped as tiny bubbles in the dough; heat and steam expand the air pockets. Sodium bicarbonate breaks down to carbon dioxide in the presence of acidic ingredients like sour milk or cream of tartar. Baking powder is a blend of calcium acid phosphate, cream of tartar or other acids, and sodium bicarbonate, which together generate gas when moistened. Baking (heating) releases more carbon dioxide from baking powder. Yeast contains enzymes that ferment glucose, a starch breakdown product, to carbon dioxide and alcohol. Heat evaporates alcohol and inactivates yeast enzymes. Leavening agents are generally considered safe food additives. Baking soda and baking powder add considerable sodium to breads, rolls, and crackers. Together, these foods contribute 25 percent of the sodium in the American diet. Only 2 percent of the sodium comes from salty snack foods like potato chips.

lecithin (phosphatidyl choline) The best-known phosphorous-containing lipid related to triglycerides (fats and oils). As an important building block of cell membranes, lecithin builds healthy cells, and helps carry fat and CHOLESTEROL as part of the lipid transport particles of the blood: LOW-DENSITY LIPOPROTEIN (LDL), HIGH-DENSITY LIPOPROTEIN (HDL), VERY LOW-DENSITY LIPOPROTEIN (VLDL), and CHYLOMICRONS. In BILE, lecithin acts like a soap to dissolve fats and soluble VITAMINS for digestion and absorption.

Lecithin contains GLYCEROL, a product of glucose metabolism, CHOLINE, a nitrogen-containing base, and two long-chain FATTY ACIDS. Lecithin is synthesized by the body, but it also occurs in a wide variety of foods. Good sources include SOYBEANS, liver, CAULIFLOWER, egg yolks, and CABBAGE. (The name lecithin is taken from the Greek word egg yolk.) Commercially, soybeans are the predominant source. As a food additive, lecithin acts as a stabilizer and EMULSIFIER in MARGARINE, CHOCOLATE, frozen desserts, salad dressings, and baked goods.

Lecithin Supplements

Using lecithin supplements, together with cutting down on unsaturated fat, may lower blood cholesterol for some people, and it may raise high-density lipoprotein, the desirable form of cholesterol (HDL), thus protecting against heart disease. Lecithin seems to protect experimental lab animals from developing liver CIRRHOSIS with an alcohol-laden diet. Patients taking certain antipsychotic drugs may eventually develop TARDIVE DYSKINESIA, marked by involuntary facial movements; choline and lecithin supplements can suppress such symptoms in some patients. Lecithin may help with short-term memory in certain elderly patients, but it has not been shown to prevent or cure ALZHEIMER'S DISEASE or other age-related dementia. Purified lecithin works best to lower blood choline levels and to help with memory loss. Most lecithin supplements are impure and may contain only 30 percent lecithin; it is questionable whether typical health food store pills will help with memory. Side effects can occur with large doses of lecithin; some people experience an upset stomach, sweating, and a loss of appetite.

Canty, D. J., and S. H. Zeisel. "Lecithin and Choline in Human Health and Disease," *Nutrition Reviews* 52, no. 10 (1994): 327–339.

leek (*Allium porrum*) A close relative of the ONION, leeks are native to Central Asia and have been an important vegetable in Europe since the Middle Ages. The leaves and stem are eaten, rather than the small, narrow bulb. Served raw, leeks can be chopped and mixed with cream cheese or COTTAGE CHEESE. They add flavor to soups and stews and are an important ingredient of quiche and vichyssoise, a creamy potato soup served cold. Leeks are also braised or broiled and served with butter or cheese sauces. Leeks are milder than onions and remain crunchy when cooked. They provide more nutrients than an equivalent serving of onions. In folk traditions, leeks have been used to stimulate appetite, protect against infection, and limit swelling due to water retention. Leeks (1 cup, 124 g) provide 76 calories; protein 1.9 g; carbohydrate, 17.5 g; fiber, 1.9 g; calcium, 73 mg; iron, 2.6 mg; vitamin C, 14.9 mg; thiamin, 0.074 mg; riboflavin, 0.037 mg; niacin, 0.50 mg.

legumes A large plant family characterized by seed-bearing pods. Common members are eaten as dried seeds: LENTILS, BEANS (kidney, fava or broad, navy, bush, string, lima, Windsor, SOYBEANS), PEAS, including CHICKPEAS or garbanzos, and PEANUTS. The roots of most legumes harbor bacteria that convert nitrogen in air to nitrogen compounds used by their hosts; therefore, legumes often grow well in depleted soils.

It is believed that legumes were among the earliest plants to be cultivated. This occurred around 10,000 B.C. in Southwest Asia, around 8000 B.C. in the Middle East, and 4000 B.C. in the New World. About 13,000 species are classified as legumes, and many are cultivated for food. Chickpeas, fava beans, and lentils probably originated in the Middle East. Soybeans represent roughly 55 percent of the world's legume production; peanuts, 12 percent; dry peas, 9 percent; dry beans, 7 percent; and chickpeas, 5 percent. More than one-third of the world legume production is supplied by the United States. Washington, Idaho, Michigan, and California are the major producers.

Legumes supply the same calories as grains, but they provide two to four times as much protein. This protein is low in calories and is both fat and cholesterol free. Legume protein is deficient in the essential sulfur-containing amino acid METHIONINE while containing adequate amounts of another essential amino acid, LYSINE. The amino acid composition of legume protein complements that of CEREAL GRAINS, which are low in lysine but contain adequate methionine. Thus the combination of both foods provides dietary protein that more closely meets protein requirements than either food eaten alone. As an example, a three-quarter-cup serving of cooked legumes provides 11 g to 13 g of protein, which would need to be supplemented with 1.5 cups of cooked cereal and three to four slices of whole-grain BREAD to provide adequate, balanced protein. Other foods also complement legume protein; nuts and small amounts of fish or poultry or egg white overcome amino acid deficiency. Soybean is the most complete protein and does not require complementing. Because legumes are less rich protein sources than meat or dairy products, strict vegetarians would need to eat relatively more legumes than people who eat animal foods.

Lentils, beans, and peas contain relatively large amounts of FIBER, nondigested carbohydrate. They lower the rate at which BLOOD SUGAR rises, decrease the need for the hormone INSULIN and therefore increase GLUCOSE TOLERANCE. These legumes also contain substances that protect against breast, colon, and prostate CANCER. Several of these substances are classified as protease inhibitors; they block certain enzymes that seem to promote cancer. Soybeans contain a group of compounds called isoflavones that are modified in the body and transformed into substances that may block the entry of the female hormone estrogen into cells. This may decrease the risk of breast and ovarian cancer.

Dried legumes are softened during cooking. Soaking legumes overnight speeds the cooking process. As an alternative, dry beans can be placed in water, heated to boiling for two minutes, and allowed to soak for an hour. Boiling softens the seed coating, allowing water to penetrate more rapidly. (See also COMPLETE PROTEIN; FOOD COMBINING; FOOD COMPLEMENTING; GLYCEMIC INDEX.)

Kleiner, Susan M. "A Hill of Beans: the Latest on Legumes," *The Physician and Sports Medicine* 23, no. 6 (June 1995): 13–14.

lemon (*Citrus limon*) A yellow, sour citrus fruit that originated in Southeast Asia between China and India. The Romans grew lemons in southern Italy, and citrus trees were cultivated by the Persians and the Arabs. Lemons rank among the top 12 fruit crops in the world and are the sixth leading fruit crop in the United States. Lemons and limes were established in Florida by the 1700s. California, Arizona, and Florida contribute most of the U.S. lemon crop because of the lemon's sensitivity to frost.

Lemons are excellent source of VITAMIN C. Lemons and LIMES were recognized for their anti-SCURVY properties by European seamen in the 17th century. However, issuance of lemon juice to sailors was not decreed in the British navy until the late 18th century.

The most common varieties of lemons are Eurekas and Lisbons. Lemons are usually picked before they are mature and have a yellow to green color. Ripening is accelerated by exposing the unripened fruit to ethylene, a nontoxic gas produced by many ripening fruit. At least half of the U.S. lemon crop is processed to lemon juice, frozen juice concentrate, and lemon-flavored soft drinks. Lemon pulp and rind are used to prepare lemon oil. PECTIN (a water-soluble FIBER) and (plant-based pigments that enhance the effects of vitamin C). Lemón and lime peels and citrus oil contain limonene, an oil that can cause skin irritation. This poses a problem because some commercial lemon-flavored beverages contain peel and peel extracts. They also contain psoralens, which can make the skin sensitive to sunlight and cause inflammation. In addition, lemons contain limonin, the bitter chemical found in the white, spongy part of the rind, which, together with other compounds, can activate defensive enzyme systems in the liver to defend against foreign compounds. Fresh lemon juice (1 cup) provides 60 calories; protein, 0.9g; carbohydrate, 21.1 g; fiber, 0.85 g; potassium, 303 mg; vitamin C, 31 mg; thiamin, 0.07 mg; riboflavin, 0.02 mg; niacin, 0.24 mg. (See also ALLERGY, FOOD.)

lentil (*Lens esculenta*) A small, disc-shaped legume that is one of the oldest cultivated plants; archaeological evidence indicates that they were cultivated in the Near East about 8000 B.C. Lentils are now widely cultivated in the cool season in the tropics and subtropical regions and in the summer season of mild temperate regions. Leading producers of lentils are India, Turkey, and Syria, Varieties range from orange to green.

Lentils contain 7.4 percent PROTEIN, more than cereal grains. Lentil protein is deficient in the sulfur-containing AMINO ACIDS: METHIONINE and CYSTEINE. Methionine is a dietary essential amino acid. Protein from cereal grains supplies ample sulfur amino acids. Therefore, the amino acid patterns of lentils and grains complement each other; mixtures of the two foods contain a higher quality protein than either by itself. Lentils are a low-fat food. Only 4 percent of calories comes from fat.

Cooked lentils are frequently served with other vegetables in casseroles, soups, and stews. Lentils contain soluble FIBER, nondigestible plant carbohydrate that causes starches to be digested slowly. Slow digestion produces a small rise in BLOOD SUGAR than simple sugars or highly refined carbohydrates; therefore, lentils are said to have a low GLYCEMIC INDEX. Lentils in Indian cuisine (dal) are prepared without the skin of the seed, and therefore contain much less fiber.

Cooked lentils, 1 cup (200 g), provide 215 calories; protein, 16 g; carbohydrate, 38 g; fiber, 10 g; fat, 1 g; calcium, 50 mg; iron, 4.2 mg; potassium, 498 mg; thiamin, 0.14 mg; riboflavin, 0.12 mg; niacin, 1.12 mg. (See also BIOLOGICAL VALUE; COMPLETE PROTEIN.)

leptin A hormone produced by fat cells that helps regulate fat storage. From the latin word *leptos,* which means "thin," leptin was discovered in the mid-1990s when researchers discovered it was instrumental in helping the body manage fat stores. Leptin travels from fat cells, where it is produced, to the hypothalamus, which regulates hunger. As fat cells increase, more leptin reaches the hypothalamus, telling it to "switch off" the hunger signal.

In 1995 researchers discovered that when genetically engineered leptin was administered to mice who could not make leptin on their own, the hormone regulated their eating behavior and overall body fat. Given those results, researchers hoped that leptin would prove helpful in treating obesity in people. However, experiments in which leptin was given to human subjects did not produce the desired results; the leptin doses did not always suppress hunger.

In 2001 researchers discovered that people who made long-term lifestyle changes to lose weight and lower obesity-related blood pressure by reducing their fat consumption and increasing their activity levels significantly lowered their leptin levels. The effect of leptin on metabolism and weight loss is an active area of research given the potential health benefits it could provide to the millions of Americans who are overweight or obese. In 2002 a study of people who had recently lost weight showed that those who were given small amounts of leptin were able to keep the weight off more easily than were those who did not receive additional amounts of the hormone. Researchers cautioned that additional clinical trials would be needed to be confirm the study's results. (See also DIET; FAT; METABOLISM; OBESITY; WEIGHT MANAGEMENT.)

Reseland, J. E. et al. "Effect of Long-Term Changes in Diet and Exercise on Plasma Leptin Concentrations," *American Journal of Clinical Nutrition* 73, no. 2 (2001): 240–245.

lettuce (*Lactuca sativa*) A green VEGETABLE with a leafy head that may be compact or loose. Lettuce belongs to the sunflower family, and it may have been cultivated in ancient Egypt or Persia. Lettuce is a popular salad vegetable in the United States. California is the leading lettuce-producing state, followed by Arizona, Florida, Colorado, Texas, and New Mexico. Lettuce is the major salad vegetable produced in the United States; about 30 pounds of lettuce are consumed per person annually. Although tomato production far exceeds that of lettuce, less than 20 percent of tomatoes are consumed fresh, as in salads.

Crisp-headed lettuce, also known as iceberg lettuce, constitutes the majority of commercially produced lettuce. Butterhead (Bibb, Big Boston, or White Boston) varieties bruise easily and are more likely to be grown for local markets. Romaine lettuce (cos lettuce) has long, dark-green leaves and is broad-ribbed, with a narrow head. Romaine is flavorful and crisp and has a higher nutrient value than iceberg lettuce. The darker the leaves, the more nutritious the salad green. Thus, Romaine lettuce contains six times as much vitamin C and five to 10 times as much beta-carotene as iceberg lettuce. Browning of lettuce at salad bars was once retarded with sulfite preservatives. Now sulfites are forbidden on fresh produce. VITAMIN C derivatives and other products are now used to keep salad lettuce fresh-looking and crisp.

All types of lettuce have a high water content (94 percent to 96 percent). The nutrient content of one head of Boston lettuce (163 g) is 21 calories; protein, 2.1 g; carbohydrate, 3.8 g; fiber, 2.7 g; calcium, 52 mg; iron, 0.49 mg; potassium, 419 mg; vitamin A, 158 retinol equivalents; thiamin, 0.1 mg; riboflavin, 0.1 mg; niacin, 0.49 mg. (See also SULFITES.)

leucine (Leu, L-leucine) A dietary essential AMINO ACID. Leucine is one of the 20 amino acids required to build proteins. Leucine is classified as branched-chain amino acid. This group of amino acids possesses hydrophobic (water-repelling) carbon chains that cannot be synthesized by animals. Adults require 14 mg per kilogram body weight daily of leucine in the diet. In the body, leucine stimulates protein synthesis in muscles, and it may stimulate the release of the insulin to trigger glucose and amino acid uptake from the bloodstream.

Leucine and other branched-chain amino acids are degraded by skeletal muscle in order to produce energy. Unlike many other amino acids, leucine cannot be converted to GLUCOSE by the LIVER and is therefore considered a "ketogenic" amino acid. During excessive fat breakdown that accompanies starvation, branched-chain amino acids including leucine yield KETONE BODIES, acidic by-products. A rare genetic defect in the ability to break down branched-chain amino acids leads to maple syrup urine disease, characterized by mental retardation, convulsions, and coma. This condition is treated by limiting the dietary intake of branched-chain amino acids. (See also ISOLEUCINE; KETOSIS; VALINE.)

leukocytes (polymorphonuclear leukocytes, white blood cells) Cells in the blood that are products of the IMMUNE SYSTEM. Leukocytes differ significantly from the numerous red blood cells. White blood cells possess nuclei and lack HEMOGLOBIN (the red oxygen transport protein of blood) unlike red blood cells, which lack nuclei but contain large amounts of hemoglobin.

There are several types of leukocytes: white cells with cytoplasmic particles (granular leukocytes) and those without grains (agranular leukocytes). Among granular leukocytes are three subclasses called neutrophils, eosinophils and basophils according to how they react to certain stains under the microscope.

Nearly 60 percent of leukocytes are neutrophils. They help defend the body against disease-causing bacteria, yeast, fungi, and viruses. Neutrophils can enter tissues by passing through capillaries, so that they can engulf invaders. Eosinophils stain orange-red easily; these cells play a role in allergic reactions, and high levels are often associated with allergic attacks and with some parasitic infections. Basophils stain blue-black. They represent less than 1 percent of the leukocytes.

Agranular leukocytes represent the largest population of white cells and originate from lymphatic tissue and bone marrow. Lymphocytes represent 20 percent to 40 percent of leukocytes, and they both regulate the immune system and carry out key defensive roles. Lymphocytes consist of B cells, T cells, and natural killer cells. B cells lead to antibody production. Antibodies are proteins released into the bloodstream to help bind and destroy foreign substances. T cells attack virus-infected cells, transplanted tissue, and cancer cells. One class of T cells (T helper cells) helps increase the immune response, while another class of T cells (T suppressor cells) helps limit the immune response. Natural killer cells destroy virus-infected cells and cancer cells by engulfing them and by producing chemicals that help destroy these altered cells. Monocytes also belong to the family of lymphocytes and function as scavengers; they mature into macrophages, a type of cell that cleans up infected areas of the body. (See also LYMPH.)

leukotrienes Powerful inflammatory agents. Leukotrienes are products of ESSENTIAL FATTY ACIDS that increase inflammation and mucus secretion and contract the muscles surrounding blood vessels and the intestines. Extremely powerful substances, leukotrienes are about 10,000 times more potent than HISTAMINE, a noted stimulant of INFLAMMATION. Leukotrienes play a role in immediate allergy attacks and in heart attacks. They constrict lung air passageways, especially the BRONCHI, in asthma attacks. They constrict coronary arteries, which deliver blood to the heart.

They are synthesized by various white blood cells; by mast cells (cells found in connective tissue that participate in inflammation and immune reactions); and by brain, heart, lung, and spleen. Leukotrienes (C_4, D_4, E_4) contain the sulfur amino acid CYSTEINE. Another leukotriene called LTB_4 attaches white cells to the site of infection or inflammation. LTB_4 is implicated in such diseases as RHEUMATOID ARTHRITIS.

Leukotrienes are linear compounds synthesized from a polyunsaturated FATTY ACID called ARACHIDONIC ACID, itself derived from the essential fatty acid, LINOLEIC ACID. The conversion of arachidonic acid to leukotrienes is not inhibited by ASPIRIN or other nonsteroidal anti-inflammatory drugs. Therefore, these pain relievers do not remedy asthma attacks. (See also IMMUNE SYSTEM.)

levulose See FRUCTOSE.

licorice (*Glycyrrhiza glabra*) A small shrub used to produce natural licorice flavoring. The roots and runners of the licorice plant are used in botanical medicine. Licorice extracts contain a steroid-like molecule called GLYCYRRHIZIN or glycyrrhizic acid that is 50 to 100 times sweeter than table sugar. It has been used in mouthwashes and toothpastes because it inhibits plaque growth and because of its pleasing flavor.

Licorice has been used for thousands of years in both Western and Eastern medical traditions. In Chinese medicine it has been used to treat stomach ulcers, asthma, and lung infections, among other conditions. Licorice inhibits inflammation due to allergic reactions to bacterial toxins. Licorice stimulates mucus secretion, which partially explains its utility in treating stomach and intestinal ulcers. It also supports the health of intestinal cells. Glycyrrhizin has also been used to treat viral hepatitis.

Licorice flavoring is used in beverages, candy, and baked goods. Most commercial licorice in the United States contains anise as flavoring agent.

If natural licorice is eaten as a steady diet, it often causes salt retention, water retention (EDEMA), swollen ankles, and puffy eyes—and thus weight (though not fat) gain. In children excessive licorice consumption can result in hormone imbalance, diarrhea, vomiting, high blood pressure, low potassium levels, and water retention. The regular use of licorice also interferes with certain medications such as DIURETICS, vasodilators, and digitalis. The active agent of licorice (glycyrrhizin) can mimic the adrenal hormone aldosterone and slow the disposal of this hormone by the liver. Glycyrrhizin also raises blood pressure. Licorice should not be used by patients with high blood pressure, kidney failure, or those who are taking medications for heart conditions.

Licorice extract, from which glycyrrhizin has been removed (deglycyrrhizinated licorice), can help heal ulcers, apparently without side effects.

life expectancy The number of years the average person can be expected to live. Life expectancy for the U.S. population reached a record high of 76.9 years in 2000 according to preliminary statistics analyzed by researchers at the Centers for Disease Control and Prevention. Mortality rates declined for several leading causes of death, including cancer and heart disease, which account for more than half of all U.S. deaths annually. The infant mortality rate also dropped to its lowest level in 2000, to 6.9 infant deaths per 1,000 live births. Wise lifestyle choices, appropriate nutrition, and exercise favor a longer, more productive and satisfying life. (See also AGING.)

life extension The hypothesis that VITAMINS and other supplements can extend the life span. The eternal quest for youth leads to the question of whether supplements can help people live longer. There is no complete answer to this question. It is clear that there are no secret formulas, no "magic bullets," and no fountain of youth. Experts suggest that a more basic question is, how can a person's health, the sense of well-being and happiness, be improved, given his or her unique inheritance and environmental challenges of living in the 21st century?

Optimal nutrition can minimize the impact of DEGENERATIVE DISEASES. Studies of groups of people throughout the world who are reported to have longer life spans, such as the Masai of Africa, Mormons, Seventh-day Adventists, and the Chinese, suggest that the healthiest people in the world:

- eat fresh fruit, fresh vegetables, and minimally processed foods regularly and drink unpolluted water;
- limit consumption of caffeinated beverages, fatty foods, refined starches like white flour, sugar, strong alcoholic beverages, and potentially harmful drugs;
- avoid excess calories and obesity;
- avoid smoking;
- engage in regular, moderate to vigorous physical EXERCISE;
- live harmoniously with their families and social groups.

(See also AGING; ANTIOXIDANTS; ILLNESS; STRESS.)

Lee, I. M. et al. "Exercise Intensity and Longevity in Men: the Harvard Alumni Health Study," *Journal of the American Medical Association* 273, no. 15 (April 19, 1995): 1,179–1,184.

light foods Foods with "light" or "lite" designation on a FOOD LABEL. The U.S. FDA food label regulations that took effect in August 1994 allow food manufacturers to use new terms, each with a specific definition of a food. "Light" or "lite" can be used to describe foods containing one-third fewer calories or half the FAT of a reference food. Alternatively, if the food contains 50 percent or more of its calories as fat, then the reduction in fat must be 50 percent. "Light" or "lite" can also refer to a low calorie—low sodium food in which the sodium content has been reduced by 50 percent of the reference food. All other uses of the term light must specify the sensory quality it describes; for example, its color or texture. (See also ADVERTISING; FOOD LABELING.)

lignin A noncarbohydrate constituent of FIBER that forms protective and structural components of plant cell walls. Lignin is a complex plastic-like material (polymer) that is insoluble and resistant to chemical breakdown. Crude fiber that remains after acid digestion of plant materials is primarily lignin. Unlike carbohydrate-based fiber, lignin is not degraded by digestive enzymes or gut microbes but passes through the digestive tract intact. It does, however, have important effects on the digestive tract: Lignin decreases the risk of CONSTIPATION by increasing the movement of stools, and it binds BILE salts. This is believed to minimize microbial degradation of these substances and hence decrease exposure of the intestine to toxic derivatives. Decreased exposure is believed to lower the risk of colon CANCER. By binding both bile salts and CHOLESTEROL and moving them out of the body as feces, blood cholesterol levels may be lowered, decreasing the risk of heart disease. Excessive fiber, including lignin, can block mineral absorption. Certain lignin constituents released by the intestine are modified in the body. Such "animal lignins" apparently interact with tissues, weakly mimicking the effects of ESTROGEN, the female sex hormone. Lignin may have a therapeutic role in lowering the risk of breast CANCER. (See also CELLULOSE; PECTIN.)

lima bean (*Phaseolus lunatus*) One of the most common BEANS in the U.S. diet, this legume is believed to have originated in Peru between 7,000 and 8,000 years ago. Spanish and Portuguese traders took beans to the Philippines, Africa, and other warm regions. Lima beans grow well in the tropics and are an important crop in Africa and Asia. Most U.S. production is in California. Green lima beans grown in the United States are mainly processed (canned and frozen).

The common varieties of green lima beans are butter beans (Fordhooks) and baby limas. Green lima beans are cooked the same way as green peas. Dry lima beans are used in soups, casseroles, and bean salads.

Certain varieties of lima beans, especially colored varieties native to the Caribbean, contain harmful substances (cyanoglycosides). Enzymes produced by intestinal microorganisms release cyanide, a potential poison, from these materials. However, the varieties of lima bean grown in the United States contain negligible amounts of these toxins.

Uncooked beans in general contain a TRYPSIN inhibitory protein that can block the action of this digestive enzyme. They also contain hemagglutinins, proteins that coagulate red blood cells. These proteins are generally inactivated during cooking. Furthermore, soaking dried beans, followed by cooking, renders these agents inactive. Mature beans contain oligosaccharides, short chains of sugars that are not digested but instead are degraded by colon bacteria and may cause gas and bloating. Soaking beans before cooking, and discarding the soak water, lessens the problem.

Thick-seeded lima beans (cooked from frozen beans; 1 cup, 171 g) contain 225 calories; protein, 15 g; carbohydrate, 41 g; fiber, 15.4 g; fat, 0.8 g; calcium, 47 mg; iron, 2.9 mg; potassium, 608 mg; thiamin, 0.43 mg; riboflavin, 0.05 mg; niacin, 0.9 mg. (See also CYANOGEN.)

lime (*Citrus aurantifolia*) A green-colored citrus fruit, smaller than a lemon. Limes originated in Southeast Asia. Arabs introduced limes into Egypt in 900 A.D., and into Spain by 1200 A.D. With the settlement of the New World, limes were introduced rapidly in the Caribbean Islands, the Florida Keys, and Mexico. Today, Florida supplies about 10 percent of the world's lime crop. A cold-resistant variety is grown in India, Mexico, Egypt, the West Indies, and other tropical regions. Nearly 50 percent of the U.S. lime crop is processed as lime juice, lime-based beverages, marmalades, syrups, and lime oil.

As with lemon, some people are allergic to lime peel. The oil of lime peel (oil of bergamot) can cause skin to blister when exposed to sunlight .

The active ingredient (psoralens) is found in the peel and to a lesser degree in carrots, celery, figs, parsley, fennel, and anise. Lime juice or beverages flavored by limes may contain lime peel and extracts. Limes are excellent sources of VITAMIN C. This explains their use by 18th-century navies to prevent scurvy on long voyages.

Lime juice (fresh, 1 cup) contains 65 calories; protein, 1.1 g; carbohydrate, 22.2 g; fiber, 1.0 g; potassium, 268 mg; vitamin C, 72 mg; thiamin, 0.05 mg; riboflavin, 0.03 mg; niacin, 0.25 mg.

linoleic acid A dietary ESSENTIAL FATTY ACID. Polyunsaturated fatty acids such as linoleic acid help maintain the flexibility of cell membranes, which is essential for their normal function. Therefore, linoleic acid is essential for normal growth and development.

Certain details of the molecular structure are important in order to understand its role. This 18-carbon acid contains two double bonds in which pairs of carbons are deficient in hydrogen atoms. Therefore, it is classified as polyunsaturated FATTY ACID. It belongs to the omega-6 family of fatty acids because the first double bond begins six carbon atoms from the end of the fatty acid.

Linoleic acid is classified as a dietary essential because the body is unable to insert double bonds in fatty acids at the sixth carbon of this long chain fatty acid. While the body cannot manufacture linoleic acid, it can convert linoleic acid to longer, more complex fatty acids, especially ARACHIDONIC ACID. In turn, the body transforms arachidonic acid to a class of PROSTAGLANDINS of the PG_2 series, hormone-like substances that stimulate inflammation, pain, BLOOD CLOTTING, smooth muscle contraction, elevated blood pressure, and other physiological processes. Other derivatives of arachidonic acid, hence of linoleic acid, are called LEUKOTRIENES. These are extremely powerful inflammatory agents.

Linoleic acid is the raw material for more complex lipids. The body converts linoleic acid to a close relative called gamma linoleic acid by an enzyme (delta 6 desaturase) as the first step in the synthesis of longer fatty acids from which regulatory substances like prostaglandins are made. This critical step is slowed by AGING, hormonal imbalance, and dietary factors such as zinc deficiency, ALCOHOLISM, excessive sugar consumption, and conditions like DIABETES.

Symptoms of essential fatty acid deficiency include severe, resistant ECZEMA, hair loss, and impaired wound healing. The deficiency in animals causes retarded growth and development. Deficiencies have been reported in infants fed nonfat milk, which lacks linoleic acid.

Many polyunsaturated seed oils supply linoleic acid in the typical American diet. SAFFLOWER oil, SOYBEAN oil, SUNFLOWER oil, CORN OIL, and MARGARINE prepared from these oils are typical sources. Linoleic acid consumption typically ranges from 5 percent to 10 percent of calories when American diets supply 25 percent to 50 percent of the daily calories as fat. Dietary recommendations generally specify that for a healthy adult the total polyunsaturated fat intake should be about 6 percent to 7 percent of daily calories, not to exceed 10 percent. Research suggests that linoleic acid should represent 5 percent of calories or 14 g/day. There is no RECOMMENDED DIETARY ALLOWANCE for this or any other polyunsaturated fatty acid, yet. Note that a high intake of polyunsaturated oils increases the need for a fat-soluble ANTIOXIDANT like VITAMIN E because polyunsaturates are more susceptible to oxidation and destruction.

A modified form of linoleic acid, called CONJUGATED LINOLEIC ACID, can offer protection against breast cancer in lab animals. Conjugated linoleic acid occurs in animal products like meat and dairy products. However, it should be noted that these animal products contain large amounts of unsaturated fat and cholesterol, which are risk factors for heart disease. (See also ALPHA LINOLEIC ACID; FAT METABOLISM.)

Holmes, M. D. et al. "Association of Dietary Intake of Fat and Fatty Acids with Risk of Breast Cancer," *JAMA* 281, no. 10 (1999): 914–920.

linseed oil See FLAXSEED OIL.

lipase A family of ENZYMES that degrade fats and oils to release free FATTY ACIDS. Three classes of lipase are important.

Pancreatic Lipase The PANCREAS secretes lipase in addition to other digestive enzymes. The free fatty acids are absorbed by intestinal cells, where they are resynthesized back into fat molecules, then packaged in fat transport particles called CHYLOMICRONS, released into the LYMPH and ultimately enter the bloodstream.

Lipoprotein Lipase This lipase occurs in capillary walls, where it breaks down fat being transported in the bloodstream by chylomicrons. Lipoprotein lipase also releases fatty acids from VERY LOW-DENSITY LIPOPROTEIN (VLDL), a particle that transports fat synthesized by the liver. Free fatty acids migrate into ADIPOCYTES (fat cells), to be stored as fat. They are also absorbed by muscle cells to be burned for energy.

Hormone-sensitive Lipase This lipase occurs in fat cells. In response to EPINEPHRINE (adrenaline), a stress hormone from adrenal glands, hormone-sensitive lipase rapidly breaks down stored fat to release fatty acids into the bloodstream. Muscle cells can then absorb the fatty acids from the blood and burn them for energy. (See also DIGESTION; FAT METABOLISM.)

lipids Fatlike, waxy, or oily chemicals that repel water and dissolve chemical solvents like petroleum, oils, ether, and benzene. The only property all lipids have in common is their insolubility in water. Common lipids in the body include CHOLESTEROL, FAT, and oils (collectively called TRIGLYCERIDES), waxes, phosphorous-containing lipids (PHOSPHOLIPIDS) like LECITHIN, as well as VITAMIN A, VITAMIN D, VITAMIN E, VITAMIN K, and BETA-CAROTENE. Lipids tend to be stored in fat tissue. Certain pollutants are also lipids: industrial chemicals like PBB, PCB; solvents like benzene, toluene, methylene chloride; cleaning solvents; and PESTICIDES like DDT.

Fat is not cholesterol. Confusion arises because these lipids occur together in MEAT, and cholesterol dissolves in the fat released during cooking because it is fat-soluble. Therefore removing fat from meat decreases the cholesterol content. Generally, a low-cholesterol diet will also be a low-saturated fat diet. A high saturated fat diet can increase BLOOD cholesterol in susceptible people due to an effect on cholesterol formation by the liver.

Serum Lipids

Fat and cholesterol are transported by the blood. However, for simplicity in diagnostic lab testing, serum (the cell-free fluid remaining after blood clots) is usually used for analysis. Thus, serum lipids consist of fat (serum triglyceride) and serum cholesterol. Following a meal, serum triglyceride levels rise for a short time only, as blood distributes fat absorbed from digested food. High serum triglyceride levels between meals may increase the risk of CARDIOVASCULAR DISEASE for people with high serum cholesterol. To evaluate the risk of heart disease, it is often more meaningful to analyze individual forms of serum cholesterol, rather than simply determining total cholesterol. This more detailed analysis measures the amounts of

LOW-DENSITY LIPOPROTEIN (LDL), the undesirable form of cholesterol; HIGH-DENSITY LIPOPROTEIN (HDL), the desirable form; and serum triglycerides separately. Elevated LDL levels and depressed HDL levels may increase the risk of clogged arteries (ATHEROSCLEROSIS).

Lipids, including cholesterol and unsaturated fatty acids, are sensitive to oxidation. Highly reactive forms of oxygen called FREE RADICALS can extract electrons from these cell constituents to make up for their own deficiency, and in the process they leave behind damaged molecules called lipid peroxides. These, in turn, are unstable and break down to products yielding more free radicals, as well as chemicals that cause mutations (mutagens) and cytotoxic (cell-killing) agents. Some of these decomposition products are responsible for the smell of rancid fat. Oxidized LDL is implicated in the origin of plaques that can clog arteries and cause heart disease. (See also CHLORINATED HYDROCARBONS; FAT METABOLISM; HYPERTRIGLYCERIDEMIA.)

lipogenesis The synthesis of fat in the body, chiefly by the LIVER and by ADIPOSE TISSUE (fat tissue). Lipogenesis occurs primarily after a high carbohydrate meal. Fat is formed from smaller building blocks, three FATTY ACIDS, and GLYCEROL, an alcohol from glucose metabolism. The process requires ATP, the energy currency of the cell, and BIOTIN. The hormone INSULIN signals lipogenesis in fat tissue, which converts surplus calories to stored fats. Unlike adipose tissue, the liver cannot store fat and must package it in order to transport it to fat cells. To accomplish this task, the liver releases newly formed fat packaged as submicroscopic particles called VERY LOW-DENSITY LIPOPROTEINS (VLDL) into the bloodstream. This represents emulsified fat, which can be distributed in blood. (See also ANABOLISM; CATABOLISM; FAT DIGESTION; FAT METABOLISM; LIPASE; LIPOLYSIS.)

Mc Devitt, R. M. et al. "De Novo Lipogenesis During Controlled Overfeeding with Sucrose or Glucose in Lean and Obese Women," *American Journal of Clinical Nutrition* 74 (2001): 737–746.

Schaefer, Ernest. "Lipoproteins, Nutrition, and Heart Disease," *American Journal of Clinical Nutrition* 75, no. 2 (2002): 121–212.

lipoic acid (alpha-lipoic acid, thioctic acid) A sulfur-containing ANTIOXIDANT involved in CARBOHYDRATE degradation that occurs naturally in the body. The body synthesizes this fat-soluble COENZYME; consequently it is not classified as a dietary essential. Lipoic acid is not a VITAMIN, nor is it derived from a vitamin. Nonetheless, it plays a critical metabolic role. Lipoic acid functions in the oxidation of carbohydrate by the MITOCHONDRIA, subcellular particles devoted to energy production. It is sometimes called the universal antioxidant because it deactivates both fat- and water-soluble FREE RADICALS and can cross the blood–brain barrier. Alpha lipoic acid has been shown to increase the effectiveness of other antioxidants, including VITAMIN E and VITAMIN C. It prevents cell damage, helps to stabilize blood sugar, and helps the liver remove toxins.

It is used to treat a variety of diseases and conditions, including chronic hepatitis, glaucoma, STROKE, and DIABETES MELLITUS. Studies have shown that alpha lipoic acid helps to eliminate blood sugar (GLUCOSE) and reduce pain, itching, and numbness in diabetic patients. It is used widely in Germany to treat diabetic neuropathy, a degenerative nerve condition that affects the nerves leading to the arms and legs.

Foods that are good sources of alpha lipoic acid include SPINACH, BROCCOLI, YEAST, and BEEF kidney and heart.

Key chemical transformations require lipoic acid: the oxidation of pyruvic acid (a small acid from glucose breakdown) to an activated form of ACETIC ACID called acetyl coenzyme A and the oxidation of alpha ketoglutaric acid, a product of the KREB'S CYCLE, which is the central energy-yielding pathway of the cell. CARBON DIOXIDE released in both oxidations represents a major portion of the carbon dioxide expired by the lungs as a metabolic waste product. To accomplish such oxidations, lipoic acid must work together with four vitamin-related coenzymes: thiamin pyrophosphate, derived from THIAMIN (vitamin B_1) FAD (FLAVIN ADENINE DINUCLEOTIDE), derived from RIBOFLAVIN (vitamin B_2); NAD (NICOTINAMIDE ADENINE DINUCLEOTIDE), derived from NIACIN (vitamin B_3); and COENZYME A, derived from PANTOTHENIC ACID (vitamin B_5). Lipoic acid is emerging as a versatile antioxidant. In the reduced form it is able to protect lipids from oxidation due to free radical attack and may protect vitamin E. It quenches superoxide and reactive oxygen compounds generated in the body during inflammation and it may play a role in regulating oxidation-reduction balance of cells. (See also CARBOHYDRATE METABOLISM.)

Packer, J. et al. "Neuroprotection by the Metabolic Antioxidant Alpha-Lipoic Acid," *Free Radical & Biologic Medicine* 22 (1997): 359–378.

lipolysis The degradation of fat to its building blocks, FATTY ACIDS and GLYCEROL. In fats and oils, three long-chain fatty acids are normally attached to glycerol, an alcohol derived from glucose breakdown. Lipolysis occurs when stored fat is degraded in response to specific hormone signals that food is not supplying enough energy, or when a stress response is triggered: EPINEPHRINE (adrenaline) from adrenal glands, GLUCAGON from the islet tissue of the PANCREAS, and CORTISOL from the adrenal glands. Skipping meals, as well as exercise, long-term FASTING, physical trauma, STARVATION, low-calorie diets, and ALCOHOLISM, favor lipolysis.

Fat is degraded by a family of enzymes called LIPASES. Epinephrine signals a hormone-sensitive lipase within adipose cells to attack stored fat and release fatty acids and glycerol into the bloodstream. There, fatty acids bind to serum ALBUMIN, a major blood protein, for transport to tissues like muscles to be oxidized for energy production. Glycerol travels to the liver, where it is converted to BLOOD SUGAR. (See also FAT METABOLISM; GLUCONEOGENESIS; LIPOGENESIS.)

lipoprotein A submicroscopic particle composed of LIPIDS and proteins that transports lipids (water-insoluble materials) through the BLOOD and LYMPH. These fluids are essentially water, yet FAT, CHOLESTEROL, and fat-soluble vitamins such as VITAMIN A repel water. The problem is fundamental: Water and oils do not mix. To accomplish the difficult task of distributing lipids in water, cells package lipids as tiny droplets of PROTEIN and PHOSPHOLIPID called MICELLES for transport in the bloodstream.

There are four major classes of serum lipoproteins:

Chylomicrons Manufactured by the intestine to transport absorbed fat to tissues. The intestine releases chylomicrons to the lymph, which drains into the blood for general distribution. Chylomicrons carry a protein called apoliprotein CII (Apo CII) that activates LIPASE, a fat-splitting enzyme located in CAPILLARIES. The released fatty acids are readily absorbed by fat cells and reincorporated into fat for storage; they are also taken up by muscle cells to be burned for energy.

Very Low-Density Lipoprotein (VLDL) Produced by the liver to transport newly synthesized fat to ADIPOSE TISSUE for storage. VLDL deposits its fatty acids on fat cells as described for chylomicrons, above. VLDL remnants are processed to become a cholesterol carrier, LOW-DENSITY LIPOPROTEIN (LDL); surplus lipid and protein are removed and cholesterol is added. Excessive VLDL is indirectly linked to an increased risk of cardiovascular disease.

Low-Density Lipoprotein (LDL) Transports cholesterol out of the liver to other tissues. It is derived from VLDL as described above. LDL contains a single protein called apolipoprotein B (ApoB). This protein is a recognition key that allows LDL to attach to specific docking sites (receptors) on cells. Once LDL binds to the cell surface, it is engulfed and its cholesterol is deposited within the cell.

Excessive LDL cholesterol appears to be linked to cardiovascular diseases through oxidation and free radical damage. When LDL cholesterol becomes oxidized, it can deposit in arterial walls, a process that can eventually clog arteries. Therefore LDL is sometimes referred to as "bad" cholesterol.

High-Density Lipoprotein (HDL) Manufactured by the liver to scavenge cholesterol from tissues and carry it back to the liver for disposal. It is sometimes called "good" cholesterol because high levels correlate with a reduced risk of HEART DISEASE. A marker protein, apolipoprotein A (Apo A), characterizes this particle. Its name is derived from the fact that HDL is the most dense lipoprotein due to its high protein content. HDL is involved in the processing of other types of lipoprotein particles. It shuttles Apo CII from spent chylomicrons and spent VLDL to newly formed chylomicrons, and VLDL and HDL transfer cholesterol between different lipoproteins. (See also DIGESTION; FAT METABOLISM; PLAQUE.)

Sacco, R. L. et al. "High-Density Lipoprotein Cholesterol and Ischemic Stroke in the Elderly (The Northern Manhattan Stroke Study)," *Journal of the American Medical Association* 285 (2001): 2,729–2,735.

lipotrope (lipotropic factor) Nutrients that may help prevent fat accumulation in the liver. The most commonly studied are METHIONINE, an essential AMINO ACID containing sulfur; CHOLINE, a nitrogen-containing building block of the phospholipid LECITHIN; the B vitamins; FOLIC ACID and VITAMIN B_{12}; and INOSITOL, a complex alcohol related to GLUCOSE. Those nutrients promote the synthesis of phospholipids, building blocks of lipoproteins, to transport lipids out of the liver.

A change in liver metabolism during STARVATION can lead to fat deposition. Abnormal fat buildup occurs in the LIVER after damage by viral HEPATITIS, ALCOHOL, solvents, PESTICIDES, HERBICIDES, drugs, steroid hormones, and even oral contraceptives. Over time, this leads to permanent liver scarring (CIRRHOSIS). Lipotropes have been shown to be effective in preventing fatty liver in experimental animals; however, they do not prevent fatty liver due to ALCOHOLISM. (See also FAT METABOLISM.)

liquid diets DIETS that range from clear liquids to complete liquefied foods. Whatever their formulation, the use of liquid diets requires medical supervision.

Clear liquid diets include only clear liquids such as carbonated beverages; COFFEE and coffee substitutes; flavored gelatins; strained fruit juices; fat-free broths of MEAT, FISH, and POULTRY; BOUILLON; and consommé. They are used before intestinal surgery or X rays of the gastrointestinal tract; and for oral feeding of critically ill patients. They also help maintain FLUID BALANCE.

ELEMENTAL DIETS, also called semi-synthetic diets, are free of FIBER and contain easily absorbed, refined carbohydrates such as simple SUGARS; VEGETABLE OIL as a source of FAT; AMINO ACIDS supplied as purified powders or as hydrolyzed CASEIN (milk protein) or hydrolyzed ALBUMIN (egg protein); and purified MINERALS and VITAMINS. Elemental diets aid DIGESTION and minimize food residues in the colon. They are used before GASTROINTESTINAL TRACT surgery, and in cases of intestinal disease, severe malnourishment, and critical illnesses.

Full liquid diets provide liquefied foods, including meat, fish, MILK, and strained cottage cheese; custard and pudding rather than whole EGGS; as well as strained vegetables, strained juices, and pureed fruits. Berries with small seeds are excluded, as are strongly flavored vegetables; dry cereals; bread; high-fat, chunky soup, stews; desserts (with nuts or other solid foods) and strongly flavored seasonings, condiments, and spices. These diets are used for patients who cannot chew or swallow whole foods; as meal replacements when incorporated into a weight loss program; or as supplemental feeding programs. Liquid diets are usually deficient in fiber and certain nutrients; hence supplements may be recommended.

INFANT FORMULAS are commercially produced and can replace breast-feeding of young infants. They are usually based on cow's milk or a milk substitute such as soy protein that contains added minerals, vitamins, vegetable oil, and LACTOSE (milk sugar) to meet specific food and drug administration requirements to assure adequate infant nutrition.

liquid protein diets See DIETS: VERY LOW CALORIE.

listeriosis A food-borne illness that may cause no symptoms in healthy people but that is particularly dangerous to fetuses or newborns, the elderly, and people with damaged immune systems. There are about 2,500 cases of serious listeriosis each year; of these, 500 patients die.

Listeriosis is caused by one species in a group of bacteria called *Listeria monocytogenes* found in cow's milk, animal and human feces, soil, and leafy vegetables. In the 1990s there were several outbreaks that were linked to the ingestion of deli lunch meats and soft cheeses (such as feta, some types of Mexican cheeses, Camembert, and blue-veined cheeses). One study found that 20 percent of hot dogs tested contained the bacterium *L. monocytogenes.*

Once thought to be exclusively a veterinary problem, it was identified as a human disease in 1981 when a Canadian outbreak was linked to tainted coleslaw made from cabbage grown in soil fertilized with *Listeria*-infected sheep manure. Four years later another outbreak was traced to Mexican-style soft cheese in California. This outbreak sickened 150 people, including many pregnant women, and resulted in newborn deaths. In the 1990s, the U.S. government recalled a wide variety of cooked products contaminated with *Listeria,* including hot dogs, bologna, and other luncheon meats; chicken and ham salad; sausages; chicken; sliced turkey breast; and sliced roast beef.

The bacteria are remarkably tough and resist heat, salt, nitrite, and acidity much better than many other organisms. It can survive on cold surfaces and can multiply slowly at temperatures as low as 34° F. (Refrigeration at 40° F or below stops the multiplication of many other food-borne bacteria.) Freezing food stops the bacteria from multiplying, and commercial pasteurization eliminates the organism in dairy products. *Listeria* does not change the taste or smell of food. When the bacteria are found in processed products, the contamination probably occurred after processing, due to poor heating or pasteurizing.

Listeria also can be spread through sexual contact, although it is not known how common this is. Babies can be born with listeriosis if their mothers ate contaminated food during pregnancy. Pregnant women are 20 times more likely than other healthy adults to get listeriosis; about one-third of all cases happen during pregnancy. However, it is newborns rather than their mothers who suffer the most serious effects of infection during pregnancy.

Patients with AIDS are 300 times more likely to get listeriosis than are healthy people. Others at increased risk include those with cancer, diabetes, kidney disease, and the elderly. While healthy adults and children sometimes become infected, they rarely become seriously ill.

Healthy adults may not have any symptoms at all or may experience a flulike illness with fever, muscle aches, and nausea or diarrhea. If infection spreads to the nervous system, it can cause a type of meningitis. If a pregnant woman develops the infection, she may experience fever, tiredness, headache, sore throat, dry cough, or back pain.

To avoid *Listeria* cross-contamination, food preparers should wash their hands, all utensils, and cutting boards that have touched raw meat and poultry. Raw vegetables should be scrubbed well before eating. Hot dogs and chicken should be cooked thoroughly.

Hurd, S. et al. "Morbidity and Mortality Weekly Report: Multistate Outbreak of Listeriosis," *Journal of the American Medical Association,* 49 (2000): 1,129–1,130.

lite See FOOD LABELING.

lite salt See SODIUM.

lithiasis The formation of stones in the body. GALLSTONES and KIDNEY STONES are the most common examples. (See also CALCIUM.)

lithium A nonessential mineral used in the treatment of bipolar disorder. Lithium is closely related to sodium and to potassium. Studies of animals maintained in controlled environments and on very restricted dietary lithium have revealed slowed growth and decreased reproduction. If there is a nutritional requirement for lithium, it seems likely to be easily satisfied by widespread occurrences of lithium in water and plant foods.

In therapeutic doses, lithium is used to normalize mood swings in people with bipolar disorder; and alcoholics. Lithium can also affect the THYROID GLAND. Overdose can cause DIARRHEA, nausea, vomiting, muscle weakness, and, in extreme cases, convulsions and coma. Excessive lithium can block hormonal control of kidneys, leading to excessive water loss (DIABETES INSIPIDUS). Nonsteroidal and anti-inflammatory agents increase lithium toxicity. (See also MINERALS; TRACE MINERALS.)

liver The largest organ of the body that performs many physiologic processes. The adult liver weighs 3 to 5 pounds. Blood from the intestines carries nutrients absorbed after DIGESTION directly to the liver via the portal vein. Certain nutrients such as fat-soluble vitamins and VITAMIN B_{12} are absorbed in the liver. Other nutrients are sent on to other parts of the body. Toxic materials are normally inactivated and then excreted.

The liver also:

Produces Bile Bile contains BILE ACIDS, synthesized from CHOLESTEROL; they act as detergents to dissolve dietary FAT and facilitate fat digestion.

Maintains Blood Sugar The liver functions as a "glucostat" to maintain BLOOD SUGAR within a normal range. For example, it absorbs excess blood sugar (GLUCOSE) after a carbohydrate meal when blood sugar is high and converts it to a storage substance called GLYCOGEN. Conversely, the liver breaks down glycogen to glucose when the blood sugar level drops too low. When the need for glucose is very high, as during fasting and crash dieting, the liver can manufacture it from noncarbohydrate substances, including most AMINO ACIDS, LACTIC ACID, PYRUVIC ACID, and several acids derived from the central pathways for energy production from fat and carbohydrate oxidation (KREB'S CYCLE).

Synthesizes Lipids The liver synthesizes cholesterol and fat from glucose under conditions of glucose excess. It forms particles, VERY LOW-DENSITY LIPOPROTEIN (VLDL) and HIGH-DENSITY LIPOPROTEIN (HDL) and, indirectly, LOW-DENSITY LIPOPROTEIN (LDL), which permit transporting these LIPIDS in the bloodstream.

Detoxifies Products of Metabolism, As Well As Many Foreign Substances The liver converts toxic AMMONIA, a by-product of protein breakdown, to the safe, excretable end product, UREA. Steroid hormones are often oxidized and attached to sulfate to increase their water solubility and thus may facilitate excretion. Some by-products are excreted in bile; the BILE PIGMENT, biliburin, is an example. Poisons, environmental pollutants, and medications such as birth control drugs can be oxidized or degraded by Phase I enzymes, including CYTOCHROME P450 enzymes. A second set of enzymes called transferases (Phase II enzymes) attach amino acids (GLYCINE, TAURINE), sugar derivatives (glucuronic acid), or other, highly water-soluble compounds like glutathione to further increase the water solubility of the modified toxins and ease their excretion by the kidneys and bile.

Synthesizes Blood Plasma Proteins The liver synthesizes most of the soluble proteins that occur with blood: serum ALBUMIN, the major soluble protein of blood; blood-clotting factors; transport proteins, such as TRANSFERRIN (used for iron transport); in addition VLDL, HDL, and LDL mentioned above.

Oxidizes Alcohol The liver is the major site for disposing of ALCOHOL. The enzymes are called ethanol oxidizing systems.

Activates Vitamins The liver converts BETA-CAROTENE, the precursor of vitamin A that occurs in plants, to VITAMIN A as needed.

Stores Many Essential Nutrients The liver stores fat-soluble nutrients like VITAMIN A, VITAMIN D, and VITAMIN K, as well as nonlipid nutrients like IRON and VITAMIN B_{12}

Helps Dispose of Aged Red Blood Cells While the liver serves as a major "garbage disposal unit" of the body, the risk of liver damage increases with excessive exposure to PESTICIDES, alcohol, hydrocarbons, toxic heavy metals like LEAD and MERCURY, solvents like carbon tetrachloride, spray paints and degreasers. Liver diseases such as hepatitis (liver inflammation) and CIRRHOSIS (liver scarring) can profoundly affect metabolic processes.

Calf liver in the diet is an excellent source of B complex vitamins, including vitamin B_{12}, VITAMIN B_6, FOLIC ACID, and RIBOFLAVIN; trace minerals like iron and ZINC, and vitamin A. It contains little calcium like most meat; the cholesterol content is high. Fried beef liver (3 oz., 85 g) provides 185 calories; protein, 23 g; carbohydrate, 7 g; fat, 7 g; cholesterol, 410 mg; calcium, 9 mg; iron, 5.3 mg; vitamin A, 9,120 retinol equivalents; thiamin, 0.18 mg; riboflavin, 3.52 mg; niacin, 12.3 mg. (See also CARBOHYDRATE METABOLISM; DETOXIFICATION; GLUCONEOGENESIS; HOMEOSTASIS.)

liver cirrhosis See CIRRHOSIS.

liverwurst Also called liver sausage, this is a German-style seasoned luncheon meat made from at least 30 percent pork liver mixed with other meats. The word in German, *leberwurst,* means "liver sausage." It is high in both iron and fat, with a texture that runs the gamut from coarse to creamy. Liverwurst is most often sliced for use as a sandwich meat or spread on bread or crackers as a snack food. Braunschweiger, the most popular type of liverwurst, is smoked and enriched with eggs and milk. Its name is derived from a town in Germany (Braunschweig). An 18 g serving of liverwurst provides calories, 58.5; protein, 2.5 g; fat 5 g; sodium, 155 mg. (See also SAUSAGE.)

lobster (*Homarus*) A crustacean belonging to the same family as crabs and shrimp. Crustaceans have rigid exoskeletons or shells with jointed bodies and legs. Lobsters are the largest shellfish. The European lobster is found off the coast of Norway and

Britain; its color is violet blue and green. The northern lobster is found in coastal waters of the east coast of Canada and the United States. Most lobster is harvested in the summer and fall in Canada, Massachusetts, and Maine.

The average lobster is a foot long (30 cm) and weighs up to 3 pounds (450–1,250 g). Its claws and tail are full of meat. Its abdomen has seven sections; it terminates in a fan-shaped tail that is also full of meat. Spring (rock) lobsters come from the southeastern United States and Pacific waters. These lack the large pincer claw of the northern species, and most of the meat is in the tail. Cooked lobster tails are usually imported from Australia, New Zealand, and South Africa.

A live lobster can be identified by a reflex action of the eyes. Lobsters can be killed humanely by cooling them for two hours and then plunging them into boiling water. When cooked, lobster turns red. They should be cooked to 165°. The small legs should pull off easily. There are many lobster dishes: Newburg, Thermidor, grilled, and roasted lobster. Souffles and mousses are also popular.

Shellfish generally are low in calories and in both total fat and saturated fat. A 3-oz. (85 g) serving of lobster provides 77 calories; protein, 16 g; fat, 0.76 g; calcium, 26 g; sodium, 272 mg; cholesterol, 81 mg; thiamin, 0.37 mg; riboflavin, 0.04 mg; niacin, 1.23 mg. (See also SEAFOOD.)

locust bean gum (carob bean gum) A GUM obtained from the bean of the carob tree that is produced in Greece, Italy, Portugal, and Spain, and used as a thickening agent and texturizer for ICE CREAM, salad dressing, pie filling, and barbecue sauce. When added to dough, it makes baked goods retain their shape. It improves the consistency and palatability of gels and other thickeners (CARAGEENAN). In large amounts, locust bean gum acts as a mild LAXATIVE. Locust bean gum is considered a safe FOOD ADDITIVE.

lopid See CHOLESTEROL-LOWERING DRUGS.

lovage (*Levisticum officinale*) A perennial aromatic HERB related to PARSLEY and CELERY that originated in Persia. It grows to a height of 5 to 7 feet; its leaves resemble celery and the greens have a celery-like flavor. Leaves and seeds can flavor many types of dishes, such as meats, salads, and soups. The dried root is sometimes used as a condiment. Lovage seeds are used as a flavoring in candy manufacturing. (See also SPICE.)

low-density lipoprotein (LDL) The lipid-protein particle that transports CHOLESTEROL from the LIVER to other tissues via the bloodstream. LDL carries 60 percent to 80 percent of the cholesterol found in serum (the clear fluid remaining after blood has clotted and blood cells are removed). LDL consists of an envelope of PHOSPHOLIPID, a fat-like substance that acts like a detergent to surround and dissolve oily cholesterol droplets. LDL is absorbed by muscle and fat cells, where it is captured by specific docking sites on cell surfaces. A unique protein called apolipoprotein B on the LDL provides a recognition site or "zip code" for docking sites on target cells. Once absorbed by cells, LDL is destroyed and its cholesterol is either incorporated in cell membranes or is stored. Interference with LDL uptake causes blood cholesterol levels to rise, increasing the risk of ATHEROSCLEROSIS.

Elevated LDL is considered to be an approximate or rough index of cardiovascular risk among U.S. men. Because elevated LDL is believed to increase the risk of heart disease, LDL has often been called "bad" or "undesirable" cholesterol. Even borderline-high LDL cholesterol levels (130 to 159 mg per 100 ml [dl] of serum) have been linked to an increased risk of clogged arteries and of heart attacks among American men. Accordingly, a target level for LDL-cholesterol is less than 130 mg/dL; for people with heart disease, the levels of LDL should be 100 mg/dL or less.

A second important form of blood cholesterol is called HDL (HIGH-DENSITY LIPOPROTEIN). HDL can be thought of as a scavenger, transporting cholesterol from tissues like muscle back to the liver for disposal.

Both LDL cholesterol and HDL cholesterol can be measured by routine lab tests. In general, a lowered LDL and an elevated HDL are desirable. HDL cholesterol should be greater than 35, for men (or 50 for women) and values greater than 65 can protect against diseased arteries. More accurate assessments of cardiovascular risk are based on measurements of LDL and HDL and LDL/HDL ratio. The most specific way of assessing LDL/HDL ratios relies on laboratory tests that measure apolipoprotein B (Apo B), the marker substance for LDL, and apolipoprotein A (Apo A), the specific protein marker for HDL.

The level of LDL cholesterol and the associated risk of heart disease depend on many factors, including inheritance, the amount of fat in the diet, and how a person chooses to live. Factors that raise LDL (and lower HDL) levels include: a high saturated fat diet; cigarette smoking; a lack of exercise; obesity; excessive alcohol consumption; and a family history of high blood cholesterol. Factors that lower LDL include: regular aerobic exercise; POLYUNSATURATED OILS and MONOUNSATURATED OILS substituted for saturated fat in the diet; adequate fiber in the diet, including soluble FIBER such as PECTIN and oat BRAN; and weight management and stress management.

Oxidized LDL represents a dangerous form of cholesterol and it is the most active blood lipid in promoting atherosclerosis. Oxidized LDL is present in clogged arteries as deposits called PLAQUE. Macrophages, scavenger cells in artery walls, may oxidize excessive LDL, or they may selectively take up oxidized LDL to become cholesterol-filled "foam" cells in arteries. Foam cells seem to set the stage for plaque buildup. Other lines of evidence support this hypothesis. Antibodies against oxidized LDL appear in patients with advanced atherosclerosis. Oxidized LDL attracts more cells (monocytes) from the blood to enter the artery wall and become resident macrophages. Furthermore, oxidized LDL helps immobilize those macrophages, thus trapping them inside arteries. Oxidized LDL can itself damage cells and possibly injure arterial walls. It is thought that the resulting damage to the arterial lining causes the release of growth factors that stimulate the migration and growth of muscle cells at the damaged area in the arterial wall. These processes may continue over years, leading eventually to plaque buildup, narrowed arteries and, ultimately, to blocked arteries and heart attack or stroke.

The exact mechanisms by which LDL is oxidized and a definition of the details of plaque formation are being actively investigated. It is known that oxidative damage in the body occurs by FREE RADICALS and other reactive forms of oxygen. These highly reactive molecules readily attack sensitive molecules in the cell, such as DNA, lipids, and protein. Antioxidant drugs can inhibit atherosclerosis in lab animals with elevated blood cholesterol levels that are susceptible to this disease. A growing body of evidence links the protective effects of antioxidant nutrients such as VITAMIN E, vitamin C, beta-carotene and carotenoids, selenium and zinc to decreased lipid oxidation and lowered risk of CARDIOVASCULAR DISEASE. (See also HYPERCHOLESTEROLEMIA; LIPOPROTEINS.)

Islam, S. et al. "Association of Apolipoprotein A Phenotypes and Oxidized Low-Density Lipoprotein Immune Complexes in Children," *Archives of Pediatric Adolescent Medicine* 153, no. 1 (1999): 57–62.

low-fat cheese See CHEESE.

low-fat diets Diets that drastically reduce the consumption of fats, oils, and fatty foods. The unmodified PRITIKIN DIET limits fat intake to approximately 10 percent of total calories, while the MACROBIOTIC DIET, based on grains, vegetables, legumes, and condiments, also entails a similar low-fat intake. A lifestyle change program has been developed for patients with heart disease that offers an alternative to bypass surgery to stop the progression of the disease. The program involves a vegetarian diet providing 10 percent fat, together with moderate exercise, stress management, and group support.

Ultra-low-fat diets are more difficult to follow than other diets because fats and oils satisfy hunger both by slowing the emptying of the stomach after a meal and by providing pleasing flavors ("mouth feel"). People generally are more successful in reducing their fat calories to 20 percent than any lower. Heredity may determine how people will respond to low-fat diets. Those who inherit small, dense versions of LDL ("bad CHOLESTEROL") and who also have low levels of HDL ("good cholesterol") may respond better to low-fat diets. Sharply reducing saturated fat intake may cause a drop in HDL. This can be minimized by losing excess weight or by regular aerobic exercise.

Current federal guidelines and the American Heart Association recommend lowering fat intake to less than 30 percent of calories because excessive fat is linked to heart disease, cancer, and obesity. Other experts are recommending reduction to 20 percent or 25 percent of calories to obtain a greater benefit and decreased risk. (See also HEART DISEASE; FAT METABOLISM.)

luncheon meats Highly processed meat typically served for sandwiches and hors d'oeuvres. BOLOGNA and salami are typical examples. Characteristically, luncheon meats contain significant FAT, saturated fat, SALT, and NITRITE. Nutrition information on the food label is based on the size of the slice. As with any food listing ingredients by the serving size, multiply the nutrient content per serving (provided by the food label) by the number of servings you actually eat to determine calories, fat, and so on.

Beef and pork luncheon meats are often highest in calories and fat. However, turkey salami, turkey bologna, and chicken may contain as many calories as cold cuts made from beef or pork, due to fat, for example, from added skin. Most luncheon meats provide about 20 mg of cholesterol per slice. Sodium nitrite is used to cure meats and to preserve their color. The sodium content can range from a low of 80 mg to a high of 400 mg of sodium per slice. DIETARY GUIDELINES FOR AMERICANS recommends choosing a diet low in fat, sodium, and cholesterol. Fat should be less than 30 percent of calories.

Turkey breast, turkey ham, and chicken breast are low-sodium, low-fat alternatives to bologna, meat loaf, or salami, which are high-fat fare. In contrast, skinless turkey or chicken breast is considered lean meat. (See also FOOD PROCESSING.)

lupus erythematosus An inflammatory disease in which defense proteins of the IMMUNE SYSTEM (ANTIBODIES) form complexes with tissue proteins, leading to tissue damage. A disease in which the body attacks itself is classified as an AUTOIMMUNE DISEASE.

Systemic lupus erythematosus, the most common type of lupus, typically develops during the 20s, 30s, or 40s—but about 15 percent to 17 percent of people with systemic lupus first notice symptoms during childhood or adolescence. Most of these are children 10 years or older; it is extremely rare in children under age five. Experts estimate between 5,000 and 10,000 children in the United States have SLE.

A healthy immune system produces proteins called antibodies that normally protect the body against bacterial and viral infections. In people with lupus, the immune system is unable to distinguish between foreign substances and the body's own cells, and it makes antibodies that target the patient's cells, sparking inflammation and pain. Systemic lupus, which can be mild or life-threatening, can affect many organs in the body. Lupus symptoms include a red facial rash, intermittent fever, severe joint pain, and bouts of extreme fatigue. The disease may affect different regions of the body, including the skin, the joints, the heart and blood vessels, the lungs, the brain, and the kidneys. Women are 10 times more prone than men; lupus affects two U.S. women per thousand. This serious disease is sometimes fatal. Common signs and symptoms include fever, arthritis damage to the nervous system, weight loss, sensitivity to light, and possibly heart disease and kidney failure. A lab test (ANA, antinuclear antibody tests) is used to monitor SLE.

Early intervention can control lupus and reduce the risk of irreversible kidney damage. Standard treatment involves the use of drugs (corticosteroids) and immune suppressants to limit INFLAMMATION. Lupus is associated with low stomach acid production (HYPOCHLORHYDRIA). Food allergies may be correlated with the incidence of SLE and should be checked. The relationship between SLE and CANDIDA YEAST overgrowth remains controversial. Two steroid homes, DHEA and testosterone, may help normalize immune function and they have been used to treat autoimmune disease. Gotu kola (*Centilla asiatica*), a medicinal herb long used in China and India, has been reported to alleviate lupus. VITAMIN B_6 sometimes relieves symptoms. FISH OILS may play a role in treating a variety of autoimmune diseases, including lupus; possible benefits of fish oil for lupus are derived from animal studies and anecdotal reports. Omega-6 fatty acids, as found in black current, borage, and evening primrose oils are helpful. In 1997 researchers discovered a genetic marker for lupus that predisposes people to the disease. It is hoped that this discovery will lead to better understanding of the disease and possible treatments or a cure. (See also MAST CELL.)

Tsao, B. P. et al. "Evidence for Linkage of a Candidate Chromosome 1 Region to Human Systemic Lupus Erythematosus (SLE)," *Journal of Clinical Investigation* 99 (1997): 725–731.

lutein A CAROTENOID found in egg yolks and many FRUITS and VEGETABLES, especially those of the dark green leafy variety such as spinach, kale, and broccoli. Lutein is a member of the xanthophyll family of pigments, which includes ASTAXANTHIN. In the body lutein is found in its highest concentrations in the macula region of the eye, directly in front of the cones of the retina. It is believed that lutein's ANTIOXIDANT properties protect the delicate eye tissues from damage by CANCER-causing FREE RADICALS, and that it may act as a light filter, preventing harmful blue light from the sun from reaching inner eye structures. Some studies support the conclusion that eating foods rich in lutein can help prevent eye disease, such as macular degeneration, a condition that causes loss of central vision and that affects one in six Americans over age 55.

Another study revealed that lutein may help prevent arteries from being clogged by plaque (ATHEROSCLEROSIS), a condition that causes heart attacks and strokes. In one study of 480 adults between the ages of 40 and 60 who had no history of heart disease, researchers noted that those subjects who had the highest levels of lutein in their blood at the study's start showed no increase in the growth of arterial plaque 18 months later. In contrast, those subjects who had the lowest lutein levels showed the greatest increase in plaque growth.

Other studies involving lutein show that this carotenoid may be helpful in preventing or battling breast and skin cancer and in reducing the risk of cataracts. Given these promising initial studies, many health professionals are recommending that patients increase their consumption of lutein-laden foods.

Purified lutein and lycopene are now available as supplements, although it is not known if they offer the same benefits as other carotenoid-rich foods.

Dwyer, James H. et al. "Oxygenated Carotenoid Lutein and Progression of Early Atherosclerosis," *Circulation* 103 (2001): 2,922–2,927.

Snodderly, D. "Evidence for Protection Against Age-Related Macular Degeneration by Carotenoids and Antioxidant Vitamins," *American Journal of Clinical Nutrition* 62 (1995): 1,448–1,461.

lycopene The principal pigment responsible for the color of TOMATOES, PAPRIKA, and pink GRAPEFRUIT. Structurally, this red plant pigment resembles BETA-CAROTENE and belongs to the carotene family of yellow-orange plant pigments (carotenoids). Unlike beta-carotene, however, lycopene lacks VITAMIN A activity; the body cannot transform it to the vitamin. Lycopene is prevalent in the testes and in the plasma, where it occurs at a greater concentration than beta-carotene. Population studies suggest the consumption of 6 mg lycopene daily from tomatoes and tomato products reduces the risk of prostate cancer. Ingesting 12 mg or more each day from food reduces the risk of lung cancer in nonsmoking men. For women risk reduction is seen at 6.5 mg daily.

Lycopene and related carotenoids can function as antioxidants to quench FREE RADICALS (highly reactive molecules generated in the body that can damage tissues and promote aging and disease). Carotenoids complement the antioxidant activity of beta-carotene, and together they help reduce inflammation, maintain healthy cell membranes, and modulate the synthesis of families of prostaglandins and leukotrienes, fatty acid derivatives that stimulate inflammation. (See also CAROTENOIDS.)

lymph The protein-rich fluid that escapes from blood vessels (capillaries) and flows between cells. Lymph has a composition resembling blood PLASMA, the fluid remaining after blood has clotted. While lymph contains ELECTROLYTES (dissolved minerals), GLUCOSE and other nutrients and certain proteins from blood, it also contains fat from digestion when it drains the intestinal tract. Lymph flows into lymphatic ducts leading to major ducts (the thoracic duct and the right lymphatic duct) that drain into large blood veins above the heart.

lymphatic system A system of vessels and organs that helps defend against infection consisting of lymphatic vessels (narrow tubes that transport a watery colorless fluid through tissues to the bloodstream). Unlike the CIRCULATORY SYSTEM (the heart and blood vessels), the lymphatic system is not a "closed loop" because it is a network of one-way roads, consisting of increasingly larger ducts (channels) that ultimately drain into the bloodstream. Diffuse lymphatic tissue and lymph nodules occur in the tissue lining passageways of the body, especially the gastrointestinal tract.

The lymphatic system can be considered a specialized connective tissue that contains defensive cells of the IMMUNE SYSTEM. Cells in lymphatic tissue, lymphocytes, help protect the body against foreign cells and cancer cells. Lymph nodes are checkpoints along the lymphatic highway; they filter the lymph and destroy foreign materials and microorganisms. The infection-fighting cells are called lymphocytes. Certain nodules such as tonsils, Peyers patches in the ileum of the small intestine, and nodules in the appendix consist of large aggregates of lymphatic tissue. (See also ALLERGY, FOOD.)

lymphocyte See IMMUNE SYSTEM.

lymphokines (cytokines) A large family of specialized proteins that regulate the immune system. Lymphokines are chemical signals mainly produced by T cells, white blood cells that help regulate the immune response, especially to combat infection by viruses, fungus, parasites, and certain cancers. Lymphokines activate antibody-producing cells (B cells). Certain lymphokines called interleukins act as growth promoters to stimulate the growth of T cells, while others destroy targeted diseased cells (tumor necrosis factor) or they can activate macrophages. Another type of lymphokine called interferon acts as a defensive protein to inhibit the production of viruses.

Lymphokines can direct lymphocytes, sensitized to a foreign invader, to destroy invading agents according to the following scenario. In the first stage, defensive cells called macrophages engulf foreigners and in turn release a lymphokine called interleukin-1, when they meet a foreign substance (ANTIGEN). If the antigen is a food, interleukin-1 may help trigger a food allergy. Interleukin-1 then stimulates T cell production. In the next stage, activated T cells release a second lymphokine, interleukin-2, which further stimulates T cell formation and the production of cytotoxic T cells, specialized in destroying invaders. (See also ALLERGY, FOOD; AUTOIMMUNE DISEASE; INFLAMMATION.)

lysine (Lys, L-lysine) A dietary essential AMINO ACID and a required building block of proteins. Lysine cannot be fabricated in the body and must be supplied by the diet. It is the only essential amino acid with two amino groups (nitrogen bearing groups). It is positively charged in body fluids and is classified as a basic amino acid because it can function chemically as an alkaline substance.

Sources of lysine (high lysine/arginine content) include red meat, fish, poultry, eggs, peanuts, soybeans, milk, brewer's yeast, and potatoes. Of the various essential amino acids in grain proteins, lysine is usually present in limited amounts; consequently, plant breeding programs have developed high lysine strains of BARLEY, SORGHUM, and CORN. Food processing and baking at high temperatures tend to destroy lysine because during extensive heating or prolonged storage, lysine in cereal protein reacts with carbohydrate, yielding an inactive complex. About a third of the lysine in dry breakfast cereals is unusable by the body for this reason. The adult daily requirement is 12 mg per kilogram of body weight per day.

Some evidence suggests that lysine supplements lessen outbreaks of herpes virus infection and diminish related symptoms, especially when supplemented with VITAMIN B_6 and MAGNESIUM. It may be beneficial to restrict consumption of ARGININE, another basic amino acid required for protein synthesis that may be a dietary essential in serious disease states and liver damage. Excessive lysine supplements may antagonize arginine. (See also AMINO ACID METABOLISM.)

lysosome A small particle, found in the cytoplasm of many types of cells, that is responsible for degrading cellular debris. Lysosomes contain powerful degradative enzymes to completely break down proteins, as well as bacteria that are engulfed by cells. Lysosomes also recycle components of worn-out organelles and cellular structures so that amino acids, cholesterol and fatty acids can be reused. A typical LIVER cell can recycle about half of its contents per week. LOW-DENSITY LIPOPROTEIN (LDL), the cholesterol transport particle in the blood, is absorbed by muscle and fat tissue and degraded by their lysosomes. This is the way cholesterol is deposited within cells.

Normally, lysosomal enzymes are confined within lysosomes to prevent indiscriminate DIGESTION of the cell. However, during tissue repair, lysosomal enzymes released from damaged cells help digest any cellular debris and prepare the area for repair and wound healing.

M

maca (*Lepidium peruvianum, Lepidium meyenii*) The dried root of a cruciferous vegetable related to the radish, maca is native to Peru, where it has been used as a food staple and a medicine by the indigenous people for thousands of years. Maca's principle constituents include protein (about 11 percent), calcium (about 10 percent), magnesium, and potassium. Other nutrients include iron, silica, iodine, manganese, zinc, and copper. It is available in dry powder, liquid extract, and capsule form.

Although unproven, claims of maca's health benefits center on its alleged ability to balance the body's hormone levels. Advocates say maca eases the symptoms of menopause, including hot flashes and vaginal dryness; enhances libido in both men and women; strengthens bones; promotes healthy skin, nail and hair growth; increases fertility; and elevates mood.

macaroni A form of PASTA in which pieces of wheat dough are formed into various shapes and dried. Macaroni includes pasta strands (such as spaghetti), shells (conchiglie), or tubes (cannelloni, elbow macaroni, or ziti), and it can be bent, corrugated, straight, or spiraled. Macaroni is composed of flour from durum wheat (a "hard wheat" rich in protein), farina (a coarsely ground endosperm of other wheats), and SEMOLINA, the coarsely milled, starchy endosperm of durum wheat after bran and germ have been removed. Semolina, farina, and durum wheat flour can be used in any combination or they can be used separately. Semolina is high in protein, which gives dough the strength to hold up to the mechanical processing needed to make pasta. A small amount of disodium phosphate is added to make pasta cook more quickly. Since January 1998 all enriched pasta, flour, rice, cornmeal, and other cereal grain products in the United States have been fortified with folic acid to help reduce the incidence of neural tube defects in newborn babies. Products marked "enriched" must contain specific amounts of certain vitamins and minerals: 4 to 5 mg of THIAMIN; 1.7 to 2.2 mg of RIBOFLAVIN; 27 to 34 mg of NIACIN; and 13 to 16.5 mg of IRON per pound. Eggs are an optional ingredient in macaroni. Other pasta variations include whole wheat, beet, spinach, and soy macaroni products. (See also BREAD; COMPLEX CARBOHYDRATE; FOLIC ACID.)

mackerel (*Scomber scombrus*) A saltwater predatory fish related to tuna, with a very streamlined body. This important food fish is typically 14 in (35 cm) in length. The Atlantic mackerel ranges from Labrador to Cape Hatteras. The king mackerel, *Scomber omovus cuvalia*, is found in coastal waters from the Carolinas to Brazil. Mackerel is an oily fish and represents one of the richest sources of marine oils, EICOSAPENTAENOIC ACID and other omega-3 fatty acids. These fatty acids lower blood lipids and may reduce the risk of ATHEROSCLEROSIS, and they help reduce symptoms of autoimmune diseases like RHEUMATOID ARTHRITIS. By decreasing the tendency of blood clot formation, they lower the risk of STROKE and HEART ATTACK. The outer layers of mackerel meat are red; the interior layers are lighter in color. Most commercial mackerel is canned; fresh mackerel is very perishable. The nutrient content of 3 oz. (85 g) provides 174 calories; protein, 15.8 g; fat, 11.8 g; cholesterol, 60 mg; calcium, 10 mg; thiamin, 0.15 mg; riboflavin, 0.265 mg; niacin, 7.72 mg. (See also OMEGA-3 FATTY ACIDS; SALMON; SEAFOOD.)

macrobiotic diet A DIET emphasizing plant foods and complex carbohydrates (STARCH and FIBER). The macrobiotic diet was introduced by George Ohsawa in the 1960s in California and it continues to be popular. The macrobiotic diet encompasses more than foods; the belief that DIGESTION and assimilation are aided by eating slowly in a peaceful, harmonious atmosphere is fundamental. In its earliest form it was an imbalanced diet emphasizing RICE and GRAINS. Brown rice was considered an optimal balance of "yin" and "yang" forces. The rigorous application of macrobiotic principles frequently caused MALNUTRITION, with ANEMIA, slowed growth, RICKETS, even kidney damage, especially in children. The modified macrobiotic diet used today, which can vary with personal needs, is wholesome and tasty and includes locally produced foods and whole grains. Animal products are used as condiments, rather than as main dishes. The diet varies with the climate and season, to minimize use of chemical preservation and unnecessary food processing. Meals consist of 50 percent to 60 percent whole grains. The macrobiotic diet supplies about 73 percent of total carbohydrate; only 15 percent to 20 percent of the CALORIES are fats and oils (from whole grains and vegetable oils). Brown rice, MILLET, OATS, RYE, BUCKWHEAT, couscous, whole WHEAT, LEGUMES, VEGETABLES, FRUITS, NUTS, and seeds complete the foundation. Legumes supply 5 percent to 10 percent of calories in the form of adzuki, lima, kidney, navy, mung, pinto, and soy beans. Bean sprouts are useful adjuncts. Sea vegetables like arame, hijiki, kombu, nori, and wakame provide texture, flavor, and essential nutrients. Seafood and poultry are incorporated according to dietary goals or preferences. (See also HIGH COMPLEX CARBOHYDRATE DIET; VEGETARIAN.)

macronutrient Nutrients required by the DIET in amounts ranging from a fraction of a gram to more than a gram. The major minerals, CALCIUM, MAGNESIUM, SODIUM, POTASSIUM, CHLORIDE, and PHOSPHORUS are considered macronutrients. These balance body fluids and build bones and teeth. CARBOHYDRATE, FAT, OIL, and PROTEIN, together with WATER, are considered other macronutrients. Together they make up the bulk of food. Fat and carbohydrate must be eaten in large amounts daily because they provide the fuel that keeps the body's machinery operating. Proteins supply building blocks to replace worn out and damaged proteins. The recommended distribution of calories looks like this: For an adult requiring 2,000 calories daily, less than 600 calories (less than 30 percent of the total) should come from fat (67 grams or 4 tablespoons). How much less than 30 percent is optimal debatable. Fifty grams of protein (1.75 oz.) supplies 200 calories (20 percent of the total). The remaining 1,200 calories (60 percent) would come from carbohydrates, preferably COMPLEX CARBOHYDRATES as found in whole grains, LEGUMES, and VEGETABLES (roughly 300 g or two-thirds of a pound).

Fat is a concentrated form of ENERGY because it provides more than twice as many calories per gram as do carbohydrate or protein. The typical American diet provides about 40 percent of total calories as fat. Some 15 percent to 25 percent of calories as fat and oils may be more appropriate to reduce the risk of CANCER, HEART DISEASE, and OBESITY. Current dietary guidelines recommend choosing a diet reduced in total fat, saturated fat, and cholesterol, with oils and fats to be used sparingly.

For the average American, carbohydrate supplies about 40 percent to 45 percent of the total calories, with sweeteners like SUCROSE, FRUCTOSE, and CORN SYRUP representing about half of this (about 130 to 150 pounds per year per person). U.S. dietary goals publicized in the 1970s called for cutting SUGAR consumption by two-thirds while doubling STARCH intake with whole vegetables and grains. Current guidelines are less specific. They call for eating ample amounts of vegetables, fruit, and grain products daily: with six to 11 servings of bread and grain products; three to five servings of vegetables; and two to four servings of fruits, with sweets to be used sparingly.

Food supplies amino acids for building the thousands of proteins of the body. An adult needs to eat only 40 to 50 grams of protein a day, though the typical diet supplies twice this amount. The body treats surplus amino acids as excess fuel: They are either converted to fat or they are burned for energy.

Drinking the equivalent of two quarts of water each day replaces water lost due to waste disposal, urine, and feces, and to perspiration. Water is essential as a coolant and as the fluid of cells and tissues needed for their normal operation. (See also DIETARY GUIDELINES FOR AMERICANS; ELECTROLYTES.)

macrophage See IMMUNE SYSTEM.

mad cow disease See BOVINE SPONGIFORM ENCEPHALOPATHY.

magnesium A major mineral nutrient. The body contains 20 to 28 g of magnesium; 40 percent is found in tissues like MUSCLE and 60 percent occurs in BONE and teeth, where it is combined with phosphate. Among soft tissues the liver and muscles contain the highest levels. Within cells magnesium is the second most prevalent type of positively charged ion (cation) after potassium. Magnesium is required for all major metabolic processes involving ATP, the chemical energy currency of the cell. More than 300 enzymes are activated by magnesium and magnesium-ATP complexes. It functions in energy-consuming processes like biosynthesis of protein and of DNA and RNA; sugar breakdown (GLYCOLYSIS); and ATP-dependent transport of materials into the cell. Magnesium is essential for the transmission of nerve impulses; for electrical potentials of cell membranes; muscle contraction; ATP formation; and maintenance of blood vessels.

Possible Roles in Maintaining Health

Magnesium is essential for normal calcium metabolism. In muscle contraction, magnesium balances the effects of calcium, which stimulates contraction. Thus, magnesium regulates calcium uptake by cells to activate functions like heartbeat. Magnesium may also:

- protect against CARDIOVASCULAR DISEASE. It can help reduce high BLOOD PRESSURE, lower CHOLESTEROL as LOW-DENSITY LIPOPROTEIN (LDL) and increase HIGH-DENSITY LIPOPROTEIN (HDL) cholesterol;
- protect against lead poisoning;
- protect against migraine and DEPRESSION;
- help maintain normal heart function and prevent irregular heartbeat (cardiac dysrhythmia). The imbalance between calcium and magnesium may increase the risk of cardiovascular disease, and magnesium deficiency increases the risk of severe disruptions of cardiac rhythm;
- help alleviate PREMENSTRUAL SYNDROME, when used with ZINC and VITAMIN B_6 in certain cases;
- prevent KIDNEY STONES;
- alleviate convulsions associated with preeclampsia and ECLAMPSIA, a syndrome in pregnancy characterized by high blood pressure and protein in the urine. In serious cases, eclampsia can lead to convulsions and coma.

Sources

Magnesium is found in MEAT (especially liver); POULTRY; FISH and SEAFOOD; green vegetables like BROCCOLI; dairy products; hard water; TOFU; AMARANTH; wheat germ; pumpkin seeds; instant COFFEE; PEANUTS, CASHEWS, BRAZIL NUTS; BREAKFAST CEREALS; cocoa powder; BLACKSTRAP MOLASSES; and YEAST. Magnesium is lost during FOOD PROCESSING.

Requirements

The adult Recommended Dietary Allowance (RDA) for magnesium is 350 mg per day for men and 280 mg for women.The typical American diet provides about 120 mg per 1,000 calories. Thus a person consuming 1,500 calories or less is likely to be magnesium deficient. Factors that increase the need for magnesium due to limited uptake or increased losses include high dietary FIBER; too much phosphate (as soft drinks) and alcoholic beverages; high psychological stress; some DIURETICS (water pills) and regular, strenuous EXERCISE. Excessive calcium in supplements may compete with magnesium. Disease and conditions that cause magnesium depletion include MALABSORPTION, MALNUTRITION, ALCOHOLISM, and intravenous feeding using nutrient mixtures that do not contain enough magnesium. Marginal deficiency is very common among teenagers and people who diet; diabetics; pregnant and lactating women; those who drink heavily; elderly persons with poor eating habits; those taking diuretics and digitalis; athletes; women with osteoporosis; and individuals with severe kidney disease and severe DIARRHEA.

Early symptoms of magnesium deficiency are vague, including a loss of appetite, upset stomach, and diarrhea making diagnosis of a mild deficiency difficult. Symptoms of long-term deficiency relate to the nervous system: confusion apathy, depression, irritability, irregular heartbeat, muscle weakness, tremors, convulsions, and poor coordination, as well as a lack of APPETITE, listlessness, nausea, and vomiting. Measurement of white blood cell magnesium can be used to help assess the nutritional status of this mineral.

Safety

Excessive use of the home remedies Epsom salts and milk of magnesia leads to deficiencies of other minerals, even toxicity. Overdose with magnesium antacids (1,500 mg or more daily) is indicated by low blood pressure, drowsiness, nausea, slurred speech, and unsteadiness. Magnesium toxicity can occur when the kidneys cannot clear large overloads. While magnesium appears to be safe, it should not be taken by patients with kidney disease or by those with heart problems (atrioventricular blocks). A physician should be consulted prior to using supplements. (See also TRACE MINERALS.)

Seelig, M. "Review and Hypothesis: Might Patients with the Chronic Fatigue Syndrome Have Latent Tetany of Magnesium Deficiency?," *Journal of Chronic Fatigue Syndrome* 4, 2 (1998): 203–205.

***maitake* mushroom (*Grifola frondosa;* hen of the woods)** An edible fungus indigenous to Japan also found in parts of northern Europe and North America. Its rippling shape gives it the appearance of butterflies. In Japanese, *maitake* means "dancing butterfly." Some people say the fungus got its name because foragers who came upon it in the woods would dance with joy knowing they were in for a delicious treat.

Maitake, which (unlike many other types of MUSHROOM) has no cap at the end of its rippling stems, grows in clusters at the foot of mature oak trees. Individual specimens can grow to more than 50 pounds, which is why it is sometimes called the "king of mushrooms." The flesh is firm and has a "woody" taste.

Maitake has been used by herbalists in Japan for years to treat a variety of illnesses, including digestion problems, stress, and hemorrhoids. Research has shown that polysaccharides (including beta-glucan) strengthen the immune system and may be effective in fighting cancer. Some studies have shown that *maitake* consumption may help slow the progression of the AIDS virus. In other studies cancerous tumors in mice that were fed *maitake* extract decreased in size. Other animal studies indicate that *maitake* shows promise in treating high blood pressure, diabetes, and OBESITY.

Maitake are often sold dried. They add an earthy flavor to soups, salads, and pilafs and can be used in almost any recipe calling for firm mushrooms. Safety data are inadequate for pregnant and breast-feeding women.

Borchers, A. T. et al. "Mushrooms, Tumors and Immunity," *Proceedings of the Society of Experimental Biological Medicine* 221, no. 4 (1999): 281–293.

malabsorption Symptoms related to long-term inadequate nutrient absorption. A person can eat a BALANCED DIET' and still be malnourished if the intestines cannot absorb nutrients or if DIGESTION is incomplete. The most common nutritional deficiencies involve minerals like CALCIUM and IRON, and vitamins such as FOLIC ACID, VITAMIN B_6, or VITAMIN A.

Symptoms are varied, depending on the kind of nutrient that is deficient. Fatigue and lowered resistance to infection are common indicators. Vitamin and mineral deficiencies alter metabolism and lower immunity. Vitamin and iron deficiencies can cause ANEMIA, "tired blood." Chronic low calcium intake leads to OSTEOPOROSIS. B complex vitamin deficiency leads to a sore tongue.

Some Causes of Malabsorption

- rapid transit time (diarrhea)
- inadequate chewing
- inadequate digestion caused by low stomach acid production (HYPOCHLORHYDRIA), one of the consequences of aging
- impaired absorption due to an unhealthy intestinal lining. Severe food allergies, sensitivities and inflammation (such as CELIAC DISEASE and Crohn's disease) injure the absorptive surface of the intestine (MICROVILLI)
- inadequate intestinal digestive enzymes. Enteropeptidase is required to activate pancreatic enzymes. Disaccharidases are required to break down sugars such as lactose (milk sugar) and sucrose (table sugar). Parasitic infection can damage the intestinal lining and decrease production of these enzymes. Lactose deficiency is

age-related among most adults worldwide. Those of Northern European extraction often continue to make ample lactase enzyme throughout their lives

- bacterial overgrowth of the small intestine, which can block absorption and limit digestion
- impaired pancreatic output. Low stomach acid or more serious conditions like pancreatitis can decrease the output of digestive enzymes
- lowered bile production, which reduces fat digestion and the uptake of fat-soluble vitamins (A, D, K, and E)
- materials that absorb minerals and may prevent their uptake by the intestine. FIBER, PHYTIC ACID, and OXALIC ACID in VEGETABLES, GRAINS, and LEGUMES are examples;
- competition by drugs. Certain drugs can block the absorption of minerals and vitamins
- excessive minerals in the diet: for example, too much ZINC blocks copper uptake
- inadequate INTRINSIC FACTOR. Paralleling low stomach acid production, the stomach may produce too little intrinsic factor to facilitate VITAMIN B_{12} uptake.

(See also BIOAVAILABILITY; DEFICIENCY, SUBCLINICAL; DRUG-NUTRIENT INTERACTION; GLOSSITIS.)

maladaptation See TOLERANCE TO TOXIC MATERIALS.

malnutrition Impaired health due to imbalanced diet or to abnormal physiologic processes required to absorb and use optimal amounts of nutrients. Thus, malnutrition can reflect the failure to obtain enough nutrients (undernutrition), or it may mean excessive amounts of nutrients (overnutrition), or both. Reliance on highly processed foods can lead to simultaneous overnutrition and undernutrition.

Overnutrition The major dietary problems in the Western world reflect too much food, rather than too little. Excessive CALORIES, refined CARBOHYDRATE, FAT, saturated fat, and sodium set the stage for modern diseases such as CANCER, CARDIOVASCULAR DISEASE, DIABETES, HYPERTENSION, and OBESITY.

Undernutrition Primary undernutrition refers to ingesting inadequate amounts of nutrients to sustain normal growth or health. Populations in developing nations often suffer from chronic undernutrition. Being significantly underweight shortens the life span and takes an immense toll in human suffering. STARVATION represents severe undernutrition; the diet does not provide enough major nutrients (protein, carbohydrate, and fat) to maintain the body. The physiological results are the same as for prolonged fasting. Other symptoms include dry skin, sores that do not heal, swelling, inflamed tongue, flabby muscles, slow growth and development, and FATIGUE and apathy. Prolonged starvation wastes the body because it must literally consume itself to survive. ANEMIA and a failure to grow are severe consequences. Inadequate body stores of vitamins and minerals generally lead to a decreased immunity and a greater risk of infection.

Other symptoms are common: slowed knee reflexes; abnormal pigmentation of eye membranes (conjunctiva), redness of eyes and eyelids; dull, brittle hair that is easily plucked and sometimes lighter in color than normal; swollen, bleeding gums; receded gum line; swollen parotid glands and THYROID GLANDS; chapped, red, or cracked lips; brittle, rigid nails; rapid heartbeat; high blood pressure and enlarged liver in children.

Secondary undernutrition refers to the body's inability to efficiently use nutrients. This situation can be caused by poor digestion, inadequate uptake due to an unhealthy intestine, or by competition of nutrients with each other or with drugs. Mild malnutrition without major deficiency symptoms is much more common than severe undernutrition in the United States, but it is much harder to detect. The most common symptom is fatigue.

The deaths of more than 6 million children in developing countries who are under the age of five are attributable to malnutrition. According to the U.S. Department of Agriculture's 1994–96 Continuing Survey of Food Intakes by Individuals, only 3 percent of all Americans meet four of the five recommendations for daily consumption of grains, fruits, vegetables, dairy products, and meats. According to a survey conducted by the Nutrition Screening Initiative, a national project to promote routine nutrition screening and better nutrition among older people, one in four elderly patients suffers from malnutrition.

The elderly are prone to malnutrition because of poverty, isolation, loss of TASTE, loss of teeth and GINGIVITIS, multiple medications, constipation and MALABSORPTION, poor eating habits, reliance on PROCESSED FOODS, skipping meals, chronic disease and physical impairments that limit the ability to shop for or cook food, and a lack of concern about nutrition.

Malnutrition in Children

Poverty and malnutrition go hand in hand, and children suffer the most worldwide. Mild undernutrition is much more common worldwide than starvation, although famine is endemic in certain regions of Africa. Marginal intake of vitamins, minerals and/or amino acids in a child's diet can lead to lowered immunity and a decreased ability of white cells to fight off infections, as well as slowed mental and physical development.

The failure of babies to thrive most often results from an inadequate diet. MARASMUS refers to the form of starvation occurring when the diet does not supply enough calories. The skeletal image usually associated with starvation reflects marasmus. Muscle wasting supplies the body with energy. Children with marasmus adapt by slowing their growth rates, which can have severe, long-term effects on mental and physical development. KWASHIORKOR is the form of starvation occurring when the diet supplies enough carbohydrate to meet daily calorie needs, but lacks adequate PROTEIN. The starving child may appear puffy and swollen because of severe edema.

Malnutrition among children of affluent, well-educated parents is a recent phenomenon in the United States. Some well-intentioned, well-educated parents apply their low-fat diets to their children to decrease the risk of childhood obesity and of heart disease later. Children grow rapidly, and low-calorie, low-fat diets can retard their growth and development. Parents should consult a specialist before putting a child on a diet. (See also BIOAVAILABILITY; CHOLESTEROL; DEFICIENCY, SUBCLINICAL.)

Salama, Peter et al. "Malnutrition, Measles, Mortality, and the Humanitarian Response During a Famine in Ethiopia," *JAMA* 286 (2001): 563–571.

malt A product of germinated BARLEY used in brewing beer. To prepare malt, germinated barley is bleached and dried to prevent further sprouting. During germination, seed enzymes cleave STARCH to the sugar, maltose, and split cell wall FIBER (hemicelluloses) into fermentable simple sugars. Other GRAINS, such as RYE and WHEAT, can also be malted. Malted milk is prepared by combining whole milk with the filtrate from a mixture of barley milk and wheat flour.

Malt is fermented by yeast to ALCOHOL when beer is brewed. Malting and brewing were among the earliest discoveries of civilization. Egyptians have brewed beer since 5000 B.C. Beer is prepared by first warming malt and nonmalted grains (a mixture called a "mash"). Mash is then filtered to obtain a sugar-rich liquid, which is boiled with hops, then fermented by adding yeasts. Whiskey manufacture depends on fermentation of mashes without filtration, then distilling the alcohol and other volatile materials.

maltase The ENZYME that digests maltose, a sugar from starch DIGESTION. The small intestine produces maltase to degrade maltose. This sugar is produced by the action of AMYLASE, the starch digestion enzyme found in saliva and in pancreatic secretions. Because maltose is too large to be absorbed by the intestine, it must be degraded to its building block, the simple sugar GLUCOSE, which is readily absorbed. Therefore, maltase plays a critical role in carbohydrate digestion. (See also CARBOHYDRATE METABOLISM; LACTASE; SUCRASE.)

maltol A FOOD ADDITIVE used as a FLAVOR ENHANCER. Maltol accentuates the flavor of CHOCOLATE, VANILLA, and fruit-flavored beverages and foods. A closely related compound (ethyl maltol) is a more powerful flavor enhancer. Both are used in gelatin desserts, ICE CREAM, jams, and baked goods with fruit flavors. Because ethyl maltol tastes sweet, its use allows the sugar content of a food to be reduced by 15 percent. Ethyl maltol masks the bitter taste of the artificial sweetener saccharin. Levels of maltol added to foods range from 15 to 250 mcg per gram (parts per million); ethyl maltol is added at considerably lower levels. Small amounts of maltol occur naturally in bread, coffee, cereals, soybeans, and malt products. Heated condensed milk, whey, and soy sauce also produce maltol. Maltol and ethyl maltol are considered safe food additives. (See also ARTIFICIAL SWEETENERS; NATURAL SWEETENERS.)

mandarin orange (*Citrus reticulata*) A citrus fruit with a unique sweet flavor related to the sweet orange. Mandarin oranges have a loose skin that is easily peeled. Certain red varieties are called TANGERINES, although the term *tangerine* is not a botanical classification. Apparently, mandarin oranges originated in Southeast Asia. Many varieties may have been developed in India, China, and Japan. Mandarin and hybrid strains are grown in most subtropical and even tropical regions throughout the world. Florida is the major domestic producer of tangerines. The original strains have been improved and crossbred with other citrus fruit. (For nutrient content, see ORANGE.)

manganese A trace mineral nutrient. Manganese is needed for normal brain and muscle function, building bones, BLOOD CLOTTING, CHOLESTEROL synthesis, fat synthesis, and DNA and RNA synthesis. Manganese activates the enzyme responsible for the formation of urea, the waste product of protein degradation. In carbohydrate metabolism, manganese is required for the synthesis of glucose from noncarbohydrate substances (GLUCONEOGENESIS). Manganese assists the action of SUPEROXIDE DISMUTASE, which degrades superoxide, a free radical and a highly damaging form of oxygen. In addition, manganese is required to synthesize components of mucopolysaccharides (GLYCOSAMINOGLYCANS), components of connective tissue. A manganese-dependent enzyme of the brain synthesizes the AMINO ACID, GLUTAMINE, as a way of removing AMMONIA, a toxic product of nitrogen metabolism. Conditions possibly associated with manganese deficiency include OSTEOPOROSIS, RHEUMATOID ARTHRITIS, LUPUS ERYTHEMATOSUS, allergies, ALCOHOLISM, and diabetes.

Sources

Good sources of manganese are NUTS, TEA, whole grains, BRAN, dried fruit, and leafy green vegetables. Their manganese content varies, depending on the manganese content of the soil. Eighty-six percent of manganese is lost in prepared white flour. DAIRY PRODUCTS, FISH, MEAT (other than organ meats), and POULTRY are poor sources of manganese. Inadequate absorption of manganese from plant sources may be a problem because digestion of plant food releases only a small fraction of the manganese it contains. Manganese supplements are best taken as a balanced multi-mineral preparation.

Requirements

The body contains low levels of manganese, and only minute amounts are required each day to maintain this level. The manganese concentration in tissues is stable primarily due to carefully controlled excretion.

There is no RECOMMENDED DIETARY ALLOWANCE for manganese. Instead, the Food and Nutrition Board has estimated a safe and adequate daily intake as 2 to 5 mg for adults. Symptoms of manganese deficiency in experimental animals include pancreatic pathology and diabetes-like symptoms, impaired growth, reproductive abnormalities, skeletal abnormalities, convulsions, and ataxia (abnormal muscle movements). Certain groups might be deficient in manganese: women, especially those on weight loss diets; anyone on a calorie-restricted diet; aged people; and VEGETARIANS.

Safety

While manganese is relatively nontoxic, too much manganese can interfere with the absorption of other minerals like IRON. High manganese intake can cause nerve damage, immune system malfunction, and damage to PANCREAS, LIVER, and KIDNEY. Excessive calcium supplements can interfere with manganese and iron uptake because they all use the same entry mechanism into intestinal cells. (See also ALLERGY, IMMEDIATE FAT METABOLISM.)

mango (*Mangifera indica*) A tropical FRUIT with an oval shape, produced by a tropical evergreen. Mangoes are green when unripe; the ripened fruit is yellow-orange and the juicy pulp is sweet and tangy. Although not a popular fruit in North America, mangoes are an important fruit crop in the tropics, and they rank seventh among the most popular fruit crop worldwide. Mangoes seem to have originated in the broad region between Thailand and India, and they have been cultivated since 5000 B.C. They are now grown in most tropical countries. India remains the largest producer of mangoes.

The ripe fruit is eaten raw or used in jams, preserves, and juices; unripened fruit is used in chutneys, a popular condiment in India. Mangoes can be seasoned with turmeric for this purpose. Nutrient content of one mango, raw (207 g), is 135 calories; protein, 1.1 g; carbohydrate, 35.2 g; fiber, 2.9 g; folic acid, 0.6 g; potassium, 323 mg; vitamin A, 806 retinol equivalents; vitamin C, 57 mg; thiamin, 0.12 mg; riboflavin, 0.12 mg; niacin, 1.21 mg.

manioc See CASSAVA.

mannitol A NATURAL SWEETENER used in chewing gum, soft candy, BREAKFAST CEREALS, frosting, and sugarless diet foods. It is also used as an antisticking agent for chewing gum because it does not absorb moisture. It occurs naturally in ASPARAGUS, OLIVES, PINEAPPLES, and SEAWEED. Commercially it is synthesized from the simple, common sugar GLUCOSE. Mannitol is classified as a sugar alcohol, but is not a sugar. It is not used efficiently by the body, nor does it raise blood sugar rapidly. Mannitol supplies only about half the calories of glucose and has about 70 percent of the sweetness of table sugar, and is considered a safe FOOD ADDITIVE. It is not metabolized to acids by oral bacteria. Tooth decay is caused by these organic acids, and, therefore, this additive may help prevent tooth decay.

Mannitol's rather poor absorption by the intestine results in osmotic DIARRHEA when large amounts are ingested. It is a LAXATIVE at a dose of 10 to 20 g daily. Such huge doses can worsen kidney disease. The U.S. FDA requires that the ingredient label warn of the laxative effect with excess consumption when daily ingestion of mannitol could reach 20 g. Mannitol may increase urination because much of it is eliminated unchanged by the kidneys. It has been used to prevent the kidneys from shutting down during major surgery. (See also ARTIFICIAL SWEETENERS; DENTAL CARIES; SORBITOL.)

mannose A simple SUGAR found in CARBOHYDRATE-containing proteins. In the body, mannose is formed from glucose and is used to form short chains of sugars (oligosaccharides) that are attached to certain proteins (GLYCOPROTEINS). When attached to certain proteins, mannose may function as a recognition marker that governs the cellular distribution of the protein and its metabolic rate within tissues. Mannose is much less common than glucose (BLOOD SUGAR) and does not occur free in foods. Mannose contains six carbon atoms and belongs to an important family of sugars (the aldohexoses) of which glucose is a member. (See also MANNITOL.)

MAO inhibitors Monoamine oxidase inhibitors are used to treat depression and high blood pressure. Examples include Marpian, Nardil, and Parnate. They block a key enzyme required to form DOPAMINE and norepinephrine, synthesized by nerve cells to conduct nerve impulses between cells.

Foods containing TYRAMINE, a degradation product found in fermented foods, are dangerous when taking MAO inhibitors because tyramine in the presence of MAO inhibitors drastically increases blood pressure. This effect may be severe enough to cause a STROKE or a HEART ATTACK. Symptoms of tyramine–MAO inhibitor interactions include vomiting, severe headaches, and nosebleed. Tyramine-containing foods to avoid include; aged CHEESES (such as Brie, Camembert, cheddar, processed American), cured MEAT (like pastrami), anchovies, AVOCADOS, BANANAS, BEETS, caffeinated beverages, chicken liver, CHOCOLATE, canned FIGS, MUSHROOMS, pickled herring, RAISINS, sausages, sour cream, chianti wine, sherry, and yeast extract. (See also DRUG-NUTRIENT INTERACTION; NEUROTRANSMITTER.)

maple syrup A syrup prepared from the sap of the sugar maple tree (*Acer saccharum*), native to eastern North America. This sweetener contains sugars like SUCROSE, glucose, and FRUCTOSE and has a distinctive flavor. During winter, starch is converted to sugar in tree roots, and it is carried up the trunk in the spring. Spring sap contains 4 percent to 10 percent sugar. It is collected in spring when the sap begins to flow and before buds open. The collected sap is concentrated by boiling down, which develops the characteristic flavor of maple syrup. The maple flavor is not present in the sap itself.

The province of Quebec remains the largest producer of maple syrup (over 20 million gallons yearly). U.S. production is about 5 percent that of Quebec. In the United States, Vermont and New York produce the most maple syrup. Commercial maple syrups are often blends of maple syrup and other less expensive syrups.

Maple syrup should be considered a REFINED CARBOHYDRATE with little nutrient content other than CALORIES. It contains only traces of CALCIUM and POTASSIUM. To prevent crystallization and molds, it should be refrigerated, but not frozen. Maple syrup can be contaminated with LEAD if it is collected in or stored in metal containers with soldered seams. Suppliers should use stainless steel during preparation. (See also NATURAL SWEETENERS.)

marasmus A progressive wasting and emaciation due to chronic deprivation of PROTEIN and CALORIES. Symptoms include wasting of MUSCLES and body fat, dry skin, low body weight, lethargy, sunken eyes, severe DIARRHEA, MALABSORPTION, and low body temperature. Diarrhea causes DEHYDRATION and losses of minerals like SODIUM, POTASSIUM, and CHLORIDE, causing ELECTROLYTE imbalance. This in turn leads to brain, kidney, and heart disorders. If left untreated, death may result. Decreased immunity promotes disease. In adapting to STARVATION, the body consumes tissue, protein, and FAT, accompanied by reduced protein synthesis and retarded growth in many tissues. All muscles, including the heart, atrophy.

Causes of marasmus include inadequate food intake; prolonged malabsorption, caused, for instance, by severe diarrhea in infants; and child neglect. Marasmus occurs in infants and children in regions of the world where low-income populations are prone to undernutrition due to an inadequate supply of protein-rich foods, especially animal protein. Dietary protein may be deficient in essential AMINO ACIDS, or the total food intake may be inadequate. In either case, consumed protein is used for energy rather than being used to supply essential amino acids for protein synthesis and maintenance.

Marasmatic children need physical and emotional warmth as well as improved nutrition. Treatment is based on an early digested diet with meals supplemented with 1 gram of high-quality protein and 50 to 60 calories per pound of body weight. (See also IMMUNE SYSTEM; KWASHIORKOR; MALNUTRITION.)

margarine A nondairy product resembling BUTTER and prepared from hydrogenated (hardened) VEGETABLE OIL. Since 1950, Americans have eaten more margarine per person a year as butter consumption has declined.

Margarine is usually manufactured from CORN OIL, SAFFLOWER oil, SOYBEAN oil, COTTONSEED OIL, PALM OIL, and PEANUT oil, and the amount of saturated fat that margarines contain varies. Small amounts of animal FAT may be added by manufacturers. Unless animal fat is added, margarine does not contain cholesterol. Margarine incorporates partially HYDROGENATED VEGETABLE OIL. Most vegetable oils contain polyunsaturated fats, which are deficient in hydrogen atoms and which are liquid at room temperature. Hydrogenation, a chemical process, adds variable amounts of hydrogen to polyunsaturates, making them more saturated and harder at room temperature. In the last steps, oil is emulsified with emulsifying agents and chilled to solidify the oil and trap water. Additives include salt, yellow coloring (BETA-CAROTENE), VITAMIN A, preservatives, and butter flavoring.

It is believed that saturated fat, rather than polyunsaturated fat, promotes clogged arteries. Although margarine is more saturated than vegetable oils like corn, safflower, and soybean oils, it is much less saturated than coconut, palm, or palm kernel oils.

Margarine contains more TRANS-FATTY ACID than butter. Trans-fatty acids are by-products of hydrogenation. The molecular shape of normal unsaturated fatty acids is bent, while saturated fats are straight molecules. Trans-fatty acids are also straight. Like saturated fatty acids, they can pack together more closely, making them more solid at room temperature. Trans-fatty acids raise cholesterol and therefore increase the risk of heart disease. Fried foods, such as french fries and doughnuts from fast food chains, are often cooked with vegetable shortening. Vegetable shortening is laden with trans-fatty acids. Food labels do not list the amount of trans-fatty acids in foods. Margarine and partially hydrogenerated vegetable oils contribute more than 80 percent of the trans-fatty acids Americans consume.

Types of Margarine

Liquid margarine is the least hydrogenated and contains a high fraction of unsaturated oil. Whipped margarine contains air to increase volume and to make the product spread more evenly; the air reduces calories by 40 percent. Stick margarine is higher in saturated fat than tub margarine or liquid margarine and may contain animal fat (BEEF TALLOW). "Diet" (low-cal) margarine contains one-half to one-third the calories of regular margarine because it contains much more water. Due to the high water content, it cannot be substituted for stick margarine or butter in recipes. Salt-free margarine is available for individuals on sodium-restricted diets.

Both margarine and butter contain the same number of calories and salt. Margarine is usually colored with beta-carotene to make it look like butter, which derives its color naturally from beta-carotene. Margarine contains no cholesterol; butter contains 32 milligrams/tsp. Margarine has 2 g of saturated fat/tsp; butter has 7.5 g. Margarine has 4 g of polyunsaturated fat/tsp.; butter has a half-gram. The PROTEIN, fat, CALCIUM, SODIUM, and VITAMIN A contents are comparable. Stick margarine contains 47 percent monounsaturated fatty acids, 53 percent polyunsaturated fatty acids and 30 percent saturated fatty acids. And margarine contains high levels of trans-fatty acids; per tablespoon, margarines contain 1 to 3 g.

Cholesterol-Lowering Margarine

Cholesterol-lowering margarines are the latest addition to this food category. These products contain either sterol esters (from vegetable oils, soybean, and corn) or stanol esters (from wood pulp). When used in combination with a heart-healthy diet, these margarines can help lower LOW-DENSITY LIPOPROTEIN (LDL) cholesterol (the "bad" cholesterol) in some patients. Elevated levels of LDL cholesterol are strongly linked to a greater risk of heart disease. In one study children who were genetically predisposed to early heart disease and who ate margarine containing sterol esters for three months reduced their LDL cholesterol levels by 18 percent. Adult relatives of the children who participated in the study also experienced some decrease in LDL cholesterol levels.

The American Heart Association does not recommend cholesterol-lowering margarine for patients who have not been diagnosed as having elevated levels of LDL cholesterol. The American Cancer Society recommends that patients eat less fat of all kinds—margarine, butter, cooking oils, vegetable shortening, or lard—to lower the risk of cancer and heart disease. Patients should avoid margarines that do not list liquid vegetable oil first on the label, and avoid those listing coconut oil, palm or palm kernel oil, or lard as ingredients in order to reduce consumption of saturated fat. Patients should buy margarines with higher levels of polyunsaturates and choose diet ("light") margarine to reduce the intake of trans-fatty acids. Margarine labels list saturated fat content but do not include trans-fatty acids. Therefore, they reveal only a portion of the content of the fat that raises LOW-DENSITY LIPOPROTEIN (LDL) cholesterol.

Nutrient content of 1 tbsp (14 g) of regular 80 percent-fat margarine, 100 calories; protein, 1.1 g; fat, 11.4 g; sodium, 153 mg; vitamin A, 140 retinol equivalents; and no water-soluble vitamins.

Miettinen, T. A. et al. "Reduction of Serum Cholesterol with Sitostanol-Ester Margarine in a Mildly Hypercholesterolemic Population," *New England Journal of Medicine* 333, no. 20 (1995): 1,308–1,312.

marjoram (*Origanum Majorana hortensis;* sweet marjoram) An HERB of the mint family. Marjoram is related to OREGANO. It has light-green oval leaves with a mild sage-like flavor. It is used in salads, meat, game, poultry, and vegetables, and with tomato-based dishes, including lentils and beans. Marjoram has been used in folk medicine to ease cramps and stomach upsets. Wild marjoram is more commonly known as oregano. (See also SPICES.)

marshmallow A spongy confection. Marshmallows are a common sweet in the United States.

They are prepared with whipped GELATIN or GUM ARABIC, corn syrup, flavoring, and table sugar. Marshmallows are used in frosting and in sauces.

Marshmallow is also a medicinal plant, *Althaea officinalis,* that has sweet roots. The root mucilage was formerly used to make marshmallows. In folk medicine it has been used externally to help heal wounds. It is used in ointments for chapped skin. Marshmallow helps decrease inflammation associated with intestinal infections and infections of the urinary tract and genital tissues, and with respiratory infections and asthma. It is also used in cough syrup and cough lozenges. Safety data are inadequate for pregnant and breast-feeding women. (See also CANDY; EMPTY CALORIES; SUCROSE.)

mast cell Immune cells in connective tissue that release inflammatory agents when stimulated. Mast cells contain SEROTONIN and HISTAMINE, which cause tiny blood vessels (CAPILLARIES) to dilate and become porous. In an inflammatory response, fluid and defensive cells leak into the tissue and the increased blood flow leads to heat, redness, and swelling. Defensive substances in the blood such as antibodies, defensive cells, and clot-forming substances can then enter the injured area. In particular, scavenger (phagocytic) white blood cells pass more easily to the site of injury. Mast cells are also abundant along blood vessels, where they produce HEPARIN, a substance that acts as an anticoagulant (prevents blood from clotting). FLAVONOIDS, plant antioxidants, can decrease inflammation by desensitizing mast cells. (See also IMMUNE SYSTEM; INFLAMMATION.)

mastication The act of chewing. Food is ingested through the mouth, where it is pulverized. Teeth grind food particles and mix them with saliva for lubrication and to initiate digestion. The tongue moves chewed food to the throat in order for it to be swallowed. Adequate chewing prepares food for efficient DIGESTION in the stomach and intestine. Chewing sends signals to the brain to prepare the gastrointestinal tract to release digestive enzymes. Inadequate chewing can cause choking, and gulping food can lead to HEARTBURN. (See also DEGLUTITION; DIGESTIVE TRACT.)

mayonnaise A spread prepared from egg yolks and oil. Mayonnaise is used in salads, vegetables, a variety of recipes, and as a sandwich spread. Mayonnaise is generally prepared from SOYBEAN oil and VINEGAR. Other ingredients include lemon or lime juice, SALT, NATURAL SWEETENER (usually sugar), MUSTARD and other spices, and MONOSODIUM GLUTAMATE. LECITHIN, a fatty substance in egg yolk, suspends (emulsifies) the vegetable oil. Emulsification is not a chemical treatment nor does it alter the nature of the oil. One tablespoon of mayonnaise contains 9 to 10 mg of cholesterol (from egg yolk) and 100 calories.

Imitation mayonnaise contains about one-third the calories and four times the amount of water as regular mayonnaise. Although homemade mayonnaise is considered a risk for food poisoning, food poisoning is not usually the result of mayonnaise spoilage because the acidic contents retard bacterial growth. Low-fat substitutes for mayonnaise include YOGURT or low-fat COTTAGE CHEESE and BUTTERMILK, seasoned with lemon juice, mustard powder, horseradish, ginger, garlic, and herbs.

meal planning See BASIC FOOD GROUPS; EXCHANGE LISTS; FOOD GUIDE PYRAMID.

meal timing See DIETING.

measures (metric to English) The 8-oz. cup and the tablespoon are standard measures for recipes. The problem is that nutrition uses the metric system, a scientific notation with liters (close to a quart) and milliliters (ml, 1/1,000 of a liter). It uses grams and milligrams (mg) instead of ounces.

The table below offers metric equivalents for common household measures.

Household Measures	Metric Measure
1 cup (8 oz. or 16 tsp)	224 grams or 240 ml
1/8 cup (1 oz. or 2 tsp)	28 grams
1 tsp	4 grams or 5 ml
1 tbsp	14 grams or 15 ml
1/4 tbsp	1 gram
1 pound (16 oz.)	454 grams
1 quart	0.95 liter
1 fluid ounce	30 milliliters

meat The flesh of animals used as food. BEEF, VEAL, LAMB, and PORK are standard fare in the United States; in 2002, the average American ate 66 pounds of beef, 51 pounds of pork, and about one pound of lamb. However, beef's popularity has steadily declined since the late 1970s as CHICKEN and FISH have become more popular. In 2000 Americans ate about 80 pounds of chicken per person annually. Much of this change in taste is due to consumer concerns about CHOLESTEROL and FAT. Nonetheless, meat production has a large economic and environmental impact. Livestock graze on one-third of the land of North America. Half of U.S. crops such as corn go to livestock feed, especially for cattle. Directly and indirectly, through fodder irrigation, farm animals account for a major part of the water consumed in the United States. Half the antibiotics produced are used for livestock.

Meat contains 20 percent to 23 percent PROTEIN, variable amounts of fat and approximately 60 percent water. The fat content depends on the type of meat, the nutritional state of the animal, the degree of trimming, and the method of preparation. Meat and dairy products supply half of the total fat, all of the cholesterol and 75 percent of the saturated FATTY ACIDS of the standard American diet. Lean meat and fat meat contain about the same cholesterol, 70 to 80 mg per 3 oz. serving of lamb, beef, chicken, or pork. Although beef and chicken contain about the same amount of cholesterol, beef fat is much more saturated than chicken fat.

Meat is an excellent source of protein, B complex vitamins and certain trace minerals like ZINC and IRON. Meat supplies about 90 percent of VITAMIN B_{12} in the U.S. diet, 70 percent of protein, 66 percent of RIBOFLAVIN, 54 percent of VITAMIN B_6, 46 percent of NIACIN and 36 percent of iron, but only 3 percent of calcium. Therefore, meat is not a very good source of calcium. Meat protein is "high quality," that is, it provides ample amounts of all of the essential AMINO ACIDS that cannot be synthesized by the body. A little animal protein with a meal increase iron uptake from plant food. Fish, poultry and shellfish are flesh and constitute the rest of the meat group, one of the four basic food groups developed in the 1950s to help design a balanced diet. In the food guide pyramid, they represent the protein group with meat, poultry, fish, dried beans, eggs, and nuts. Two to three servings of this group is recommended daily.

There are several concerns with a high meat diet:

1. Meat contributes about 35 percent of the saturated fat to the typical American diet. In particular, red meat contributes about 49 grams of fat per person per day and accounts for about 30 percent of total fat consumption. Excessive fat is associated with an increased risk of OBESITY, elevated blood cholesterol and increased risk of heart disease and of CANCER. In contrast, POULTRY and fish, provided they are not breaded and fried, add little to the total fat consumption.
2. Excessive protein consumption is generally a bigger problem in the United States than inadequate dietary protein. Protein quality is not generally an issue except in the case of a VEGETARIAN who does not eat a variety of plant protein sources. Too much protein causes calcium loss and promotes bone loss (OSTEOPOROSIS).
3. A high-protein diet may interfere with kidney function, especially in diabetics.
4. Meat is often contaminated with traces of PESTICIDES, growth promoters, drugs, and antibiotics. Their long-term effects on health are not known.

Grading Meat

The USDA has defined various grades of beef according to fat content. The cut of meat is more important than the grade of meat, which depends on the texture and the amount of visible fat. For example, top round is leaner than rib roast. Regulations apply to beef, mutton, lamb, calf, veal, and pork, but government grading of meat is not compulsory. Still, more than half the beef is graded, either Prime, Choice, Select, Standard, Commercial, Utility, Cutter, or Canner for beef. Pork is graded No. 1, No. 2, No. 3, No. 4., and Utility.

Light or "lite" meat refers to cuts of meat that have at least 25 percent less fat than standard cuts for that grade of meat. USDA nutritional beef, also known as Natural Beef, refers to meat that has been minimally processed. Growth stimulants, antibiotics, and other additives to fatten the animals have been avoided. USDA Light Select, Light Choice, and Light Prime contain 25 percent less fat than the corresponding cuts.

The order in going from least-fat to most-fat grades is as follows: Light Select (or Good), Select (or Good), Light Choice, Choice, Light Prime, and Prime. Most ungraded meat is Select (Good); it corresponds to supermarket brands of lean beef. "Extra lean" meat contains less than 5 percent fat. About half the USDA Select meat cuts fall in this category. NFF1 refers to meat containing less than 3.5 percent fat. FEF2 refers to cuts of meat with less than 6 percent fat.

Pork is the flesh of hogs; ham refers to the rear leg muscle or rear quarter. Ninety-five percent "fat-free ham" refers to ham containing 5 percent of the weight of the ham as fat. Caloriewise, 20 percent to 30 percent of the calories in these hams can be derived from saturated fat, so they are not free of fat. Pork is a high-fat food, although some cuts of pork, trimmed of visible fat, have less fat. For example, center loin provides 8.9 g of fat per 3-oz. serving. The same cut untrimmed contains 19 g of fat. Only a small fraction of pork is graded.

Meat Labeling

Labels for processed meat and poultry products are required to provide the nutrient content, amount of fat and number of calories. The listing of fat composition, sodium content, and other nutritional information is voluntary. This information can be made available in notebooks or on placards in grocery stores. Ground beef can be called "lean" only if a 3.5 oz. serving contains less than 10 g of fat, less than 4.5 g of saturated fat and less than 95 mg of cholesterol.

Ground beef can be labeled "extra lean" if it contains less than 5 g of fat, less than 2 g of saturated fat and less than 95 mg of cholesterol. The 2002 Farm Act amends the Agricultural Marketing Act of 1946 to require retailers to inform consumers of the country of origin for muscle cuts of beef, lamb, and pork and ground beef, ground lamb, and ground pork, among other foods. The 2002 act states, with few exceptions, a retailer may use a "United States country of origin" label if the product is from an animal that was exclusively born, raised, and slaughtered in the United States.

Safety

Federal inspection of animal products relies on the USDA to evaluate the quality, characteristics, yield or proportion of important cuts of meat. Freedom from damage, proper labeling, and absence of adulteration and disease are key aims of meat inspection. In 1967 Congress passed the Wholesome Meat Act, which required all meat sold in the United States to be inspected according to either a federal program or an equivalent state cooperative program. After several outbreaks of *E. coli* poisoning through hamburger and two through roast beef in the early 1990s, consumers became increasingly concerned about the safety of eating meat. Then, in January 1993, an outbreak of *E. coli* 0157:H7 led to more than 700 reported illnesses and the deaths of four children in Washington State, Idaho, and Nevada. In 1996 President Clinton announced a new initiative to improve meat and poultry inspection. Under these new guidelines meat and poultry processors must follow a system of safety checks throughout processing, meet certain standards for *Salmonella* contamination, test for generic *E. coli* bacteria, and identify and control sanitation risks.

In 2000 the government completed implementation of its landmark rule on Pathogen Reduction and Hazard Analysis and Critical Control Point (HACCP) systems, which was published in the *Federal Register* on July 25, 1996. Implementation was phased in based on plant size. Under the regulations each meat and poultry plant must develop and implement a written plan for meeting its sanitation responsibilities and an HACCP plan that systematically addresses all significant hazards associated with its products. In addition, all slaughter plants must regularly test for generic *E. coli* to verify their procedures for preventing and reducing fecal contamination. Raw products from slaughter plants and plants that grind meat and poultry are subject to *Salmonella* testing by the government in an effort to reduce microbial contamination over time.

With the Pathogen Reduction and HACCP final rule, the government has shifted its regulatory approach for meat and poultry to include not only the product but also the process. A system under which potential food safety problems are identified and prevented is replacing a system that focused largely on detecting problems at the end of the production line.

Safe handling instructions are available for ground meat and all raw meat products as a measure to combat food poisoning linked to uncooked or partially cooked meat, especially due to a strain of the bacterium *Escherichia coli* 0157:H7. The safe handling instructions notify the consumer that food products may contain bacteria that can cause illness if mishandled or improperly cooked.

Cooking meat can create several classes of carcinogenic agents. Charring meat, poultry, or fish produces polycyclic aromatic compounds, especially when fat drippings deposit soot on charcoal-broiled food. Scraping off the charred portion can remove these materials. Another class is called heterocyclic amines (HCAs). A combination of longer cooking time and high temperature determines the extent of formation; HCAs tend to form within meat and cannot be scraped off. Once eaten, the liver activates HCAs, which can alter DNA, a first step in cancer development. Precooking hamburger for two minutes drives off some of the raw materials for HCAs, and, when barbecued, such hamburger produces much less cancer-causing material than hamburger exclusively grilled.

Red meat need not be excluded for a fat-restricted diet to reduce fat consumption. Patients should eat small portions of lean cuts of meat and trim visible fat before cooking. Roasted meat contains less fat than broiled or braised meat. To avoid producing cancer-causing agents during cooking, meat should not be overcooked or charred. Low-fat meat (5 percent to 15 percent fat), include Light Select (Good), Select (Good), or Light Choice grades.

Meat in Prepared Foods

Food producers are required to meet FDA standards for meat content in a variety of prepared foods. The amount of meat permitted in different foods varies immensely. This is important to keep in mind if meat or protein content is a concern.

The following is a partial listing of FDA standards for meat contents:

Meat Product	Percent Meat
meatballs	65
beef enchiladas	15
beef tacos	15
chili con carne	40
gravy with beef	35
ham salad	35
pizza with meat	15
spaghetti and meatballs	12
chicken with broth	43

(See also BOVINE SPONGIFORM ENCEPHALOPATHY; DIETARY GUIDELINES FOR AMERICANS; FOOD POISONING; HAMBURGER; HOT DOG; MEAT, PROCESSED; MEAT CONTAMINANTS; MEAT SUBSTITUTES; STANDARDS OF IDENTITY; TOXOPLASMOSIS.)

Key, Timothy J. "Mortality in Vegetarians and Nonvegetarians: Detailed Findings from a Collaborative Analysis of Five Prospective Studies," *American Journal of Clinical Nutrition* 70 (1999): 516S–524S.

meat, processed Meat that has been modified by chemical treatment and extensive manipulation. This category includes BACON, PASTRAMI, SALAMI, LIVERWURST, HAM, HOT DOGS, hot SAUSAGES, LUNCHEON MEATS, cold cuts, BOLOGNA, and Polish sausage. Sausages and processed meats are some of the fattest foods available. Salami, bologna, and liver sausage contain especially large amount of FAT, and up to 80 percent of their calories can come from fat. This level is equivalent to a huge 15 to 17 g per 2 oz. serving. Processed meats often contain high levels of SODIUM (500 to 1,000 mg per serving). Furthermore, sodium NITRITE is sometimes added as a preservative, or it is added to enhance the color or flavor of the product.

Low-fat processed meat provide 2 to 3 g of fat per slice, a reasonably low value for a processed meat. Chicken or turkey breast and products made only from these are leaner than red meat. Generally, the serving size is one ounce (28 g). If a smaller serving size is used, it will have fewer calories. (See also CONVENIENCE FOOD; PROCESSED FOOD.)

meat alternatives Nonmeat or nonanimal protein foods. Consumers choose MEAT alternatives to lower animal protein intake, to decrease FAT consumption and to better utilize plant protein sources. All LEGUMES, whether BEANS, LENTILS, or PEAS, contain high levels of protein. No plant source contains cholesterol unless animal fat has been added. "High quality" protein is found in most animal protein and in several plant sources such as soybean and AMARANTH. Such protein provides

COMPARISON OF FAT AND CHOLESTEROL IN MEAT AND NONMEAT PRODUCTS

Protein Item (grams)	Fat (grams)	Calories	Percent Cals as Fat	Cholesterol
Meat products:				
(28 g) beef & pork bologna	8	89	81	16 mg
(45 g) beef & pork hot dog	13.1	145	81	23 mg
(85 g) hamburger (regular)	17.8	245	65	76 mg
(13 g) pork sausage	4	50	72	11 mg
Typical non-meat (soy-based) products:				
(18 g) nonmeat bologna	21	320	60	none
(30 g) nonmeat hot dog	18	345	47	none
(17.5 g) nonmeat burger	16	219	56	none
(10 g) nonmeat sausage	8	175	41	none
(14 g) nonmeat turkey	1	80	11	none

AMINO ACIDS that cannot be manufactured by the body in appropriate ratios to provide enough protein building blocks to support growth and maintain health.

Nonmeat products can be prepared from eggs or egg whites and grain protein. GLUTEN, the protein fraction of wheat, may also be used regardless of its source. Although tofu and soybean protein are low-fat foods, their conversion to meatless burgers, hot dogs, and sausages requires extensive processing. Food additives are frequently added along the way. Nonmeat alternatives often contain high levels of fat, although most of this is polyunsaturated rather than saturated, as found in red meat. Deep-fat-fried products will be highest in fat; SODIUM is often high as well.

Soybean protein is a common meat alternative because it provides a favorable balance of essential amino acids. Soy protein can easily be processed to resemble meat in texture and taste. Two forms, TEMPEH and TOFU, have long been used in traditional diets in Japan, Indonesia, and China. They easily absorb flavors and require little cooking. Tempeh utilizes whole soy beans, including FIBER, and contains somewhat less fat than tofu. A typical 4-oz. serving of tofu provides 5 to 7 g of fat and 80 to 100 calories, and tempeh provides 4 to 5 g of fat and 150 calories. By comparison, 4 oz. of uncooked, extra lean ground beef provide about 18 g of fat and 290 calories. (See also FATTY ACIDS; FOOD PROCESSING; MEAT SUBSTITUTES.)

meat contaminants Foreign substances, tissue contaminants, or excessive amounts of growth-promoting compounds that are present in MEAT. Antibiotics, growth promoters, PESTICIDES, and THYROID glands are examples of substances that may contaminate meat and POULTRY. More than 20,000 animal drugs are in use and, according to the FDA, 500 to 600 synthetic chemicals are present in beef alone; most are probably harmless. However, 42 are suspected of causing cancer and another 20 are suspected of causing birth defects. Some of these chemicals have been found in meat at levels higher than those set by the FDA. Since January 1989, European nations have banned U.S. beef with growth-promoting hormones. In the United States, there is no way to know which meats, poultry, or animal products are even slightly contaminated. U.S. consumers frequently have a choice of buying organic beef and organic poultry, supposedly grown without growth promoters and excessive drugs.

Growth Promoters

Hormones and growth promoters are often given to animals to speed weight gain; occasionally these are misused. Steroid growth promoters can increase the risk of cancer. DIETHYLSTILBESTROL (DES) is an example of a HORMONE-like drug once used to promote growth in beef. It is now banned in the United States, although residues occasionally show up in spot checks of meat. The degree of risk of long-term exposure to low levels of hormone analogs and other drugs in meat is unknown.

Antibiotics

Antibiotics are used as feed additives that promote growth in livestock. However, their use in feed can lead to drug-resistant bacteria, which theoretically could infect people who eat the contaminated meat or dairy products. Antibiotic residues also may contaminate meat. As an example, sulfamethazine, a sulfa drug used to treat bacterial infections in cattle, pigs, sheep, and poultry, is used as a growth promoter for pigs. Research indicates it causes cancer in lab animals. This drug cannot be given to livestock close to the time of slaughter and cannot be given to milk cows because it is a forbidden contaminant in milk. Nonetheless, there may be significant meat and milk contamination; spot checks have found sulfa drugs in veal and pork and milk from various metropolitan areas in the United States.

Contaminated Feed

In the 1990s reports of people in Europe who developed a rare but deadly neurological disorder, variant Creutzfeldt-Jakob Disease (vCJD), raised public concerns about the safety of eating beef. In 1996 10 people in the United Kingdom began exhibiting unusual symptoms, including leg pain, difficulty walking, hallucinations, and slurred speech. Eventually, the patients could not walk, speak, or feed themselves. Within two years they had all died. Autopsies revealed that the victims' brain tissue had disintegrated, giving it the sponge-like appearance similar to the brains of cattle infected with BOVINE SPONGIFORM ENCEPHALOPATHY (BSE).

The patients' symptoms were like those seen in people who suffered from a rare, fatal neurological disorder called Cruetzfeldt-Jakob Disease (CJD). Most victims of that disease die in their late 60s after years of suffering lingering dementia, but the patients diagnosed with vCJD were all in their 20s. Researchers suspect these patients contracted vCJD after eating the flesh of cattle that had BSE.

The source of the BSE outbreak is unknown, but evidence suggests it was spread, in part, by feeding meal to cattle that combined ground meat and bone from BSE-infected cattle. Scientists believe the disease may be caused by either a virus or prion, an abnormal partially proteinase K–resistant protein that causes normal prion protein in the host to change and form more abnormal protein. The BSE agent is highly resistant to heat, ultraviolet light, ionizing radiation, and disinfectants that usually kill viruses or bacteria.

The British government took several steps to contain the disease, including slaughtering thousands of animals that were suspected of infection and banning the use of meat-and-bone meal. The measures were successful, reducing the number of confirmed cases in the United Kingdom from 36,680 in 1992 to fewer than 1,500 in 2000.

Pesticides

Beef and pork are generally contaminated with trace amounts of a variety of pesticides. Fortunately, the levels are generally very low. Cow's milk is likewise contaminated. Herbicide contamination occurs when animals graze on land contaminated with dioxin-containing herbicides (such as Silvet and 2-4-5T).

Thyroid Gland

Occasionally, meat is contaminated by thyroid glands from carcasses improperly trimmed by meat packers. This could be a problem for patients with heart disease. Symptoms (insomnia, DIARRHEA, nervousness) disappear when the contaminated meat is no longer eaten.

Animal Drugs

Drugs such as clorsulon administered to prevent liver flukes in cattle are potential cancer-causing agents. Gentian violet causes cancer, but it is still permitted in animal feed to prevent it from molding. Traces of these chemicals show up in meat, eggs, and poultry. (See also ANTIBIOTIC-RESISTANT BACTERIA IN FOOD; CARCINOGEN; MAD COW DISEASE; TOXOPLASMOSIS.)

meat curing A treatment designed to preserve and to add flavor to meat. In the United States, this term pertains primarily to pork. Salt (sodium chloride) has been used since ancient times to preserve meat. It is added to processed meats as a preservative and a flavoring agent; it is also added to cause meat particles in products like bologna and hot dogs to stick together. The salt content is high enough to make salted meat products unsuitable for persons restricted to low-salt diets.

Sodium NITRITE, sodium NITRATE, and potassium nitrate help prevent a particularly deadly form of food poisoning called BOTULISM. Nitrite is the primary preservative. Nitrites and nitrates also help develop the flavor and texture of cured meats. However, nitrite can combine with AMINES, common nitrogen-containing compounds in food, to form NITROSOAMINES, which are potential cancer-causing agents (CARCINOGEN). As a partial solution to this problem, sodium nitrite can be combined with sodium and potassium ascorbate (VITAMIN C) to inhibit nitrosoamine formation. Garlic also limits nitrosoamine formation.

Smoked meat and fish have been prepared since ancient times. Smoking dries meat, adds materials that act as preservatives, and adds characteristic flavor. Smoking may introduce trace amounts of carcinogens (cancer-causing agents), however. Meat packers often use liquid smoke or synthetic smoke for flavoring. "Liquid smoke" is made from wood smoke treated to remove certain dangerous constituents; "synthetic smoke" is a synthetic mixture of chemicals that create a pleasing flavor.

Phosphate is among the most common food additives in cured meat products. Phosphate promotes water uptake by meat, increasing its juiciness. Federal regulations specify that the phosphate level cannot exceed 0.5 percent and the amount must be listed on the label.

meatless meat See MEAT SUBSTITUTES.

meat packing The slaughter of livestock and preparation of meat for transport and sale. Following slaughter, dressed beef carcasses are chilled at 32° F in a humid atmosphere for a week or so to permit enzymatic breakdown of muscle tissue. Bacteria within the carcass provide a characteristic flavor to beef. (Lamb is not aged.) Beef can be tenderized by injecting cattle with a mixture of plant-derived, protein-degrading enzymes (PROTEOLYTIC ENZYMES) minutes before slaughter. Less tender cuts may be tenderized by blade insertion. Electrically shocked meat is more tender than unshocked meat. Applying an electrical current to the carcass after slaughter prevents rigor mortis and muscle contraction. Consequently, less chilling and less aging time are required.

Mechanical deboning salvages meat left on bones after hand trimming. Ground bones are pressed through a screen to separate bone fragments from tissue. Mechanically deboned meat finds use in SAUSAGE, BOLOGNA, and other luncheon meat products. Deboned meat need not be indicated on a food label. Because it contains bone fragments, the calcium content is significantly higher than regular meat. The amount of calcium per serving must be shown on the label in order to provide the consumer with an estimate of the bone content.

meat substitutes Fabricated foods that resemble MEAT in texture and amino acid (PROTEIN) content but are essentially devoid of meat or POULTRY. The most common meat substitutes are primarily either single cell protein or soy protein based. Meat substitutes offer several advantages over meat: They are less expensive; they are convenient to use; they meet dietary restrictions, such as in low-cholesterol diets. Certain meat substitutes approach beef in fat content, however; the fat ranges from 6 g of fat per serving for meatless chicken (36 percent calories from fat) to 16 g of fat per serving for meatless bologna (51 percent calories from fat).

Single-cell Protein (SCP)

Protein that is obtained from single-celled organisms such as YEAST, bacteria, or algae can be used as food. Brewer's yeast and torula yeast, produced from fermenting wood residues and other cellulose sources, are used as animal feed. FUNGUS is the source of a protein produced in Britain. This product is high in FIBER and low in fat and CHOLESTEROL. Its texture and flavor are easily changed to resemble beef or poultry and it is used in frozen meatless pies. The potential for single-cell protein production is huge. One thousand pounds of single-cell organisms can produce 50 tons of protein per day, while a thousand-pound steer produces only 1 pound of protein a day and an equal weight of SOYBEANS can produce 80 pounds of protein a day. Among problems in converting single-cell protein to food are: PALATABILITY, protein quality (balanced amino acid content) and digestibility, as well as a high content of NUCLEIC ACID and possible toxins.

Soybean Protein

Soybean protein is the most common vegetable meat substitute, marketed as grits, flour, soy protein concentrate (which contains 70 percent or more soybean as protein), and isolated soy protein (90 percent protein). These basic forms can be extruded or spun. Spun soy protein is most often used as meat analogs, simulated (meatless) bacon bits, ham chunks, chicken chunks, hamburger patties, sausages, bacon slices, and turkey chunks, which look and taste like the authentic food but with a different texture. Soy protein meal analogs generally contain fat (partially hydrogenated vegetable oils), artificial coloring and flavoring (possibly monosodium glutamate), soy sauce, and salt. They may be enriched with several vitamins. Soy protein is a nutritious source of protein without cholesterol. It is low in trace minerals like IRON and ZINC, however. (See also TEXTURIZED VEGETABLE PROTEIN.)

meat tenderizer Mixtures of powdered protein-digesting ENZYMES used to make tough MEAT more tender. The enzymes may come from PAPAYA (papain), PINEAPPLE (bromelain), FIGS (ficin), bacteria (subtilisin), and FUNGI. These powerful enzymes degrade fibrous protein of connective tissue and MUSCLE and are destroyed during cooking. Most commercial tenderizers include seasonings, SALT, and MSG (MONOSODIUM GLUTAMATE). Meat tenderizers are considered safe additives. (See also FOOD ADDITIVES.)

medications See ALCOHOL/DRUG INTERACTIONS; DRUG/NUTRIENT INTERACTION.

medicinal plants It is likely that all cultural groups have used plants as therapeutic agents since prehistoric times. China and India have recorded descriptions of medicinal plants as early as 2700 B.C. Egyptian, Greek, Roman, and Arab physicians described medicinal properties of plants. Indigenous people of Central America, South America, North America, and Africa have further contributed to the knowledge of medicinal plants.

Research led to the isolation and characterization of the active principles of many botanical medicines now manufactured or isolated by pharmaceutical firms. Among them are morphine (from poppy); reserpine (a tranquilizer from snakeroot); curare (a muscle relaxant from the curare vine); quinine (the first malarial treatment, from the bark of the cinchona tree); digitalis (heart stimulant from foxglove); atropine (pupil-dilating drug from deadly nightshade); and others. Medicinal plants are currently being screened for anticancer and antiviral constituents on which to base new drugs. With the appearance of antibiotic-resistant bacteria, medicinal plants offer the promise of new treatment.

A set of terms describing the use of plant remedies and ailments for which they are employed predates pharmacology. The following is a brief description of key terms used in botanical medicine.

Alteratives Produce a gradual change in the body, normalizing body functions. Examples include DANDELION, ECHINACEA, GINSENG.

Anodynes Relieve pain. Examples include hops and wintergreen.

Appetite Stimulants Examples include ALFALFA, ANISE, CHAMOMILE, CELERY, dandelion, ginseng, mint, PARSLEY, ROSEMARY, savory.

Astringents Contract certain tissues and decrease mucous discharge. Examples include bayberry; BLACKBERRY; witch hazel.

Carminatives Reduce FLATULENCE (gas). Examples include aniseed, CAPSICUM, CARDAMOM, CUMIN, FENNEL seed, GINGER root, LOVAGE root, NUTMEG, PEPPERMINT, spearmint, valerian root.

Cathartics Relieve CONSTIPATION. Examples include CHICORY, dandelion.

Demulcents Oily or mucilaginous materials that soothe digestive upsets. Examples include BORAGE, chamomile, ginger root, sassafras.

Diaphoretics Induce sweating. Examples include borage, chamomile, ginger root, sassafras.

Diuretics Induce frequent urination. Examples include alfalfa, buchu leaves, celery, chicory, corn silk, dandelion, horehound, parsley (root), wild carrot.

Expectorants Loosen phlegm, mucous secretion from lungs and windpipe. Examples include angelica, GARLIC, horehound, LICORICE.

Febrifungis Antipyretics that lower body temperature during episodes of fever. Examples include angelica, BALM, borage, dandelion.

Nervines Counterbalance stress and fatigue by calming, soothing the body. Examples include chamomile, hops, passion flower, valerian root.

Stimulants Examples include angelica, bayberry leaves, capsicum, cardamom, sarsaparilla root, wintergreen.

Tonics Stimulate appetite, invigorate. Examples include celery seed, ginseng, goldenseal, hops.

There are several caveats in using medicinal plants:

- A number of plant species may be harmful (such as comfrey, lobelia, sassafras root).
- Allergic reactions may occur in susceptible people.
- Safe and adequate doses depend on many variables. Often it is difficult to standardize herbal preparations because of variation in harvesting, storage, and growth conditions. Furthermore, doses tolerated in adults may be harmful to children.
- Often claims like "blood purifier" are used without definition. Professional medical advice is prudent for any chronic symptoms.

(See also HERBS.)

Mediterranean Diet Pyramid A food guide based on the traditional diet of Greece, Crete, and southern Italy. These areas are noted for their low incidence of heart disease, cancer, and other chronic diseases, possibly due to the low consumption of saturated fat during the 1960s or earlier. The Mediterranean Diet Pyramid was publicized in 1994 by the Oldways Preservation and Exchange Trust, the Harvard School of Public Health, and the World Health Organization Regional Office for Europe.

The foundation of the Mediterranean Diet Pyramid is the daily consumption of bread, pasta, rice, couscous, bulgur and other grains, potatoes, large amounts of fruits and vegetables, with beans, legumes, and nuts as a source of protein. The Mediterranean diet also recommends small daily servings of yogurt and low-fat cheese, as well as olive oil in place of butter and other oils, cheese, pastries, and meat. Cheese and yogurt are limited to one half-ounce (1 tablespoon) of cheese and one cup daily, respectively. Sweets and eggs can be eaten once or twice a week; poultry and fish are limited to two or three servings weekly. Red meat is limited to a few times a month. Unlike other guides, this food guide allows for wine in moderation (one glass per day for women, two glasses for men). It also calls for regular physical exercise.

There are several points to consider when using this food guide. Eating more fats and oil regardless of source can increase the risk of weight gain, especially for overweight diabetics. Healthy southern Italian men in the 1960s consumed 30 percent of their calories as fats and oils. The pyramid cautions that consuming more than 35 percent of calories as fat may be satisfactory for active individuals without weight problems. It is not recommended to drink alcohol to decrease the risk of heart disease, because there are safer ways, such as increasing the exercise level and stopping tobacco use. (See also CARDIOVASCULAR DISEASE; FOOD PYRAMID.)

Willet, W. C. et al. "Mediterranean Diet Pyramid: a Cultural Model for Healthy Eating," *American Journal of Clinical Nutrition* 61, no. 6, supp. (1995): 1,402S–1,406S.

medium-chain triglycerides (MCTs) Fats derived from COCONUT OIL and palm kernel oil. Coconut oil contains 60 percent MCT. MCTs are prepared commercially by synthesis using saturated fatty acids containing six to 12 carbon atoms. In contrast, the fatty acids commonly found in fats and oils contain carbon chains with 16 or 18 carbon atoms. Saturated fats are filled up with hydrogen atoms. MCTs provide 8.3 calories per gram while fat provides 9 calories per gram; therefore, MCTs cannot be classified as "diet" foods.

MCTs are more easily absorbed than the usual animal fats and vegetable oils. They are broken down to free fatty acids and directly enter the bloodstream, where they can be used immediately for energy production by the LIVER and MUSCLE. They are not as readily stored in fat. In contrast, the usual dietary fats and oils must be packaged as particles called CHYLOMICRONS by intestinal cells, released into the lymphatic system, and subsequently broken down in capillaries before their fatty acids can be taken up by tissues.

MCTs are used in oral and intravenous feeding formulas as a quick source of energy for patients requiring nutritional support, such as premature infants and patients with fat maldigestion (such as CELIAC DISEASE and CROHN'S DISEASE) or severe trauma. They have also been used in a variety of nutritional supplements as a source of quick energy and to aid in weight control by increasing heat production (thermogenesis). However, research has yielded mixed results on this last point. MCTs tend to lower serum cholesterol levels more than unsaturated vegetable oils. They may cause abdominal cramping and bloating. In excess they can be converted to KETONE BODIES, acids that accumulate in the blood and disrupt acid-base balance. (See also FAT DIGESTION; FAT METABOLISM.)

Bach, A. C. "The Usefulness of Dietary Medium-Chain Triglycerides in Body Weight Control: Fact or Fancy?" *Journal of Lipid Research* 37 (1996): 708–726.

megadose A relatively large amount of a nutrient not easily obtainable by eating food. There is no fixed definition for the megadose of a VITAMIN or MINERAL. As a rule of thumb, a megadose can be defined as being greater than 10 times the RECOMMENDED DIETARY ALLOWANCE (RDA). Megadoses of nutrients can therefore range from milligram to gram quantities, depending upon the particular nutrient. The extent to which vitamin and mineral supplements taken in excess of the RDA have a beneficial effect on health remains controversial. There is a consensus that supplements even at high levels can help remedy conditions due to obvious nutrient deficiencies. Subtle deficiencies that do not cause deficiency diseases are less well recognized, more common, and less often treated. Complicating the picture is the fact that individual nutrient requirements are a function of inherited tendencies toward disease, health history, and environmental factors at home and work, as well as lifestyle choices. Thus, the level of supplements effective for one individual may be ineffective for another.

Certain nutrients taken in excess can cause side effects; the levels of vitamins causing toxicity vary considerably among individuals. Certain trace minerals may cause adverse effects at levels only five to 10 times the RDAs, and fat-soluble vitamins such as VITAMIN A and VITAMIN D accumulate in the body with excessive consumption and cause toxic symptoms. On the other hand, vitamins in reasonable amounts are generally far safer than most prescription drugs and even over-the-counter medications like aspirin or cortisone creams. (See also BIOCHEMICAL INDIVIDUALITY; HYPERVITAMINOSIS; ORTHOMOLECULAR MEDICINE.)

Blanchard, J. "Pharmacokinetic Perspectives on Megadoses of Ascorbic Acid," *American Journal of Clinical Nutrition* 66 (1997): 1,165–1,171.

megaloblastic anemia A condition resulting from a deficiency of normal RED BLOOD CELLS in which the blood contains primitive red blood cells called megaloblasts. These large nucleated cells are found in the bone marrow as parents to normal, mature red blood cells, which lack nuclei. Megaloblastic anemia occurs in cases of severe deficiencies of B vitamins, VITAMIN B_{12}, and FOLIC ACID, which are required to produce new cells, including red blood cells.

megavitamin therapy See ORTHOMOLECULAR MEDICINE.

melatonin A hormone produced by the pineal gland, which lies deep within the brain. During the day, light enters the eye and triggers nerve signals that shut down melatonin production. In the dark, melatonin is released into the bloodstream where it helps coordinate hormonal activity with the NERVOUS SYSTEM. It may even help regulate the sleep cycle and help overcome jet lag. Melatonin may regulate complex processes including fertility.

There are hints that melatonin may influence AGING. In experimental animals, melatonin has been shown to increase the life span, although long-term effects in humans are unknown. Melatonin may slow down wear and tear throughout life. It can act as an ANTIOXIDANT to help clear the body of oxidative damage accumulated during the daytime due to normal metabolism, as well as exposure to pollutants like cigarette smoke and ozone. Several degenerative diseases, including heart disease and cancer, have been linked to oxidative damage. In addition, melatonin can increase immunity and delay the age-dependent shrinkage of the thymus gland in lab animals. The thymus is the home of T cells, key white blood cells that fight infection. Although synthetic melatonin is available in health food stores, this supplement is clearly a hormone. It is not a nutrient in the sense of a vitamin or other building block for the body, and it should be used judiciously. (See also ENDOCRINE SYSTEM; FREE RADICAL; IMMUNE SYSTEM.)

Reiter, R. J. et al. "Melatonin: Its Intracellular and Genomic Actions," *Trends in Endochronology Metabolism* 7, no. 1 (1996): 22–27.

melon The sweet, juicy FRUIT of several plants of the cucurbit (gourd) family, which includes SQUASH and CUCUMBERS. CANTALOUPE, CASABA, HONEYDEW, musk crenshaw, Persian, and WATERMELON are typical representatives. Most melons originated in the Middle East and were cultivated by the ancient Egyptians and the Romans. Watermelon originated in Africa and in North America. Various types of melons are imported from Central America, Chile, and New Zealand. Florida, Texas, Georgia, California, and Arizona supply the domestic U.S. market of cantaloupes, watermelons, honeydew melons, and the like.

Melons are round or oblong fruit grown from either climbing or trailing vines. The pulp may be white, green, yellow, pink, or red. All melons are about 90 percent water. They are good sources of POTASSIUM and VITAMIN C. When the pulp is deep orange, they are an excellent source of vitamin A, in the form of BETA-CAROTENE.

menadione A synthetic form of VITAMIN K used as a supplement. Unlike natural vitamin K, this analog is smaller and has no side chain attached. It is processed by the LIVER. Vitamin K is required in the formation of certain clotting proteins of the BLOOD and in the formation of several proteins found in BONE, blood, and kidneys. While large amounts of vitamin K are not generally toxic, excessive menadione can cause hemolytic ANEMIA and excessive production of BILE PIGMENT and JAUNDICE in newborn infants.

Menkes' syndrome A rare genetic disease caused by the inability of the intestine to absorb COPPER adequately. Copper is an essential TRACE MINERAL nutrient, and copper malabsorption leads to progressive mental retardation, low body temperature, skeletal abnormalities, abnormal hair development, and degeneration of connective tissue structures such as the aorta and other vessel walls. A copper dependent ENZYME (lysyloxidase) stabilizes collagen fibers incorporated in vessel walls. Progressive nerve damage associated with Menkes' syndrome often causes death at a very early age. (See also COLLAGEN; LYSINE.)

menopause Cessation of monthly, menstrual periods. As women reach middle age their bodies begin to produce less estrogen. At some point the level declines sharply, triggering the onset of menopause. The abrupt change in hormone levels causes most women to suffer uncomfortable and sometimes disorienting side effects, including hot flashes, headaches, mood swings, forgetfulness, and night sweats.

After menopause, women face a much higher risk of OSTEOPOROSIS and HEART DISEASE. If a woman has not consumed sufficient amounts of calcium throughout her life, her bones may become brittle and prone to fractures. The problem is magnified after a woman goes through menopause because estrogen helps to maintain bone strength.

To lessen the negative side effects of menopause, many women in recent decades opted to undergo hormone replacement therapy (HRT), which involves taking the hormone drugs estrogen and progestin. Women who took the drugs were much less likely to suffer osteoporosis-related fractures.

However, in 2002 a study of hormone replacement therapy in 16,000 postmenopausal women was halted when researchers discovered that the hormone drugs caused a slight but significant increase in the risk of invasive breast cancer and also increased the risk of heart attack, stroke, and blood clots. Although researchers reported that the risk to any individual woman was small, they cautioned that the drugs' risks outweighed their benefits. After these results were announced many women who had been on HRT stopped taking hormone medication.

To decrease the risk of osteoporosis, any postmenopausal woman who is not taking hormone replacements should consume 1,500 mg of calcium daily. Women who have opted to continue with HRT should consume 1,000 mg of calcium daily. Foods that are high in calcium include milk and milk products such as cheese and yogurt, canned fish with bones (like sardines), green leafy vegetables, and tofu.

Menopausal and postmenopausal should also be careful to get enough VITAMIN D, which helps with calcium absorption. Again, milk and milk products are rich in this vitamin. The body can also manufacture vitamin D when it is exposed to sunlight.

As a woman's body ages, and especially after she has reached menopause, her metabolism slows, and fatty tissue begins to replace muscle tissue. This, in turn, increases the risk of heart disease and diabetes. Therefore, older women should eat fewer fatty and sugary foods and increase their consumption of lean meats, vegetables, and fruits.

Some foods contain compounds that have estrogen-like qualities. These phytoestrogens are found in soybeans and other legumes and in lesser amounts in carrots, corn, apples, and oats. By mimicking estrogen these phytoestrogens may lower the risk of menopause-related symptoms.

Moquette, Magee E. *Eat Well for a Healthy Menopause: The Low-Fat, High Nutrition Guide.* New York: Wiley, 1996.

mercury A toxic HEAVY METAL and an environmental pollutant. Chemically combined mercury is a widespread industrial waste; combustion pollutants may be a primary cause of mercury pollution. Once released into the environment, mercury can combine with carbon to create a more toxic form of mercury called methylmercury, which accumulates in the FOOD CHAIN because it is fat soluble and concentrates in fatty tissues. Predatory fish at the top of the aquatic food chain possess the highest levels. The average American adult consumes 2 to 3 mcg of mercury daily. Mercury levels (in parts per million) for popular fish are as follows: TUNA (0.32), shark (0.46), and swordfish (1.0), King mackerel (0.73), grouper (0.43), and lobster (0.31). The allowable amount of mercury in commercial fish is 1.00 part per million. One bite of a tuna sandwich may be equivalent to the amount of mercury released in the average person's fillings in a day.

Because many rivers and lakes are polluted by industrial wastes, domestic freshwater fish are often contaminated with mercury. The high levels of methylmercury in fish has triggered health advisories for many lakes in the United States and Canada. Native Americans subsisting on locally caught fish or on game animals eating those fish, are also at risk. In communities relying on fish for food, people can consume 200 times the federally designated tolerable level. Health departments in at least 21 states, including Michigan, Minnesota, and Wisconsin, have established advisories for mercury contaminated freshwater fish.

Methylmercury acts as a nerve poison and the brain is susceptible to mercury toxicity. Adults eating fish containing substantial amounts of methylmercury can suffer irreversible nerve and brain damage. The fetus is extremely sensitive to methylmercury. Low doses can lead to retardation due to severe brain damage. Whether mercury causes heart disease has not been established.

To minimize consumption of mercury, patients should avoid tuna and swordfish if pregnant. Patients should also eat saltwater fish like salmon, rather than freshwater fish harvested from polluted water and avoid eating freshwater fish from polluted waters more than two to four times a month.

In July 2002 an advisory panel to the FDA broadened that recommendation, adding that pregnant women should eat no more than two cans of tuna a week. If pregnant women ate any other fish, they should eat no more than one can of tuna a week. Because the FDA does not oversee locally caught fish in lakes and rivers—which some experts say carry even higher levels of mercury in some cases—pregnant women should get their doctor's advice about locally caught freshwater fish.

Mercury was named as a possible cause for a dramatic increase in the 1990s in the number of U.S. children diagnosed with neurological disorders, including autism and autism spectrum disorder. During the 1990s many of the vaccines that children received at regular doctors' visits during the first five years after birth contained a preservative called thimerosal, which is 49.6 percent mercury by weight. In 1999 the FDA announced that "infants who receive thimerosal-containing vaccines at several visits may have been exposed to more mercury than recommended by federal guidelines" and asked vaccine manufacturers to remove thimerosal from all childhood vaccines. In 2001 the National Institute of Medicine reported that while there was no proof that thimerosal exposure was related to autism, the connection was medically plausible. The subject is currently being studied. (See also AMALGAM FILLINGS; BIRTH DEFECTS; BREAST-FEEDING.)

Ball, Leslie et al. "An Assessment of Thimerosal Use in Childhood Vaccines," *Pediatrics* 107, no. 5 (2001): 1,147–1,154.

Lorscheider, Fritz L. et al. "Mercury Exposure from 'Silver' Tooth Fillings: Emerging Evidence Questions a Traditional Dental Paradigm," *FASEB Journal* 917 (April 1995): 504–508.

metabolic acidosis Excessive acid in body fluids, especially the blood. This condition may be the result of the production of acids like KETONE BODIES during excessive fat breakdown; the loss of BICARBONATE, a blood BUFFER; or the loss of essential ELECTROLYTES due to kidney disease. The accumulation of ketone bodies accompanies STARVATION, FASTING, crash DIETING, uncontrolled diabetes, and chronic ALCOHOLISM. Aspirin poisoning can contribute to ACIDOSIS. Excessive acid production can cause severe mineral loss and DEHYDRATION due to increased urine volume. (See also FAT METABOLISM.)

metabolic alkalosis See ALKALOSIS.

metabolic pathway A series of ENZYMES that function together like an assembly line to degrade larger molecules or to manufacture larger molecules from raw materials. The final product of a metabolic pathway is thus the result of many chemical modifications, mostly carried out one step at a time.

Many hormones regulate metabolic pathways. GLUCAGON and EPINEPHRINE (adrenaline) are hormones that make fuel available for tissues. They raise blood sugar levels by activating enzymes that break down liver GLYCOGEN, the storage form of glucose, to release glucose and raise blood sugar. In addition, epinephrine stimulates enzymes that break down body fat to release fatty acids, thus raising blood fatty acid levels. (See also ANABOLISM; CATABOLISM; INHIBITION; METABOLISM.)

Metabolic Syndrome (Syndrome X) A complex, diverse collection of signs and symptoms associated with increased blood sugar, blood lipids, and blood pressure during aging. Sedentary lifestyles lead to weight gain and abdominal (apple-shaped) obesity during aging. Each of these traits is a risk factor for cardiovascular disease in general and, specifically, coronary heart disease, but the combination of these traits dramatically increases the risk. Insulin resistance is also related to type 2 (adult onset) diabetes. Insulin resistance, in which high levels of insulin are secreted to lower blood sugar levels, is an underlying imbalance in metabolic syndrome. High blood insulin levels signal the body to make more fat from glucose, thereby increasing the levels of blood triglycerides and LDL-cholesterol (low-density lipoprotein), the "bad" form of cholesterol, while decreasing blood HDL-cholesterol (high-density lipoprotein), the beneficial form.

Significantly, each of the risk factors associated with metabolic syndrome can be reduced by lifestyle changes such as diet. To decrease the risk of metabolic syndrome and related disorders, middle-aged people should exercise regularly and reduce daily calories to lose extra weight and improve blood pressure. Obesity triggers insulin resistance, therefore weight management is a key. Shifting from a diet high in saturated fat to one enriched in monounsaturated fats, such as olive oil and canola oil can also improve insulin sensitivity and reduce high blood pressure.

metabolic water WATER produced by reactions carried out in the cell. An average of 13 ml of water is formed for every 100 calories of food completely oxidized to carbon dioxide. The complete oxidation of 100 g of carbohydrate to carbon dioxide yields 60 ml of water; 100 g of protein yields 40 ml and 100 g of fat yields 110 ml. Consequently, a typical American diet produces about 200 ml of water daily. However, this is still only a fraction of the water needed to replenish water lost in urine, feces, and respiration. About 2 liters per day are required to replenish water losses. (See also DEHYDRATION; ENERGY; METABOLISM; OXIDATION.)

metabolism The sum of chemical reactions performed by cells. In metabolism, ENZYMES, the protein catalysts of cells, work together like assembly lines. Such functional systems are called METABOLIC PATHWAYS. Metabolism is conveniently broken down into two categories: CATABOLISM and ANABOLISM.

Catabolism

Catabolism refers to enzyme systems that oxidize fuel nutrients (carbohydrates, amino acids, and fat) to ENERGY and to waste products, CARBON DIOXIDE and WATER. Catabolism traps chemical energy as ATP in the MITOCHONDRIA, the cell's powerhouse. Catabolism also includes the degradation of nutrients and more complex structures to provide smaller, simpler molecules for cellular building blocks for the cell.

Catabolic pathways include:

- UREA CYCLE, which produces the major nitrogenous waste, UREA, excreted in urine.
- KREB'S CYCLE, the central energy-yielding pathway of the cells, producing carbon dioxide by degrading fat, amino acids, and carbohydrate.
- GLYCOLYSIS, which breaks down GLUCOSE (blood sugar) and smaller oxidation products (pyruvic acid, lactic acid) while delivering energy to the cell independently of oxygen.
- OXIDATIVE PHOSPHORYLATION, the formation of ATP accompanying a sequential series of oxidation-reduction reactions leading ultimately to the reduction of oxygen to water.

Anabolism

Anabolism refers to enzyme pathways that build up cellular components, rather than tear them down. Anabolism produces all of the machinery to operate and reproduce cells. Anabolic precursors require chemical energy, most of which is provided in the form of ATP, the energy currency of the cell produced by catabolism.

Anabolism is stimulated by INSULIN after meals containing carbohydrates. This HORMONE stimulates cells to store surplus chemical energy as fat (from fatty acids) and glycogen (from glucose). Over a longer period of time, anabolism occurs when the body is growing, as during pregnancy, childhood, adolescence, body building, and fat accumulation.

Anabolic pathways include:

- Fatty acid and fat synthesis, for energy storage.
- Cholesterol synthesis; cholesterol functions in membranes and serves as a hormone precursor.
- DNA and RNA synthesis; DNA stores information while RNA functions in guiding the synthesis of proteins.
- Protein synthesis, which includes synthesizing enzymes and certain non-steroid hormones.
- Glycogen synthesis, the formation of the storage carbohydrate glycogen by muscle and liver.
- Amino Acid synthesis; formation of 10 of the 20 amino acids.

Health and maintenance of body weight require a balance between the opposing processes of anabolism and catabolism. When anabolism exceeds catabolism, synthetic processes prevail. In this situation the body's overall metabolism shifts to building protein and to storing energy as fat and glycogen. When the body requires more energy than is provided by food, catabolism exceeds anabolism, breakdown and degradation exceed synthesis, and the body burns carbohydrate, fat, and protein. The body switches to a CATABOLIC STATE during illness, surgery, and starvation. (See also AMINO ACID METABOLISM; BASAL METABOLIC RATE; CARBOHYDRATE METABOLISM; FATTY ACIDS.)

Bjorntorp, P. "The Regulation of Adipose Tissue Distribution in Humans." *International Journal of Obesity* 20 (1996): 291–302.

metabolite A chemical produced by enzyme-catalyzed reactions. Metabolites may be products of degradation: Metabolites of GLUCOSE degradation include simple acids like LACTIC ACID, PYRUVIC ACID, and ACETIC ACID coupled to a carrier molecule called COENZYME A. Metabolites of amino breakdown include AMMONIA and UREA as nitrogen-containing waste products, and acids like alpha ketoglutaric acid and OXALOACETIC ACID. Bilirubin or BILE PIGMENT is a primary metabolite of hemoglobin, the oxygen-transporter of red blood cells. Metabolites are also products of synthetic reactions of the cell. For example, the brain chemicals (NEUROTRANSMITTERS) DOPAMINE and norepinephrine are metabolites of the amino acid TYROSINE. Bile acids for fat digestion are metabolites of CHOLESTEROL. Drugs and medications are metabolized (altered chemically) by the liver so they can be inactivated and excreted.

metalloenzyme An ENZYME or protein catalyst that requires a metal ion to complete its catalytic site where reactions occur. Many trace mineral nutrients function as enzyme helpers:

Copper A variety of enzymes require COPPER: Lysyloxidase helps assemble connective tissue; cytochromic oxidase transfers electrons to reduce oxygen to water in the final step of oxidation of fuels; and a type of SUPEROXIDE DISMUTASE destroys superoxide, a potentially damaging form of oxygen.

Iron Most IRON-containing enzymes are involved in oxidations and reductions: CYTOCHROMES transport electrons in the oxidation of fuel molecules to liberate energy and in the oxidation of potentially damaging materials to increase their water solubility, hence decrease their toxicity. A variety of oxidases perform one-step oxidations.

Zinc More than 100 different enzymes require ZINC, including DNA polymerase, the enzyme that synthesizes DNA chains, and RNA polymerase, which synthesizes RNA. DNA and RNA synthesis is required for cell multiplication. Zinc is required by superoxide dismutase, and CARBOXYPEPTIDASE, a digestive enzyme.

Magnesium Many enzymes that utilize ATP, the cellular form of chemical energy, are activated by MAGNESIUM-ATP combinations.

Manganese Superoxide dismutase and pyruvate carboxylase require MANGANESE. The enzyme that initiates liver synthesis of glucose from amino acids during fasting requires manganese.

Selenium GLUTATHIONE PEROXIDASE, a SELENIUM-containing enzyme, destroys two types of potentially damaging compounds: HYDROGEN PEROXIDE and LIPID peroxides, produced when lipids are attacked by oxygen.

Molybdenum Two important enzymes require MOLYBDENUM: Xanthine oxidase is involved in the synthesis of the waste product URIC ACID; sulfite oxidase destroys SULFITES.

Cobalt The only known role for COBALT is its function as part of an enzyme helper derived from VITAMIN B_{12}. It is required by at least two different human enzymes. (See also COENZYME; TRACE MINERALS.)

methanol The simplest type of ALCOHOL also known as wood alcohol or methyl alcohol. Methanol is derived from wood processing and is highly toxic, unlike ETHANOL, which comes from the fermentation of grains. As little as 20 milliliters can cause permanent blindness or even death. Treatment of methanol poisoning involves administering ethanol. Ethanol competes with liver enzymes and prevents them from converting methanol to a toxic by-product, formaldehyde. Most cases of methanol poisoning are due to ingestion of methanol in lieu of alcoholic beverages and liquors. (See also INHIBITION.)

methionine (Met, L-methionine) An essential AMINO ACID that contains sulfur. The body cannot manufacture methionine; therefore it must be supplied by digesting food PROTEIN. Methionine is a critical building block for cellular proteins, and this versatile amino acid plays many roles. It functions as the raw material for the sulfur-containing amino acid CYSTEINE; for the formation of acetylcholine, a NEUROTRANSMITTER (chemical synthesized by the nervous system for transmitting impulses between cells); for the hormone EPINEPHRINE (adrenaline); and for CHOLINE, required to form LECITHIN, a FAT lipid substance containing phosphorus. Lecithin functions as a building block of the lipid carriers in the bloodstream, like LOW-DENSITY LIPOPROTEIN (LDL) and VERY LOW-DENSITY LIPOPROTEIN (VLDL) to transport fat and CHOLESTEROL. Methionine is converted to sulfate, used by the LIVER to solubilize toxic chemicals and waste products so they can be excreted. TAURINE, a compound used to form BILE salts for fat digestion, is a nonprotein amino acid derived from methionine. Methionine is converted to HOMOCYSTEINE, a simplified sulfur amino acid that eventually is transformed to CYSTEINE, a sulfur amino acid commonly used by the body, via vitamin B_6 dependent steps. Methionine can be regenerated from homocysteine via steps dependent on FOLIC ACID. With folic acid and VITAMIN B_6 deficient diets, blood levels of homocysteine rise. Population studies have demonstrated that elevated homocysteine levels increase the risk of CARDIOVASCULAR DISEASE.

Sources of methionine include: MEAT, FISH, POULTRY, GARLIC, ONIONS, BEANS, and legumes. Grains are generally low in sulfur amino acids. Infants require 58 mg of sulfur amino acids per kilogram of body weight daily; adults require 13 mg. A chronic protein deficiency leads to inadequate intake of dietary essential amino acids, including methionine, and produces stunted growth, EDEMA, fragile hair, loss of muscle mass and hormonal irregularities. Homocystinuria, an inherited disease due to incomplete breakdown of methionine, can lead to CARDIOVASCULAR DISEASE. One person in 200 carries this genetic trait. (See also DETOXIFICATION; KWASHIORKOR; LIPOPROTEIN; LIPOTROPE.)

methylene chloride An organic solvent sometimes used to manufacture decaffeinated COFFEE. Methylene chloride is classified as a chlorinated hydrocarbon because it contains chlorine and carbon. Such compounds have been linked to CANCER. Although the U.S. FDA concluded this solvent causes cancer, it considers the level remaining in decaffeinated coffee so low that the health risk of exposure is negligible. Habitually drinking large amounts of decaffeinated coffee could pose a problem, however. Other manufacturers use ethyl acetate, a nontoxic solvent, or water extraction to remove most of the caffeine from roasted coffee. (See also CARCINOGEN; FOOD ADDITIVES.)

micelle A microscopic particle that permits the suspension of insoluble liquids in water. Micelles require detergent-like molecules (dispersing agents), which possess a characteristic molecular structure. They have a fat-soluble region at one end of the molecule to interact with the lipid-soluble material being dispersed, and a water-attracting region to interact with water at the opposite end. The result of combining dispersing agents and lipids is a stable suspension of microscopic droplets. The body forms a variety of micelles to transport lipids via the lymph and blood. Typical examples include CHYLOMICRONS, which transport dietary fat from the intestine to other tissues, and LOW-DENSITY LIPOPROTEIN (LDL), which transports CHOLESTEROL from the liver to peripheral tissues. (See also HIGH-DENSITY LIPOPROTEIN; VERY LOW-DENSITY LIPOPROTEIN.)

microgram A very small metric unit of weight, abbreviated mcg. One microgram is one-millionth of a gram, or one-thousandth of a milligram. Certain trace nutrients are required daily in only microgram amounts, as illustrated by the following adult RECOMMENDED DIETARY ALLOWANCES (RDAs): VITAMIN B_{12}, 1.6–2.0 mcg; VITAMIN D, 5 mcg; VITAMIN K, 65 to 80 mcg; FOLIC ACID, 180 to 200 mcg; and IODINE, 150 mcg. (See also MEASURES; TRACE MINERALS; VITAMIN.)

micronutrients Nutrients that are required by the body in trace amounts—milligrams (thousandths of a gram) or micrograms (millionths of a gram). Although only tiny amounts of certain VITAMINS and MINERALS are required, they nonetheless serve extremely important roles. Inadequate trace nutrients is a major health issue for certain populations both in the United States and throughout the world, for several reasons. Micronutrients are most likely to be lost or destroyed because of their instability in highly processed foods; thus, refined foods and synthetic foods are likely to be deficient in many micronutrients. Only a few micronutrients are added to processed foods by enrichment programs.

Vitamins The weight of all B vitamins needed by the average person daily amounts to no more than 10 staples. The reason such small amounts are required is that they serve as enzyme helpers (coenzymes). Enzymes function as chemical catalysts; they are used repeatedly before wearing out and are needed in only small amounts. In contrast with B vitamins, VITAMIN C does not function as an enzyme helper. While trace amounts of this vitamin will prevent the vitamin C deficiency disease of scurvy, much more is needed for tissue repair, wound healing, toxic chemical disposal, and to maintain a strong immune system. Low amounts of fat-soluble vitamins are required daily and their functions are diverse: VITAMIN A forms a visual pigment and is needed for normal tissue development; VITAMIN K assists blood clotting; VITAMIN E is an ANTIOXIDANT; and VITAMIN D forms a hormone.

Trace Minerals Together the quantities of minerals like ZINC, IRON, CHROMIUM, COPPER, IODINE, MANGANESE, and MOLYBDENUM required daily would be a pill weighing a fraction of a gram. These micronutrients generally serve as enzyme helpers (cofactors). Iodine is required in the formation of thyroid hormones and chromium supports the blood-lowering effects of INSULIN. The daily requirements of major minerals (CALCIUM, PHOSPHORUS, SODIUM, CHLORIDE, and POTASSIUM) are thousands of times larger. (See also JUNK FOOD; NUTRIENT DENSITY.)

microvilli Minute, hair-like extensions of the surface of cells lining the small INTESTINE and used to absorb nutrients. The inside of the small intestine resembles a wrinkled shag carpet. VILLI are analogous to the shag and make up the "brush border" of the intestinal surface. Cells that make up the villi are themselves covered with still thinner fibers called microvilli, visible only through an electron microscope. The villi and microvilli provide the intestine with a huge surface area: If its fuzzy inner surface were flattened out, the total surface area of the intestine would be the size of a baseball diamond.

AGING, health, diet history, and FOOD SENSITIVITIES can lead to a flattening of microvilli and villi. Loss of this rough surface drastically reduces the amount of nutrients that can be absorbed by the body during DIGESTION. Thus, aging and food sensitivities can lead to MALNUTRITION even when consuming a BALANCED DIET. An extreme example of food sensitivity is CELIAC DISEASE, a severe sensitivity to grain protein that destroys intestinal villi. Celiac disease may cause severe malnutrition and retard growth of children. (See also DIGESTIVE TRACT; MALABSORPTION.)

microwave cooking A rapid heating technique that generally requires one-quarter to one-half the cooking time of an electric oven. Microwave COOKING entails heating foods by means of electromagnetic energy; microwaves are like FM radiowaves. Microwaves cook by causing water molecules in food to vibrate rapidly, which creates heat in the interior of food quickly.

To avoid microwave exposure consumers should make sure the door of the microwave oven closes properly and that the seal on the door is not damaged. Seals should be kept clean and free of obstruction. Any oven can leak radiation if the interlocking system does not work. Patients should avoid standing in front of a microwave oven when it is running. Newer pacemakers have shields that protect against microwave interference. People with pacemakers from 1990 or earlier should stand at least five feet away from a working microwave oven. Metal twist ties, leaded glass, or metal-trimmed porcelain can create arcing and cause fires.

Because foods cooked in microwave ovens require less time and less water, microwave cooking removes fewer minerals and vitamins than conventional cooking, especially when food is reheated. Microwave cooking does not brown food. Cooking at high temperatures, like baking, produces compounds that can cause cancer in experimental animals; microwaving food virtually eliminates this hazard. Microwave cooking generally does not heat MEAT hotter than boiling water.

It is important to stir foods during microwave cooking. Microwaves may not penetrate a roast or CHICKEN uniformly; consequently, uncooked portions of meat may contain bacteria such as SALMONELLA, which can cause FOOD POISONING, and in PORK, parasites causing TRICHINOSIS. Therefore, when microwaving POULTRY, pieces should be turned or rearranged at least once during the cooking interval to ensure even and complete cooking. Microwaved bacon contains much less NITRITE than fried bacon, and therefore produces much less NITROSOAMINE than fried bacon. Nitrosoamine is a cancer causing agent formed when the preservative sodium nitrite is heated with meat.

It is recommended to microwave meat on paper, not on a platter because meat touching a ceramic surface can become hot enough to create materials that can cause DNA damage (mutagens). (See also FOOD IRRADIATION.)

microwave popcorn Microwave popcorn accounts for two-thirds of the popcorn market. Microwaving is a quick and easy method of making popcorn, although it may not be as nutritious as air-blown popcorn. Microwavable popcorn can contain 50 percent to 60 percent of its calories as added FAT. Partially hydrogenated VEGETABLE OIL, COCONUT OIL, or PALM OIL, can double the calories. Another disadvantage: Microwavable popcorn contains excessive amounts of SALT. The label will show whether a brand contains added salt, ARTIFICIAL FLAVOR or coloring, or synthetic ANTIOXIDANTS (BHA and BHT). Garlic powder, yeast, chili powder, or Parmesan CHEESE will stick to the popcorn if misted with a spray bottle of water first. Popcorn should not be microwaved in a brown paper bag; it could catch fire. (See also COOKING.)

migraine headache A severe form of recurrent headache that causes throbbing pain, light sensitivity, vomiting, diarrhea, and altered visual perception. The causes of migraines are not entirely understood. Some experts thought TYRAMINE-containing foods and beverages were implicated in perhaps 10 percent of cases. These foods include CHOCOLATE, aged cheeses, and red wine, and avoiding these may be helpful.

However, experiments using tyramine alone have failed to substantiate its primary role in causing migraine headaches. Double-blind administration of tyramine to patients who benefited from a low-tyramine diet did not provoke attacks of migraine.

The problem with many food–headache studies has been an overly simplistic view of the pain-causing sequence. In general, any food that can imitate or release mediator substances in the bloodstream may produce pain. Any food that is capable of producing an allergic response can cause headache; this means that staple foods containing milk, wheat, eggs, soy, fish, and other foods can cause headaches. Thus, the solution to a chronic headache problem involves complete diet revision and not simply the exclusion of one or two foods.

Migraine has many causes; it is a disease that may be induced by ingesting large amounts of chemical mediators in some individuals or through an allergic reaction to foods in others, but the exact way in which foods cause the migraine is not clear. Some food-allergic reactions are triggered by a hypersensitivity reaction in the gut.

Eliminating offending foods can also alleviate symptoms. Magnesium deficiency is also associated with migraines. Intravenous treatment with MAGNESIUM and VITAMIN B_6 can also be beneficial. Magnesium counters muscle spasm, and it acts like certain calcium-channel blockers used in conventional treatment to reduce symptoms. (See also ALLERGY, FOOD.)

milk Liquid secreted by mammals to nourish their young. Milk from goats, sheep, buffalo, and cows is consumed in different parts of the world and is converted into a diverse group of products, including BUTTER, CHEESE, dried milk, YOGURT, KEFIR, and ICE CREAM. Goat's milk accounts for about 3 percent of the world milk supply, yet in Asia and Africa goat's milk represents an important part of the diet. Goat's milk resembles cow's milk in composition, although its droplets are smaller and remain suspended during storage. In contrast, cow's milk will separate upon standing, and in the United States most cow's milk is homogenized. Milk and milk products comprise one of the basic four food groups, a system long used in meal preparation guidelines in the United States. Dairy products contribute a substantial part of the typical American diet (15 percent to 20 percent).

In 2001 the National Institutes of Health (NIH) reported that only 13.5 percent of girls and 36.3 percent of boys age 12 to 19 in the United States were consuming the recommended daily amount (RDA) of calcium, thereby increasing their risk for osteoporosis and other bone diseases. Nearly 90 percent of adult bone mass is established by the end of this age range. The NIH attributed this in part to children drinking less milk and more soft drinks and noncitrus drinks. To respond to this "calcium crisis," the NIH instituted a nationwide campaign called "Milk Matters" to educate consumers about the importance of calcium in children's diets and to promote milk consumption by children.

Whole cow's milk is prominent in European and North American diets, although many other adult populations of the world cannot tolerate it because they have lost the childhood ability to digest milk sugar (LACTOSE INTOLERANCE). Cow's milk contains about 88 percent water. Solids include CARBOHYDRATE, PROTEIN, MINERALS, and VITAMINS; the exact composition is affected by the season, the type of feed, the environmental temperature and the breed of dairy cattle. In the typical American diet, milk provides about 10 percent of the daily allowances of ENERGY, 11 percent of fat intake, 20 percent of the protein, 72 percent of CALCIUM, 30 percent of PHOSPHORUS, and 12 percent of VITAMIN A. In the United States, all milk except raw milk is fortified with vitamins A and D. Typically, the amounts are relatively small: One cup of milk contains 20 percent of the DAILY REFERENCE INTAKE (RDI) of VITAMIN D and 10 percent of the RDI of VITAMIN A. Milk typically provides 36 percent of the RDA of RIBOFLAVIN. However, when milk is stored in plastic bottles, fluorescent lighting can destroy riboflavin and vitamin A within a day. Riboflavin in milk packaged in cardboard containers is stable.

Whole milk contains 4 percent fat because most of milk is water. Milk fat represents about 48 percent of the calories in milk, far above the 30 percent fat calories recommended for daily consumption by dietary guidelines. Milk fat is considered saturated fat. Whole milk contains 22 mg of CHOLESTEROL per cup. Reduced cholesterol milk contains about 25 percent of the original cholesterol content.

Whole milk contains 3.3 percent protein in the form of whey and CASEIN. Casein accounts for about 80 percent of the milk protein and gives milk its white color. Whey protein remains after casein and fat have been removed from milk for cheese manufacture. The proteins in milk enhance the uptake of the B vitamin FOLIC ACID in the INTESTINE.

Potential Problems with Cow's Milk

As a Food for Children Cow's milk evolved to support the growth of a calf, and it differs from human milk in important ways. Cow's milk is low in CARNITINE, an amino acid used in energy production that is very high in human milk. Manufacturers of INFANT FORMULAS now add carnitine. Cow's milk contains little IRON. Infants fed cow's milk alone can become iron-deficient and grow slowly. Once the baby's body has become iron deficient, mental development slows even after iron supplements have been given to remedy the iron deficiency.

Parents should not substitute breast milk or formula with cow's milk until the baby is a year old. Although breast milk and formula contain plenty of fat to support the infant's growth, cow's milk does not supply enough fat for the infant. Finally, there is a potential for allergies and milk intolerance when cow's milk is given to young children too early in their development. Although skim milk is lower in fat than whole milk and is a desirable option for adults, a baby's kidneys may not be able to handle skim milk's very concentrated protein.

As a Food for Adults Humans are the only species that drink milk as adults. Milk is an excellent source of calcium and vitamins; however, it is a high-fat food. Butterfat is a highly saturated fat, and high consumption of saturated fat promotes clogged arteries. Milk may contain a variety of low-level contaminants because grain-fed cattle can be exposed to pesticides and environmental pollutants like PCB and PBB, which cattle eliminate through their milk. As an example, the pesticide heptachlor extensively contaminated milk produced in Hawaii in 1982. ANTIBIOTICS and growth promoters added to livestock feed are also eliminated through milk. The levels of contaminants are generally quite low, though amounts vary. Rarely, the antibiotic penicillin has been detected in milk at high enough levels to cause a reaction in sensitive people. The veterinary antibiotic sulfamethazine is not approved for use in dairy cattle feed. This drug causes tumors in lab animals. Nonetheless, this substance has periodically been found to contaminate milk. U.S. FDA intervention has decreased this occurrence. Milk boosts the production of stomach acid so it is no longer recommended for ulcers. Recent studies suggest that milk partially blocks the anti-ulcer medication cimetidine.

Bovine Growth Hormone About one-third of U.S. dairy farms inject their cattle with Recombinant Bovine Growth Hormone (rBGH), which is a genetically engineered duplicate of a hormone produced by dairy cows. Milk production in cattle that receive these injections increases by 10 percent to 15 percent. The FDA approved use of rBGH in 1993. Some studies have linked this hormone with an increased risk of diabetes and breast, prostate, and colorectal cancer. Based on these concerns, Canada rejected use of the hormone in milk production in that country in 1999. The FDA maintains that the use of rBGH in dairy cattle poses no risk to the health of humans.

Milk Processing

To prevent cream from separating from fresh milk, butterfat is broken up into tiny droplets, too small to rise to the top of a milk carton. This homogenization is accomplished by forcing the milk through a nozzle at high pressure. No law requires milk to be homogenized.

Milk is heated, or pasteurized, to kill certain disease producing bacteria. Besides killing harmful bacteria, pasteurization kills the lactic acid bacteria responsible for souring milk. Pasteurized milk will nonetheless eventually spoil, since not all bacteria are killed. Ultra-high temperatures used to sterilize milk are normally reserved for canned milk or packaged milk stored at room temperature. Pasteurization does not destroy nutrients.

Comparison of Nutrient Contents

Whole milk (1 cup, 8 oz.) provides 210 calories; protein, 7.9 g; carbohydrate, 11.4 g; fat, 8.2 g; cholesterol, 33 mg; calcium, 290 mg; vitamin A, 76 retinol equivalents; thiamin, 0.09 mg; riboflavin, 0.41 mg; niacin, 0.22 mg. Other milk preparations contain similar amounts of protein, carbohydrate, calcium, thiamin, riboflavin, and niacin. Vitamin D and vitamin A are added.

Low-fat milk (2 percent fat) contains half the fat content of whole milk. However, it is not a low-fat food. Though it contains 2 percent fat by weight, this amount is equivalent to 30 percent of the total calories. Sometimes low-fat milk is fortified with nonfat dry milk solids. One cup of 2 percent milk provides 121 calories; protein, 8.1 g; carbohydrate, 11.7 g; calcium, 297 mg; fat, 4.8 g; cholesterol, 22 mg; vitamin A, 140 retinol equivalents; thiamin, 0.1 mg; riboflavin, 0.4 mg; niacin, 0.21 mg. One percent milk supplies 1 percent fat by weight. Only 21 percent of its calories come from fat. One cup provides 105 calories; protein, 8 g; carbohydrate, 11.7 g; fat 2.5 g; cholesterol, 10 mg; calcium, 300 mg; vitamin A, 145 retinol equivalents; thiamin, 0.1 mg; riboflavin, 0.42 mg; niacin, 0.21 mg. Skim milk contains less than 0.2 percent fat but is also homogenized. A cup contains 86 calories; protein, 8.3 g; carbohydrate, 11.9 g; fat 0.44 g; cholesterol, 4 mg; calcium, 302 mg; vitamin A, 149 retinol equivalents; thiamin, 0.09 mg; riboflavin, 0.34 mg; niacin, 0.22 mg.

Powdered Whole Milk

To remove water, milk is sprayed in a drying oven to dry milk droplets. The exposure to hot air can oxidize fat and cholesterol. Oxidized forms of these lipids are potentially harmful; oxidized cholesterol is thought to contribute to ATHEROSCLEROSIS. Powdered skim milk contains very little fat or cholesterol and lacks the oxidized lipids prevalent in powdered whole milk. A cup of powdered nonfat milk provides 244 calories; protein, 23.9 g; carbohydrate, 35.5 g; fat, 0.51 g; cholesterol, 12 mg; calcium, 837 mg; vitamin A, 483 retinol equivalents; thiamin, 0.28 mg; riboflavin, 1.19 mg; niacin, 0.61 mg.

Skim Milk and Children's Diets; Raw Milk

Malnourished young children have been observed in American families whose parents restricted their fat consumption, including substituting skim milk or nonfat milk for whole milk out of fear of childhood OBESITY. Baby obesity is probably a function of total calorie intake, not just fat intake. Adequate fat is essential to support the rapid growth and development required by young children. Parents should use caution when decreasing a child's caloric intake and seek medical advice about fat restrictions for children.

Certified raw milk—commercially available, unprocessed milk that has not been heated—is certified by states that assure strict sanitary conditions have been met in its production. Consumers selecting this type of milk believe it is more nutritious than homogenized, pasteurized milk. Nonetheless, there is a very real risk of developing food poisoning (SALMONELLA) unless milk is pasteurized, and the FDA has banned interstate sales of raw milk. Raw milk production is tightly controlled through state certification procedures. Many first-time users of raw milk develop gastrointestinal disease. Infants and elderly persons are especially at risk. People who habitually drink raw milk develop immunity to at least some of the disease-causing bacteria in raw milk. (See also ALLERGY, FOOD; DIETARY GUIDELINES FOR AMERICANS; MILK ALLERGY.)

Binkley, K. E. "Allergy to Supplemental Lactase Enzyme," *Journal of Allergy and Clinical Immunology* 97, no. 8 (1996): 1,414–1,416.

milk-alkali syndrome A condition resulting from high calcium levels in the BLOOD. Milk-alkali syndrome can occur during long-term high consumption of MILK together with alkaline substances such as ANTACIDS. Excessive calcium may contribute to kidney stones, or it may be deposited in soft tissue and harden them. Symptoms include vomiting, gastrointestinal bleeding and hypertension. (See also ACIDOSIS; ALKALOSIS.)

milk allergy A reaction of the immune system to milk and milk products. The immune system recognizes milk proteins as foreign and overreacts by triggering an allergic attack. Allergies to COW'S MILK and to milk products are among the most common food allergies in the United States. A milk ALLERGY may show up quickly, with symptoms such as hives and asthma or more severe symptoms (immediate hypersensitivity), or it may show up hours after contact (delayed hypersensitivity), with symptoms ranging from ringing ears to joint pain.

The best way to avoid an allergic attack is to avoid milk and milk products. Patients should examine food labels carefully to see whether the milk protein products CASEIN or whey have been added. For delayed reactions, milk and milk products should be avoided long enough for the body to recover (up to several weeks). Once symptoms have declined, patients should try eating the suspected food and monitor carefully how their bodies respond. Depending on the response, patients may be able to eat dairy products occasionally (perhaps once a week or two) after the IMMUNE SYSTEM recovers. (See also BREAST-FEEDING; ELIMINATION DIET; LACTOSE INTOLERANCE; ROTATION DIET.)

milk intolerance See LACTOSE INTOLERANCE.

milk thistle (*Silybum marianum*) A thistle used in botanical medicine to treat liver disorders that grows in Europe and in the United States. Extracts of leaves, seeds, and fruit have been used in folk medicine for jaundice and to trigger milk production in nursing mothers.

Extracts of milk thistle are now used in pharmaceutical preparations to prevent liver damage and increase liver function. Silymarin extract is a mixture of complex substances that prevent liver damage due to FREE RADICALS (highly reactive molecules that can attack cells and damage their membranes and their DNA). Silymarin helps the liver detoxify foreign substances by increasing the production of GLUTATHIONE, the cells' own antioxidant. Glutathione also aids in the detoxification of many substances, ranging from hormones to toxic chemicals. Silymarin also helps the liver by blocking the production of LEUKOTRIENES, very potent agents that trigger inflammation. Silymarin may help improve symptoms of CIRRHOSIS, hepatitis, and alcohol- and diabetes-induced liver damage, as well as psoriasis. Most studies were performed with a milk thistle extract containing standardized amounts of silymarin. Silymarin also may decrease insulin resistance in diabetics and patients with alcoholic cirrhosis.

Safety data are inadequate for pregnant and breast-feeding women. (See also BOTANICAL EXTRACTS; HERBAL MEDICINE; MEDICINAL PLANTS.)

millet (*Panicum miliaceum*) A cereal GRAIN that is a food STAPLE in parts of India, Africa, China, and elsewhere. Millet has been cultivated since prehistoric times in regions of North Africa and Central Asia, though its origin is obscure. Most millet is produced in Asia and Africa. In Europe and the United States, millet is grown mainly as forage for poultry and as bird feed. Pearl millet, the major type produced for human consumption, is sold as whole grain and can be cooked like other grains.

Millet contains an average of 10 percent to 12 percent PROTEIN. While its protein is superior to that of WHEAT or CORN in terms of content of essential AMINO ACIDS, it nonetheless contains less than half the amount of the essential amino acid LYSINE that is found in high-quality protein sources such as meat. Millet lacks GLUTEN, the wheat protein that makes dough prepared from wheat flour elastic; thus millet flour is not suitable for leavened breads. Millet flour is used in making flat cakes and breads. The whole grain is used in soups, stews, or as a cooked cereal; millet is also popped, roasted, or sprouted. It is used in steamed dishes and deep-fried doughs. Millet (cooked, 1/2 cup, 95 g) provides 54 calories; protein, 1.4 g; carbohydrate, 10.8 g; fiber, 1.3 g; iron, 1.1 g; thiamin, 0.1 mg; riboflavin, 0.06 mg; niacin, 0.4 mg. (See also AMARANTH; BUCKWHEAT; QUINOA; RICE; SORGHUM.)

milligram A metric measure of weight equivalent to one one-thousandth of a gram; 28 grams equal one ounce. (See also MEASURES.)

milliliter A metric measure of volume, equivalent to one one-thousandth liter, which is roughly one quart. A milliliter is about one-thirtieth of an ounce. (See also MEASURES.)

mineralocorticoids Hormones of the ADRENAL GLANDS (adrenal cortex) that regulate WATER and SODIUM excretion in urine. ALDOSTERONE is the primary mineralocorticoid: It increases the recovery of sodium in KIDNEY tubules while losing POTASSIUM. An increase in blood potassium level and a large increase in blood sodium stimulate mineralocorticoid release. The pituitary regulates mineralocorticoid release from the adrenals via the hormone corticotropin. Mineralocorticoid deficiency leads to excessively dilute urine (DIABETES INSIPIDUS), severe dehydration and fluid imbalances, because of the body's inability to concentrate urine. Diabetes insipidus causes the danger of severe DEHYDRATION and ELECTROLYTE imbalance.

Symptoms of mineralocorticoid insufficiency include muscle weakness, abnormal cardiac function, and hypertension. LICORICE root has MINERAL corticoid activity; licorice extract is used in some licorice candy and chewing tobacco. (See also FLUID BALANCE; GLUCOCORTICOID.)

mineral oil See LAXATIVE.

minerals Inorganic (noncarbon containing) NUTRIENTS. Minerals are elements remaining after a food is burned completely to ash. Minerals cannot be formed in the body and must be obtained from the diet. Mineral nutrients are either positively charged (cations) or negatively charged (ANIONS). Cations are derived from metals, including CALCIUM, cobalt, CHROMIUM, COPPER, IRON, MAGNESIUM, MANGANESE, MOLYBDENUM (as molybdate), POTASSIUM, SELENIUM (as selenate), SODIUM, and ZINC. Nonmetallic elements yield anions: IODINE as iodide; sulfur as sulfate; phosphorus as phosphate; chlorine as CHLORIDE; and fluorine as FLUORIDE. Combinations of anions and cations yield salts such as sodium chloride, calcium phosphate, and sodium iodide.

Minerals serve diverse functions. They provide the building blocks of teeth and bones and are components of connective tissue. They activate enzymes and are responsible for the transmission of nerve impulses and muscle contraction. They help regulate physiologic processes like the pH (hydrogen ion concentration) and blood volume.

The body requires at least 21 different minerals. Seven of these are required in large amounts and are classified as "major" minerals, or macrominerals. The amounts of macrominerals required daily range from a fraction of a gram to several grams. Calcium, phosphate, and magnesium are bone builders and metabolic helpers. Potassium, sodium, sulfate and chloride are the major electrolytes (ions) in body fluids. These ions help regulate the acid-base balance of body fluids and balance charged chemicals in the blood. They are partially responsible for osmotic pressure in blood vessels and cells.

TRACE MINERALS, or microminerals, are needed in much smaller amounts. The levels needed per day vary from micrograms (millionths of a gram) to milligrams (thousandths of a gram). Trace minerals include cobalt, iron, manganese, copper, selenium, molybdenum, and zinc, which assist the action of enzymes. Chromium and iodine play roles in hormone function, while fluoride helps build teeth and bones. Other trace minerals, including BORON, SILICON, and VANADIUM, play unspecified roles.

Macrominerals and trace minerals originate in soil and water. Essential minerals can be depleted by intensive cultivation of a single crop year after year. On the other hand, overfertilizing can kill microorganisms needed to make soil minerals soluble for crop uptake or alter the chemical composition of the soil so that certain minerals become insoluble and cannot be taken up readily. Soils may be naturally deficient in cobalt, copper, molybdenum, and phosphorus; other soils contain excessive amounts of selenium, yielding high-selenium grains and forage. Water supplies contain minerals. "Hard" water contains calcium, magnesium, and sometimes iron and fluoride, and "soft" water contains more sodium and potassium and less calcium, magnesium, and iron. Drinking water can therefore provide significant amounts of minerals.

Mineral Antagonists in Food

Excessive plant FIBER can bind minerals in food, thus limiting their efficient absorption. CELLULOSE and HEMICELLULOSE, from BRAN, fruits, and vegetables, and LIGNIN may increase excretion of calcium, potassium, zinc, and other minerals. PHYTIC ACID, a phosphorus-containing compound present in the outer layers of grains, binds calcium, iron, and zinc. In terms of supplementation, excessive amounts of one mineral can inhibit the uptake or upset the metabolism of another; zinc and copper, calcium and phosphorous, magnesium and calcium, iron and copper are examples of minerals that can compete with each other. (See also MALABSORPTION.)

minimal daily requirement (MDR) An outdated reference for judging the adequacy of nutrient intake that is now seldom used. The MDR is based on a model developed in the 1940s that a minimal amount of a vitamin is required to prevent a full-blown vitamin deficiency disease. The MDR is not suitable for either meal planning or DIET analysis.

The MDR is not equivalent to the RECOMMENDED DIETARY ALLOWANCE (RDA), which correlates with the amount of a nutrient estimated to be necessary to maintain the health of most Americans. The RDA was developed to replace the MDR and is used in diet planning and analysis of groups of people. (See also RECOMMENDED DAILY INTAKE; USRDA.)

mitochondria Small particles that function as the cell's powerhouse to produce energy. Most cells (except red blood cells) contain between 50 and several thousand mitochondria. Mitochondria oxidize nutrients with molecular oxygen and trap ENERGY as chemical energy (ATP) in a process called cellular RESPIRATION. Mitochondria provide more than 95 percent of ATP required by cells. ATP is a "high energy" compound universally used by organisms to drive reactions and energy-requiring processes such as muscle contraction, conduction of nerve impulses, cell division, and the transport of nutrients into cells. Fuel molecules are oxidized in a sequence of chemical reaction to carbon dioxide and water. These oxidation steps account for more than 90 percent of the oxygen used by cells. (See also AMINO ACID METABOLISM; CARBOHYDRATE METABOLISM; OXIDATIVE PHOSPHORYLATION; PEROXISOME.)

modified cornstarch A FOOD ADDITIVE used as a thickener. Cornstarch has traditionally been used, but chemically modified cornstarch is more stable and is often used in processed and frozen foods. Short-term safety studies with lab animals have indicated no harmful effects of modified cornstarch, and the effects of lifetime exposures are unknown. Before 1985, modified starch was used extensively in baby foods. Much of the industry has reformulated its products without any added starches. (See also INFANT FORMULAS.)

molasses A thick syrup that is a by-product of cane or beet sugar manufacture. Molasses contains high levels of table sugar (SUCROSE). Because it is less pure than table sugar, it contains small amounts of other materials such as TRACE MINERALS and VITAMINS. Nonetheless, molasses is classified as a refined SWEETENER and provides primarily CARBOHYDRATE-TYPE CALORIES. Blackstrap molasses, the least refined type of molasses, provides variable amounts of iron and chromium. When cane juice is evaporated to remove excess water, sugar crystallizes and solid sugar can be removed. Blackstrap molasses is the molasses remaining after repeated boilings and removal of crystallized sugar. Most molasses produced in the United States is used in animal feed, in yeast production and in fermentation processes such as rum production. The baking industry uses molasses to impart flavor and to maintain freshness in baked goods. It is also used to flavor caramel candy. In home cooking, molasses is also used in baked beans and in glazes on sweet potatoes and HAM. Nutrient contents of 100 g of medium molasses is 250 calories; protein, 2.4 g; carbohydrate, 60 g; calcium, 290 mg; potassium, 1,063 mg; iron, 6 mg; thiamin, 0.10 mg; riboflavin, 0.10 mg; niacin, 1.2 mg. (See also NATURAL SWEETENERS.)

mold A type of fungi that degrades stored food and causes spoilage. Molds in the home or workplace may cause environmental sensitivity. Molds characteristically form a network of filaments or threads (mycelium) and spore masses. Some molds produce toxic materials called mycotoxins. Moldy grain can be hazardous because of the production of such toxins, which are linked to cancer and have caused death in many livestock who have ingested moldy corn. Moldy wheat contains toxins called trichothecenes that apparently weaken the immune system and increase susceptibility to disease. One of these (deoxynivalenol) has been studied extensively. Low levels have been reported in common U.S. foods such as BREAKFAST CEREAL, BREAD, and even baby food. The U.S. FDA has suggested limiting the level to one part per million in wheat; Canada, Romania, and Russia have set limits for this type of mycotoxin in grain.

The most widely studied mycotoxin is AFLATOXIN, a toxin that causes liver cancer in animals. It is produced by a storage mold that infests damp grains. Aflatoxin is formed by peanuts and corn contaminated by the mold ASPERGILLUS. Aflatoxin does not contaminate sweet corn, such as frozen corn. Among PEANUT butters, aflatoxin contamination is found to be highest in the fresh, ground varieties. Animal feed ingredients are major sources of aflatoxin in other foods. The amount of aflatoxin permitted by the U.S. FDA in foods is 20 parts per billion, although levels as low as one part per billion cause cancer in experimental animals. Its toxicity in humans is less well established. Still other molds produce the toxin ochratoxin A, which is linked to kidney cancer in lab animals. Surveys have found low levels in a tiny percent of wheat samples.

Patients should avoid eating moldy, shriveled or discolored nuts or any nuts that taste bad. In general, patients should discard moldy food, rather than cut out the moldy section. Molds and fungi send out filaments beyond the immediately obvious moldy area; thus, toxins may remain in the food. Aflatoxin is not destroyed by cooking. (See also *CANDIDA ALBICANS*; FUNGUS.)

molecule A stable assembly of atoms, tightly bonded together in a predictable fashion. Most nutrients and components of cells are either molecules or groups of molecules. A few simple molecules play key roles. Thus, WATER, which possesses only three atoms, is the most common molecule of the body. OXYGEN (with two atoms) is required to burn fuels in the body for energy production. Somewhat larger molecules include fuels like sugars (GLUCOSE with 24 atoms) and FATTY ACIDS (56 atoms for stearic acid). Vitamins are somewhat more complex molecules, roughly 10 to 30 times larger than water molecules. The most complex molecules are very long chains (polymers) of simple molecules bound together. Thus, 20 AMINO ACIDS, the building blocks of protein, are linked together like beads on a chain; proteins are typically chains of 50 to 1,000 amino acids. Thousands of glucose molecules are linked to form STARCH. RNA and DNA, the cellular machinery for manufacturing protein and for storing genetic information, are chains of simple molecular building blocks composed of phosphate, simple sugars called ribose or deoxyribose, and just four nitrogen-containing ring compounds. Lipids such as CHOLESTEROL and fat are other common molecules constructed from simple raw materials, in this case the simple acid, ACETIC ACID. Inorganic compounds formed by MINERALS are not classified as molecules because they separate into charged fragments called ions when dissolved in body fluids. (See also CYTOPLASM; METABOLITE.)

molybdenum A trace mineral NUTRIENT present in all body tissues. Only minute amounts of this mineral are required for health. Molybdenum possibly helps to retard DEGENERATIVE DISEASES, CANCER, and AGING. A molybdenum-containing enzyme of the liver (sulfite oxidase) destroys SULFITE, used as a preservative in foods and drugs. In this role, molybdenum acts as a detoxification agent. The production of URIC ACID from the degradation of purines (building blocks of RNA and DNA) requires molybdenum.

Good sources of molybdenum include LIVER, whole GRAINS, green leafy vegetables, and LEGUMES. A recommended dietary allowance has not been determined for molybdenum, and the requirement for optimal health is not known. A safe and adequate daily intake for adults is estimated to be 75 to 250 mcg. People who rely on a diet of refined and processed foods, who have high levels of uric acid and are prone to GOUT-like symptoms, or who are copper deficient can potentially be deficient in this TRACE MINERAL. High copper intake antagonizes molybdenum uptake; very high levels of molybdenum increase copper losses. (See also MINERALS.)

monoglycerides Food additive oils used to improve the taste of margarine. Monoglycerides are normal products of fat digestion and occur in foods, where they comprise about 1 percent of normal fat intake. PEANUT butter contains small amounts of monoglycerides (and the related diglycerides), which contain zero fatty acids rather than a single fatty acid chain. Monoglyceride is also used to make cakes fluffier by trapping air bubbles and helps prevent BREAD from becoming stale.

Monoglyceride derivatives are also used in processed foods. Ethoxylated monoglyceride is a dough conditioner. Acetylated monoglyceride, a waxy substance, is used as a coating on jelly beans and in chocolate coatings on frozen desserts. (See also FOOD ADDITIVES; LIPIDS.)

monosodium glutamate (MSG) A flavor enhancer for MEAT, POULTRY, SEAFOOD, and VEGETABLES, especially in Asian foods, restaurant foods, and processed foods. MSG is a form of the common amino acid glutamic acid, which the body synthesizes and obtains from the diet. Glutamic acid is a product of digestion of food proteins. The body uses glutamic acid as a fine-tuner of brain function, as well as a protein building block.

Producers frequently add MSG to seasoned salt, soy sauce, BOUILLON, gravy mixes, meat bases, cheese dips, CRACKERS, dried and canned soups, pre-cooked and frozen packaged foods, mayonnaise, and salad dressing. MSG is frequently added to processed foods like frozen entrees, FRANKFURTERS, and canned meat. Labeling laws require manufacturers to list monosodium glutamate when it is added to foods. Although HYDROLYZED VEGETABLE PROTEIN can contain from 8 percent to 40 percent MSG, when added to foods, the label can simply note "natural flavor" or "natural flavoring," without mentioning the MSG content. The U.S. FDA has proposed that the phrase "contains glutamate" be added to labels following hydrolyzed protein in ingredient lists.

Side Effects

MSG has long been considered a safe food additive, but, the long-term effects of consuming many grams of MSG are unknown. The amount of MSG in a bowl of won ton soup (3 g) can cause a reaction in sensitive people. Excessive MSG may cause MSG RELATED SYNDROME (Chinese restaurant syndrome) with transient symptoms such as numbness of chest, back and neck; worsening of ASTHMA; tingling or burning sensation; heart palpitations; anxiety; frequent urination; thirst; stomachache; or vomiting. MSG reactions generally pass shortly after they are induced. (See also FLAVOR ENHANCERS; FOOD ADDITIVES; FOOD PROCESSING.)

monounsaturated oils (*monounsaturates,* oleic oils) A type of plant oil that is more healthful than saturated FATS. The most common monounsaturates include OLIVE OIL, AVOCADO oil, ALMOND oil, CANOLA OIL (a form of rapeseed oil), and certain SUNFLOWER oils. The latter two oils come from hybrid plants whose oils closely resemble olive oil. In terms of their chemical makeup, monounsaturated oils contain predominantly monounsaturated FATTY ACIDS, which simply lack a pair of hydrogen atoms and contain one double bond. These oils contain comparatively less polyunsaturated fatty acids and saturated fatty acids than other oils. As an example, olive oil contains 72 percent monounsaturated and 9 percent polyunsaturated fatty acids, while avocado oil and almond oil contain 69 percent and 68 percent monounsaturated fatty acids, respectively.

Monounsaturated oils have been recommended as safer and more healthful cooking oils than other oils and fats. They help lower blood CHOLESTEROL, LDL-cholesterol (LOW-DENSITY LIPOPROTEIN, the less desirable kind of cholesterol), while maintaining —or slightly increasing—HDL-cholesterol (HIGH-DENSITY LIPOPROTEIN, the desirable kind of cholesterol). Monounsaturates resist rancidity. When heated during cooking, monounsaturates form fewer FREE RADICALS, highly reactive chemical fragments, than do POLYUNSATURATED OILS like safflower oil or corn oil. When reading food labels, look for the words "oleic oil, monounsaturated" and "unrefined" as a guide to those oils resembling olive oil. (See also HYDROGENATED VEGETABLE OIL; VEGETABLE OIL.)

mood See FOOD AND THE NERVOUS SYSTEM.

mouth The oral cavity. The mouth is defined by four structures: the hard palate, the bony structure that is the roof of the mouth; the soft palate, the arch-shaped structure at the back of the mouth composed of muscle; the uvula, the cone-shaped structure hanging down from the soft palate; and the tongue and its muscles, which form the floor of the mouth.

The teeth and the tongue are accessory structures of the mouth. The tongue functions to move chewed food to the back of the mouth. It has a characteristic rough surface due to small structures called papillae. Taste buds are microscopic nerve endings within the papillae.

Teeth are locked into the socket of the lower and upper jaw. By the time a person reaches the age of 17 to 24 he or she will usually have a full set of 32 teeth. The function of biting off pieces of food and pulverizing it during chewing is aided by saliva, fluid secreted by glands in or around the mouth. Up to a liter of saliva is secreted daily to lubricate food particles and to initiate starch digestion. (See also DIGESTIVE TRACT; ESOPHAGUS; STOMACH.)

MSG related syndrome (Chinese restaurant syndrome) A reaction to food seasoned with MONOSODIUM GLUTAMATE (MSG). MSG is widely used as a FLAVOR ENHANCER in processed foods, meat, poultry, seafood, and vegetables, especially in Oriental cooking. Excessive MSG can be associated with symptoms in susceptible people: a tingling or burning sensation (face, upper back, neck, or arms); heart palpitations; anxiety, excessive urination and thirst; stomachache; vomiting; attacks mimicking epileptic seizures in children; asthma; and possibly depression. Migraine headaches can result from consumption of food treated with MSG. Generally the symptoms are transitory. Women are more likely to experience this syndrome than men.

The details of how MSG causes these effects are not known. Caffeine and vitamin B_6 may counteract the effects in some people. Some research suggests that MSG related syndrome is the result of histamines found in shrimp paste, soy sauce and other fermented flavorings. It is very important for individuals who develop tightness of the chest to seek medical advice, to be certain more serious problems are not overlooked. (See also FOOD ADDITIVES.)

Tarasoff L., and M. F. Kelly. "Monosodium L-glutamate: a double-blind study and review," *Food and Chemical Toxicology* 31, no. 12 (1993): 1,019—1,035.

MSM (methylsulfonylmethane) A naturally occurring sulfur compound. All living things require sulfur to survive. In fact, it is one of the four most abundant minerals in the human body; the other three are magnesium, phosphorus, and calcium. By far the largest percentage of sulfur in the body is the form of sulfate, SO_4.

Sulfur as the amino acid cysteine helps to maintain cell structure, supports the immune system balance, and aids in ridding the body of toxins. Sulfur is essential in the production of collagen, which the body needs to make cartilage and connective tissues. Symptoms associated with sulfur deficiencies include a poorly functioning immune system, gastrointestinal problems, allergies, arthritis, and nail, hair, and skin problems. Dietary source of cysteine and sulfate are usually more than adequate.

MSM, which in its natural form is an odorless and nontoxic white crystalline powder, occurs in low levels in raw and unprocessed foods, especially fruits and cruciferous vegetables, including broccoli, cabbage, and brussels sprouts. Other MSM-rich foods include garlic, onions, raw nuts and seeds, peppers, and asparagus. MSM is lost during processing, cooking, or storing of food. MSM is now available in nutritional supplements.

Sulfur compounds have long been credited with anti-inflammatory properties. Some people claim that supplementing the diet with MSM can relieve pain, especially pain and inflammation associated with rheumatoid arthritis and osteoarthritis. However, there is as yet no credible scientific support for these claims or for claims that MSM can alleviate other ailments, including gastrointestinal problems, allergies, and chronic fatigue. Reliable data on the safety of MSM are lacking.

mucopolysaccharide See GLYCOSAMINOGLYCANS.

mucous membrane The tissue lining the tubular surfaces within the body such as the lungs, digestive tract, urinary, tract and reproductive tract. The mucous membrane includes a supporting, connective tissue layer (*Lamina propria*) and layers of smooth muscle. Frequently, it is covered by a layer of MUCUS to form a front-line defense against potential toxic agents. Mucous membranes of the digestive tract both protect the body against foreign intruders and selectively absorb nutrients. They provide a capillary network and a network of lymphatic vessels to distribute the absorbed nutrients. Certain regions of mucous membranes are further specialized with GLANDS that secrete mucus, DIGESTIVE ENZYMES and MINERALS, and binding factors for nutrient assimilation and hormones. The mucosal surface of the small intestine is highly folded to provide an extensive surface area to increase nutrient absorption. (See also DIGESTION; MICROVILLI; VILLI.)

mucus A slippery, sticky secretion from the mucous glands of moist surfaces within the body. Mucus also lubricates food particles, assisting in their smooth movement through the digestive tract. Mucus forms a thick barrier and protects the lining of the stomach from strong stomach acid, and protects the INTESTINE from toxic materials and disease-causing microorganisms. (See also DIGESTIVE TRACT; SALIVA.)

muffin A small, round bread traditionally eaten at breakfast. Muffins are now eaten for lunch, dinner, and for snacks. They are frequently high-CALORIE, high-FAT foods, however, and the fat content can range from less than 0.5 g to 16 g. The percentage of calories from fat can range from less than 2 percent to more than 50 percent. A majority of commercially available muffins incorporate HYDROGENATED VEGETABLE OIL. Such oils are "saturated"; excessive saturated fat is linked to an increased risk of CARDIOVASCULAR DISEASE. Diet guidelines call for Americans to decrease their consumption of saturated fat from all sources. CHOLESTEROL in muffins comes from whole MILK, whole EGGS, and lard (when used). A muffin made from whole eggs may contain 20 mg of cholesterol. Fat-free muffins are usually made with egg whites and nonfat milk or skim milk in place of whole eggs and whole milk.

To minimize fat, sodium, and cholesterol contributed by muffins, patients should:

- avoid eating muffins listing sugar or fat (oil or shortening) as the first or second ingredient. Cheese and chocolate additions increase calories.
- select fat-free muffins. Muffins using CANOLA OIL, SUNFLOWER oil, and the like are preferable to hydrogenated fat.
- choose muffins made from whole grain flour, BRAN, FRUIT, and vegetables, which are generally more healthful.

Nutrient contents for a commercial blueberry muffin (45 g) are 140 calories; protein, 2.7 g; carbohydrate, 22 g; fiber, 1.25 g; fat, 4.9 g; cholesterol, 45 mg; sodium, 225 g; thiamin, 0.11 mg; riboflavin, 0.13 mg; niacin, 1.17 mg. (See also BISCUIT; CRACKER.)

multiple sclerosis See AUTOIMMUNE DISEASES.

mung bean (*Phaseolus aureus*) A LEGUME usually consumed in America as bean sprouts. Mung beans probably originated in India and were cultivated in China and Southeast Asia for centuries. More recently, mung beans were introduced into Africa, the West Indies, and the United States. India and Pakistan account for most of the world production. In India and Pakistan mung bean flour is prepared from dried beans. For sprouting, moistened beans are allowed to begin growing (germinate) in the dark for four to seven days. A pound (0.45 kg) of mung beans yields six to eight pounds of sprouts (2.7 to 3.6 kg). Sprouts are used in salads or can be stir-fried with CELERY, green PEPPER, beans, ONIONS, MEAT, FISH, or POULTRY. Sprouts can be used in quiches, chow mein, and chop suey. Nutrient content of 1 cup of mung beans (104 g) is: 32 calories; protein, 3 g; carbohydrate, 6 g; fiber, 0.84 g; vitamin A, 22 retinol equivalents; thiamin, 0.09 mg; riboflavin, 0.13 mg; niacin, 0.78 mg; vitamin C, 14 mg.

muscle Tissues of the body whose cells have the ability to contract, and therefore to perform physical work. Muscles contract or relax in response to nerve impulses.

Muscle cells shorten their elongated form through the action of contractile proteins called MYOSIN and actin. This complex process utilizes ATP as the energy source; actin interacts with myosin, CALCIUM, and ATP. Myosin is the major component of muscle filaments. ATP supplies the energy for contraction of actin-myosin filaments. Energy liberated from ATP is responsible for work and the generation of heat associated with chemical work.

The three basic muscle types are the smooth muscles (found in the walls of internal organs) like the digestive tract and blood vessels; cardiac muscles of the walls of the heart; and skeletal muscles, which are attached to bones.

Smooth muscles surround most internal organs such as the gastrointestinal tract and even blood vessels. Neither smooth muscles nor cardiac muscles can be consciously controlled.

Skeletal muscles are attached to the 206 bones of the body. Their contraction and relaxation determine the movement of the body. They are voluntary; that is, they are consciously controlled. Under the microscope, skeletal muscles are banded; hence they are also called striated muscles. Nerve impulses stimulate skeletal cells to contract. Muscles require a rich supply of nutrients and oxygen from the bloodstream; they also require efficient waste elimination and an efficient cooling system. An abundant supply of blood to muscle cells meets both requirements.

The amount of ATP in skeletal muscle available at a given moment permits vigorous physical activity lasting only a few seconds. Therefore ATP must be regenerated within the muscle cell. Unlike other tissues of the body, skeletal muscles alternate between periods of inactivity and great activity. To help meet these needs, they contain a high energy molecule called phosphocreatine, which is used to supplement ATP for a few more seconds. Phosphocreatine and ATP combined provide enough energy for muscles to contract maximally for only about 15 seconds. Therefore ATP must be replenished by the oxidation of fuels. One of these fuels is the simple sugar GLUCOSE, which is available from blood glucose or it is released from muscle GLYCOGEN, the storage form of glucose. During strenuous EXERCISE, when the need for ATP exceeds the oxidative capacity of the muscle, muscles break down glucose to LACTIC ACID to produce ATP without the participation of oxygen. Lactic acid diffuses out of muscle cells to be absorbed by the bloodstream. During starvation, skeleton muscle is degraded to amino acids, which are converted to glucose by the liver to fuel the brain.

Fatty acids absorbed from the bloodstream represent the second major energy source. During low to moderate exercise, fatty acids supply half the energy required by skeletal muscles. Fat becomes the major fuel during medium to intense exercise, lasting more than 1.5 hours; thus fat can supply as much as 70 percent of the calories needed during moderate exercise lasting four to six hours. (See also AEROBIC; CARBOHYDRATE METABOLISM; GLYCOLYSIS; OXYGEN DEBT; STARVATION.)

mushroom A diverse family of fungi sometimes used as food. Basidiomycetes represent certain club fungi characterized by fleshy fruiting bodies (toadstools). They grow in soil containing organic matter and also can grow on living trees or on dead wood. Cup fungi (Ascomycetes) such as truffles are also often classified as mushrooms.

Together, Basidiomycetes and Ascomycetes include about 10,000 species of mushrooms. Currently about 853 million pounds of mushrooms are harvested commercially each year in the United States. The five most popular cultivated mushrooms are: *Agaricus bisporus,* which is the light-colored, mild mushroom most common to Americans. Oyster mushrooms (*Pleurotus ostreatus*) resemble oysters in shape and color. The oyster mushroom is common in the Far East and in Europe. Padi straw mushrooms (*Volvariella volvaeae*) are produced in the Orient where they are grown in rice paddies and are usually sold dried. Truffles (*Tuber melanosporum*) are the most expensive mushrooms. This cup FUNGUS grows underground in association with beech and oak trees. Truffles are produced primarily in France and Italy.

MAITAKE (*Grifola frondosa*) grows at the foot of mature oak trees. Native to Japan, this mushroom has no cap at the end of its rippling stems. Individual specimens can grow to more than 50 pounds. The flesh is firm and has a woody taste.

Shiitake (*Letinus edodes*) has a smoky flavor and grows on hardwood logs. It is grown mainly in China and Japan and is exported in canned, dried, or pickled forms. Shiitake is also currently grown in California. These mushrooms can be stir-fried or sautéed with onions. Other popular types of mushroom include oyster, wood ears, and portabellas.

Several wild mushrooms are also popular. Chanterelles are deep yellow-orange and used in soups, casseroles, and stews. The morel has a nutty flavor. This mushroom, which is shaped like a pine cone, is used in soups, casseroles, stews, and sautéed dishes.

Raw mushrooms contain hydrazines, which are substances shown to cause cancer in experimental animals. Many hydrazines can be eliminated or destroyed by cooking or drying.

Poisonous Mushrooms There is no completely foolproof way of distinguishing safe from unsafe wild mushrooms; many wild varieties are poisonous. The severity of mushroom poisoning varies with the amount and the type of mushroom eaten, as well as with the season. As a rule of thumb, if symptoms appear within two hours after eating the mushroom, the illness probably will not be severe. If symptoms develop more than two hours after eating the mushroom, emergency treatment may be required.

Nutrient content of common mushrooms ($^1/_2$ cup, cooked from raw, 78 g) is 21 calories; protein, 1.7 g; carbohydrate, 1.6 g; fiber, 0.77 g; potassium, 278 mg; thiamin, 0.06 mg; riboflavin, 0.23 mg; niacin, 3.5 mg. (See also AMANITA; MOLD.)

Wasser, S. P., and A. L. Weis. "Therapeutic Effects of Substances Occurring in Higher Basidiomycetes Mushrooms: A Modern Perspective," *Critical Reviews in Immunology* 19 (1999): 65–96.

mustard A popular condiment prepared from ground mustard seeds. White mustard (*Brassica hirta*), brown mustard (*Brassica nigra*), and Ethiopian mustard (*Brassica carinata*) are used in the United States. Brown mustard is also known as Indian mustard; it is grown for its leaves as well as for its seeds. These species originated in different regions of Eurasia: White mustard apparently came from the eastern Mediterranean; brown mustard from India; black mustard from Asia Minor; Ethiopian mustard is a hybrid. Brown mustard has been used for at least 5,000 years. Mustard powder is ground mustard seed; it is also marketed as a paste.

The hot ingredients are liberated by enzymatic action when mustard powder is moistened. The typical condiment is a mixture of mustard seed powder, salt, vinegar, and SPICES, and it may contain wine and acidic preservatives (tartaric acid and CITRIC ACID). Though low in CALORIES, the commercial product is high in SODIUM. In folk medicine, mustard is used in a poultice to relieve lung congestion due to colds and to relieve the pain associated with arthritis. Mustard can irritate the skin of some people.

mustard greens (*Brasicca juncea*) A dark-green leafy vegetable that belongs to the cabbage family and resembles kale. Oriental mustard greens are a milder tasting variety. Mustard greens are cooked before eating; steaming and sauteeing are common methods of preparation. The greens can be served with cheese or white sauce. Alternatively, the greens can be included in casseroles, omelets, or soups. Mustard greens provide (cooked, 1 cup) 21 calories; protein, 3.2 g; carbohydrate, 2.9 g; fiber, 2.9 g; calcium, 104 mg; iron, 1.7 mg; vitamin A, 424 retinol equivalents; thiamin, 0.06 mg; riboflavin, 0.09 mg; niacin, 0.61 mg.

mutagen Agents that produce permanent changes in gene structure. Mutagens alter genes by chemically altering the structure of DNA, the genetic material of cells. They produce new traits, passed from one generation to the next. Most mutagens are also CANCER-causing agents (CARCINOGENS). Sample mutagens include tobacco smoke, asbestos, PESTICIDES, industrial chemicals like formaldehyde and vinylchloride, and solvents like benzene. Some mutagens occur in food naturally. Examples include hydrazines in mushrooms. Grilled, fried, or broiled fish, poultry, and meat contain mutagens. Other types of mutagenic agents include ultraviolet light, X rays, gamma rays, and radiation from radon seepage into basements from soil.

Certain substances are not themselves mutagens; rather they are converted to mutagens in the body. NITRITE, a food preservative, is converted in the stomach to NITROSOAMINES, reactive nitrogen-containing compounds that are mutagens and carcinogens. Benzopyrene in soot deposited on BARBECUED MEAT and certain pesticides are activated by the liver to highly reactive compounds that can attack DNA and cause mutations.

DeRisi, J. L. et al. "Exploring the Metabolic and Genetic Control of Gene Expression on a Genomic Scale," *Science* 278 (1997): 680–686.

mutation A permanent alteration in the structure of DNA, the genetic material of a cell. The alterations in DNA can be passed on from one generation to the next unless repaired. Cells possess elaborate mechanisms to repair damaged DNA by environmental influences (mutagens) as well as within cells by wear and tear. One theory of AGING proposes that, over time, an individual's DNA repair system becomes less capable of performing its task and DNA damage accumulates, leading ultimately to CANCER. Appropriate nutrition can support DNA synthesis and repair, as well as minimizing the impact of agents that can cause mutations. Key to countering the latter agents are ANTIOXIDANTS, compounds that either destroy highly reactive chemicals called FREE RADICALS or prevent further oxidative damage. Antioxidant nutrients include VITAMIN C, VITAMIN E, and BETA-CAROTENE (pro-vitamin A), as well as SELENIUM and other TRACE MINERALS. (See CANCER PREVENTION DIET; GENE.)

myelin The fatty material that covers certain nerve fibers and acts as an insulator. Many axons lying beyond the brain and spinal cord are surrounded by this multiple-layered, lipid-rich segmented covering. Myelin increases the speed of nerve impulse conduction and helps maintain the integrity of the axon. Myelin is responsible for the white color of nerve tissue. Myelin contains complex lipids called sphingomyelin as well as PHOSPHOLIPIDS such as LECITHIN. VITAMIN B_{12} is essential for healthy myelin; severe vitamin B_{12} deficiency can lead to irreversible nerve damage. Diseases like multiple sclerosis are related to myelin destruction. (See also AUTOIMMUNE DISEASES; NERVOUS SYSTEM; NEUROTRANSMITTER.)

myosin The major protein responsible for muscle contraction. It comprises about 65 percent of the total muscle protein. Myosin chains combine to form thick filaments (myofilaments). ATP is degraded by myosin; in the presence of CALCIUM, myosin shifts to a bent, low-energy configuration. This pulls along the attached actin chain (an intracellular protein chain), thus contracting muscle fibers. (See also EXERCISE.)

myxedema A condition resulting from low THYROID function. Myxedema is characterized by a low rate of metabolism and decreased heat production. The symptoms include apathy; exhaustion and chronic FATIGUE; drowsiness; sensitivity to cold; coarse, thickened skin; and swelling due to fluid accumulation. Myxedema can be caused by a deficiency of IODINE, atrophy of thyroid gland, or excessive use of anti-thyroid drugs. Depressed thyroid function can be due to autoimmune attack in the thyroid gland. (See also HYPOTHYROIDISM.)

N

N-acetylcysteine (NAC) A derivative of the sulfur-containing amino acid CYSTEINE that occurs naturally in the body, N-acetylcysteine is used to produce the powerful cell ANTIOXIDANT GLUTATHIONE. This sulfur compound delivers cysteine to cells. It has been used medicinally to reduce mucus buildup in people suffering from respiratory ailments such as chronic bronchitis and asthma, and adult respiratory distress syndrome. NAC may help reduce the risk of heart attack in patients with unstable chest pain. It is also helpful as an IV treatment in ridding the body of toxic levels of the nonsteroidal anti-inflammatory drug (NSAID) acetaminophen.

Now also available as a DIETARY SUPPLEMENT, N-acetylcysteine is promoted as an aid in boosting the body's immune system, preventing heart disease and cancer and slowing the progression of Parkinson's disease and multiple sclerosis. Initial studies indicate N-acetylcysteine shows promise in treating some or all of the conditions. However, additional research is needed to confirm these preliminary studies. Because N-acetylcysteine is sold as a dietary supplement for treating these conditions and not as a drug, its safety and efficacy has not been tested by the U.S. Food and Drug Administration (FDA) or any other government agency. Breast-feeding women should avoid NAC. Pregnant women should use it only with a doctor's prescription.

Grandjean, E. M., P. Berthet, R. Ruffmann, et al. "Efficacy of Oral Long-Term *N*-acetylcysteine in Chronic Bronchopulmonary Disease: A Meta-Analysis of Published Double-Blind, Placebo-Controlled Clinical Trials," *Clinical Therapy* 22 (2000): 209–221.

naphthoquinone See VITAMIN K.

narcotics See ADDICTION.

National Cholesterol Education Program See CHOLESTEROL.

National Marine Fisheries Service Organization that is part of the National Oceanic and Atmospheric Association (NOAA), responsible for overseeing fisheries management in the United States. Under the federal Agricultural Marketing Act of 1946, NOAA administers a voluntary Seafood Inspection Program to ensure that seafood sold in the United States complies with applicable food regulations, including the Hazard Analysis and Critical Control Point (HACCP, pronounced "has-sip") regulations implemented by the U.S. Food and Drug Administration (FDA) in 1997. This program requires seafood processors, repackers, and warehouses that supply seafood for sale in the United States to have in place a food safety program to identify and eliminate sources of food-borne illnesses. The aim of the HACCP system is to prevent problems before they start by conducting spot checks of manufacturing processes and random testing of seafood products. Retailers are exempt from HACCP requirements.

National Research Council (NRC) The branch of the National Academy of Sciences promotes the effective use of scientific information and advises the federal government on scientific and technical matters. The NRC provides services for following policies set by both the National Academy of Sciences and the National Academy of Engineering in meeting the needs of government, the public, and scientists. It is administered by these academies, as well as by the Institute of Medicine.

Among the many responsibilities of the NRC is the development and evaluation of nutrient standards for good health. In 1941, the Food and Nutrition Board of the NRC published the Recommended Dietary Allowances (RDAs), the benchmark of nutritional adequacy in the United States, with revised editions generally appearing every five years. The 10th edition was published in 1989. Since then the Food and Nutrition Board, in cooperation with Health Canada, has been gradually replacing the RDAs with DIETARY REFERENCE INTAKES (DRIs), which incorporate more recent science that has broadened our understanding of the role of nutrients in human health. (See also DIETARY GUIDELINES FOR AMERICANS; NUTRIENT; VITAMIN.)

National School Lunch Program See SCHOOL LUNCH PROGRAM.

natural flavors See FLAVORS.

natural food Foods that have been minimally processed and grown without the use of synthetic fertilizers and pesticides. Other than for meat and poultry, the term *natural* has not been defined legally and therefore has many interpretations. The "natural" food label is a strong selling point, and food producers have capitalized on consumer interest. Thus the word *natural* may be used to describe PROCESSED FOODS and synthetic food and beverages, which sometimes are highly processed and contain preservatives and artificial coloring. A beverage labeled "natural" might be completely synthetic, with only the lemon flavor as a nonsynthetic ingredient; a product labeled "Natural Juice Apple Pie" may indicate only the juice is natural. Natural food also has the connotation of being free from additives like PRESERVATIVES, EMULSIFIERS, and thickeners. Under current U.S. FDA regulations, an entire food cannot be labeled natural if it contains synthetic ingredients, ARTIFICIAL FLAVORS, or ARTIFICIAL FOOD COLORS.

Natural Meat

According to the USDA, MEAT or poultry labeled "natural" has not been processed more than in usual kitchen practice. This refers to procedures that can be performed in the kitchen: washing, shredding, chipping, grating, grinding, chopping, mixing, and cooking. Natural meat must come from animals raised without hormones or at least not exposed to feedlot growth stimulants (such as antibiotics) to fatten livestock later than 60 days before slaughter. The "natural beef" label doesn't guarantee the meat is absolutely free of antibiotics and growth factors because some producers feed hormones and antibiotics up to 60 days before slaughter. This time may be inadequate to completely clear chemical residues from some animals. (See also FOOD ADDITIVES; ORGANIC FOODS.)

natural sweeteners Naturally occurring CARBOHYDRATES or compounds related to SUGARS that are used as sweeteners. Carbohydrate sweeteners contribute four CALORIES per gram (less than half as much as fat). The most common are the simple sugars or materials that are primarily sugars: FRUCTOSE and high fructose corn syrup; GLUCOSE (known in the food industry as DEXTROSE); CORN SYRUP; various forms of SUCROSE, including MOLASSES, brown sugar, table sugar, turbinado sugar, and cane sugar; BARLEY MALT; HONEY; fruit concentrates; and ground dates (date sugar). Amasake is a sweetener prepared from fermented rice. Each provides carbohydrate with only a few other nutrients; therefore the content of VITAMINS, minerals, and FIBER, as compared to that found in whole foods, is low (EMPTY CALORIES).

Sugar alcohols taste sweet and are not as easily metabolized as sugars. MANNITOL, related to the sugar mannose, is poorly utilized. XYLITOL, derived from the sugar xylose, while degraded, contributes fewer calories than sugar. SORBITOL, related to sorbose, is the most widely used sugar alcohol and is only slowly absorbed by the intestine. Relative to table sugar, fructose is 1.7 times as sweet; glucose, 0.7; mannitol, 0.7; and sorbitol, 0.6.

Potential Problems with High Sugar Consumption

Undernutrition Sugars supply empty calories because they provide low or negligible amounts of key nutrients. CARBOHYDRATE METABOLISM requires B vitamins like THIAMIN and minerals like ZINC, CHROMIUM, and MAGNESIUM. Excessive concentrated sweeteners displace more nutritious food and increase the body's burden for these nutrients. Few people relying on a junk food diet increase their consumption of high-quality foods to make up the difference.

Overnutrition Excessive consumption of sugar and refined carbohydrate represents excessive calories. Surplus calories are converted to FAT, regardless of their source. It should be noted that starches and sugars are not in themselves inherently fattening unless they represent excess calories.

Blood Sugar Imbalances The excessive consumption of simple sugars and sucrose can cause BLOOD SUGAR levels to fluctuate. In contrast, STARCHES in vegetables and legumes are often slowly digested and glucose is absorbed slowly, permitting a more balanced control of blood sugar.

Cavities Excessive sugar consumption leads to more cavities and contributes to soaring dental costs.

U.S. DIETARY GUIDELINES FOR AMERICANS call for eating less sugar and more complex carbohydrate, starch, and fiber (whole foods) as vegetables, fruits, and legumes. The FOOD GUIDE PYRAMID, the most recent meal planning guideline, specifies eating sweets sparingly. (See also ADDICTION AND SUGAR; INVERT SUGAR; MAPLE SYRUP; NUTRIENT DENSITY; TEETH.)

Anderson, G. H. "Sugars, Sweetness and Food Intake," *American Journal of Clinical Nutrition* 62, supp. 1 (1995): 195S–202S.

Wolever, T. M., and J. B. Miller. "Sugars and Blood Glucose Control," *American Journal of Clinical Nutrition* 62, supp. 1 (1995): 212S–221S.

natural vitamins See VITAMIN.

nectar A FRUIT drink made with fruit juice and fruit pulp. Typical nectars are made from APRICOT, GUAVA, MANGO, PEACH, and other fruit. Ingredients are specified by the STANDARDS OF IDENTITY established by the U.S. FDA. These are standard recipes long used by the food industry. Nectars include various combinations of fruit juice, SUGAR, and other natural sweeteners, together with fruit puree, fruit pulp, VITAMIN C, and CITRIC ACID. The term *nectar* also refers to a sweet, syrupy fluid secreted by flowers and collected by bees to produce HONEY.

nectarine (*Prunus persica*) A subspecies of PEACH with a smooth skin and a distinctive flavor. The close similarity between nectarines and peaches is demonstrated by the fact that nectarines occasionally mutate to peaches and vice versa. Nectarines and peaches are believed to have originated in China. There are more than 150 varieties of nectarine, differing slightly in taste, shape, size, and skin coloring. Fantasia, Summer Grand, Royal Giant and May Grand are popular varieties. The United States is a major producer, and California produces most of the domestic crop. Hard nectarines can be softened by storing them in a paper bag at room temperature for several days. The mature fruit does not get very much sweeter, but it can become softer and juicier.

Nutrient contents of one raw nectarine, without pit, is 67 calories; protein, 1.3 g; carbohydrate, 16 g; fiber, 3.13 g; fat, 0.6 g; potassium, 288 mg; vitamin A, 100 retinol equivalents; vitamin C, 7 mg; thiamin, 0.02 mg; riboflavin, 0.06 mg; niacin, 1.35 mg.

nephron The functional unit of kidneys that filters the blood. The nephron further modifies filtered fluid from the blood to produce urine. Nephrons are composed of two structures: renal tubules and the glomerulus, a cluster of CAPILLARIES. WATER, MINERALS, GLUCOSE, VITAMINS, AMINO ACIDS, very small proteins, nitrogenous wastes, and small molecules migrate from the capillaries of the glomerulus and enter the renal tubule, which draws urine from the kidneys.

As the filtrate moves down the tubules, nearly 99 percent of the water is reabsorbed into the blood. Only 1.5 liters (1 percent leaves as urine daily. By reabsorbing most of the materials, the body can retain essential nutrients, while disposing of wastes like UREA. For example, normally all of the glucose filtered by the glomerulus is reabsorbed, thus, maintaining blood glucose levels. So much liquid is filtered by the kidney that if nutrients were not reabsorbed back into the bloodstream, the blood would be drained of these materials within half an hour.

The region of the tubule adjacent to the capsule (proximal tubule) reabsorbs glucose, amino acids, SODIUM, CHLORIDE, BICARBONATE, POTASSIUM, and water. Farther down the tubule, sodium, chloride, urea, and water are reabsorbed. Sodium and water are controlled by the hormone ALDOSTERONE. The kidney releases potassium and AMMONIA to maintain ELECTROLYTE balance and water balance of the blood. In order to maintain blood pH close to 7.4 (neutral pH) and to maintain acid-base balance, sodium is reabsorbed while hydrogen ions are released.

The kidney plays a role in VITAMIN D metabolism as well. Tubules of the kidney activate vitamin D by converting a partially modified form (called hydroxycholecalciferol) to the fully active hormone, called calciferol. (See also GLOMERULAR FILTRATION.)

nervous system A primary communication system consisting of the brain, spinal cord, and nerve fibers radiating to all parts of the body. The brain and spinal cord occupy a central position in the body and are called the "central nervous system" (CNS). The nervous system transmits information via electrical nerve impulses conducted between nerve cells. Impulses are generated by changes in the body's internal or external environment.

Specialized cells of the nervous system are called neurons and neuroglia. Neuroglia are connective tissue cells supporting the neurons, while neurons are specialized cells of the nervous system that conduct nerve impulses. The nervous system is composed of billions of neurons. With age, neurons are progressively and irreversibly lost.

Sensory neurons transmit impulses to the spinal cord and brain from all regions of the body, while motoneurons transmit impulses away from the brain and spinal cord to muscles and glands. Interneurons lie within the gray matter of either the brain or spinal cord and conduct impulses from sensory neurons to motoneurons. A fatty layer called MYELIN insulates nerve fibers, bundles of neurons.

Neurons contain a cell body with nucleus, CYTOPLASM and MITOCHONDRIA. Each neuron possesses many dendrites, highly branched extensions of the cell body that are the "receiving" parts of neurons and conduct a nerve impulse toward the cell body; and an AXON, a single, long cytoplasmic extension that conducts nerve impulses away from the cell body to another cell. Axons contain mitochondria but no protein synthesizing machinery; they vary in length from a few millimeters up to a meter or more. The ends of axons terminate in bulb-like structures that store NEUROTRANSMITTERS. These chemicals determine whether an impulse will pass onto the next cell. Nerve fiber refers to any process projecting from the cell body. Typically, sensory neurons transmit impulses from the skin, sense organs, muscle joints and viscera to the spinal cord and the brain. Motoneurons convey impulses from the brain and spinal cord to either muscles or glands. Connecting neurons (intraneurons) carry impulses from sensory neurons to motor neurons and occur in the brain and spinal cord.

Many nutrients support nerve function, and the following minerals are critical. CALCIUM is required for nerve transmission; when blood calcium levels fall, nerves become hypersensitive, and the result is frozen muscles (tetany). High calcium concentrations depress nerve irritability. The amount of neurotransmitters (serotonin, acetylcholine, norepinephrine) released is proportional to the calcium concentration in the nerve terminus. POTASSIUM and SODIUM are important in nerve transmission. Stimulation of a nerve causes potassium to migrate out of the neuron and sodium to migrate inward, altering the membrane potential (electrical current) and conducting a nerve impulse down the axon.

Individual nerve cells communicate at specialized gaps called synapses by means of chemical messages called neurotransmitters. When a nerve impulse reaches the end of an axon it triggers the release of neurotransmitters that migrate across the gap and stimulate a nerve impulse or other response in the receiving cell. Neurotransmitters are often derived from AMINO ACIDS. Dopamine and norepinephrine are derived from the amino acid TYROSINE, while TRYPTOPHAN supplies SEROTONIN. Cholinergic nerve fibers release the neurotransmitter ACETYLCHOLINE and are derived from the nitrogen-containing nutrient CHOLINE.

The peripheral nervous system contains sensory nerves. These carry information from organs like the skin to the brain. Motor nerve fibers carry impulses from the brain to specific regions such as skeletal muscles.

The automatic nervous system adapts the body to change. It consists of two functional parts. The sympathetic nervous system responds to stress, and adaptations include dilation of bronchi and increased heart rate. The PARASYMPATHETIC NERVOUS SYSTEM returns the body to the normal, unstressed state, counterbalancing the sympathetic nervous system. It restores energy during rest and recuperation.

The average human brain weighs about three lbs (1.4 kg) and contains 11 billion cells. Although it represents only 2 percent of the total body weight, it consumes 20 percent to 30 percent of the GLUCOSE from digestion and CARBOHYDRATE METABOLISM. The thalamus of the forebrain is an egg-shaped mass that relays sensory information to other regions of the brain. It seems to help with concentration. Lying beneath the thalamus is the HYPOTHALAMUS, which regulates eating, drinking, sexual behavior, heat production, and emotions. It also controls the ENDOCRINE SYSTEM, a system of hormone-secreting glands located throughout the body.

Twelve pairs of nerves are attached at the under surface of the brain. Several are important in regulating eating and digestion. Their fibers conduct pulses between the brain and the head, neck, thorax, and abdominal cavity. The olfactory nerve is responsible for the sense of SMELL. The trigeminal nerve functions in the sensations involving the face, teeth, and chewing. The facial nerve is responsible for TASTE. The glossopharyngeal nerve controls taste, swallowing, salivation, and sensations in the throat region. The vagus nerve also regulates swallowing, sensations of throat and larynx, and of the abdominal regions; for example, it regulates PERISTALSIS. The hypoglossal nerve regulates tongue movements (swallowing).

It is now known that brain peptides, such as ENDORPHINS, are synthesized in the intestine, while hormones bind to targets in the brain and affect its function. The nervous system can activate the immune system, while chemicals released by the immune response can affect the central nervous system. The gastrointestinal tract is surrounded by an elaborate network of nerves so that the stomach and intestines are directly linked to the brain. The ability of the digestive system to monitor food has important ramifications for WEIGHT MANAGEMENT, SATIETY, and hunger. With the discovery that the hormonal system (endocrine system) as well as the immune system can affect the brain and alter behavior and mood, and that the nervous system can alter the immune response and hormone balance, has come a new appreciation of the interdependency of these three systems in maintaining a balance among all systems of the body (HOMEOSTASIS). This synthesis has spawned a new scientific discipline, psychoneuroimmunology.

In addition to supplying energy, primarily as glucose, food can alter the nervous system in important ways. One focus has been in the formation of neurotransmitters, chemicals manufactured by nerves to help transit nerve impulses. Two amino acids that serve as the raw materials for the manufacture of neurotransmitters are tryptophan and tyrosine. Tryptophan forms the neurotransmitter serotonin, used to regulate relaxation and sleepiness. Low blood levels of tryptophan are linked to depression, and some clinical studies suggest that tryptophan supplementation can lessen depression. Tryptophan tends to make normal people drowsy, and it has been sold as a mild sleep inducer. However, the U.S. FDA has banned its sale because of deaths associated with contaminated tryptophan. Foods low in protein and rich in carbohydrate can raise brain levels of tryptophan, probably because they stimulate the release of insulin, which lowers the blood levels of most amino acids, except for tryptophan. According to one hypothesis, tryptophan in the blood competes with more abundant, branched chain amino acids, which also possess lipid-like properties, for entry into the brain. The amount of tryptophan reaching the brain increases after eating starchy or sweet foods. On the other hand the more numerous amino acids can displace tryptophan for entry into the brain after eating a protein-rich meal. As a result, brain tryptophan levels may drop. The observation is that normal healthy adults can feel relaxed, sleepy, or more calm or lethargic within two hours following a high-carbohydrate meal. Another possibility is that glucose from carbohydrate digestion can affect the brain's activity.

The amino acid tyrosine is converted to the neurotransmitter norepinephrine, which helps maintain mental alertness. The brain level of norepinephrine drops with stress. Tyrosine supplements may help combat fatigue and improve the ability to perform mental tasks. A light lunch or snack increases mental functioning and decreases the error rate in tasks, and seems to sharpen the mind.

Certain B vitamins help in the manufacture of serotonin and norepinephrine: VITAMIN B_6, VITAMIN B_{12}, and FOLIC ACID. Deficiencies of any of these vitamins can promote depression, senility, and decreased ability to concentrate. Correction of the B vitamin deficiency can ease these symptoms. Even in healthy elderly people without obvious deficiency symptoms, a lower level of folacin and vitamin B_{12} has corresponded to lower scores on reasoning tests. Surveys have shown that between 20 percent and 66 percent of healthy people over the age of 65 possess low levels of vitamin B_6, vitamin B_{12}, and folic acid. (See also ADDICTION; DIGESTIVE TRACT; FOOD AND THE NERVOUS SYSTEM; MOUTH.)

Duthie, S. J. et al. "Homocystine, Vitamin B Status, and Cognitive Function in the Elderly," *American Journal of Clinical Nutrition* 75, no. 5 (2002): 908–913.

net protein utilization (NPU) An index used to estimate the ability of a food PROTEIN to supply indispensable AMINO ACIDS. Only retained nitrogen is measured. The NPU is based on the ratio of the amount of dietary protein converted to body protein divided by the amount of protein eaten. Thus, a poorly digested protein would have a low NPU score. In this respect, it differs from the BIOLOGICAL VALUE, which does not account for digestibility of food. Frequently, proteins are measured for their growth-promoting effect on young animals or for their ability to maintain nitrogen equilibrium, a balance between protein nitrogen consumed and the amount lost daily (NITROGEN BALANCE). Since only retained nitrogen is measured, NPU does not specifically assess the inefficiency of digestion. Thus, a poorly digested protein would have a low NPU score. (See also CHEMICAL SCORE.)

neural tube defects (NTD) Congenital disorders related to the incomplete development of the neural tube. Neural tube defects contribute to infant mortality throughout the world. Anencephalus is the absence of brain and spinal cord. In spina bifida, the spinal cord is pushed through the wall of the spinal canal between vertebrae. Encephalocele refers to the protrusion of the brain through a cranial opening. Both genetic and environmental factors are implicated. Several studies have confirmed that women who take the B vitamin FOLIC ACID before becoming pregnant and during the first two months of pregnancy greatly reduce the risk of bearing a child with a neural tube defect. Consequently, the Centers for Disease Control and Prevention (CDC) recommends that all women of childbearing age take a multivitamin that contains at least 400 mcg of folic acid daily. In 1998 the U.S. FDA began requiring all enriched grain products, including cereals, breads, pasta, and rice, to be fortified with folic acid at the rate of 140 mcg per 100 g of grain. This action was taken based on studies that showed that only about 25 percent of women of childbearing age in the United States regularly consumed enough folic acid. In 2001 the CDC reported that the number of children born with these defects had dropped by 19 percent since the enrichment program began. (See also BIRTH DEFECTS; HOMOCYSTEINE; VITAMIN.)

Honein, Margaret A. "Impact of Folic Acid Fortification in the U.S. Food Supply on the Occurrence of Neural Tube Defects," *JAMA* 285 (2001): 2,981–2,986.

neuron See NERVOUS SYSTEM.

neuropathy, peripheral Disease of the peripheral nerves (the nerves feeding into the spinal column and brain). Nutritional deficiencies can cause peripheral nerve degeneration. Severe deficiency of the B vitamin THIAMIN, a disease whose chief characteristic is BERIBERI, also leads to neuropathy. Certain toxic chemicals like plasticizers and several medications such as Isoniazid also cause neuropathy. Diseases affecting the entire body like diabetes, certain AUTOIMMUNE DISEASES like Guillain-Barre syndrome, and a variety of rare hereditary diseases are associated with peripheral neuropathy. Neuropathy can be caused by HEPATITIS, infectious mononucleosis, ALCOHOLISM, and lead poisoning. (See also DEFICIENCY DISEASE; HEAVY METALS; NERVOUS SYSTEM.)

McLeod, J. G. "Investigation of Peripheral Neuropathy," *Journal of Neurological and Neurosurgical Psychiatry* 58 (1995): 274–283.

neurotransmitter A chemical required to transmit nerve impulses between nerve cells. Unlike an electrical network, nerves are not continuous; the end of a nerve cell does not touch its target. Instead, individual nerve cells are separated by a microscopic gap called a synapse. In response to a nerve impulse traveling down the nerve cell, the nerve ending releases neurotransmitter molecules, which then diffuse across the gap and bind to the adjacent cell. Depending on the nature of the receiving cells, this contact can stimulate or inhibit the target cell.

At least three classes of neurotransmitters respond to diet: Catecholamines (DOPAMINE and norepinephrine) come from the AMINO ACID, TYROSINE. Eating a protein-rich meal can increase blood tyrosine levels and increase levels of this amino acid in the brain. Elevated brain tyrosine increases dopamine and norepinephrine production, promoting wakefulness and alertness.

On the other hand, SEROTONIN tends to induce relaxation and sleep. Serotonin comes from the essential amino acid-TRYPTOPHAN. Eating a meal high in carbohydrates is believed to increase indirectly brain tryptophan levels. Elevated blood sugar stimulates insulin release; this hormone stimulates the uptake by muscle of amino acids that compete with tryptophan for uptake by the brain, allowing more tryptophan into the brain. This in turn leads to higher serotonin formation in the brain, promoting a state of relaxation. Amino acid research in humans is still considered preliminary.

ACETYLCHOLINE is manufactured from CHOLINE, a nitrogen-containing nutrient and raw material for neurotransmitter synthesis. The body can synthesize choline, and it comes also from dietary lipids, particularly LECITHIN, a common phosphate-bearing lipid found in most foods. Acetylcholine participates in many brain functions, including memory. Victims of ALZHEIMER'S DISEASE have low levels of acetylcholine in their brains. (See also ENDORPHINS; NERVOUS SYSTEM.)

neutral fats See FAT; VEGETABLE OIL.

NHANES (National Health and Nutrition Examination Survey) In 1956 Congress passed the National Health Survey Act, which authorized the federal government to conduct a continuing survey that would produce statistics on the amount, distribution, and effects of illness and disability in the United States. During the next decades nutrition began to play a greater role in the understanding of sickness and disability.

In 1970 a special task force reporting to the Department of Health, Education, and Welfare recommended that future surveys include clinical observation and professional assessment as well as recording of dietary intake patterns. Since then the U.S. Center for Health Statistics has been conducting regular National Health and Nutrition Examination Surveys.

NHANES I provided statistics between 1971 and 1975; NHANES II between 1976 and 1980; and NHANES III between 1988 and 1994. A Hispanic Health and Nutrition Examination survey was conducted from 1982 to 1984.

Since 1999 NHANES has been conducted annually. Beginning in 2002 it merged with the U.S. Department of Agriculture's Continuing Survey of Food Intakes (CSFII), to produce the National Food and Nutrition Survey (NFNS). This integrated survey provides comprehensive information on the health and nutrition intakes of the U.S. population. (See also EATING PATTERNS.)

Kleges, R. C., L. H. Eck, and J. W. Ray. "Who Underreports Dietary Intake in Dietary Recall? Evidence from the Second National Health and Nutrition Examination Survey," *Journal of Consultative and Clinical Psychology* 63, no. 3 (1995): 438–444.

niacin (nicotinic acid, vitamin B_3) A heat-stable member of the B VITAMIN complex needed by the body to extract ENERGY from FAT, CARBOHYDRATE, and PROTEIN. Tissues convert niacin to two closely related COENZYMES (enzyme helpers): NICOTINAMIDE ADENINE DINUCLEOTIDE (NAD) and nicotinamide adenine dinucleotide phosphate (NADP). NAD functions as an oxidizing agent used in processes that "burn" fuels to produce energy in the cell. These include the oxidation of GLUCOSE (GLYCOLYSIS) and of FATTY ACIDS. NAD transfers electrons to the mitochondrial ELECTRON TRANSPORT CHAIN, which ultimately reduces OXYGEN to water. This process liberates vast amounts of chemical energy trapped as ATP as well as releasing heat. NADP is generated from the oxidation of glucose (pentose phosphate pathway). The reduced form of NADP, NADPH, is used as a reducing agent in biosynthetic reactions rather than for energy production. CHOLESTEROL, fatty acids, and other important compounds require NADPH for their synthesis. NADPH is also the basis of a powerful antioxidant system (GLUTATHIONE) to protect most cells from the damaging effects of highly reactive molecules called FREE RADICALS. NADPH also functions in the synthesis of DEOXYRIBOSE, the sugar building block of DNA.

Possible Roles of Niacin in Disease

PELLAGRA is a severe niacin deficiency disease that mimics schizophrenia. Skin rashes, DIARRHEA, and mouth sores are prevalent in pellagra. At the turn of the century, pellagra was epidemic in the southern United States among people whose diet was based on corn. By 1937, research demonstrated that niacin cured pellagra-like symptoms in dogs and, shortly thereafter, that niacin treatment cured pellagra. Niacin has been used in food fortification since 1941.

Niacin is effective in the treatment of elevated (hyperlipidemia) blood lipids that does not respond to dietary intervention alone, and it has been approved by the USFDA for this treatment. It may also reduce the risk of a second heart attack in men. Niacin is effective in lowering high blood triglycerides and elevated LDL-cholesterol, the "bad" form, and raising HDL-cholesterol, the beneficial form. Niacin is generally considered an adjunct therapy, used in conjunction with cholesterol-lowering drugs, such as statins and bile binding resins. As an example, niacin in combination with bile-binding agents may effectively slow the progression of atherosclerosis in men with existing cardiovascular disease.

The use of niacin to treat schizophrenia and DEPRESSION is controversial. Generally negative results have been reported for patients with long-standing schizophrenia. Some clinicians reported improvement in patients with schizophrenia using megavitamin treatment with niacin or niacinamide, VITAMIN B_6 and VITAMIN C and in patients with depression using niacinamide and tryptophan, together with taking steps to improve the diet. The American Psychological Association disapproved the use of niacin in the treatment of mental disorders in 1979.

Niacin when taken in combination with cholesterol-lowering "statin" drugs may prevent HEART ATTACKS.

Niacin seems to increase the production of PROSTAGLANDINS. These hormone-like chemicals are produced locally within tissues to help control many physiologic processes such as BLOOD CLOTTING and INFLAMMATION.

Large doses of niacin may alleviate noninflammatory ARTHRITIS, while low doses of niacin can relieve migraine headaches. Niacin supplements may help normalize blood sugar in patients with hypoglycemia. Large doses of niacin may prevent harmful effects of chemical pollutants, drugs, and alcohol, and may help during recovery and drug rehabilitation (the mechanism is not known). This is a promising area of research, but niacin cannot be claimed to be a broad-spectrum detoxification agent.

Sources

Good sources of niacin are EGGS, MEAT (especially liver), fish, POULTRY, and unprocessed food, including peanuts and potatoes. COFFEE provides about 3 mg per cup. Niacin is one of the commonly fortified nutrients; consequently, enriched flour and cereals are good sources. MILK and CHEESE are good sources because they contain large amounts of the essential AMINO ACID, TRYPTOPHAN, which is partially converted by the body to niacin. Protein-deficient diets are often related to pellagra. This explains why diets incorporating milk can prevent or cure pellagra.

The form available from animal foods is NIACINAMIDE, a derivative of niacin; plant foods provide niacin itself. Niacin is one of the most stable of the B vitamins: It resists most cooking procedures and can be stored in the dry state indefinitely without loss. Canning, DEHYDRATION, and exposure to air or light cause little destruction.

Up to 70 percent of the niacin in most cereal grains, including corn, is present as a bound form called niacytin. It is not released during digestion and therefore is poorly absorbed. Traditionally, corn tortillas are prepared from corn pretreated with lime water to improve dough consistency, a treatment that also frees niacin. Pellagra is uncommon in Mexico, Central America, and South America, where corn is soaked in lime. Niacin deficiency and pellagra are common only in certain regions of

Africa and Asia, where corn is a major source of protein. Because niacin is so prevalent in high-quality protein, only alcoholics and heavy drinkers are likely to be deficient in the United States. Symptoms of mild deficiency include apathy, headache, irritability, and memory loss.

Requirements

The RECOMMENDED DIETARY ALLOWANCE for health adult men is 19 mg; for nonpregnant, nonlactating women it is 15 mg. The daily niacin requirement varies with the number of calories burned daily (the energy expenditure) and the protein intake. One niacin equivalent equals 1 mg of preformed niacin or 60 mg of dietary tryptophan.

Niacin can be synthesized in the body from the essential amino acid tryptophan. Tissues can form an average of 1 mg of niacin from 60 mg of tryptophan provided by dietary protein. Consequently, a high-quality protein diet supplies substantial tryptophan for niacin synthesis. On the other hand, a protein-deficient diet or a diet relying on low tryptophan protein increases the dietary requirement for niacin. Most animal protein contains 1.4 percent tryptophan; vegetable protein, 1 percent; and corn protein, only 0.6 percent.

Safety

Niacin (but not closely related niacinamide) expands CAPILLARIES and can lead to itching and flushing at doses commonly used in multivitamin supplements (100 mg or more). While nausea, diarrhea, and flushing may accompany niacin usage, these side effects are not considered dangerous. Excessive niacin can cause irregular heartbeat, cramps, headache, and liver inflammation. "Sustained release" niacin may cause less flushing, but some preparations may be more toxic to the liver. Other forms, such as inositol hexaniacinate, may improve niacin therapy. Large doses of niacin can increase BLOOD SUGAR in diabetics, increase the risk of GOUT, and aggravate ulcers. Niacin supplements are not recommended for those with PEPTIC ULCERS, COLITIS, ASTHMA, liver disease, GOUT, or erratic heartbeat. Using niacin therapeutically (1,000 mg or more per day) requires medical supervision; liver function and blood sugar need to be monitored. (See also CARBOHYDRATE METABOLISM; CHOLESTEROL-LOWERING DRUGS; FAT METABOLISM; FORTIFICATION.)

Brown, B. G. et al. "Simvastatin and Niacin, Antioxidant Vitamins, or the Combination for the Prevention of Coronary Disease," *New England Journal of Medicine* 345, no. 22 (2001): 1,583–1,592.

niacinamide (nicotinamide) A derivative of the water-soluble vitamin NIACIN. Niacinamide is readily formed in the body from niacin and incorporated into two important COENZYMES (enzyme helpers): NICOTINAMIDE ADENINE DINUCLEOTIDE (NAD) and its phosphate-containing analog, nicotinamide adenine dinucleotide phosphate (NADP). By assisting in oxidation-reduction reactions, NAD performs an essential role in energy production from nutrients. NAD is required by all cells in many aspects of metabolism, including CARBOHYDRATE, FATTY ACID, and AMINO ACID degradation. The reduced form of NADP, NADPH, participates in reductions required for biosynthesis.

Niacinamide is the most prevalent form of this vitamin in animal products and MEAT, although niacin is more prevalent in plant foods. Niacinamide lacks the capillary-expanding (skin-flushing) activity of niacin and is somewhat safer than niacin; hence it is more often used when large amounts of the vitamin are required. Side effects of niacinamide include nausea, headache, fatigue, sore mouth. Large amounts can injure the liver (jaundice). (See also ANABOLISM; B COMPLEX; DETOXIFICATION; GLUTATHIONE.)

nickel A possible TRACE MINERAL nutrient. Nickel is now known to be an essential trace mineral nutrient of all higher plants, including cereal grains and legumes, which require nickel for seeds to grow. Nickel helps plants liberate nitrogen from soil and absorb IRON. Nickel also seems to be a trace mineral nutrient for some animal species, though its function is unknown. Diets that exclude nickel slow growth in sheep, goats, cows, and rats. Nickel deficiency decreases red blood cell production in these animals as well. Nickel-deficient chickens develop abnormally. Human requirements, if any, are unknown. A typical American diet supplies an estimated 0.3 to 0.6 mg of nickel daily.

Like many trace minerals, minute amounts may be essential nutrients, though high-level exposure is hazardous. Because nickel is an industrial waste, it has emerged as an environmental pollutant. The toxicity of high doses of nickel is well documented; for example, nickel carbonyl is a hazardous industrial chemical, and exposure in the workplace is regulated. Nickel allergies are linked to jewelry; once a person is sensitized, nickel allergies are long-lasting.

nicotinamide See NIACINAMIDE.

nicotinamide adenine dinucleotide (NAD, NADH) An enzyme helper (COENZYME) that functions in oxidation/reduction reactions of cells. NAD contains the B vitamin NIACIN. NAD assists dehydrogenases, a family of enzymes that remove hydrogen atoms from substances (oxidation). Lactate dehydrogenase is a typical dehydrogenase: This enzyme oxidizes LACTIC ACID to PYRUVIC ACID as an intermediate step in the formation of GLUCOSE, the dominant sugar used by the body. Other dehydrogenases oxidize fatty acids and perform oxidation steps in the KREB'S CYCLE, the central energy yielding pathway of the cell.

Nicotinamide Adenine Dinucleotide Phosphate (NADP, NADPH)

NADP closely resembles NAD in structure and function. As the second coenzyme based on niacin it contains an additional phosphate group. The reduced form, NADPH, is used in biosynthetic pathways, including fatty acid and cholesterol synthesis. NADPH is produced by the oxidation of glucose (the pentose phosphate pathway). NADPH supports GLUTATHIONE PEROXIDASE, an important ANTIOXIDANT system for neutralizing oxidative damage to lipids and membranes. (See also B COMPLEX; CARBOHYDRATE METABOLISM; FATTY ACID; OXIDATIVE PHOSPHORYLATION.)

nicotinic acid See NIACIN.

night blindness (nyctalopia) A condition resulting from a chronic deficiency of VITAMIN A. Vitamin A is required to form "visual purple," the pigment required for vision in dim light. With vitamin A deficiency, inadequate pigment causes an abnormally slow adaptation in going from vision in strong light to dim light. Hereditary factors may contribute to night blindness as well.

nightshade family A plant family that includes TOMATOES, POTATOES, EGGPLANT, PEPPERS, and tobacco. Anecdotal reports have been interpreted by some to suggest that eating vegetables from this family may promote joint inflammation in susceptible people. However, no carefully controlled studies have been conducted, and the hyptothesis remains unproven. Arthritic symptoms may diminish by avoiding contact with foods that cause reactions. (See also ARTHRITIS; FOOD SENSITIVITY.)

nitrate An inorganic, nitrogen-containing ion used as a FOOD ADDITIVE for processed MEAT and meat products. Meat can legally contain 91 mg added sodium or potassium nitrate per pound. Chopped meat can contain 778 mg per pound, and dry, cured meat can contain 991 mg per pound. Its role in meat is not clear, though nitrate seems to provide a reservoir for bacterial conversion to nitrite, which acts as an antimicrobial agent. Nitrite can be converted to a potential cancer-causing agent called NITROSOAMINE.

Nitrate occurs naturally in food. Green VEGETABLES are a major source of nitrates and BEETS, SPINACH, and LETTUCE are likely sources. The level depends on the plant species and variety, the part of the plant consumed, the stage of maturity, levels of fertilizers in the soil, and the rate of plant growth. The estimated-typical daily intake of nitrate is 6 mg from vegetables; 9.4 mg from cured meats; 2 mg from bread; and 1.4 mg from FRUIT and fruit juices. Drinking water supplies an average of 0.7 mg daily. High levels of nitrate can occur in well water in rural areas, due to contamination from feed lots and run-off from fertilizer-affected fields. A limit of 10 mg of nitrate per liter has been set by the U.S. Public Health Service.

Nitrate in well water used to prepare formula can be a hazard for infants. Up to six months after birth, stomach acid production in infants is low, which permits bacteria in the intestine to convert nitrate to nitrite. Nitrite can disable infants' hemoglobin and induce a condition called methenoglobinemia, in which nitrite-modified hemoglobin cannot transport adequate oxygen. In older children, nitrate is absorbed in the stomach before it can reach intestinal bacteria that could reduce it to nitrite. Infants drink proportionately much more water (in formula) than adults do, and their hemoglobin is also more sensitive to nitrite attack. Formula prepared from distilled water is safer. (See also PROCESSED FOOD.)

nitric oxide A small, potentially toxic, compound of oxygen and nitrogen that is also a FREE RADICAL. Nitric oxide is different from laughing gas, nitrous oxide, N_2O. Nitric oxide serves multiple functions in the body as a freely diffusible messenger molecule. It is synthesized by specific enzymes, nitric oxide synthases, from the amino acid ARGININE.

Nitric oxide serves as a NEUROTRANSMITTER in the brain and other parts of the nervous system and perhaps plays a key role in memory. Neurotransmitters are chemicals that transmit nerve impulses between the gaps that exist between cells. When MACROPHAGES, phagocytic cells of the immune system, are stimulated to respond to foreign invaders and immune activators, they produce large amounts of nitric oxide to wage chemical warfare against viruses and bacteria. Nitric oxide is produced by endothelial cells lining blood vessels where it relaxes blood vessels and helps maintain blood pressure.

Too little nitric oxide may play a role in hypertension and angina. It also is involved in penile erection and may be a factor in impotence. Nitric oxide also interacts with blood platelets to decrease platelet aggregation, thus lowing the risk of blood clots. Red blood cells rapidly inactive nitric oxide by converting it to nitrate for excretion. Excesses of nitric oxide may be a factor in strokes and inflammatory bowel disease. In stroke, too much calcium can enter cells, causing nitric oxide overproduction to toxic levels when oxygen supply is restored. Nitric oxide combines with SUPEROXIDE, another free radical produced in the body, to form peroxynitrite. This powerful oxidizing agent may account for some of the cellular damage that occurs with prolonged inflammation and could contribute to tissue damage in colitis and other conditions.

nitrite (potassium nitrite, sodium nitrite) A common food additive to processed meat. Nitrites are added to cure MEATS, like LUNCHEON MEATS, liverwurst, SALAMI, BACON, BOLOGNA, HAM, and HOT DOGS to prevent them from turning gray and to create a meaty flavor. Cured white meat does not need a pink color, so nitrite is not usually added to it. Nitrite decomposes to nitric oxide, which reacts with pigments in meat to form an appealing pink color. Nitrites can inhibit bacterial growth, and one argument for continuing to use sodium nitrite is that it prevents spoilage and BOTULISM. Dry cured meat may contain 283 mg of nitrite per pound, while chopped meat can contain 71 mg per pound. Dietary vegetables supply 0.20 mg daily, while cured meats supply several milligrams daily. Until the late 1970s, nitrite was needlessly added to BABY FOOD. Yielding to consumer pressure, baby food manufacturers have stopped this practice. Bacterial action on nitrate in saliva and in the intestine can produce several milligrams of nitrite daily.

Safety

Nitrite-containing bacon, when fried, yields NITROSOAMINES, a family of nitrogen-containing, cancer-causing chemicals. Furthermore, significant levels of nitrosoamines appear in cooked SAUSAGE and cured meats. Specific nitrosoamines have caused CANCER in all animals tested. Under conditions present in the stomach, nitrite also can react with AMINES found in protein-containing foods to form nitrosoamines. Population studies have linked nitrite intake and cancer. Although nitrites and nitrates come from vegetables, this does not necessarily lead to nitrosoamines because VITAMIN C and similar chemicals in the food block nitrosoamine formation. The FDA has approved the use of nitrites since they themselves do not cause cancer. Furthermore, VITAMIN C (ascorbic acid) or similar agents must be added to cured meats in order to reduce the risk of nitrosoamines. Nitrite is now listed on food labels. Nitrite-free meat is increasingly available. (See also CARCINOGEN; NITROGEN CYCLE; PRESERVATIVE.)

nitrogen One of the four major elements used to assemble the carbon-based molecules of life. The other three building blocks are hydrogen, carbon, and OXYGEN. Nitrogen is a key constituents of AMINES, alkaline substances found in cells. In all cells, nitrogen appears in the amino acids, which are incorporated into protein, including enzymes; in purines and pyrimidines, the building blocks of DNA and RNA, the information molecules of the cell; in PHOSPHOLIPIDS, the structural elements of membranes; in certain HORMONES; and in brain chemicals (NEUROTRANSMITTERS) synthesized by nerve cells to carry nerve impulses. Nitrogen contributes to the function of HEME (the oxygen-binding pigment of the oxygen-transport protein, HEMOGLOBIN); THIAMIN (vitamin B_1); RIBOFLAVIN (vitamin B_2); NIACIN (vitamin B_3); VITAMIN B_6; and VITAMIN B_{12}. The nitrogen-containing waste product of protein metabolism is urea, excreted in the urine.

In the NITROGEN CYCLE, atmospheric nitrogen is reduced to ammonia by bacteria residing in the roots of legumes like beans or alfalfa. The ammonia is readily taken up by the plant and can be used to fabricate all nitrogen-containing cell building blocks, including chlorophyll. Animals eat these plant materials primarily as amino acids in food proteins. Cells are generally able to adapt this nitrogen source to their own nitrogen-containing compounds. Thus, ultimately plants are the source of nitrogen in animal cells. Lightning can oxidize atmospheric nitrogen to NITRATE, which leaches into soil as rainfall. Alternatively, nitrate, ammonia, or urea fertilizers are applied during crop cultivation. Nitrate is rapidly absorbed by plants, while urea breaks down to ammonia. Plant tissues can reduce nitrate to ammonia, which is more readily used. When plant or animal tissue decomposes, bacteria can oxidize nitrogen to nitrate, which can then be reabsorbed by plants to reinitiate the cycle. Denitrifying bacteria are able to transform nitrate back to atmospheric nitrogen (N_2).

nitrogen balance A measure of the nutritional state of an individual that pertains to PROTEIN and AMINO ACID consumption. Nitrogen balance compares the level of dietary nitrogen, as represented by amino acids of food protein, with the amount of their nitrogen waste products, lost in urine, feces, and perspiration.

Proteins of every tissue are constantly being replaced, as they wear out due to chemical changes and are degraded to amino acids. The released amino acids may be reused, or they may be degraded for energy, their nitrogen excreted primarily as UREA. If incoming protein just balances the need for amino acids to compensate for wear and tear, the individual is considered to be in "nitrogen equilibrium." Healthy adults maintaining a steady body weight are generally in this state.

Negative Nitrogen Balance When the diet lacks adequate amino acids for growth and maintenance, demand exceeds supply. To compensate, the body breaks down its own protein to supply amino acids. FASTING, ILLNESS, diabetes, fever, surgery, STARVATION, ALCOHOLISM, severe weight loss programs, and crash DIETING place the individual in negative nitrogen balance.

Positive Nitrogen Balance When the body accumulates protein and new tissue is being built, more nitrogen is stored as protein than is lost as waste. Positive nitrogen balance occurs during rapid periods of growth during childhood, adolescence and pregnancy.

nitrogen cycle The movement of nitrogen from the atmosphere through organisms. Nitrogen (N_2) as a gas represents about 80 percent of the atmosphere. Though very abundant, it cannot be used by higher organisms and must be chemically modified to be a nutrient for plants and animals. Bacteria that live symbiotically in the roots of legumes such as PEAS, BEANS, and ALFALFA initiate the process. They convert atmospheric nitrogen to the simplest nitrogen compound, AMMONIA (NH_3), via a process called nitrogen fixation. Alternatively, lightning bolts energize nitrogen to react with oxygen in the air to create NITRATE. Plants incorporate both ammonia and nitrate into AMINO ACIDS, which form PROTEIN. When ingested by animals, plant proteins are broken down to amino acids and incorporated into animal protein. The most useful dietary form of nitrogen for humans is protein: It is digested to release amino acids. Most other nitrogen-containing cell components, like DNA and RNA, can be constructed from amino acids. Animals excrete nitrogenous wastes like UREA, the end product of protein metabolism. Soil bacteria can convert waste nitrogen compounds back to atmospheric nitrogen and ammonia, to be reincorporated into plants. Bacteria, fungi and molds decay plant and animal tissues to help recycle key nutrients. (See also GREEN REVOLUTION; HUNGER; LEGUMES; NITROGEN BALANCE.)

nitrosoamine A cancer-causing agent formed from the common FOOD ADDITIVE NITRITE. Nitrite is a common additive in highly processed meat products and cured meats. Mice, rats, hamsters, pigs, dogs, monkeys, and fish develop CANCER when exposed to several nitrosoamines, which can modify DNA in test tube experiments. In the stomach and intestine they can react with amines, nitrogen-containing compounds present in many foods. Nitrosoamines have been detected in cooked SAUSAGE and BACON, tobacco smoke, cured meats, PESTICIDES, smoked fish, powdered milk, alcoholic beverages, and several types of industrial plants, as well as new car interiors. The level of exposure constituting a health hazard to humans is unknown. VITAMIN C and GARLIC inhibit nitrosoamine formation. (See also FOOD PRESERVATION.)

nondairy creamer (nondairy whitener) A synthetic liquid or powder replacement for milk or cream in coffee. Consumers who choose a nondairy creamer may wish to choose to avoid the calories, CHOLESTEROL, and FAT of cream. However, cream replacements contain 0.7 g of fat per teaspoon in the form of emulsified COCONUT OIL, palm kernel oil, or partially HYDROGENATED VEGETABLE OIL. Not only does a nondairy creamer contain as many fat calories as cream, coconut oil is the most saturated fat available, and a high intake of saturated fat promotes elevated blood fat and cholesterol levels. Nondairy creamers do not contain cholesterol because vegetable oils do not contain cholesterol. On the other hand, they may contain CORN SYRUP as a sweetener, whey and sodium caseinate as protein emulsifiers, sodium aluminosilicate as a stabilizer, as well as artificial flavoring and coloring. Nondairy creamers are nutritionally inferior to milk and are not a milk substitute for children. (See also IMITATION FOOD.)

nonfat dry milk See MILK.

nonheme iron See IRON.

nonprotein nitrogen NITROGEN sources other than protein that can be used to build proteins of the body. Though dietary protein supplies most of the nitrogen for protein synthesis as amino acids, other nitrogen sources can contribute nitrogen. AMMONIA can be reincorporated into amino acids and hence proteins. Individuals on low-protein diets utilize alternative sources of nitrogen more effectively than those who are well fed.

noodles Strings or ribbons of unleavened baked dough. The U.S. FDA defines all pastas as either noodles or MACARONI. Noodles must contain one or more of the following: milled durum WHEAT flour, farina (coarsely ground wheat endosperm from less-hard wheat), or semolina (a granular product of milled durum wheat), together with 5.5 percent egg. (Macaroni need not contain egg.) Noodles have been a mainstay of Asian cookery since ancient times. RICE flour and MUNG BEAN flour are popular in Southeast Asia. Today, noodles are stir-fried, pan-fried, or used in soups and sauces. Specific examples include:

- Mung bean thread noodles (transparent noodles or jelly noodles) resemble silver threads. They soften rapidly in water and are a staple in China, Indonesia, Malaysia, and Japan.
- Rice noodles are thin and wiry when dry. When soaked in water and cooked, they soften and form the basis of many dishes. Rice noodles are popular in Burma, Cambodia, Indonesia, and Vietnam.
- Soba noodles are made from BUCKWHEAT.
- Udon noodles are thick noodles prepared from wheat flour without eggs. They can be either flat or round.
- Bean curd noodles, also called soy noodles, resemble typical egg noodles except they are somewhat thicker and may be grayish in color.

(See also SOYBEAN.)

nori See SEAWEED.

nucleic acids Substances that function as the genetic material and the PROTEIN synthesizing machinery of all cells. DNA is the genetic blueprint. Each species possesses a unique DNA that guides all of a cell's structure and functions; it has been called the cell's "master plan." Alterations in DNA lead to altered inheritance.

RNA is considerably smaller than DNA and does not function as a genetic blueprint of the body. RNA serves as a messenger by which information for building proteins can be translated in the cytoplasm. Thus, RNA directs the assembly of proteins from amino acid raw materials. Special types of RNA form ribosomes, upon which proteins are constructed, and messenger and transfer RNA to translate genetic codewords into amino acids. Both DNA and RNA are assembled from building blocks: a simple sugar, DEOXYRIBOSE, phosphate, and nitrogen-containing cyclic bases called purines and pyrimidines.

The overall composition of RNA is similar to DNA. Each contains a phosphate, a simple sugar—ribose in RNA and deoxyribose in DNA. RNA and DNA contain four nitrogen-containing ring compounds. Three of these are identical: ADENINE, GUANINE, and cytosine. In addition, RNA contains uracil, while DNA contains thymin. (See also FREE RADICALS; MUTAGEN; MUTATION.)

"nursing bottle" syndrome Extensive dental decay in babies due to sucking sweetened beverages for a long period of time. When a baby falls asleep with JUICE-filled bottle or a bottle filled with a sweet drink (even milk) in its mouth, reduced active sucking and reduced saliva flow allow sugar to bathe the upper teeth and lower back TEETH. This favors bacterial growth, cavity formation, and, eventually, extensive dental decay. This syndrome can be avoided by not allowing the infant or young child to fall asleep with a bottle of juice or milk. (See also BREAST-FEEDING; INFANT FORMULA.)

nut A seed typically enclosed by a tough woody shell. Nuts are products of trees; ALMONDS, CHESTNUTS, and HAZELNUTS are typical examples. The PEANUT is an example of a nut that is usually the pod of a LEGUME (member of the pea family). Certain varieties of ALMONDS and PECANS may have soft as well as hard shells. The COCONUT is the leading nut crop worldwide, followed by peanuts; together they account for 94 percent of the world nut production. Nonetheless, nut production is small when compared with the yield of GRAINS and LEGUMES, which are major food items.

Nuts have been a staple in hunter-gatherer societies since prehistoric times. Ancient civilizations cultivated almonds, PISTACHIO nuts, and WALNUTS in Asia. BRAZIL NUTS, peanuts, and cashews originated in South America. Acorns were eaten by Native Americans, who soaked the crushed nuts in water to remove toxic, bitter materials (TANNINS). Though nuts are still harvested in America from wild trees, often nut tree orchards permit more efficient means of production, including mechanical harvesting.

Nuts contain high levels of FAT, CARBOHYDRATE, and PROTEIN to nurture the sprouted seedling until it can perform PHOTOSYNTHESIS. Typically, one ounce ($^1/_8$ cup) of most nuts contains 13 to 18 g of fat, representing an average of 160 fat calories, and 70 percent to 90 percent of calories come from fat. Because of their high fat content, nuts contain 140 more calories per ounce than grains and legumes. On the other hand, the fat in unroasted nuts is unsaturated and unprocessed, an advantage over vegetable shortening or animal fat, which are saturated fats. Brazil nuts, hazelnuts, hickory nuts, peanuts, pecans, pistachios, and walnuts provide 4.7 to 10 g of the ESSENTIAL FATTY ACID, LINOLEIC ACID, per ounce (28 g). Americans who eat nuts frequently seem to have a lower risk of heart attack and coronary disease.

COMPARISON OF UNSATURATED FATTY ACID CONTENT IN TYPICAL NUTS

Calories/oz.	Monounsaturated Fat	Polyunsaturated Fat
almonds (167)	68%	22%
pecans (187)	66%	26%
pistachios (162)	71%	16%
peanuts (164)	52%	33%
walnuts (182)	24%	70%

COCONUT OIL has the highest percentage of saturated fatty acid of the common vegetable oils and resists rancidity. Snack nuts (roasted nuts) are usually roasted in palm kernel oil or coconut oil, increasing their saturated fat content. They are also often heavily salted. A cup of roasted peanuts contains 1,000 mg of sodium, one-third of the suggested daily intake. Dry roasted nuts are not cooked in oil, though they may be salted. Nut butters, such as almond butter or peanut butter, can be used as snacks. If unsweetened and if no additives are used, nut butters are equivalent to a typical nut snack. Although usually eaten as a snack food, chopped nuts can be added to fruit salads, yogurt, pancakes, pilaf, and baked goods for a pleasing variety.

Macadamia nuts contain 72 percent fat; they are fried in deep fat and sold as high-calorie snacks or used for confections. Pecans contain a similar high fat level. Chestnuts differ from other nuts in that they contain three to four times more carbohydrate and less fat and protein than other nuts, and their overall nutrient profile resembles that of dry corn or rice products.

In general, shelled nuts are sold vacuum-packed to increase their shelf life; they should be refrigerated or frozen to slow rancidity due to their high unsaturated oil content. Nuts typically contain 20 percent protein by weight, similar to that found in legumes and about twice as much as found in GRAINS. Peanuts contain 26 percent protein, the highest protein content among commonly available nuts. Defatted nut meal such as almond meal and peanut flour is used as a protein-rich flour. Nut protein contains higher amounts of most essential AMINO ACIDS when compared to grains, but less than legumes. Nuts contain less LYSINE, an essential amino acid. Mixtures of grains and cereals with nuts provide a complementary mixture of essential amino acids that more nearly matches dietary requirements than either alone.

Nuts are generally good sources of the B complex vitamins (like NIACIN, RIBOFLAVIN, and THIAMIN), VITAMIN E, PHOSPHORUS, and MAGNESIUM. Roasting destroys thiamin. Most nuts provide other important trace minerals, including CHROMIUM, MANGANESE, ZINC, and SELENIUM. Typically, nuts contain up to seven times the amounts of these minerals as found in other unprocessed foods. Nuts also provide CHOLINE, a nutrient required for fat transport and nerve function. (See also AFLATOXIN; COMPLETE PROTEIN; PROTEIN QUALITY.)

Kris-Etherton, P. M. et al. "Nuts and Their Bioactive Constituents: Effects on Serum Lipids and Other Factors that Affect Disease Risk," *American Journal of Clinical Nutrition* 70 (1999): 504S–511S.

Nutrasweet See ASPARTAME.

nutraceutical Foods or food-derived ingredients that have the potential of treating or preventing chronic disease. Many ingredients in foods, particularly those derived from plants, possess the ability to benefit health. Vegetables, fruits, nuts, legumes, spices, and teas contain substances that possibly help prevent many of the chronic, degenerative diseases that characterize aging in populations of developed nations. In terms of anticancer effects, the various chemicals in foods could affect the two stages of development of cancer. They could prevent damage to healthy cells' DNA, that is, prevent mutations. These agents may block the activation of carcinogens, stimulate the levels of protective enzymes that detoxify carcinogens, or trap carcinogens.

FLAVONOIDS are complex substances widely distributed in vegetables and fruits, often associated with pigments (such as anthocyanins). They are strong antioxidants, linked with cancer prevention, increased immunity, and lowered risk of cardiovascular disease. Common sources include red wine, apples, onions, and tea. ISOFLAVONES (such as genistein) from soy possess weak estrogen activity and apparently lower the risk of breast cancer. Organosulfur compounds in GARLIC and ONION, including allicin, dially disulfide, and ajoene, in a addition to saponins and flavonoids, possess strong antibacterial and antiviral properties as well as anticancer properties. Vegetables of the cabbage family (cruciferous vegetables) produce SULFORAPHANE and ISOTHIOCYANATES, sulfur-containing chemicals, as well as indoles that can protect against cancer by selectively raising the levels of liver detoxifying enzymes so that the liver can rid the body of potentially mutagenic substances more readily. Many dark green leafy vegetables and orange fruits and vegetables contain orange pigments called CAROTENOIDS that enhance the immune system and function as antioxidants, preserve vision, and inhibit tumor growth. Ellagic acid from GRAPES and STRAWBERRIES deactivates potential carcinogens. Turmeric provides curcuminoids that also inhibit the growth of cancer cells. Regardless of the source, food-derived preparations need to be standardized (that is, the identities and levels of key active ingredients should be known). (See also PHYTOCHEMICALS.)

nutrient An ingredient of foods that can be used by the body for growth and maintenance of health. Foods are mixtures of nutrients, and the relative amounts of the various nutrients in a given food depend on conditions of growth, storage, degree of processing, and method of cooking. DIGESTION releases nutrients from foods, which can then be absorbed by the intestinal tract. Certain nutrients must be supplied by the diet because the body cannot manufacture them. More than 50 different kinds of nutrients have been identified; 40 are definitely required for human growth, development, and health. They include WATER, CARBOHYDRATE, 10 AMINO ACIDS, two types of ESSENTIAL FATTY ACIDS from OILS and FAT, 13 VITAMINS and 15 MINERALS. These nutrients are used for energy, to supply building blocks to replace worn out cell constituents, and for normal cell and tissue function.

Carbohydrates, fat, and PROTEIN, together, represent hundreds of grams (approximately a pound) in the adult diet. Distribution of calories among these three MACRONUTRIENTS varies with the culture and the sub-population. Fat and carbohydrate are the major fuels. Dietary protein is the primary source of amino acids used to fashion the body's own proteins. Major minerals like SODIUM chloride; plant structural materials like FIBER; and WATER are also classified as macronutrients because large quantities are needed. Minerals represent ELECTROLYTES and bony, hard structures. The body represents about 65 percent water; weight-wise, the diet must supply more water than any other nutrient.

Vitamins and trace minerals are classified as MICRONUTRIENTS because they are needed in only minute amounts, ranging from micrograms (1/1,000 gram) to milligrams (1/1,000,000 of a gram). They can form enzyme helpers (the B COMPLEX, trace minerals like ZINC and COPPER); they may build hormones (like VITAMIN D or IODINE); or they may serve a protective role as an ANTIOXIDANT to reduce chemical damage to cells (VITAMIN C, SELENIUM, among others).

Requirements

A majority of essential nutrients are sufficiently well characterized to warrant recommendations for daily allowances, whatever their source. Nutrient allowances need to provide a reasonable margin of safety to account for factors such as age, STRESS, lifestyle habits, gender, pregnancy and lactation. The Food and Nutrition Board of the National Research Council formulated RECOMMENDED DIETARY ALLOWANCES (RDA) estimated to meet the needs of 95 percent of healthy Americans. Nutrient recommendations rely upon biochemical research, clinical case histories of nutrient-deficient individuals, human experimentation with suboptimal diets, animal growth experiments and examination of nutrient intake of healthy people. Reduced nutrient intake as well as excessive nutrient consumption can lead to MALNUTRITION. A BALANCED DIET supplies all nutrients in adequate amounts to maintain health. Reliance on foods containing high levels of fat or calories—as sweets, fatty snack foods, and many highly processed foods—crowds out micronutrients like vitamins and trace minerals. (See also COENZYME; COFACTOR; DIETARY GUIDELINES FOR AMERICANS; FOOD PROCESSING; VITAMIN E.)

nutrient density The relative concentration of nutrients in a food as compared to the calories found in wholesome, unprocessed food. Fruit has a higher nutrient density than fruit juice because fruit contains higher proportions of nutrients like VITAMINS, MINERALS, PROTEIN, and FIBER, and fruit juice has a higher nutrient density than soda pop. This concept is especially useful in evaluating PROCESSED FOODS. The higher the nutrient density, the closer the food is to the initial unprocessed food and the more key nutrients it has. Thus, JUNK FOOD and many highly processed food products made from bleached FLOUR, and manufactured meal products, often have a low nutrient density. Excessive calories contribute significantly to the problem of overweight facing many Americans. The ENRICHMENT and fortification of foods and beverages, the addition of vitamins and minerals, especially to cereal grain products like BREAKFAST CEREALS, flour and BREAD, together with MILK, attempts to improve the nutrient density of these popular foods. (See also DIETARY GUIDELINES FOR AMERICANS; FAST FOOD; FOOD ADDITIVES; FOOD PROCESSING; OBESITY.)

nutrition The science of FOODS, NUTRIENTS, and their relationship to health and disease. (See also NUTRITIONIST.)

nutritional equivalency Characteristic of a substitute or manufactured food, simulating a basic food and containing as much of the essential nutrients, as defined by the U.S. recommended daily allowances (USRDA), as the basic food. Thus a food can be considered nutritionally equivalent if it is not nutritionally inferior. There are important limitations to the U.S. FDA's definition of nutritional equivalency. A product can be declared nutritionally equivalent though it contains excessive amounts of any of the 20 nutrients for which USRDAS exist or if it contains different nutrient-to-calorie ratios. A food that provides fewer fat calories but equal levels of essential nutrients can be regarded as nutritionally superior. A substitute food can be classified nutritionally equivalent to its traditional counterpart even though it does not contain essential nutrients such as VITAMIN K and many minerals—CHROMIUM, SELENIUM, MOLYBDENUM, MANGANESE, FLUORIDE—as well as MACRONUTRIENTS, SODIUM, POTASSIUM, and CHLORIDE.

The legal definition excludes other factors in foods. For example, dietary FIBER is not considered a component of nutritional equivalency, and uncharacterized materials in vegetables apparently reduce the risk of some forms of cancer and are excluded. Finally, the definition of nutritional equivalency does not generally deal with BIOAVAILABILITY, that is, the degree to which nutrients in food can be absorbed and used. Digestibility, nutrient uptake and interrelationships among nutrients influence nutrient availability in fabricated foods. Functional laboratory tests measure an attribute that reflects nutrient use. As an example, PROTEIN EFFICIENCY RATIO (PER) is a standardized functional test that accesses protein utilization of foods. (See also FOOD LABELING; IMITATION FOOD.)

nutritional supplements See VITAMIN.

nutritional status An assessment of the adequacy of the diet in meeting individual nutrient needs. Nutritional assessment entails a comprehensive health evaluation: Medical history, diet analysis, physical exam, and measurement of height and weight can reflect nutrient status. This evaluation may require laboratory tests to determine the tissue and fluid levels of specific VITAMINS and MINERALS, or measurement of biochemical markers of nutrient adequacy, such as serum FERRITIN, to assess IRON status.

Many factors can influence a person's nutrient status, and sorting them out can be a challenge. An illness can cause appetite loss or difficulty in swallowing or chewing; it can interfere with DIGESTION or assimilation of food or alter nutrient usage or excretion of wastes. An elderly patient may not be able to purchase or prepare adequate food because of physical limitations. Diminished taste with aging may lead to the selection of salty foods. Dentures can make chewing difficult, while diminished stomach acid output can decrease VITAMIN B_{12} absorption as well as mineral absorption and digestion in general. A lack of EXERCISE can contribute to problems of excessive weight. Overmedication can lead to DEPRESSION and disinterest in food, MALNUTRITION and weight loss. (See also ASSESSMENT, NUTRITION; DIET RECORD; DIETITIAN; MALABSORPTION; OBESITY.)

nutritional yeast See BAKER'S YEAST; BREWER'S YEAST; *CANDIDA ALBICANS*.

nutritionist A professional who specializes in nutritional counseling. Currently, training is not uniform from state to state. Nutritionists' backgrounds range from mail order credentials to Ph.D.s from accredited universities. Most nutrition programs require training in food science and the biological sciences. A number of states have legislation that licenses nutritionists if they are registered DIETITIANS or if they have an advanced degree from a recognized college or university. A graduate of a program in nutrition, nutrition education, or dietetics is likely to be qualified. A number of professional organizations offer certification programs that assure high standards and are open to qualified health care professionals, such as the International and American Associations of Clinical Nutritionists and the Certification Board of Nutrition Specialists.

nutrition labeling See FOOD LABELING.

O

oats (*Avena sativa*) A common cereal GRAIN grown in temperate regions, particularly in North America and northern Europe. There are six species, including common oats and cultivated red oats, that are grown in the Americas. Oats are classified as winter and spring varieties, according to their planting time. Only about 5 percent of the U.S. crop is used as a food crop; most ends up as livestock feed. An inedible, loose, pithy hull surrounds the kernel, or groat, and must be removed for human consumption.

Pure oats and pure oat BRAN are the least processed form of oats. Oat flakes, prepared by steaming and flaking whole kernels, are the basis for porridge. Oatmeal is prepared by cutting kernels to small granules with a mealy texture. Consumption of old-fashioned oatmeal as a BREAKFAST CEREAL has declined with the increased popularity of ready-cooked oatmeal cereals. Rolled oats, prepared by crushing oats with still rollers, are used in breakfast food, cookies, breads, and GRANOLA, which is a mixture of rolled oats, honey, nuts, raisins, or dates. Milling produces oat flour. Oat flour contains a natural ANTIOXIDANT that increases the stability of oat flour in storage.

Oat Bran

Oat bran is derived from an outer layer of oat kernels by milling. It is a good source of SILICON, a trace mineral needed for healthy joints, and a form of FIBER called beta-glucan. The fiber in oat bran is water soluble and differs from water-insoluble WHEAT bran, the kind usually found in bran-enriched breakfast cereals. Eating oat bran daily in muffins and a bowl of hot oatmeal—together with daily exercise and eating less animal FAT as found in red MEAT and BUTTER—can lower blood fat and CHOLESTEROL even in diabetics. Oat bran alone has a modest effect in lowering elevated levels of the less desirable LOW-DENSITY LIPOPROTEIN (LDL) cholesterol. Oat bran has been used as a fat substitute to reduce fat in beef and pork sausage products. A mixture of oatmeal and oat flour has been developed by the USDA as a fat-substitute called Oatrim or "hydrolyzed oat flour." Oatrim contains one calorie per gram, as compared with nine calories per gram of fat and four calories per gram of STARCH. This fat substitute is used in baked goods and processed meats, and other products are under development.

Oatmeal

Hot oatmeal is a traditional breakfast, and its emergence as an important source of fiber has caused a resurgence in popularity. Steel cut, rolled, or quick-cooking oats all contain the same amount of fiber. However, processed, cold oat breakfast cereals contain much less fiber (about 2 g per serving). Dry oatmeal contains about 14 percent protein, but cooked oatmeal is only about 2 percent protein.

Nutrient content of regular cooked oatmeal or rolled oats, (1 cup fortified) is: 145 calories; protein, 6 g; carbohydrate, 25.2 g; fiber, 9.23 g; fat, 2.3 g; iron, 1.6 mg; sodium, 285 mg; vitamin A, 453 retinol equivalents; thiamin, 0.53 mg; riboflavin, 0.29 mg; niacin, 5.9 mg.

obesity An excessive accumulation of body fat for a given body size based on muscle and bone (frame size). In 1998 the federal government adopted new standards for determining whether a person is overweight or obese. Before then, people were considered overweight if their weight was at least 10 percent to 20 percent over optimal body weight. Obesity was defined as being more than 25 percent over the optimal body weight for men and 30 percent over the optimal body weight for women.

Under the new standards, a person with a BODY MASS INDEX (BMI) of 25 or more is considered overweight. The BMI is determined by dividing a person's weight in kilograms by the square of his or her height in meters. A healthy BMI falls between 19 and 25. A person with a BMI of 30 or above is considered obese. According to statistics compiled by the World Health Organization, obesity is increasing worldwide—an estimated 1.2 billion people in the world are overweight. Its rapid increase among Americans during the 1990s (12 percent in 1991 to 17.9 percent in 1998) prompted some health officials to conclude that it had reached epidemic proportions. In 2001 27 percent of adults between the ages of 20 and 74 were obese. The rate of overweight among children was 13 percent.

Based on these figures, a former U.S. surgeon general, David Satcher, concluded that overweight and obesity may soon cause as much preventable disease and death as cigarette smoking. The conditions were already responsible for as many as 300,000 premature deaths each year, costing the nation an estimated $117 billion. The prevalence varies among groups. The average American adult gains a pound a year through middle age.

Childhood obesity has increased dramatically since 1965 in the United States, reflecting an increased prevalence of obesity among children in Western countries. The rising rate of overweight and obesity among young people is of special concern because childhood and adolescence is often a time in life when people are the most active and therefore least likely to gain excessive weight. Also, unhealthy nutrition and lifestyle habits that lead to overweight and obesity developed during this time have a good chance of continuing into adulthood.

The number of obese Americans has increased, despite a national preoccupation with dieting. The fear of being fat has become an American obsession. U.S. society places a premium on being slender and most women and some men have dieted at least once. Being obese or overweight often brings a profound social stigma affecting personal life, life insurance premiums, and employment opportunities. Nevertheless, in the 1980s the renewed interest in healthy lifestyles in America apparently affected a limited number of people. Sedentary lifestyles continue to prevail.

Types of Obesity

Hyperblastic obesity is characterized by an excessive number of fat cells. Increased fat cell size is classified as hypertrophic obesity, and individuals with hyperblastic-hypertrophic obesity have increased numbers of enlarged fat cells in their adipose tissue. Hyperblastic obesity is usually associated with childhood, while hypertrophic obesity develops later in life and is associated with diabetes and other aspects of metabolic imbalance.

Obesity as a Health Hazard

It has been noted that the death rate increases 2 percent for each pound over a person's healthy weight. For persons who are 40 pounds overweight, the death rate is estimated to be 80 percent higher during the next 25 years of their life. Lean men survive longer than overweight men in the United States. Obesity increases the risk of HEART DISEASE, diabetes, GOUT, ARTHRITIS, CANCER of the liver and esophagus, GALLSTONES, hernia, intestinal blockage, kidney disease, and TOXEMIA of pregnancy. In the United States, obesity increases the risk of angina, high blood pressure (HYPERTENSION), high blood fat, elevated (LOW-DENSITY LIPOPROTEIN) LDL, and sudden death from heart disease. One clue to understanding the relationship between obesity and elevated blood fat is the observation that obese people have higher insulin levels, which seems to promote higher blood lipids.

The location of fat accumulation makes a difference in health risks. Male-patterned obesity, with fat deposited primarily in the abdomen and trunk, is called android obesity (the "spare tire" or "apple" profile). Android obesity in men or women is associated with an increased risk for CARDIOVASCULAR DISEASE, hypertension, elevated BLOOD SUGAR, and gallstones. The greater the proportion of abdominal fat, the greater the risk. Abdominal fat may be more readily converted to cholesterol than fat deposited elsewhere. Pear-shaped people, with fat accumulation around the hips, do not experience as much diabetes or high blood pressure or as many heart attacks as those whose fat is around the middle.

Possible Mechanisms for Regulating Body Weight

Complex mechanisms involving the NERVOUS SYSTEM, the ENDOCRINE SYSTEM, and the DIGESTIVE SYSTEM, and adipose tissue regulate eating, energy balance, and thus obesity. Regions of the brain, such as the HYPOTHALAMUS and the brain stem, help regulate food intake, body weight, body size, and body fat content. The hypothalamus plays a critical role in eating and balancing energy requirements with intake. The lateral hypothalamus controls eating activity; the paraventricular nucleus regulates nutrient balance and the ventromedial hypothalamus regulates energy balance by regulating the sympathetic nervous system, which helps the body adapt to stress. The hypothalamus regulates the ENDOCRINE SYSTEM (hormone secreting system). It activates the PITUITARY GLAND, which signals the adrenal gland to release GLUCOCORTICOIDS. In turn, these STEROID hormones regulate the nervous system, appetite, and fat metabolism. Obesity is linked to altered function of the brain stem and hypothalamus and to changes in the autonomic nervous system, which regulates energy expenditure and regulates thermogenesis. At the molecular level, altered production of NEUROTRANSMITTERS, chemicals required to transmit nerve impulses, brain peptides, and brain hormones, may alter critical control and feedback mechanisms that maintain body weight.

Several hypotheses link food intake and energy balance to regulate body weight through an interplay between the endocrine system and the nervous system. A hypothetical very general control system involves the following components: A proposed "controller" resides in the brain. Signals leaving the brain regulate heat production, physical activity, food intake, energy storage as fat, and metabolism for doing work and producing heat. These factors stimulate the release of hormones. Nutrients and hormones from various glands and fat cells are then carried back to brain centers that in turn generate signals that are interpreted by the hypothalamus to diminish eating. Stomach distension triggers the nervous system to create a feeling of fullness. The action of GLUCOSE (blood sugar), fat, and protein in the intestines on receptors could also send signals back to the brain to diminish eating behavior.

In 2002 researchers reported that the recently discovered "hunger hormone" ghrelin might be a significant factor in determining why some people become obese and why most people find it hard to keep weight off once it is lost. A study of a small group of obese people revealed they had much higher blood levels of ghrelin, which is produced by stomach cells, after they lost weight through diet control and exercise. In contrast, people who lost weight after gastric bypass surgery, which reroutes the flow of food, had low levels of ghrelin. The extremely low levels of ghrelin in people who had undergone gastric bypass surgery might explain why these people were usually more successful in keeping weight off. Researchers cautioned that the results were preliminary and that ghrelin is probably only one of many tools the body uses to regulate body weight.

Another hypothesis predicts a "set point" that tends to keep body weight at a constant level. According to the "set point" hypothesis for body weight, each person has a biologically determined body weight, believed to be inherited. In some obese individuals, the set point may be too high. When fat cells decrease in size (for example, after DIETING) they could indirectly signal the brain to increase food consumption. Thus, an obese person with large numbers of fat cells could crave food, leading to excessive eating after dieting. According to a related hypothesis, some obese people earlier in their lives, perhaps during early childhood, ate much more than their bodies needed during their formative years. According to this proposal, this event patterned the body for burning energy and storing fat. Once overweight, obesity in these individuals could be sustained even when consuming an average amount of food.

Insulin insensitivity (resistance to the action of insulin) correlates with obesity; increasing tissue sensitivity to insulin is hypothesized to lower the body's set point. Recent discoveries shed light on the relationships among obesity, satiety, and non-insulin dependent diabetes. Fat cells normally secrete a protein called LEPTIN that induces satiety. Leptin signals the brain to reduce consumption of fatty foods and possibly to increase the basal metabolism of fat cells. Therefore, leptin helps regulate body weight by limiting body fat accumulation. Mice with mutations on the gene coding for leptin become obese. Researchers now believe obese people often make more than enough leptin, but the brain does not respond effectively to shut down eating because its binding sites or cell signaling mechanisms are defective. A region of the brain likely to be affected by leptin is the HYPOTHALAMUS, which integrates many functions of the body. Specifically, the region known as ventromedial nucleus, which regulates satiety, may be involved. Leptin could shut off signals in the brain that direct feeding (hunger signals), including neuropeptides. One possibility is neuropeptide Y, which induces lab animals to eat more carbohydrate and fat. In the set point model, leptin could act like a thermometer: When the body gets too thin, less leptin is made, more food is eaten, and less energy is consumed. When the body gets too fat, more leptin is made, less food is consumed, and more energy is burned.

A variety of mutations in other genes link obesity and diabetes. As an example, mutations in a protein called beta$_3$-adrenergic receptor, an attachment site which binds a NEUROTRANSMITTER (norepinephrine), increase the risk of middle-age weight gain and diabetes. Under normal conditions norepinephrine produced by the sympathetic nervous system stimulates fat cells to burn stored fats. The implication is that with a faulty neurotransmitter attachment site in fat tissue, the body burns less fat efficiently and calories accumulate. As an alternative to the set point hypothesis, the "settling point" theory proposes that body weight is not fixed, but that it is maintained according to feedback loops that are determined by an interplay between genes and environment. Systems controlling hunger and satiety respond rapidly to dietary protein and carbohydrate, but the feedback from a fatty meal may be too slow to prevent overconsumption. Thus, increased dietary fat could alter the body's equilibrium and shift body fat upward. The number of fat cells in the body is a determining factor. Fat cells are added during childhood and it could very well be that how much fatty food is consumed and how many calories are burned before adulthood has a major impact for the risk of obesity.

Human obesity is a complex phenomenon with many causes. Inheritance as well as diet and medical history can contribute to excessive weight gain and many questions about the detailed interrelationships remain unanswered. Apparently, many genes interact to control weight, it is therefore unlikely that any single pharmacologic agent related to a gene product will substitute for changing the diet and exercising regularly to maintain desired weight. In any event, very extensive clinical experience suggests that diets—that improve insulin sensitivity and glucose tolerance by emphasizing VEGETABLES and LEGUMES and minimizing sugary or high fat foods—together with regular physical exercise can support long-term weight loss and reduce the risk of cardiovascular disease.

Causes of Obesity

Many adults achieve an energy balance in which caloric intake matches energy expenditure. Body fat does not change very much under these conditions. Excessive body fat could be related to eating more calories or to small energy expenditure, or both. Energy expenditure refers to the calories spent for body functions, physical activity, digestion, and food metabolism. Both heredity and the environment play a part in obesity and, therefore, there is no single approach to treatment. Overeating, differences in metabolism, AGING, genetic predisposition, and excessive food consumption during early childhood have been implicated.

Overeating Clearly the prolonged consumption of excessive calories, when energy intake exceeds energy expenditure, leads to obesity. Energy expenditure refers to the calories spent for body functions, physical activity, digestion, and food metabolism. Body fat can be reduced only when energy expenditure exceeds caloric intake. The body adapts to excessive food consumption—whether excessive PROTEIN, CARBOHYDRATE, fat, or ALCOHOL—by storing the surplus calories as body fat. Many reports have suggested that obese people eat the same, or sometimes less than nonobese people. Using new research methods based on ingesting double-labeled water, that is, water containing a "heavy" form of oxygen (O^{18}) and "heavy" hydrogen (deuterium), investigators have demonstrated that, on the average, obese people generally eat more, but they habitually underreport their food consumption.

Differences in Energy Expenditure Although obese people are generally less active than nonobese people, they tend to use the same amounts of energy because they weigh more. Sedentary lifestyles contribute to obesity. About 70 percent of adult Americans fail to exercise 20 minutes or more three times a week as recommended. Most people will lose weight if such an exercise program is coupled with consuming no more than 1,500 calories daily. Individuals who exercise regularly, or who exercise before and after a high-calorie meal, lose more energy as heat after eating than those who do not exercise.

Differences in Metabolism This picture is unclear. Very rarely do glandular imbalances lead to obesity. Cushing's syndrome, excessive production of glucocorticoids, a form of adrenal hormone, is an example of hormone imbalance that can promote obesity. Obese people do not have unusually slow metabolisms. When resting metabolic rates are compared based upon the muscle/bone mass, there is not a significant difference between metabolic rates of nonobese and obese individuals. Formerly obese individuals preferentially store fat rather than burn it, and studies suggest that overweight and obese people tend to eat more fat and less carbohydrate. In general, the body consumes calories more slowly after weight is lost, and it burns calories more rapidly when weight is gained, for fat as well as for thin people. One hypothesis contends that people adjust their metabolism to maintain a "set point" weight. Thus someone who has lost significant amounts of fat (10 percent of their body weight) will burn fewer calories when exercising than someone who has maintained his or her weight without a weight-loss program. Apparently, the body adjusts its metabolism by altering the efficiency of muscles in burning calories. Recently, a type of prostaglandin has been shown to act as a hormone to trigger the production of fat cells from immature cells.

Aging In the United States, both men and women tend to become fatter with increasing age. This could be due to a decreased metabolic rate (a lower BASAL METABOLIC RATE) and a sedentary lifestyle coupled with an easy access to high-calorie food.

Meal Frequency The frequency of meals and meal composition may be a factor in obesity. Eating fewer meals may increase fat deposition, while smaller, more frequent meals, with more food at breakfast and less at supper, may promote weight loss.

TV Watching Excessive TV watching correlates with overeating. Reduced physical activity, lowered metabolic rates, as well as visual cues to eating high-fat snack foods and drinking alcoholic beverages, contribute to the increased prevalence of overweight. Dietary fat, which provides nine calories per gram, is more fattening than either protein or carbohydrate, which provide four calories per gram. Fat calories in food differ from calories in carbohydrate: Fat in food is more easily converted to body fat than is carbohydrate.

Inheritance One broad generalization can be made: Obesity persists over a life span. Fat children tend to become fat adults, suggesting a predisposition to being overweight. Early adulthood is an important period for the development of lifelong patterns. The question remains, to what degree is obesity the product of genetics? Studies with twins suggest that between 50 percent and 70 percent of the variability in relative body weight represents genetic variability. Current research focuses on locating specific obesity genes. Genes influence both metabolism and behavior. Many genes regulate hunger and satiety. A flurry of recent research has yielded impartial genetic discoveries: gene *OB* causes fat cells to produce a satiety protein called lepin. A gene then codes for the receptor of this hormone in the brain. Still another gene codes for a hormone-producing enzyme (carboxypeptidase E). A gene that codes for a neurotransmitter receptor (binding site; Beta$_3$-adrenergic receptor) for norepinephrine is also implicated in maintaining weight. Mutations of these genes can increase the risk of obesity and diabetes in lab animals and possibly in people. There will be more to add to this unfinished story as more discoveries are made.

Successful Weight Loss

A Willingness to Change Therapeutic approaches to obesity and weight management have met with only modest success. Only 2 percent to 10 percent of Americans who diet to lose weight and participate in weight loss programs will keep the pounds off more than several years. Most of the lost fat is regained within a few months after the dieter discontinues the diet regimen. Dieting without a long-term commitment to changing daily habits is destined to fail.

Attitude is perhaps the most prominent factor in changing behavior. Regarding overeating, understanding underlying feelings for which overeating compensates seems essential for permanent weight loss. Eating can provide immediate gratification, but this seldom resolves deep-seated emotional issues. After short-term sensory satisfaction, emotional pain or longing often returns. For example, responding to feelings of low self-esteem by crash dieting does not solve the underlying issue, and too often the dieter returns to old eating habits. Counselors recommend beginning with an inventory of talents and qualities that fill your life with the most satisfaction and choosing activities and relationships that bring satisfaction and a sense of well-being.

Slow Weight Loss Successful long-term weight control requires the slow loss of body fat without cyclic, on-again, off-again dieting (YO-YO DIETING). Losing a pound a week helps maintain muscle (LEAN BODY MASS) while preferentially losing fat.

Exercise Exercising for life helps keep the body engine "revved up," so that more calories are burned by muscle and less insulin is required to dispose of elevated blood sugar following meals.

Improved Diet A high-fat, high-calorie, low-fiber diet is thought to be the major dietary factor in obesity in the United States. Therefore the recommended diet might be low in fat, high in fiber and complex carbohydrates (60 percent to 70 percent of calories), with adequate protein (10 percent to 15 percent of calories). Emphasis on natural, whole foods simplifies this task of avoiding the pervasive high-calorie foods that fill the American food landscape. Another approach to obesity and overweight focuses on helping people through advocacy and social support with the premise that being overweight can be part of an enjoyable, fulfilling life: The Association for the Health Enhancement of Large People and the National Association to Advance Fat Acceptance are two such groups.

Weight Loss Drugs

Like diets, anti-obesity drugs tend to be effective only as long as the patient follows the prescription. When drugs are withdrawn, weight lost usually returns unless permanent behavior changes have been made. Amphetamines have adverse side effects: They have the potential for addiction and tolerance (more drug is required to get the same effect with chronic use). Another class of drug promotes nutrient malabsorption so that patients taking these drugs do not absorb calories efficiently.

Two appetite suppressants, fenfluramine and dexfenfluramine, were taken off the market by the U.S. FDA in 1997 when it was discovered that thousands of patients who took these drugs developed potentially deadly primary pulmonary hypertension and heart valve abnormalities. Dexfenfluramine was shown to cause these injuries when taken alone, and fenfluramine was linked to valve problems in patients who combined it with the drug phentermine in a mixture popularly known as "fen-phen." Both fenfluramine and dexfenfluramine helped patients lose weight by increasing serotonin levels in the blood stream, which provided a sense of well-being and satiety. The problem, researchers discovered after the drugs were removed from the market, was that the drugs destroyed the body's ability to control the amount of serotonin circulating in the blood. Excessive amounts of serotonin can cause cell damage to cardiopulmonary structures.

In late 2000 the FDA issued a public health advisory warning patients about phenylpropanolamine hydrochloride (PPA). This drug is widely used in both over-the-counter and prescription-only nasal decongestants and for weight control in some over-the-counter drug products. The warning was issued after medical researchers published a study showing that phenylpropanolamine increases the risk of hemorrhagic stroke (bleeding into the brain or into tissue surrounding the brain) in women. Men may also be at risk. Since then the FDA has taken steps to remove PPA from all drug products. No drug is both entirely safe and effective for weight loss, nor is it certain that taking current medications for many years is better than being fat. Drugs that suppress appetite are not recommended for those who wish to lose only 5 to 10 pounds of fat.

Childhood Obesity

An estimated 13 percent of U.S. children six to 11 years old and 14 percent of adolescents 12 to 19 years old are overweight. The number of obese children and adolescents in the United States doubled between 1982 and 2002. Obesity is recognized as a U.S. epidemic affecting children. Low-income minority children face even higher rates of obesity. An overweight adolescent between age 10 and 14 who has at least one overweight or obese parent has a 79 percent likelihood of being overweight as an adult.

Childhood obesity is linked to many of the factors that cause adult obesity:

Heredity As in adult obesity, genes play a role. Children born to obese mothers are more likely to be obese. If both parents are obese, the probability of their children becoming obese is very high.

Overfeeding Some babies have more fat cells than usual. If they are also overfed, they are more likely to become obese children. In addition, overfeeding a child may lead to larger, not more, fat cells. This may make controlling weight more difficult as an adult. (It should be pointed out that plump babies do not necessarily become obese adults.)

Lower Metabolism Infants who become overweight during their first year have a lower basal metabolic rate than usual. Their mechanism for regulating body weight might be lower than average.

Eating Too Much Fatty Food The more JUNK FOOD is consumed, the more likely the child will be obese. Bogalusa Heart Study is an ongoing population study to examine risk factors for cardiovascular disease in children. Results from this study reveal that children who consume more than 30 percent of their calories from fat were more likely to eat less CALCIUM, IRON, MAGNESIUM, and vitamins like RIBOFLAVIN, NIACIN, THIAMIN, VITAMIN B_6, VITAMIN B_{12}, and VITAMIN E.

Too Much TV and Not Enough Exercise The odds of becoming obese increase with the number of hours of TV viewed each day. Children's basal metabolic rate decreases, and they get less physical activity. Children who watch TV eat more of the high-calorie, highly processed food they see advertised, and parents fill the role of food "gate keepers." Children eat what is available to them, whether it is candy, soft drinks, or fatty convenience foods, or fruit, low-fat foods, and sugar-free beverages.

The home environment and parents present the model for a child's eating habits. A child's shift to a more healthful lifestyle needs to be nurtured by parents to become permanent. As with overweight adults, regular exercise is extremely important in children's health and maintaining a desirable weight.

However, overzealous dietary restrictions by parents can encourage self-imposed dieting and eating disorders, a prevalent problem among children and adolescents in the United States. As many as 80 percent of 10-year-old girls suffer from a fear of body fat; some already show signs of dieting, bingeing, overeating, and anorexia. The message they are receiving is that any accumulation of body fat is socially unacceptable. However, among white, middle-class, healthy girls in the United States, weight before and during puberty does not seem to be a predictor of weight gain at middle age. On the other hand, weight gained after puberty (during early adolescence) has correlated with weight gain as adults. For boys, prepuberty weight appears to be a good predictor of adult obesity. A physician should be consulted before talking to children about weight. Periodic increases in fat, especially among girls, are a normal occurrence. Weight maintenance, after the child has grown into his or her own weight, is preferable to dieting. Generally, children can be taught to prefer lower fat foods by exposure and availability. (See also MALNUTRITION; WEIGHT MANAGEMENT.)

Asayama, Kohtaro et al. "Increased Serum Cholesterol Ester Transfer Protein in Obese Children," *Obesity Research* 10 (2002): 439–446.

Cummings, D. E. et al. "Plasma Ghrelin Levels After Diet-Induced Weight Loss or Gastric Bypass Surgery," *New England Journal of Medicine* 346, no. 21 (May 23, 2002): 1,623–1,630.

octacosanol A complex alcohol that is a normal constituent of wheat germ and wheat germ oil. Other sources include whole grain cereals, seeds and NUTS, and many plant oils and WAXES. Persistent claims that octacosanol supplementation has a positive effect on physical endurance and muscular strength have not been substantiated by research. The Federal Trade Commission concluded that wheat germ oil did not improve endurance or stamina. Octacosanol seems to improve reaction time. (See also ERGOGENIC SUPPLEMENTS.)

oil See VEGETABLE OIL.

oil palm (***Elaeis guineensis***) A palm that is a major source of edible oil. The oil palm yields more oil per acre than any other plant. It originated in West Africa, and plantations now exist in Malaysia, China, and Indonesia, as well as Tanzania, the Ivory Coast, Nigeria, and other regions. Palm oil is prepared from fibrous pulp of the fruit, and palm kernel oil is obtained from the seed or kernel, which contains about 50 percent oil. Palm kernel oil is used for margarine production and food manufacture. It is among the most SATURATED FATS, containing 86.7 percent saturated FATTY ACIDS, 1.6 percent polyunsaturated fatty acids, and 11.7 percent monounsaturated fatty acids. (See also COCONUT OIL; TROPICAL OILS.)

okra (***Hibiscus esculentus; Abelmoschus esculentus***) A vegetable that bears seeds in edible pods whose ancestors may have been widely distributed from Africa to India. Okra now grows in regions with a moderate climate, including the southern states of the United States. Much of the U.S. okra crop is frozen or canned. Okra contains a mucilage that acts as a thickener in soups and stews. Because okra changes to an unappetizing color when cooked in utensils containing iron, copper, or brass, glass or stainless steel containers are used. Okra's slippery mucilage is balanced by acidic foods like tomatoes and lemons and by vinegar. Okra, long considered part of Deep South cuisine, is also part of Indian, Caribbean, South American, and African recipes.

Nutrient content of okra (8 pods, 85 g, cooked) is: 27 calories; protein, 1.6 g; carbohydrate, 6.1 g; fiber, 2.75 g; calcium, 54 g; iron, 0.38 mg; potassium, 274 mg; vitamin C, 14 mg; thiamin, 0.11 mg; riboflavin, 0.05 mg; niacin, 0.74 mg.

oleic acid A nonessential FATTY ACID and a common constituent of FATS and OILS found in foods and fat synthesized by the body. Oleic acid is distinguished from the other common fatty acids, the energy-rich building blocks of fats and oils. It contains 18 carbon atoms and a single double bond, is deficient in hydrogen atoms, and thus is classified as a monounsaturated fatty acid. In contrast, saturated fatty acids are building blocks filled up with hydrogen atoms and polyunsaturated fatty acids possessing two or more double bonds and are more unsaturated than oleic acid. Oils rich in oleic acid are called monounsaturated oils. VEGETABLE OILS like olive oil, AVOCADO oil, and CANOLA OIL contain high amounts of oleic acid. Oleic acid-rich vegetable oils seem to lower the less desirable forms of blood CHOLESTEROL, LOW-DENSITY LIPOPROTEIN (LDL) with high fat intake, and to increase more desirable forms of cholesterol, HIGH-DENSITY LIPOPROTEIN (HDL). Olive oil is more stable to oxidation than polyunsaturates such as safflower oil or corn oil. The recommendation is to decrease fat and oil consumption generally, and to use more monounsaturates in cooking, rather than saturates (butter, lard, shortening, coconut oil, or palm oil) or polyunsaturates (such as CORN OIL, SAFFLOWER oil, and SOYBEAN oil).

Olestra (sucrose polyester, imitation fat [Olean]) A noncaloric fat substitute approved for use in snack foods such as crackers, potato chips, and other chips. Olestra tastes like LARD and VEGETABLE OILS; it is neither digested nor absorbed by the body. By comparison, FAT and oils contain 126 calories per tablespoon. Olestra resembles the structure of fat, except that it has a molecule of sucrose at its core to which are attached eight fatty acids, rather than three. Because it possesses a new substance, sucrose polyester had to be approved by the U.S. FDA. All products containing Olestra are labeled to notify the consumer that Olestra may cause abdominal cramping and loose stools and that it inhibits the uptake of certain nutrients. Vitamins A, D, E, and K have been added. The question of malabsorption of CAROTENOIDS has not been addressed.

In addition to these potential safety problems, animal studies suggest Olestra can cause liver damage, birth defects, and cancer. More complete studies are needed to establish its safety. Regardless of their source, fat substitutes cannot replace the need to eat less high-fat food and to change eating habits. (See also WEIGHT MANAGEMENT.)

olive (***Olea europaea***) The oil-rich fruit of a semitropical evergreen adapted to hot, dry climates. Olives were probably first cultivated in the Eastern Mediterranean region as early as 6000 B.C. There are now more than 60 varieties. Mediterranean countries remain major producers; together, Italy and Spain produce more than half of the world's olives and 60 percent of the world's olive oil production. Olives are also grown in Australia, China, Greece, Turkey, and France, as well as in the United States. Spanish colonists introduced olives to California in the 18th century; that state continues to be a major domestic supplier. At maturity, ripened olives contain 15 percent to 35 percent oil, and OLIVE OIL is a major cooking oil. The oil content varies according to soil conditions, climate, and time of harvest.

Olives must be processed for consumption. In the Spanish method, green (unripe) olives are first treated with alkali, then fermented, and canned or bottled. The alkali destroys a bitter constituent called oleuropein. In the American method, half-ripe, reddish fruit are cured in lye (strong alkali). Olives darken as pigments oxidize. They are rinsed and then placed in fermentation tanks containing BRINE. In the Greek method, fully mature olives are harvested and soaked in brine to remove the bitter components. Ripe, pitted olives (10.47 g) provide 50 calories; protein, 0.4 g; carbohydrate, 2.9 g; fiber, 1.4 g; fat, 4.5 g; calcium, 42 mg; iron, 1.5 mg; sodium, 410 mg; and traces of B vitamins.

olive leaf extract The extracted juice of the leaf of the olive tree. This substance has been used for centuries as an herbal remedy for a variety of ailments, especially infection and fever. In the mid-1800s Dr. Daniel Hanbury reported that olive leaf extract was effective in reducing fever associated with an epidemic of malaria on a Mediterranean island.

In recent decades researchers have discovered that eleuropein, an ingredient in olive leaf extract, has antibacterial, antiviral, and anti-inflammatory properties and may help reduce the risk of CORONARY ARTERY DISEASE by lowering LOW-DENSITY LIPOPROTEIN (LDL) CHOLESTEROL. Laboratory studies conducted in the 1960s revealed than an active ingredient in eleuropein (elenolic acid) either killed or inhibited the growth of a number of pathogenic organisms, including bacteria, yeasts, and viruses, but because the compound rapidly binds to proteins in the blood, rendering it ineffective, attempts to develop a marketable drug from the substance were abandoned.

There is limited clinical evidence suggesting that olive leaf may help lower high blood pressure. However, reliable clinical studies on human beings that confirm the safety and potential health benefits of olive leaf extract do not yet exist. Nevertheless, nonscientific literature is filled with anecdotal accounts of the extract's ability to heal. It has been available as a dietary supplement in the United States since the mid-1990s.

Ruiz-Gutierrez, V. et al. "Oleuropein on Lipid and Fatty Acid Composition of Rat Heart." *Nutrition Research* 15, no. 1 (1995): 37–51.

olive oil An oil extracted from ground olives. Spain is currently the world's leading producer of bulk olive oil; Italy is a leading producer of bottled olive oil. The International Oil Agreement was negotiated through the U.N. to ensure olive cultivation and olive oil production in the Mediterranean region.

To produce olive oil, crushed olives are mechanically pressed several times. The temperature for olive oil extraction can be 50° to 110° F. There is no legal definition of "cold-pressed" oil, but the hotter the pressing, the more oil is extracted.

Olive oil is classified as a monounsaturated fat because it contains large amounts of OLEIC ACID, a monounsaturated FATTY ACID with one double bond and lacking two hydrogen atoms—in contrast with polyunsaturates, containing polyunsaturated fatty acids with two or more double bonds and lacking several pairs of hydrogen atoms, and saturates, containing predominantly saturated fatty acids (no double bonds and completely filled up with hydrogen atoms). Because olive oil is more stable to oxidation and rancidity, olive oil is not chemically stabilized (partially hydrogenated). Olive oil, like all oils, provides 14 g of fat per tablespoon, equivalent to 120 calories.

Proposed Grades of Oil

An independent U.S. FDA analysis of 30 imported olive oils revealed that five were not olive oil and 18 were mislabeled as "extra virgin" oil.

"Extra virgin olive oil" is prepared from mechanical pressing and is filtered without refining. "Virgin olive oil" is not highly refined and has a golden color and a unique flavor and taste. The acid content is no more than 1 percent. Virgin olive oil is filtered after pressing and is unrefined; the oil has a rather fruity flavor, and its acid content is less than 2 percent. Oil labeled "olive oil" is usually listed as being "100 percent pure." It is actually a blend of refined and unrefined olive oil and accounts for about 70 percent of U.S. olive oil consumption. Refining involves extraction at high temperatures and with solvents, neutralization of acids, and bleaching.

Potential Health Benefits of Olive Oil

People who eat predominantly olive oil have lower blood fat and cholesterol and a reduced risk of clogged arteries. Olive oil seems to lower blood levels of the less desirable form of CHOLESTEROL, LOW-DENSITY LIPOPROTEIN (LDL), while raising the level of HIGH-DENSITY LIPOPROTEIN (HDL), the more desirable kind of cholesterol. If the intake of polyunsaturates increases substantially above 7 percent of daily calories, the current average, polyunsaturated oils lower LDL (a desirable effect) but also lower HDL (an undesirable effect). By following current dietary guidelines that call for eating less fat (less than 30 percent of total calories) and less saturated fat (less than 10 percent of calories), people necessarily increase their consumption of unsaturates. Substituting monounsaturated oils for saturates and polyunsaturated fats and oils may be desirable while decreasing total fat consumption because high consumption of polyunsaturates is more likely to promote the oxidation of LDL cholesterol, the less desirable form, thus increasing the probability that oxidized LDL will be taken up by blood vessels and create plaque in arteries. Furthermore, animal studies suggest polyunsaturates can increase the risk of some forms of cancer. Cooking with olive oil instead of polyunsaturated vegetable oils (safflower oil, corn oil, etc.) may be advantageous because olive oil does not break down as readily when heated. (See also ATHEROSCLEROSIS; CARDIOVASCULAR DISEASE; FAT METABOLISM.)

"Special report: olive oil," *UC Berkeley Wellness Letter,* 11, no. 9 (June, 1995): 6.

omega-3 fatty acids See ESSENTIAL FATTY ACIDS; FLAXSEED OIL.

omega-6 fatty acids See ESSENTIAL FATTY ACIDS.

onion (*Allium cepa*) A vegetable with an underground bulb closely related to GARLIC and leeks, belonging to the lily family. Onions apparently originated in prehistoric central Asia, and were grown in ancient Egypt, Greece, and Rome, as well as China. There are more than 500 varieties; all of the edible species possess a pungent bulb. Europeans introduced onions to the Americas. Today, China, the United States, and India produce the largest yields, and onions rank sixth among vegetable crops worldwide.

Green onions may be harvested before the onion has matured. Alternatively, mature onion bulbs can be harvested. The length of time that dried bulbs can be stored ranges from several days to months, depending on the variety, their stage of maturity, and temperature and humidity during storage.

There are two types of dry onion. Flat onions, elongated Spanish onions, and Bermuda onions are usually mild flavored. They do not store as well as globe or late-crop onions, which frequently possess a stronger flavor. The latter store well and can be marketed throughout the year. Onions can be canned, dehydrated, frozen, or pickled.

Onions and their relatives possess a complex family of sulfur compounds related to the sulfur-containing amino acid cysteine. Once their layers are cut, the sulfur-containing compounds come into contact with an enzyme called allinase that releases volatile (gaseous) compounds that can irritate eyes. Cooking onions and GARLIC modifies these sulfur compounds, and they are not so irritating after cooking.

The medicinal properties of onions and garlic have been known for thousands of years, and recorded use includes treatment of wounds and infections, tumors, worms and parasites, weakness, FATIGUE, and asthma. Onions resemble garlic in terms of active ingredients and therapeutic effects. The consumption of garlic and onions correlates with lowered blood cholesterol levels. Generally, the higher the dose of garlic and onions, the greater the reduction. Onions also seem to lower blood CHOLESTEROL by helping to block cholesterol synthesis. Onions and garlic contain a variety of pungent, sulfur-containing compounds. One of these lowers BLOOD SUGAR; another counteracts blood platelet stickiness and reduces the tendency for blood to clot and, at the same time, raises HIGH-DENSITY LIPOPROTEIN (HDL), the desirable form of cholesterol that protects against cardiovascular disease. Onions help decrease elevated blood sugar levels in diabetics, possibly by slowing the breakdown of insulin, the hormone responsible for stimulating sugar uptake from the blood. They may also increase insulin secretion.

Onions as well as garlic contain compounds that block the production of inflammatory agents. For example, onions contain a FLAVONOID called QUERCETIN, a plant pigment known to reduce INFLAMMATION.

Both onions and garlic have antibiotic properties and have been shown to be effective against fungi and parasites as well. Furthermore, onions and garlic contain substances that block tumor growth in animals. Sulfur compounds apparently induce enzyme systems in the LIVER that detoxify potentially harmful compounds. Flavonoids are ANTIOXIDANTS that block damage due to free radical attack. Free radicals are highly reactive molecules that avidly attack cells. Flavonoids play a role in the anticancer properties of onions and garlic because free radical damage is linked to cancer.

Raw, chopped onions (1 cup, 160 g) provide 54 calories; protein, 1.9 g; carbohydrate, 11.7 g; fiber, 2.64 g; iron, 0.59 mg; potassium, 248 mg; vitamin C, 13 mg; thiamin, 0.1 mg; riboflavin, 0.02 mg; and niacin, 0.16 mg. (See also CARCINOGEN; HEART ATTACK.)

orange (*Citrus sinensis*) An orange-colored CITRUS FRUIT, that is the most popular fruit crop in the United States. Orange trees grow in semi-tropical regions and probably originated in Southeast Asia and Southern China. Spanish explorers and colonists brought the orange to the New World in the 16th century. In the United States, oranges are cultivated in Arizona, California, Texas, and Florida.

The three principal varieties of orange include the sweet (common, China orange), *C. sinensis;* the loose-skinned orange, *C. mobilis;* and the sour, bitter Seville orange, *C. aurantium.* Sweet oranges are represented by the blood orange, the navel orange and the Valencia (Spanish) orange, in addition to the Hamlin, Jaffa, and Pineapple varieties. Only sweet oranges are grown commercially in the United States.

The color of the orange peel does not necessarily indicate maturity because most oranges are picked green and exposed to ethylene gas at warm temperatures to enhance the orange color. Sour oranges, such as the Seville, are grown in Spain for marmalade and orange liqueurs.

Three quarters of U.S. orange production is processed and 80 percent of this ends up as frozen orange juice concentrate. Oranges and orange juice contain large amounts of VITAMIN C, and this contributes a substantial percentage of the vitamin C intake in the typical U.S. diet. The white inner portion of the peel is a good source of FLAVONOIDS, plant substances that act as antioxidants to prevent oxidative damage.

Certain individuals may be allergic to components in the orange peel and neither the peel nor products made from it should be eaten by such people. Citrus peel also contains citral, a compound that blocks the action of vitamin A. Organic orange peels have not been sprayed with pesticides. One orange (131 g) provides 60 calories; protein, 1.2 g; carbohydrate, 15.4 g; fiber, 2.97 g; potassium, 237 mg; vitamin C, 70 mg; thiamin 0.11 mg; riboflavin, 0.05 mg; and niacin, 0.37 mg.

Orange Juice

Fifteen percent of the U.S. orange crop is used for fresh orange juice. Commercial orange juice may contain up to 10 percent mandarin orange juice and up to 5 percent sour orange juice. Frozen orange juice concentrate contains up to four times higher concentrations of nutrients than fresh juice. Orange juice can be used to enhance the flavor of root vegetables and can be added to jams and marmalades. Orange juice is a good source of vitamin C and POTASSIUM. Most 100 percent orange juices provide 60 mg of vitamin C or more and 80 to 100 calories per cup. The current REFERENCE DAILY INTAKE (formerly the USRDA) for vitamin C is 60 mg. Vitamin C is readily oxidized upon exposure to the air to an inactive form. Fresh-squeezed orange juice loses 60 percent of its vitamin C when stored for 24 hours at room temperature, or 20 percent when orange juice is refrigerated.

Once prepared, orange juice should be kept chilled in a sealed container to reduce loss of vitamin C. In comparison with fresh orange juice, canned orange juice has been heated, reducing the levels of vitamin C. Up to 10 percent of U.S. frozen orange juice concentrate was estimated to be adulterated with sugar, orange solids, or chemical extenders in 1993. Some of the modifications have been subtle and difficult to detect. One cup of freshly squeezed orange juice provides 111 calories; 1.7 g protein; carbohydrate, 25.8 g; fiber, 0.5 g; potassium, 496 mg; vitamin C, 124 mg; thiamin, 0.22 mg; riboflavin, 0.07 mg; niacin, 0.78 mg.

Orange Drinks

Orange drinks and sodas are not orange juice. Their orange color is due to ARTIFICIAL FOOD COLORS. They represent empty calories because they are usually low in vitamin C and potassium and contain added SUCROSE, high FRUCTOSE CORN SYRUP, or ASPARTAME as SWEETENERS.

oregano (*Origanum vulgare;* wild marjoram) An herb used in cooking. The flavor of oregano's dark-green leaves resembles that of THYME and sweet MARJORAM, but is more pungent. The dried herb possesses a stronger flavor than fresh leaves. Oregano is often used to season Mexican and Italian dishes (PASTA and PIZZA), beans, meat such as lamb or poultry, and tomato soups. Before refrigeration, oregano was used to retard food spoilage. The essential oils of oregano possess a wide range of antifungal and bacterial activities.

organelle A subcellular particle or membrane component within cells that possesses a specialized metabolic function. Examples include MITOCHONDRIA, the nucleus, LYSOSOMES, and ENDOPLASMIC RETICULUM.

Each type of cell, with the exception of RED BLOOD CELLS, contains up to several hundred small, bean-shaped structures known as mitochondria. They are about the size of bacteria and contain their own DNA and protein synthesizing machinery. Mitochondria are called the powerhouses of the cell because they provide the enzymes that convert fuels such as FAT and CARBOHYDRATE to ENERGY, yielding metabolic end products, WATER, and CARBON DIOXIDE. In the typical cell, mitochondria produce more than 90 percent of the cell's chemical energy in the form of ATP.

Most cells, except red blood cells, contain a nucleus that houses DNA, the genetic blueprint of the cell, together with the machinery for synthesizing (replicating) DNA. The nucleus also contains enzymes needed to repair damage to DNA. DNA directs the formation of RNA molecules, which guide protein synthesis in the cytoplasm.

Lysosomes function as the cell's garbage disposal units. They degrade worn-out, damaged structures and PROTEIN whose components will be recycled. Endoplasmic reticulum is a complex membrane that houses enzymes that deactivate drugs and chemicals; that activate the B vitamin FOLIC ACID; elongate fatty acids; and synthesize specialized products for secretion, like digestive enzymes of the PANCREAS. (See also DNA; GENE; LIVER; METABOLISM.)

organic foods Foods that have been grown without chemical fertilizers and synthetic PESTICIDES. In the case of MEAT and dairy products, organic refers to animals raised without the use of growth promoters like hormones, antibiotics, and other substances that are added to animal feed. Any packaging or processing has been carried out without the use of synthetic compounds.

In 1990, the U.S. Congress passed the Organic Foods Production Act. This law required the U.S. Secretary of Agriculture to develop a National Organic Program (NOP), administered by the AGRICULTURAL MARKETING SERVICE, to establish uniform standards of organic food production as well as organic farming management. A 15-member National Organic Standards Board (NOSB) advises the Secretary of Agriculture on all aspects of the NOP and creates a list of approved and prohibited substances and ingredients in organic food production and handling. Among the substances prohibited: ash from manure burning, arsenic, lead salts, sodium fluoaluminate (mined), strychnine, and tobacco dust. As of October 21, 2002, organic farmers and organic food handlers seeking to be recognized as "organic" and to use the "organic" label must meet national standards through certification procedures.

Organic farming emphasizes animal manure, cultivation of legumes (plants that add nitrogen back to the soil), and biological pest control. A product can be "certified organic" if it contains at least 95 percent organic ingredients. The manufacturer needs to list the percentage of organic ingredients on the food label, or on the information panel, unless the food is 100 percent organic.

Labeling is voluntary; food producers who meet the government standards do not have to include the word *organic* on their products, but if they do, the labeling must meet certain requirements. Single-ingredient foods, such as pieces of fruit, will display a small "USDA organic" sticker. The seal also appears on packages of meat, cartons of milk or eggs, and cheese. Products that include organic ingredients, such as BREAKFAST CEREAL, fall into one of four categories. Those with 100 percent organic ingredients can include a statement saying that on the front of the package as well as the "USDA organic" seal. Products that are at least 95 percent organic can display the seal on the package front. If only 70 percent of the ingredients are organic, the package may indicate the product is "made with" the organic ingredients, and these must be listed on the side panel. Products with less than 70 percent organic ingredients cannot make any "organic" claims on the front of the package, but may list organic ingredients on the side. The Organic Food Production Act outlines uniform national certification criteria for organic growers and producers. This plan requires the accreditation of individual organic certifiers, to be defined by the NOSB. There are about 50 certification agencies in the United States and Canada, including the CALIFORNIA CERTIFIED ORGANIC FARMERS (CCOF) and Quality Certification Services.

Organic foods may be more costly, depending on the season, because more hand labor is involved when synthetic pesticides are omitted, and organic farming carries greater business risks. Organic food may not look as attractive as nonorganic produce because some chemicals that create a cosmetic effect have not been used. Nutrient-depleted soils will produce crops with decreased levels of trace nutrients, and good soils increase the nutritional quality of produce. There is evidence that organic produce may be more nutritious than produce from conventional farms, in terms of boron, calcium, chromium, copper, iodine, iron, magnesium, manganese, potassium, silicon, selenium, and zinc. For example, comparisons of trace minerals in organic and conventionally grown apples, corn, peas, potatoes, and wheat purchased over a two-year period suggested that the average nutrient content of organic foods can average twofold greater than that of conventional commercial produce. One explanation is that synthetic fertilizers of nitrate, phosphates, and other minerals do not enrich soils with a broad spectrum of nutrient minerals. Commercially grown food contained more aluminum, lead, and mercury.

Organic farming provides environmental dividends as well. It requires less energy, minimizes groundwater pollution, and reduces soil erosion. Manure benefits the soil by building loam and increasing water holding capacity. Legumes increase soil nitrogen for crops. Farm worker safety is also a consideration because synthetic pesticides pose the greatest risk to farm workers. The high crop yields of modern agriculture result partially from the use of chemical fertilizers and synthetic pesticides. The tonnage of pesticides applied to U.S. farms has grown 33-fold since World War II, and pesticide toxicity has increased tenfold. The decreased use of synthetic pesticides, together with crop rotation and biological pest control, in combination with organic farming methods and judicious use of certain synthetic pesticides and fertilizers and conservation, seems a realistic approach to preserve resources.

The organic food market is growing rapidly. According to the AGRICULTURAL RESEARCH SERVICE, one in four Americans buys organic foods. Retail sales of organic products, which reached $7.8 billion in 2000, increased by 20 percent annually between 1995 and 2001. (See also CERTIFIED ORGANIC VEGETABLES; NATURAL FOOD.)

Brown, James E. *Organic Gardening, Vegetable Growing in Simple Terms.* New York: Simon & Schuster, 1999.

organic meat MEAT grown without growth promoters like hormones, antibiotics, and other substances that are added to animal feed. (See also ANTIBIOTIC-RESISTANT BACTERIA IN FOOD; ORGANIC FOODS.)

organ meat MEAT that represents internal organs such as the LIVER, kidney, heart, and brains. In contrast, nonorgan meat is comprised primarily of muscle and connective tissue. Sweetbreads are derived from the thymus gland of young cattle. (See also PROCESSED FOOD.)

ornithine A nonessential AMINO ACID required in the formation of UREA, the end product of PROTEIN metabolism. Ornithine is made by the body. Although not incorporated into proteins, ornithine helps the LIVER convert the toxic nitrogen waste AMMONIA to urea via the UREA CYCLE, the enzyme system responsible for urea formation. Urea is eliminated by the KIDNEYS in urine. Ornithine is converted by the body to ARGININE, an amino acid that functions as a protein building block. Ornithine also forms polyamines, a family of nitrogen-containing chemicals that play a role in cell differentiation and growth.

Ornithine Supplements

Ornithine, as well as arginine, has found its way into health food stores. Body builders and athletes use ornithine out of the belief that it stimulates the production of GROWTH HORMONE.

Growth hormone causes muscle growth in normal animals. Moderate amounts of arginine and ornithine do not seem to affect growth hormone levels. Very large oral doses of ornithine may stimulate the release of growth hormone; however, the evidence that it can selectively burn fat and build muscle remains skimpy. Ornithine's beneficial effects for athletes may be partially due to its role in eliminating nitrogen waste products. In addition, in lab animals ornithine seems to stimulate the THYMUS GLAND, thus boosting immunity. Consumption of large amounts of single amino acids over time may cause potentially dangerous side effects. Seizures have been reported to occur with high doses of ornithine, and the long-term effects of a high dosage of ornithine are not known. Ornithine supplements are not recommended for patients with kidney or liver conditions. Safety data are inadequate for pregnant and breast-feeding women. (See also AMINO ACID METABOLISM; EXERCISE; LYSINE.)

orthomolecular medicine The use of NUTRIENTS and naturally occurring materials to treat illness and disease due to inherited enzyme deficiencies. Human nutrition has moved beyond treating disease to preventing illness and improving the quality of life and using large amounts of VITAMINS. Megavitamin therapy is one strategy to treat deficiencies that are the result of increased needs due to inheritance, though it continues to be controversial. The basis for this approach is the variability in enzyme levels and efficiencies among individuals. Mutant enzymes can require much larger amounts of vitamins than usual in order to function optimally. Vitamin and mineral therapy has successfully been used to treat disease and to improve health in some cases. Furthermore, evidence points to a biochemical imbalance in neurological disorders and learning disabilities, among others.

There is a growing awareness that mild deficiencies of minerals and vitamins play a role in chronic diseases. Deficiencies of antioxidant vitamins are linked to CARDIOVASCULAR DISEASE and certain forms of CANCER, for example. Nutrient malabsorption can lead to deficiencies with aging and therapeutic doses of vitamins and minerals may be required to prevent such common conditions as osteoporosis. Environmental stress in the form of air pollutants, drugs, viral infections, and reliance on convenience foods increases vitamin needs, and supplementation can be an effective strategy in these situations.

Conditions where large amounts of vitamins (more than 10 times the Recommended Dietary Allowance) are well recognized clinically include treatment of elevated cholesterol with B vitamin niacin, and of skin disorders with vitamin A derivatives. On the other hand, the use of vitamins to treat conditions other than well-established deficiency diseases is still considered unorthodox in some medical circles.

Megavitamin treatment is not always effective. The literature on megavitamin therapy also contains exaggerated claims of cure based on misinterpretations of data from case studies of treated individuals. Vitamins are generally safer than most synthetic drugs and they are less expensive, but most experts believe that supplements are no substitute for a wholesome diet. Excessive amounts of any nutrient can lead to possible side effects and toxicity. (See also MALABSORPTION.)

Challem, J. "Beta-Carotene and Other Carotenoids: Promises, Failures, and a New Vision," *Journal of Orthomolecular Medicine* 12 (1997): 11–19.

ossification The process of bone formation. Ossification requires CALCIUM, MAGNESIUM, and PHOSPHORUS as primary building blocks. Many trace nutrients are needed for bone building: MANGANESE, BORON, VITAMIN D, VITAMIN K, VITAMIN C, VITAMIN A, FLUORIDE, COPPER, ZINC, and SILICON. The rate of bone growth is controlled by hormones such as GROWTH HORMONE from the PITUITARY GLAND and steroid hormones produced by the ovaries and testes. The growth of the SKELETON requires increased intake of calcium over the amount lost (positive calcium balance) until adult size is reached, usually by the late teens or early twenties. Lengthwise bone growth in women is generally completed earlier than in men.

Osteoblasts are cells that form calcified deposits to make up bony structure. They secrete the connective tissue protein COLLAGEN, which forms filaments that in turn form a matrix. Osteoblasts connect with another type of cell called osteocytes, which are bone cells that are surrounded by crystallized minerals and lie deep within bone. Thus, osteocytes and osteoblasts remain connected with each other and maintain bone structure. Throughout life, bone is constantly being reabsorbed and reformed. Adult bone replacement amounts to about 18 percent per year. (See also OSTEOMALACIA; OSTEOPOROSIS; RICKETS.)

osteoarthritis A chronic, degenerative joint disease and the most common form of ARTHRITIS. Cartilage may be destroyed and bone spur formation can limit joint function. Weight-bearing joints such as ankles, hips, spine, and knees are often affected. A point is reached at which repair mechanisms can no longer keep up with wear and tear. Joints may be stiff and sore due to damage through prolonged usage. Most Americans over the age of 50 experience a degree of osteoarthritis. Osteoarthritis may follow infections or joint injury. STRESS, excessive weight, poor posture, imbalanced musculoskeletal system, even poor muscle tone aggravate the condition. Physical therapy, structural alignments and exercise may aid in treating early degenerative joint disease.

It is important to curtail INFLAMMATION. Scavenger cells (MACROPHAGES), summoned to the damaged area release substances that destroy cell debris and can damage surrounding healthy tissue. In addition, FREE RADICALS (extremely reactive oxidants) cause chronic inflammation when produced at joints. ANTIOXIDANTS such as vitamin E, VITAMIN C, BETA-CAROTENE, and related carotenoids and FLAVONOIDS can quash free radicals and reduce inflammation. Flavonoids are natural antioxidants found in the pulp of citrus fruit, most vegetables and fruits. High levels of fish and fish oil and seed oils from flax, borage, and black currant lessen pain and may help arthritic patients. These oils belong to the omega-3 class of fatty acids, known to blunt inflammation. They give rise to a family of PROSTAGLANDINS (PG_3) fat-derived hormones that control inflammation.

Food allergy and food sensitivity can aggravate inflammation in degenerative joint disease. A diet that eliminates food allergens may minimize overreaction of the immune system in food-sensitive people. Niacinamide has been used to improve the range of joint motion and to help lessens pain and swelling. Some studies have shown that CHONDROITIN (a complex CARBOHYDRATE), when taken with the amino sugar GLUCOSAMINE, can significantly relieve symptoms of osteoarthritis. In the body chondroitin acts like a magnet, drawing nutrient-filled fluids into tendons, ligaments, and cartilage. This helps make the cartilage more shock absorbent.

As a dietary supplement chondroitin can reduce joint pain and inflammation and may help maintain or repair cartilage. It is still unclear how this is achieved. However, patients who have taken chondroitin supplements show increased levels of hyaluronic acid, a primary component of the fluid that lubricates joints. These benefits seem to increase when chondroitin is taken in combination with glucosamine, an amino sugar needed by the body to form connective tissue. Patients suffering from osteoarthritis who took chondroitin and glucosamine supplements showed reduced pain and improved joint mobility.

The long-term safety of these supplements has not yet been determined. There are some indications that glucosamine can increase blood sugar levels, so people with diabetes should avoid taking supplements that mix chondroitin with glucosamine unless done under a doctor's supervision. (See also ESSENTIAL FATTY ACIDS; OSTEOPOROSIS; RHEUMATOID ARTHRITIS.)

McAlindon, Timothy E. et al. "Glucosamine and Chondroitin for Treatment of Osteoarthritis: A Systematic Quality Assessment and Meta-Analysis," *Journal of the American Medical Association* 283 (2000): 1,469–1,475.

osteomalacia (adult rickets) An adult bone disease caused by chronic VITAMIN D deficiency or by a deficiency of CALCIUM or PHOSPHORUS. In osteomalacia, bones do not calcify properly; they become soft and flexible, leading to a distortion of the pelvis, spine, and rib cage. Symptoms include pain in these regions and progressive weakness. When the diet contains adequate calcium and phosphorus, osteomalacia can easily be prevented with extra VITAMIN D during the winter months. Vitamin D is manufactured in the skin when exposed to sunshine; it has been commonly added to milk and milk products since the 1940s. (See also OSTEOPOROSIS.)

osteoporosis A chronic degenerative disease due to the loss of bone mass or increased bone porosity. The term *osteoporosis* means, literally, porous bones. The affected bones are deficient in CALCIUM, phosphorus, and other minerals, and they contain less structural protein. In contrast, another bone disease, OSTEOMALACIA, results from soft bones due to altered mineral ratios. Osteoporosis is the most common bone disorder in America. It occurs much more frequently in women than in men. Men have larger bones, eat more calcium and get more exercise than women, although alcoholic men are an exception. Mineral loss from bones typically begins in the 20s, and 50 percent of the bone loss in women occurs before menopause. Postmenopausal osteoporosis (type I) is the most common form; type II osteoporosis occurs with AGING. In both men and women, symptoms include curved spine, loss of height, and brittle, accident-prone bones, particularly the spin and hip. Calcium is preferentially lost from the long bones of the legs, the spine, the jaw bone, the wrists and the ankles when there is not enough calcium in the diet, or when it is poorly absorbed. Loss of bone of the spine can lead to compression fractures and a loss in weight frequently associated with aging. With reduced bone support, gums may be damaged and teeth may be lost.

The social and economic impact of osteoporosis is enormous. An estimated 10 million Americans have this disease, and another 34 million people are estimated to have low bone mass, placing them at increased risk for osteoporosis. About 1.5 million fractures due to weakened bones occur each year in the United States. With osteoporosis, fractured bones mend slowly.

Most fractures associated with this disease occur in the spine, hips, wrists, and ribs. The risk that a woman will suffer a hip fracture during her lifetime is the same as her combined risk for developing breast, uterine, and ovarian cancer. Half of all women and a third of all men will suffer an osteoporosis-related fracture after their 50th birthday.

Hip fractures can be especially debilitating and even deadly. One-fourth of patients who could walk before a hip fracture are unable to do so once the fracture heals. About a quarter of those who suffer hip fractures after the age of 50 die within a year after their injury.

The rate at which bone is lost also affects the risk of osteoporosis. Contrary to common belief, bone is a dynamic tissue; it is constantly being formed and broken down. Until the early 20s, more bone is made than broken down as growth progresses. Bone mineral content of the spine and wrist reaches a maximum density in the late 30s and early 40s. After peak bone loss has been reached, there is little change until the 40s, when the balance between synthesis and degradation shifts to favor degradation. Bone loss accelerates at menopause and continues at a high rate for about 10 years. Afterward, bone is lost at a rate of 0.2 percent to 0.5 percent per year. Typically, a U.S. female will lose between 30 percent and 50 percent of her cortical bone (the spongy interior bone structure). It has often been assumed that menopause triggers bone loss. However, the rate of bone loss increases rapidly between the ages of 40 and 44, much earlier than menopause, which in the United States occurs at an average age of 52.

Osteoporosis is a complex disease involving both genetic and environmental factors, including such nonmodifiable factors as gender, ethnic background, body build, family history of osteoporosis, and age. Nevertheless, osteoporosis is one of the most preventable of the degenerative diseases.

Medical history affects the risk of osteoporosis as follows:

- Hormone imbalance. Because hormones maintain bone structure, hormonal imbalances can lead to osteoporosis. Examples include deficiencies of estrogen due to surgical removal of ovaries, and to postmenopause; Cushing's syndrome (excessive production of GLUCOCORTICOIDS by the adrenal glands); conditions that lead to excessive glucocorticoids, as chronic stress or overmedication with hydrocortisone; and overproduction of hormones from the pituitary gland; and cortisone and thyroid medications;
- Certain rare genetic diseases (Marfan's syndrome, homocystinuria);
- RHEUMATOID ARTHRITIS;
- Conditions that promote ACIDOSIS, such as chronic obstructive lung disease and possibly diabetes;
- Milk sensitivity or milk allergy;
- Anorexia nervosa;
- Conditions that lead to severe calcium malabsorption. These include excessive use of medications, such as certain anticonvulsant drugs and anticancer drugs that block calcium uptake; low stomach acid production (hypochlorhydria, achlorhydria); stomach surgery, and anti-ulcer drugs, like cimetidine, which blocks stomach acid production and limits calcium digestion).

Lifestyle factors play a major role in determining the risk of osteoporosis, including:

- A lack of physical, weight-bearing exercise (sedentary lifestyle, being bedridden). Exercise such as walking, jogging, and dancing increases bone density and delays bone loss at all ages. On the other hand, strenuous exercise such as running a marathon can disrupt hormone balance and increase bone loss.
- Excessive alcohol consumption contributes to malnutrition and increased bone loss.
- Cigarette smoking increases bone degradation and limits bone rebuilding.
- Stress, both emotional and physical—fear, trauma, dehydration, surgery, and the like—can lead to bone loss in many elderly persons, depending upon the degree of calcium malabsorption, the absorbability of dietary calcium and other lifestyle influences.

Various dietary factors affect bone strength and bone turnover. These include a deficiency of calcium, trace minerals, and vitamin D. High bone density is a major factor in decreasing the risk of bone loss, and strong bones require adequate dietary calcium. Bones can be thought of as a bank account: The larger the bone and the more calcium it has, the more it can tolerate slow withdrawal as the body ages. With age, the ability to absorb calcium declines; this difference is made up by increased production of hormones that promote mineral loss from bone. Calcium deficiency is linked to osteoporosis.

The RECOMMENDED DIETARY ALLOWANCE (RDA) for calcium in the United States is 800 mg for adult women. The RDA for girls and young women between the ages of 12 and 19 is 1,200 mg; they generally get only 900 mg of calcium daily. American women generally consume less than 500 mg of calcium daily after menopause, which increases the risk of osteoporosis. The National Institutes of Health recommends that postmenopausal women not taking estrogen, and men over 65, consume 1,000 to 1,500 mg of calcium daily. The extra 1,000 mg they need to add could come from any one of the following: supplementation with about 1,000 mg of calcium; consuming three cups of milk, two cups of nonfat yogurt, four ounces of cheese, nine ounces of sardines, or four to five cups of cooked broccoli or kale daily. These portions of canned fish and vegetables are much more of these foods than most people want in a day. Furthermore, many women decrease their intake of dairy products due to milk sensitivity and lactose intolerance therefore, many may opt for calcium supplements.

MAGNESIUM is also quite important in maintaining bone strength. Supplementation with magnesium together with calcium may help prevent bone thinning and actually help rebuild bone in postmenopausal women with osteoporosis. A mild magnesium deficiency increases the risk of osteoporosis. Magnesium deficiency is associated with lowered levels of calcitriol, the active form of VITAMIN D (see below). Magnesium may help the secretion of PARATHYROID hormone, required for the formation of adequate calcitriol.

In addition to major mineral nutrients, calcium, and magnesium, many trace mineral nutrients support calcium uptake and contribute to bone strength. BORON deprivation increases urinary excretion of calcium, and adequate dietary boron may cut the bone loss associated with menopause. Boron may affect parathyroid hormone and the activation of estrogen and vitamin D to calcitriol. Adequate boron seems to diminish bone losses associated with menopause. COPPER plays a role in calcium assimilation; it is required to stabilize COLLAGEN, the structural proteins that help form the matrix for calcification. Osteoporosis occurs with copper deficiency; the bones of copper-deficient animals are fragile. Fluoride was once thought to be helpful in preventing osteoporosis, but a 1999 study by the Centers for Disease Control and Prevention found no evidence to support that theory.

Vitamins

Vitamin D is required for calcium absorption. It is converted to the hormone calcitriol, which stimulates the production of calcium uptake proteins. Vitamin D is formed in the skin and is also obtained from the diet, though milk and fortified cereals are the only major sources. The liver and kidneys process the vitamin to calcitriol. This activated form of vitamin D is 10 times more effective in stimulating calcium absorption than vitamin D. Studies show that elderly patients who remain indoors during the winter without exposure to sunlight or its equivalent run the risk of decreased calcium uptake.

VITAMIN C is required for normal collagen fiber formation, and presumably for normal calcification. Low VITAMIN B_6, FOLIC ACID, and VITAMIN B_{12} deficiencies may contribute to the risk of osteoporosis. These vitamins play a role in the metabolism of sulfur-containing AMINO ACIDS, METHIONINE, and CYSTEINE. The accumulation of a by-product of methionine degradation, HOMOCYSTEINE, may occur with deficiencies, and this buildup is implicated in osteoporosis as well as other degenerative diseases. VITAMIN K plays a role in the formation of a calcium-binding protein, osteocalcin. Proper mineralization requires adequate levels of this protein. Vitamin K is abundant in green leafy VEGETABLES, a possible factor in the protection against osteoporosis afforded by a vegetarian diet.

Other dietary factors increase the risk of osteoporosis. Crash dieting or severe caloric restriction leads to mineral malnutrition, including calcium deficiency. Close examination of the typical American diet reveals a high protein intake but frequent deficiencies of trace minerals required for bone building. Urinary calcium losses appear to increase with high-protein diets, irrespective of dietary calcium. High-protein diets are also high-phosphate diets, and excessive phosphate also increases calcium excretion.

Vegetarian diets correlate with decreased prevalence of osteoporosis, although initial bone mass of vegetarians may be equivalent to that of meat eaters. Vegetarian diets provide less protein and phosphorus but more boron. Each of the following factors increases bone loss.

- Excessive sugar consumption increases calcium excretion.
- Excessive coffee and caffeine intake appear to increase calcium excretion. Generally, the more coffee that is consumed, the less milk. Women who drink milk throughout their adult lives may be able to counter the bone-thinning effects of coffee.
- Excessive soft drinks containing phosphate. A high phosphate diet with limited calcium limits calcium absorption and increases bone degradation.
- Excessive sodium has been linked to increased risk of osteoporosis and increased urinary losses of calcium.
- Decreased estrogen production after menopause increases bone loss. Theoretically, estrogen stimulates vitamin D to increase calcium intake; it slows calcium loss by the kidneys; and it increases production of a hormone to store calcium in bone. With estrogen deficiency, osteo-

clasts, cells that break down bone, are more sensitive to parathyroid hormone, causing increased bone breakdown. While estrogen therapy for elderly women stops further bone loss and decreases the risk of fractures of thinned bones after menopause, alone it may not prevent osteoporosis.

Recommendations

Patients should:

- consume enough calcium and magnesium. Girls and young women can take calcium supplements and eat calcium-rich foods to build up their bone density during their growth years. A daily consumption of up to 1,000 mg of calcium before menopause and 1,500 mg daily after menopause is recommended. People who are susceptible to kidney stones need to consult their physician before calcium supplementation. Several hundred mg of magnesium are generally well tolerated; more can lead to diarrhea.
- obtain enough vitamin D from fortified milk and milk products to deposit calcium into bones. Adequate sunshine enables the skin to make vitamin D.
- obtain enough manganese, copper, and zinc. These minerals help with calcium utilization for bone building.
- avoid excessive fiber supplements, high-protein diets, and soft drinks with phosphate.
- stop smoking.
- exercise regularly throughout life. Walking daily, cycling, dancing, bike riding, and similar exercises are most beneficial in retaining calcium in bone.
- avoid excessive amounts of antacids that contain aluminum. Aluminum can interfere with normal calcium absorption and assimilation.
- consult a specialist regarding estrogen replacement therapy after menopause. For calcium to reverse osteoporosis after menopause, a woman may need to take low doses of estrogen and to exercise daily in addition to calcium supplementation. Who should not take estrogen? Women who are obese, who have a history of breast cancer or blood clotting problems. Estrogen therapy requires medical supervision because of potential side effects. (See also OSTEOARTHRITIS.)

Marchigiano, G. "Calcium Intake in Midlife Women: One step in Preventing Osteoporosis." *Orthopaedic Nursing* (September/October 1999): 11–20.

ovalbumin The major egg PROTEIN. Ovalbumin represents about 25 percent of the total protein of EGG white.

Overeaters Anonymous (OA) An organization that provides support groups based on the Twelve Step Program of Alcoholics Anonymous. These groups can help people deal with issues surrounding compulsive eating, bingeing and purging. There are no dues, and participation is voluntary. It is run entirely by volunteers.

Members of OA focus on getting control of their own lives and identifying underlying emotional issues, not on DIETING, nor on losing weight, nor even on food. There are no weigh-ins and no guarantees of weight loss. Eating disorder programs managed by hospitals and clinics often send their participants to OA to strengthen their own behavior modification strategies. (See also OBESITY; WEIGHT MANAGEMENT.)

overweight In 1998 the federal government adopted new standards for determining whether a person is overweight or obese. Before then people were considered overweight if their weight was at least 10 percent to 20 percent over optimal body weight. Obesity was defined as being more than 25 percent over the optimal body weight for men and 30 percent over the optimal body weight for women.

Under the new standards a person with a BODY MASS INDEX (BMI) of 25 or more is considered overweight. The BMI is determined by dividing a person's weight in kilograms by the square of his or her height in meters. A healthy BMI falls between 19 and 25. A person with a BMI of 30 or above is considered obese. (See also DIETING; FAT; IDEAL BODY WEIGHT; WEIGHT MANAGEMENT.)

ovo-vegetarian One who eats plant-derived foods and eggs. A lacto-ovo-vegetarian is one who eats plant-derived foods, milk products, and eggs. (See also VEGETARIAN.)

oxalic acid/oxalate An acid found in a variety of vegetables that binds CALCIUM very tightly. Oxalic acid forms salts called oxalates with minerals, making them less available for absorption. SPINACH, beet greens, CHIVES, RHUBARB, and PARSLEY contain significant amounts of calcium, but they also contain high levels of oxalic acid. However, oxalic acid does not block calcium uptake of IRON or of the calcium in other foods. It is not clear whether cooking greens makes calcium more available. Even with oxalates, these green leafy vegetables will supply significant TRACE MINERALS, plus VITAMINS and FIBER, and should be part of a BALANCED DIET.

Oxalic acid may be a potential by-product of vitamin C consumption in excess of amounts achievable from dietary sources in cases of kidney disease and of those prone to the formation of calcium oxalate KIDNEY STONES, based on anecdotal reports in a small number of cases.

Oxalic acid consumption may be a problem for people who are prone to kidney stones, or those who eat a lot of BRAN for fiber and whose diets are high in oxalates and low in calcium. MAGNESIUM increases the solubility of calcium oxalate and decreases the probability of kidney stones, and VITAMIN B_6 reduces oxalate production. Getting enough VITAMIN K is also important: Vitamin K assists in the formation of a urinary protein that inhibits calcium oxalate precipitation and helps inhibit kidney stone formation. (See also MALABSORPTION.)

oxaloacetic acid An acid that is both the starting point and final product of the KREB'S CYCLE. This cycle plays a central role in the oxidation of FAT, CARBOHYDRATES, and AMINO ACIDS for energy production by the body. Oxaloacetic acid receives incoming carbon atoms to form CITRIC ACID. Sequential oxidation steps release these carbon atoms as CARBON DIOXIDE, the ultimate end product, while regenerating oxaloacetic acid. Oxaloacetic acid serves a second role: It can accept nitrogen to generate the acidic AMINO ACID, ASPARTIC ACID. It is also required to synthesize GLUCOSE (BLOOD SUGAR) from amino acids to fuel the brain during STARVATION. (See also CARBOHYDRATE METABOLISM; GLUCONEOGENESIS.)

oxidation The primary chemical reaction by which chemical ENERGY is released from food for use by cells. The oxidation of fuel molecules in foods involves the addition of oxygen atoms to carbon atoms and the removal of hydrogen atoms. The ultimate oxidation product of carbon compounds is CARBON DIOXIDE. Indeed, carbon dioxide in expired air comes from the direct oxidation of FAT, CARBOHYDRATE, PROTEIN, and other fuel molecules by cells in the body.

Most oxidation takes place in small particles in the cytoplasm known as mitochondria. These cellular powerhouses consume more than 90 percent of the oxygen that the cells use. They oxidize most of the fuels to carbon dioxide, while producing ATP. This form of chemical energy is readily used to power energy-requiring operations of the cell. The total energy released by oxidations occurring in cells is the same as when substances are burned in a test tube. The difference lies in the fact that within cells oxidation proceeds in small steps, speeded up by ENZYMES, in order to capture chemical energy efficiently. About 40 percent of the potential energy trapped in the simple sugar GLUCOSE, for example, is captured as ATP.

Cellular oxidations require electron carriers called COENZYMES as enzyme helpers. The most important are NICOTINAMIDE ADENINE DINUCLEOTIDE (NAD), derived from the B vitamin NIACIN, and FLAVIN ADENINE DINUCLEOTIDE (FAD), derived from the B vitamin RIBOFLAVIN. In this process oxygen is reduced to water (METABOLIC WATER), also produced by mitochondria, which generate about 200 ml daily.

Many degradative enzymes function together as METABOLIC PATHWAYS. Important energy-yielding pathways oxidize glucose (GLYCOLYSIS) and carbohydrate, fatty acids and amino acids (KREB'S CYCLE). Most ATP formation occurs in mitochondria via a pathway called OXIDATIVE PHOSPHORYLATION. (See also AMINO ACID METABOLISM; CARBOHYDRATE METABOLISM; FAT METABOLISM.)

oxidative phosphorylation The oxygen-dependent process of trapping chemical ENERGY released by the OXIDATION of fuel molecules. Oxidative phosphorylation occurs in MITOCHONDRIA, small particles in cells that function as powerhouses. Cellular oxidations in mitochondria release electrons that are transported to oxygen. Their passage to oxygen is performed by a sequence of electron carriers and enzymes known collectively as the ELECTRON TRANSPORT CHAIN. When electrons are transported from one electron carrier to the next and ultimately to oxygen, a portion of the released energy is trapped as ATP; the remainder is lost as heat. ATP is a chemical form of energy universally used by cells to drive energy-requiring processes, from the contraction of muscle fibers and the transport of nutrients into cells to the biosynthesis of cellular constituents for cell growth and maintenance. Only mitochondria possess the enzyme machinery for coupling the flow of electrons to the reduction of oxygen to water, and simultaneously to synthesize ATP.

Electron transport and ATP production can be uncoupled, that is, oxidations can occur with decreased ATP production. Various chemicals alter the structure of mitochondria and act as uncouplers; certain environmental pollutants, poisons, and drugs can interfere with ATP production, with potentially disastrous effects on cellular metabolism. Poisons like cyanide block electron transport, hence ATP production, in cells. The drug dinitrophenol was once marketed as a weight loss aid because it allowed more fuel to be burned with less ATP production. But the use of dinitrophenol led to excessive heat production, and it was banned. Even large amounts of normal products such as BILE PIGMENT, bilirubin, and fatty acids can act as uncouplers. Certain patches of body fat called brown fat possess mitochondria that can be hormonally uncoupled to produce heat to protect newborn mammals, including infants. Thyroid hormone and the nervous system can regulate the efficiency of ATP production to a limited extent.

oxygen The element that accounts for approximately 21 percent of Earth's atmosphere and is essential for aerobic organisms. Animals require ample oxygen to oxidize food to ENERGY. Carbon atoms are oxidized to CARBON DIOXIDE, the first metabolic waste product. Oxygen acts as the ultimate oxidizing agent of fuel molecules, and it is reduced to WATER, the second waste product.

Oxygen taken up from air in the lungs must be distributed throughout the body to all cells via the circulatory system. Thus, oxygen is absorbed into the bloodstream at the lungs, where it binds to the oxygen carrier protein in RED BLOOD CELLS called HEMOGLOBIN. Oxygenated red blood cells are pumped to tissues and oxygen is released in capillaries in response to acidic waste products and carbon dioxide from cellular metabolism, and to a low oxygen concentration. Oxygen molecules simply diffuse (migrate) into cells to participate in cellular oxidations.

Oxygen can be partially reduced by enzymes to form highly reactive molecules. Thus, activated phagocytic cells (neutrophils, macrophages) produce the FREE RADICAL superoxide, which can destroy invading microorganisms. Overproduction of superoxide during chronic INFLAMMATION can readily damage cellular components like proteins, lipids, and DNA. Cells possess defense mechanisms to combat such agents. COPPER, MANGANESE, and ZINC activate the enzyme SUPEROXIDE DISMUTASE, which neutralizes superoxide. (See also ANTIOXIDANT.)

oxygen debt The amount of OXYGEN required to support the physiologic response to strenuous physical activity. Oxygen debt is characterized by rapid or labored breathing (hyperventilation) and increased metabolic rate that continues when EXERCISE ceases. During mild physical exercise, oxygen delivered by the bloodstream is adequate for muscles to oxidize GLUCOSE (BLOOD SUGAR) completely to CARBON DIOXIDE. The liberated energy powers muscle contraction. However, during vigorous exercise, oxygen delivery to muscle cells becomes too slow to produce enough ATP from the oxidation of glucose and fatty acids to meet the increased demand of muscle contraction. In this case, additional ATP can be generated by the incomplete oxidation of glucose through a process called anaerobic GLYCOLYSIS.

Glycolysis is the initial stage of carbohydrate oxidation, which oxidizes glucose to a fragment called PYRUVIC ACID and produces ATP without the participation of oxygen. In muscle cells, the increased need for ATP outstrips the cells' ability to oxidize pyruvic acid during strenuous exercise. In this case pyruvic acid is converted to LACTIC ACID, which diffuses into the bloodstream to be processed to glucose by the liver. Panting at the end of strenuous exercise provides additional oxygen, which is used to replenish cellular ATP and to rebuild GLYCO-

GEN (stored glucose) in muscle fibers. Lactic acid accumulation may be partially responsible for the fatigue and stress that accompany strenuous exercise. During the recovery period, the oxygen debt is repaid, lactic acid buildup is disposed of, energy stores are replenished, and the breathing rate normalizes. (See also ANAEROBIC; CARBOHYDRATE METABOLISM.)

oyster (*Ostrea spp.*) A saltwater shellfish belonging to the family of bivalve mollusks. Although indigenous to many parts of the world, oysters are now farmed to avoid depletion and to minimize their contamination from polluted water. East Coast and West Coast varieties are available in the United States. In oyster cultivation, small seed oysters are first attached to a stationary support. As they grow in size they are transferred to beds, where their growth can be supervised. Traditionally it was recommended that oysters and clams be harvested only in months containing an "r" (September through April) to avoid contamination by blooms of "red tide" microorganisms. These organisms produce a toxin that accumulates in oysters and mussels and can cause food poisoning. State health departments monitor shellfish and may restrict harvest in other months. A marine bacterium, *Vibrio vulnificus,* can infect warm, brackish waters and infest shellfish such as oysters. The bacterium can cause blood poisoning in individuals with a weakened immune system.

Fresh oysters are traditionally eaten raw with lemon juice or sauce. However, the consumption of raw or partially and cooked shellfish substantially increases the risk of food poisoning and of diseases transmitted by sewage, such as hepatitis A and Norwalk virus. Cooked oysters are far safer. They can be poached, browned, cooked on skewers, or used in soups and sauces. Oysters canned in oil contain more calories than fresh oysters. Oysters are an excellent source of ZINC, though different varieties contain differing amounts. One oyster, cooked (100 g), provides 90 calories; protein, 5 g; carbohydrate, 5 g; fat, 5 g; cholesterol, 35 mg; calcium, 49 mg; iron, 3 mg; zinc, 9 mg; thiamin, 0.15 mg; riboflavin, 0.29 mg; niacin, 2.1 mg.

oyster shell A common CALCIUM supplement that is not a recommended calcium source because it contains variable amounts of LEAD, a widespread environmental pollutant. Lead resembles calcium and is incorporated into the bone and shells of many organisms. (See also HEAVY METALS; SEAFOOD.)

P

PABA (para-aminobenzoic acid) A bacterial growth promoter. Bacteria use PABA to manufacture FOLIC ACID. In humans and animals, folacin is a B VITAMIN required for cell multiplication and growth; humans cannot convert PABA to folacin, so PABA is not a vitamin. In animals like rats and mice, PABA can stimulate intestinal bacteria to produce enough folic acid to meet the animals' needs. This explains why PABA was once considered a vitamin. PABA is widespread in foods; GRAINS, wheat germ, and organ meats are noteworthy.

Some people have reported that oral doses of PABA reduced hair loss and symptoms of ARTHRITIS. However, if taken orally, PABA may cause nausea and diarrhea. PABA can accumulate in tissues and damage the liver. Until recently, PABA was a common ingredient in sunscreen to block ultraviolet radiation, which ages the SKIN. Applied to the skin, PABA can cause rash in susceptible people. When taken orally, PABA may make the skin more sensitive to sunburn and increase the risk of skin cancer, and it can increase bacterial resistance to sulfa drugs. PABA has been used as a pharmaceutical agent to treat rickettsial infections. Rickettsia are microorganisms that cause diseases such as typhus and Rocky Mountain spotted fever. Safety data for oral use are inadequate for pregnant and breast-feeding women. (See also ANTIMETABOLITE; ULTRAVIOLET LIGHT.)

packaging The container used to store and display food items. In addition to storing a food safely, in the context of marketing, packaging refers to the visual impact of a packaged food, an important factor in sales. Many brands of food must compete with similar products on a store shelf in order to catch the consumer's eye. Food choices in U.S. SUPERMARKETS have more than doubled during the last 20 years, yet consumers spend an average of 30 minutes per visit to a supermarket, the same length of time as earlier.

The shapes, sizes, colors, designs, letters, and pictures, even the information on the food labels, can prompt a shopper to buy one product over the next. For example, brown and gold and country scenes can be used to promote more wholesome products like whole wheat bread. Packages can also project a calculated image to target a specific consumer group. Thus, children are targeted for presweetened cold BREAKFAST CEREALS. The packing image may reflect a health consciousness or it may play upon consumer fears, desires for acceptance, success, romance, or even a desirable lifestyle.

Plastic Food Containers

Plastics generally decompose very slowly because they are resistant to microbial attack, oxidation, and light degradation. Newer types of plastics are less resistant to environmental exposure. Starch can be added to produce biodegradable plastics, making them more easily broken down by soil organisms. Photodegradable plastics break down when exposed to the ultraviolet light in sunlight. PVC food containers are made with polyvinyl chloride: they release minute amounts of cancer-causing vinyl chloride used to make this plastic. After reviewing the safety of PVC, the U.S. FDA approved the use of PVC food packaging while setting a limit for vinyl chloride. Manufacturers responded by minimizing vinyl chloride in containers. (See also ADVERTISING; PRODUCT PLACEMENT.)

pagophagia The medical term for an insatiable desire for ice cubes. Often other crunchy materials like celery stalks, raw carrots, and seeds are craved. The cause of this behavior is not known; pagophagia may be a symptom of a mineral deficiency. Pagophagia can be distinguished from PICA, a CRAVING for materials not considered food, such as clay, dirt, plaster, and starch.

palatability The degree to which FOODS are pleasing or acceptable, based on physical characteristics. Foods can be rejected or accepted on the basis of their sensory properties; visual appearance, flavor, and aroma contribute to food preferences. The social environment plays a role, and acceptance of foods can be a learned response. Certain ingredients can make a food more acceptable. FAT contributes to the palatability and popularity of many foods: MEAT; fried foods, including stir-fried foods; baked goods like chips, CRACKERS, and pastry; and CONVENIENCE FOODS.

The palatability of a food also relates to physiologic responses including SMELL, texture in the mouth ("mouth feel"), temperature of the food and TASTE sensations of sweet, sour, salty, and bitter. Taste sensitivity diminishes with age, with smoking and with certain diseases. As an example, cancer patients often experience a metallic, bitter taste that alters their desire for red meat. Smell and taste of foods are closely linked. When a substance is smelled, olfactory organs in the nose interact directly with odor molecules. (Merging olfactory sensations with taste sensations gives rise to the distinctive flavors of foods.)

palm See OIL PALM.

palmitic acid A saturated FATTY ACID that is a common constituent of FAT and coconut oil. Palmitic and related fatty acids are classified as saturated because their carbon atom building blocks are fully occupied by hydrogen atoms. The body produces palmitic acid, consequently it is not a dietary essential fatty acid. Palmitic acid containing 16 carbon atoms is readily converted to other common fatty acids—stearic acid, and a saturated fatty acid with 18 carbons, and OLEIC ACID, the most common monounsaturated fatty acid. Oleic is formed from stearic acid by the removal of two hydrogen atoms to create one double bond.

Palmitic acid is a predominant component of dietary saturated fat, including COCONUT OIL and BUTTERFAT. High consumption of saturated fats, especially those containing large amounts of palmitic acid, correlates with elevated serum CHOLESTEROL and an increased risk of CARDIOVASCULAR DISEASE among American men. Saturated fats seem to promote the formation of blood clots; possibly palmitic acid reduces the formation of substances that reduce the stickiness of blood PLATELETS, particles that promote clot formation.

Recent dietary recommendations to lower the risk of cardiovascular disease suggest reducing overall fat consumption to less than 30 percent of daily calories. Some experts recommend a more drastic reduction to less than 25 percent and a decreased consumption of saturated fats (less than 7 percent of calories) and modest increases in consumption of polyunsaturated fats and monounsaturated fats. (See also ATHEROSCLEROSIS; DIETARY GUIDELINES FOR AMERICANS; FAT METABOLISM.)

palm oil (palm kernel oil) Oil obtained from a variety of palm used in cooking and in food processing. Palm oils are among the most common FOOD ADDITIVES because they are inexpensive and contribute a satisfying taste in processed foods like potato and corn chips, cookies, and CRACKERS, as well as popcorn sold at movie theaters. As food additives they contribute surplus calories to convenience foods.

Palm oils are a source of SATURATED FAT, which are fats whose carbon atoms are filled up (saturated) with hydrogen atoms. This distinction is important because of the link between increased saturated fat consumption and an increased risk of high blood CHOLESTEROL and heart disease in susceptible people. Palm oil is more saturated (49 percent) than LARD (41 percent), though less saturated than BUTTERFAT (62 percent). At 82 percent saturated FATTY ACIDS, palm kernel oil is second only to COCONUT OIL, the most saturated fat. Excessive consumption of palm oil by Americans is believed to carry the same risks of HEART DISEASE for susceptible people as does animal fat. (See also FATTY ACIDS; OIL PALM; TROPICAL OILS.)

pancreas An elongated, tapered gland that functions both as a source of hormones (endocrine function) and as a source of digestive ENZYMES (exocrine function). The pancreas is about 8 in long and lies adjacent to the stomach within the first bend of the small intestine. The tail of this gland extends to the spleen. Its ducts drain into the upper reaches of the intestine (DUODENUM).

Endocrine Function

Nestled within pancreatic tissue are about a million small clusters of cells called pancreatic islets (islets of Langerhans). The clusters are composed of three kinds of cells: alpha cells, which secrete GLUCAGON, a hormone that raises BLOOD SUGAR; beta cells, which secrete INSULIN, the hormone that lowers blood sugar; and delta cells, which secrete somatostatin, a hormone that blocks the release of insulin and glucagon. Capillaries surrounding each islet take up these hormones for distribution by the bloodstream. The release of glucagon and insulin is regulated by feedback systems. When blood sugar falls below a threshold level, chemical sensors in alpha cells stimulate glucagon release. When blood sugar rises above normal, sensors in beta cells stimulate insulin release. In juvenile DIABETES MELLITUS (insulin-dependent diabetes mellitus) the insulin producing cells are destroyed and the patient must rely on insulin injections.

Exocrine Function

The bulk of cells in the pancreas are devoted to producing digestive enzymes. Digestive enzymes are secreted by specialized clusters of cells called acinar cells into small ducts that drain into larger ducts and on into the intestine. Pancreatic duct cells secrete BICARBONATE to neutralize STOMACH ACID. Ultimately secretions leave the organ via large ducts that empty into the SMALL INTESTINE.

The pancreas secretes between 1.2 and 1.5 liters of pancreatic juice daily. This fluid contains digestive enzymes capable of degrading all major fuel nutrients in foods, together with bicarbonate, electrolytes (ions) like CHLORIDE and SODIUM, and water. Pancreatic enzymes include PROTEASES, which digest PROTEIN; LIPASE, which digests fat; phospholipase, which degrades PHOSPHOLIPIDS; and AMYLASE, which digests starch. Proteases and phospholipase are synthesized and released as inactive precursors (ZYMOGEN) to prevent these powerful enzymes from degrading pancreatic tissue. Premature activation, as in PANCREATITIS, leads to painful inflammation and, ultimately, to tissue damage. When pancreatic zymogens reach the intestine, they are converted to active enzymes. An intestinal enzyme called ENTEROPEPTIDASE first activates TRYPSIN, itself a powerful protein-degrading enzyme. Trypsin in turn activates other protein-degrading enzymes, in a cascade of activations. Most digestive enzymes are themselves broken down to constituent amino acids, which are absorbed and recycled. This represents a considerable savings because the pancreas secretes 20 to 30 g of protein daily that otherwise would be lost.

Pancreatic enzyme secretion is regulated by the PARASYMPATHETIC NERVOUS SYSTEM via the vagus nerve, the branch of the nervous system regulating involuntary actions, and by hormones. SECRETIN, released by the intestine when it contacts partially digested food (CHYME) from the stomach, regulates bicarbonate secretion. Secretion of digestive enzymes is signaled by CHOLECYSTOKININ, a hormone secreted when the small intestine contacts fat or protein released by the stomach. (See also DIGESTION; ENDOCRINE SYSTEM.)

pancreatin A digestive aid generally prepared from hog pancreas. Pancreatin contains major pancreatic enzymes, chiefly AMYLASE for starch digestion, proteolytic enzymes for protein digestion, and LIPASES for fat digestion. The potency of a given preparation varies depending on the producer. Pancreatic enzymes are inactivated by the strong acidic environment of the stomach; therefore, coated tablets can permit active enzymes to reach the intestine, where the protective coating dissolves and the enzymes digest food at the relatively neutral pH of the intestine. Alternatively, pancreatin can be protected by taking sodium bicarbonate simultaneously to neutralize stomach acid. (See also DIGESTION; DIGESTIVE ENZYMES.)

pancreatitis Inflammation of the PANCREAS causing a spectrum of symptoms ranging from mild to severe. Acute pancreatitis may lead to tissue damage, characterized by sudden, intense abdominal pain, vomiting, and shock, and can be life threatening. About 0.2 percent of U.S. general hospital admissions represent acute pancreatic necrosis (tissue death). Acute pancreatitis usually occurs at midlife and is generally caused by ALCOHOLISM or by bile duct obstruction (GALLSTONES). The damage appears to be caused by premature activation of DIGESTIVE ENZYMES, either due to release within pancreas cells or leakage of enzymes out of blocked duct systems. FREE RADICAL damage also has been linked to pancreatitis. Chronic alcohol consumption is believed to lead to obstruction of pancreatic ducts. When it is necessary to minimize pancreatic secretion during medical treatment, oral intake of food is stopped and the patient is fed intravenously.

Mild (subclinical) pancreatitis can lead to progressive tissue damage but is not usually preceded by a severe attack. Recurrent pain may occur at intervals for years. Attacks can be precipitated by alcohol abuse, overeating or by the use of prescription drugs. The most likely cause of mild pancreatitis is alcoholism, and typically MALNUTRITION plays a role. Diagnosis is difficult because of the wide range symptoms that may not appear until late in the disease process. (See also CIRRHOSIS.)

pancreozymin See CHOLECYSTOKININ.

pangamic acid (calcium pangamate, Vitamin B_{15}) Generally, a mixture of chemicals including a compound called dimethylglycine, claimed to increase athletic performance. Pangamic acid is not really a VITAMIN, and it has no known essential function in animals or humans. However, manufacturers are able to bottle a variety of substances under the name of vitamin B_{15}. The material is widely distributed in foods ranging from BREWER'S YEAST to LIVER. Dimethylglycine is itself formed from the essential AMINO ACID methionine and is related to the simple amino acid glycine.

Very few studies outside the former Soviet Union have shown any beneficial effect in athletic performance. There, pangamic acid was used to treat ALCOHOLISM, FATIGUE, diabetes, heart disease, HEPATITIS, and AGING. Available evidence indicates pangamic acid does not increase oxygen utilization, or cardiovascular response to EXERCISE.

Pangamic acid could potentially serve as a source of methyl groups to help reuse METHIONINE. It could also help protect against fatty liver in experimental animals, and it may help the body use fat. CHOLINE is a safer alternative, however. Evidence for the effectiveness of pangamic acid in cancer treatment is mixed: Pangamic acid may cause CANCER in some experimental animals, while inhibiting cancer in others. Its use is considered experimental. Dimethylglycine has been used to treat cataracts and epilepsy. (See also ERGOGENIC SUPPLEMENTS.)

pantothenic acid A widely distributed water-soluble VITAMIN and a member of the B complex. The name is derived from the Greek word PANTOTHEN, meaning "everywhere." Indeed, pantothenic acid is present in all plant and animal cells. The commercially available form is calcium pantothenate.

Pantothenic acid plays a pivotal role in energy production from FAT, CARBOHYDRATE, and PROTEIN. Pantothenic acid forms the core of COENZYME A, the enzyme helper that carries FATTY ACIDS throughout metabolism, including fat synthesis and fat degradation. The oxidation of carbohydrates, fatty acids and amino acids eventually yields the very simple acid, ACETIC ACID, bound to coenzyme A as acetyl coenzyme A. In turn, acetyl coenzyme A feeds the metabolic machinery (KREB'S CYCLE) of the cell's powerhouse, the MITOCHONDRIA, where the carbons of acetic acid are oxidized to CARBON DIOXIDE to produce useful chemical ENERGY in the form of ATP. Furthermore, coenzyme A helps synthesize certain important compounds like CITRIC ACID; most LIPIDS, including CHOLESTEROL; STEROID hormones; and KETONE BODIES, fat derivatives made during starvation. Coenzyme A is required in the synthesis of the important NEUROTRANSMITTER, ACETYLCHOLINE, a chemical required for nerve transmission. Other functions of coenzyme A include the synthesis of HEME for the formation of the red blood cell protein HEMOGLOBIN.

Pantotheine (pantothine), a daughter molecule of pantothenic acid, contains the additional sulfur amino acids CYSTEINE. It may lower serum cholesterol and TRIGLYCERIDES in those with elevated levels, while pantothenic acid has little effect. Animal studies indicate that heart levels of pantotheine decline when oxygen supply is limited. It may be easier to convert pantotheine to coenzyme A than pantothenic acid, and therefore pantotheine may be a more effective therapeutic material in certain instances.

Good sources of pantothenic acid include LIVER, dried BEANS and PEAS, whole GRAINS, wheat germ, dark-green VEGETABLES, NUTS like peanuts, EGGS, and YEAST. Lesser amounts occur in MILK and other vegetables. Refined, heavily processed foods and fruits contain little pantothenic acid, and pantothenic acid is partially destroyed by food processing. Beneficial INTESTINAL FLORA contribute pantothenic acid.

Possible Roles in Maintaining Health

Anecdotal reports attest to the claim that pantothenic acid can increase athletic performance, but studies have yielded mixed results. Pantothenic acid blood levels are significantly lower in patients with RHEUMATOID ARTHRITIS, and preliminary clinical trials suggest that pantothenic acid may alleviate pain and joint stiffness in such patients. Pantothenic acid supplementation speeds wound healing in experimental animals; whether this occurs in humans is unknown. Preliminary evidence suggests that pantothenic acid can boost the liver's ability to oxidize alcohol. Studies with experimental animals suggest antibody production decreases with pantothenic acid deficiency, and pantothine supplementation may stimulate the IMMUNE SYSTEM. Pantothenic acid deficiency causes gray hair in animals, but supplements apparently do not reduce graying hair in people.

The levels of pantothenic acid required for optimal health remain unknown, and there is no RECOMMENDED DIETARY ALLOWANCE (RDA). It is estimated that 4 to 7 mg per day is safe and adequate for healthy people. The REFERENCE DAILY INTAKE is 10 mg per day. Deficiencies are rare, though anyone relying on a diet of highly processed foods can be at risk.

Outright deficiency symptoms have rarely been reported and occur only among severely malnourished people. However, pantothenic acid deficiencies have been produced in experimental animals. Symptoms of prolonged pantothenic acid deficiency include sore feet, burning pain in heels, vomiting, cramps, fatigue, insomnia, and respiratory infections.

Advocates believe that daily supplements in moderate amounts are reasonable as a preventive measure for healthy people. Pantothenic acid as well as vitamin C have been recommended to support adrenal glands during stress. Side effects of megadoses (10 to 20 g) include diarrhea, sleepiness, depression or nausea. There is no known toxicity for this versatile vitamin. However, long-term safety research has been inadequate. (See also AGING; CARBOHYDRATE METABOLISM; FAT METABOLISM.)

papain A protein-degrading enzyme obtained from PAPAYA leaves and from the sap of the green fruit. Commercially, papain powder is used as a MEAT TENDERIZER. To be effective, it must penetrate the meat; sprinkling the surface of MEAT with tenderizer should be followed by piercing with a fork. Papain is sometimes injected into cattle before slaughter to tenderize meat and during meat packing. When added to beverages, it breaks down protein particles that create cloudiness. As a food supplement, papain is used as a digestive aid. Cooking destroys papain, though it resists stomach acid. In medicine, papain digests dead tissue, and it has been used as a "biological scalpel" in the treatment of herniated lumbar disks. Papain preparations have also been used to treat stomach problems. (See also CARBOHYDRATE METABOLISM; DIGESTION; FAT METABOLISM; FOOD ADDITIVES.)

papaya (*Carica papaya*) The melon-like fruit of a small, palm-like evergreen that probably originated in Central America, papaya is now cultivated in tropical regions worldwide. India, Indonesia, Chile, Mexico, and Zaire rank among the top producers. Papayas also come from Hawaii, Florida, Puerto Rico, and Central and South America. The fruit may weigh up to 20 lb. Ripe papaya is yellow-orange on the outside, with a sweet, red-orange pulp. It may be round or elongated depending on the variety. The most common variety in U.S. markets is the Solo; Mexican papayas are much larger. Papayas are usually eaten fresh, in salads, and in sherbets, or juiced, pickled, and candied.

Papaya leaves and fruit contain PAPAIN and chymopapain, powerful protein-degrading enzymes that are used as digestive acids and MEAT TENDERIZERS. Papaya is a good source of potassium and vitamin C. Nutrient content of whole fruit (304 g, edible portion) is: 117 calories; protein, 1.9 g; carbohydrate, 29.8 g; fiber, 5.2 g; potassium, 780 mg;

vitamin A, 612 retinol equivalents; vitamin C, 188 mg; thiamin, 0.08 mg; riboflavin, 0.10 mg; niacin, 1.03 mg. (See also PROTEASE.)

paprika A red seasoning prepared from grinding a sweet red PEPPER into a powder. Paprika has a high VITAMIN C content. Paprika's flavor is enhanced when cooking with onions and is often used in stews, chilis, lentils, and curry dishes. Nutrient content of 1 tsp (2.1 g) is: 6 calories; protein, 0.3 g; carbohydrate, 1.3 g; fiber, 0.5 g; fat, 0.3 g; vitamin C, 1.4 mg; thiamin, 0.01 mg; riboflavin, 0.04 mg; niacin, 10.35 mg. (See also CONDIMENT.)

parasites Potentially harmful microorganisms that capture their nourishment from their host. Many parasites that infect the gastrointestinal tract are single-cell animals (protozoa). They often involve complex life cycles, such as maturation in different parts of the body and in different hosts, and they may form very stable cysts that persist in the environment. Among protozoa that have been recently associated with contaminated water or food are *Giardia lamblia, Cryptosporidium parvum, Cyclospora cayetanensis, Dientamoeba fragilis,* and *Entamoeba histolytica.* Raw fish may be contaminated with roundworms, tapeworms, and flukes.

Giardia is found throughout the world and it is among the most commonly diagnosed intestinal parasites, causing diarrhea, abdominal pain, flatulence, diarrhea, and weight loss (GIARDIASIS). Giardia may become dormant, with no obvious symptoms, although patients can still transmit the disease. Giardia contaminates water supplies in many parts of the United States and giardiasis is often linked to poor sanitation. People drinking untreated water from streams and wells are most likely to get this intestinal infection. Outbreaks have been attributed to contaminated municipal water supplies in regions of Oregon, Colorado, Utah, Washington, New Hampshire, and New York. Patients who have weakened immune systems are at risk for giardiasis. People living in close quarters, children, and campers also can become infected with this parasite.

Cryptosporidium causes cryptosporidiosis with watery diarrhea, cramping, and anorexia. If diarrhea has persisted for more than two weeks, patients may require fluid and electrolyte replacement. The parasite is common in the environment, and animal-to-person and waterborne transmission have been observed. Person-to-person transmission occurs through fecal contamination, especially in day care centers and hospital settings. An outbreak in 1993 in Milwaukee due to contaminated municipal water supply caused diarrhea in some 400,000 people. Drinking apple cider and exposure to contaminated water at water parks have also been linked to outbreaks. Ingesting as few as 30 cysts can cause infection. For people with compromised immune systems, cryptosporidiosis can be life threatening. Neither standard filtration systems nor chlorination destroy cryptosporidium, thus, most water treatment facilities do not eliminate the parasite.

Cyclospora has only recently become a public health concern in the U.S., although the distribution of this parasite is worldwide. Travel to developing countries increases the risk of infection. Cyclospora infects the intestine, causing cramps, vomiting, weight loss, and explosive diarrhea lasting one to three weeks. It was first identified in the United States in 1990, and caused 1,000 cases in 14 states in 1996.

D. fragilis is widely distributed in the United States and surveys have detected an incidence of 1.4 percent to 19 percent for a given population. Institutionalized people and children in day care centers are commonly infected. The mode of transmission is not known. *D. fragilis* causes intermittent diarrhea, abdominal pain, nausea, fatigue, and elevated white cell counts. Symptoms may persist over long periods until treatment is begun.

E. histolytica causes amoebic dysentery and is most prevalent in the tropics and subtropics. The usual mode of transmission is through the oral-fecal route, although disease can be transmitted sexually. *E. histolytica* infection is common in many areas, however, few individuals develop clinical symptoms, which include persistent bloody diarrhea with pain and cramping. Symptoms can mimic ulcerative colitis. The parasite can become dormant and the patient may not exhibit any symptoms. On the other hand, in 2 percent to 8 percent of cases, the parasite penetrates the intestinal wall and invades other organs such as the liver, possibly causing jaundice. The severity of the disease is related to the strain of the infecting organism and the patient's immune status. Symptoms may last indefinitely until treated.

Specific antiparasitic drugs are typically used to eradicate these parasites. Boiling water at least one minute or using a filtration device that removes particles less than one micron in diameter can remove parasites. Bottled water that has been distilled or purified by reverse osmosis is the safest type. A high standard of personal hygiene is warranted to avoid cross-infection among family members and those living in close quarters. (See also FOOD POISONING.)

parasympathetic nervous system A division of the autonomic NERVOUS SYSTEM that regulates involuntary processes to conserve energy, balance systems of the body and return the body to normal operation after it has responded to an injury or threatening situation. The autonomic nervous system regulates activities of smooth muscles of internal organs (viscera), heart muscle, and certain glands. It is composed of two divisions that complement each other. The parasympathetic portion counterbalances the sympathetic nervous system, which responds to stressful events and expends energy.

The parasympathetic nervous system originates from nerves in the brain stem and in the lower portion of the spinal cord. It contracts the pupil, iris, ciliary muscles (which results in clear vision), lungs, salivary glands, the heart, INTESTINE, LIVER, STOMACH, KIDNEY, PANCREAS, spleen, bladder, rectum, and reproductive organs. Parasympathetic nerve impulses to digestive glands and to the gastrointestinal tract stimulate DIGESTION and absorption of nutrients, for example. (See also HOMEOSTASIS; STRESS.)

parathyroid glands Small HORMONE-secreting glands embedded in the THYROID GLAND. Usually two parathyroids are attached to each side of the thyroid gland. They release a single hormone called parathyroid hormone (parathormone, PTH) into the bloodstream; the hormone increases blood levels of CALCIUM and MAGNESIUM. Parathormone secretion is regulated without participation of the PITUITARY GLAND, the master endocrine gland. When the level of calcium in the blood drops, more PTH is released. When the calcium level of the blood rises, less PTH is secreted, and CALCITONIN is released by the thyroid gland to lower blood calcium levels.

PTH stimulates the uptake of calcium, phosphate, and magnesium by the intestine when adequate levels of VITAMIN D are present. It does this by stimulating the activation of vitamin D to calcitrol D_3 and by activating BONE-degrading cells (osteoclasts) and stimulating their production. Osteoclasts then release calcium and phosphate in the blood. In addition, PTH directs the kidneys to excrete phosphate in the urine. (See also ENDOCRINE SYSTEM.)

parenteral nutrition Introducing nutrients into the body by means other than the mouth when patients cannot eat or drink. Parenteral nutrition is used to bypass the INTESTINE and DIGESTION by feeding nutrients intravenously, by injection under the skin or into muscles (parenteral hyperalimentation). Nutrients adequate to meet caloric requirements can be delivered intravenously. Solutions containing water, ELECTROLYTES, and sugar GLUCOSE (dextrose) as an energy source are commonly administered via a peripheral vein on the arm or leg. Other nutrients like VITAMINS, minerals, and fats may be included.

Peripheral parenteral nutrition provides about 2,500 calories per day, with 90 g of AMINO ACIDS. Patients who might receive this form of nutrition include those who need short-term support (one to two weeks), those with normal energy needs and normal kidney function, those who need additional nutrients beyond the amounts from oral or tube feeding, and patients for whom insertion of a catheter into a central vein could be a problem.

Total parenteral nutrition (TPN) refers to administering high-concentration nutrients in adequate concentrations to meet total caloric needs via a catheter into a large, rapidly flowing vein, typically flowing into the heart to assure rapid mixing and dilution with blood. Even so, it is much easier to maintain nutrient status by TPN than it is to replenish depleted nutrient stores by TPN. TPN is the most expensive method of feeding. In either peripheral parenteral nutrition or TPN, the patient's response to parenteral formulas needs to be carefully monitored, particularly in terms of caloric needs and nitrogen balance.

TPN is indicated when long-term parenteral nutrition is required, when nutrient requirements are high or when patients are starved or severely malnourished. Typical conditions that may warrant TPN by the central veins include extensive surgery, burns, or physical trauma; prolonged vomiting or diarrhea; ANOREXIA NERVOSA; CANCER; and severe digestive conditions like pancreatitis (inflamed pancreas), INFLAMMATORY BOWEL DISEASE, kidney failure, liver failure, and others.

Complete parenteral solutions include all essential amino acids, electrolytes, vitamins, MINERALS, and energy sources such as glucose, the traditional energy source, and emulsified FAT. Fatty acids may be combined with LECITHIN, a natural emulsifier, to increase their solubility, or MEDIUM-CHAIN TRIGLYCERIDES may be used directly for energy by cells. Fat emulsions are a concentrated form of energy, and a 10 percent solution provides 1 calorie per milliliter or 1,000 calories per liter. Fat does not irritate veins as easily as amino acids and glucose. Fat emulsions also provide essential fatty acids. Potential problems with intravenous fat emulsions include backaches, allergic reactions, excessive lymphocytes, blurred vision, or other symptoms. Historically, inadequate parenteral nutrition has produced deficiency symptoms and revealed the necessity of essential fatty acids and certain trace minerals. (See also CATABOLIC STATE.)

parietal cells (oxyntic cell) Stomach cells that secrete both hydrochloric acid (STOMACH ACID) and INTRINSIC FACTOR, a protein needed to bind VITAMIN B_{12} and absorb this vitamin in the INTESTINE. Hydrochloric acid activates the protein-digesting enzyme pepsin. Low stomach acid production contributes to maldigestion, while low production of intrinsic factor correlates with vitamin B_{12} deficiencies ranging from subclinical (mild) deficiencies with no obvious symptoms to severe illness with PERNICIOUS ANEMIA. (See also ACHLORHYDRIA; DIGESTION.)

Parkinson's disease (PD) An incurable neurological disorder leading to muscle rigidity, muscle weakness, slowed movements, tremors, and a characteristic halting gait and loss of balance. Parkinson's disease often develops slowly over years and currently affects more than 1 million U.S. citizens, most 50 or older. There is a progressive loss of brain cells that produce DOPAMINE, a type of NEUROTRANSMITTER or brain chemical that helps nerves communicate. Perhaps as many as 30 percent of children and adolescents who take antipsychotic (neuroleptic) drugs develop Parkinson symptoms (secondary Parkinsonism). These drugs are often prescribed for childhood conduct disorders and to control aggression and violent behavior. The symptoms can persist for months after treatment has stopped.

The cause of cell death associated with Parkinson's disease is unknown, although environmental toxins and an inherited inability to deal with toxins are hypothetical factors. The use of an herbicide (paraquat) correlated with the development of Parkinson's disease in Quebec. Viral infection has not been ruled out, though viruses have not been identified with the disease. There are hints that nutrition can play a role in the development of Parkinson's disease. This disease could be the result of FREE RADICAL damage in some cases. Free radicals are chemical fragments produced in the body that can be very destructive. Antioxidant nutrients prevent free radical damage; whether VITAMIN C and VITAMIN E supplementation may lessen the effects of this disease remains to be proven.

Drugs can control symptoms of Parkinson's disease in some cases. However, their effectiveness becomes sporadic with prolonged treatment, and the drugs currently employed can cause severe side effects, including mental disturbances and loss of balance. Levodopa (L-dopa) was introduced in the 1960s; this raw material can be taken up by the brain and converted to dopamine. In combination with a synthetic compound called carbidopa to inhibit levodopa breakdown, it is possible to use less of the drug, reducing its side effects. Often, there are problems dealing with long-term use of levodopa medication, such as involuntary movements. No anti-Parkinsonian drug slows the natural progression of the underlying disease.

Deprenyl, a monoamine oxidase inhibitor, may offer protection against nerve damage. TRYPTOPHAN and TYROSINE are amino acids that have been used with imapramine, an anti-Parkinsonian drug. Tryptophan was withdrawn from the market by the U.S. FDA in 1989.

Digesting PROTEIN yields both tyrosine and PHENYLALANINE, amino acids that compete with anti-Parkinson's drugs for admission through the brain's protective barrier (BLOOD-BRAIN BARRIER); many patients may become immobilized for several hours after eating protein. To reduce this competition, protein can be limited to dinner, although this may limit the drug's effectiveness in the evening. An alternative strategy calls for eating carbohydrate and protein in a ratio of seven to one in meals throughout the day. This is more balanced than a high-carbohydrate/low-protein diet. Legumes, especially broad beans (fava beans), contain L-dopa. Taking smaller drug doses every two to three hours and just before meals may be effective; controlled-release formulations may also help maintain constant blood levels during the day. (See also AMINO ACID METABOLISM; MAO INHIBITORS; NERVOUS SYSTEM.)

parsley (*Petroselinum crispum*) A biennial HERB used as a seasoning. There are more than 30 varieties of parsley, the most common herb in the United States. The parsley family of vegetables includes CARROTS, CELERY, and PARSNIPS, as well as other herbs (angelica, CARAWAY, CHERVIL, coriander, CUMIN, DILL, FENNEL, LOVAGE). Parsley originated in the Mediterranean region and has been cultivated for at least 2,000 years. It was apparently first used as an herbal medicine and later as a food. Parsley leaves are used as a flavoring and as a garnish, either dried or fresh, in soups, meat dishes, poultry, fish, and stuffing, as well as in vegetable dishes and salads. Parsley can be added to spreads and to butter. Parsley has been used in herbal medicine as a laxative and as a diuretic agent (to increase urination), and it has antimicrobial properties. Folk medicine has a tradition of using parsley to treat jaundice and liver conditions.

parsnip (*Pastinaca sativa*) A root vegetable that resembles CARROT, to which it is related. Parsnips were developed in the Middle Ages from wild plants growing in the Mediterranean area and for centuries was a staple in Europe until it was displaced by potatoes. It is not a major vegetable crop in the United States. Parsnips are white to yellow, while carrots are orange and possess a distinctive nutty taste. The flavor becomes sweeter after exposure to frost and when stored starch is broken down to sugar. Parsnips can be used in place of turnips. Cooked parsnips can be pureed or mashed with potatoes and can be fried, candied, roasted with meat or baked.

Nutrient content of 1 cup of cooked parsnips (156 g) is: 125 calories; protein, 2.1 g; carbohydrate, 30.4 g; fiber, 4.36 g; fat, 1.4 g; potassium, 573 mg; thiamin, 0.13 mg; riboflavin, 0.08 mg; niacin, 0.15 mg.

pasta A basic food made from a dried paste of wheat flour. Pasta comes in hundreds of forms and is used in recipes from Asia to America. *Pasta* is the Italian word for "paste." To prepare pasta, flour and water are mixed and the dough is extruded through die plates to shape it, the cut into ribbons, tubes, or strings, which are dried. Most commercially available pasta is prepared from SEMOLINA, a refined flour from durum WHEAT. Durum wheat contains a high percentage of GLUTEN, the sticky protein that holds the dough together. Pasta can be prepared from whole wheat flour as well as white flour. Pastas from whole wheat contain about 5 g of fiber per 3.5-oz. serving. Japanese pasta is prepared from soft whole wheat with a lower gluten content than semolina. In this case, dough is generally rolled into flat sheets, then cut.

Although various shapes of pasta bear Italian names, the U.S. FDA defines pasta either MACARONI or NOODLES. Macaroni is made without eggs and contains three basic ingredients: semolina; farina, a coarsely ground starchy flour that contains less protein than durum wheat; and/or flour from durum wheat. Noodles contain in addition a minimum of 5.5 percent egg (by weight). Consequently, noodles provide fat and cholesterol. Rather than being a fattening, calorie-rich food, pasta is a good source of COMPLEX CARBOHYDRATE. For example, 82 percent of the calories in spaghetti comes from carbohydrate, the rest from protein. Pastas can be fattening when oil, CHEESE, BUTTER, heavy cream, or fatty meats are added. These contain far more calories. Corn, quinoa, and rice pasta are also available; they are as healthful as wheat pasta. They must be labeled "pasta substitutes" on the food label because they do not conform to federal definitions for pasta. (See also BREAD.)

O'Neill, Molly. "So It May Be True After All: Eating Pasta Makes You Fat," *New York Times*, February 8, 1995, B1, B7.

pasteurization A method of FOOD PROCESSING that involves heat to destroy harmful microorganisms and microorganisms that cause spoilage. Louis Pasteur discovered the process that bears his name when he found that WINE and BEER could be preserved by heating above 57.2° C (135° F). Now MILK, CHEESE, egg products, wine, beer, and fruit juices are generally pasteurized at temperatures between 60° C and 100° C (212° F). Products are cooled rapidly after the heat treatment to prevent being cooked.

Milk is pasteurized by heating at 62° C for 30 minutes or by flash heating, a process that involves heating at high temperatures for a short time. These processes kill 97 percent to 99 percent of nonspore-forming, pathogenic bacteria, including tuberculosis bacteria, salmonella, and streptococcus. Pasteurization does not kill all microorganisms in a food or beverage, however. The growth of surviving organisms may be retarded by additional procedures such as chilling. Pasteurization can kill microorganisms that would otherwise compete with a pure starter strain of a bacterium or yeast used in food processing, such as in cheese making. Pasteurization is effective in destroying certain disease-producing microorganisms in milk without altering the overall quality of the product; this process is appropriate to destroy heat-susceptible organisms such as yeasts in fruit juices. (See also FOOD PRESERVATION.)

pastrami A spiced and smoked deli meat usually made from beef brisket trimmed of fat. It is prepared by rubbing the fresh meat with several spices, including garlic, black pepper, allspice, and cinnamon. The meat is then cured, smoked, and cooked slowly. Pastrami is usually sliced thin and served either hot or cold, usually in sandwiches, such as the popular reuben. A 2-oz. serving provides calories, 80; sodium, 610 mg; fat, 4 g; protein, 10 g.

pastry A sweet dessert or baked good with a flour-based crust. Pastries are often filled with fruit, creme, or some other confection.

pau d'arco See LA PACHO.

PCBs See POLYCHLORINATED BIPHENYLS.

pea (*Pisum arvense* and *P. sativum*) A LEGUME that ranks among the 10 most important VEGETABLE crops worldwide. Peas were cultivated by the Chinese in 2000 B.C., and dried peas have been uncovered in Egyptian tombs. Garden peas are treated as fresh vegetables, while dried peas, such as chickpeas and split peas, require long cooking times. Dry green peas are the main pea crop in the United States; Idaho and Washington produce most of the domestic dry peas. Dried peas are used in canned soups and dehydrated pea soup. Dried split peas cook in about 25 minutes while quick-cooking peas can be cooked within 15 minutes because they have been pretreated with enzymes and steamed. The United States produces more fresh green peas than any other country. Most of the U.S. crop is either frozen or canned; frozen green peas represent the leading frozen vegetable in America. They retain their flavor and color. Most canned peas contain added salt and sugar. Snow peas are meant to be eaten with the pod intact.

Peas provide FIBER, IRON, and the B COMPLEX vitamins. As a source of minerals, peas contain much less CALCIUM and PHOSPHORUS than BEANS. Like other legumes, peas contain substantial protein, however, pea protein is deficient in the sulfur amino acids CYSTEINE and L-METHIONINE, and it contains sufficient amounts of another dietary essential amino acid, LYSINE, to complement the low lysine content in grain protein, so that combining legume protein with grain protein (cereal products) yields a mixed protein with a higher quality than that obtained by eating either alone.

P. arvense is the field pea, grown for its seeds. It grows wild in the Republic of Georgia and probably originated in central Asia and Europe. Its seeds are gray-brown, while the garden pea produces green seeds. Field peas are not used for food in the United States. Generally, they are grown to fertilize fields and to provide animal fodder. Like other legumes, this vegetable can grow in nitrogen-depleted soils because its roots possess nodules that contain bacteria that convert atmospheric NITROGEN to nitrogen compounds readily absorbed by the plant.

Nutrient content of cooked green peas (1/2 cup from frozen peas, 80 g) is: 63 calories; protein, 4.1 g; carbohydrate, 11.4 g; fiber, 7.7 g; iron, 1.25 mg; potassium, 134 mg; thiamin, 0.23 mg; riboflavin, 0.14 mg; niacin, 1.18 mg. (See also FOOD COMPLEMENTING.)

peach (*Prunus persica*) A juicy, sweet FRUIT produced by a tree related to APRICOT, CHERRY, and PLUM. The peach is classified as a drupe, that is, a fruit whose hard seed or pit is enclosed by a soft pulp with a thin skin. The peach probably originated in China, where it is described in writings from 2000 B.C. Colonists brought the peach to North America, and now it is grown in 32 states and in Canada. The United States and Italy are the world's major producers of peaches and the related NECTARINE. California produces over 60 percent of the domestic peach crop, and peaches are the third most popular fruit grown domestically. There are thousands of varieties, though relatively few are important commercially. Peaches can be classified as either cling peaches, if the stone is difficult to remove from the flesh (Fortuna, Gaume, Johnson, Paloro and Sims), or freestone, if the pit comes free easily (Elberta, J. H. Hale, Redhaven, Hiley, and Golden Jubilee). Peach fuzz is removed mechanically after harvest. U.S. peaches are sold fresh, frozen, or canned. The fresh fruit contains modest amounts of potassium and vitamin C. Nutrient contents of one whole peach, fresh, peeled, and pitted (87 g), is: 37 calories; protein, 0.6 g; carbohydrate, 9.6 g; fiber, 2.0 g; potassium, 171 mg; vitamin C, 6 mg; thiamin, 0.01 mg.; riboflavin, 0.04 mg; niacin, 0.86 mg.

peanut (*Arachis hypogaea;* ground nut, goober, ground pea, earth nut) An annual legume that produces an underground pod with two or more edible kernels. Peanuts are not true NUTS. Peanuts were cultivated by ancient peoples of Mexico and South America. Colonists took peanuts to Africa and other countries, and they are now a major crop in India, the People's Republic of China, the United States, Africa (Sudan, South Africa, Senegal), the Far East (Indonesia), and South America (Argentina, Brazil). Southern states such as Georgia, Alabama, the Carolinas, Virginia, Florida, and Mississippi lead the United States in peanut production.

Peanuts are dried after harvesting and stored until processing. Most nuts sold in pods represent a variety called large-seeded Virginias. Small seeded varieties or runners are used primarily to make PEANUT BUTTER. Spanish peanuts are used in candies, peanut butter, and salted nuts. During processing, unshelled peanuts are cleaned, whitened, and polished before marketing. Shelling reduces the shelf life by about 70 percent. The skin and seed coat are removed by blanching. Peanuts are dry-roasted for candy, peanut butter, and baked goods. Nuts may also be roasted in oil and served as a snack food. Roasted whole peanuts are soaked in saltwater, dried, and then roasted in the shell. Roasting increases the flavor of peanuts by increasing the amounts of free AMINO ACIDS and SUGAR in kernels. Raw peanuts are cooked like beans. Peanuts can be defatted by roasting them in VEGETABLE OIL under pressure to remove 60 percent to 80 percent of the oil. Worldwide, peanuts are mainly processed for their oil or converted to peanut flour. The protein content is 26 percent and, like most legumes, peanut protein is somewhat low in the essential amino acid LYSINE. In developing nations, peanut flour is mixed with other protein sources like fish, flour, sesame, and millet to increase the overall protein quality. Nutrient contents of 1 cup (oil roasted, salted, 145 g) provides: 841 calories; protein, 38.8 g; carbohydrate, 26.8 g; fiber, 11.7 g; fat, 71.3 g; calcium, 125 mg; iron, 2.7 mg; potassium, 1,020 mg; sodium, 626 mg; thiamin, 0.42 mg; riboflavin, 0.15 mg; niacin, 2.15 mg.

Peanut Oil

Nearly 70 percent of the world peanut crop is used for oil product, and peanut oil accounts for 20 percent of the total vegetable oil consumption. Peanuts are rich in oil: 100 pounds of whole nuts yields 32 pounds of oil, and small podded varieties contain 50 percent oil. The oil contains 76 percent to 82 percent unsaturated FATTY ACIDS, that is, fatty acids with double bonds. Monounsaturated fatty acids represent 48.4 percent of the total; polyunsaturated fatty acids, 33.6 percent; and saturated fatty acids, 18 percent. Peanut oil is used as a cooking oil because it has a high smoke point (that is, it produces smoke only at high temperatures). The oil is also used in salad dressing, vegetable shortening, and MARGARINE. (See also AFLATOXIN.)

peanut butter Due to its popularity, half the U.S. peanut crop ends up as peanut butter. The annual U.S. consumption of peanut BUTTER is about three pounds per person. Peanut butter is prepared by grinding dry roasted peanuts and may contain added SALT, SUGAR, flavors, HYDROGENATED VEGETABLE OIL, and ANTIOXIDANTS to retard spoilage. By law, at least 90 percent of the content must be peanuts in order for a product to be labeled as "peanut butter." Peanut butter is an excellent source of protein; however, it is also a high-FAT food. About 80 percent of its calories come from fat. One tablespoon contains about 95 calories.

Peanut butter often contains traces of a mold toxin, AFLATOXIN, which is produced by a storage mold called ASPERGILLUS that often infests damp nuts and grains. In experimental animals, aflatoxin is a very powerful liver CARCINOGEN (cancer-causing agent). Industry monitors aflatoxin levels in peanut butter carefully, and spot-checks have rarely detected levels higher than the legal limit of 15 parts per billion. Levels as low as 1 part per billion can cause cancer in certain species. There is little compelling evidence that eating peanut butter with traces of aflatoxin in amounts usually encountered in the Western diet causes cancer. However, it seems prudent not to eat peanut butter as a steady diet. When making peanut butter, stale, discolored, or shriveled peanuts should be avoided. Freshly ground peanut butter should be refrigerated to retard spoilage. Nutrient contents of peanut butter (one tablespoon, 16 g) is: 95 calories; protein, 4.6 g; carbohydrate, 2.5 g; fiber, 1.2 g; fat, 8.2 g; iron, 0.29 mg; sodium, 75 mg; thiamin, 0.02 mg; riboflavin, 0.02 mg; niacin, 2.15 mg. (See also SATURATED FAT.)

pear (*Pyrus spp.*) A popular, juicy FRUIT related to the APPLE and QUINCE that originated in Asia and cultivated as early as 1000 B.C. They are now grown in temperate zones worldwide. Thousands of varieties of pears have been developed. Pears are round or bell-shaped; the neck may be long or practically indistinguishable. The flesh has a sandy texture due to "grit" cells. The taste ranges from sweet to acidic. Pears grown in North America are the common European pear, *P. communis* (Bartlett, Bosc, Comice, for example); and the Asian pear, *P. pyrifolia.* Crosses between the two species are blight-resistant and possess a desirable texture and taste. Hybrid varieties include Kieffer, LeConte, and Garber. The Anjou is the most popular winter pear; the Bartlett is the leading summer pear. Italy, the United States and China are leaders in pear production. Pears are grown in most U.S. states: California, Washington, Oregon, New York, and Michigan are among the top producers.

Over 60 percent of the pear crop is processed (canned or dried). Pears are picked green because the immature fruit is firm and can be transported more easily without bruising. As pears ripen, starch is converted to sugar and the flesh softens. Pears stored in sealed plastic bags will turn brown due to limited oxygen. Lemon juice spread on freshly sliced pears will prevent their darkening. Much of the carbohydrate content is simple sugars (fructose, GLUCOSE, and others). When eaten with the skin, pears are a good source of fiber. Most vitamin C is also concentrated in the skin. One Bartlett pear (raw, 166 g) provides 98 calories; protein, 0.7 g; carbohydrate, 25.1 g; fiber, 5.0 g; fat, 0.7 g; potassium, 208 mg; vitamin C, 7 mg; thiamin, 0.07 mg; riboflavin, 0.17 mg; niacin, 0.17 mg.

pecan (*Carya illinoensis*) The seed of the pecan tree, a species of hickory. Pecans are native to the southern United States and the Mississippi River Basin. Georgia alone produces about 40 percent of the U.S. crop. Nearly 90 percent of pecans are sold as shelled nuts. Pecans contain 70 percent oil, a fat content higher than peanuts and most other nuts. Shelled pecans should be refrigerated or stored in the freezer to minimize rancidity. When frozen, nuts in the shell can be kept for two years. Pecans are used in baked goods, ice cream, candy, salads, desserts, and vegetable dishes. The nutrient value of dried pecans (1 cup, unsalted, shelled, 108 g) is: 720 calories; protein, 8.4 g; carbohydrate, 19.7 g; fiber, 6.5 g; fat, 73.1 g; calcium, 39 mg; iron, 2.3 mg; potassium, 423 mg; thiamin, 0.92 mg; riboflavin, 0.14 mg; niacin, 0.96 mg.

pectin An important type of water-soluble FIBER. Dietary fiber represents the nondigested carbohydrate that strengthens plant cells and acts as an intercellular "cement." Pectin differs from BRAN, which is a common form of insoluble fiber. Pectin is composed of branched carbohydrate chains containing an acidic sugar (galacturonic acid), together with the simple sugars (galactose or arabinose).

Pectin affects health in several ways. Pectin, not bran, lowers BLOOD PRESSURE and blood CHOLESTEROL, and regularly eating soluble fiber as fruit, oat bran, and legumes may significantly lower blood cholesterol. Pectin also helps maintain normal BLOOD SUGAR. Pectin softens stools to help prevent bulges in the colon (DIVERTICULOSIS) and hemorrhoids and helps reduce the risk of colon CANCER. Pectin heals COLITIS in experimental animals. A possible explanation is that pectin is broken down by gut bacteria to SHORT-CHAIN FATTY ACIDS, which promote healthy epithelial cell lining of the intestine.

Good sources of pectin include many fruits like APPLES and berries, VEGETABLES, seeds, BEANS, split peas, LENTILS, SQUASH, CARROTS, and OAT bran. Pectin is virtually absent from whole grains. Apple peel contains 15 percent pectin, while onion skins are 11 percent to 12 percent pectin. When extracted from plant material, pectin is a white powder that readily forms gels when dissolved in water. Lemon, lime, grapefruit, and orange rinds contain up to 30 percent pectin and are a commercial source of pectin. As a FOOD ADDITIVE, pectin is used for jellies and jams because it gels in the presence of sugar and acid. It is used to thicken barbecue sauces, YOGURT, cranberry sauce, and canned frosting. Pectin is classified as a safe additive. (See also COMPLEX CARBOHYDRATE.)

pectinase A family of enzymes occurring in plants and microorganisms that degrade PECTIN, a form of dietary fiber that causes gel formation. Pectinase softens plant tissue and FRUIT and destroys the gelling capability of many fruit JUICES. Commercially, pectinase is extracted from certain bacteria and plant products and is added by the food industry to clarify fruit juice concentrates, WINE, VINEGAR, syrup, and JELLY. (See also FOOD ADDITIVES.)

pellagra A disease due to a chronic deficiency of the B vitamin NIACIN. In the early 1900s, pellagra was widespread in the southern United States when people relied on CORN as their main PROTEIN source. With niacin and RIBOFLAVIN enrichment of grain products and flour in the 1920s, pellagra practically disappeared in Europe and North America. It is associated with chronic ALCOHOLISM and still occurs in other parts of the world in populations with nutritionally inadequate diets relying on corn. The body converts about 2 percent of the daily intake of the essential amino acid TRYPTOPHAN to niacin. Therefore, diets that provide minimal animal protein and are low in tryptophan, promote pellagra. Niacin deficiency leads to sore tongue (GLOSSITIS), skin disorders like DERMATITIS, bloody DIARRHEA, and inflammation of the GASTROINTESTINAL TRACT. Pellagra affects the NERVOUS SYSTEM, causing DEPRESSION, anxiety, and psychosis. Pellagra readily responds to treatment with niacin or its counterpart, NIACINAMIDE. (See also ENRICHMENT; FORTIFICATION; MALNUTRITION.)

pentose A family of simple sugars that are key building blocks of DNA, the genetic material, and RNA, the mechanism guiding protein synthesis. Unlike hexoses like glucose, which contain six carbon atoms, pentoses contain five carbon atoms; ribose and DEOXYRIBOSE are the most common. Both ribose and deoxyribose are synthesized from GLUCOSE (BLOOD SUGAR) and are not required nutrients. Pentoses do not occur free in foods but instead are building blocks of many plant polysaccharides (sugar polymers) as FIBER. For example, D-xylose and L-arabinose are common constituents in fruits and root vegetables. (See also CARBOHYDRATE.)

pepper (*Capsicum spp.*) A green or red VEGETABLE belonging to the capsicum family. Peppers are native to the New World, where they were harvested in Mexico before 5000 B.C. and were domesticated independently along the Peruvian coast. European explorers introduced peppers to the Old World, where they spread rapidly. Peppers are customarily classified as CHILI PEPPERS (*C. frutescens*) when they possess a strong flavor, and as sweet peppers (*C. annum*) when their large fruit possesses a mild flavor. Peppers now rank among the top 20 important vegetable crops, with China, Nigeria, Spain, Italy, Turkey, and Mexico among the leading pepper-producing nations. Florida and California produce most domestic sweet peppers. Much of the U.S. crop is sold as a fresh vegetable. However, peppers may be canned, pickled, dehydrated, or frozen. In addition to salads, fresh as well as processed peppers can be used in relishes and garnishes for fish, meats, and poultry. Sweet peppers can be stuffed and baked. They add zest to omelets, pizzas, and stews. Sweet peppers are an excellent source of vitamin C, and the red varieties contribute vitamin A. Peppers belong to the nightshade family, which includes EGGPLANT, TOMATOES, and POTATOES.

The most popular pepper in the United States is bell pepper, a sweet pepper. Bell peppers can be green, yellow-orange, or red, depending on their stage of ripeness. Bell peppers lack the ingredient in chili peppers that gives hot peppers their bite; instead they have a mild flavor. Other types of sweet peppers include banana, Cubanelle, and pimento.

Hot peppers contain CAPSAICIN as the active ingredient. This material affects digestion by stimulating salivation, stomach acid production, and perhaps PERISTALSIS. Capsaicin also kills bacteria. Capsaicin may also help prevent blood clot formation. Hot chili peppers may contain sufficiently high levels of capsaicin to burn mucous membranes, and irritating, volatile oil may be released during frying. Leading varieties are marketed fresh, dried, or canned: Anaheim, ancho, cascabel, cayenne, cherry, habanero, jalapeño, poblano, and serrano.

Hot peppers provide important seasonings. These include:

- Cayenne pepper—a hot seasoning prepared from dried chili peppers.
- Chili powder—a hot seasoning prepared from ground red chili peppers. Chili powder often contains cumin, salt, oregano, and garlic powder as well.
- Paprika—a mild seasoning prepared from ground, mild-flavored types of sweet pepper.
- Red pepper—a hot seasoning prepared from ground dried red chili peppers.

One sweet green pepper (raw, 74 g) provides 18 calories; protein, 3.9 g; carbohydrate, 1.3 g; fat, 0.3 g; iron, 0.94 mg; potassium, 144 mg; vitamin C, 95 mg; thiamin, 0.06 mg; riboflavin, 0.04 mg; niacin, 0.41 mg. Sweet red peppers contain more vitamin A (570 retinol equivalents) and more vitamin C (141 mg).

peppermint (*Mentha piperita*) A perennial HERB with a refreshing flavor. Peppermint is a popular choice of herb tea. Peppermint leaves are used as a flavoring in sauces, fruit salads, drinks, and punches. Peppermint oil is extracted from dried plants and is used to flavor CHEWING GUM, CANDY, and other consumer goods like toothpaste. Peppermint has a long history in folk medicine for treating digestive problems. Peppermint oil possesses anti-inflammatory and anti-ulcer activity and relieves symptoms associated with severe indigestion, gastritis, and enteritis (inflammation of the stomach and intestine, respectively). Peppermint oil stimulates bile secretion and normalizes gastrointestinal functions. It also possesses antimicrobial activity. (See also SPICE.)

pepsin A digestive ENZYME produced in the STOMACH that, together with STOMACH ACID, initiates protein DIGESTION. Pepsin originates in CHIEF CELLS of pyloric glands (gastric glands). Pepsin requires an acidic environment for full activity. It is manufactured as an inactive form called pepsinogen to prevent destruction of the glands. After secretion into the stomach, stomach acid rapidly activates pepsinogen to pepsin, where it breaks down food proteins into fragments, setting the stage for the powerful, pancreatic enzymes to complete the digestion of proteins to amino acids. Hydrochloric acid supplements, such as glutamic acid hydrochloride, usually contain pepsin. (See also PROTEASE.)

peptic ulcer A sore or erosion in the lining of the stomach or upper portion of the intestine. Stress, cigarette smoking, food allergy, low-fiber diets, and overdosing with ASPIRIN are linked to an increased risk of ulcers. Most peptic ulcers are associated with recurrent pain in the abdominal area after a meal, which may be called HEARTBURN. Consumption of ANTACIDS to neutralize stomach acid usually relieves the pain. Drugs that block stomach acid secretion and antacids are used in treatment. However, they have side effects and disrupt DIGESTION. Relapse rate is high with the drug cimetidine because it alters the lining of the stomach and the intestine. Raw cabbage juice and a component of LICORICE have been used in healing ulcers. Chronic infection by the bacterium *HELICOBACTER PYLORI* has been shown to cause a form of stomach inflammation called atrophic gastritis, and the bacterium is probably a cause of stomach ulcers as well. Researchers recently discovered that BROCCOLI and broccoli sprouts contain a chemical, SULFORAFANE, that kills *H. pylori* in mice. Similar studies on humans are ongoing. (See also DUODENAL ULCER; GASTRIC ULCER.)

peptide A molecule composed of a chain of amino acids. Amino acids form chains by linking up in a "head to toe" fashion so that the amino group of one amino acid binds to an acid group of another amino acid.

The antioxidant glutathione, manufactured in cells from the amino acids glutamic acid, cysteine and glycine, is classified as a tripeptide because it contains three linked amino acids. Certain HORMONES, like OXYTOCIN and ANTIDIURETIC HORMONE, which contain nine amino acids, are classified as nonapeptides. Other peptides are biologically important. Enkephalins are brain peptides composed of five amino acids that decrease sensitivity to pain. Peptides are produced during DIGESTION, and are in turn degraded to amino acids and absorbed.

Proteins are polypeptides, long chains assembled from 20 different amino acids and ranging in size from 50 or 60 amino acids to a thousand or more. The characteristic properties of each type of polypeptide reside in the unique sequence of its amino acids. When peptides are digested by peptidases and proteolytic ENZYMES, they yield their constituent amino acids.

perch (*Perca*) A large family of freshwater game and food fish characterized by spiny fins that are widely distributed in lakes and streams, and even in brackish water. *P. flavescens*, the North American perch (yellow perch), is found in the United States and Canada; *P. fluviatilis* lives in central Europe. The walleye pike and yellow perch, important game fish, belong to a closely related genus. Saltwater fish such as sea bass and rockfish families are not true perch. Perch is a lean fish with a firm white meat and mild flavor. Perch is sold as fillets or whole, dressed, and can be poached, broiled, or sauteed. With less than a gram of fat per serving, perch is classified as a lean fish. Nutrient content of 3 oz. (85 g) is: 80 calories; protein, 15.8 g; fat, 1.4 g; calcium, 91 mg; cholesterol, 36 mg; thiamin, 0.08 mg; riboflavin, 0.094 mg; and niacin, 1.7 mg. (See also SALMON.)

periodontal disease A progressive disease of gums supporting the bone of TEETH. Several stages have been identified: GINGIVITIS refers to swollen, inflamed gums that bleed easily. There may be bad breath. Periodontitis is a more serious condition, in which gums recede and deep pockets form, harboring disease-producing bacteria, and inflammation erodes the ligament binding the tooth to the jaw bone. As the infection progresses, deep tissue is damaged and teeth become loose.

The culprit of gum disease is plaque, a sticky film produced by bacteria that provides a haven for further bacterial growth. If not removed by daily brushing, plaque accumulates at the gum line and can cause gum inflammation. Plaque can become calcified or harden into tartar. Plaque deposits beneath the gum line favor the growth of pathogenic bacteria. The IMMUNE SYSTEM attacks the infection by causing INFLAMMATION. This process releases tissue-destroying enzymes to enable defensive cells to attack the site of infection. Thus inflammation leads to further tissue destruction.

The most important tactic in preventing periodontal disease is to keep teeth clean, especially along the gum line. This means careful brushing, flossing, and regular prophylactic cleaning by professionals. Most often, periodontitis can be controlled with personal and professional cleaning together with procedures that remove deep pockets of plaque and tartar and remove tooth layers with toxic bacteria. The risk of gum disease increases with pregnancy and with the use of oral contraceptives (which raises hormones that increase gum sensitivity); cigarette smoking (which slows healing); alcohol consumption (which reduces the flow of saliva); a depressed immune system; and medications that dry the mouth (antidepressants, antihistamines, antihypertensives, decongestants, and muscle relaxants, among others). Children whose family history includes periodontal disease are at greater risk for this condition. (See also DENTAL PLAQUE; TEETH.)

peristalsis The sequential wave-like contraction and relaxation of smooth muscles that moves food through the digestive tract. Once chewed, food enters the ESOPHAGUS, the passageway leading to the stomach. Powerful, involuntary muscular contractions propel food in its various stages of disintegration and DIGESTION. Circular muscular contractions constrict the walls of the esophagus, stomach and INTESTINE and squeeze the food forward. Passage of food into the stomach generally requires four to eight seconds. After food enters the stomach, slower peristaltic waves mix food with GASTRIC JUICES to produce a liquefied food (CHYME). Food may remain in the stomach an hour or so. Peristalsis then propels the chyme through the intestine, where the contractions are weaker than in the stomach and esophagus. Food remains in the small intestine for three to five hours. In the colon, slow peristalsis (three to 12 contractions per minute) moves the chyme downward. Finally, strong peristaltic waves drive the contents of the colon toward the rectum. Food ALLERGY and FOOD SENSITIVITY can contract smooth muscles, slowing transit through the digestive tract (a situation called hypomotility), leading to CONSTIPATION, or they may cause rapid peristalsis (hypermotility) leading to DIARRHEA. Hypermotility may interfere with digestion and absorption of nutrients. (See also DIGESTIVE TRACT.)

pernicious anemia A deficiency of normal RED BLOOD CELLS due to inadequate uptake of VITAMIN B_{12}. In this disorder, vitamin B_{12} cannot be absorbed because the stomach fails to secrete adequate amounts of vitamin B_{12} binding protein, INTRINSIC FACTOR, required for absorption of vitamin B_{12}. Chronic vitamin B_{12} deficiency limits the ability of BONE MARROW to produce red blood cells, causing anemia, characterized by a progressive decrease in the number of red BLOOD cells and the appearance of giant red blood cells, together with gastrointestinal disturbance, weakness, and nerve damage. Pernicious anemia can be treated by vitamin B_{12} injections. (See also MALABSORPTION; MALNUTRITION.)

peroxidase Antioxidant ENZYMES that form part of the body's defense against highly reactive and damaging forms of oxygen (peroxides). Peroxidases readily destroy HYDROGEN PEROXIDE, an oxidizing agent produced by metabolism, and lipid peroxides. Peroxides are potentially hazardous to cells because they generate FREE RADICALS. These chemical fragments can rapidly damage cellular proteins, membranes and genetic material. Peroxidases belong to a large family of iron-containing enzymes that carry out oxidation. (See also CATALASE.)

peroxides Highly reactive oxidation products, especially of lipids and fat. Fats, oils, and cholesterol react with oxygen in the presence of metal ions when heated to form peroxides. POLYUNSATURATED OILS like safflower oil are particularly sensitive to peroxidation because of their chemical structure, with multiple bonds. The resulting lipid peroxides are dangerous because they spontaneously decompose into FREE RADICALS and other unstable chemical species that may attack DNA, producing mutations and causing cancer; or they may kill cells outright. Lipid peroxides also trigger inflammation.

The body's defense system can destroy free radicals before they can attack cells and peroxidases (GLUTATHIONE PEROXIDASE) can disarm lipid peroxides to prevent further damage. The required nutrients include SELENIUM, GLUTATHIONE, and VITAMIN C. Other antioxidants, including VITAMIN E and BETA-CAROTENE, can quench free radicals produced by lipid peroxide breakdown. However, the reserve capacity to destroy peroxides can be overwhelmed with continuous exposure to free radicals, especially when the nutritional status is compromised by a diet based on highly processed food. Lipid peroxides occur in fatty foods that have been highly processed, as when the fat is heated and exposed to air, such as in deep fat-fried foods and in polyunsaturated vegetable oils exposed to heat, light, and traces of iron or other metal ions. Whole or minimally processed foods contain ANTIOXIDANTS like vitamin E and carotenoids, which protect these foods.

To minimize peroxide formation in fats and oils, lower cooking temperatures and OLIVE OIL should be used instead of polyunsaturated oils like CORN OIL or SAFFLOWER oil (monounsaturated fat is less easily oxidized). Cooking oils should be refrigerated in sealed containers to reduce their oxidation. (See also GLUTATHIONE PEROXIDASE; RANCIDITY.)

peroxisome A small particle found in the CYTOPLASM of most cells that perform a variety of oxidations. Peroxisomes operate independently of MITOCHONDRIA, the primary oxidative powerhouse of the cell, to degrade FATTY ACIDS, including the by-products of the chemical processing of vegetable oils called TRANS-FATTY ACIDS, with the production of HYDROGEN PEROXIDE. The oxidase enzymes of peroxisomes also break down unusual amino acids (D-amino acids) derived from microbial and plant sources. They degrade the toxic agent hydrogen peroxide. (See also FAT DIGESTION.)

pesco-vegetarian A person who consumes a diet based on plant foods that includes fish and milk and egg products, but no other animal protein. (See also VEGETARIAN.)

pesticides Substances used to control or destroy undesirable organisms, especially rodents, insects, weeds, and molds. Pesticides may be synthetic chemicals or they may be made of natural materials. Rodenticides are used to control mice and rats; insecticides control insects, mites, spiders, and ticks. Other classes of pesticides control slugs, snails, and nematodes that attack root vegetables in particular. Herbicides control weeds; these may contain agents that change plant growth or alter leaf physiology. Fungicides control the growth of MOLD and fungus on produce.

The United States alone uses over a billion pounds of pesticides yearly, and the use of pesticides provides considerable benefits in crop production throughout the world. These chemicals protect against the natural threats of blight and insect pests that in times past decimated crops. Fifty percent of the dollars spent in pest control goes to weed control, and this has been a major factor in making farming less labor intensive. The increased availability of food has lowered food costs. Prior to 1950, consumers spent on the average 24 percent of the family budget on food; by 2001, consumers spent 13.4 percent on food. The cogent argument is made that the use of pesticides has dramatically lowered the cost of fruits and vegetables, making them more affordable and increasing their consumption as recommended by governmental agencies to reduce the risk of chronic illness.

The first pesticides were natural products, which continue to be important agricultural materials. As an example, large-scale production of biopesticides, living organisms or their by-products, has been successful in some instances. The soil bacterium *Bacillus thuringiensis* produces a protein toxin (poison) that specifically affects certain moths and caterpillars without affecting other insects, animals, or humans. Aerial spraying programs have used this procedure to destroy infestations of the Asian gypsy moth. This biopesticide is approved for about 200 crops in the United States. However, in Hawaii, Florida, and New York, as well as in the Philippines, Thailand, and Japan, moths have evolved a resistance to this toxin. An alternative strategy relies on baiting traps with pheromones, chemicals that act as sex attractants for the male or female moth. Genetic engineering and biotechnology continue to be applied to develop safer, more effective biopesticides.

Synthetic chemical pesticides are recent creations (post-World War II) and played a role in launching the GREEN REVOLUTION. Among the first was DDT, an extremely potent pesticide that kills insects by altering the ability of their nerve cells to conduct nerve impulses. There are almost 900 EPA registered pesticides. The federal Insecticide, Fungicide and Rodenticide Act (1972) prohibits the use of cancer-causing pesticides, and the DELANEY CLAUSE prohibits the addition of cancer-causing agents to foods. This was superseded by the Food Quality Protection Act of 1996, which established a single health-based standard for pesticide residues in all foods.

The U.S. FDA monitors pesticide levels in foods and the EPA establishes upper limits for the amounts of registered pesticides in foods called "maximum residue limits."

Natural Pesticides

Natural pesticides are widespread, apparently because plants defend themselves against predators, fungi, molds, and infection by producing toxins, and it seems likely that each plant species produces its own characteristic set of toxins. Humans eat an estimated 5,000 to 10,000 natural pesticides and related compounds and consume about 1.5 g of these substances daily. For example, lima beans produce 23 toxins and cabbage yield 49 toxins and related compounds. Twenty-seven natural pesticides found to be rodent carcinogens are present in foods ranging from APPLE, basil, and BRUSSELS SPROUTS to CELERY, EGGPLANT, fennel, horseradish, and potato.

At the same time, vegetables like ONIONS, CRUCIFEROUS VEGETABLES, including BROCCOLI and CAULIFLOWER, and most fresh FRUITS contain many nutrients and substances that counterbalance these natural pesticides and offer protection against cancer. The following is a brief listing.

- GARLIC and onions contain allylic sulfides and other organosulfur compounds that may stimulate a DETOXICATION enzyme in the liver.
- Parsley, CARROTS, squash, sweet POTATOES, CANTALOUPE, kale, and turnip greens contain beta-carotene and related carotenoids that can act as antioxidants to prevent cellular damage.
- Green TEA and berries contain TANNINS that also act as antioxidants.
- Most fruits and vegetables contain FLAVONOIDS that act as antioxidants and some may also block the target sites of estrogen that can promote certain cancers.
- Cabbage and related vegetables, including broccoli, as well as squash, yams, tomatoes, PEPPERS and SOY provide plant sterols that help maintain normal differentiation. The cabbage family contains indoles that increase the production of protective enzymes.
- Mustard, horseradish, and cabbage-family vegetables like broccoli contain ISOTHIOCYANATES, which also induce protective enzymes.
- Citrus fruits contain limonoids that stimulate the production of protective enzymes in the liver.
- TOMATOES and red grapefruit contain the red pigment LYCOPENE, which acts as an antioxidant to protect cells against damage.
- Parsley, carrots, cruciferous vegetables in addition to squash, yams, tomatoes, peppers, mint, basil, and cucumber, among others, contain monoterpenes that inhibit the metabolism of tumors, act as antioxidants, and stimulate the production of protective enzymes.
- Parsley, carrots, vegetables of the cabbage family, eggplant, pepper, citrus fruit, whole grains, and berries provide polyphenols (tannins) that inhibit the formation of nitrosoamines, a cancer-causing agent; act as antioxidants; and increase levels of protective enzymes.

Safety Issues Regarding Synthetic Pesticides

The long-term effects of pesticides on health are a controversial area. One position is that foods containing legal levels of pesticide residues generally pose no health risk to adults or children, provided they eat foods produced in the United States. Because they are so prevalent in plants, some investigators contend that natural toxins in foods provide a greater hazard than synthetic pesticide residues.

A number of potential problems with pesticide use have been identified.

1. Little is known about the safety of long-term exposure to low levels of multiple pesticide residues and to related compounds like PCBs (polychlorinated biphenyls) and PBBs (polybrominated biphenyls). Studies have linked the herbicide 2,4-D to non-Hodgkins lymphoma, a cancer of the lymphatic system, and PCBs and pesticides like DDT with breast cancer.
2. When screening pesticides, the EPA does not test whether they can imitate estrogen, a human female reproductive hormone. As an example, endosulfan, a pesticide used on carrots, lettuce, spinach, and tomatoes among 40 other vegeta-

bles, possesses estrogen-like properties, comparable to DDT. Exposure to such pesticides and chemicals like PCBs can disrupt the endocrine system, possibly by mimicking hormones, thus altering fertility and sexual development in animals and perhaps in humans, and increasing the risk of breast cancer.

3. Certain pesticides, environmental pollutants and antibiotics alter the integrity of MITOCHONDRIA, the energy powerhouses of the cell. The purpose of mitochondria is to produce ATP, the chemical currency of cells. Normally about three ATP are generated for each oxygen atom consumed. However, toxic chemicals can lower this ratio, significantly decreasing ATP output. This phenomenon is called uncoupling. An individual whose mitochondria are partially uncoupled has compromised health and is susceptible to other environmental insults such as viral infection or damage from oxygen.
4. More imported food is contaminated with pesticides than domestic produce. Imported fruit and vegetables may be sprayed with pesticides banned in the United States (DDT, endrin, heptachlor, aldrin, and chlordane). The FDA randomly tests imported food for pesticide residue. Samples are collected at the point of entry. All imported foods must meet the same maximum residue limits as does domestic foods. In 1999 the FDA analyzed 9,438 samples of domestic and imported food products for pesticide residue. Some 61 percent of the domestic samples and 46 percent of the imported food were contaminated.
5. An estimated 25 percent of the currently used pesticides enter both plants and animals and cannot be easily removed.
6. Pests are increasingly resistant to pesticides, so that larger amounts have to be applied.

To minimize consumption of pesticide-contaminated food patients should:

- Buy certified organically grown fruit and vegetables (produce grown without chemicals, including pesticides). Most nonorganic fruits and certain vegetables often contain higher than usual amounts of pesticides. These include tomatoes, eggplant, pepper, peach, and artichoke.
- Grow produce. The home gardener can either choose not to use pesticides or to use the safer varieties. Some pesticides are water-soluble and easily wash off from produce and decompose.
- Thoroughly wash produce with soap and water. The outer layers of lettuce, cabbage, carrots, peaches, cucumbers, and apples should be peeled off. Pesticides adhering to the skin or outer leaves can be removed; but neither strategy will remove the estimated 40 percent of pesticides that are "systemic" (contained within the fruit or vegetable). Wax that may contain fungicides cannot be washed off.
- Buy locally grown produce in season because it is less likely to be treated with fungicides. Buy domestic rather than imported produce; it is less likely to contain residues. Be aware that perfect-looking fruit may be a sign that chemicals have been used to improve its cosmetic appearance.
- Eat a wide variety of foods.
- Trim fat off meat and poultry. Use skim milk and discard fat and drippings from cooking. Pesticides such as aldrin and chlordane accumulate in animal fat.

Food Quality Protection Act of 1996

The Food Quality Protection Act of 1996 reforms the FEDERAL FOOD DRUG AND COSMETIC ACT and supersedes the DELANEY CLAUSE. It also amends the federal Insecticide, Fungicide and Rodenticide Act by establishing a single health-based standard for pesticide residues in all foods. The new safety standard to apply to pesticides is based on being reasonably certain that a given pesticide's residue will not harm the consumer. This act allows the use of additives that pose a negligible health risk, based on modern risk assessment methods, for both raw and processed foods. Other provisions prohibit states from setting tolerances stricter than federal standards, unless approved by the EPA. It also allows economic considerations to be weighed. Thus there could be continued use of some products that could exceed the negligible risk standard if they are required to assure an adequate food supply. The EPA has the authority to require chemical manufacturers to disclose information about their pesticides. Prior existing pesticides are being reviewed in light of the new standard and all existing tolerances for pesticides will be reviewed by

2006. Provisions to ensure the safety of children, infants, and pregnant women are included. When the evidence for safety is questionable, then the allowable levels are lowered to permit up to tenfold more protection. The act also requires distribution of health information about pesticides in foods by food stores nationwide. (See also CERTIFIED ORGANIC VEGETABLES; GREEN REVOLUTION; RISK DUE TO CHEMICALS IN FOOD AND WATER.)

phagocyte A defensive cell capable of engulfing bacteria, foreign materials, and cellular debris. The macrophage, a type of WHITE BLOOD CELL, is an important phagocyte of the body's IMMUNE SYSTEM. Macrophage engulf bacteria and foreign materials and release powerful chemicals, including the FREE RADICAL superoxide, HYDROGEN PEROXIDE, and NITRIC ACID to kill the invader, then digest the dead bacteria. Phagocytic cells patrol blood vessel surfaces, weeding out dead and dying cells. They avidly take up oxidized LOW-DENSITY LIPOPROTEIN, the major cholesterol carrier in the blood, and become engorged with lipid. In so doing, they become "foam" cells, which congregate on arterial walls. These events are believed to participate in the buildup of lipid deposits, leading to clogged arteries. (See also ATHEROSCLEROSIS; FREE RADICALS.)

pharynx The medical term for the throat, the tube connecting the nose and mouth to the ESOPHAGUS, the tube leading down to the STOMACH. The pharynx also connects the nose to airways leading to the lungs. The pharynx guides masticated food into the esophagus. Unchewed food can become lodged in this region, causing choking. The walls of the pharynx contain important lymphoid tissues such as adenoids and tonsils. (See also DIGESTIVE TRACT; LYMPHATIC SYSTEM.)

phenylalanine (Phe, L-phenylalanine) An essential AMINO ACID that serves as a general protein building block. Phenylalanine is incorporated into brain proteins and smaller amino acid chains (neuropeptides) such as GROWTH HORMONE and enkephalin. The body cannot synthesize phenylalanine; it must be supplied by dietary protein. The typical U.S. diet supplies about 5 g of phenylalanine daily. An adult typically requires about 1 g of phenylalanine plus TYROSINE per day. In foods, phenylalanine occurs in both animal and plant protein. Good sources of phenylalanine include any animal protein, including meat, fish, poultry, and dairy products. For comparison, a cup of GRANOLA contains 0.65 g of phenylalanine; a cup of COTTAGE CHEESE, 1.70 g; 3 oz. of hamburger, 0.53 g; and 1 can of tuna, 1.91 g.

Phenylalanine is converted to the nonessential amino acid, tyrosine. In turn, tyrosine is transformed by the NERVOUS SYSTEM into a family of NEUROTRANSMITTERS (chemicals that allow nerve impulses between cells): DOPAMINE, norepinephrine, and EPINEPHRINE. The adrenal glands also convert tyrosine to epinephrine, which functions as a stress hormone (adrenaline). Eating a protein meal raises blood levels of phenylalanine and tyrosine and allows large amounts of these amino acids to enter the brain, which in turn leads to higher levels of dopamine and norepinephrine. Phenylalanine and tyrosine metabolism require many supportive nutrients: IRON, COPPER, VITAMIN B_6, NIACIN, and VITAMIN C.

Phenylalanine Supplements

Phenylalanine (and tyrosine) supplements are claimed to increase alertness, to diminish pain and to improve mood, and helps regulate the intestinal hormone CHOLECYSTOKININ (CCK). This hormone stimulates the pancreas and gallbladder to release digestive juices and signals the brain to turn off hunger signals.

However, tyrosine and phenylalanine supplements can raise high blood pressure to dangerous, even deadly levels, especially in patients taking MAO INHIBITORS as antidepressants. People with high blood pressure should consult their doctor before using phenylalanine.

Phenylalanine aggravates migraine headaches in some patients, and produces toxic effects in patients with PHENYLKETONURIA (PKU), a genetic disease based on the inability to break down phenylalanine. ASPARTAME, an ARTIFICIAL SWEETENER, contains phenylalanine as a major ingredient. Because phenylalanine is a major constituent of aspartame, individuals with PKU are warned of foods and beverages containing this additive, and they should avoid phenylalanine supplements.

In general, amino acids are powerful agents in the body and amino acid research in humans is still considered preliminary. In many cases the long-term effects and safe doses of phenylalanine, tyrosine, or other amino acids are not known.

A synthetic form of phenylalanine, D-phenylalanine is the mirror image of the naturally occurring form of phenylalanine, L-phenylalanine. D-phenylalanine is rarely found in nature. It is not used by the body for proteins or neurotransmitters, nor is it a nutrient. D-phenylalanine seems promising as a treatment of chronic pain, particularly back pain, and dental pain. It apparently works by blocking the breakdown of ENDORPHINS, the brain's own pain killers (opiates), and also has anti-inflammatory effects. Naturally occurring phenylalanine (L-phenylalanine) does not behave in this fashion. (See also DEPRESSION; DRUG/NUTRIENT INTERACTION.)

phenylketonuria (PKU) A rare genetic disease caused by the inability to degrade the essential AMINO ACID, PHENYLALANINE. PKU patients lack a critical enzyme called phenylalanine hydroxylase, which converts phenylalanine to tyrosine, a nonessential amino acid. In PKU patients, surplus phenylalanine is converted instead to phenylketone, a breakdown product that is excreted in the urine. Excessive phenylalanine and phenylketones can cause severe mental retardation within one to two years after birth unless the diet is corrected to lower phenylalanine intake.

Although PKU is rare, states require that babies be screened for it by blood tests at birth. Children with PKU are fed a diet that restricts phenylalanine. Since phenylalanine cannot be manufactured in the body and is required for growth, the diet must supply enough to support growth while avoiding excess. As the child grows, the diet is modified to meet changing needs. The restrictive diet can often be relaxed as children mature, and they usually can go on to lead healthy lives as adults. (See also BIRTH DEFECTS.)

Waisbren, S. E. et al. "Neonatal Neurological Assessment of Offspring in Maternal Phenylketonuria." *Journal of Inherited Metabolic Disorders* 21 (1998): 39–48.

phenylpropanolamine Before 2001, this drug was the major active ingredient in diet pills, as well as in many medications for colds and allergies. In November 2000 the U.S. FDA asked all drug companies in the United States to stop using phenylpropanolamine in their products in the wake of a study that showed that it increased the risk of hemorrhagic stroke, especially in women. After reviewing the results of this study, the FDA's Nonprescription Drugs Advisory Committee concluded that phenylpropanolamine was not safe for use. (See also DIETING; DRUG/NUTRIENT INTERACTION.)

phosphatidylserine (PS) A phospholipid related to lecithin found in all cells in the human body, PS is found in its highest concentrations in the outer membrane of brain cells. Phosphatidylserine supports the fluidity of these membranes, which increases their ability to transmit electrical impulses passed from one cell to another. It is believed that as a person ages, nerve cells lose fluidity and cannot conduct electrical impulses as effectively as they once did; this is one reason why many older people have impaired memory function and find it harder to think and reason. PS also increases the nerve cells' ability to accumulate, store, and receive substances necessary to transmit electrical currents. It may also protect cells from the damage of FREE RADICALS.

Several clinical studies showed that taking PS supplements can improve cognitive and memory function, especially in older people. Subjects in several studies who took oral supplements of 300 mg of the nutrient (derived from cows' brains) had improved memory and concentration. Subjects in other studies who took PS supplements experienced relief from depression and had lowered stress levels.

Small quantities of PS can be found in many foods, including rice and green leafy vegetables such as cabbage. Because of health concerns related to BOVINE SPONGIFORM ENCEPHALITIS, soy lecithin rather than cows' brains is now used to make PS supplements. Experts disagree on whether this soy-based PS is as effective as the PS derived from cows, which was used in the clinical trials that showed such success in promoting memory and cognitive function among the elderly. Safety data are inadequate for pregnant and lactating women. (See also AGING; ALZHEIMER'S DISEASE.)

Brambilla, F., M. Maggioni, and A. E. Panerai et al. "Beta-Endorphin Concentration in Peripheral Blood

Mononuclear Cells of Elderly Depressed Patients: Effects of Phosphatidylserine Therapy," *Neuropsychobiology* 34 (1996): 18–21.

phospholipid A class of LIPIDS related to FATS. Phospholipids contain PHOSPHATE, while fats do not. In addition, phospholipids contain a nitrogen-containing compound such as SERINE or CHOLINE, or a carbohydrate-like molecule, INOSITOL. The body can manufacture its own phospholipids, and phospholipids occur in all foods.

The most common phospholipid, LECITHIN, contains choline. In practice, dietary lecithin is the major source of choline, needed for cell membrane function and the formation of NEUROTRANSMITTERS, chemicals that help transmit nerve impulses. Many nerve fibers, especially those outside the brain and spinal cord, are insulated with a white segmented covering called myelin. This lipid covering contains phospholipids and serves as insulation. Phospholipids have the ability to emulsify fat and other water-insoluble materials. As a constituent of BILE, phospholipids emulsify cholesterol and help prevent gallstone formation, and they speed up fat digestion and absorption. Phospholipids help form LOW-DENSITY LIPOPROTEIN (LDL), HIGH-DENSITY LIPOPROTEIN (HDL), and CHYLOMICRONS, lipid carriers that transport cholesterol and fat in the bloodstream.

Phospholipids also have the ability to form double lipid layers, which are the foundation of all cell membranes. As major membrane building blocks, phospholipids form protective barriers that define the cell boundary as well as the internal structures of the cell, like the nucleus, where genetic information is stored, and MITOCHONDRIA, where energy is produced.

Phospholipids incorporated into cell membranes possess polyunsaturated FATTY ACIDS. Because these fatty acids are bent molecules they do not pack together easily, and they contribute to membrane flexibility. Membrane phospholipids serve as a reserve of fatty acids for the synthesis of hormone-like fatty acid derivatives, PROSTAGLANDINS. A cascade of events leading to INFLAMMATION begins with the liberation of ARACHIDONIC ACID, a polyunsaturated fatty acid and a precursor of proinflammatory agents, from membrane phospholipids. (See also ESSENTIAL FATTY ACIDS.)

phosphorus A major mineral nutrient found primarily in bones and teeth. Phosphorus is the most common mineral in the body after CALCIUM and accounts for nearly 1.5 pounds of an adult's weight. Phosphorus exists in the body as phosphate, an inorganic, negatively charged ion. Phosphate and calcium metabolism are linked. They are withdrawn together from bone to maintain normal blood levels; vitamin D is required for both calcium and phosphate uptake. Calcium phosphate forms hydroxyapatite, the mineral deposit of bones and teeth, which represents 80 percent of the total phosphorus in the body. The remainder occurs in blood and soft tissues.

In blood, phosphate acts as a BUFFER to help maintain acid/base balance. The phosphate level in blood is increased by PARATHYROID hormone from the parathyroid gland and decreased by calcitonin, a hormone from the thyroid gland. The KIDNEY also helps to regulate phosphate. If blood phosphate levels rise, kidneys excrete phosphate; when dietary phosphate is low, they excrete less.

Tissues incorporate phosphate as PHOSPHOLIPIDS. These relatives of FAT form cell membranes and form lipid protein particles to transport fat and CHOLESTEROL through the circulation. Phosphate comprises part of the backbone structure of DNA and RNA. These substances store genetic information and control protein synthesis, cell division and growth and maintenance of the body.

Phosphate forms a building block of many COENZYMES, enzyme helpers derived from VITAMINS: NIACIN, RIBOFLAVIN, PANTOTHENIC ACID, THIAMIN, VITAMIN B_{12}, and VITAMIN B_6. ATP (adenosine triphosphate) contains phosphate groups in a form representing large amounts of potential energy that can be tapped to drive biosynthetic reactions. The formation and utilization of ATP present extremely important aspects of energy utilization by all life forms.

Sources of Phosphate

Major food sources of phosphate include: FISH, MEAT, MILK and milk products, POULTRY, EGGS, NUTS, BEANS, and PEAS. Though meat is a good source of phosphorus, it is a poor source of calcium; cheese is rich in calcium but low in phosphorus. Soft drinks are a major dietary source of this nutrient. Juices, fruit, and vegetables such as lettuce, celery, and carrots provide negligible phosphorus. Cereal grains and grain products contain phosphorus. However, much of the phosphorus in cereal grains is in the form of PHYTIC ACID, which is not readily digested. More than 20 FOOD ADDITIVES contain phosphorus, including phosphoric acid, sodium hydrogen phosphate, pyrophosphate, and POLYPHOSPHATES. These additives find use as pill stabilizers, acidifiers, chelating agents to bind up unwanted metal ions, leavening agents in baked goods, and emulsifiers in CHEESE.

Requirements

The RECOMMENDED DIETARY ALLOWANCE for phosphorus is 1,000 mg for adults. The standard U.S. diet is phosphate-rich and deficiencies are unlikely. When the ratio of calcium to phosphorus is approximately equal, phosphorus uptake is adequate. An excess of dietary phosphorus over calcium can decrease calcium uptake.

People who chronically ingest excessive amounts of ANTACIDS, patients with bone fractures, and strict vegetarians eating high-fiber foods grown on phosphorus-depleted soil may become deficient in this mineral. Symptoms include loss of appetite, weakness, and pain. Certain bone diseases, RICKETS in children, and OSTEOMALACIA in adults, are caused by chronic deficiencies of VITAMIN D, calcium, and phosphorus, or by an imbalance of calcium and phosphorus. Excessive levels of phosphorus can cause low blood calcium, with tetany and convulsions. (See also MACRONUTRIENT.)

photosynthesis The process by which plants trap the energy in sunlight and use it to convert atmospheric CARBON DIOXIDE into CARBOHYDRATE. Photosynthesis represents a nonpolluting and renewable resource. Because all foods come directly or indirectly from plants, plants form the foundation of the FOOD CHAIN. Animals and fish eat plants, which in turn serve as human food sources.

About 2 percent of the energy in sunlight actually reaches the ground and 1 percent of this is transformed into plant products by photosynthesis. Photosynthesis relies on the trapping of energy by the green plant pigment chlorophyll. In the first stage, or the light reaction of photosynthesis, water molecules are split into OXYGEN and hydrogen atoms. Oxygen is released to the atmosphere and energy is trapped in the form of ATP. In the second phase, or the dark reaction, carbon dioxide reacts with hydrogen atoms to form carbohydrate. The ATP generated by the light reaction drives this conversion. The overall process requires six molecules of carbon dioxide and six molecules of water plus sunlight to produce a single molecule of GLUCOSE, a simple sugar, plus six molecules of oxygen. The resulting glucose is converted to all other carbon compounds needed by the plant, including STARCH, CELLULOSE, FAT and other water-insoluble lipids, AMINO ACIDS and PROTEIN, and even DNA, the genetic material. Most materials produced by plants are indigestible; generally only 5 percent of a plant is suitable for human nutrition. (See also CARBOHYDRATE METABOLISM; NUTRIENT.)

pH regulators Food additives used to adjust the degree of acidity or alkalinity of a food or beverage. The pH scale refers to the acidity scale for water solutions and is based on the concentration of hydrogen ions. The scale runs from pH 0 to pH 14. The lower the pH and the more concentrated the acid, the higher the hydrogen ion concentration. A pH less than 7 is acidic; pH 7 is neutral (neither acidic nor basic); and a pH greater than 7 is alkaline (basic). The pH scale is a logarithmic scale: A pH of 3 is 10 times more acidic than a pH of 4 and 100 times more acidic than a pH of 5. Put another way, small changes in pH reflect large changes in hydrogen ion concentration.

STOMACH pH is normally about 2, due to hydrochloric acid, a very strong mineral acid produced in the stomach. Vinegar has a pH of about 5 and is somewhat acidic. Venous blood pH normally ranges between 7.36 and 7.41, slightly alkaline. A blood pH below 6.8 (severe ACIDOSIS) or above 7.8 (severe ALKALOSIS) is usually fatal. Urinary pH ranges from 5 to 8.

The final products of metabolism of fruits and vegetables, which are rich in potassium, tend to make the body more alkaline. Foods that make the body more alkaline include LEGUMES, SQUASH, members of the CABBAGE family, and dark green leafy vegetables. Meat, dairy products (high-protein foods), refined carbohydrate and sugar tend to acidify the body because they produce an acidic residue. Vegans (strict vegetarians) tend to produce more alkaline end products than meat eaters.

Because most enzymes and cellular processes operate effectively at pHs close to neutral, the body possesses many elaborate systems that regulate the pH of the body fluids. All physiologic processes, from cell division to nerve transmission, rely on enzymes, and they are exquisitely sensitive to pH for optimal activity. The KIDNEYS, lungs, and RED BLOOD CELLS are especially involved in the regulating process. Together, they help maintain a constant internal environment (HOMEOSTASIS).

pH considerations are also important in packaged foods and beverages. Excessively acidic or alkaline conditions can alter the appearance, taste and nutrient quality of prepared foods and beverages. Therefore, food additives called pH regulating agents are used to control the degree of acidity or alkalinity of commercially prepared foods and beverages. Examples include CITRIC ACID and various forms of phosphates like sodium dihydrogen phosphate in SOFT DRINKS. (See also ACID INDIGESTION; BUFFER.)

physical activity See EXERCISE.

physical fitness See FITNESS.

phytic acid/phytate A plant compound containing phosphate bound to a carbohydrate-like compound called INOSITOL. Phytic acid occurs in unsprouted GRAINS, seeds, and LEGUMES and is particularly rich in BRAN, the outer layer of grains. Although these foods often have a high phosphorus content, the phosphate in phytates is not released by digestion. Phytic acid can bind minerals very tightly, and in the intestine, phytic acid will bind IRON, MAGNESIUM, and ZINC, limiting their uptake. When bread is leavened by YEAST, yeast enzymes degrade phytic acid, and yeast-leavened bread poses no threat to mineral absorption. Phytic acid is also destroyed by baking and FOOD PROCESSING. A balanced diet emphasizing minimally processed foods does not pose a problem, but wheat bran added to supplement a diet relying on high-sugar, high-fat processed food may interfere with mineral absorption. (See also MALABSORPTION.)

phytochemicals A very broad class of chemicals derived from plants that have a beneficial effect on health. In the broad sense, phytochemicals include VITAMIN C and compounds like BETA-CAROTENE, which can be converted to VITAMIN A. However, phytochemicals include thousands of other substances; some are not well characterized and their effects are poorly understood. Many others remain to be identified. Inadequate consumption of phytochemicals may well be a major contributing factor in the chronic diseases prevalent in most Western societies. Much of what is currently known about phytochemicals is the result of recent research. Most attention has focused on the possible effects of phytochemicals in the development of cardiovascular disease and of cancer. Often, conclusions are based on studies with isolated cells or laboratory animals. How far such findings can be applied to humans is frequently not clear. Recent research has focused on several important classes that profoundly affect health. They occur in vegetables, fruits, seeds, legumes, tea, medicinal plants, spices, culinary herbs, and even edible mushrooms. Phytochemicals are conveniently classified into the following groups: FLAVONOIDS, PHYTOSTEROLS, CAROTENOIDS, indoles, coumarins, organosulfur compounds, terpenes, saponins, lignans, and ISOTHIOCYANATES. The accompanying table includes sources and possible actions of primary phytochemicals. The following examples are noteworthy.

Flavonoids Over 5,000 flavonoids have been identified. Plants evolved this large class of compounds to protect themselves against oxidative damage. Flavonoids consist of multiple ring structures; the purple, blue, and red color of fruits and berries represent flavonoids. Flavonoids act as ANTIOXIDANTS to squelch very reactive chemicals called FREE RADICALS, which are generated by pollutants as well as from oxygen by the body's own processes. Flavonoids can stabilize connective tissue and capillaries, and seem to work together with vitamin C in this regard. They also decrease inflammation by several mechanisms. They inhibit the infiltration of immune cells that cause inflammation (neutrophils). They block enzymes that generate inflammatory prostaglandins and leukotrienes, fatty acid derivatives with hormone-

PHYTOCHEMICALS THAT MAY BENEFIT HEALTH

Phytochemicals	Typical Source	Possible Roles
Flavonoids		
Polyphenols like quercetin, kaempferol anthocyanin	Fruits, berries, vegetables, kale, bark stems, wine	Antioxidant. May stimulate detoxication enzymes and protects liver. Strengthens capillaries. Blocks inflammation. May inhibit tumor formation.
Phytosterols		
Isoflavones like Genistein	Soybeans, lentils, peas	May inhibit estrogen-promoted cancers and lower high blood cholesterol to decrease the risk of atherosclerosis.
Carotenoids		
Carotenes like alpha-carotene and beta-carotene	Carrots, yams, cantaloupe, butternut squash	Antioxidant. May protect against heart disease and stroke.
Lycopene	Tomatoes, red grapefruit	Antioxidant. May protect against cancers of the cervix, stomach, bladder, colon, and prostate.
Xanthophylls	Dark green leafy vegetables	Antioxidant. May protect against heart disease and stroke.
Indoles	Cruciferous vegetables, such as broccoli, cabbage, and brussels sprouts	May protect against breast cancer.
Coumarins	Citrus fruit, tomatoes	May prevent blood clotting and may stimulate detoxication enzymes in the liver.
Organosulfur Compounds		
Diallyl disulfide, S-allylcysteine, others	Garlic, onions, leeks, shallots, chives	May block carcinogens and suppress carcinogenic changes in cells. May stimulate detoxication enzymes.
Terpenes		
Monoterpenes	Citrus fruit, caraway seeds	May block action of carcinogens.
Triterpenes	Licorice root, citrus fruit	May inhibit hormone related cancers.
Saponins	Soybeans, many vegetables, herbs	May have anticancer activity. May lower high blood cholesterol.
Lignans	Flaxseed, wheat, barley	An antioxidant. May protect against cancers.
Isothiocyanates		
Sulforaphane and others	Cruciferous vegetables, including broccoli, watercress, cabbage, mustard, horseradish	May protect against breast cancer, stimulate detoxication enzymes, and protect against cigarette smoke.

like qualities, and they desensitize mast cells, a type of immune cell embedded in tissues that release inflammatory agents like histamine when they encounter a foreign invader. Various flavonoids decrease the ability of platelets to form dangerous blood clots. Flavonoids can either activate or inhibit detoxication enzymes of the liver that help dispose of wastes and toxic materials. Such phytochemicals in wine, onions, apples, and tea are believed to reduce the risk of CORONARY ARTERY DISEASE.

Isothiocyanates The cabbage family (Brassica vegetables) possesses sulfur compounds that protect against some forms of cancer. SULFORAPHANE is an example. Isothiocyanates seem to act on detoxication mechanisms, speeding up the inactivation and disposal of potentially harmful compounds like pollutants from the body.

Phytoestrogens A group of compounds found in soybean and other legumes. Saponins and isoflavones possess very weak estrogen activity. Estrogen is a female sex hormone, and by mimicking estrogen, phytoestrogens may lower the risk of certain cancers, including breast cancer.

Carotenoids Yellow-orange pigments that occur in dark green leafy vegetables and orange vegetables and fruits. Carotenoids act as antioxidants and they bolster the immune system. Beta-carotene is the most famous example.

Organosulfur Compounds Onions, leeks, and garlic supply a host of sulfur-containing compounds, such as dialyl sulfide and allicin, that serve the body in many ways. They strengthen the immune system, serve as antimicrobial agents, and help the body's ability to process potentially harmful substances.

A well balanced diet will provide ample amounts of phytochemicals. However, in the United States most people do not consume the minimum recommended five servings of fruits and vegetables daily. A serving is considered only half a cup. If this trend continues, it seems likely that the inadequate consumption of phytochemicals will have a profound negative impact on health in future decades.

American Dietetic Association. "The Position of the American Dietetic Association: Phytochemicals and Functional Foods," *Journal of the American Dietetic Association* 95 (1995): 493.

phytoesterols (plant sterols, plant stanols, sterol esters) Plant extracts that inhibit the body's absorption of CHOLESTEROL. Phytoesterols such as sito stanol are found in vegetable oils, especially soybean oil, as well as many fruits, nuts, and cereals. Excess cholesterol in the body, especially the "bad" type, LOW-DENSITY LIPOPROTEIN (LDL), can cause the build up of plaque in arteries, which increases the risk of heart attack and stroke.

In one study children who were genetically predisposed to early heart disease and who ate MARGARINE that contained sterol esters for three months reduced their LDL cholesterol levels by 18 percent. Adult relatives of the children who participated in the study also experienced some decrease in LDL cholesterol levels. The U.S. Food and Drug Administration recently gave companies that produce foods, such as certain margarines, containing amounts of phytoesterols that have been proven to lower cholesterol levels permission to claim that consuming these foods can lower the risk of heart disease. Safety data are inadequate for pregnant and breast-feeding women.

Hallikainen, M. A. et al. "Plant Stanol Esters Affect Serum Cholesterol Concentrations of Hyphercholesterolemic Men and Women in a Dose Dependent Manner," *Journal of Nutrition* 130, no. 4 (2000): 767–776.

phytoestrogens Plant products related to cholesterol that to a limited extent mimic ESTROGENS (female sex hormones). Phytoestrogens are found in a variety of medicinal HERBS with a long history in folk medicine, such as DONG QUAI (angelica), LICORICE, BLACK COHOSH, and FENNEL as well as soy foods. The estrogen-like activity of phytosterols is low, perhaps only 0.25 percent of the activity of estrogen. They can counteract high estrogen levels or they can cause an increase in estrogenic activity, depending on the circumstances. Phytoestrogens may compete with estrogen, thus minimizing the effects of excessive estrogen. Phytoestrogens may help relieve some of the symptoms of menopause and lower the risk of OSTEOPOROSIS, a bone-thinning disease. However, some experts warn that women at risk for inherited breast cancer should avoid excess phytoestrogens. Two broad classes of compounds describe photoestrogens: ISOFLAVONES and saponins. Isoflavones are a type of FLAVONOID found in high levels in soybeans, genestein is a primary example. Saponins are cholesterol-like molecules that can mimic steroid hormones because they possess a similar molecular shape. Saponins are widely distributed in legumes, including soybeans; chickpeas, mung beans, and kidney beans. Saponins have the ability to lower blood cholesterol, to serve as antioxidants, to inhibit viruses, and to inhibit certain forms of cancer. Safety data for use of therapeutic amounts of isoflavones are inadequate for pregnant and breast-feeding women. (See also ENDOCRINE SYSTEM.)

pica An abnormal CRAVING for nonfood materials. These may be STARCH, clay, dirt, wood, or chalk. Clay eating among tribal peoples could have its origins in the ability of clay to bind toxic materials. Iron deficiency may be the cause of pica in some cases. Animals and livestock eat dirt when they become mineral deficient. (See also PAGOPHAGIA.)

pimento (*Pimento dioaca*) A sweet red PEPPER that is three to four inches long and about two inches wide. *Pimento* is similar to *pimienta,* which means "pepper" in Spanish, and is the name of the semiwild tree on which the pepper grows. Spanish explorers gave the tree its name shortly after arriving in the Caribbean Islands. The pimento tree is indigenous to those islands, where most of the world's crop grows. Berries that grow on the tree are harvested, dried, and sometimes ground to create allspice, a spice similar in taste to nutmeg. Marinated pimento slices are often used as a condiment or as a stuffing for pitted green olives. Most of the annual crop is harvested to make PAPRIKA, a mild seasoning used to flavor a variety of foods, including soups, stews, and many Indian dishes. Two tablespoons of marinated pimentos (25 g) provides: calories, 5; sodium, 5 mg.

pineapple (*Ananas comosus*) A tropical plant with stiff, spiny leaves that yields a single large FRUIT. The pineapple originated in Brazil and then spread to the Caribbean. Europeans took the pineapple to Australia, South Africa, and Hawaii. China, Hawaii, the Philippines, India, Brazil, and Mexico are the leading producers. Most fresh pineapple marketed in the United States comes from Puerto Rico, Hawaii, and Mexico. Pineapples weigh from one to 20 pounds depending on the variety. A typical Hawaiian pineapple, the Smooth Cayenne variety, can weigh several pounds. This cone-shaped pineapple is the most popular fresh pineapple in the United States.

Pineapple contains about 15 percent sugar. Unlike many fruits, pineapple does not ripen at home. The fruit can be eaten fresh or can be cooked. Pineapple juice is canned or frozen as a concentrate. Pineapple is also used in ice cream, baked goods, and salads, and is served with meat. Fresh pineapple cannot be used with gelatin-based desserts and salads because it contains BROMELAIN, a protein-degrading enzyme that breaks down jelled protein. Canning destroys the activity. Bromelain is used in meat tenderizers, in certain plant-based digestive aids, and as a beer clarifier. Pineapple is an excellent source of VITAMIN C. Nutrient content of 1 cup (155 g), raw, is: 76 calories; protein, 0.6 g; carbohydrate, 19.2 g; fiber, 2.95 g; fat, 0.7 g; potassium, 175 mg; vitamin C, 124 mg; thiamin, 0.14 mg; riboflavin, 0.06 mg; niacin, 0.65 mg.

pinocytosis The process by which a cell feeds itself by enveloping fluid and substances in its environment. Pinocytosis allows molecules that would normally be excluded by the outer membrane to enter the cell; most cells carry out pinocytosis. In receptor-mediated endocytosis, docking sites (receptors) on the cell surface bind external molecules or particles. As an example, large particles such as LOW-DENSITY LIPOPROTEIN (LDL), which transfers CHOLESTEROL to tissues, attach to the outer cell surface at specific receptor sites. The membrane at the point of attachment forms a pit; the pit deepens and eventually pinches off. The adhered material is engulfed, forming a membrane-bound sac, or vesicle, as the cell membrane reseals itself. The pinched-off vesicles migrate to LYSOSOMES, particles distributed throughout the cytoplasm that digest cellular debris and engulfed particles. Lysosomes then release AMINO ACIDS and cholesterol from degraded LDL to be recycled. Intestinal cells can absorb food proteins, peptides, and bacterial products that have escaped digestion. The uptake of such foreign materials contributes to the burden confronting the body's immune system.

Pinocytosis differs from phagocytosis (cell eating), in which the cell sends out projections that envelope large particles like bacteria and form a sac enclosing the particle. Solid material inside the vesicle is digested by lysosomes. Few cells carry out phagocytosis. (See also ALLERGY; DIGESTION; FOOD SENSITIVITY.)

pistachio (*Pistacia vera*) The edible seed of a small, tropical evergreen tree of the cashew family. The pistachio is native to the Mediterranean area and Asia. Major nut-producing areas are Iran, Syria, Turkey, and the United States (California). The seed occurs within a small fruit. The pale green meat is used as coloring and flavoring for candy, ice cream, and baked goods. Salted nuts are eaten as snack food. Imported pistachios are often dyed red. The nutrient contents of 1 oz. (28 g, dried, shelled nuts) provide 164 calories; protein, 5.9 g; carbohydrate, 7 g; fiber, 1.3 g; fat, 13.7 g; sodium, 221 mg; thiamin, 0.22 mg; riboflavin, 0.05 mg; niacin, 0.31 mg.

pituitary gland The "master gland" that regulates many other hormone-secreting (endocrine) glands. This gland is located deep in the skull beneath the region of the brain called the HYPOTHALAMUS and is about the size of a pea. It possesses two lobes, each of which produces hormones. The anterior lobe (adenohypophysis) produces GROWTH HORMONE, which regulates the METABOLISM and growth of muscle and bone. It also produces a range of stimulating factors: thyroid-stimulating hormone, which stimulates the THYROID GLAND to release thyroxine to regulate the rate of metabolism in all tissues; follicle-stimulating hormone and luteinizing hormone to regulate ovulation; PROLACTIN, which stimulates milk production; adrenocorticotropic hormone (ACTH), which activates the outer region of the ADRENAL GLAND (adrenal cortex) to secrete glucocorticoids to raise BLOOD SUGAR and mineralocorticoids to regulate sodium and water balance.

The posterior lobe (neurohypophysis) secretes OXYTOCIN, which regulates milk production and uterine contractions, and ANTIDIURETIC HORMONE (vasopressin), which conserves WATER and SODIUM in the kidney. Oxytocin and vasopressin are first synthesized in the hypothalamus and travel to the pituitary to be secreted. The pituitary and hypothalamus represent a direct link between the NERVOUS SYSTEM and the ENDOCRINE SYSTEM. The hypothalamus is that region of the brain that controls involuntary responses that regulate the internal environment: body temperature, blood pressure, and water balance, among others. The pituitary gland receives signals from the hypothalamus in the form of trophic hormones. (See also HOMEOSTASIS.)

pizza A flat, circular bread baked with a variety of toppings. The word *pizza* is Italian for "pie." The average American eats about 23 pounds yearly. Pizza dough is rolled or pressed flat, traditionally topped with TOMATOES, tomato paste, and herbs, and baked. The American variety of pizza is topped with mozzarella or Parmesan CHEESE, various types of SAUSAGE, MUSHROOMS, OLIVES, VEGETABLES, spices, and anchovies, among other toppings. Pizza is often high in FAT, CALORIES, and SODIUM. Cheese and MEAT toppings like pepperoni contribute the fat.

Frozen pizza is usually highly processed; it contains imitation cheese as well as FOOD ADDITIVES. It may be labeled as containing imitation cheese or cheese substitute. Nutrient content of one slice (120 g) of a typical cheese pizza made with vegetable shortening is: 290 calories; protein, 15 g; carbohydrate, 39 g; fiber, 2.2 g; fat, 9 g; cholesterol, 56 mg; calcium, 220 mg; sodium, 700 mg; thiamin, 0.34 mg; riboflavin, 0.29 mg; niacin, 4.2 mg. (See also CONVENIENCE FOOD; PASTA; PROCESSED FOOD.)

PKU See PHENYLKETONURIA.

placebo In general, a sugar pill or treatment that does not contain an active substance or effective material associated with a cure. Placebos may also be therapeutic procedures that lack specific effects. Placebos have a wide range of effects on human physiology and can decrease pulse rate; decrease serum cholesterol and fat levels; lower BLOOD SUGAR in diabetic patients; heal DUODENAL ULCERS; decrease stomach acid production; lower elevated blood pressure; reduce pain associated with ARTHRITIS, ACID INDIGESTION, ulcers, labor pain, and PREMENSTRUAL SYNDROME, among other conditions. Placebo effects have been observed in surgery and drug therapy.

Placebo Effect

The placebo effect refers to positive changes produced by placebos that may aid in recovery. (If the placebo has a deleterious effect in the healing process, the result is called a nocebo effect.) Belief, hope, or faith in a cure to alleviate a disease or symptoms can mobilize the body's ability to heal itself. Thus, the relationship between physician and patient has an immediate impact on the effectiveness of a therapeutic intervention. It is ancient wisdom that a large percentage of people will get better simply after talking with someone they trust, or when they visualize wellness, in prayer, meditation, or ritual. Placebos gained prominence in the 1960s when careful medical experimentation frequently incorporated double-blind, placebo-controlled studies. In these studies, neither the doctor nor the patients knew who was getting the therapeutic dose or who was receiving a neutral control (placebo) until after the treatment or experiment had been completed.

Apparently, the expectation of relief even from a sugar pill stimulates the brain to release painkiller chemicals called ENDORPHINS. The NERVOUS SYSTEM is tightly coupled with the IMMUNE SYSTEM (the body's defense system), as well as with the ENDOCRINE SYSTEM (hormone-producing system). Thus, endorphins can alter antibody production, white cell production, natural killer cell function and other important aspects of immunity. In some cases, levels increase; in others, levels decline. The autonomic nervous system, regulating involuntary processes and hormones, seems to participate in the healing process as well. (See also CLINICAL TRIAL; RISK DUE TO CHEMICALS IN FOOD AND WATER.)

plantain (*Musa paradisiaca*) The FRUIT that resembles a large green BANANA. The plantain is native to India and today is cultivated worldwide in tropical areas. Plantains become more palatable when baked, fried, or otherwise cooked like a vegetable. Plantains contain more STARCH and less SUGAR than bananas and are made into a flour in tropical regions of the world, where they are a staple food. Powdered plantains may heal PEPTIC ULCERS. Cooking may destroy the anti-ulcer components, however. Plantains can be baked like potatoes or sliced and used in stir-fries or stews and soups. Nutritionally, plantains resemble bananas. Nutrient contents of 1 cup (148 g) is: 181 calories; protein, 1.9 g; carbohydrate, 47.2 g; fiber, 0.74 g; fat, 0.55 g; potassium, 739 mg; vitamin C, 27.2 mg; thiamin 0.077 mg; riboflavin, 0.08 mg; niacin, 1.0 mg.

plaque, arterial Plaques on the inner surface of arteries. They contain mineral deposits, connective TISSUE, and waxy deposits enriched in cells containing LIPIDS and CHOLESTEROL. In certain cases, plaque is related to the uptake of oxidized cholesterol from the blood. These deposits contribute to stiffened, obstructed arteries and restricted blood flow and play a major role in CARDIOVASCULAR DISEASE. (See also ATHEROSCLEROSIS; LOW-DENSITY LIPOPROTEIN.)

plaque, dental Deposits on teeth that consists of a sticky mass of oral bacteria, carbohydrate secreted by bacteria and minerals. Such deposits promote tooth decay by holding bacteria close to the tooth surface. They can harden over time as more mineral is deposited. Plaque contributes to tooth decay and gum disease. (See also PERIODONTAL DISEASE.)

plasma The clear, cell-free fluid of BLOOD. Plasma contains the soluble proteins of blood, including clotting proteins, HORMONES, NUTRIENTS like glucose, gamma globulin (ANTIBODIES), nutrients like glucose and soluble waste products such as UREA, but not RED BLOOD CELLS or white blood cells. Plasma represents about 50 percent of the volume of the blood. It is prepared by centrifuging whole blood to remove red blood cells and white blood cells. In laboratory testing, plasma is used to measure levels of nutrients such as AMINO ACIDS and ESSENTIAL FATTY ACIDS. (See also HEMATOCRIT; SERUM.)

platelets (thrombocytes) Small cell fragments in the blood that help initiate blood clot formation. They are oval or round discs and lack a nucleus. Platelets are produced by the fragmentation of a large precursor cell called mega-karyocyte produced on BONE marrow. Platelets are normally maintained at a concentration of 250,000 to 750,000 per milliliter of blood. Platelets plug damaged blood vessels in the following way. When they come into contact with damaged vessel walls, they attach to COLLAGEN exposed by injury and form clumps. Platelets develop irregular projections to increase cell-cell contact and then release thromboxane, a hormone-like lipid, and other factors that make platelets more sticky to help form a blood clot and seal the wound. Platelets release SEROTONIN, which causes blood vessels to contract, to further reduce bleeding. Platelet aggregation is limited by polyunsaturated FATTY ACIDS in FISH and FISH OIL. These dietary components may decrease the rate of BLOOD CLOTTING and lower the risk of

STROKE. (See also CARDIOVASCULAR DISEASE; EICOSAPENTAENOIC ACID.)

plum (*Prunus spp.*) An oval or round FRUIT related to APRICOTS, CHERRIES, and PEACHES. The Japanese plum originated in China, and plums have been grown in Europe for thousands of years. There are more than 140 varieties of plum. *P. americana* is native to North America; *P. domestica, P. mexicana,* and *P. salicina* are common species that originated in Europe and China. The smooth skin ranges in color from yellow or green to shades of red and purple. Ripe plums have a higher sugar content than most other fruits, and the flesh is usually yellow or red.

Top plum producers worldwide include Romania, the United States, China, and Germany. California leads other states in domestic plum production. Plum varieties include Bearly, Burbank, Burmosa, Casselman, Duarte, Empress, French, Friar, Italian, Kelsey, Queen Rosa, President, Red Beaut, Santa Rosa, Simka, and Wickson. Hard plums will ripen when placed in a closed paper bag for several days at room temperature. The nutrient contents of one raw plum without its pit (66 g) are: 36 calories; protein, 0.5 g; carbohydrate, 8.6 g; fiber, 1.45 g; fat, 0.4 g; vitamin C, 6 mg; thiamin, 0.03 mg; riboflavin, 0.06 mg; niacin, 0.33 mg.

Prunes

Most plums are dried as prunes or are canned; only 20 percent to 30 percent of plums are marketed fresh. In June 2000 the U.S. Food and Drug Administration granted a request by the California Prune Board to use the term *dried plums* as an alternative to *prunes,* and on November 29, 2000, the California Prune Board became the California Dried Plum Board. The board wanted to increase awareness that prunes are dried plums and change the image of prunes from "old and laxative" to healthy and contemporary. Research conducted by the board had shown that younger consumers were more likely to try "dried plums" than "prunes." Regardless of their name, prunes are an excellent fat-free substitute for butter, margarine, and oil in baked products and are a good source of vitamin A and fiber.

The most common variety used for prunes is the California French. California supplies almost all domestic prunes. The tree-ripened fruit is carefully dried. Prunes are a high-fiber food, containing more fiber than most other fruits and vegetables. Prune juice is rich in potassium. One cup contains 3 mg of iron, 473 mg of potassium and 182 calories. Because of its high sugar content it can be substituted for sugar in beverages, sauces, or salads. Prune juice is a by-product of prune dehydration in prune production.

PMS See PREMENSTRUAL SYNDROME.

pollock (*Pollachius virens*) A saltwater bottom fish similar to cod in size, shape, and quality of flesh. Pollock is classified as a lean fish. The North Pacific pollock fishery is a $1 billion-a-year industry and represents the world's single most profitable fishing industry. Most pollock is converted to fish sticks and to SURIMI, a bland fish protein mixture. Surimi forms the basis of imitation crab meat and other imitation seafoods. Pollock can be baked, broiled, poached, or used in chowders. The nutrient content of 3.5 oz. (100 g) of steamed pollack is; 99 calories; protein, 23.3 g; fat, 0.9 g; cholesterol, 75 mg; potassium, 350 mg; thiamin, 0.12 mg; riboflavin, 0.26 mg; niacin, 4 mg.

polybrominated biphenyls (PBBs) A synthetic flame-retardant that has been banned for many years in the United States. PBBs were once used to coat roofs and to treat fabric. PBBs are related to POLYCHLORINATED BIPHENYLS (PCBs); both are long-lasting environmental pollutants.

PBBs belong to the class of halogenated hydrocarbons that are generally toxic and potentially cancer-causing agents. The long-term effect of chronic, low-level exposure to PBBs is unknown. Symptoms of severe exposure include memory loss, poor hand coordination, swollen joints, abdominal pain, diarrhea, and acne. PBBs cause CANCER, in addition to impaired immunity and liver malfunction in experimental animals. In humans, acute exposure to PBBs is related to headaches and nervous disorders.

PBBs are compounds containing two benzene rings, with bromine atoms attached to various positions on the rings. PBB is a generic term referring to a family of closely related compounds. Attention was drawn to the toxicity of PBBs when a Michigan chemical company packed PBBs in bags labeled as a mineral supplement that were used as a feed additive for livestock. It was inadvertently shipped to farms, and by 1973 it had caused widespread damage to dairy herds. PBBs contaminated wildlife, Great Lakes fish, poultry, and cattle, and gradually spread so that most Michigan residents were contaminated.

PBBs resist degradation in the environment by light, heat, and oxygen and are only slowly broken down by microbes. As fat-soluble substances. PBBs accumulate in the fatty tissues of organisms that consume them because they are relatively resistant to cellular processes. Animals at the top of the FOOD CHAIN, like predatory fish and birds and omnivores like humans, tend to collect the highest levels of PBBs and other stable, fat-soluble pollutants. Most Americans now carry trace amounts of PBBs in their tissues. PBBs accumulate in human fat and are released through breast milk. In spite of widespread contamination of breast milk by traces of pollutants, authorities agree that the advantages of BREAST-FEEDING outweigh the disadvantages. (See also PESTICIDES; RISK DUE TO CHEMICALS IN FOOD AND WATER.)

polychlorinated biphenyls (PCBs) A widely distributed industrial pollutant that were formerly manufactured for use as insulators in electrical transformers, paints, adhesives, and caulking compounds. PCBs are one of the first examples presented of environmental chemical hazards from nonPESTICIDE industrial chemicals. PCBs were first detected as environmental pollutants in Sweden in 1966. In 1968 more than a thousand Japanese were affected with Yusho (rice-oil) disease, due to PCB contamination of cooking oil. Since that time, PCBs have been detected in foods such as MILK, EGGS, MEAT, and FISH in many regions of the world. In 1977, polar bears from Arctic were shown to contain significant levels of PCBs, indicating this pollutant had spread through the global FOOD CHAIN. Production of PCBs in the United States was halted in 1977.

PCBs belong to the class of CHLORINATED HYDROCARBONS, carbon compounds that generally are toxic and are potentially cancer-causing agents. PCBs are double–ring structures with chlorine atoms attached to various positions on both rings. There are over 40 different forms (isomers) in this family. They resist environmental degradation by sunlight, heat and exposure to air. Gradual microbial degradation occurs; bacteria have been isolated that remove chlorine atoms permitting PCB oxidation. Nonetheless, the rates of degradation in the environment are slow, and PCBs persist a long time. Being fat-soluble, PCBs accumulate in the cell membranes and fatty tissues of all organisms that digest them because they are relatively resistant to metabolic conversions.

By 1980, the EPA estimated that more than 90 percent of Americans carried PCB residues in their fatty tissues. PCB residues remain widespread. Exposure has come via many accidental routes. The most important food sources of PCBs are freshwater fish, notably from the Great Lakes, and bottom-feeding fish from waters near industrial areas, such as striped bass in the Hudson River. For 30 years PCBs were discharged into the Hudson River (New York State) as waste from capacitor plants, contaminating fish. Widespread PCB population of Great Lakes fish was detected only after mink, who were fed fish from Lake Michigan, developed severe reproductive abnormalities or died. In 1979, contamination by PCBs in Billings, Montana, led to the destruction of hundreds of thousands of CHICKENS, eggs, and thousands of pounds of PORK. In other instances, fodder stored in silos painted with PCB-containing paint led to contaminated dairy herds and thus contaminated milk and milk products.

Symptoms of severe exposure include a form of severe acne (chloracne), visual disturbances, spasms, headaches, FATIGUE, nausea, and numbness. The long-term effects of chronic low-level exposures are unknown. Chronic exposure may be linked to an increased risk of CANCER because PCBs are linked to liver tumors and reproductive problems in experimental animals. Environmental contaminants, including PCBs and by-products of the pesticide DDT, were found in higher levels in the breast fat of women who had breast cancer than in the breast tissue of women without cancer. Dioxin, PCBs, and other industrial chemicals can change fertility and sexual behavior in animals, fish, and perhaps humans. These substances may alter the endocrine system by mimicking the action of the feminizing HORMONE estrogen.

Some studies show that pregnant women who consume fish contaminated with low levels of PCBs give birth to low birth weight babies with developmental abnormalities. In 1979, cooking oil contaminated with PCBs caused mass poisoning in Taiwan. Children born to Taiwanese women exposed to PCBs were more likely to have delayed development, abnormal lungs and skin, and more neurological complaints than normal children. Traces of PCBs are routinely detected in the BREAST MILK of American women. Nonetheless, the World Health Organization (WHO) and La Leche League recommend breast-feeding, agreeing that the advantages of breast-feeding outweigh the disadvantages. (See also RISK DUE TO CHEMICALS IN FOOD AND WATER.)

Pijnenburg, A. M. et al. "Polybrominated biphenyl and diphenylether flame retardants: analysis, toxicity, and environmental occurrence," *Reviews of Environmental Contamination and Toxicology* 141 (1995): 1–26.

polydipsia Excessive thirst that occurs after extensive loss of body fluids. (See also DEHYDRATION; DIABETES MELLITUS.)

polyglycerol esters Synthetic compounds resembling fat that are used to emulsify oils in foods. A key ingredient of these lipids is glycerol, a small triple alcohol that is the backbone of fat molecules. Polyglycerol esters contain several linked glycerol units, to which are attached various fatty acids. The fatty acids can be short- or long-chain, unsaturated or saturated, to create oils or solid fats. The polyglycerol esters may be either water-soluble or water-insoluble, depending on the ingredients used in their fabrication. As "hybrid" fats, they provide 80 percent of the calories of true fats and oils. (See also FAT SUBSTITUTE; FOOD ADDITIVE.)

polyneuropathy A disease affecting groups of peripheral nerves. These nerves exclude the brain (cranial nerves) and the spinal column (spinal nerves). Polyneuropathy is caused by toxic exposure, nutritional deficiency, or metabolic abnormality. Both sides of the body are affected; symptoms involve leg pain, muscle weakness, numbness, and even partial paralysis. Both motor reactions (movement) and sensory responses (touch, response to pain) may be affected. Chronic, severe deficiencies of the B vitamins, THIAMIN, PANTOTHENIC ACID, and VITAMIN B_6, cause polyneuropathy. Such deficiencies can occur in alcoholics and are associated with MALNUTRITION as well as maldigestion. Uncontrolled DIABETES MELLITUS in older patients causes peripheral nerve damage due to damaged capillaries feeding peripheral tissue. Lead poisoning also causes a progressive neuropathy. (See also ALCOHOLISM; BERIBERI.)

polypeptide See PEPTIDE.

polyphosphates FOOD ADDITIVES used to bind unwanted metal ions. Polyphosphates aid in curing meats and in enhancing meat flavors. Polyphosphates are chains of three or more phosphates, the nutrient form of PHOSPHORUS. The combined forms contain potassium, sodium, or other minerals. They are readily broken down to phosphate and are considered safe food additives. (See also CHELATE.)

polysaccharides A large family of CARBOHYDRATES that possess long chains made up of many building blocks of simple sugar (monosaccharides) or sugar derivatives. Polysaccharides can be branched or unbranched. They may contain a single type of carbohydrate building block, or they may contain several types, including sugar amines such as glucosamine (nitrogen-containing sugars) or sugar acids like galacturonic acid or glucuronic acid. Polysaccharides are classified as complex carbohydrates because they are complex molecules compared to simple sugars.

The physical and chemical properties and biological function of polysaccharides depend on the number, the kind, and the sequence of sugars within the complex carbohydrates. Most polysaccharides found in food are either plant FIBER or STARCH. Fiber represents a mixture of different kinds of polysaccharides, each composed of different sets of sugars. They strengthen plant cell walls and plant tissue. Common examples are CELLULOSE, PECTIN, GUMS, and HEMICELLULOSE made from modified glucose and other sugars. The primary structural polysaccharide of plants is cellulose, an insoluble fiber. Pectin represents a water-soluble form of fiber. Fiber is not digested in the small intestine, but is more or less broken down by colonic bacteria to provide important fuels for cells lining the colon.

Starch is the principal plant storage of carbohydrate and contains only GLUCOSE. It is common in grains like WHEAT, CORN, and RICE, and in starchy vegetables like potatoes. Animals make several polysaccharides. The liver and skeletal muscles store glucose in the form of long, branched chains called GLYCOGEN. Muscles release glucose from glycogen for quick energy, while the liver releases glucose from its stored glycogen into the blood stream to help maintain steady BLOOD SUGAR levels between meals. Mucopolysaccharides (GLYCOSAMINOGLYCANS) create slippery surfaces in joints, structural materials that hold together cells (connective tissue) and the protective linings of the stomach and intestines. (See also CARBOHYDRATE DIGESTION; CARBOHYDRATE METABOLISM.)

polysorbates Synthetic polymers added to emulsify (suspend) oils and flavors in frozen desserts, bread dough, artificial whipped cream and nondairy creamer, beverages, CANDY, and ICE CREAM. Polysorbates are prepared by combining FATTY ACIDS with SORBITOL, a sugar alcohol, then linking many sorbate molecules together in long chains. The most prevalent form is polysorbate 60. The fatty acids are released by digestion and absorbed, and the remaining polymer is eliminated. Polysorbates have been used with patients to increase fat assimilation. Levels up to 5 percent have been fed to experimental animals and do not appear harmful. They have been in use since the 1940s and are apparently safe additives. (See also EMULSIFIERS; FOOD ADDITIVES.)

polyunsaturated fatty acids See FATTY ACIDS.

polyunsaturated oils Liquid FATS that contain a relatively high percentage of polyunsaturated FATTY ACIDS as building blocks. These bent molecules contain multiple double bonds. Because they are bent, they do not stick together tightly and thus do not solidify as easily as do SATURATED FATS, which possess straight chains. Fats containing more than 45 percent of their acids as polyunsaturated fatty acids are oils at room temperature and are classified as polyunsaturates. Vegetable oils like COTTONSEED OIL, CORN OIL, SAFFLOWER oil, and SOYBEAN oil contain LINOLEIC ACID, the omega-6 ESSENTIAL FATTY ACID with two unsaturated bonds; safflower oil is one of the richest sources of linoleic acid. A second essential fatty acid, ALPHA LINOLENIC ACID, contains three unsaturated bonds and represents the omega-3 family of fatty acids. FLAXSEED OIL is an important plant source. Neither linoleic acid nor alpha linolenic acid can be synthesized by the body; they must be supplied by the diet. It is important to note that not all vegetable oils are polyunsaturates: PALM OIL and COCONUT OIL are classified as saturated fats; OLIVE OIL and canola oil are monounsaturates because they contain monounsaturated fatty acids. Fish oils are another source of polyunsaturated oils. These oils contain high levels of EICOSAPENTAENOIC ACID, a polyunsaturated fatty acid with five unsaturated bonds, and docosahexaeonic acid, with four unsaturated bonds. Flaxseed oil and fish oil supply polyunsaturated fatty acids belonging to the omega-3 family that can help reduce inflammation, reduce levels of blood triglycerides (fats) and help lower the risk of stroke and heart attack by reducing the tendency to form blood clots.

A large body of evidence indicates that replacing dietary saturated fatty acids with polyunsaturated or monounsaturated oils decreases LOW-DENSITY LIPOPROTEIN (LDL), the less desirable form of blood CHOLESTEROL, in healthy people and in those with inherited cardiovascular disease. However, monounsaturates do not lower HIGH-DENSITY LIPOPROTEIN (HDL), the beneficial form of blood cholesterol, and are preferable to polyunsaturated oils, which lower HDL at levels greater than 7 percent of total daily calories. Health concerns relating to high intakes of polyunsaturated fatty acids include possible promotion of tumors and suppression of the immune system in animals; elevated blood fats; increased susceptibility to oxidation by free radicals; and increased risk of GALLSTONES. The typical American diet provides 37 percent of calories as fat. Nearly 14 percent is derived from saturated fatty acids; 16 percent from monounsaturates; and 7 percent from polyunsaturates. General recommendations are to reduce consumption of fats, especially saturated fats; to increase consumption of COMPLEX CARBOHYDRATES from FRUITS and vegetables and LEGUMES; to replace part of the saturated fat with olive oil or canola oil; and to consume fatty cold water fish like SALMON and MACKEREL several times a week to increase intake of the omega-3 polyunsaturates.

The ratio of polyunsaturated fatty acids to saturated fatty acids (P/S ratio) has been used as an index of polyunsaturated fatty acid intake. Current dietary intakes for North Americans provide a P/S ratio of about 2/1, and a ratio of 1/1 has been recommended. The P/S ratio is too simplistic for measuring the risk of blood clot formation or atherosclerosis because the polyunsaturates represents both omega-6 and omega-3 fatty acids, each responsible for different, multiple effects. (See also FAT METABOLISM.)

polyunsaturated vegetable oils See POLYUNSATURATED OILS.

popcorn A variety of CORN characterized by kernels with a tough coat. When heated, the water content within popcorn turns to steam, and the resulting pressure causes kernels to "explode." As a snack food, popcorn offers many advantages: It contains high levels of complex carbohydrate and provides six times the amount of fiber as an equivalent amount of broccoli. Air-popped popcorn is virtually oil free; one cup provides only 30 calories and 0.4 g of fat. Oil- or butter-popped corn is not low-fat fare, however. One cup, salted and with butter, provides 154 calories and 14 g of fat. MICROWAVE POPCORN usually contains saturated fat (coconut oil, palm kernel oil, or shortening). Even the "lite" version derives 40 percent to 50 percent of its calories from added fat. Movie theater popcorn is often buttered in addition to being cooked in shortening (hydrogenated canola shortening), which is saturated fat. Added salt can increase salt intake appreciably. (See also CONVENIENCE FOOD.)

pork A red meat from hogs. Together with BEEF, pork represents an important component of the standard American diet. Annual U.S. pork consumption is about 47 pounds per person, less than beef. Consumption of both types of red meat has declined over the last 20 years, in part due to consumers' concerns about pork and pork products being high-fat, high-SATURATED FAT, and high-CHOLESTEROL foods. In response, breeders and farmers now produce hogs that yield pork that is about 30 percent lower in fat content.

Fresh pork is divided into various cuts—shoulder (pork roasts), loin (top loin, sirloin, tenderloin), side (spare ribs)—that determine the fat content. Two-thirds of pork marketed in the United States is cured and smoked to preserve flavor. Bacon refers to cured pork belly from the side of a hog after spare ribs have been removed. Canadian bacon represents cured pork loin, a less fatty alternative to bacon. HAM describes rear leg cuts of hog meat; most are sold fully cooked.

Traditionally considered a source of high-fat meat, hogs have been bred to accumulate massive amounts of fat. A broiled pork chop is 63 percent fat, while a lean cut of a pork rib roast is 45.2 percent fat. Processed pork products include sausage and hot dogs, traditional high-fat products. Pork fat (lard) is somewhat less saturated than beef fat (tallow). Unlike beef, there is no grading system for pork. Low-fat cuts of pork are comparable to the leanest cuts of beef; only the leanest cuts of pork approach skinless turkey or chicken breast. Loin supplies the leanest cuts: Tenderloin supplies 26 percent of its calories from fat. For comparison, ham provides 46 percent of its calories as fat, and extra-lean ham supplies 33 percent of its calories as fat.

Bacon is cured by injecting brine into a pork belly; smoke flavor may also be injected or the bacon may be smoked after curing. Most hams are cured in brine. Pork legs are injected with a solution containing salt, sodium nitrate, and sugar. Hams that are dry cured are rubbed with a mixture of salt, sodium nitrite, sodium nitrate, and seasoning. These "country hams" are drier, and their color is darker than well-cured hams.

The nutrient contents of 3.1 oz. (87 g) of broiled pork chops (with bone) are: 275 calories; protein, 23.9 g; fat, 19.2 g; cholesterol, 84 mg; calcium, 4 mg; thiamin, 0.82 mg; riboflavin, 0.24 mg; niacin, 4.35 mg. Pork roast—roasted, lean, 3 oz. (85 g)—provides 187 calories; protein, 24 g; fat, 9.4 g; cholesterol, 80 mg; calcium, 6 mg; thiamin, 0.59 mg; riboflavin, 0.3 mg; niacin, 4.2 mg. (See also PROCESSED FOOD.)

postprandial Following a meal. Postprandial HYPOGLYCEMIA refers to low BLOOD SUGAR after eating; postprandial hypertriglyceridemia refers to increased TRIGLYCERIDES (FAT) in the BLOOD after eating fatty foods. Overnight fasting is required when measuring serum lipids such as fat and CHOLESTEROL in order to avoid interference by dietary lipids.

potassium A mineral nutrient found primarily within cells. Potassium is a positively charged ELECTROLYTE (cation) and serves an important role in skeletal muscle contraction, heart muscle contraction, transmission of nerve impulses, and the release of ENERGY from FOOD.

Potassium in the blood helps maintain normal BLOOD PRESSURE. A variety of population studies link high-potassium diets with a decreased risk of essential HYPERTENSION (elevated blood pressure), the most common form of which has no explanation. Certain hypertensives may be helped by increasing their potassium intake, although calcium or magnesium supplementation seem effective in other cases. Adequate potassium in the diet may reduce the risk of stroke independent of effects on hypertension.

Sources

Potassium is found in many foods; good sources of potassium are fruits such as BANANAS, CANTALOUPE, GRAPEFRUIT, WATERMELON, dried fruit (RAISINS, APRICOTS, FIGS), and fruit juices; dried PEAS and BEANS; fresh FISH; beef liver; and MILK. For vegetable sources consider AVOCADO, baked POTATOES, winter SQUASH, kidney beans and mustard greens, and BRUSSELS SPROUTS. Processed foods generally contain less potassium and more sodium than unprocessed, whole foods. Thus a slice of white enriched bread provides 28 mg of potassium and 129 mg of SODIUM, in comparison with a piece of cake (71 mg of potassium and 269 mg of sodium). A baked potato with skin contains 844 mg of potassium and 16 mg of sodium, as compared to 14 potato chips (28 g) with 369 mg of potassium and 133 mg of sodium. Low-sodium salt and SALT SUBSTITUTES contain potassium chloride together with other ingredients in order to mask the metallic taste of potassium chloride.

Requirements

The recommended intake viewed as safe and adequate is 1,875 to 5,625 mg daily. The amounts needed are fairly high, similar to the sodium requirement. Potassium is excreted in urine, and excessive renal loss can be caused by DIURETICS (water pills) used to treat high blood pressure. Patients treated with diuretics generally require an extra 1,500 mg of potassium daily, and their potassium status should be monitored regularly. Symptoms of deficiency include weakness, nausea, loss of appetite, altered mental states such as fear and sleepiness, and impaired heart function. Mild potassium deficiency due to diuretic therapy can be counterbalanced by eating potassium-rich foods. Metabolic imbalances leading to the accumulation of organic acids in the blood, such as untreated diabetes, can cause METABOLIC ACIDOSIS (the accumulation of acids in the blood) associated with the excessive excretion of potassium. Prolonged DIARRHEA, vomiting, and excessive use of laxatives also promote potassium losses. Potassium deficiency may also occur in patients with liver disease or who take digitalis, a medication.

Large doses of potassium can lead to electrolyte imbalances and toxic effects, especially for people with kidney disease, diabetes, or heart problems. Side effects of excessive potassium include diarrhea, vomiting, and irregular heartbeat in normal people. Rarely, extended-release potassium tablets and capsules can cause ulcers, bleeding, and heartburn. People with kidney failure need medical advice before eating potassium-rich foods and potassium supplements.

potassium bromate A food additive used to age flour. When added at levels between 5 and 75 parts per million, this potassium compound improves the texture of dough for baking. Heating converts bromate to bromide, which is excreted by the kidneys and is considered safe. (See also FOOD ADDITIVES; WHEAT.)

potato (*solanum tuberosum*) A starchy underground tuber that belongs to the nightshade family, which includes TOMATO and red and green PEPPER. The most widely cultivated vegetable, there are about 2,000 varieties of potato, although only eight are cultivated worldwide. Potatoes are grown in temperature regions of North America and Europe. Potato production ranks fourth in the United

States, after WHEAT, RICE, and CORN. Potatoes originated in the Andes Mountains of South America between 4,000 and 7,000 years ago. The Spaniards brought potatoes to Europe, and European settlers introduced potatoes to North America in the 18th century. The four leading U.S. procedures of potatoes are Idaho, Washington, Maine, and Oregon. Major varieties of white potatoes include Katahdin, Cobbler, Kennebec, California Long White, and White Rose. Red varieties include Russet, Burbank, Red Pontiac, Red La Soda, and Red McClure. Most Idaho baking potatoes are Russet and Burbanks. Only freshly harvested potatoes can be labeled "new." Special varieties appear in farmer's markets and food cooperatives; the Finnish yellow wax variety has an appealing buttery taste.

Baked potatoes, especially with skins, are recommended as a whole, unprocessed vegetable. Potatoes are also broiled, steamed, microwaved, and mashed. Contact with aluminum or iron will discolor them; stainless-steel pots and cutlery are more suitable. Potatoes are used in soups, stews, and cold salads. A potato supplies 20 percent of the RECOMMENDED DIETARY ALLOWANCE (RDA) for VITAMIN C. In the United States potatoes represent about 37 percent of all fresh vegetables, about 126 pounds per person per year. Because so many potatoes are eaten, they supply a substantial amount of the vitamin C requirement for Americans. Potatoes are excellent sources of POTASSIUM as well. With skins, they supply fiber. Whole potatoes are also a low-fat fare. However, added fat can change this. A plain potato with skin (200 g) provides about 200 calories, but adding a tablespoon of butter adds 100 calories. Furthermore, this increase is due to cholesterol-promoting saturated animal fat. Typical toppings like gravy, CHEESE, MARGARINE, MAYONNAISE, and bacon bits offered at fast-food establishments increase both the fat and the sodium content significantly. About 65 percent of potatoes consumed in the United States are in the form of convenience foods like french fries, which represent increased fat and sodium content.

The nutrient content of one whole potato (with skin, baked, 202 g) is: 220 calories; protein, 4.7 g; carbohydrate, 51 g; fiber, 4.4 g; potassium, 884 mg; vitamin C, 26 mg; thiamin, 0.22 mg.; riboflavin, 0.07 mg; niacin, 3.32 mg.

Toxins in Potatoes

Greening due to exposure to sunlight or bruising causes accumulation of a toxic, bitter substance called solanine. Small amounts are normally present and account for the characteristic potato flavor. Solanine concentrates in the eyes of the potato and in blemished, bruised and green areas or in potatoes stored at high temperature. Solanine also occurs in the green leaves and stems of the potato plant, which are not edible. Excessive solanine can cause headache, diarrhea, nausea, and cramps. Solanine buildup can be minimized by storing potatoes in a dry, cool place and discarding soft potatoes or potatoes with sprouts or a greenish tinge.

Processed Potato Products

The United States consumption of processed potatoes has risen steadily in recent decades. Potato chips are a popular snack food. They are produced by deep-fat frying. To reduce water content, processing incorporates a drying step.

Instant potatoes (dehydrated potatoes) are prepared from cooked mashed potatoes that are filtered and treated with synthetic ANTIOXIDANTS like BHA and BHT and then bleached. Powdered cellulose derivatives contribute fluffiness; EMULSIFIERS contribute mixing qualities; milk solids are sometimes added; and VITAMINS like NIACIN, THIAMIN, and RIBOFLAVIN may be added for fortification. The product is cooked and granulated.

Frozen french fries are prepared from sliced, blanched potatoes that have been fried in hot oil briefly, cooled, and then frozen. The partially cooked slices may be coated with cellulose gum or modified starch to maintain color during frying.

Potato flour is also available. It resembles the flour of cereal grains but lacks GLUTEN and is not suitable for bread dough. (See also CASSAVA; CONVENIENCE FOOD; SWEET POTATO.)

poultry Birds bred and raised for human consumption. Poultry and EGGS have been basic to the diet for thousands of years, and few societies exclude poultry from the diet. In contrast, several religions exclude various types of red MEAT. CHICKEN, TURKEY, ducks, and geese are the most common types of poultry. Other kinds of poultry include guinea fowl, pigeons, and quail. Wild ducks, pheasants, and the like are considered game birds, not poultry.

A staple throughout the world, chicken can be roasted, broiled, grilled, poached, sauteed, baked, and stir-fried. In the United States, chicken and turkey consumption has climbed steadily over the last two decades. Consumers have moved away from BEEF due to concerns about SATURATED FAT and CHOLESTEROL as risk factors for HEART DISEASE. Roasted chicken and turkey can be low-FAT fare. White meat chicken contains 23 percent calories as fat. When cooked, white meat without skin provides 30 percent to 80 percent fewer fat calories than cooked beef, depending on the type of cut. Dark meat chicken provides 20 percent more calories as white, with about 14 g of fat (3.5 oz.). Turkey breast contains the least fat of any meat, with less than 1 g of fat per 3.5 oz. serving. As with chicken, most of the fat is attached to the skin. Dark meat contains more fat than white. White meat turkey contains 14 percent fat calories. By comparison, lean steak provides 37 percent calories as fat. Both turkey and chicken are processed for roasts, pot pies, sausage, hot dogs, and cold cuts like turkey ham, bologna, pastrami, salami, and the like. Often these contain as much fat as their beef counterparts. Sugar, salt, monosodium glutamate (MSG), and nitrites (potential cancer-causing agents) represent common additives.

Consumers often choose ground chicken and ground turkey over HAMBURGER, expecting a lower fat content. However, there are currently no government standards regulating their fat content, as there are for ground beef. Ground poultry can contain as much fat as is found in the whole bird. Thus, ground poultry may be low fat or high, depending on the proportion of skin and dark meat added.

The United States and Canada are among the leading consumers of poultry. Many reasons account for the popularity of poultry and eggs. Because hens lay eggs regularly, poultry are a ready food source; and the poultry industry can adjust more easily to market and production factors than the cattle and other livestock industries. Furthermore, poultry and poultry products are generally less expensive than red meat.

Poultry fat is less saturated than beef fat. Chicken provides 32 percent saturated fatty acids and 26 percent polyunsaturates; turkey provides 40 percent saturates and 35 percent polyunsaturates; while beef provides 45 percent to 46 percent saturates and only 3.6 percent polyunsaturates.

Most turkey and chicken production is part of an integrated industry in which a relatively small number of corporations control production and marketing. Poultry farms can be considered meat factories rather than farms in which chickens are mass-produced and grown in small compartments. Advocates believe that free-ranging chickens that have ample space to grow can be healthier than their mass-produced counterparts. Organically grown chicken and turkey, raised without the use of synthetic growth promoters, are available at some markets and health food stores.

Turkeys and chickens are bred to grow faster and to be fatter than their forebears. However, much of the fat lies close to the skin, and trimming this visible fat and removing the skin substantially lowers the fat content. Growth promoters and antibiotics also play a role in poultry production, and these residues may be present. With mass production has come an increased risk of bacterial contamination. Between 25 percent and 33 percent of chicken and turkey carcasses are contaminated with SALMONELLA, a disease-producing (pathogenic) bacteria, due to fecal contamination during processing. Other dangerous species of bacteria, including campylobacter, are also present. Thorough cooking kills such pathogenic bacteria; however, consumers must be aware of the potential hazards of raw meat. Poultry must be kept refrigerated or frozen after purchase to avoid microbial growth. Meat juice and flesh should not contact other foods like raw vegetables. To avoid cross-contamination, everything that comes in contact with raw turkey or chicken, including hands, utensils and cutting board, must be washed. Preparers should never partially cook, then store poultry; this promotes the growth of disease-causing bacteria. Stuffing should be cooked outside the bird.

The nutrient content of 1 cup (140 g) of chicken (roasted, both dark and light meat) is: 266 calories; protein, 40.5 g; fat, 10.4 g; cholesterol, 125 mg; calcium, 21 mg; iron, 1.7 mg; thiamin, 0.1 mg; riboflavin, 0.25 mg; niacin, 12.8 mg.

The nutrient content of 1 cup (140 g) of turkey (roasted, both dark and light meat) is: 240 calories;

protein, 41 g; fat, 7 g; cholesterol, 106 mg; calcium, 35 mg; iron, 2.5 mg; thiamin, 0.09 mg; riboflavin, 0.26 mg; and niacin, 7.62 mg. (See also BEEF TALLOW; VEGETARIAN.)

powdered cellulose See IMITATION FOOD.

powdered milk See MILK.

ppb (parts per billion) An extremely small amount equivalent to one-billionth of a gram of material. One part per billion is equivalent to 0.0000001 percent of a gram, or 1 mg per kilogram. Parts per billion can be visualized as one one-thousandth of an inch in 16 miles or one cent in $10 million. PESTICIDE and CARCINOGEN contamination in food can be measured in parts per billion.

ppm (parts per million) A very small amount of material equivalent to one-millionth of a gram (1 mcg). One part per million can be interpreted as 0.0001 percent or as one inch in 16 miles. TRACE MINERALS and VITAMINS can exist in these concentrations in foods and in the body.

prawn See SHRIMP.

prebiotics Nondigestible nutrients in foods or dietary supplements that help to maintain balance among the more than 400 strains of bacteria that live in the gastrointestinal tract. Some of these bacteria, such as lactobacillus and bifidobacter, are considered helpful, or "friendly." Others, such as pathogenic *Escherichia coli* and salmonella, can be harmful, but they all play a role in the digestive process and the intestinal ecology.

Many illnesses are caused or worsened by an imbalance in the types and amount of the bacteria that are present naturally in the stomach, intestines, and especially in the colon. When added to the diet, prebiotics may help restore balance by providing more of the nutrients that friendly bacteria feed on. Prebiotic foods include Jerusalem artichokes, onions, honey, blueberries, and leeks, although the amount of prebiotics in these foods is low. Supplements provide much higher concentrations.

One of the largest groups of prebiotics is FRUCTOOLIGOSACCHARIDES (FOS), composed of sugar (GLUCOSE and FRUCTOSE) molecules that are bonded together in such a way that they cannot be broken down by digestive enzymes. Consequently, they pass intact through the stomach and small intestine. Once they reach the large intestine or colon, they are fermented to short-chain fatty acids and lactic acid, which are consumed by friendly bacteria. Safety data are inadequate for pregnant and breast-feeding women. (See also DIGESTIVE TRACT.)

Gibson, G. R., and M. B. Roberfroid. "Dietary Modulation of the Human Colonic Microbiota: Introducing the Concept of Prebiotics," *Journal of Nutrition* 125 (1995): 1,401–1,412.

pregnancy and nutritional requirements Normal conception, embryonic development, and fetal development depend on the medical history, lifestyle, and nutritional state of the mother. While healthy babies can be born to women who are poorly fed, pregnancy and lactation often leave the mother with drained reserves and jeopardized health, and there is a greater probability of a high-risk birth.

According to the Food and Nutrition Board of the National Academy of Sciences, weight gain during pregnancy is now viewed as 25 to 35 lb. for women of average weight for height. A desirable weight gain should be worked out between the pregnant woman and her physician. The weight gain aids fetal growth and lowers the risks of low birth weights, infant mortality, and developmental problems. A large amount of new tissue is built and major changes occur in the mother's body to accommodate growth and developmental problems. A large amount of new tissue is built and major changes occur in the mother's body to accommodate growth and development of the placenta and fetus. Of the weight gained, one-third is converted to fetal tissue (6 to 8 lb.; the remainder forms the placeta (1 to 5 lb.), extra blood (3 to 4 lb.), enlarged breasts (1 to 2 lb.), enlarged uterus (2 lb.) and increased maternal fat stores (about 10 lb. [4.5 kg]). The weight gained during pregnancy is distributed among protein, fat, water, and blood.

Protein The rate of protein synthesis remains high throughout embryonic and fetal development, although most of the fetal growth occurs in the last three months of pregnancy. Tissues like the brain, heart, and liver are composed mainly of protein (excluding water). New protein represents a net gain that is a positive NITROGEN BALANCE. There is an apparent correlation between maternal low blood protein levels and the risk of TOXEMIA of pregnancy, which is associated with high blood pressure and protein loss in the urine.

Fat A gain of nearly 10 lb. of body fat is equivalent to 47,500 calories. This provides an ample energy reserve for the mother and fetus and for lactation.

Water Typically, about 60 percent of the gained weight is water. All new tissues require water because it is the principal constituent of the body and body fluids. Water is also stored as a fluid reserve to compensate for blood loss at childbirth. About 40 percent of pregnant women will retain excess water. The maternal blood volume increases by 30 percent, and the number of RED BLOOD CELLS increases by 18 percent. Maternal blood supplies the embryo and fetus with nutrients, including amino acids for protein synthesis and glucose and fatty acids for energy.

Nutritional Requirements

Protein Dietary protein supplies amino acids, the raw materials for new protein. An estimated 1.3 g, 6.1 g, and 10.7 g of protein/day are required for the first, second, and third trimesters, respectively. Therefore, an additional 10 g/day above the adult requirement of 50 g/day throughout pregnancy is thought to meet the needs of most healthy pregnant women. The RECOMMENDED DIETARY ALLOWANCE (RDA) for protein during pregnancy is 60 g per day.

Calories Metabolic changes occur that favor weight gain. Hormonal balance changes to maintain high blood GLUCOSE, amino acids, and FATTY ACIDS to store fat while slowing maternal utilization.

Calcium, Phosphorus, and Vitamin D The RDA for CALCIUM is 1,200 mg daily; the RDA for phosphorus is 1,200 mg and the RDA for vitamin D is 10 mcg. The rate of calcium absorption jumps in the last two months of pregnancy to accommodate skeletal growth of the fetus; an infant at birth possesses nearly 30 g of calcium, mainly in bone. Dietary calcium may be better absorbed during pregnancy. However, it is important that the mother receive enough dietary calcium from conception until the end of lactation, and a calcium intake of 1,200 mg/day is advised. Although the amounts of phosphorus required for health are unknown, the total allowance should match that of calcium (1,200 mg/day). Vitamin D is required for calcium uptake and assimilation. Whether pregnancy increases the vitamin D requirement is not proven; however, the RDA for vitamin D is set at 10 mcg/day for pregnant and lactating women. Early deposition of this fat-soluble vitamin provided in a balanced diet provides a reserve for later use when growth is very rapid.

Iron Extra iron is required during pregnancy for increased production of RED BLOOD CELLS, to supply the fetus and placenta and to cope with blood loss during delivery. In the first trimester, cessation of menstruation compensates for additional needs of iron. To assure adequate iron throughout pregnancy, women need at 30 mg/day; this represents an additional 15 mg above the normal adult level. This high amount of iron cannot be supported by the usual American diet or by stored iron, so iron supplements are required. Because women do not menstruate during breast-feeding, iron requirements during lactation are essentially the same as those for nonpregnant women.

Folic Acid Pregnancy increases the risk of deficiency when the intake of this fragile, water-soluble vitamin is marginal. The RDA for folic acid is 400 mcg during pregnancy. To meet this requirement, vigilance is necessary in selecting foods. Evidence indicates that folic acid supplementation before conception and during the first months of pregnancy significantly reduces the risk of NEURAL TUBE DEFECTS. (Federal agencies now recommend that women who are considering pregnancy as well as those who are pregnant consume 400 mcg of folic acid daily.) During the first six months of lactation, the maternal RDA is 280 mg/day. The requirements for certain other nutrients also increase during pregnancy and breast-feeding (the following comparisons are made relative to the RDAs for nonpregnant adult women):

Vitamin A Although the RDA does not increase during pregnancy, a 1.6-fold increase in the RDA during lactation is recommended (total of 1,300 mcg of retinol).

Vitamin E A 20 percent increase in the RDA during pregnancy, to 10 mg/day, is recommended. A 1.6-fold increase during the first six months of lactation, to 12 mg/day, is recommended.

Vitamin C Pregnancy calls for a 17 percent increase in the RDA to 70 mg/day. The RDA during lactation is 95 mg/day.

Thiamin A 50 percent increase in the RDA during pregnancy has been set at 1.5 mg/day. The RDA during lactation is about the same, 1.6 mg/day.

Riboflavin There is a 23 percent increase during pregnancy to 1.6 mg/day. A 38 percent increase in riboflavin intake to 1.8 mg/day during lactation is recommended.

Niacin Pregnancy entails a 13 percent increase in the RDA of niacin to 17 mg/day. A 23 percent increase during lactation to 20 mg/day is recommended.

Vitamin B_6 The RDA increases by 38 percent during pregnancy, to 2.2 mg per day. During lactation RDA increases to 2.6 mg per day.

Magnesium The RDA increases to 300 mg daily during pregnancy. During lactation the RDA is 355 mg/day.

Zinc The RDA increases by 25 percent during pregnancy to 15 mg per day. During lactation the requirement is 19 mg/day.

Iodine The RDA increases by 17 percent to 175 mcg daily. During lactation the RDA is 200 mcg.

Selenium The RDA increases by 18 percent to 65 mcg/day. During lactation, the RDA is 75 mcg.

Possible nutrition-related problems during pregnancy are:

- Anemia: Inadequate functional red blood cells are the end product of a chronic deficiency, most frequently of iron, though deficiencies of protein, COPPER, and vitamins like folic acid, vitamin B_6, vitamin E, vitamin C, or vitamin B_{12} may cause ANEMIA.
- CONSTIPATION: A decrease in muscle tone and the pressure of the growing fetus can cause constipation. Adequate water intake and fiber, in the form of vegetables, whole grains, and fresh fruit, are recommended.
- Diabetes: Certain hormones increase during pregnancy that counteract INSULIN, the hormone that lowers blood glucose, promoting glucose uptake by tissues. This can lead to gestational diabetes, which can cause placental malfunction, oversized infants, and labor complications.
- Excessive weight gain: There is no ideal body weight and weight does not indicate nutritional status. Too rapid weight gain can be caused by high-fat, high-calorie food that is low in important nutrients. Food choices need to be nutrient dense, that is, they need to contain a high percentage of vitamins, minerals, and fiber relative to calories. A major effort to lose weight during pregnancy can cause abnormal mental development in infants.
- Preeclampsia: This disorder affects about 7 percent of women in the third trimester of pregnancy. Water retention (EDEMA), elevated blood pressure, and passage of protein in urine are signs of the more dangerous condition, toxemia, which threatens both the mother and fetus. Salt restriction and the use of DIURETICS can be hazardous and require medical supervision. The incidence of toxemia has declined with better prenatal care. High-quality protein is essential during pregnancy.
- Heartburn: STOMACH ACID may be forced up into the esophagus by the enlarged fetus. Small, frequent meals may help avoid this problem. Pregnant women should avoid foods that cause digestive problems.
- Inadequate weight gain: Mothers whose nutritional deficiencies are corrected are more likely to have normal-term pregnancy and normal births.
- Drug and alcohol use; smoking: Studies of FETAL ALCOHOL SYNDROME suggest that there is no safe dose of ALCOHOL during pregnancy. It has been suggested that alcohol may be one of the most common cause of BIRTH DEFECTS and mental retardation in the United States. The use of cocaine, heroin, and addictive drugs during pregnancy leads to drug addicted infants who experience severe withdrawal symptoms at birth. Mental disturbances such as irritability and problems with social adjustment can continue throughout childhood and into adult life. Smoking is associated with reduced birth weight because carbon monoxide in cigarette smoke reduces the oxygen supply to the fetus. Many

medications pass through the placenta and adversely affect the fetus. No medication or nutritional supplement should be taken during pregnancy without medical supervision. (See also DIETING; EDEMA.)

Allen, Lindsay. "Anemia and Iron Deficiency: Effects on Pregnancy Outcome," *American Journal of Clinical Nutrition* 71 (2000): 1,280S–1,284S.

premenstrual syndrome (PMS) An array of symptoms associated with menstruation based on hormonal patterns, now regarded as a major issue in women's health. Between 30 percent and 40 percent of American women report premenstrual symptoms; as many as 10 percent may experience severe forms. Most women with PMS are over 30 years of age. Typically, signs and symptoms recur one to two weeks before menstruation. A woman with PMS may experience symptoms such as bouts of irritability, DEPRESSION, tension, altered sex drive, breast pain, abdominal bloating, swollen ankles, and constipation. Symptoms often occur seven to 10 days before menses and progressively worsen until the onset of menstruation, when symptoms disappear.

There is considerable debate about the causes of PMS and why some women are affected more than others. Changes in hormone levels associated with the menstrual cycle seem to be the key. PMS is divided into four categories based on symptoms of hormonal patterns.

PMS-A The most common form of PMS, which causes anxiety with nervous tensions, mood swings, and insomnia. Women with PMS-A have imbalanced hormones with elevated ESTROGEN, (a major female hormone) and lowered PROGESTERONE, a hormone that rises sharply in the second half of the menstrual cycle. Women with PMS-A may consume excessive amounts of dairy products and refined CARBOHYDRATES. Excess estrogen seems to alter nervous system chemistry and change the levels of important NEUROTRANSMITTERS: increased amounts of EPINEPHRINE, norepinephrine, and SEROTONIN, and decreased amounts of DOPAMINE and phenylethylamine. Such changes could explain certain symptoms. Epinephrine triggers anxiety, norepinephrine induces irritability, while high levels of serotonin lead to nervous tension and inability to concentrate. Elevated estrogen may also affect mood by reducing serotonin synthesis and reducing the effectiveness of blood sugar regulation. Furthermore, estrogen stimulates the production of the pituitary hormone PROLACTIN; excessive prolactin causes symptoms similar to those of PMS-A and PMS-H. Elevated estrogen may lower ENDORPHIN activity in the brain. (Endorphins are brain opiates that improve mood.)

PMS-C Symptoms include a craving for sweets, increased APPETITE, FATIGUE, dizziness, headache, and heart palpitations. Women with PMS-C have altered glucose tolerance, suggestive of overproduction of INSULIN, and their MAGNESIUM levels may be low. Magnesium is required for many metabolic steps associated with energy production and neurotransmitter synthesis, and it is essential for the transmission of nerve impulses. Symptoms of long-term deficiency relate to the NERVOUS SYSTEM: weakness, apathy, depression, and low pain threshold. Decreased PROSTAGLANDIN synthesis (PGE_1) may be implicated in some cases. Prostaglandins are hormone-like derivatives of ESSENTIAL FATTY ACIDS that help regulate many processes of the body.

PMS-D The key symptom is depression. Crying, confusion, mood swings, forgetfulness, and insomnia are also reported. This form is less prevalent. Some women show signs of toxic lead accumulation, while others produce abnormally high levels of serum progesterone and low estrogen during the last two weeks of the menstrual cycle. Excess stress can increase adrenal steroid hormone production, including progesterone and androgens, hormones that promote masculine traits. These hormones could inhibit ovarian estrogen production. Still another possibility is an increased rate of breakdown of key neurotransmitters in affected women. Progesterone is a widely used therapeutic agent for PMS; however, results of treatment have been mixed. As with other approaches, progesterone may be effective only for certain individuals.

PMS-H Symptoms include cyclic weight gain and swelling of hands and feet. Bloating can cause breast tenderness. PMS-H is one of the more prevalent subgroups. Women retain water and SODIUM due to excessive production of the hormone ALDOSTERONE, produced by the adrenal glands, which increases water and sodium retention. Stress is known to stimulate adrenal hormone production, including aldosterone. Alternatively, estrogen excess causes increased secretion of ANGIOTENSIN II. This hormone, in turn, triggers fluid retention in the kidneys.

Nutritional Considerations

PMS is a condition with many possible causes; consequently, no single treatment or supplement is likely to be a cure. Nonetheless, nutritional modifications can improve mood, help correct neurotransmitter imbalances, assist in optimizing blood sugar regulation and remedy nutritional deficiencies. Comparisons of women with and without PMS symptoms reveal that PMS patients often consume more refined carbohydrate (including SUGAR) more MILK and milk products, more sodium, but fewer trace minerals like ZINC, IRON, and magnesium. Various supplements may be effective in some cases.

Magnesium levels in PMS patients may be significantly lower than in women without symptoms. Magnesium deficiency can lead to elevated aldosterone levels and fluid retention. Low magnesium may reduce serotonin activity. Magnesium supplementation may reduce nervousness and breast tenderness.

VITAMIN B_6 supplementation may be effective in treating PMS in some cases, but not all, suggesting other factors may be involved. After reviewing nine published clinical trials in which PMS patients were given supplements of vitamin B_6, a group of British researchers concluded that a 50 mg of vitamin B_6 daily is likely to be beneficial to patients with PMS symptoms, especially breast tenderness and PMS-related depression. There does not appear to be an increase in benefit with higher doses of vitamin B_6. Vitamin B_6 deficiency also reduces the ability of the kidney to secrete sodium and promotes fluid retention. Vitamin B_6 has been recommended for anxiety and depression, and many women report relief. Serious side effects such as nerve damage can occur with high doses of vitamin B_6 consumed over a long time. VITAMIN A via its precursor BETA-CAROTENE may reduce PMS symptoms in some cases. VITAMIN E supplementation has been used to reduce PMS symptoms, including breast tenderness, with mixed results. There are few studies in this area.

Supplemental plant seed oils can be used to balance essential fatty acids. EVENING PRIMROSE OIL, BORAGE oil and BLACK CURRANT OIL contain GAMMA LINOLENIC ACID, which may promote the formation of a prostaglandin (PGE_1), a hormone-like substance that can help normalize certain responses, including insulin secretion and control of blood sugar.

Reduced consumption of sugar, sweets, and bakery goods with white flour helps normalize BLOOD SUGAR regulation. A balanced diet based on minimally processed foods is a powerful strategy for promoting health generally. Highly processed foods, CONVENIENCE FOODS, and snack foods provide fewer trace minerals, less fiber, and more salt, sugar, and fat. An increased consumption of complex carbohydrates and fiber with fruit and vegetables helps normalize blood sugar levels and reduces the likelihood of constipation.

Studies suggest that decreasing FAT in meals to 15 percent of daily calories and increasing complex carbohydrates with vegetables and grains may decrease breast swelling and soreness. This represents a severe cutback in fat for most people, who average more than 30 percent of their calories from fat. Eating less SALT before typical onset of symptoms may reduce water retention and swelling. Women who drink large amounts of COFFEE are more likely to suffer from PMS. Excess CAFFEINE increases the level of epinephrine (adrenaline), a stress hormone. ALCOHOL is a depressant and can worsen depression. Regular physical EXERCISE has a long history in helping to manage stress and improve a sense of well-being. (See also ENDOCRINE SYSTEM.)

Bendich, A. "The Potential for Dietary Supplements to Reduce Premenstrual Syndrome," *Journal of the American College of Nutrition* 19 (2000): 3–12.

Shamberger, R. J. "Nutritional and Clinical Observations in Premenstrual Syndrome," *Journal of Advancement in Medicine* 8, no. 2 (1995): 131–145.

Wyatt, K. M. et al. "Efficacy of Vitamin B-6 in the Treatment of Premenstrual Syndrome: Systemic Review," *British Medical Journal* 318 (1999): 1,375–1,381.

preservation of food See FOOD PRESERVATION.

preservative A chemical added to food to minimize chemical alteration or microbial degradation. Preservatives therefore increase the shelf life, safety, palatability, and sensory appeal of foods. Preservatives fall into two general categories. ANTIOXIDANTS reduce the rate of oxidation of foods by OXYGEN and FREE RADICALS, extremely reactive chemical fragments that promote RANCIDITY and discoloration. Examples of antioxidant preservatives are BHA and BHT. Antimicrobial preservatives inhibit the proliferation of bacteria, yeasts, and molds but do not necessarily destroy all microbes. Sodium NITRITE, CITRIC ACID, and CALCIUM PROPIONATE are typical of this group. (See also FOOD ADDITIVES; FOOD PRESERVATION; PROPYL GALLATE.)

pressor amines Nitrogen-containing compounds that constrict blood vessels and increase blood pressure. TYRAMINE and HISTAMINE are pressor amines that occur in certain foods. Tyramine is a degradation product of the amino acid TYROSINE, while the amino acid HISTIDINE yields histamine. Pressor amines are fermentation by-products and occur in CHEESE, CHOCOLATE, WINE, and pickled herring, among other foods. These substances can trigger severe high blood pressure in patients taking antidepressant medications called monoamine oxidase inhibitors, like isocarboxazid and phenelzine. (See also HYPERTENSION; NERVOUS SYSTEM; VASOCONSTRICTION.)

pressure cooking Heating foods under pressure to cook them at a high temperature. Pressure cookers are containers that generate steam under tight lids and with a safety valve. With increased pressure, the boiling point of water increases. This means that foods can be cooked at higher temperatures than those attainable without a sealed utensil. Pressure cookers are used commercially to produce canned meat and canned vegetables. At higher elevations water boils at a lower temperature, therefore, pressure cooking is often used at high altitudes to shorten cooking times. (See also FOOD PROCESSING.)

pretzel A type of brittle CRACKER made from twisted strands of dough used as a snack food. The name originated from the Latin *brachiatus,* meaning "with branch-like arms." Pretzels can be hard or soft. The dough contains wheat flour, salt, yeast, vegetable shortening and malt. By dipping the pretzel in very hot coconut oil, pretzels become sealed, a process that greatly increases their shelf life. Nutrient contents of a Dutch twist pretzel made with enriched flour (16 g) are: 65 calories; protein, 1.5 g; carbohydrate, 12.8 g; fiber, 0.36 g; fat, 0.6 g; sodium, 258 mg; thiamin, 0.05 mg; riboflavin, 0.04 mg; niacin, 0.7 mg. (See also CONVENIENCE FOOD.)

prickly pear cactus (*Opuntia fiscus-indica, O. tuva;* Indian fig) The most common edible cacti, characterized by large flat fleshy stems with spines. The prickly pear supplies an edible fruit called cactus pear as well as pads that are used as a vegetable. Native to deserts of the Southwestern United States and Mexico, the prickly pear cactus has spread to many warm regions, and cactus pears are a common food in many countries. Mexico, in particular, and Sicily produce large amounts of this fruit. Cactus pears are oval fruit that formed after blossoming. They are usually less than 3 inches in diameter, with a rigid husk that can be green to magenta in color. The coarse flesh is sweet and mild-tasting and contains small, coarse seeds. The skin of cactus pears must be peeled off before fruit can be eaten. Cactus pads or leaves are eaten as vegetables. They are despined and the "eyes" are removed; then the pads are sliced into strips and cooked like green beans. The flavor is reminiscent of bell peppers. They are used as a side dish, or with tomatoes, chili peppers, and corn.

Pritikin diet A high complex carbohydrate, very low-fat diet coupled with regular aerobic exercise. The Pritikin diet is a low-cholesterol, low-sodium diet in which fat accounts for only 5 percent to 10 percent; protein, 10 percent to 15 percent; and complex carbohydrate, 80 percent. Sugar, animal fat, salt, alcohol, and coffee are omitted. The diet emphasizes whole grains, beans and legumes, fresh vegetables, fruits, nonfat dairy products, and small amounts of lean meat, fowl, and fish in six to eight small meals throughout the day. The diet was a part of a supervised program to decrease the risk of cardiovascular disease. The unmodified diet revealed a number of defects. It did not provide adequate levels of essential fatty acids from fish and from seed oils. Ultra-low-fat diets are more difficult than other diets to follow because fats and oils satisfy hunger and provide flavor and "mouth feel" that make food satisfying. People generally have more success with reducing their fat to 20 percent to 25 percent of their calories. (See also DIET; DIETING; HIGH COMPLEX CARBOHYDRATE.)

probiotics Organisms such as lactobacillus and bifidobacterium that are considered "friendly" bacteria and reside naturally in the digestive tract, especially the colon, where gut bacteria can account for several pounds of fecal matter. Probiotic organisms limit the growth of disease-causing bacteria and other harmful organisms in the intestinal tract that can cause digestive problems such as DIARRHEA, CONSTIPATION, and FLATULENCE. They degrade fiber to short-chain fatty acids which support the growth and development of colonic cells.

Limited clinical evidence suggests that oral Lactobacillus supplements may prevent antibiotic-associated diarrhea in children, diarrhea in children from all causes, traveler's diarrhea, and atopic eczema in infants allergic to cow's milk. There is preliminary evidence that intravaginal use of some lactobacillus species might reduce the risk of urinary tract infections.

Fermented milk products such as yogurt and kefir contain probiotics. They are also available as DIETARY SUPPLEMENTS. Many companies that promote probiotic supplementation claim they can reduce the risk of cancer, boost the immune system, and cure inflammatory bowel disease. No long-term reliable studies to confirm these claims have yet been published in reputable scientific journals. Because dietary supplements are not subject to the same strict federal governmental testing as are drugs, the safety and efficacy of probiotic supplements have not been proven. Safety data are inadequate for pregnant and breast-feeding women. (See also *CANDIDA ALBICANS;* INTESTINAL FLORA; *LACTOBACILLUS ACIDOPHILUS;* PREBIOTICS.)

Bengmark, S. "Colonic Food: Pre- and Probiotics," *American Journal of Gastroenterology* 95, Supp. 1 (2000) 1: S5–7.

processed food Food that has been treated by physical and chemical procedures to increase its edibility, safety, nutrient content, convenience, or attractiveness. Minimally processed foods have been treated using operations found in the typical home kitchen. Chopping, grinding, sieving, mixing, juicing, and blending are examples of physical changes that produce minimally processed foods. Baking, boiling, steaming, broiling, BRAISING, and FERMENTATION bring about chemical changes in food, but nutrient content is not usually drastically altered by these steps. The United States Department of Agriculture defines "minimally processed" to mean that meat or poultry has been handled only during slaughter, cleaning and cutting. No grinding, breading, or curing is involved in minimally processed meat.

Commercial processing of foods employs more drastic changes to prevent spoilage, increase ease of storage and increase consumer appeal through increased convenience or visual appeal. Highly processed foods differ significantly from their sources in terms of appearance, nutritional value, structure, texture, and taste. Grinding, milling, extruding, bleaching, extracting, exposure to acids and bases, and curing are common procedures. Highly processed foods contain fewer nutrients in smaller amounts than the foods from which they were derived and are said to have a low nutrient density. Commercial processing tends to concentrate STARCH, PROTEIN, FAT, and OILS at the expense of MINERALS, VITAMINS, FIBER, and ESSENTIAL FATTY ACIDS. Often, extensive chemical treatment destroys fragile nutrients like water-soluble vitamins, particularly VITAMIN C, FOLIC ACID, and THIAMIN. This means that the ratio of nutrients like vitamins and minerals to calories is usually lower than in the original food.

The following examples illustrate this point. Canned vegetables lose 57 percent to 77 percent of vitamin B_6. Losses of this vitamin in curing meats is about 40 percent. Losses of VITAMIN B_6 in CORN and RICE products, breads and flour is extensive: 86 percent for corn flakes; puffed rice, 66 percent; bran flakes, 25 percent. The loss of nutrients in refining whole WHEAT to white flour is also significant: thiamin, 77 percent; RIBOFLAVIN, 80 percent; NIACIN, 81 percent; vitamin B_6, 72 percent; PANTOTHENIC ACID, 50 percent; folacin, 67 percent; and VITAMIN E, 86 percent. Similarly, 40 percent to 89 percent of trace minerals are removed in preparing white flour. For example, white bread is lower in chromium by 71 percent, zinc by 77 percent and copper by 70 percent than whole wheat bread.

ENRICHMENT of white flour replaces a few of the more than 20 nutrients, such as CALCIUM, riboflavin, and thiamin, depleted during extensive food processing. Fortification adds nutrients that may not originally be present, such as VITAMIN A and VITAMIN D. This is only a partial solution because foods are not enriched or fortified with vitamin B_6, folic acid, zinc, chromium, manganese, magnesium, among other vitamins and minerals.

Examples of Processed Foods

Cereals Cold BREAKFAST CEREALS are processed grain products. Refined flour from corn, oats, and wheat is molded into a huge variety of shapes and flavors for breakfast cereals, yet the basic ingredients remain essentially unchanged since they were first introduced about a hundred years ago. Many cereal products and baked goods contain extra fat, salt, and sugar far beyond the levels found in the original unprocessed food.

Dairy Product Substitutes Many traditional egg and milk products have been substituted for by extensively modified or synthetic foods. Ice cream substitutes, imitation cheese, imitation eggs, MARGARINE, and NONDAIRY CREAMER are a few of the many processed foods in this category. In these foods, traditional animal FAT may be replaced with VEGETABLE OIL and a wide range of thickeners, EMULSIFIERS, GUMS, binders, and fillers are used to create textures analogous to the foods they replace or to create new foods.

Meat, Fish, Poultry, and Seafood Substitutes TEXTURIZED VEGETABLE PROTEIN is soy protein that has been treated chemically, extruded, and colored to resemble meat or seafood. SURIMI is fish protein that has been mashed and pulverized, extruded and blended with small amounts of shellfish to create a wide range of imitation seafoods that taste like authentic shellfish.

Baked Goods Wheat, corn, and rice, as well as POTATOES, are the basis for a growing variety of highly processed foods. Examples include potato chips, corn chips, and frozen pizza. These foods contain high amounts of fat, SODIUM, and SUGAR, and an extensive array of FOOD ADDITIVES, including ARTIFICIAL FOOD COLORS, ARTIFICIAL FLAVORS, ANTIOXIDANTS like BHA and BHT to prevent rancidity; preservatives; partially hydrogenated vegetable oil, coconut, or palm kernel oil; SWEETENERS like dextrose, maltodextrins, and corn syrup solids.

Meal Replacements Beverage powders and sweetened bars are designed to be eaten with water or milk, rather than the mixture of foods that typify a complete meal. The nutrients of these preparations often represent combinations of sugars, soy derivatives, peanut butter, white flour, vegetable oil like coconut oil or palm kernel oil, and salt. Federal regulations specify that certain key nutrients must be present at levels equivalent to 25 percent of the U.S. RECOMMENDED DIETARY ALLOWANCE.

Potential Problems with Processed Foods

A major concern regarding highly processed foods is that they are an increasingly large part of the typical U.S. diet, already characterized by too much sodium, too many calories, too much saturated fat, too much sugar, and too much phosphate. Highly processed foods may lack as yet unrecognized, nutritionally important factors that occur in whole or minimally processed foods. Ingredients of dark green leafy vegetables, of vegetables of the cabbage family and in fruits that seem to protect against CANCER are only partially understood or identified. Furthermore, several nutrients may work together to create a greater effect than when simply added together as whole or minimally processed foods are eaten (synergistic effect). (See also CONVENIENCE FOOD; DIETARY GUIDELINES FOR AMERICANS; FOOD GUIDE PYRAMID; JUNK FOOD.)

produce Fruits and vegetables and other agricultural products. These are usually perishable items with a limited shelf life.

produce freshener Chemicals added to fruits and vegetables to prevent browning and wilting. After the governmental ban of SULFITES from use as a preservative on fresh fruit and vegetables, several products have been developed for use by restaurants and fast food franchises to keep precut fruit and salads from browning. These products are odorless, tasteless, safe, and "fully natural," with ingredients like VITAMIN C and SUGAR. (See also FOOD ADDITIVES; PRODUCE WASH.)

produce wash A liquid mixture of natural ingredients such as baking soda, grapefruit oil, and citric acid designed to remove unwanted residues, including pesticides and wax coatings, from fruits and vegetables. The first of these products appeared in the produce aisles of grocery stores in 2000. Since then several companies, capitalizing on increasing consumer awareness that fresh produce can carry a host of unhealthy and sometimes deadly substances, have introduced competing brands. Some early product labeling included claims that produce wash could rid produce of pesticides, but these statements were removed after the products' makers learned the claims would subject the products to registration as pesticides by the U.S. EPA.

No federal agency has tested these products for effectiveness, but at least two universities have conducted these examinations. In these studies fresh produce was contaminated with SALMONELLA and then sprayed with a liquid containing similar ingredients to those found in commercial produce washes. The tests revealed that the produce washes were more effective than was water alone in reducing bacteria, but washing with water is still an effective way of eliminating much of the unwanted residue on produce. The American Dietetic Association recommends that consumers:

- Wash produce in water or with a produce wash using a scrub brush and rinsing thoroughly.
- Discard the outer leaves of leafy vegetables like lettuce and cabbage.
- Scrub and rinse the outside of melons with water or a produce wash product before cutting rinds.
- Waxed produce should be washed with water or a produce wash; alternatively, the skin should be peeled.
- Vegetables should be cut on a clean cutting board or surface, not one that was just used for raw meat, using a clean knife.
- Produce should be stored on a shelf or drawer above raw meat in the refrigerator to avoid raw meat juices dripping on the produce below.
- Refrigerator produce drawer should be kept clean and sanitary.

proenzyme (zymogen) An inactive form of a digestive enzyme. Digestive enzymes that break down PROTEINS and membrane constituents, PHOSPHOLIPIDS, are first synthesized in massive amounts as inert precursors by several tissues, especially the pancreas and the stomach lining. Premature activation of digestive enzymes can lead to cellular damage and, ultimately, tissue destruction.

During the normal course of events, the proenzyme is secreted into the digestive tract, where it is specifically activated either by acid-induced changes (pepsinogen to PEPSIN in the stomach); by a specific activator enzyme (trypsinogen to TRYPSIN by intestinal ENTEROPEPTIDASE); or by self activation (autoactivation). The new enzyme is able to carry out its digestive function safely outside the tissue or organ. Other examples include the pancreatic products chymotrypsinogen, which is converted to CHYMOTRYPSIN (protein digestion); prophospholipase which is converted to phospholipase (phospholipid digestion). (See also DIGESTION; PROTEASE.)

progesterone A steroid HORMONE from the ovaries and ADRENAL GLANDS that prepares the lining of the uterus for implantation of the fertilized egg during the latter half of the menstrual cycle. Progesterone promotes the development and maintenance of the placenta during pregnancy. Progesterone also is a developmental hormone, regulating the maturation of mammary glands.

The ovaries synthesize estrogen, a female sex hormone, and progesterone in a cyclic pattern. At menstruation, levels of both hormones plummet, then progesterone levels again rise after ovulation. Imbalances of progesterone production are implicated in the occurrence of PREMENSTRUAL SYNDROME. Like all steroid hormones, progesterone is synthesized from CHOLESTEROL. The adrenal glands synthesize the progesterone needed to make ALDOSTERONE, a hormone regulating sodium excretion and water balance. Progesterone is also secreted by the corpus luteum and the placenta. (See also ENDOCRINE SYSTEM.)

prolactin (lactogenic hormone) A HORMONE produced by the anterior portion of the PITUITARY GLAND that stimulates breast development. Alone, prolactin has little effect on mammary glands. After childbirth, prolactin stimulates lactation, together with the hormone OXYTOCIN, produced by the posterior pituitary gland. Lactation requires concerted actions by: ESTROGENS, female hormones; steroid hormones of the ADRENAL GLAND; GROWTH HORMONE, also from the anterior pituitary; thyroxine from the THYROID GLAND; and INSULIN from the PANCREAS.

Prolactin functions in the menstrual cycle as well. Prolactin inhibiting factor from the hypothalamus (brain) blocks prolactin release at the beginning of the cycle. When estrogen and progesterone levels fall in the late phase of the cycle, production of the inhibiting factor diminishes; the pituitary releases more prolactin and the blood level of prolactin increases. This increase may temporarily cause breast tenderness before menstruation. When the cycle begins again, the blood level of estrogen rises and prolactin again drops. In males prolactin supports luteinizing hormone to stimulate TESTOSTERONE production. Testosterone is the primary masculinizing hormone. (See also PREMENSTRUAL SYNDROME.)

prolamines Major plant proteins that occur in cereal GRAINS. Prolamines contain a large amount of the AMINO ACID, PROLINE. Prolamines of WHEAT include GLUTEN. It is this fraction of wheat to which patients with CELIAC DISEASE are sensitive. Gliaden is the subfraction of wheat that contains very high levels of GLUTAMINE as well as proline. Wheat contains approximately 40 percent to 50 percent prolamine; RYE, 30 percent to 50 percent; OATS, 10 percent to 15 percent; maize (CORN), 50 percent to 55 percent; and MILLET, 50 percent to 60 percent. Millet contains prolamines with antigenic activity similar to the gluten of wheat. (See also FOOD SENSITIVITY.)

proline (Pro, L-proline) One of the 20 amino acids that function as a protein building block. Proline is not a dietary essential amino acid because it can be readily synthesized by the body from another amino acid, GLUTAMIC ACID. Of 20 amino acids that serve as protein building blocks, only proline possesses a nitrogen atom bound in a ring. Its unique structure confers a distinctive structure to proteins in which it occurs in appreciable amounts. As a predominant constituent of COLLAGEN, it confers a unique helix to this very important connective tissue protein structure, allowing a characteristic rigidity. (See also AMINO ACID METABOLISM; HYDROXYPROLINE.)

proof Refers to the alcohol (ethanol) content in alcoholic beverages. The value assigned to proof corresponds to double the actual alcohol content. Thus 100 proof vodka contains 50 percent grain alcohol. (See also BEER; WINE.)

propionic acid A low molecule weight organic acid formed by the microbial FERMENTATION of CARBOHYDRATE. Propionic acid is a SHORT-CHAIN FATTY ACID containing three carbon atoms. The short-chain FATTY ACIDS, acetic acid, propionic acid and BUTYRIC ACID, are normal products of fermentation of fiber by intestinal bacteria, and they are important fuels for the colon. Propionic acid is a natural preservative in Swiss cheese; it also occurs in milk. Propionic acid is also a normal breakdown product of AMINO ACIDS and fatty acids in the body and is readily oxidized for energy production.

Sodium and calcium propionate are common preservatives that retard the growth of mold and bacteria and are considered safe FOOD ADDITIVES. (See also INTESTINAL FLORA.)

propyl gallate A synthetic FOOD ADDITIVE used as a PRESERVATIVE to increase shelf life. Propyl gallate acts as an ANTIOXIDANT to reduce unwanted oxidations that cause fat decomposition (RANCIDITY), leading to altered color and texture in foods. It is used with BHA and BHT to preserve FAT, LARD, VEGETABLE OIL, meat products, soup bases, chewing gum, and cold breakfast cereals. Propyl gallate is often used in food packaging; it can migrate from the packaging lining into foods like cereals and potato flakes. The safety of propyl gallate has been questioned because it is linked to tumors in experimental animals. (See also CANCER.)

prostaglandins (PG) Derivatives of ESSENTIAL FATTY ACIDS that serve as local, short-lived hormones. Prostaglandins (and related compounds—thromboxanes and LEUKOTRIENES) regulate most physiologic processes in the body, including INFLAMMATION, especially in joints, skin, and eyes;

pain and fever; blood pressure; production of blood clots; female reproductive cycle functions like inducing labor; stomach acid secretion; pituitary responses to brain signals; contraction of bronchial tubes and other smooth muscles; and fat degradation for energy production. Rather than circulating in the bloodstream to alter the function of a distant organ, prostaglandins affect cells and tissue in the immediate vicinity of origin. They are apparently synthesized by all mammalian cells, except red blood cells. In contrast, hormones originate only from specialized ENDOCRINE GLANDS. Prostaglandins are rapidly inactivated by oxidation and by structural modification.

Three families of prostaglandins designated by letters of the alphabet (PGA, PGE, PGI) play prominent roles. More than 30 different prostaglandins have been isolated, each with a specific function or functions. All possess 20 carbon atoms, a ring, and two side chains. They differ in the number and position of double bonds. A numerical subscript designates the number of double bonds in their side chains, thus PG_1, PG_2, and PG_3 have one, two, or three double bonds, respectively. This distinction is important because each type comes from a different FATTY ACID precursor. PG_1 and PG_2 are derived from the omega-6 family of essential fatty acids, based on LINOLEIC ACID. The PG_3 series is derived from alpha linolenic acid, of the omega-3 family of essential fatty acids.

Prostaglandins of the PG_1 Series

The PG_1 series, with a single double bond in a side chain, is synthesized from the essential fatty acid, linoleic acid, and its product, GAMMA LINOLEIC ACID. These prostaglandins tend to return body systems toward normal functioning (HOMEOSTASIS). As an example, PGE_1 decreases the stickiness of blood platelets, small particles in blood necessary for blood clotting, thus decreasing the tendency of clots to form. Series 1 prostaglandins thus help minimize the risk of heart attack and stroke. They also stimulate water excretion by the kidneys to counteract edema and they activate various types of T lymphocytes, the generals and foot soldiers that comprise cellular immunity. PGE_1 dilates (opens up) blood vessels, thus improving circulation and reducing blood pressure. It reduces tissue inflammation as found in ARTHRITIS. Nutrients that support the conversion of gamma linolenic acid to PGE_1 include VITAMIN B_6, ZINC, NIACIN, and VITAMIN C.

Prostaglandins of the PG_2 Series

PG_2 prostaglandins are derived from ARACHIDONIC ACID, a highly unsaturated fatty acid supplied by the diet in animal fat and also produced from linoleic acid. PGE_2, a well-characterized member of this series, promotes BLOOD CLOTTING through increased platelet aggregation and induces sodium and water retention by the kidneys, leading to edema, and stimulates inflammation and associated pain.

Understanding how PG_2 prostaglandins are synthesized has shed light on the ways anti-inflammatory drugs operate in the body. To begin PG_2 synthesis, arachidonic acid must first be liberated from membrane lipids by a specific lipase (fat splitting enzyme). Next, the "cyclic" pathway of arachidonic acid metabolism forms ring structures, characteristic of prostaglandins. ASPIRIN blocks pain and inflammation by inhibiting the enzyme (cyclooxygenase) that forms the prostaglandin ring, thus preventing PGE_2 formation. Steroid medications like hydrocortisone are effective anti-inflammatory agents because they reduce inflammation by reducing the rate of arachidonic acid production.

Prostaglandins of the PG_3 Series

The PG_3 prostaglandins are derived from EICOSAPENTAENOIC ACID (EPA), a major ingredient of fish and FISH OILS. The PG_3 prostaglandins counterbalance the PG_2 prostaglandins and return the body to normal functioning. Thus PGE_3 decreases platelet stickiness and decreases the risk of clot formation. EPA also blocks the conversion of arachidonic acid to thromboxane (TXA_2), a compound that promotes blood clotting. A diet high in fish and fish oil provides EPA and favors the production of PGI_3, another potent inhibitor of blood clotting. PGE_3 causes blood vessel dilation (vasodilation), while PGE_2 causes vessel constriction (vasoconstriction). The ultimate precursor of EPA is alpha linolenic acid, the second essential fatty acid. This is found in high levels in certain seed oils such as FLAXSEED OIL and walnut oil, and in dark green leafy vegetables.

Several health conditions and nutrients affect the transformation of fatty acids to prostaglandins. The following factors reduce the body's ability to form the counterbalancing PG_1 series of prostaglandins: excessive CHOLESTEROL and dietary saturated fatty acids, excessive TRANS-FATTY ACIDS from processed vegetable oil, high alcohol consumption, zinc deficiency, uncontrolled DIABETES, high sugar consumption, and aging.

During normal conditions, the formation of prostaglandins and related substances appears to draw on dietary polyunsaturated fatty acids. The synthesis of arachidonic acid from linoleic acid is normally quite slow, and the PG_1 prostaglandins would predominate. However, during injury, prostaglandins are derived from stored fatty acids in membranes. The principal fatty acid released in response to injury is arachidonic acid, leading to excessive PG_2 prostaglandins and inflammatory conditions. It has been suggested that diets high in saturated fatty acids, or diets with a high omega-6/omega-3 polyunsaturates ratio, facilitate PGE_2 and thromboxane (TX_2) production and promote blood clotting and inflammation. (See also IMMUNE SYSTEM.)

Harris, W. S. "n-3 Fatty Acids and Serum Lipoproteins: Human Studies," *American Journal of Clinical Nutrition* 65 (1997 Suppl.): 1,645–1,654.

prostatic hyperplasia (benign prostatic hyperplasia, BPH) Prostate enlargement. The prostate gland is a walnut-sized gland surrounded by a portion of the urethra (tube draining the bladder through the penis). The only apparent function of the gland is to secrete fluid that both nourishes sperm and carries it through the penis. Prostate enlargement begins in many men by the age of 40. At least 50 percent of men up to the age of 50 have this condition, and it affects 75 percent of men over 70. Symptoms include a frequent, urgent need to urinate; urination at night can interrupt sleep. Urination is intermittent or delayed and has a weakened stream. Urine retained in the bladder through incomplete urination can cause urinary tract infections.

Aging processes in men favor the development of prostate problems. In the first place, prostatic enlargement represents abnormal male hormone metabolism. After the age of 50, levels of dihydrotestosterone, a potent derivative of TESTOSTERONE, increase in the prostate and stimulate tissue growth. Increased levels of PROLACTIN increase the uptake of testosterone by the prostate and elevated estrogen levels block enzymes that would normally dispose of testosterone and dihydrotestosterone.

The Role of Nutrition

Prolactin levels in men increase with stress and with alcohol consumption. ZINC supplements have been reported to reduce the size of the prostate and reduce symptoms. This trace mineral nutrient inhibits the enzyme that converts testosterone to dihydrotestosterone, and it also inhibits testosterone uptake, conditions favoring increased excretion of these hormones. Furthermore, zinc inhibits prolactin secretion. Extracts of saw palmetto berries can inhibit the buildup of dihydrotestosterone and can help men with enlarged prostate.

In some patients prostatic hyperplasia reflects an imbalance in ESSENTIAL FATTY ACIDS, FLAXSEED OIL, SOYBEAN oil, and EVENING PRIMROSE OIL may help correct essential fatty acid deficiencies. Extra vitamin E is needed when consumption of unsaturated fatty acids in significantly increased. Environmental pollutants like PCBs, PBBs, DIOXIN, hexachlorobenzene and pesticides can stimulate dihydrotestosterone formation and act as weak estrogens. This suggests that reduced exposure to such agents may be beneficial. A BALANCED DIET with minimally processed foods can also support the liver's ability to dispose of surplus testosterone and estrogen hormones.

Men should have regular physical exams after the age of 50. A digital exam, a blood test for prostate specific antigen, and ultrasound can help determine whether a tumor is involved. If examination rules out prostate CANCER, a problem with urination may be managed by cutting down on fluid intake in the evening. Alcoholic beverages and CAFFEINE stimulate urination, and these should be avoided. Certain medications can aggravate urinary problems. These include diuretics, tranquilizers, antidepressants, and certain anticonvulsive agents. Antihistamines and decongestants promote urine retention and should be avoided. (See also ENDOCRINE SYSTEM; KIDNEYS.)

Ripple, M. O. et al. "Prooxident-Antioxidant Shift Induced by Androgen Treatment of Human Prostate Carcinoma Cells," *Journal of the National Cancer Institute* 89 (1997): 40–48.

protease (proteolytic enzyme) An enzyme capable of digesting proteins. Proteases play important roles in digestion by breaking down food proteins to small fragments (PEPTIDES) and free AMINO ACIDS that can be absorbed by the small intestine.

PEPSIN is a protease produced in the STOMACH that initiates protein digestion and requires stomach acid for maximal activity. The PANCREAS produces a battery of powerful proteases to finish protein digestion in the small intestine. These include TRYPSIN, CHYMOTRYPSIN, and carboxypeptidase. MEAT TENDERIZERS contain mixtures of plant proteases from pineapple (BROMELAIN) and papaya (PAPAIN) and from microorganisms (subtilism).

A deficiency of digestive proteases can cause MALNUTRITION because protein digestion is faulty. Inadequate digestive ENZYMES can be caused by an unhealthy stomach lining, by low stomach acid production, by pancreatic disease, by a damaged intestinal lining and by blockage of the common duct that carries juices of the pancreas and bile from the gallbladder to the intestine. (See also PANCREATITIS.)

protein A complex polymer of amino acids; the most common material in the body. The word protein is derived from the Greek word *proteios,* meaning "foremost" or "of primary importance." Perhaps as many as 100,000 different types of proteins make up 50 percent of the dry matter of the body. All life forms—bacteria, fungi, viruses, plants, and animals—rely on proteins for structure and the function of processes essential for growth and reproduction, for converting fuel to energy and using the released energy for maintenance, and for disposal of waste. Integration of organs and tissues ultimately relies on proteins.

Each type of protein contains a unique sequence of amino acids, similar to multicolored beads on a chain. By varying the numbers of different amino acids and their sequences, the body creates proteins of SKIN, BLOOD, MUSCLE, hair, BONE, and nails, as well as ENZYMES, the catalysts that speed up chemical reactions of cells.

Despite this immense diversity, only 20 different amino acids are generally recognized as building blocks. It also seems likely that a SELENIUM derivative of the sulfur-containing amino acid CYSTEINE, called selenocysteine, is used occasionally as a protein precursor, making the total 21. All amino acid building blocks contain NITROGEN; therefore, proteins are a dietary source of nitrogen and amino acids. The nitrogen content of protein is about 16 percent; crude protein content can be estimated from the nitrogen content of a food. To form proteins, amino acids are bound together by a special linkage called a peptide bond; a general name for proteins is "polypeptide." Breaking peptide bonds by acids, by alkali or by enzymes yields the constituent amino acid. It is worth pointing out that certain amino acids do not survive harsh conditions such as exposure to strong acids or alkalis or heat. GLUTAMINE and ASPARAGINE are broken down to GLUTAMIC ACID and ASPARTIC ACID, respectively.

Although 20 amino acid building blocks are incorporated into proteins, proteins may contain more than 20 different amino acids. This is explained by the fact that certain amino acids are modified after they have been linked up in mature proteins. Examples of modified amino acids formed in proteins include: PROLINE, converted to HYDROXYPROLINE, and LYSINE, converted to hydroxylysine (in connective tissue); glutamic acid, to gamma carboxyglutamic acid (in blood clotting proteins); SERINE and THREONINE, to phosphoserine and phosphothreonine (in regulatory proteins). Cysteine is oxidized to cystine to stabilize many proteins, such as KERATIN in hair.

Protein Structure

Protein chains fold up to form either condensed (globular) structures analogous to a ball of string; or they align themselves to form chains and fibers or sheet-like structures. Generally, proteins that serve a dynamic role are globular structures. Enzymes, HORMONES, ANTIBODIES, HEMOGLOBIN, and serum proteins like ALBUMIN are globular. The blood-clotting protein, fibrinogen, is transformed from a globular to a fibrous structure, FIBRIN, when blood-clotting is activated. Other fibrous proteins serve structural functions: COLLAGEN, elastin, and keratin are fibrous proteins of skin, connective tissue and hair. Altering the unique three-dimensional structure of a protein usually causes a loss in biological function. This process is called denaturation. Denaturing agents include acidic and alkaline conditions, heat, and heavy metals like MERCURY and LEAD.

Protein Digestion

Digesting dietary proteins supplies essential amino acids that cannot be made in adequate amounts by the body. The dietary amino acids are used to assemble the body's own proteins. Any surplus is burned for ENERGY or converted to FAT. Most Americans eat more than enough protein to meet their amino acid needs.

Protein denaturation plays an important role in DIGESTION. Cooking foods denatures and partially breaks down proteins, making them more accessible to DIGESTIVE ENZYMES. Highly crosslinked proteins of hair, feathers, and skin do not break down in the digestive tract because the protein chains cannot be attached to digestive enzymes.

Protein digestion normally begins in the stomach where the strong acid (hydrochloric acid) unfolds protein in food, rendering it more accessible to attack by the digestive enzymes of the stomach. The initial phase of protein digestion yields fragments called PEPTIDES, rather than individual amino acids. Digestive enzymes of the pancreas further break down protein fragments to free amino acids. Final stages of protein digestion require intestinal enzymes called peptidases that convert small fragments to free amino acids. Ultimately, individual amino acids are absorbed through the intestine and then distributed via the bloodstream to all cells of the body.

Protein Synthesis

A key question in understanding metabolism is how the cell achieves the precision required to assemble structures as complex as proteins without error. Much of the cell's exquisite machinery is devoted to this process. Life has evolved a template process for ordering amino acids in the proper sequence. The sequence is locked away in the nucleus of the cell in the form of a nucleic acid called DNA, the most complex molecules made by the cell. This genetic material stores information about protein structure as a sequence in code words. Prior to protein synthesis, copies of the genetic messages must be transported to the cytoplasm, where protein synthesis occurs. The vehicle for this transfer is a second type of NUCLEIC ACID called messenger RNA. This molecule bears the code words defining the amino acid sequence of a single protein. The messenger combines with cytoplasmic particles called ribosomes, protein synthesizing factories of cells. A third kind of RNA, called transfer RNA, transport each type of amino acid to the ribosome, matches up with appropriate code words in messenger RNA, and aligns amino acids in their proper sequence. The amino acids are then "zipped" together to construct the new protein. Energy for protein synthesis is generated by the oxidation of fuels.

Classification of Proteins

Proteins can be classified according to their functions:

- Carrier proteins, such as hemoglobin of red blood cells, serum lipoproteins LOW-DENSITY LIPOPROTEIN (LDL) and HIGH-DENSITY LIPOPROTEIN (HDL), which transport CHOLESTEROL in the blood.
- Structural proteins like collagen, found in skin, cartilage, and scar tissue.
- Regulators, such as hormones (INSULIN, GLUCAGON, GROWTH HORMONE, and ENDORPHINS, the brain's own painkillers).
- Contractile proteins, such as actin and MYOSIN of muscle.
- Defensive proteins, such as antibodies (gamma globulins) and blood clotting proteins.
- Enzymes, catalysts of the chemical changes that occur in the body. Examples are PEPSIN and TRYPSIN (digests proteins), LIPASE (digests fat), and AMYLASE (digests STARCH). Other enzymes synthesize many materials, including DNA and RNA; GLYCOGEN to store glucose; fat to store energy and even BLOOD SUGAR. Still other enzymes oxidize fat and carbohydrate to produce energy.

Simple proteins are also classified according to their solubilities.

- Albumins are water soluble. They occur in serum, milk, and eggs.
- Globulins are poorly soluble in water, but their solubility increases in salt solutions. They occur in serum, the fluid from clotted blood. Gamma-

globulin, the fraction of blood containing antibodies, is representative.

- Albuminoids are highly insoluble proteins found in hair, collagen, and connective tissue.
- Glutelins are soluble in dilute acid or alkaline. These proteins occur in cereal grains. The GLUTEN of wheat contains glutelins.
- PROLAMINES are soluble in organic solvents such as alcohols. ZEIN in corn and GLIADEN in wheat are prolamines. They are rich in the amino acid proline.

Certain proteins are coupled with nonprotein components.

- LIPOPROTEINS are complexes of phospholipids and fat and cholesterol. LDL (the less desirable form of cholesterol) and HDL (the more desirable form of cholesterol) are examples.
- Metalloproteins are complex metal ions. As an example, the serum protein transferrin binds COPPER, IRON, and ZINC in blood.
- FERRITIN is an iron storage complex. It is measured to assess iron nutritional status.
- Mucoproteins and GLYCOPROTEINS contain carbohydrate chains of differing length and composition. They are produced by moist membranes that line the body cavities, such as the gastric intestinal tract. Mucins serve as lubricants.
- Nucleoprotein are protein complexes with RNA and DNA: Chromatin of the cell nucleus is an example of these complexes.
- Phosphoproteins, such as the milk protein CASEIN, contain phosphate.
- Flavoproteins contain COENZYMES (enzyme helpers) derived from the B vitamin RIBOFLAVIN. Flavoproteins occur in fat oxidation in energy-yielding pathways like the KREB'S CYCLE.

Dietary Protein Requirements

Worn-out proteins are degraded and replaced by new ones. A steady input of essential amino acids is therefore required even when the body is at a stable weight. The RECOMMENDED DIETARY ALLOWANCE (RDA) of 0.75 g protein per kilogram of body weight for adults was established based on long-term and short-term studies of humans. Thus, an adult male weighing 174 lb. requires 63 g of protein daily; and an adult female weighing 138 lb. requires 50 g daily. Protein requirements were determined for individuals with a routinely high protein intake. Over time, people can adapt to low protein intake and achieve nitrogen balance without necessarily depleting their protein stores.

Children require relatively more protein than adults to support their rapid growth. The protein in an infant's body increases up to 15 percent during the first year. An intake of 2.2 g/kg of body weight is required per day up to the first five months of age; 1.2 g/kg from one to three years; 1.1 g/kg from four to six years; and about 1 g/kg from seven to 14 years. During pregnancy, protein needs increase dramatically to meet the needs of the placenta, fetus, and maternal tissues. Consequently the RDA is 60 g of protein throughout pregnancy—an increase of 10 g/day over the adult RDA. Breast milk is a protein-rich food that requires extra dietary protein to sustain its production. The protein RDA during lactation is between 62 and 65 g/day. These allowances are based on the requirements of healthy people consuming high-quality protein. The DAILY REFERENCE VALUE used by the FDA for food labels is 50 g except for children: one to four years, 16 g; infants under one year, 14 g; pregnant women, 60 g; lactating mothers, 65 g. The typical U.S. diet supplies much more protein than is required. Thus, the average protein intake for U.S. men is 75 percent above the RDA, and for women it is 35 percent more. Consequently, few people need protein supplements.

Nonetheless, certain groups of Americans may be at risk for protein deficiency: chronic dieters, elderly persons, persons with low incomes and especially low-income pregnant women. People with intestinal malabsorption disorders such as CROHN'S DISEASE and CELIAC DISEASE may need special protein or amino acid mixtures. Athletes who participate in high endurance training, such as cyclists, cross-country skiers, and long distance runners, need more protein than sedentary people. Weight lifters and body builders also need somewhat more protein than sedentary people as they increase muscle mass. Weight-conscious women athletes who diet may not obtain enough protein from the food they eat.

Protein Malnutrition

Protein deficiency in its extreme form in children is called KWASHIORKOR. In developing nations, children after weaning may be fed an unbalanced diet of starchy foods that are low in essential amino acids, such as BANANAS, YAMS, and CASSAVAS. Mental development and functioning may be severely altered in infants following severe protein deficiency.

With inadequate dietary protein, yet with adequate calories, less muscle wasting occurs than with malnutrition due to a lack of both protein and energy sources because protein is not broken down so extensively. One reason is that less glucocorticoid is released by the adrenal glands. This hormone family switches the body into a degradative mode (CATABOLIC STATE) and causes muscle wasting to supply energy. Glucocorticoids tend to maintain blood sugar levels and increase blood amino acid levels at the expense of muscle protein.

Protein synthesis in glands and tissues is dramatically affected by a lack of essential amino acids. Digestive enzyme secretion by the PANCREAS and the intestine declines. Atrophy of all intestinal lining can lead to malabsorption, which in turn increases the risk of DIARRHEA, mineral loss and ELECTROLYTE imbalance, and dehydration. Protein deficiency reduces liver function; inadequate processing of fatty acids leads to the accumulation of fat in the liver due to the inability to transport fat out of the liver. Depleted serum protein synthesis by the liver adversely affects fluid balance. With less protein and electrolytes in the circulation, more water resides in tissue, causing EDEMA. ANEMIA can result from chronic protein deficiency because of inadequate supply of amino acids to manufacture red blood cells. With decreased dietary protein, antibody production is limited, leaving the individual prone to infection. Protein malnutrition causes apathy and irritability.

Problems with Excessive Protein Consumption

Excessive consumption of red meat correlates with a high saturated fat intake, and excessive saturated fat is linked to cardiovascular disease and to problems of overweight. Red meat contains 35 percent to 50 percent saturated fat. In contrast, chicken is 25 percent saturated and fish is 20 percent saturated. Vegetables and fruit contain almost no saturated fat.

The surplus waste products from burning excess protein place an extra burden on the kidneys. This can be a problem for diabetics and for those with kidney problems. Surplus protein drains CALCIUM from the body, perhaps contributing to OSTEOPOROSIS. Excess animal protein may increase the risk of liver cancer in lab animals. Consumption of milk, egg and meat protein raises blood cholesterol in rabbits, while soy bean protein does not have this effect.

Dietary Recommendations

To lower intake of animal fat and hence the risk of heart disease, patients should move away from the belief that meat should be eaten every day. Instead, meat should be considered a condiment. A two-ounce serving of lean meat a day provides the RDA for most healthy adults. Patients should replace red meat with fish or poultry, reduce consumption of fatty meat like sausage, hot dogs, and luncheon meat, and eat a variety of vegetables to obtain low-fat, balanced protein in place of red meat. Grains and vegetables provide important fiber and complex carbohydrates along with their protein.

Assessment of Protein Quality

Protein quality refers to the degree to which a food protein supplies needed amino acids. It is evaluated by several different procedures.

1. BIOLOGICAL VALUE (BV) measures the efficiency of utilization of absorbed nitrogen made under carefully standardized conditions and provides a comparison with a protein-free diet. However, few animals besides rats will consume protein-free diets long enough for such a study, limiting its usefulness. For less digestible protein, or high-fiber foods, BV is inadequate.
2. NET PROTEIN UTILIZATION (NPU) measures the efficiency of overall utilization of ingested nitrogen (from amino acids of digested protein). For completely digestive proteins, NPU equals BV.
3. PROTEIN EFFICIENCY RATIO (PER) evaluates protein quality while allowing for the body's needs for maintenance. It is based on the weight gained by lab animals fed a test diet compared to the amount of protein consumed by those animals.
4. Nitrogen balance index is used to estimate human protein needs. When proteins supply adequate amino acids, nitrogen balance is positive, that is, the amount of nitrogen provided by

food is greater than the amount lost in urine and feces.

5. CHEMICAL SCORES are derived by comparing the amino acid composition of a test protein as compared with the amino acid composition of a reference protein that provides essential amino acid to meet the requirements of children. Egg protein and human milk are typically used. The content of an amino acid in the reference protein is assigned a value of 100 percent. Typically, chemical scores of 70 or higher are considered adequate protein sources.

(See also AMINO ACID METABOLISM; HUNGER; STARVATION.)

Hu, F. B. et al. "Dietary Protein and Risk of Ischemic Heart Disease in Women," *American Journal of Clinical Nutrition* 70 (1999): 221.

protein complementation Combining different types of protein in order to make up for any AMINO ACID deficiencies when each is eaten separately. Vegetables proteins often contain less than optimal amounts of certain essential AMINO ACIDS such as lysine or methionine. Making the appropriate match creates a complete protein mixture that more nearly matches a high-quality protein providing ample amounts of the essential amino acids. Eating such a mixture with each meal does not seem necessary. Eating a variety of selected, whole, minimally processed plant protein foods throughout the day can supply the body with adequate essential amino acids.

Traditional meals throughout the world often incorporate complementary proteins. Grains complement BEANS, PEAS, and LENTILS; examples are rice and bean casseroles, lentil curry and rice, wheat bread and baked beans, corn tortillas and beans. Seeds like SESAME and SUNFLOWER complement peas, beans, and lentils: roasted nuts with soybeans; sesame seeds in bean soap; hummus (garbanzo beans plus sesame seeds). Milk products complement grains: pasta and cheese, cheese sandwich. (See also PROTEIN QUALITY.)

protein efficiency ratio (PER) A measure of PROTEIN quality. PER is one of the most commonly used procedures to assess the adequacy of a food protein in providing ample amounts of all dietary essential amino acids to meet the needs for maintenance and growth. In the United States, PER is a basis for regulations governing protein content in food labeling and RECOMMENDED DIETARY ALLOWANCES (RDA). PER is defined as the weight (in grams) gained by growing animals divided by the protein intake (in grams) over a period of time. Studies usually use young rats over a 10-day feeding period. This procedure has important drawbacks. It assumes that all dietary protein is used for growth; no allowance is made for maintenance. Furthermore, the amino acid requirements for rats are not the same as for humans.

The PER for CASEIN (milk protein) is taken as a reference point for the protein RDA. For food labels, 50 g of a protein with a PER value comparable to casein is considered to meet 100 percent of the DAILY REFERENCE VALUE for nonpregnant nonlactating adults. When the PER is less than casein, at least 65 g of food protein is required to meet 100 percent of the USRDA. When consumption of FAT or CARBOHYDRATE is inadequate to meet energy requirements, dietary protein will not support growth regardless of its ability to supply essential AMINO ACIDS as a high-quality protein, because a minimum amount of carbohydrate is required in the diet to fuel the nervous system and maintain health.

protein quality The degree to which a food protein supplies all dietary essential AMINO ACIDS. A high-quality food protein provides ample amounts of all amino acids the body cannot make in sufficient amounts to support growth and maintenance. Such a protein source is designated as "complete." Partially complete proteins can maintain life but cannot support growth. Low-quality protein is deficient in one or more essential amino acids and by itself cannot support growth and maintenance. Incomplete proteins neither maintain growth nor sustain life and lead to wasting of tissue protein.

Animal protein is generally high-quality protein because ample amounts of all dietary essential amino acids are represented. GELATIN is an exception. This degraded form of COLLAGEN lacks the essential amino acids TRYPTOPHAN and METHIONINE.

Good sources of complete protein are MEAT, FISH, POULTRY, and dairy products like EGGS. Red meat is the favored source of high-quality protein in the

United States. However, these same sources provides excess cholesterol and saturated fat and lack fiber. On the other hand, meat is an exceptional source of zinc, iron, and VITAMIN B_{12}.

Vegetable protein, with some exceptions, is lower in quality than animal protein because most plant proteins are generally low in at least one essential amino acid. Grains are usually low in lysine (corn, wheat, rye) while legumes are equally low in sulfur-containing amino acids methionine and cysteine. The proteins of SOYBEANS, dried BEANS, AMARANTH, and QUINOA contain relatively large amounts of all essential amino acids and are of higher quality than other plant protein sources. Because flesh in all forms—red meat, poultry, and fish—is so common in the Western diet, obtaining adequate protein is generally not a problem in these countries except for strict vegetarians. By eating a variety of minimally processed vegetables, grains, nuts, and legumes each day, an individual can readily obtain vegetable protein to supply ample amino acids to meet daily needs. (See also PROTEIN COMPLEMENTATION; VEGETARIAN.)

protein-sparing fast See DIET, VERY LOW CALORIE.

proteolytic enzyme See PROTEASE.

provitamin A See BETA-CAROTENE.

prudent diet See CHOLESTEROL.

psoralen A chemical found in FIGS, CELERY leaves, and PARSLEY that can increase sensitivity to sunlight. Psoralen is a potential MUTAGEN (an agent that causes mutations) and CARCINOGEN (cancer-causing agent). It can be activated by exposure to ultraviolet light in sunlight to attack cell membranes and the genetic material (DNA). Because of its ability to kill cells (cytotoxicity), it has been isolated and used therapeutically to treat psoriasis and certain types of cancer.

psychoneuroimmunology The study of the relationship between emotions, the NERVOUS SYSTEM, and the IMMUNE SYSTEM. Recent research reflects the renewed interest in examining a key assumption of ancient medicinal traditions, that mental states can affect the body's ability to fight illness. Modern research has demonstrated that the linkage between the brain and the immune system exists at the cellular and biochemical level. Excessive physical and emotional STRESS have been shown to decrease immune function as well as imbalance the endocrine (HORMONE) system. Proponents believe this sets the stage for DEGENERATIVE DISEASE.

The immune system is strongly affected by signals sent from the brain via at least two pathways. In the first, the HYPOTHALAMUS, the region of the brain that integrates fundamental processes, including heartbeat, digestion, body temperature, blood pressure, appetite, and emotions, regulates hormone release. Neurotransmitters, brain chemicals that help carry nerve impulses, regulate the hypothalamus, so the brain can either activate or retard the immune system. In the second pathway, the autonomic nervous system, the branch of the nervous system that acts as the "autopilot" of the body, also regulates immunity. In the first pathway, the hypothalamus sends chemical signals to the PITUITARY GLAND, the "master gland." Under stressful conditions, the hypothalamus releases a chemical called corticotropin-releasing factor that signals the pituitary to secrete ACTH (ADRENOCORTICOTROPIC HORMONE), the hormone that activates the adrenal glands. In turn, the adrenal glands release steroid hormones, glucocorticoids, into the bloodstream. High levels of glucocorticoids tend to shut down the immune response, especially the T cells, the foot soldiers of the immune system. On the other hand, low levels of glucocorticoids can stimulate immune cells.

In a second pathway linking brain and immunity, the nerves of the autonomic nervous system are closely linked to the lymphatic tissues—the spleen, lymph nodes, bone marrow, thymus gland—where many types of immune cells reside. Thus, nerves send signals via neurotransmitters directly to tissues responsible for immune activity. In turn, lymphatic tissues act as an endocrine (hormone-secreting) gland. They produce many proteins—including ENDORPHINS, ACTH, LYMPHOKINES, and thymosins from the thymus—that are secreted into the bloodstream and facilitate two-way communication with the brain. These developments emphasize that research into causes of disease needs to evaluate contributions of both the brain and the immune system. (See also PLACEBO.)

Nee, L. E. "Effects of Psychosocial Interactions at a Cellular Level" *Social Work* 40 (March 20, 1995): 259–262.

psyllium A natural FIBER used to relieve CONSTIPATION. Psyllium is an annual herb grown in India and southern Europe. Its seeds contain high levels of a water-soluble fiber (gum), a nondigested plant carbohydrate. Psyllium fiber has long been marketed as a BULKING AGENT and LAXATIVE. Recent research suggests psyllium fiber may help lower blood CHOLESTEROL levels significantly when a typical dose is taken over several weeks. Other sources of soluble fiber, including GUAR GUM, OAT bran, and PECTIN, also lower blood cholesterol levels. Food rich in soluble fiber might lower blood cholesterol an additional 5 percent if the level is already below 200, or if the person is already on a low-fat diet. Diet and exercise are the first strategies to lower blood cholesterol. Psyllium fiber can cause gas and intestinal upset in some people due to its fermentation by gut bacteria. Excessive amounts can block the absorption of fat-soluble VITAMINS and of MINERALS. In addition, some individuals may be allergic to psyllium gum. Chronic constipation can indicate a serious underlying problem, and a qualified health care provider should be consulted.

pulses Edible seeds of LEGUMES. Pulses commonly used as food include LENTILS, BEANS, CHICKPEAS, cowpeas, field peas, PEANUTS, and SOYBEANS. These seeds and nuts possess a higher protein content than grains; their protein contains adequate lysine, an essential amino acid often found in low amounts in other plant protein. However, pulses generally are deficient in sulfur-containing amino acids CYSTEINE and METHIONINE. Soybeans are an exception. (See also PROTEIN COMPLEMENTATION.)

pumpkin (*Cucurbita* spp.) A member of the gourd and squash family. Pumpkins are large orange fruit with coarse, sweet, strongly flavored flesh. The flesh, seeds, and flowers are eaten. Pumpkins originated in Central America and Mexico; ancient Aztec and Inca gardeners cultivated varieties that had sweet flesh. By the time Europeans arrived in the New World, pumpkins had spread throughout Mexico, North America, southeastern Canada, and the Caribbean. Pumpkins are canned and frozen and are baked in pies, cakes, and custards. Pumpkin is a rich source of vitamin A (beta-carotene). The nutrient contents of 1 cup (canned, 245 g) are: 83 calories; protein 2.7 g; carbohydrate, 19.8 g; fiber, 5.6 g; fat, 0.7 g; iron, 3.4 mg; potassium, 504 mg; vitamin A, 5,400 retinol equivalents; vitamin C, 12 mg; thiamin, 0.08 mg; riboflavin, 0.19 mg; niacin, 1.0 mg.

purified cellulose See FLOUR SUBSTITUTE.

purine A nitrogen-containing compound that is a building block of DNA and RNA, substances that store information and guide protein synthesis in the cell. The most common purines are ADENINE and GUANINE, and they have a double ring structure. Together with THYMINE cytidine and uracil, they are the building blocks that define the genetic code. Purines are synthesized in the body and are not essential nutrients. Adenine is also linked up with the simple sugar ribose and phosphate to form ATP, the energy currency of the cell and the basis for most energy-requiring processes in cells. Degradation of purines ultimately yields URIC ACID, which is excreted in the urine. People who are susceptible to GOUT or who have abnormal purine metabolism may need to limit their intake of purine-rich foods; these include fish like ANCHOVIES, HERRING, and SARDINES; organ meat like brains, kidney, and liver; yeast and mushrooms. (See also DNA; RNA.)

Pycnogenol (maritime pine bark; pine bark extract) A plant extract from a pine tree that grows along the coast of France. Pycnogenol contains the same compounds as found in grape seed extract. Considered a FLAVONOID, this compound is sold as a DIETARY SUPPLEMENT in the United States, where it is promoted as a powerful ANTIOXIDANT.

Some studies done decades ago indicated Pycnogenol's antioxidant properties showed promise in reducing the risk of CARDIOVASCULAR DISEASE. There is some clinical evidence that pycnogenol can help reduce symptoms of varicose veins, and improve certain eye conditions. It is also credited with promoting good circulation and reducing "bad" LOW-DENSITY LIPOPROTEIN cholesterol levels that can cause buildup of arterial plaque, increasing the risk of heart disease. No recent long-term studies in humans to confirm these claims have been published in reputable scientific or medical literature. Because Pycnogenol is sold in this country as a dietary supplement and not a drug, its safety and efficacy have not been tested by the federal government. Safety data are inadequate for pregnant and breast-feeding women. (See also PHYTOCHEMICALS.)

pygeum (African plum tree) An evergreen tree native to central and southern Africa, where it grows at high altitudes. Its powdered bark has been used on that continent for thousands of years as a treatment for disorders of the urinary tract.

Initial studies indicated that this DIETARY SUPPLEMENT can reduce urinary tract problems, including difficulty voiding and infections, associated with enlarged prostate, a condition that affects millions of men over 40. The National Institutes of Health are conducting randomized, controlled clinical trials to test this theory.

Ishani, A. et al. "Pygeum Africanum for the Treatment of Patients with Benign Prostatic Hyperplasia: A Systematic Review and Quantitative Meta-analysis," *American Journal of Medicine* 109 (2000): 654–664.

pyramid See FOOD GUIDE PYRAMID.

pyridoxamine See VITAMIN B_6.

pyridoxine See VITAMIN B_6.

pyrimidine A widely distributed family of nitrogen-containing compounds. Three of the most common pyrimidines are THYMINE, its analog uracil, and cytidine. Together with the PURINES, ADENINE, and GUANINE, they constitute the alphabet of the genetic code. The pyrimidines and purines of DNA and RNA are synthesized by the body and are not required nutrients. Unlike purines, which are degraded and excreted as URIC ACID, pyrimidines are readily broken down to easily disposed waste products, AMMONIA and simple acids. Mutagens (agents that cause MUTATIONS) often chemically alter pyrimidines and purines in DNA. (See also GENE.)

pyruvic acid A simple organic acid that is an end product of GLUCOSE degradation. Glucose is the widely used simple sugar of the cell that serves as fuel, and is particularly necessary to the brain and nervous system. The breakdown of glucose to pyruvic acid initiates energy production from major dietary carbohydrates by a sequence of enzymes collectively called GLYCOLYSIS. With plentiful oxygen, pyruvic acid migrates from the cytoplasm into the cell's powerhouses, the MITOCHONDRIA, where the elaborate enzyme system of the KREB'S CYCLE completely oxidizes pyruvic acid to CARBON DIOXIDE and WATER. Energy released in this oxidation is trapped as ATP, the energy currency of the cell that drives biosynthetic reactions, muscle contractions, transport of materials into cells, and nerve conduction.

When the access to oxygen is limited in skeletal muscle during strenuous exertion, pyruvic acid is converted to LACTIC ACID rather than being oxidized by mitochondria. Lactic acid must be shipped to the liver for disposal. Pyruvic acid readily acquires nitrogen to form the simple amino acid ALANINE; therefore, alanine is a nonessential amino acid. (See also CARBOHYDRATE METABOLISM; GLYCOGEN; OXYGEN DEBT; TRANSAMINATION.)

Q

quercetin A widely distributed plant pigment that is classified as a FLAVONOID. It is found in fruits like APPLES, vegetables like ONIONS, and in TEA. A typical Western diet supplies about 25 mg of quercetin daily. Onions, apples, kale, sweet cherries, grapes, red cabbage, and green beans are good sources.

Quercetin produces a broad range of effects in the body. It can function as an ANTIOXIDANT to quench highly reactive chemicals called FREE RADICALS. Together with VITAMIN C, quercetin helps strengthen fragile capillaries and connective tissue. It can inhibit tumor formation and modulate enzymes in the liver that degrade drugs, pollutants, and cancer-causing agents. Quercetin can reduce inflammation by blocking the formation and the release of inflammatory agents, and it possesses antimicrobial activity as well. (See also PHYTOCHEMICALS.)

quince (*Cydonia cydonia*) A yellow, pear-shaped FRUIT harvested from the cydonia tree, native to Iran and the Caucasus. The flesh is hard and extremely tart, preventing it from being eaten raw. Quince contains high levels of pectin, a gel-forming fiber. It is used in marmalades, jellies, jams, fruit preserves, and syrup as a thickening agent. One quince (151 g) provides 53 calories; protein, 0.37 g; carbohydrate, 14 g; fiber, 1.6 g; potassium, 181 mg; vitamin C, 14 mg; thiamin, 0.018 mg; riboflavin, 0.028 mg; niacin, 0.18 mg. (See also CITRUS FRUIT.)

quinoa (chenopodium) A grain-like product unrelated to true grains. A cousin to spinach and swiss chard, quinoa produces edible greens in addition to its seeds, which form large clusters at the end of the stalk. Domesticated and grown in South America for 5,000 years, quinoa was cultivated by the Incas. This hardy plant grows well at high elevations that experience little rainfall.

Quinoa is imported from South America. Domestic supplies come from the Rocky Mountain region (Colorado). The seeds are protected by a resin-like layer (saponin), which must be removed by treatment with alkali to be edible. The cleansed grain resembles millet. Quinoa has a high protein content. Quinoa protein is well balanced in essential AMINO ACIDS and has substantial amounts of lysine, unlike cereal grains. Quinoa also contains more iron than other grains and contains substantial amounts of other trace minerals and calcium, as well as B complex vitamins. The cooking time for quinoa is shorter than for rice or millet. Its delicate taste combines well with other grains in pilaf or baked grain casseroles.

The nutrient content of 3.5 oz. (100 g) of dry grain is 374 calories; protein, 13 g; carbohydrate, 69 g; fat, 6 g; potassium, 740 mg; iron, 9 mg; thiamin, 0.2 mg; riboflavin, 0.4 mg; niacin, 3.0 mg.

quinone A family of lipids that readily undergo oxidation-reduction reactions. Two important quinone derivatives occur in the body: VITAMIN K and COENZYME Q. Vitamin K serves as a cofactor in the synthesis of several proteins required for BLOOD CLOTTING, while coenzyme Q functions as an electron carrier in MITOCHONDRIA, the cell's powerhouses. Coenzyme Q participates in the transfer of electrons to convert OXYGEN to water. At the same time ENERGY is trapped as ATP, a chemical form used by the cell. (See also ELECTRON TRANSPORT CHAIN; OXIDATIVE PHOSPHORYLATION.)

quorn A meat substitute made from the fungus *Fusarium venenatum*. To make quorn the fungus is grown in large fermentation vats, producing a microprotein. The substance is then spun at high velocity in a centrifuge to remove water. The remaining material (quorn) is then mixed with other ingredients, including flavor enhancers and egg whites, to create a substance that looks and tastes like meat. Pound for pound, quorn contains fewer calories and less saturated fat and cholesterol than do chicken or beef.

Quorn has been sold in Great Britain since 1985 and has become the most popular meat substitute in Europe. In 2001 the U.S. FDA allowed quorn to be marketed to U.S. consumers as a "generally recognized as safe" (GRAS) food. Since then some consumer groups have raised concerns about the labeling and safety of quorn. Critics say that statements on quorn products that claim it is derived from the "mushroom family" are false and misleading. Some consumers have reported allergic and other adverse reactions to eating quorn. One serving of quorn "chicken" nuggets (100 g) provides 212 calories; protein, 9.4 g; fat, 9.4 g; cholesterol, 0 g.

Miller, S. A., and J. T. Dwyer. "Evaluating the Safety and Nutritional Value of Mycoprotein," *Food Technology* 55, no. 7 (2001): 42–47.

R

radiation preservation of food See FOOD IRRADIATION.

radiation therapy (radiotherapy) Using carefully aimed doses of radiation to shrink or destroy certain types of CANCER, especially tumors that cannot be removed safely with surgery. During treatments highly calibrated equipment bombards cancerous tumors with high doses of radiation without exposing neighboring healthy tissue. Typically a patient undergoes daily treatments for two to nine weeks.

As with other cancer treatments such as chemotherapy, radiation therapy can cause negative and sometimes dangerous nutrition-related side effects, including nausea, vomiting, mouth sores, appetite loss, heartburn, difficulty swallowing, bloating, and diarrhea. Inadequate nutrition during radiation therapy can slow healing and recovery.

During this time most patients need to make sure they eat enough and that they get the right balance of nutrients to keep up their strength, decrease the risk of infection, and promote healing. Some helpful tips include eating a small meal about an hour before each treatment; eating small, frequent meals throughout the day; and supplementing meals with liquid meal replacements to increase caloric and protein intake. Patients should consider seeking the support of a nutritionist to ensure they are getting the right amount and combination of nutrients during radiation therapy.

Chase, Daniella et al. *What to Eat When You Have Cancer.* New York: Contemporary Books, 1996.

radioactivity See CARCINOGEN.

radish (*Raphanus sativus*) A root vegetable with a distinctive sharp flavor; related to broccoli, kale, and cabbage. These cruciferous vegetables possess anticancer properties. The radish probably originated in western Asia and was used by Babylonians and ancient Egyptians. It was introduced to China around 500 B.C., where new varieties were developed with a tangy flavor. According to the variety, radishes may be round, tapered, or oblong, and the color can be white, red, yellow, purple, or black. The Oriental radish, daikon, can weigh up to 5 lb. (2.3 kg). The common radish (red globe) is usually eaten raw as a condiment and as a salad vegetable. Black radishes are the size of turnips; their flesh is white and very pungent. Radishes can be cooked as a vegetable, added to soups, or pickled. The nutrient contents of 10 radishes (raw, 45 g) is 7 calories; protein, 0.27 g; carbohydrate, 1.6 g; fiber, 0.24 g; vitamin C, 10 mg; riboflavin, 0.02 mg; niacin, 0.135 mg.

radon See CARCINOGEN.

raisin A dried form of several varieties of grapes. Half of the world's supply of raisins comes from the San Joaquin Valley of California. Muscat, Sultana, Thompson Seedless, and Zante Currant represent the principal varieties of grapes suitable for raisins. Ripe grapes are dehydrated either mechanically or are sun-dried so that raisins contain 17 percent water, compared to about 80 percent for grapes. Nutrients like sugar are much more concentrated in raisins than in the fresh fruit, and raisins are a good source of iron, potassium, B vitamins, dietary fiber, and carbohydrate (calories). Golden raisins are dried Thompson Seedless grapes that have been treated with sulfur dioxide then dehydrated in forced dry air. Other varieties include currants (from Black Corinth grapes); Sultanas (from a large green grape), popular in Europe; Muscat raisins (from green Muscat grapes), which are fruity flavored and often used in fruit cakes. Unopened packages of raisins can be stored a year when refrigerated, longer when frozen. The nutrient content of 1 cup (seedless, 145 g) is: 435 calories; protein, 4.7 g; carbohydrate, 115 g; fiber, 9.6 g; fat, 0.7 g; iron, 3.0 mg; potassium, 1,089 mg; vitamin C, 5 mg; thiamin, 0.23 mg; riboflavin, 0.13 mg; niacin, 1.29 mg.

rancidity The process by which fats and oils become oxidized through exposure to air. Rancid fat has an "off" flavor and a disagreeable odor. In meat, iron-containing protein react with oxygen to produce free radicals that cause loss of flavor accompanying fat decomposition. The oxidation of fats usually occurs spontaneously, though slowly, at room temperature. Exposure to heat, light, and trace metals like IRON greatly speeds the reaction of oxygen. Rancidity lowers the content of other lipids, including VITAMIN A and VITAMIN E. Thus, the rancid foods are less wholesome and less nutritious than fresh foods.

At a molecular level, oxygen and a reactive chemical species called FREE RADICALS, molecules that are electron deficient, can attack unsaturated FATTY ACIDS in fats and oils. Unsaturated fatty acids contain double bonds that lack pairs of hydrogen atoms. These bonds are fragile and susceptible to chemical modification, leading to the formation of PEROXIDES, which are potent intermediates in fat oxidation. Lipid peroxides can trigger INFLAMMATION and spontaneously decompose into more free radicals plus fragments that are both cytoxic (cell killing) and mutagenic (causing mutations).

Most cells contain an antioxidant enzyme system called GLUTATHIONE PEROXIDASE that converts unstable oxidized lipids (lipid peroxides) to harmless fatty acids that can be used for energy.

A growing family of FOOD ADDITIVES called ANTIOXIDANTS is used to control or prevent oxidation of processed vegetable oils and processed foods containing fats and oils in order to increase their stability during storage. Ascorbic acid (VITAMIN C) and vitamin E prevent oxidative damage, and additives like CITRIC ACID can bind metal ions that could otherwise catalyze a reaction with oxygen. Synthetic antioxidants, including BHA, BHT, and PROPYL GALLATE, are designed to disarm free radicals before they can cause damage. Because of the safety concerns raised about synthetic antioxidants, the food industry has studied naturally occurring antioxidants that can be added to foods and fats and oils to stabilize them. As an example, rosemary extracts have proven effective in stabilizing vegetable oils. (See also FOOD PRESERVATION.)

rapeseed (*Brassica napus; B. campestris*) One of the five most important oil-producing seed crops and the only oil seed successfully grown worldwide. The origins of rapeseed are obscure, although reference to it is made in 3,000-year-old Sanskrit writings. The seed contains 40 percent to 50 percent oil. Rapeseed oil typically contains erucic acid, a fatty acid analog that interferes with FAT METABOLISM in experimental animals when consumed in large amounts. New strains of rapeseed that contain little of this acid or another antinutrient, glucosinolate, were developed in Canada and Europe. The oil derived from the new strains of rapeseed, CANOLA OIL, contains significantly more OLEIC ACID, the monounsaturate of OLIVE OIL. The fatty acid composition of canola oil resembles olive oil and it too is classified as a monounsaturate. Canola oil is used in SHORTENING, MARGARINE, salad oil, MAYONNAISE, and as a cooking oil. It contains 6.9 percent saturated fatty acids; 34.6 percent polyunsaturated fatty acids; and 58.5 percent monounsaturated fatty acids. (See also VEGETABLE OIL.)

raspberry (*Rubus spp.*) The FRUIT of a family of brambles (Rosaceae) that includes BLACKBERRY and loganberry. Raspberries resemble blackberries, except the berry core remains on the vine when raspberries are picked. Each fruit is composed of tiny drupes, each of which can be considered a fruit. Raspberries apparently originated in eastern Asia. They now grow wild from the Arctic Circle to northern South America. Cultivation was probably initiated in Europe in the 16th century. Red raspberries are the most common variety in America, but they may be yellow, black, or purple as well. Oregon and Washington are major raspberry producers. Ninety percent of the U.S. crop is processed, and most is quick frozen because it has a short shelf life. Most red or dark blue-purple berries contain pigments (ANTHOCYANINS) that have beneficial effects on connective tissue and inflammation. These and related berries contain ellagic acid, a substance that may help prevent some forms of cancer. Raspberries are good sources of FIBER, POTASSIUM, and VITAMIN C. The nutrient contents of 1 cup (raw, 123 g) are: 60 calories; protein, 1.1 g; carbohydrate, 14.2 g; fiber, 9.1 g; fat, 0.7 g; potassium, 187 mg; vitamin C, 31 mg; thiamin, 0.04 mg; riboflavin, 0.11 mg; niacin, 1.11 mg. (See also FLAVONOIDS.)

raw fish See SEAFOOD.

raw meat disease See TOXOPLASMOSIS.

raw milk See MILK.

raw shellfish See SHELLFISH.

raw sugar See SUCROSE.

RD See DIETITIAN.

RDA See USRDA.

recommended daily allowances See USRDA.

Recommended Dietary Allowances (RDA) The Food and Nutrition Board of the U.S. National Academy of Sciences has periodically published recommended average daily intakes for several nutrients selected as adequate to meet the dietary needs of most healthy Americans. Generally, the RDAs were reviewed every five years or so, the most recent edition being 1989. RDAs were established for the following categories:

- ENERGY;
- fat-soluble VITAMINS: VITAMINS A, VITAMIN D, VITAMIN E, VITAMIN K (added in 1989);
- water-soluble VITAMINS: VITAMIN C, FOLIC ACID, NIACIN, RIBOFLAVIN, THIAMIN, VITAMIN B_6, VITAMIN B_{12};
- macrominerals: CALCIUM, MAGNESIUM, PHOSPHORUS;
- trace minerals: IODINE, IRON, ZINC, MAGNESIUM, SELENIUM (added in 1989).

The RDAs have been replaced by a new set of dietary recommendations called DIETARY REFERENCE INTAKES (DRI). These are meant to shift nutritional focus from deficiency to lowering the risk of disease. They reflect the latest research on what levels of nutrition are best to combat diseases such as cancer, osteoporosis, and CORONARY ARTERY DISEASE.

The DRIs incorporate the RDAs along with three other nutrient-based reference values: the estimated average requirement (the daily intake estimated to meet the nutrient requirements of people in a specific age or gender group); the adequate intake (when an estimated average requirement is not available, this intake level is determined based on observing what amount of nutrients sustain health in a specific group of people); and the tolerable upper intake level (the daily nutrient intake that is unlikely to pose risks of adverse health effects to almost all healthy people of a specific age or gender).

The RDAs are based on population needs. Groups referred to in the RDA tables include: infants; children between the ages of one and three; between four and six; and between seven and ten; males or females between the ages of 11 and 14; between 15 and 18, 19 and 22, 23 and 50; men and women over 50; pregnant women; and lactating women.

All recommendations except for energy intend that nutrient intake will exceed the requirements of most healthy people. This decision was made in order to address the problem of variability in individual nutrient needs. Mathematically, RDAs have been chosen to cover 97.5 percent of a given group of people by selecting values lying between two standard deviations above the mean nutrient requirement for a population.

The determination of the RDAs for energy differs significantly from other recommendations for specific nutrients. The allowances for energy employ the average (mean) requirement for each population reported. The mean was chosen because a higher recommended energy allowance would significantly increase the odds that many people, who have average energy needs, would become overweight.

The RDAs were selected after evaluating evidence that comes from animal as well as human studies. Nutrient requirements are generally set at levels that ensure that body stores are adequate for normal functions, growth, and development. In people, the nutrient turnover and rates of depletion of nutrient body pools are most usually unknown. Therefore experimental evidence for setting the RDAs generally relies on the following: intakes that maintain adequate blood levels; excretion of surplus doses in urine or feces; maintenance of a balance of intake and body losses; measurement of body function or metabolic process; knowledge of the amount of a nutrient needed to prevent or even cure disease in humans and sometimes in experimental animals; and examination of nutrient intakes of apparently healthy people. (See also FOOD GUIDE PYRAMID.)

King, J. "The Need to Consider Functional Endpoints in Defining Nutrient Requirements," *American Journal of Clinical Nutrition* 63 (1996): 983S–984S.

Recommended Nutrient Intakes (for Canadians) (RNI) The Canadian version of the U.S. Recommended Dietary Allowances. The RNIs are being replaced by the DIETARY REFERENCE INTAKES, established by Canadian and U.S. scientists according to a review process overseen by the Food and Nutrition Board of the U.S. National Academy of Sciences.

red blood cells (erythrocytes) The major type of cells in blood. Red blood cells transport OXYGEN to all cells of the body, and their color reflects the high content of HEMOGLOBIN, the red oxygen transport protein. The importance of red blood cells is indicated by their numbers: The average person has 35 trillion red blood cells. Males have about 5 million red blood cells per milliliter of blood and females have about 4.5 million per milliliter. Each red blood cell contains about 280 million hemoglobin (protein) molecules. The blood of the average adult male contains 14 to 16.5 g of hemoglobin per 100 ml of blood; the average adult female has 12 to 14 g per 100 ml.

Inhalation brings fresh air into the lungs where hemoglobin binds oxygen, which is then carried to tissues via arteries. Oxygen binding is reversible so

COUNCIL FOR RESPONSIBLE NUTRITION

Minerals: Historical Comparison or RDIs, RDAs, and DRIs, 1968 to Present

NUTRIENT	RDI*	1968 RDA**	1974 RDA**	1980 RDA**	1989 RDA**	DRIs***
Calcium	1000 mg	1300 mg	1200 mg	1200 mg	1200 mg	1300 mg
Phosphorus	1000 mg	1300 mg	1200 mg	1200 mg	1200 mg	1250 mg (700 adult)
Iron	18 mg	18 mg	18 mg	18 mg	15 mg	18 mg
Iodine	150 mcg	150 mcg	150 mcg	150 mcg	150 mcg	150 mcg
Magnesium	400 mg	400 mg	400 mg	400 mg	400 mg	420 mg
Zinc	15 mg	10-15 mg	15 mg	15 mg	15 mg	11 mg
Selenium	70 mcg	–	–		70 mcg	55 mcg
Copper	2 mg	–	–	2–3 mg	1.5–3 mg	0.9 mg
Manganese	2 mg	–	2.5–7 mg	2.5–5 mg	2–5 mg	2.3 mg
Chromium	120 mcg	–	–	50–200 mcg	50–200 mcg	35 mcg
Molybdenum	75 mcg	–	45–500 mcg	150–500 mcg	75–250 mcg	45 mcg

* The Reference Daily Intake (RDI) is the value established by the Food and Drug Administration (FDA) for use in nutrition labeling. It was based initially on the highest 1968 Recommended Dietary Allowance (RDA) for each nutrient, to assure that needs were met for all age groups.

** The RDAs were established and periodically revised by the Food and Nutrition Board. Value shown is the highest RDA for each nutrient, in the year indicated for each revision.

*** The Dietary Reference Intakes (DRI) are the most recent set of dietary recommendations established by the Food and Nutrition Board of the Institute of Medicine, 1997–2001. They replace previous RDAs, and may be the basis for eventually updating the RDIs. The value shown here is the highest DRI for each nutrient.

Council for Responsible Nutrition, 2001
1875 I Street N.W. Suite 400, Washington, D.C. 20006 • (202) 872-1488

COUNCIL FOR RESPONSIBLE NUTRITION

Minerals: Comparison of Current RDIs, New DRIs, and ULs

MINERAL	CURRENT RDI*	NEW DRI**	UL***
Calcium	1000 mg	1300 mg	2500 mg
Iron	18 mg	18 mg	45 mg
Phosphorus	1000 mg	1250 mg	4000 mg
Iodine	150 mcg	150 mcg	1100 mcg
Magnesium	400 mg	420 mg	350 mg#
Zinc	15 mg	11 mg	40 mg
Selenium	70 mcg	55 mcg	400 mcg
Copper	2 mg	0.9 mg	10 mg
Manganese	2 mg	2.3 mg	11 mg
Chromium	120 mcg	35 mcg	*ND*
Molybdenum	75 mcg	45 mcg	2000 mcg

* The Reference Daily Intake (RDI) is the value established by the Food and Drug Administration (FDA) for use in nutrition labeling. It was based initially on the highest 1968 Recommended Dietary Allowance (RDA) for each nutrient, to assure that needs were met for all age groups.
** The Dietary Reference Intakes (DRI) are the most recent set of dietary recommendations established by the Food and Nutrition Board of the Institute of Medicine, 1997–2001. They replace previous RDAs, and may be the basis for eventually updating the RDIs. The value shown here is the highest DRI for each nutrient.
*** The Upper Limit (UL) is the upper level of intake considered to be **safe** for use by adults, incorporating a safety factor. In some cases, lower ULs have been established for children.
# Upper limit for magnesium applies only to intakes from dietary supplements or pharmaceutical products, not including intakes from food and water.
ND Upper Limit not determined. No adverse effects observed from high intakes of the nutrient.

Council for Responsible Nutrition, 2001
1875 I Street N.W. Suite 400, Washington, D.C. 20006 • (202) 872-1488

COUNCIL FOR RESPONSIBLE NUTRITION

Vitamins: Historical Comparison of RDIs, RDAs, and DRIs, 1968 to Present

NUTRIENT	RDI*	1968 RDA**	1974 RDA**	1980 RDA**	1989 RDA**	DRIs***
Vitamin A	5000 IU	5000 IU	1000 RE (5000 IU)	1000 RE	1000 RE	900 mcg (3000 IU)
Vitamin C	60 mg	60 mg	45 mg	60 mg	60 mg	90 mg
Vitamin D	400 IU (10 mcg)	400 IU (10 mcg)	400 IU (10 mcg)	10 mcg (400 IU)	10 mcg (400 IU)	15 mcg (600 IU)
Vitamin E	30 IU (20 mg)	30 IU (20 mg)	15 IU (10 mg)	10 mg (15 IU)	10 mg (15 IU)	15 mg #
Vitamin K	80 mcg	–	–	70–140 mcg	80 mcg	120 mcg
Thiamin	1.5 mg	1.5 mg	1.5 mg	1.5 mg	1.5 mg	1.2 mg
Riboflavin	1.7 mg	1.7 mg	1.8 mg	1.7 mg	1.8 mg	1.3 mg
Niacin	20 mg	20 mg	20 mg	19 mg	20 mg	16 mg
Vitamin B^6	2 mg	2 mg	2 mg	2.2 mg	2 mg	1.7 mg
Folate	0.4 mg (400 mcg)	400 mcg	400 mcg	400 mcg	200 mcg	400 mcg food, 200 mcg synthetic ##
Vitamin B^{12}	6 mcg	6 mcg	3 mcg	3 mcg	2 mcg	2.4 mcg ###
Biotin	(300 mcg)	150–300 mcg	100–300 mcg	100–200 mcg	30–100 mcg	30 mcg
Pantothenic acid	10 mg	5–10 mg	5–10 mg	4–7 mg	4–7 mg	5 mg
Choline	–	–	–	–	–	550 mg

* The Reference Daily Intake (RDI) is the value established by the Food and Drug Administration (FDA) for use in nutrition labeling. It was based initially on the highest 1968 Recommended Dietary Allowance (RDA) for each nutrient, to assure that needs were met for all age groups.
** The RDAs were established and periodically revised by the Food and Nutrition Board. Value shown is the highest RDA for each nutrient, in the year indicated for each revision.
*** The Dietary Reference Intakes (DRI) are the most recent set of dietary recommendations established by the Food and Nutrition Board of the Institute of Medicine, 1997–2001. They replace previous RDAs, and may be the basis for eventually updating the RDIs. The value shown here is the highest DRI for each nutrient.

(continues)

COUNCIL FOR RESPONSIBLE NUTRITION *(continued)*

Historical vitamin E conversion factors were amended in the DRI report, so that 15 mg is defined as the equivalent of 22 IU of natural vitamin E or 33 IU of synthetic vitamin E.
It is recommended that women of childbearing age obtain 400 mcg of synthetic folic acid from fortified breakfast cereals or dietary supplements, in addition to dietary folate.
It is recommended that people over 50 meet the B_{12} recommendation through fortified foods or supplements, to improve bioavailability.

Council for Responsible Nutrition, 2001
1875 I Street N.W. Suite 400, Washington, D.C. 20006 • (202) 872-1488

COUNCIL FOR RESPONSIBLE NUTRITION

Vitamins: Comparison of Current RDIs, New DRIs, and ULs

VITAMIN	CURRENT RDI*	NEW DRI**	UL***
Vitamin A	5000 IU	900 mcg (3000 IU)	3000 mcg (10,000 IU)
Vitamin C	60 mg	90 mg	2000 mg
Vitamin D	400 IU (10 mcg)	15 mcg (600 IU)	50 mcg (2000 IU)
Vitamin E	30 IU (20 mg)	15 mg #	1000 mg
Vitamin K	80 mcg	120 mcg	*ND*
Thiamin	1.5 mg	1.2 mg	*ND*
Riboflavin	1.7 mg	1.3 mg	*ND*
Niacin	20 mg	16 mg	35 mg
Vitamin B_6	2 mg	1.7 mg	100 mg
Folate	400 mcg (0.4 mg)	400 mcg from food, 200 mcg synthetic ##	1000 mcg synthetic
Vitamin B_{12}	6 mcg	2.4 mcg ###	*ND*
Biotin	300 mcg	30 mcg	*ND*
Pantothenic acid	10 mg	5 mg	*ND*
Choline	Not established	550 mg	3500 mg

* The Reference Daily Intake (RDI) is the value established by the Food and Drug Administration (FDA) for use in nutrition labeling. It was based initially on the highest 1968 Recommended Dietary Allowance (RDA) for each nutrient, to assure that needs were met for all age groups.
** The Dietary Reference Intakes (DRI) are the most recent set of dietary recommendations established by the Food and Nutrition Board of the Institute of Medicine, 1997–2001. They replace previous RDAs, and may be the basis for eventually updating the RDIs. The value shown here is the highest DRI for each nutrient.
*** The Upper Limit (UL) is the upper level of intake considered to be **safe** for use by adults, incorporating a safety factor. In some cases, lower ULs have been established for children.
# Historical vitamin E conversion factors were amended in the DRI report, so that 15 mg is defined as the equivalent of 22 IU of natural vitamin E or 33 IU of synthetic vitamin E.
It is recommended that women of childbearing age obtain 400 mcg of synthetic folic acid from fortified breakfast cereals or dietary supplements, in addition to dietary folate.
It is recommended that people over 50 meet the B_{12} recommendation through fortified foods or supplements, to improve bioavailability.
ND Upper Limit not determined. No adverse effects observed from high intakes of the nutrient.

Council for Responsible Nutrition, 2001
1875 I Street N.W. Suite 400, Washington, D.C. 20006 • (202) 872-1488

that hemoglobin releases oxygen in tissues where there is a low concentration of oxygen. Elevated CARBON DIOXIDE concentration and acid production from actively metabolizing tissues also promote oxygen release from red blood cells. Released oxygen diffuses into cells where it oxidizes fuels to carbon dioxide. Red blood cells pick up carbon dioxide for the return trip to the lungs via blood vessels. Red blood cells transport about 23 percent of carbon dioxide in this manner. In the lungs red blood cells release carbon dioxide and again bind incoming oxygen.

Red blood cells are highly specialized. The disk shape presents a larger surface area than a sphere, which helps the diffusion of oxygen into the cells. Red blood cells lack a nucleus and MITOCHONDRIA and therefore cannot divide, nor use oxygen to derive energy from the oxidation of fuel molecules. Instead they rely on GLYCOLYSIS, an oxygen-independent mechanism for oxidation of glucose

(BLOOD SUGAR) to LACTIC ACID. The surface of the red blood cell possesses certain carbohydrate clusters (blood group substances) that are the basis for blood typing; for example, according to the ABO blood groups and Rh blood groups.

Formation

ERYTHROPOIESIS refers to the process of red blood cell formation. During embryonic development, red blood cells are produced by the yolk sac, liver, spleen, thymus gland, lymph nodes, and bone marrow, while in adults, red blood cells come from the bone marrow of long bones like the femur, and from the cranium, sternum, ribs, vertebrae, pelvis, and lymphoid tissues. The initial parent cells are called hemocytoblasts. These cells differentiate into proerythroblasts, an intermediate stage that eventually differentiates into reticulocytes (immature red blood cells), and finally into mature red blood cells (erythrocytes). The usual fraction of reticulocytes in blood is between 0.5 percent and 1.5 percent. The percentage increases with ANEMIA, when the number of functional red blood cells becomes inadequate; with bleeding; hemolysis (rapid breakdown of red blood cells); and in response to supplementation for IRON deficiency.

The kidney stimulates the production of the hormone, erythropoietin, which stimulates the production of red blood cells in response to lowered oxygen pressure, as experienced at high elevations. When the body suddenly needs more red blood cells, the kidneys become oxygen-deficient and release an enzyme that converts a blood protein to erythropoietin.

The levels of red blood cells represent a balance between the formation and destruction of red blood cells. Aged red blood cells are destroyed by the spleen and by the liver. The protein portion of hemoglobin is degraded to AMINO ACIDS; the red pigment, HEME, is degraded to BILE PIGMENT, bilirubin, which is excreted, and releases iron, which is reused.

A number of nutrients besides iron support cell division and protein synthesis in general, and red blood cell formation in particular: FOLIC ACID, PYRIDOXINE, VITAMIN B_{12}, and amino acids. ANTIOXIDANTS like VITAMIN E help maintain the red blood cell membrane and prevent fragility. Deficiencies of any of these nutrients can cause anemia, a condition resulting from an inadequate level of functional red blood cells. Several inborn errors of metabolism (mutations) cause abnormal hemoglobins to be formed. These in turn can alter the shape of red blood cells and shorten their life span, resulting in anemia. Sickle-cell anemia and glucose 6 phosphate dehydrogenase deficiency are the most common. (See also HEMATOCRIT; LEUKOCYTES.)

red dye numbers 2, 3, 40 See ARTIFICIAL FOOD COLORS.

red meat See MEAT.

red tide Refers to a plankton bloom often occurring in marine waters during the late summer and fall. The term *red tide* comes from the red-brown color of plankton. The plankton produce a nerve poison that can accumulate to dangerous levels in shellfish such as CLAMS and mussels although it does not affect the shellfish. Eating contaminated clams, mussels, and oysters causes paralytic shellfish poisoning. The adage of avoiding shellfish during months that end in the letter "r"—September, October, November, and December—is no longer appropriate because red tide alerts now occur in other months. Red tide warnings by county health departments can be issued as early as April.

Symptoms of paralytic shellfish poisoning includes stomach cramps, dizziness, difficulty in breathing, and tingling mouth. Symptoms can appear up to two hours after eating contaminated shellfish; in severe cases, poisoning can be fatal. There is no antidote. Immediate medical attention is mandated. (See also SEAFOOD.)

Reference Daily Intake (RDI) A replacement term for "USRDA" (Recommended Daily Allowance), a set of reference values introduced in 1973 to be used for vitamins, minerals, and protein to help consumers evaluate the nutritional content for food labels. For the time being, RDIs are identical to the USRDAs except for protein, which is adjusted to the specific needs of different age groups.

NUTRIENT	AMOUNT
Vitamin A	5,000 International Units (IU)
Vitamin C	60 milligrams (mg)
Thiamin	1.5 mg
Riboflavin	1.7 mg
Niacin	20 mg
Calcium	1.0 gram (g)
Iron	18 mg
Vitamin D	400 IU
Vitamin E	30 IU
Vitamin B_6	2.0 mg
Folic acid	0.4 mg
Vitamin B_{12}	6 micrograms (mcg)
Phosphorus	1.0 g
Iodine	150 mcg
Magnesium	400 mg
Zinc	15 mg
Copper	2 mg
Biotin	0.3 mg
Pantothenic acid	10 mg

(Based on National Academy of Sciences' 1968 Recommended Dietary Allowances.)

Additions Jan. 1, 1997	
Vitamin K	80 mcg
Molybdenum	75 mcg
Chloride	3,400 mg
Manganese	2.0 mg
Selenium	70 mcg
Chromium	120 mcg

reference protein A source of PROTEIN used as a basis for comparing food proteins according to their amino acid compositions. Reference proteins provide all essential amino acids in sufficient quantity to meet the needs of infants and children, who require substantially more protein than adults, based on their body weight, to support their higher growth rates. Another property of reference proteins is that they are highly digestible. High-quality protein sources often used as reference proteins include egg, human milk, meat, and fish. The amino acid patterns for human milk and whole egg protein are as follows:

Amino Acid	Human Milk mg/100 g	Whole Egg mg/100g
Histidine	23	24
Isoleucine	56	63
Leucine	95	88
Lysine	68	68
Methionine and cysteine	40	56
Phenylalanine and tyrosine	99	98
Threonine	46	49
Tryptophan	17	16
Valine	63	72

The CHEMICAL SCORE attempts to measure the nutritive value of food protein in comparison with a reference protein. In this case, the amount of the least abundant limiting essential amino acid in the test protein is expressed as a percentage of that amino acid in the reference protein. Thus, a good-quality protein source could have a chemical score of 70 or above. Most meat and dairy protein fall into this category. (See also BIOLOGICAL VALUE; PROTEIN COMPLEMENTATION; PROTEIN EFFICIENCY RATIO.)

refined carbohydrates Highly purified SUGARS or STARCHES. These substances occur in sweeteners and in products that are mainly starch. Each type of refined carbohydrate supplies the same four calories per gram. Purified simple sugars and starches represent EMPTY CALORIES, that is, calories lacking in VITAMINS, FIBER, PROTEIN, and MINERALS.

One of the most common refined carbohydrates is table sugar (SUCROSE), highly purified from sugar beets or sugar cane by repeated crystallization. The following sweeteners are only slightly less purified forms of sucrose: brown sugar, caramelized sugar, HONEY, MOLASSES, and turbinado sugar.

Other refined sugars besides sucrose serve as common FOOD ADDITIVES:

- Dextrose (grape sugar) is another name for the pure compound of GLUCOSE, used by food manufacturers. Dextrose occurs in corn syrup.
- Maltodextrins are starch fragments containing several glucose units. They yield glucose when digested and provide no other nutrients.
- Fructose (fruit sugar) occurs as high FRUCTOSE CORN SYRUP. This sweetener also contains glucose, but no other nutrient.
- Sugar alcohols function as sweeteners: MANNITOL, SORBITOL, and XYLITOL. None provides anything other than calories to overall nutrition.

Refined Starches

Purified starches are isolated from WHEAT, CORN, and POTATOES, among other sources. Starch is used as a thickener in many foods. White flour is a staple of the American diet. Though not pure starch, white flour and products prepared from white bread—cold BREAKFAST CEREALS, muffins, PASTRY, pancake mix, pasta (spaghetti, noodles), and the like—contain much less of the vitamins, minerals, essential oils, and fiber than are found in the whole grain from which they were derived. Milling wheat separates the starchy endosperm from the highly nutritious germ and bran (the hull of the seed or kernel).

Recent dietary guidelines have consistently emphasized minimally processed foods like FRUIT and VEGETABLES. U.S. DIETARY GUIDELINES FOR AMERICANS (2000) recommend eating sweets sparingly and suggest that whole grains, vegetables, and fruits are the foundation of a healthy diet. The 1992 FOOD GUIDE PYRAMID of the USDA recommends three to five servings of vegetables, two to four servings of fruit and six to 11 servings of rice, bread, cereal, and pasta daily, with the admonition to use sweets and added sugar sparingly. (See also CARBOHYDRATE METABOLISM; NATURAL SWEETENERS.)

reishi mushroom (*Ganoderma lucidurn, ling-zhi*) A fungus native to East Asia, where it has been used since ancient times to treat a variety of ailments and diseases, including ulcers, cancer, and insomnia. Its Chinese name, *ling-zhi,* means "herb of spiritual potency."

The fungus grows on rotting logs and stumps. The fruiting part of the fungus is a mushroom, which has been harvested by Chinese herbalists for at least 4,000 years. The mushroom's flesh can be eaten whole, but because it is hard and bitter it is more often cut up or dried for use in teas.

Few reliable studies have been done to support reishi's medicinal uses. However, researchers at a Chinese university discovered that the fungus contains a high level of polysaccharides, which are known to stimulate the body's immune system.

Safety data are inadequate for pregnant and breast-feeding women.

renin An enzyme produced by the KIDNEYS that helps increase blood pressure. In response to a drop in BLOOD PRESSURE, renin activates the HORMONE, ANGIOTENSIN, which in turn stimulates the ADRENAL GLANDS to produce ALDOSTERONE, the hormone that directs the kidneys to retain SODIUM and water. Elevated levels of renin correlate with increased risk of heart attack among people with moderate high blood pressure (HYPERTENSION). Possibly too much angiotensin can trigger reduced blood flow to the heart. (See also CARDIOVASCULAR DISEASE; PROTEASE.)

rennet An extract from the stomach of ruminants, such as calves, that contains the enzyme rennin. Cheese production relies on the action of rennin that coagulate the proteins in milk, forming solid curds (from which cheese is made) and liquid whey. (See also DENATURED PROTEIN.)

respiration, cellular The use of oxygen by cells to burn fuel nutrients for energy. OXYGEN delivered by the blood is taken up by MITOCHONDRIA, particles in the cytoplasm that function as the cell's powerhouses. Mitochondrial enzymes completely oxidize FAT, CARBOHYDRATE, and AMINO ACIDS to CARBON DIOXIDE and chemical energy released by this process is trapped as ATP. ATP is the energy currency of cells; it provides the necessary energy for the synthesis of cellular components—proteins, RNA, DNA—as well as for transmission of nerve impulses, muscle contraction and the transport of nutrients across cell membranes. Carbon dioxide diffuses out of cells into the bloodstream, which transports it to the lungs to be expired. Respiration requires specialized enzyme machinery called the terminal ELECTRON TRANSPORT CHAIN. This sequence of linked oxidation-reduction enzymes receives electrons from individual oxidation reactions of the cell and passes them on to oxygen, which is converted to water. The sequential transfer of electrons to oxygen is coupled with the generation of ATP, a process called OXIDATIVE PHOSPHORYLATION.

Certain toxins and poisons like cyanide inhibit cellular respiration, limit ATP production and may ultimately cause death. Nutrients required to support respiration include B vitamins NIACIN, RIBOFLAVIN, THIAMIN, PANTOTHENIC ACID, and trace minerals like COPPER and IRON. Another nutrient that may be required in the diet under certain conditions is COENZYME Q. This lipid helps funnel electrons into the system. (See also CARBOHYDRATE METABOLISM; FAT METABOLISM; RESPIRATORY QUOTIENT.)

respiratory chain See ELECTRON TRANSPORT CHAIN.

respiratory quotient (RQ) The ratio of the volume of expired CARBON DIOXIDE to the volume of OXYGEN consumed. This measurement can be used to determine whether PROTEIN, CARBOHYDRATE, and FAT represent the major energy sources of the body. Carbohydrate and protein are more oxidized (contain more oxygen), and less oxygen is required to oxidize them completely to carbon dioxide. Therefore, their RQ values are higher than that of fat: carbohydrate, 1.0; protein, 0.80; fat, 0.71; mixed diet, 0.82. The RQ may exceed 1.0 if large amounts of carbohydrate are being converted to fat. (See also METABOLISM.)

resveratrol A substance found in the skin of red GRAPES frequently used to make red WINE and grape juice. Resveratrol is a chemical that acts as an antibiotic in the plants that produce it. Although it is found in the components of other plants, including peanuts and eucalyptus, it appears in red grape skin in high concentrations.

Resveratrol is responsible in part for the CHOLESTEROL-lowering effect of red wine as determined by animal studies. It has also been suggested as the possible explanation for the "French Paradox," the low incidence of heart disease among French citizens who regularly eat high-fat foods and drink red wine. Additional research on humans is needed to determine whether supplementation with resveratrol would benefit patients at risk of cholesterol-related heart disease, and to establish the safety of this supplement. Several studies have confirmed that resveratrol is an effective and powerful ANTIOXIDANT. Consequently, researchers are investigating its possible role in preventing or inhibiting the growth of CANCER cells.

Kopp, P. "Resveratrol, a Phytoestrogen Found in Red Wine. A Possible Explanation for the Conundrum of the 'French Paradox'?" *European Journal of Endocrinology* 138 (1998): 619–620.

retinal The biologically activated form of VITAMIN A required to form visual purple (rhodopsin), the pigment in the retina responsible for night vision. The enzymatic conversion of vitamin A to retinal requires the trace mineral ZINC. (See also NIGHT BLINDNESS.)

retinoic acid (9-cis retinoic acid) An oxidized form of VITAMIN A, believed to be a new, fat-soluble HORMONE. Cis retinoic acid may guide normal embryonic development and regulate normal cell division and may be involved in regulating blood CHOLESTEROL levels. CANCER is characterized by uncontrolled cell division; some patients with certain kinds of cancer, such as leukemia, respond to treatments with retinoic acid. In 2002 Dartmouth Medical School researchers reported a significant discovery related to retinoic acid that may be an important step in eventually finding a cure for cancer. By studying how retinoic acid works to cause remission of acute promylocytic leukemia, a deadly blood cancer, researchers discovered that when the gene UBE1L was introduced into leukemic cells, it killed them in the same way that retinoic acid does. (See also ENDOCRINE SYSTEM.)

retinoid See BETA-CAROTENE; VITAMIN A.

retinol See VITAMIN A.

retinol equivalents (RE) See VITAMIN A.

rheumatoid arthritis (RA) A chronic inflammatory disease of the joints. Rheumatoid arthritis is characterized by overgrowth of joint tissue leading to swollen immobilized joints as a result of an overactive IMMUNE SYSTEM. Rheumatoid arthritis is classified as an AUTOIMMUNE DISEASE in which the immune system attacks the body by developing antibodies against joint tissue. An estimated 7 million people in the United States are affected by RA. The much more common ailment, OSTEOARTHRITIS, represents a joint "wear and tear" arthritis and does not involve the immune system, is not an autoimmune disease, and its cause is unrelated to rheumatoid arthritis.

Rheumatoid arthritis can begin in young or middle-aged adults. The triggering mechanisms are unproven. It seems likely there are many contributing factors. Infections, allergies, genetic susceptibility, lifestyle, and nutritional factors may play a role. There is no cure, although some medications are used to reduce INFLAMMATION (anti-inflammatory drugs). ASPIRIN is the most common drug used to relieve pain and swelling, but high doses of aspirin can cause gastrointestinal bleeding, stomach irritation, even reduced hearing. Newer anti-inflammatory medicines and less irritating nonsteroidal anti-inflammatory drugs (NSAIDS) are now available as prescription drugs. Other NSAIDS include ibuprofen and indomethicin. However, NSAIDS in general can cause intestinal inflammation and increase gut permeability to potentially harmful substances. Cortisone-related drugs can relieve inflammation. Long-term use can lead to disabling side effects. These effects include suppression of the immune system, bone demineralization, and thinning of skin.

Studies in the 1980s demonstrated that fasting often reduces symptoms of rheumatoid arthritis, but pain, swelling, and stiffness return when fasting ends. Preliminary clinical trials suggest that a gluten-free, vegan diet (no animal protein, no wheat) for three to five months followed by a lactovegetarian diet (only milk and milk products plus plant-derived foods) for the rest of the year can significantly reduce pain, improve grip strength, and reduce swelling among patients with rheumatoid arthritis. Therefore, food sensitivities should be ruled out.

Imbalanced PROSTAGLANDINS are linked to chronic conditions. These derivatives of essential fatty acids help regulate many physiologic processes, including inflammation. A growing body of evidence suggests that diet can influence prostaglandin levels. Supplemental seed oils containing the polyunsaturated fatty acid GAMMA LINOLENIC ACID, such as BORAGE oil and EVENING PRIMROSE OIL can reduce arthritic pain. Gamma linolenic acid is obtained from the ESSENTIAL FATTY ACID, LINOLEIC ACID, and leads to the formation of a set of anti-inflammatory prostaglandins. Other anti-inflammatory prostaglandins are derived from omega-3 fatty acids that occur in flaxseed oil and coldwater fish like SALMON, HERRING, SARDINES, and fish oils. These fish provide omega-3 fatty acids, such as EICOSAPENTAENOIC ACID, and diets rich in fish can decrease inflammation. Supplemental omega-3 oils (flaxseed oil and fish oil) may help decrease symptoms of arthritis.

Among the B vitamins, PANTOTHENIC ACID in large amounts has been used to relieve symptoms of rheumatoid arthritis. Vitamin K may help stabilize joint linings. Free radical and oxidative damage accompany inflammation, and the diet should provide ample ANTIOXIDANTS: SELENIUM, VITAMIN E, and VITAMIN C. ZINC, MANGANESE, and COPPER support the antioxidant enzyme, SUPEROXIDE DISMUTASE, which can protect tissues from free radical damage. Herbal preparations such as feverfew and LICORICE have been used in botanical medicine to treat rheumatoid arthritis. FLAVONOIDS such as QUERCETIN and catechin reduce inflammation by acting as antioxidants and by inhibiting mast cell degranulation, a major contributor to tissue injury. They also limit tissue destruction associated with inflammation. (See also OSTEOMALACIA; OSTEOPOROSIS.)

Toohey, Cordain L. et al. "Modulation of Immune Function by Dietary Lectins in Rheumatoid Arthritis," *British Journal of Nutrition* 83, no. 3 (2000): 207–217.

rhubarb (*Rheum rhaponticum*) A cultivated perennial with thick, typically red stalks that is classified as a fruit. Only the leaf stalks of this plant are edible because roots and leaves contain a potentially toxic material, OXALIC ACID. Rhubarb stalks are cooked in pies, sauces, rhubarb crumble, and other baked goods, jams, and preserves, and they can be fermented to produce wine. Rhubarb is extremely tart and requires the addition of sweeteners to make it appetizing. The calcium in rhubarb is poorly absorbed. Like spinach, it is not a good dietary source of calcium. Nutrient content of cooked rhubarb with added sugar (1 cup, 240 g) is: 279 calories; protein, 0.9 g; carbohydrate, 75 g; fiber, 5.3 g; calcium, 348 mg; vitamin C, 8 mg; thiamin, 0.04 mg; riboflavin, 0.06 mg; and niacin, 0.48 mg.

riboflavin (vitamin B_2) A bright yellow B complex VITAMIN. This widely distributed vitamin functions in oxidation-reduction reactions. Riboflavin works together with the B vitamins THIAMIN, NIACIN, and PANTOTHENIC ACID to oxidize FAT and CARBOHYDRATE to carbon dioxide to produce

ENERGY. The complete oxidation of these fuels occurs via the KREB'S CYCLE, a sequence of enzyme-catalyzed steps that represents the major energy-yielding pathway of most tissues. Riboflavin is the parent of FLAVIN ADENINE DINUCLEOTIDE (FAD) and flavin mononucleotide (FMN), two enzyme helpers (COENZYMES). Riboflavin participates in the body's defense system to oxidize toxins and foreign compounds. It supports glutathione reductase, an enzyme that replenishes an important cellular ANTIOXIDANT called glutathione. This system represents a major defense against oxidative damage. In addition, the production of steroid HORMONES by the ADRENAL GLANDS requires riboflavin. More generally, riboflavin is essential for successful reproduction in experimental animals, for healthy skin, eyes, and nerve function.

Possible Roles in Maintaining Health

Unlike niacin deficiency or thiamin deficiency, chronic riboflavin deficiency does not cause a distinctive human disease. ARIBOFLAVINOSIS, a riboflavin deficiency disease, occurs in association with deficiencies of other B complex vitamins. Symptoms of riboflavin deficiency include FATIGUE, delayed wound healing, sore mouth, cracks in the corners of the mouth, tongue inflammation (GLOSSITIS), blurred vision and light sensitivity, and eczema of face and genitalia.

Sources

Riboflavin is widely distributed among foods, but the levels vary greatly. Rich sources include organ meats (LIVER, kidney, and heart); dairy products (MILK, CHEESE, YOGURT); and BREWER'S YEAST. BREAKFAST CEREAL, enriched flour, almonds, lean meat, raw mushrooms, wheat bran, enriched cornmeal, soybean flour, and dark green leafy VEGETABLES are good sources. Fifty percent of the riboflavin in milk can be lost within two hours after exposure to light. Storing milk in cartons rather than in glass bottles markedly reduces the loss. Riboflavin is destroyed by light and by heat. Up to 20 percent of riboflavin is lost from milk by evaporation or by PASTEURIZATION. Raw fruits and vegetables generally provide little riboflavin.

The U.S. enrichment program for white flour was initiated in 1941. Since then, riboflavin, as well as thiamin, niacin, and iron, have been added to flour and cereal products that together account for an estimated 0.33 mg of riboflavin per day for a typical American. Riboflavin is nontoxic; excesses are excreted and turn urine yellow.

Requirements

The RECOMMENDED DIETARY ALLOWANCE (RDA) of riboflavin is 1.7 mg per day for men and 1.3 mg per day for women between the ages of 25 and 50. The requirement is somewhat higher for women who are pregnant or breast-feeding. Anyone with a severely compromised diet is prone to B complex vitamin deficiency in general. This includes children of developing countries who do not eat enough eggs, meat, and milk or enriched foods; alcoholics; elderly persons with an imbalanced diet; people on severe weight loss programs; chronic users of fiber-based laxatives or tranquilizers; and patients with HYPOTHYROIDISM. Vigorous EXERCISE also can increase the requirement of riboflavin in women. (See also CARBOHYDRATE METABOLISM; FAT METABOLISM.)

rice (*Oryza sativa*) An important cereal grain and a food staple in Asia and other parts of the world. Rice is a grass related to WHEAT, OATS, and BARLEY. Rice originated from wild species that persist in southeast Asia. Rice culture occurred in China by 2200 B.C. and in Thailand by 5000 to 3500 B.C. Worldwide, China, India, Indonesia, Bangladesh, and Thailand produce the most rice. In populations dependent on rice, it can account for 60 percent to 80 percent of total calories. In Asia the average annual consumption is 200 to 400 pounds (90 to 180 g) per person. Rice consumption in the United States has been steadily growing in the past two decades. In 2002 per capita rice consumption in this country was 26.5 pounds a year. The U.S. produces 1 percent to 2 percent of the world's crop.

There are many thousands of rice strains, including strains adapted to warm or cold climates, low or high elevations. Paddy rice is cultivated in flooded fields most of the growing season, while upland rice can grow in wet soil and doesn't require flooding. Many hardy strains of rice now used were products of the GREEN REVOLUTION, a concentrated effort of agriculture, science, and industry to improve crop productivity in developing nations. Use of these strains, better irrigation, increased use of chemical fertilizers and synthetic pesticides created a dramatic increase in grain production in Asia, South America, and Africa.

Rice is classified according to size: Short-grain rice is oval in shape, contains less AMYLOSE, a straight-chain form of STARCH, and is sticky when cooked. Medium-grain rice is more tender than long-grain rice and is used to make cold breakfast cereals. Long-grain rice has a high amylose content, and its kernels do not stick to each other when cooked. Long-grain rice accounts for more than 70 percent of the U.S. domestic production. Waxy rice cooks to a sticky paste and is used for cakes and confections. Wild rice, *Zizania aquatica,* is native to eastern North America. Though it is an annual grass, it is a distant cousin of true rice.

White or polished rice is produced by milling to remove bran, husk, and germ, which reduces the content of B vitamins. Polished rice is approximately 92 percent starch and only 2 percent additional nutrients. Notably, the content of THIAMIN in polished rice is only 18 percent of that of husked rice. Among populations subsisting primarily on white rice, the thiamin deficiency disease, BERIBERI may occur.

In the United States, white rice is enriched with thiamin, RIBOFLAVIN, NIACIN, IRON, and CALCIUM. Removing hulls from dried, rough rice yields brown rice. Brown rice resembles whole wheat in nutrient content. The protein content is lower than wheat but the quality is higher. Nonetheless, rice protein is deficient in the AMINO ACID, LYSINE, typical of most grains. Rice contains more niacin than does corn. Parboiled rice represents rough rice that has been soaked, steamed, and dried to loosen husks, which are removed by milling. Greater amounts of nutrients are retained than in white rice. Rice is used as a breakfast food (puffed rice, flakes, crispies), rice flour, flaked rice, rice-based baby food, rice oil, and rice bran. Rice bran contains fiber that can help reduce blood cholesterol levels and rice oil, which also has a cholesterol-lowering effect. Rice bran does not become sticky when cooked, unlike oat bran. Rice is commonly steamed or boiled. The more water used in cooking rice, the more nutrients are lost.

The nutrient content of 1 cup (205 g) of white, enriched rice (cooked without salt) is 223 calories; protein, 4.1 g; carbohydrate, 49.6 g; fiber, 0.82 g; fat, 0.2 g; iron, 2.9 mg; thiamin, 0.22 mg; riboflavin, 0.02 mg; niacin, 2.05 mg.

rickets A disorder of bone formation in growing children commonly due to VITAMIN D deficiency. Rickets is characterized by softening and deformation of long BONES, reflecting an interference with bone growth and altered mineralization. The bone disease in adults resulting from vitamin D deficiency is called OSTEOMALACIA. The mineral portion of bone consists mainly of CALCIUM and phosphate; thus a deficiency of either can cause rickets. Low calcium can be the result of a dietary deficiency of calcium or of vitamin D, or a problem with vitamin D's activation to the hormone form, calcitriol (1,25-dihydroxyvitamin D_3). Some people may be unable to convert vitamin D to calcitriol because of a rare genetic defect in the kidney enzyme performing the last step in the activation of vitamin D to calcitriol. Dietary vitamin D sources include fortified MILK and fish liver oils. (Alternatively, ultraviolet light converts provitamin D in the skin to vitamin D; therefore, inadequate exposure to winter sunlight, particularly in populations living in northern latitudes and in institutionalized people, can lead to vitamin D deficiency. Still other problems can be caused by malabsorption syndromes associated with CELIAC DISEASE and INFLAMMATORY BOWEL DISEASE, which can limit uptake of fat-soluble vitamins, including vitamin D, even when dietary intake is normal.

Abnormally low phosphate and calcium in children's diets can also cause rickets. Hormone imbalances, such as an increased secretion of parathyroid hormone, can trigger calcium and phosphate release from bone. This loss of mineral softens bone.

Sometimes rickets accompanies kidney disease when the kidneys fail to synthesize calcitriol. Other types of rickets can be caused by genetic abnormalities in tissues so that the hormone, though present, cannot perform its physiologic functions. (See also OSTEOARTHRITIS; OSTEOPOROSIS; SKELETON.)

risk due to chemicals in food and water The chance of injury or illness resulting from exposure to synthetic chemicals in FOOD. Logical and reasonable decisions can be made when risks are identified and their magnitude assessed. In reality, no substance is absolutely safe and there is no risk-free environment, although modern technology and policies based on simple, rapid solutions to public health problems have nurtured this common expectation.

Risk estimates are averages of populations and are not designed for individuals. Epidemiology, the study of populations, has identified several large risks for chronic diseases. In the United States, HEART DISEASE is the number-one killer, accounting for 40 percent of all deaths (death rate is 265.9 per 100,000 people). Risk increases with age, family history of heart disease, OBESITY, high blood pressure, smoking, and excessive fat intake. CANCER is the number-two killer, with 25 percent of deaths. About 77 percent of all cancers are diagnosed in people who are age 55 or older. According to the American Cancer Society, one-third of all cancer deaths in 2002 (about 185,170) were related to poor nutrition and sedentary lifestyles; about 170,000 cancer deaths were related to tobacco use; another 19,000 were related to excessive alcohol use, often in combination with tobacco use.

Stroke is the third leading cause of death, killing more than 166,000 people annually (60.2 deaths per 100,000 people).

One problem inherent in assessing cancer risk is that the delay between exposure to a cancer-causing agent (CARCINOGEN) and development of cancer can be many years. The risk of disease also depends on an individual's health history and genetic predisposition. Deficiencies in primary health care, which especially affect pregnant women, fetuses, children, and low-income people, also increase disease and death risks. Stroke accounts for 6.9 percent of deaths (death rate of 61 per 100,000). Those at greatest risk are adults over 55, particularly over the age of 65. Risk increases with age, untreated high blood pressure, DIABETES, obesity, and smoking.

Technology has posed questions about the definition of a safe level of exposure to potentially harmful agents. Sensitive analytical techniques can now readily detect traces of contaminants in foods at levels unattainable in the 1970s. Contaminant levels at parts per billion and even parts per trillion can be detected in air, water, foods, and even human milk. The long-term effects on health of chronic exposure to such low levels of multiple contaminants remain unknown.

Under the Food Quality Protection Act of 1996 the EPA is required to consider risks and benefits of agricultural chemicals. This act created a new safety standard for pesticides in food: a reasonable certainty of no harm.

Public perception of risk depends in part on the source of the risk, whether it is readily apparent, and the circumstances under which it appeared. Man-made hazards are less acceptable than natural (uncontrollable) causes. Perceived risk increases when there is no clear benefit and when the risk is unfamiliar. For example, a government agency can estimate that a pesticide may cause between 1 and 100 deaths per million; this risk may be perceived as unacceptable by some. On the other hand, traffic accidents kill about 42,000 Americans yearly (about 110 people a day) which is generally considered an acceptable modern-day risk.

Each approach to risk assessment presents strengths and weaknesses. A common experimental strategy in cancer risk assessment is based on examining cancer risk for rats and mice exposed to high levels of an agent in order to detect an observable effect. Applying these data to human populations involves assumptions that humans will behave in the same way as animals and assumptions that the effects of a low dose can be calculated from a high dose administered to the animals. Even more uncertainty is involved if comparisons are made on the basis of extreme toxicity. On the other hand, risks calculated in a similar way can be compared; thus the risk of consuming different types of carcinogens can be compared from historical data. Exposure to similar compounds can also be used as a basis of comparison. Risks of cancer due to various chlorinated hydrocarbons in chlorinated drinking water can be similarly compared.

Questions to Ask Regarding a Risk

- What is the absolute risk? Is it 1 per 1,000 or 10 per million? A tenfold increase in risk (a statement about relative risk) has different meanings in terms of the total numbers of people involved in each of these cases. Thus a tenfold increase in risk at 1 per 1,000 is 10 per thousand, or 10,000 people per million. A tenfold increase in risk at 10 per million is 100 people per million, meaning that far fewer people will be affected.

- What is the likelihood of exposure? Risk increases with amount of exposure or dosage and duration of exposure.
- What are the tradeoffs? For example, is it acceptable to use a pesticide that lowers food costs substantially, yet could increase the number of cancer deaths by one in a million? This would be an application of a so-called negligible risk standard. (See also GENETIC ENGINEERING.)

RNA (ribonucleic acid) The type of biomolecule that directs the synthesis of PROTEIN after receiving information from DNA. RNA is classified as a NUCLEIC ACID, the same chemical family as DNA. Three different types of RNA perform different functions in protein synthesis. "Messenger-RNA" represents a copy of the genetic material that carries the code words specifying the amino acid sequence characteristic of each protein. "Ribosomal RNA" occurs in ribosomes, cytoplasmic particles that combine with messenger RNA and provide the site of protein synthesis. A third family of RNA is "transfer RNA," which carries activated amino acids to assemble proteins. Transfer RNAs "read" code words in the messenger RNA, align amino acids in the proper sequence and permit amino acids to be joined together. Thus transfer RNAs help translate the language of DNA into the language of proteins in all cells.

In terms of composition, RNA consists of phosphate; the simple sugar, ribose; and four nitrogen-containing compounds (ADENINE, GUANINE, uracil, and CYTOSINE). Three of these bases occur in DNA; only uracil is unique to RNA. RNA is assembled by the body from simple nutrients, and there is no dietary requirement for RNA. The enzyme that synthesizes RNA (RNA polymerase) requires the trace mineral nutrient ZINC for activity. (See also PURINE; PYRIMIDINE; URIC ACID.)

rosemary (*Rosmarinus officinalis*) A perennial evergreen that grows as a shrub. Rosemary has long, thin leaves with a rich scent. Leaves of this pungent herb are used dried or fresh as a strong seasoning for pork, veal, lamb, and chicken. It is used with tomato sauce, marinades, soups, and ragouts. Rosemary extracts are used as an antioxidant by the food industry. The herb contains rosemaricine, which can stimulate the digestive tract, help with fat digestion and lessen joint pain. It has been used as an antiseptic mouthwash and gargle.

rotation diet A DIET plan in which related FOODS or foods within botanical families are not eaten more frequently than every four days. Studies of patients, especially children with food ALLERGIES, suggest that rotating foods and eating them in moderation reduces the tendency to develop new food allergies or to activate existing sensitivities. Rotation diets can help reduce the symptoms of food allergies and to identify problematic foods. Use of rotation diets also permits the patient to eliminate many foods. A variety of books are now available to assist in food selection, menu planning, and meal preparation. Typically, foods are listed in four columns representing days one to four and grouped according to families. Typical categories include MEAT, GRAIN, FISH, FRUIT, VEGETABLES, beverages, NUTS and seeds, NATURAL SWEETENERS, MILK or milk substitutes, thickeners, and fats and oils. Foods in one list do not appear in the other lists, in order to avoid selecting a food more frequently than every four days.

It is advisable to begin a rotation diet slowly because this type of diet represents major adjustments. One approach is to begin by rotating grains/starches by using wheat products on day one, then rice products on day two, then corn products on day three, with oats on day four. Grain alternatives such as AMARANTH, QUINOA, MILLET, or BARLEY can be substituted for any of the above grain groups. After one to two weeks, meats can be rotated, for example, beef (red meat) on day one, then turkey (poultry) on day two, then pork (red meat) on day three, then chicken (poultry) on day four. Veal, calf liver, venison, and lamb fall within the beef category because these are related. Similarly, goose and turkey fall in the turkey group, and pheasant and quail are listed with chicken. To rotate fruits, the following are options: CITRUS FRUIT on day one, followed by the apple/grape family on day two, then by MELONS on day three and berries on day four. For vegetables, options can include CARROTS, BEETS, CHARD, SPINACH, or CELERY on day one; then the LEGUMES with PEAS, BEANS, LENTILS or soy, or the squash family on day two; then nightshade vegetables, such as POTATO, EGGPLANT, or PEPPERS on day three; and the cabbage family with CAULIFLOWER, BROCCOLI, or BRUSSELS SPROUTS on day four. Symptoms may improve after several weeks of diet rotation. Often, it is easier to use a rotation diet when other family members support each other in making major dietary changes.

Vatn M. H. et al. "Adverse Reaction to Food: Assessment by Double-Blind Placebo-Controlled Food Challenge and Clinical Psychosomatic and Immunologic Analysis," *Digestion* 56, (1995): 421–428.

royal jelly A viscous liquid secreted by the salivary glands of "nurse" bees and fed to the bee larvae that will eventually develop into "queen" bees. Like BEE POLLEN, royal jelly has been marketed by food supplement manufacturers as a treatment for fatigue, digestive disorders, and cardiovascular problems. No reliable scientific studies support these claims, and the safety of royal jelly supplements has not been established. Some consumers have reported suffering allergic reactions.

rutabaga (*Brassica napobrassica;* Swedish turnip) A root vegetable that resembles a large TURNIP. It is believed to have originated in a hybrid between KALE and turnip, perhaps in medieval Europe. Rutabaga is used both as food and as livestock fodder. In the United States, it is grown mainly in the northern states. Unlike turnip greens, rutabaga leaves are not edible. The root can be baked, boiled, and mashed with potatoes, served in souffles, casseroles, stews, and soups.

Turnips and rutabagas contain small amounts of GOITROGENS, substances that block IODINE uptake. The effects of these materials can be worsened by an iodine-deficient diet and when large quantities are eaten, not a usual situation in the United States. Rutabagas are a rich source of vitamin C. The nutrient content of 1 cup (140 g) of rutabagas is: 64 calories; protein, 1.5 g; carbohydrate, 15.4 g; fiber, 1.4 g; fat, 0.28 g; vitamin A, 810 IU; vitamin C, 60 mg; thiamin, 0.1 mg; riboflavin, 0.1 mg; niacin, 0.14 mg.

rye (*Secale cereale*) A common cereal grain related to wheat. Rye was domesticated in northern Europe in the fourth century B.C., and independently in Asia and the Middle East. In medieval Europe rye became a staple bread grain. Rye flour is second only to wheat flour in terms of worldwide popularity for bread making, although it accounts for only 3 percent of the worldwide production of cereal grains and ranks eighth in the world. Northern Europe remains a major region for rye production. Popularity in the United States has declined steadily since 1920, and the United States produces 2 percent of the world rye crop. Ergot, a fungus that produces a poisonous substance that can cause convulsions, can infect rye. Limits have been established for ergot contamination.

Rye berries (groats), representing the husked whole grain, can be cooked like RICE. Whole rye flour is dark and contains most of the nutrients of rye berries. Light rye flour is a refined product, containing relatively more starch and less germ; it may be bleached. Bleached rye flour is less nutritious than dark flour. Cracked rye is crushed rye berries. It can be cooked like cracked wheat or OATS, as a BREAKFAST CEREAL. Rolled rye flakes are produced by heating rye berries until soft, and flattening them with steel rollers. Rye is used to produce crackers and rye flakes are used as a hamburger extender. Rye is also sprouted and served as a salad green. Rye is fermented to make whiskey.

Authentic rye bread is dense with a robust flavor. It is less responsive to yeast as a leavening agent; consequently, wheat flour is often added to improve dough-rising properties. Rye bread prepared with wheat flour may contain artificial coloring or other coloring to darken it. The nutrient value of rye is similar to wheat. Rye protein, like wheat protein, is deficient in the essential amino acid LYSINE. Rye flour (1 cup, dark) provides 419 calories; protein, 20.9 g; carbohydrate, 87.2 g; fiber, 3.1 g; fat, 3.3 g; calcium, 69 mg; sodium, 1 mg; thiamin, 0.78 mg; riboflavin, 0.28 mg; niacin, 3.5 mg.

S

saccharin One of the oldest ARTIFICIAL SWEETENERS, saccharin has been available for more than 100 years. It is not metabolized in humans and it provides no calories. Although saccharin is 300 to 700 times sweeter than TABLE SUGAR, it is often perceived to have a bitter or "metallic" aftertaste at high concentrations. Saccharin is generally combined with a sugar, DEXTROSE, or with ASPARTAME, another artificial sweetener, for tabletop sweeteners. The compound is stable to baking and acidic conditions; this versatility contributes to its use in many products, including baked foods, salad dressings, reduced calorie jams, toothpaste, mouthwash, and other personal care products. Saccharin can be added to chewing gum where it is used with SORBITOL, a sweet sugar analog.

In May 2000 officials at the National Institute of Environmental Health Sciences and its subdivision, the National Toxicology Program, announced that saccharin would no longer appear on their list of "cancer threats." Saccharin had officially been listed as a carcinogen in March 1977 when Canadian researchers discovered a link between saccharin and bladder tumors in male rats. This finding immediately triggered the threat of the DELANEY CLAUSE, a congressionally mandated provision that requires the U.S. Food and Drug Administration to ban any synthetic food chemical shown to cause cancer when ingested by laboratory animals. When millions of dieting Americans heard that the only low-calorie sweetener available was going to be banned (cyclamates had been banned in 1970 for similar reasons), they were upset; Congress responded by protecting saccharin from the Delaney Clause by allowing it back on the market with a health warning label. Saccharin's chances were further damaged in 1981 when the National Toxicology Program, referring again to the Canadian rat study, decided to put saccharin on its "cancer causing" list—formally declaring it an "anticipated human carcinogen."

In September 1996 the Calorie Control Council, a trade group of the diet food industry, petitioned the toxicology program to have saccharin reclassified. Subsequently, two government scientific panels that looked at the possible link between saccharin and cancer supported removal, saying that any link to cancer was weak. A third scientific panel of nongovernment experts voted 4–3 against taking saccharin off the list.

Nevertheless, in December 2000 Congress passed the Saccharin Warning Elimination via Environmental Testing Employing Science and Technology Act ("SWEETEST Act") after a National Toxicology Program review concluded that saccharin poses no health hazard to humans. The report concluded that the observed bladder tumors in rats were caused by mechanisms not relevant to humans and that no data in humans suggest that a carcinogenic hazard exists. The legislation allowed manufacturers to remove the warning labels from saccharin packages that said the sweetener had been shown to cause cancer in lab animals. (See also FOOD ADDITIVES; NATURAL SWEETENERS.)

S-adenosylmethionine (SAMe) A synthetic form of the AMINO ACID METHIONINE, S-adenosylmethionine is found in every cell in the human body. SAMe has been used in Europe since the 1960s as a prescription antidepressant and pain reliever and was introduced to the U.S. market in 1999 as a dietary supplement.

In the body SAMe normally maintains cell membranes and is involved in methylation, a process that, among other things, helps to regulate levels of the mood-lifting neurotransmitters serotonin and dopamine. Some study subjects have reported that SAMe is effective as an antidepressant. Several clinical studies have demonstrated that SAMe is better than placebo and is equivalent to nonsteroidal anti-inflammatory drugs (NSAIDS) such as ibuprofen for easing pain associated with osteoarthritis. Patients suffering from fibromyalgia have also reported significant relief from the symptoms that accompany that disease. SAMe has also shown some promise in treating patients who suffer liver diseases such as cirrhosis (liver failure) caused by alcohol abuse.

Because SAMe was introduced in the United States as a dietary supplement, it has not undergone review by the U.S. FDA for safety or efficacy, and many scientists and others in the medical community have expressed skepticism regarding its reported health benefits. These critics say the study subjects may have been reporting PLACEBO effects and that all the studies that have been done so far were for periods of time that were too short to produce statistically significant results. Additional studies are ongoing. Safety data are inadequate for pregnant and breast-feeding women.

Soekin, A. L. "Abstract: Safety and Efficacy of S-adenosylmethionine (SAMe) for Osteoarthritis," *Journal of Family Practice* 51, no. 5 (2002): 425–430.

safflower (*Carthamus tinctorius*) A thistle-like plant that produces oil-rich seeds resembling small sunflower seeds. Safflower is a late arrival in the United States, becoming an established crop only in the 1950s and 1960s as POLYUNSATURATED VEGETABLE OILS gained in popularity in response to fears about CHOLESTEROL and SATURATED FAT and their link to ATHEROSCLEROSIS. Varieties of safflower yielding 50 percent oil have been developed. Safflower is cultivated in California and Montana.

Safflower oil contains the highest percentage of polyunsaturated FATTY ACIDS and the lowest percentage of saturated fatty acids among commercially available oils. Typically, safflower oil contains 74 percent to 77 percent LINOLEIC ACID, an essential polyunsaturated fatty acid; 16.4 percent OLEIC ACID, a monounsaturated fatty acid; and 6.6 percent saturated fatty acids. Like SOYBEAN oil, it has a high smoke point (440° to 480° F) and is often used in deep-fat frying and sauteeing. Safflower oil is rich in VITAMIN E. As a polyunsaturated oil, it is susceptible to RANCIDITY (decomposition) when heated. These oils should not be reheated.

Like all commercial polyunsaturated cooking oils, safflower is partially hydrogenated to reduce its susceptibility to oxidation and decrease the rate of rancidity. Hydrogenation refers to the chemical hardening process that adds hydrogen atoms and decreases the level of saturation. Hydrogenated safflower oil yields MARGARINE, VEGETABLE SHORTENING, MAYONNAISE, and other products. Hydrogenation creates TRANSFATTY ACIDS. The safety of these unusual products has been questioned.

The consumption of polyunsaturated vegetable oils like safflower oil can lower the level of LOW-DENSITY LIPOPROTEIN (LDL), the less desirable form of cholesterol, but at the same time a high intake can lower the level of HIGH-DENSITY LIPOPROTEIN (HDL), the desirable form of cholesterol. (See also ESSENTIAL FATTY ACIDS.)

saffron (*Crocus sativus*) This small crocus produces flowers with intense yellow-orange filaments. When dried, the stamens yield a pungent spice and brilliant yellow coloring agent. Saffron is used for rice dishes, soup, and sauces, as well as certain meat dishes in Indian, Italian, and Spanish cuisine. Saffron is best dissolved in a small amount of warm water before use for uniform mixing. (See also FOOD ADDITIVES; FOOD COLORING, NATURAL.)

sage (*Salvia officinalis*) A common perennial HERB whose fresh or dried leaves add a pungent, bitter taste to foods. There are over 500 varieties of sage, including the common garden sage. It is used to flavor poultry, fatty meat like pork, veal, ham, or lamb, and in marinades, minestrone, and sauces. Sage has long been used as a medicinal herb in folk medicine. Its name comes from the Latin *salvus,* which means healthy. It possesses bacterial and antifungal properties and it has been used to aid digestion. Sage tea has been used to reduce coughing associated with colds and for irregular menstruation. As with any medicinal herb, the consumption of large amounts for long periods of time is not recommended. (See also PARSLEY.)

sago Starch from the trunk of a tropical palm. In the South Pacific, sago palm flour and starch are staple foods. They are used as food thickeners. Commercially, sago starch is used as a noncorn source of glucose from which to manufacture corn-free VITAMIN C for certain individuals who are ultrasensitive to corn products. (See also OIL PALM; PALM OILS.)

salami A deli sausage usually made from PORK or a combination of pork and BEEF and several seasonings, including salt, garlic, black pepper, and fennel. Salami is a high-fat (generally 30 percent) and high-sodium food. Some, but not all, salamis are cured and may contain preservatives such as nitrites. Several varieties are available, including cacciatore, pepperoni, and genoa. Salami is usually sliced thin for use in sandwiches or, in the case of pepperoni, on pizza. One slice of cooked salami (23 g) yields 57.5 calories; fat, 4.5 g; protein, 3 g; potassium, 45.5 mg; sodium 245 mg.

saliva The fluid secreted by glands of the MOUTH. Three pairs of salivary glands produce saliva. Parotid glands, located on each side of the face, drain through ducts opening in the inner surface of the cheek. Sublingual glands drain into the floor of the mouth. Submaxillary glands (submandibular glands) are located beneath the base of the tongue and drain in the floor of the mouth. Tiny buccal glands in the mouth also contribute saliva. The combined saliva from all these sources amounts to a quart (1 liter) of fluid daily.

In composition, saliva is 99.5 percent water. Saliva serves important functions: It acts as a lubricant, as a moistening agent and as a dissolving agent for flavors as food is chewed and swallowed. Saliva contains mucins, slippery PROTEINS that provide the lubricating action. Without water and mucins, swallowing would be very difficult. Saliva contains the digestive enzyme AMYLASE, which initiates starch DIGESTION, and chewing food thoroughly to a uniform paste assists starch breakdown by this enzyme. Saliva also contains ions (electrolytes)—SODIUM, CHLORIDE, and BICARBONATE. Chloride activates amylase. These minerals are later absorbed and recycled. For defense, saliva contains lysozyme, an enzyme that ruptures some disease-producing bacteria, and a protective ANTIBODY, secretory IgA, that can bind to foreign materials, including viruses, bacteria, and yeast, to reduce this risk of infection.

Salivation is controlled exclusively by the NERVOUS SYSTEM. Savory aromas, visual images, sounds of food preparation, and memories can stimulate salivation. Salivation also occurs in response to irritating foods and with nausea. Saliva flow after eating flushes chemical remnants out of the mouth and adjusts the acidity to neutral. Dehydration can decrease salivation. A variety of medications, such as antihistamines (diphenylpyraline and azatidine), diminish mucous secretions, including saliva. Stress stimulates the sympathetic nervous system to reduce salivation. On the other hand, dryness of the mouth promotes thirst sensations. (See also DEGLUTITION; TASTE.)

salmon (*Oncorhynchus*) A saltwater fish valued as a food fish, and as a sport fish. The word *salmon* is derived from the Latin *salmo,* which means "leaping." Salmon can weigh up to 65 lb. and measure up to 3 ft. long. Varieties include the Atlantic salmon and the five varieties of Pacific salmon: sockeye (red) salmon (*O. nerka*), both canned and sold fresh; Chinook (king) salmon (*O. tschawytscha*), the largest and fattiest variety; coho (sliver) salmon (*O. kisutch*), smaller fish, sold fresh; pink (humpback) salmon (*O. gorbuscha*), the smallest variety, bland flesh, sold canned; and chum (dog) salmon (*O. keta*), lower in fat and with pale flesh. Salmon are a migratory fish that spawn in fresh water. Young fish live in fresh water for two years before migrating to the sea. Pollution, dam construction, and overharvesting have drastically reduced the numbers of this food fish in many parts of the world. Commercial salmon comes from many countries, such as Chile, Norway, and Canada (eastern Canada and British Columbia). Imported salmon are generally pen-raised rather than wild fish. Domestic, pen-raised salmon are also readily available. In the United States, Maine, Alaska, and Washington support most major salmon fisheries, and canned salmon comes from the northern Pacific. Most Atlantic salmon comes from Canada and Norway.

Salmon is an oily fish, rich in beneficial marine lipids. Salmon fat contains 30 percent to 40 percent omega-3 polyunsaturated FATTY ACIDS, mainly EPA (EICOSAPENTAENOIC ACID) and DHA (DOCASAHEXAENOIC ACID). These polyunsaturates are believed to decrease the risk of STROKE and CARDIOVASCULAR DISEASE. They decrease the risk of blood clots by inhibiting blood platelet aggregation. Platelets are cell fragments in the blood that initiate clotting.

Pen-raised salmon are more likely to be contaminated with industrial pollutants when grown in waters near industrial areas. Consumer advocates have criticized seafood safety in the United States. PCB contamination has been detected in fresh salmon although the levels were below tolerance limits set by the U.S. FDA. Canned salmon sold in the United States comes from the Pacific off the coast of Alaska, an area less likely to be polluted by industrial waste. Salmon is smoked, poached, grilled, marinated, baked, or canned. The nutrient content of 3 oz. (85 g) of broiled salmon is: 140 calories; protein, 21 g; fat, 5 g; cholesterol, 60 mg; thiamin, 0.18 mg; riboflavin, 0.14 mg; niacin, 5.5 g. (See also FISH OIL; OMEGA-3 FATTY ACIDS; SEAFOOD.)

salmonella A bacterium that includes more than 1,300 strains that frequently causes FOOD POISONING. Salmonella does not form spores and is destroyed by heat. Its usual habitat is the intestinal tract of an animal host. Salmonella occurs in animal feed, food processing plants, and food handling, and the bacteria are easily spread by fecal contamination. Flies, rodents, and insects that contact infected fecal material may also contaminate food. Sewage-contaminated water is known to carry salmonella and cause disease.

Livestock and poultry are major sources of human infection. About one in 20,000 eggs is contaminated. Thoroughly cooking eggs destroys the bacteria. According to the U.S. Centers for Disease Control and Prevention, most cases of salmonella poisoning are caused by eating undercooked eggs in sauces, salads, and processed foods. Salmonella grows readily in milk and milk-derived dishes such as custard, egg dishes, and salad dressing. MEAT and meat products like SAUSAGE, meat pies, sandwiches, and chili can become contaminated when allowed to stand at room temperature for several hours if infected by a food handler.

salmonellosis A form of food poisoning caused by salmonella. Salmonellosis is one of the three most common food-borne diseases associated with bacteria, and it is one of the fastest growing food-borne illnesses. Every year about 40,000 cases of salmonellosis are reported in the United States. The actual number of cases may be much higher because many people who have been infected do not seek professional care and are therefore not diagnosed and reported. Illness caused by salmonella is more common during the summer months, and children are more likely to be infected. Salmonellosis can be fatal, especially in young children, the immunocompromised, and elderly people. About 1,000 persons die each year from acute salmonellosis. Some strains of salmonella resist antibiotics, and dairy cattle fed antibiotics were the likely source of a drug-resistant salmonella strain that caused a large U.S. outbreak of food poisoning, involved six states in 1985. This outbreak caused 1,000 deaths, 35,000 hospitalizations and left an estimated 125,000 people with increased risk of chronic illnesses such as ARTHRITIS, osteomyelitis, ankylosing spondylitis, and COLITIS.

Salmonellosis often causes flu-like symptoms. Fever, abdominal cramping, headache, DIARRHEA, and vomiting generally appear 12 to 36 hours after eating tainted food. Symptoms may last from two days to a week. Illness is most severe in those with weakened immune systems, commonly found in very young children and in elderly people. Maldigestion and MALABSORPTION can result from intestinal damage due to this disease.

Salmonellosis was almost unknown in the United States 40 years ago. Increased volume and speed of food production, increased drug resistance of bacteria, and relaxed enforcement by government agencies contributed to widespread contamination of food, especially POULTRY. Raw milk, raw cheese, any raw or undercooked meat, including salami and hamburger, and fresh eggs can be contaminated by feces and fecal bacteria and can thus be a potential source of contamination. Pasteurized eggs are used to prepare commercial MAYONNAISE, and it is not a carrier. Freshwater as well as marine fish caught from waters highly polluted by raw sewage may be contaminated by salmonella.

All food handlers should thoroughly wash their hands before handling food to eliminate fecal contamination. They should carefully clean all equipment used in food preparation, including cutting boards. Raw vegetables should not come into contact with utensils used to prepare raw meat and poultry. Food should be refrigerated. Salmonella is destroyed by heating at 140° F (60° C) for 20 minutes or at 149° F (60° C) for three minutes. (See also BOTULISM.)

Olsen, S. J. et al. "The Changing Epidemiology of Salmonella: Trends in Serotypes Isolated from Humans in the U.S., 1987–1997," *Journal of Infectious Diseases* 183 (2000): 756–761.

salt See SODIUM.

salt substitutes (potassium chloride, lite salt, low-sodium salt) A combination of chemicals that taste like table salt but contains less SODIUM. Excessive salt in the diet can cause HIGH BLOOD PRESSURE in hypertensive people who are sodium sensitive. Most salt substitutes are mixtures of table salt (sodium chloride) and POTASSIUM chloride. Potassium is an essential nutrient in its own right and can lower blood pressure in some people. Excessive potassium can irritate the stomach and might start an ulcer. Diseased or damaged kidneys may not be able to excrete potassium properly; a toxic excess can accumulate. Therefore, patients taking certain DIURETICS (water pills), beta blockers or non-steroidal anti-inflammatory drugs; who are diabetic; or who have kidney disease are advised to avoid such salt substitutes. The safest strategy is to cut back on salt entirely and to use herbs and spices to improve the flavor in place of table salt. There are many different herbs to choose from, each with its own different, pleasing flavor. Consider CAYENNE pepper, basil, garlic powder, mace, marjoram, SAGE, savory and thyme, or blends. (See also FOOD ADDITIVES; HYPERTENSION.)

salt tablets See SODIUM.

SAMe See S-ADENOSYLMETHIONINE.

sardine Various small saltwater fish, including alewife, Atlantic HERRING, pilchard, and sprat. The name probably originated from the small Mediterranean fish in the vicinity of the island of Sardinia. Sardines are a fatty fish. Atlantic herring is a good source of OMEGA-3 FATTY ACIDS, the essential fatty acids thought to protect against heart attacks.

Sardines are rich sources of calcium because the fish is cooked bones and all. Its soft bones contribute to a high calcium content. A 4 oz. serving of sardines provides 50 percent of the REFERENCE DAILY INTAKE (RDI) of calcium and 20 percent of the RDI or iron. Sardines contain significant levels of salt. The same 4 oz. serving provides approximately 600 mg of sodium, one-third to one-half of the amount judged safe.

Sardines are often packed in oil, which increases their calories. Sardines packed in olive oil would be preferable to those packed in soybean oil because of olive oil's greater stability and protective effects against heart disease. Norwegian sardines are often packed in sardine oil, which has a high content of omega-3 fatty acids. Blot the fish in oil with a paper towel before eating them, to remove excess oil and to lower calories. Sardines packed in water are now available. The nutrient content of 3 oz. (85 g) of sardines (canned, packed in soybean oil, drained, and including bones) is: 175 calories; protein, 20 g; fat, 9.4 g; cholesterol, 85 mg; calcium, 371 mg; iron, 2.6 mg; thiamin, 0.03 mg; riboflavin, 0.17 mg; niacin, 4.6 mg.

sarsaparilla (*Smilax sarsaparilla*) A medicinal herb native to tropical regions of South America and the Caribbean. This perennial evergreen grows as a vine; its roots are used in botanical medicine. Europeans learned of its use from Native Americans. According to folk traditions, sarsaparilla has been used as a tonic (to improve body function) and in the treatment of coughs, digestive disorders, fever, gout, skin conditions, and arthritis. Externally it has been used for burns and wounds. No toxicity has been reported, though the effects of long-term, high-level consumption are unknown.

Sarsaparilla contains a family of saponins, steroid-like molecules that appear to bind cell wall materials released by bacteria in the intestine. Endotoxins can be absorbed by the gut and pass into the bloodstream unless removed by the liver. By rendering endotoxins unabsorbable, sarsaparilla may improve liver function and decrease the burden of foreign materials. The plant does not contain testosterone, the male hormone, and does not increase muscle mass. Thus, there is little evidence to support the contention that sarsaparilla acts as a sexual rejuvenator. Sarsaparilla extracts have been routinely used to flavor beverages, candy, baked goods, and other foods.

satiety The sense of being filled up and having APPETITE satisfied, as opposed to HUNGER. Appetite is a complex phenomenon involving many psychological and biochemical factors. No single event is likely to control it. Fat and oils in foods slow emptying of the stomach and contribute to the feeling of being full. Researchers are exploring the hypothesis that depleted fat cells may signal the brain to eat and cause hunger after weight loss. LEPTIN, a recently discovered protein produced by fat cells, has been shown to enter the brain and control the consumption of fatty foods. Dietary FIBER, undigestible plant material, swells when moistened, creating a feeling of fullness. As a further benefit, fiber displaces calorie-rich foods, so fewer calories are eaten.

Mechanical contact with food triggers the stomach and intestine to release gut peptides that trigger satiety. This feedback mechanism requires 10 to 20 minutes, while signals are being sent back to the brain. As an example, the hormone CHOLECYSTOKININ signals the brain to stop sending hunger signals after eating. Whether cholecystokinin can be manipulated by dietary changes is not known for certain. Brain peptides are also probably involved in regulatory food consumption and satiety. Enterostatin decreases fat intake in experimental animals. The development of drugs to increase satiety is currently an area of active research. Strategies to promote a feeling of satiation and to curb appetite include eating a snack a half-hour before a meal, eating slowly and chewing each bite thoroughly and waiting 20 minutes before taking a second helping. These approaches give the hormone time to reach the brain and create a feeling of fullness. (See also APPETITE SUPPRESSANTS; CRAVING.)

saturated fat FAT that contains a high percentage of saturated FATTY ACIDS and exists as a solid at room temperature. Saturation is a chemical concept, referring to the fact that carbon atoms in the fatty acid molecules are bonded to a maximum number of hydrogen atoms ("filled up"). Typical sources of saturated fat are animal fat, as found in BEEF, veal, LAMB, PORK, meat products, MILK, EGGS, BUTTER, and products like ICE CREAM, milk, and CHOCOLATE. Certain plant oils are also saturated, including COCONUT OIL, PALM, and palm kernel oils. Unsaturated fat (vegetable oils) can be converted to saturated fats by a chemical process called hydrogenation, and these appear on the market as vegetable shortening.

Saturated Fatty Acids

Common building blocks of fats and oils, these organic acids contain a maximum number of hydrogen atoms and lack double bonds. Fatty acids are built of carbon chains, which may be long or short. Long-chain, saturated fatty acids include PALMITIC ACID (16 carbon atoms) and STEARIC ACID (18 carbon atoms). They are waxy solids at room temperature and can form fats that are also solids at room temperature. Typical short-chain saturated fatty acids include: acetic acid (containing two carbon atoms), propionic acid (with three carbon atoms), and BUTYRIC ACID (four carbon atoms). Medium-chain fatty acids include CAPRYLIC ACID (with eight carbons); capric acid (10 carbons); lauric acid (12 carbons); and myristic acid (14 carbons). All saturated fatty acids are readily oxidized by mitochondrial enzyme systems to produce energy with carbon dioxide and water as waste products. Fatty acids yield more than twice the amount of energy as carbohydrate and protein when they are burned. (See also ESSENTIAL FATTY ACIDS.)

saturated vegetable oils See TROPICAL OILS.

sauce A flavorful relish or liquid dressing served with foods. Sauces are usually high-FAT foods. Stroganoff and orloff usually contain butter. Hollandaise and bearnaise sauces contain butter and egg yolks; bearnaise contains undercooked raw egg yolk and so is a potential source of food poisoning. MAYONNAISE contains egg yolks, VINEGAR, and a vegetable oil. Brown sauces (bordelaise and bourguignon) may be lower in fat if fat has been skimmed off and if butter has not been added. Tartar sauce and remoulade are flavored mayonnaise.

sauerkraut Fermented white CABBAGE. Cabbage is pickled in salt, spices, and cabbage juice by lactic acid-producing bacteria. The lactic acid gives sauerkraut its characteristic sour flavor. Canned sauerkraut also has a very high sodium level (up to 780 mg per half-cup). It can be strained and rinsed to decrease the sodium content. Dill seed and onion can be used to enhance the flavor of sauerkraut. (See also FERMENTATION; FOOD PRESERVATION.)

sausage A seasoned, ground meat product usually containing high levels of SODIUM and FAT and packed in a casing. The term *sausage* is derived from the Latin *salsicius,* meaning "seasoned with salt." Most sausage contains highly seasoned, finely ground beef and pork and table salt. Any meat from a USDA-inspected carcass can be used to make sausage and animal fat can be added. Thus, blood sausage is made from blood, pork fat, and seasoning. The final product may be cured (smoked) and dry or semidry. Dry and semidry sausage may contain NITRITES as preservatives, which have been linked to an increased risk of stomach cancer if consumed in large amounts. Fresh sausage is made from raw meat and must be cooked. Semidry sausage has been smoked; dry sausage may or may not be smoked; and cooked sausage is ready to eat. Examples include BOLOGNA, braunschweiger, frankfurter, head cheese, knackwurst, LIVERWURST, salami, souse, and Vienna sausage.

Sausages contain ample protein, iron, and many B vitamins; however, they also contain almost 55 percent of their calories as fat. A few brands contain less than 40 percent of their calories as fat. Tofu and turkey sausage may contain less fat than pork or beef products. It is recommended that sausage be eaten as a condiment or flavoring with foods rather than as a main dish.

Pork sausage, cooked, can provide 72 percent of calories as fat; fat accounts for 31 percent of the weight. One link, 13 g, provides 50 calories; protein, 2.5 g; carbohydrate, 0.1 g; fat, 4 g; cholesterol, 11 mg; sodium, 168 mg; thiamin, 0.1 mg; riboflavin, 0.03 mg; niacin, 0.59 mg. (See also CHICKEN; MEAT, PROCESSED; MEAT SUBSTITUTES; POULTRY.)

sauté Refers to pan frying small strips or slices of food quickly in a hot skillet with a small amount of butter or oil. Be sure oil is hot before adding foods to minimize the amounts of oil they soak up. Pork slices, veal scallops, chicken breast, fish fillet, tofu, onions, carrots, garlic, and other vegetables and grains can be sauteed.

saw palmetto (*Serenoa repens*) A small palm tree native to South Carolina, Georgia, and Florida that produces berries with medicinal properties. Saw palmetto berries have a long history of use by Native Americans, while later European physicians used the berries to treat enlarged prostate (benign prostatic hyperplasia), genitourinary tract imbalances, and as a tonic to boost nutrient and general body functioning. Modern formulations employ a fat-soluble extract of saw palmetto berries containing large-molecular-weight alcohols and plant sterols, compounds related to cholesterol. Saw palmetto berry extracts block the conversion of the male sex hormone, testosterone, to a more potent compound, dehydrotesterone, that promotes prostatic enlargement, and promote the breakdown of the more active compound. These effects may possibly explain the saw palmetto relief of common symptoms such as decreased urination at night, increased urinary flow rates, and decreased residual urine content in the bladder. No significant side effects of saw palmetto berry extracts or berries have been noted.

School Breakfast Program A federal program to provide funds for nutritious breakfasts for children. The National School Breakfast Program was established by the Child Nutrition Act of 1966 an authorized as a permanent appropriation in 1975. Fewer children participate in the BREAKFAST program than in the SCHOOL LUNCH PROGRAM. In the 1999–2000 school year 7.6 million children participated in the breakfast program, while 27.4 million children participated in the lunch program. Usually a state's Department of Education administers this program.

The school breakfast must contain one serving of meat or meat alternative (such as eggs or peanut butter), two or more servings of different fruits or vegetables, and one serving of milk.

Factors weighed in planning school food service programs include: cultural and ethnic backgrounds of students, needs of handicapped students, as well as fitting meals to accommodate class and bus schedules. Practical nutrition education can be part of breakfast programs. Evaluation of school nutrition programs finds that most students participating in school breakfast programs are from low-income families.

Breakfast is considered the most important meal for both children and adults because of its positive impact on performance and alertness. Nonetheless, many Americans skip breakfast, especially teenagers. Students who skip breakfast have higher rates of tardiness, higher absenteeism and lower performance, and more FATIGUE. Researchers shows that low-income children who participate in the School Breakfast Program have higher standardized achievement test scores than children not in the program. (See also HUNGER; WIC.)

School Lunch Program A federal program established under the National School Lunch Program of 1946 to protect the health of U.S. children through the consumption of nutritious foods. The act authorized state grant-in-aid program to provide cash and food. The cost is shared among the USDA, state and local governments, and children's families. Household income determines whether a child will receive a reduced rate or free meal. To qualify, household income must be below 185 percent of the federal poverty level; for free meals household income must fall below 130 percent of the poverty level.

The National School Lunch Program is open to public and private schools and to residential child care institutions. Schools that participate in the program receive financial assistance, donated surplus commodities and technical assistance in equipping and managing the program. In the 1970s, the Nutrition Education and Training Program was developed to educate students about the relationship between nutrition and health, to train food service personnel in management, and to instruct teachers in nutrition education. The program was expanded due to increased need for low-cost, subsidized meals, especially among economically disadvantaged children.

On a typical day in school year 2000–2001, 15.6 million children participated in the program. The program has continued to serve nutritious school lunches to children who would not likely receive lunch from another source. Furthermore, school lunches have provided approximately 33 percent of the RECOMMENDED DIETARY ALLOWANCES (RDAs) for children of various ages. Eligibility for participation in the program is contingent upon operating on a nonprofit basis, providing free or reduced price lunches to needy children, making lunches available to all children providing dining and kitchen facilities, avoiding segregation of needy children and serving meals that conform to USDA guidelines.

School lunches must meet the DIETARY GUIDELINES FOR AMERICANS, which recommend that no more than 30 percent of a person's calories come from fat and less than 10 percent from saturated fat. The lunches should also provide one-third of the U.S. RDA of protein, iron, calcium, and vitamins A and C. In 2001 the Physician's Committee for Responsible Medicine issued a report that found that many school lunches offered in the National School Lunch Program did not meet these requirements. Only one in 12 elementary school districts substituted lower-fat, cholesterol-free plant protein in place of meat, and one-fourth were not meeting USDA nutrition requirements.

scromboid fish poisoning A type of FOOD POISONING that occurs within an hour after eating species of spoiled fish that populate tropical oceans, including TUNA, MACKEREL, skipjack, BONITO, HERRING, mahi-mahi, SARDINES, and anchovies. An important clue to contamination is that infected fish taste metallic and peppery. Symptoms of poisoning include flushing, sweating, nausea, vomiting, diarrhea, headache, and dizziness. Antihistamines relieve the symptoms. Scromboid fish poisoning can be prevented by keeping fresh fish on ice or refrigerated until it is cooked. (See also FOOD TOXINS.)

scurvy A disease caused by severe deficiency of VITAMIN C (ascorbic acid). Scurvy has been described since ancient times. Long sea voyages of the 15th through the 17th centuries frequently decimated the ranks of sailors. As early as 1593, a British admiral demonstrated that lemon juice cured the disease. A Scottish naval surgeon conducted the first controlled experiment in the treatment of scurvy in 1753, which proved that citrus fruits protected seamen and cured scurvy. Not until 40 years later were limes routinely issued to British seamen to prevent scurvy. However, scurvy continued into more recent times. It was prevalent during the American Civil War, and in 1912 half the men on Scott's expedition to the South Pole died of scurvy.

During initial stages of vitamin C deficiency, an individual may feel listless. Wounds may heal slowly and gums may bleed easily. Bruising occurs easily. Minute hemorrhages appear around hair follicles or stomach, buttocks, legs, and arms. Later stages are characterized by weight loss, weakness, painful muscles, swollen joints, spongy gums, and loss of teeth. Vitamin C plays several important roles that can be related to scurvy. Chief among these is the requirement for vitamin C in COLLAGEN. The formation of mature collagen, the major structural protein of connective tissue, relies on the availability of key building blocks called hydroxyproline and hydroxylysine. The production of hydroxyproline from proline and of hydroxyl lysine from lysine requires vitamin C. As a versatile antioxidant and key support nutrient of the immune system, vitamin C exhibits wide-ranging benefits on health. Modest deficiencies do not manifest themselves as scurvy, rather they increase the susceptibility to infections and oxidative damage leading to chronic diseases.

Infants relying on cow's milk may be prone to scurvy because much of the vitamin C is destroyed during pasteurization. Infants require proportionately higher levels of vitamin C because of their high rate of tissue growth. Breast milk contains adequate vitamin C to support infant development.

Among adults, low-income elderly persons are susceptible to scurvy if they do not eat fresh fruit and vegetables. Overcooking destroys most vitamin C in vegetables. Chronic disease, injuries, and surgery are more likely in this group, and these conditions deplete the body stores of this vitamin. (See also MALNUTRITION.)

Rajakumar, Kumaravel. "Infantile Scurvy: A Historical Perspective," *Pediatrics* 108, no. 4 (2001): e76.

seafood Edible marine fish and shellfish such as CLAMS, mussels, scallops, OYSTERS, LOBSTERS, and SHRIMP that represent an important, highly nutritious food source. It is low in saturated fat and calories and is a good source of PROTEIN, IRON, VITAMIN B_{12}, IODINE, PHOSPHORUS, ZINC, and COPPER. Fish and fish oil are particularly rich in the omega-3 family of polyunsaturated FATTY ACIDS, which help reduce INFLAMMATION in conditions like ARTHRITIS and psoriasis, as well as reducing the risk of blood clot formation, thus offering protection against HEART ATTACKS. COD LIVER OIL contains high levels of VITAMIN A and VITAMIN D, which may be toxic when consumed in large amounts. Several servings per week of the following fatty fish are recommended: bluefish, butterfish, halibut, herring, mackerel, striped bass, orange roughy, smelt, salmon, sardines, trout, and pompano.

The larva of parasitic worms may contaminate raw fish, including Pacific salmon, Pacific red snapper (rockfish), and herring; thus raw fish dishes (sushi, sashimi, CEVICHE, lomi-lomi) carry a risk of parasitic disease, such as anisakiasis. Inadequately smoked or salted fish can carry parasites. The severe abdominal pain of such a disease is due to acute intestinal inflammation. The parasite is killed by cooking marine fish thoroughly. Pregnant and nursing women, very young children, and elderly people should avoid raw fish and shellfish to minimize this risk.

Chemical Contamination

Chemical contaminants are another prominent issue in seafood safety. Fish and shellfish are generally more susceptible to chemical contamination than meat and poultry because they filter huge amounts of water through their bodies and feed on other organisms in which contaminants may be concentrated. Clams and oysters can filter 15 to 20 gallons of water daily. While thorough cooking destroys parasites and microorganisms, this does not eliminate chemical pollutants like LEAD, chlordane, DIOXIN, DDT, MERCURY, PBBs, and PCBS. Such industrial chemicals were once widely used in PESTICIDES, electrical insulation, plastics, dyes, and other products. Over decades these environmental pollutants have crept into the FOOD CHAIN because they are not readily broken down and because they tend to accumulate in plants and animals.

Varying levels of pollutants have been reported in both domestic and imported fish. While levels of detected pollutants have generally fallen below FDA tolerance limits, those limits were set when fish consumption was lower and consequently people accumulated less of these pollutants. The level of pollutant can vary with the source, but in many markets it is often difficult for the consumer to determine the source of fish sold. Pollutant levels in salmon from Pacific waters may be lower than from other sources; however, the fish the consumer buys may come from Chile, Norway, Eastern Canada, Maine, as well as from Washington, Alaska, or British Columbia.

Chemical pollutants may increase the risk of certain cancers, birth defects, and neurological damage in unborn children. However, the potential health hazards of long-term, very low-level exposure remain unknown. Because residue buildup occurs over years, it may be hard to trace a disease cause to a specific pollutant exposure.

Shellfish can accumulate disease-causing bacteria and viruses when exposed to untreated sewage. Harvesting is limited to waters that are certified as being clean, although enforcing the policy is limited by resources. Eating raw shellfish carries the risk of gastrointestinal disease with symptoms such as diarrhea, cramps, nausea, and vomiting. Shellfish also transmit hepatitis A virus. Well-cooked shellfish are safer than raw or semi-cooked shellfish.

To ensure that seafood is as safe to eat as possible, consumers should

- Buy fresh seafood. Fish and shellfish spoil easily and should be handled with care. Fresh fish should have a mild "ocean" smell; they should not smell "fishy" or smell like ammonia.
- Fresh seafood should be bought from reputable merchants who can identify their source.
- Seafood should be refrigerated at home immediately after purchase to prevent bacterial growth, minimize spoilage, and reduce the risk of FOOD POISONING. Raw seafood that will not be eaten within two days should be frozen. Most shrimp have been frozen and thawed, and should be cooked as soon as possible.
- Frozen seafood should be thawed in the refrigerator or in cold running water and not refrozen. Other raw shellfish, including lobster, should be alive when purchased.
- Cooked shellfish should be refrigerated and used on the same day.
- Mussels, clams, and oysters should be moistened and refrigerated to keep them alive rather than stored in plastic bags. They should not be stored for a long time in fresh water.
- Any shellfish that remains closed after steaming should be discarded. Raw shellfish that remain closed are dead and may have begun to decompose.
- Consumers should follow the same rules in handling raw seafood as when handling raw poultry and raw meat to avoid contaminating cooked dishes or fresh vegetables with bacteria: Wash with soap and water all utensils, countertops, cutting boards and hands that have come into contact with raw seafood.
- Consumers should eat a variety of seafoods rather than a single source to minimize overexposure to pollutants. Elderly people, young children, pregnant women, patients with compromised immune systems or with liver disease should avoid eating raw seafood.

Connor, W. E. "Importance of n-3 Fatty Acids in Health and Disease," *American Journal of Clinical Nutrition* 71 (2000): 171S–175S.

seafood inspection Fish and shellfish are among the most perishable foods, yet seafood is one of the least regulated foods; it remains the only flesh that does not undergo mandatory inspection. In contrast, meat and poultry processing facilities are inspected daily. A single-time FDA inspection of most U.S. seafood processing plants revealed a relatively low violation rate of up to 5.1 percent of plants, depending on the region.

An estimated 20 percent of food-borne illness is caused by seafood. Seafood can be contaminated by bacteria, viruses, parasites, and industrial wastes and pollutants. While the National Academy of Sciences has concluded that most seafood is safe to eat, this advisory organization has also recommended increased inspection and regulation of the industry. Fish testing in specific areas is left to state agencies, and testing for chemical contaminants remains scattered. Only very small numbers or samples of fish are monitored for chemical contaminants. The FDA established a new Office of Seafood in 1991 to address this issue. In 1994, the FDA launched a seafood safety initiative designed to keep contaminated seafood off the market shelves. Seafood processors need to maintain detailed records of safety procedures; to identify where shellfish were harvested; to catch fish only from waters the government has certified as being clean; and to store their catch at proper temperatures. Ready to eat seafood will have to be cooked and stored at safe temperatures as well.

sea salt A less pure form of table salt (SODIUM chloride). Sea salt contains low levels of certain minerals found in sea water. Using 3.5 g of sea salt would supply 22 percent of the REFERENCE DAILY INTAKE (RDI) of MAGNESIUM; 2.2. percent of the RDI of IODINE; 2.7 percent of the RDI of CALCIUM. Magnesium carbonate is the additive used to prevent caking. This is more healthful than aluminum silicate used for the same purpose in refined salt. Sea salt is not iodized and lacks iodine. As a source of sodium, sea salt carries with it the same risks for high blood pressure (HYPERTENSION) as ordinary table salt in susceptible people. (See also TRACE MINERALS.)

seaweed A large family of marine ALGAE. Edible seaweed is one of the richest sources of vitamins and minerals. Sea vegetables provide IODINE, SELENIUM, IRON, CALCIUM, PHOSPHORUS, and MAGNESIUM, as well as BETA-CAROTENE, VITAMIN E, and the B COMPLEX. Sea vegetables are not an adequate source of vitamin B_{12} because they possess substances that are inactive analogs or forms of the compound that the body cannot use. Vegetarians who do not eat milk, eggs, fish, or meat should consider taking a vitamin B_{12} supplement rather than relying on seaweed.

Traditionally, Asian diets include a variety of seaweed. The edible algae can be categorized as brown algae and red algae. Brown algae are represented by arame, hijiki, kelp, kombu, and wakame. Arame is a Japanese product; it is softened by prolonged cooking, sun-dried, and finally sliced into strands and packaged. Arame contains B complex vitamins and minerals. The calcium content is 1,170 mg per 100 g. Hijiki is found in the Far East; 100 g (dry weight) contains calcium, 1,400 mg; iron, 29 mg; plus BETA-CAROTENE and B complex vitamins. This seaweed is dried, steamed to stiffen it, again dried, then soaked in arame juice and dried for market. Kelp refers to a large family, and members are used commercially as a source of food additives, EMULSIFIERS, thickeners, and STABILIZERS. Kelp is dried and sold whole, or powdered when it is used as a flavoring. Kelp can be steamed, pickled, or boiled. It contains significant calcium and other minerals; 100 g contains calcium, 1,093 mg; sodium, 3,007 mg; and potassium, 5,273 mg.

Kombu is a general name for several species of brown algae. Dashi consists of broad strips and is used in soups, while tororo is shaved into slivers that can be marinated. Kombu is often used with root vegetables, rice, and vegetables. It provides significant beta-carotene, 430 retinol equivalents per 100 mg, as well as the B complex and vitamin C. Wakame comes from Japan. It is dried and processed for preservation. It can be added to soups, like miso soup, cooked as a vegetable, used as a garnish, or soaked and then added to salads. Wakame contains calcium, iron, and vitamins; 100 g provides calcium, 1,300 mg; iron, 13 mg; niacin, 10 mg; and vitamin C, 15 mg. Brown sea vegetables like kombu contain alginic acid and other ingredients that bind toxic heavy metals like strontium, cadmium, and radium. Alginic acid is used to treat cadmium poisoning and help remove it from the body.

Red algae include carragheen and nori. Carragheen yields a gum called CARRAGEENAN that is used in prepared foods, primarily for its ability to form gels in puddings, jellies, and the like. Carrageenan inhibits herpes simplex virus (oral and genital forms) as well as tumor-inducing RNA viruses in test tube experiments. It also provides (per 100 g): calcium, 885 mg; sodium, 2,892 mg; and potassium, 2,844 mg. Nori is a cultivated red sea vegetable. Fresh nori is washed, chopped into fragments, dried, and packaged. Sheets of nori are wrapped around rice used in sushi and California rolls. Nori provides (per 100 g): calcium, 260 mg; iron, 12 mg; high levels of beta-carotene, 11,000 retinol equivalents; thiamin, 25 mg; niacin, 10 mg; and vitamin C, 20 mg.

Seaweed has an ancient history of use in Eastern medicine, including Chinese and Indian medicine (Ayurvedic medicine). It has been used to treat intestinal parasites. GOITER, enlarged thyroid due to iodine deficiency, is effectively treated by seaweed because of its high iodine content. Certain species of seaweed have been used in folk medicine to treat high blood pressure, constipation, wounds and ulcers, GOUT, liver and kidney ailments, menstrual irregularities, and to improve digestion. Alginic acid is used in some antacids to treat ACID INDIGESTION and to treat wounds. Fucoidin is another type of complex carbohydrate (polysaccharide) from seaweed. In animals, this material inhibits chemically-induced cancers. (See also FOOD ADDITIVES; MACROBIOTIC DIET.)

Wein, Bibi. "The World's Healthiest Diet," *Lifestyles* 17, no. 3 (March 1995): 172–175.

secretin A HORMONE released by the small intestine that blocks the release of gastric juice and STOMACH ACID. Secretin slows the movement (PERISTALSIS) of material down the gastrointestinal tract. It stimulates the secretion of BICARBONATE by pancreatic duct cells to neutralize the acidic, partially digested food discharged by the STOMACH into the small intestine. To further prepare the intestine for DIGESTION, secretin stimulates bile production to aid fat digestion and the secretion of intestinal juice and digestive enzymes. Secretin release is triggered by food entering the small intestine, including partially digested carbohydrate and fat, as well as by fluids that contain high or very low concentrations of ions. (See also ENDOCRINE SYSTEM.)

selenium A TRACE MINERAL nutrient with anticancer and antiaging properties. Selenium helps protect cells against oxidative stress. As a part of the enzyme GLUTATHIONE PEROXIDASE, selenium serves as an ANTIOXIDANT by destroying highly reactive chemicals that can form FREE RADICALS. Glutathione peroxidase destroys HYDROGEN PEROXIDE, a naturally occurring chemical that is a powerful oxidizing agent. Hydrogen peroxide is produced for antimicrobial defense by macrophages, a type of white blood cell that engulfs foreign invaders, and it is a by-product of another antioxidant system (SUPEROXIDE DISMUTASE) that destroys a highly reactive form of oxygen called superoxide. Glutathione peroxidase neutralizes oxidative damage to lipids in cell membranes, thus limiting their damage due to free radical attack. Selenium may possess other antioxidant properties as well.

Selenium is generally recognized as an anticancer agent. In selenium-deficient experimental animals, LIVER cells become defective and more prone to become cancerous when activated. Studies show that populations with a low selenium intake are more prone to gastrointestinal, breast and rectal cancer. Deficiency of selenium leads to lowered glutathione peroxidase activity. Furthermore, extensive Chinese studies have suggested that selenium supplementation provides protection against hepatitis B and liver cancer. Selenium may inhibit the development of cancer by blocking the activation of certain cancer-promoting genes, by inhibiting viruses linked to cancer or by supporting healthy cell division and protecting cells against oxidative damage that could damage their DNA.

Selenium supports a healthy IMMUNE SYSTEM, where it stimulates antibody production and defensive cells (lymphocytes, macrophages and natural killer cells). Some AIDS patients may be selenium deficient. Selenium can block mercury, arsenic, and cadmium poisoning. Damaged heart muscle (cardiomyopathy) has occurred in patients fed intravenously mixtures that lacked selenium, and populations in areas of China characterized by regional selenium deficiency are more disease prone. OSTEOARTHRITIS in Chinese children has also been linked to selenium deficiency.

RECOMMENDED DIETARY ALLOWANCES (RDA) published in 1989 proposed a selenium RDA for the first time as 70 mcg/day for men and 55 mcg for nonpregnant, nonlactating women. Obtaining adequate selenium is a growing problem in the United States. Regions like the Pacific Northwest, the Great Lakes region, and some southern states (Georgia and the Carolinas) possess low soil concentrations of selenium, and vegetables and grains growing in depleted soils contain only low levels of selenium. Possibly, acid rain prevents plants from taking up this mineral from soil. The average U.S. intake is about 100 mg/day.

Good dietary sources of selenium include organ meats, such as liver and kidney; BREWER'S YEAST;

ocean FISH and SHELLFISH; and red MEAT. Vegetable sources (if grown in soil with enough selenium) are ONIONS, GARLIC, MUSHROOMS, and BROCCOLI. Asparagus, cabbage, and whole grains contain small amounts of selenium. FRUITS and most VEGETABLES and drinking water generally provide little selenium. Supplements containing inorganic selenium (sodium selenite or sodium selenate) should probably be taken separately from large amounts of vitamin C to avoid interference.

Chemically combined selenium represents the most prevalent form of the selenium in the typical diet. Selenium can replace sulfur in the amino acids CYSTEINE and METHIONINE to form the analogs, selenocysteine and selenomethionine. Selenocysteine occurs in a variety of proteins including glutathione peroxidase and is found in meat. Selenomethionine cannot be synthesized by the body and is supplied in the diet by a variety of foods. It can substitute for methionine in a variety of the body's proteins. The breakdown of methionine and selenomethionine releases cysteine and selenocysteine, respectively.

Safety

Toxicity can occur with daily consumption of 5 mg. Toxic levels of selenium occur in agricultural drainwater in some states. Certain regions are characterized by high levels of selenium (North and South Dakota and the San Joaquin Valley of California). Soils with high selenium cause unusually high levels in plants such as wheat. Symptoms of selenium toxicity include skin sores, garlic breath, fingernails with ridges and bumps, hair loss, and lethargy. Severe toxicity is indicated by fragile, black nails, metallic taste, dizziness, peripheral nerve damage, nausea, weight loss, and jaundice. Children, elderly persons and people with chronic illnesses may tolerate less selenium in their diets, while physically active people may tolerate more. Sodium selenite, the inorganic form of selenium, can cause cancer at very high doses. Organic selenium that occurs in foods is not carcinogenic.

Cammack, P. M. "Selenium Deficiency Alters Thyroid Hormone Metabolism in Guinea Pigs," *Journal of Nutrition* 125 (1995): 302–308.

self-rising flour See BAKING SODA.

semolina Milled durum WHEAT used to produce PASTA like macaroni and spaghetti. The high protein (gluten) content of durum wheat lends itself to elastic, resilient dough that is suitable for the mechanical processing involved in making pasta.

senility An old-fashioned term for memory loss associated with AGING. This phenomenon usually begins with loss of short-term memory and the ability to process new information quickly. Recollection of past events also slows down. ALZHEIMER'S DISEASE is the most common of the more than 70 types of dementia. It currently affects 4 million Americans but experts believe that will rise to 22 million by 2025.

Many of the people who appear to be suffering from dementia and forgetfulness may instead have nutritional deficiencies, including VITAMIN B_{12} deficiency due to inadequate absorption. The uptake of this vitamin declines with age, especially in those with stomach troubles. Injections of vitamin B_{12}, or taking large doses in tablet form, is a preventive measure.

Forgetfulness, learning difficulties, and problems remembering new things can frequently be caused by overmedication. Many elderly U.S citizens (65 or older) take prescription drugs they should not be using, some of which may cause confusion or amnesia. Similar problems may be due to adverse reactions to medication. As an example, DIURETICS (water pills) can cause excessive sodium loss, especially for those on a salt-restricted diet. This condition, called hyponatremia, is easily detected if the change is dramatic. However, if the change is slow, it is more difficult to detect and the symptoms match senile dementia. This condition is reversible if caught soon enough. Memory loss is also worsened by drugs blocking the formation of neurotransmitters. Drugs that fall into this category include sleeping pills and medications for reducing tremors, decreasing stomach acid and calming nerves. Other possible causes of forgetfulness include high fever, minor head injuries, DEPRESSION, loneliness, and boredom. To combat senility, exercise the brain by keeping mentally active and avoiding drugs that characteristically cause a dry mouth because this class of drugs may interfere with neurotransmitters.

Prescription drugs Hydergine, the hormone vasopressin (antidiuretic hormone), and unipocetine have been used to enhance memory. Lipids like phosphatidylserine and phosphatidylethanolamine play structural roles in cell membranes, and treatment with these substances suggests some improvement in certain patients with Alzheimer's disease. CHOLINE and LECITHIN (the phospholipid derivative of choline) may improve short-term memory in susceptible patients. However, they do not appear to alter the course of Alzheimer's disease. Treatment with phosphatidylcholine and prescription drugs like physostigmine and Hydergine have yielded mixed results. Three decades of research suggest that phosphatidyl serine benefits cognitive function, including memory and learning in elderly people. Other studies indicate that a derivative of the amino acid CARNITINE, L-acetylcarnitine, shows promise in moderating age-related depression, as well as the effects of stroke and nerve degeneration related to DIABETES MELLITUS. (See also FOOD; GINKGO; PREBIOTICS.)

Le Bars, P. L. "A Placebo-Controlled Double-Blind, Randomized Trial with a Special Extract of Ginkgo Biloba in Dementia," *JAMA* 278 (1997): 1,327–1,332.

sensitivity See FOOD SENSITIVITY.

sequestrants (chelating agents) Agents used to reduce color changes and SPOILAGE in canned foods, PROCESSED FOODS, and bottled salad dressings. Sequestrants bind metal ions like iron, which catalyze the reaction of oxygen with sensitive materials in food. Examples of sequestering agents are CITRIC ACID, malic acid, tartaric acid, and EDTA. Citric acid is used in ice cream, sherbet, fruit drinks, soft drinks, jellies, canned fruits and vegetables, and cheese. It is considered a safe additive. EDTA is widely used in salad dressings, MARGARINE, MAYONNAISE and sandwich spreads, prepared fresh fruit, potatoes, canned shellfish, beer, and soft drinks. EDTA too is considered safe. (See also FOOD ADDITIVES; MINERALS.)

serine (Ser, L-serine) A nonessential AMINO ACID required to synthesize proteins. Serine plays a role in many synthetic reactions that require FOLIC ACID, VITAMIN B_6, and NIACIN. It can be converted to the simplest amino acid, GLYCINE, and vice versa. Serine can assist in the synthesis of PURINES and PYRIMIDINES, the building blocks of DNA and RNA. Serine can be converted to ethanolamine and CHOLINE, two nitrogen-containing compounds required for phospholipid synthesis and cell membrane formation, and to certain NEUROTRANSMITTERS, brain chemicals required to transmit signals in nerves. Serine is classified as a "glycogenic" amino acid because during STARVATION it can be converted to BLOOD SUGAR to fuel the brain. (See also AMINO ACID METABOLISM.)

serotonin A chemical found in the brain and defensive cells of connective tissue. Mast cells, a type of defensive cell lodged in connective tissue, produce serotonin from the essential amino acid TRYPTOPHAN to slow blood flow in damaged areas because it acts as a powerful vasoconstrictor. In the brain, serotonin functions as a neurotransmitter, a chemical required for the transmission of nerve impulses. Serotonin is involved in inducing sleep, sensory perception, and temperature. It diminishes pain, reduces APPETITE, and has a calming effect. Certain antidepressants such as Prozac boost serotonin levels. Diet can possibly affect mood by altering brain serotonin levels. Eating carbohydrates may reduce the level of most amino acids in the blood except tryptophan, so that this amino acid can more easily penetrate the BLOOD-BRAIN BARRIER without competing with other amino acids. According to this hypothesis, as the level of tryptophan rises in the brain, more serotonin is synthesized, leading to relaxation and decreased alertness. (See also NERVOUS SYSTEM.)

serum The clear, straw-colored fluid remaining after blood has clotted. Serum contains CHOLESTEROL (serum cholesterol) in the form of LOW-DENSITY LIPOPROTEIN (LDL, the less desirable form) and HIGH-DENSITY LIPOPROTEIN (HDL, the more desirable form); fat (TRIGLYCERIDES); proteins produced by the liver such as serum ALBUMIN; ELECTROLYTES (ionic minerals like SODIUM, POTASSIUM and CHLORIDE); waste materials like UREA and URIC ACID; and nutrients such as AMINO ACIDS and BLOOD SUGAR (GLUCOSE). Serum is often used in the clinical laboratory to measure these parameters for diagnosis, rather than whole blood, which contains cells that can alter these parameters. For example, red blood cells possess their own complement of enzymes, lipids, and minerals.

serum lipids See CHOLESTEROL.

sesame (*Sesamum indicum*) An annual tropical plant grown since ancient times for its edible seed oil. Sesame was cultivated in Palestine and Syria as early as 3000 B.C. It is now cultivated in China, India, Burma, and Mexico; the United States is a major importer. Sesame seeds contain 50 percent oil by weight; the oil can be extracted from crushed, whole seeds. The seed is dehulled for human consumption because its hull contains 2 percent to 3 percent OXALIC ACID, which binds minerals and gives it a bitter flavor. The U.S. imports 70 million pounds of sesame seeds annually; most of this is used for hamburger buns. Ground sesame seeds are used in hummus and tahini (a sesame seed paste). Halvah is a confection made with ground sesame seeds. Sesame seeds are used with stir-fried vegetables and fried poultry in Asian cuisine.

Sesame oil is more saturated than VEGETABLE OILS like safflower, corn, or soybean oil, which all contain more than 50 percent polyunsaturated fatty acids. Sesame oil contains 43.8 percent polyunsaturated fatty acid (LINOLEIC ACID); 14.6 percent saturated fatty acids (mainly PALMITIC ACID and STEARIC ACID); and 41.5 percent monounsaturated fatty acids (OLEIC ACID). The oil has a strong nutty flavor and is often used in stir-fry meals. The nutrient content of sesame seeds (15 g) is: 84 calories, protein, 3.6 g; carbohydrate, 0.6 g; fat, 7.1 g; calcium, 18 mg; iron, 1.1 mg; thiamin, 0.29 mg; riboflavin, 0.03 mg; niacin, 0.8 mg. (See also HYDROGENATED VEGETABLE OIL.)

set point See DIETING; WEIGHT MANAGEMENT.

shellfish Mollusks and crustaceans that have been long used as food sources. Univalve mollusks such as abalone are enclosed in a single shell; bivalve mollusks with a two-part shell include CLAMS mussels, OYSTERS, and scallops. Cephalopods (creatures with tentacles, like squid) are a type of mollusk. Crustaceans, which possess a tough outer layer and segmented bodies and legs, include CRAB, LOBSTERS, crayfish, prawns, and SHRIMP. Shellfish provide rich sources of protein low in saturated fat and total fat, and TRACE MINERALS such as IODINE, ZINC, and COPPER. Generally, shellfish contain the usual amounts of cholesterol as found in meat. Shrimp contain somewhat higher levels, though less than found in eggs. Like ocean fish, shellfish contain omega-3 oils that offer protection against heart disease.

Raw shellfish are a major source of severe, food-borne disease. Disease organisms carried by shellfish include salmonella and hepatitis A virus. Bacteria can cause gastroenteritis (inflamed stomach and intestines) with diarrhea, nausea, vomiting, and cramps. Shellfish are bottom feeders and filter vast amounts of water, therefore they tend to accumulate waste products and disease-producing bacteria and viruses when grown in waters contaminated by sewage. Clams and oysters can filter 15 to 20 gallons of sea water daily.

FDA and state inspections are designed to make certain that shellfish are harvested from clean waters. However, regulation of the shellfish industry is spotty because few agents are available to monitor 10 million acres of approved shellfish beds in U.S. coastal waters. To meet the increased consumer demand, the fishing industry is taking fish and shellfish closer to shore, where pollution is higher and the risk of polluted SEAFOOD is higher. Raw or undercooked shellfish are the major seafood hazards. The bacterium *Vibrio vulnificus* produces a toxin causing a shellfish poisoning associated with contaminated seafood, especially oysters from the Gulf Coast. Immune compromised people and those with liver disease (cirrhosis) are most vulnerable. The toxin can cause skin ulcers and occurs as normal marine flora in warmer temperate waters. Its production is not associated with pollution.

RED TIDE is an explosive growth of a microscopic marine algae. Poisonous dinoflagellates produce neurotoxins that are not destroyed by cooking. Paralytic shellfish poisoning is caused by *Gonyaulax catenella* and *G. acetenella* along Pacific coasts and *G. tamarensis* in the Bay of Fundy and in the St.

Lawrence estuary on the North Atlantic. Symptoms begin with numbness in lips and tongue, spreading to arms and legs and respiratory distress. Red tide can cause blood poisoning and death in high-risk individuals—patients with liver disease, AIDS, or alcoholics. Mussels gradually destroy or eliminate bound poisons after an algal bloom. In general, raw oysters should be avoided during the warmer months, April to October.

Razor clams from U.S. Pacific Northwest beaches can be contaminated with domoic acid, a naturally occurring neurotoxin that causes nausea, fever, abdominal cramps, short-term memory loss, coma, and death in severe cases. This toxin is produced by marine plankton. Internal organs of Dungeness crab harvested off the coasts of California, Oregon, and Washington may be contaminated, although the crab meat itself is safe. (See also SEAFOOD INSPECTION.)

sherbet A frozen DESSERT prepared from fruit juice or fruit puree, sugar, milk, egg white, or gelatin or dipped marshmallows. In contrast, sorbets are fruit-based frozen desserts that do not contain dairy products. (See also ICE CREAM.)

shigellosis A severe type of FOOD POISONING caused by shigella, an intestinal bacterium. Symptoms include very severe DIARRHEA, lasting several days, with possible bloody stools and accompanied by fever and possibly DEHYDRATION. Most people recover fairly rapidly, even without treatment with antibiotics. However, shigellosis can be life-threatening to children and to the elderly. Shigella is carried by fecal matter, and the disease can be transmitted by food handlers with poor hygiene. State law requires that cases of shigellosis be reported to health departments. (See also SALMONELLA.)

shiitake mushroom (*Lentinus edodes;* forest mushroom) An edible MUSHROOM especially popular in Asia. Shiitake mushrooms are cultivated commercially and are available in United States markets. Shiitake contains a broad spectrum of amino acids, potassium, and ergosterol, a substance that can be converted to vitamin D in the presence of sunlight. In addition, shiitake mushrooms have been used in Asian medicine for thousands of years. Shiitake contains carbohydrate materials and polysaccharides, including lentinan, which stimulates the immune system and which has antitumor activity. Lentinan may boost white blood cells called T helper cells that gear up the immune system. Shiitake extracts also boost antiviral defenses by increasing interferon production. Extracts can lower blood cholesterol levels.

shock See ANAPHYLAXIS.

short-chain fatty acids Very small fatty acids that have an odor (volatile fatty acids). Short-chain fatty acids are produced by the anaerobic fermentation of carbohydrate by colonic bacteria. With normal digestion, typically the main source of fermentable carbohydrate is dietary FIBER, plant cell wall materials, and undigested starch. Short-chain fatty acids include ACETIC ACID (acetate, a two-carbon acid); PROPIONIC ACID (propionate, a three-carbon acid); and BUTYRIC ACID (butyrate, a four-carbon acid).

Short-chain fatty acids are readily absorbed by the colon and can be considered a major factor in human energy metabolism. It is estimated that short-chain fatty acids produced by colonic bacteria can satisfy 5 percent to 10 percent of the body's energy needs. Acetic acid and propionic acid are used by the liver, while butyric acid is a preferred fuel by cells lining the gut. Indeed, butyrate is a primary energy source for these cells. In addition, butyrate helps guide the development and maintenance of colonic cells and may decrease susceptibility to colon CANCER and colitis.

More than usual amounts of fermentable carbohydrate enter the colon with high-fiber diets and during carbohydrate MALABSORPTION and maldigestion, leading to increased production of short-chain fatty acids. The production of short-chain fatty acids lowers intestinal ammonia levels liberated through bacterial metabolism and limits the uptake of this waste product. Ammonia can induce abnormalities in intestinal cells. Short-chain fatty acids also inhibit the growth of certain pathogenic species like salmonella, and the resulting lowered colonic pH (increased acidity) favors VITAMIN K absorption, MUCUS secretion, and magnesium uptake. (See also FAT METABOLISM; INTESTINAL FLORA.)

shortening A FAT added to a food item to keep it soft during baking. By dispersing fat droplets throughout a dough, starch and grain protein do not congeal into a compact mass when cooked. BUTTER (milk fat), LARD (pork fat), and TALLOW (beef fat) are traditional shortening agents. Vegetable shortenings contain hydrogenated vegetable oils. These are solids, unlike the original oils. They are prepared from hydrogenated oils with varying melting points, and with varying degrees of softness. Vegetable shortening is often prepared from CORN OIL, COTTONSEED OIL, OLIVE OIL, PEANUT oil, PALM OIL, SAFFLOWER oil, SESAME oil, or SOYBEAN oil. Regardless of form, all fats and oils provide nine calories per gram, more than twice as much as derived from carbohydrate and protein (four calories per gram).

Shortening is used for biscuits, bread, cookies, and pie crusts. The amount of shortening varies with the recipe. Bread and rolls contain 1 percent to 2 percent shortening; cakes, 10 percent to 20 percent, and pastries, 30 percent. When shortenings are used for baking mixes, whipped topping, icing, and filling, various emulsifying agents are included. These include MONOGLYCERIDES (glycerol with only one fatty acid). Emulsifiers allow water to be mixed with the shortening without separation. (See also DIETARY GUIDELINES FOR AMERICANS; FAT METABOLISM; VEGETABLE OIL.)

shrimp A type of SHELLFISH with 10 legs that range in size from 0.5 in. to several inches. When cooked, shrimp turn red due to a chemical change in the shell pigment. Typically, the parts of cooked shrimp sold at markets are the abdominal region and tail parts, after the heads have been removed. Shrimp is a high-protein food that is also a good source of CALCIUM. Shrimp contains somewhat higher than usual levels of cholesterol, though less than found in eggs. Shrimp can be canned, converted to shrimp paste, breaded and fried, or stir-fried. The nutrient content of 3.5 oz. (100 g) is: 109 calories; protein, 23.8 g; fat, 1.5 g; cholesterol, 152 mg; calcium, 320 mg; iron, 2.2 mg; thiamin, 0.03 mg; riboflavin, 0.03 mg; niacin, 3.7 mg.

silicon The second most common element on the surface of the Earth and widely found in plants and water. Silicon is also found in the skin, BONE, and connective tissue of animals. It is an essential nutrient in animals, required for normal skeletal development of rats and chicks, for example. It seems probable that silicon is essential for humans, although this remains to be established. No RECOMMENDED DIETARY ALLOWANCE has been established for silicon. Silicon participates in the formation of connective tissue where it forms complexes between protein and acidic polysaccharide complexes. Acidic polysaccharides (GLYCOSAMINOGLYCANS) contribute to the gelatinous material that holds cells together. In humans, the silicon content of the aorta, the skin, and the thymus decreases with age.

Silicon is widely distributed in whole grains, organ meats like liver, and red meat. Most of the silicon of whole grains is lost when white flour is prepared, and highly processed foods contain little silicon. The typical diet supplies approximately 1 g per day. Within the confines of the typical diet, silicon is nontoxic. (See also SKELETON; TRACE MINERAL.)

simple carbohydrate See CARBOHYDRATE.

single-cell protein Food PROTEIN derived from cultured bacteria, YEAST, fungi, and algae. Algae (seaweed) has long been used as food. Brewer's yeast, a by-product of the brewing industry, and TORULA YEAST are widely available food supplements. The potential of cultured microorganisms serving as an edible protein source is huge. A single-cell fermenter covering 0.8 sq km (one-third of a square mile) could theoretically supply 10 percent of the protein requirement of the world's population. By-products of the food, paper, and chemical industry can be fermented by many microorganisms as inexpensive energy sources. These include methane, ALCOHOL, STARCH, MOLASSES, cellulose, and animal waste products. Even fewer requirements are needed for algae; photosynthetic organisms can be grown in illuminated ponds supplied with mineral nutrients.

Problems associated with single-cell protein have limited its development as a major food source. Most single-cell protein is not palatable unless processed to eliminate bitter or unpleasant tasting materials. Digestibility of single-cell protein varies with the sources. Cooking algae increases its digestibility, but the digestibility of yeast is little altered by processing. The high nucleic acid content of single-cell organisms leads to increased purine uptake. When purines are metabolized, uric acid output rises and increases the risk of GOUT in susceptible people. Furthermore, toxic materials and pollutants can contaminate single-cell protein. Another consideration is the fact that single-cell protein is generally deficient in the dietary essential AMINO ACIDS, LYSINE, and METHIONINE. Though the amino acid profile is more balanced than in cereal grain protein it remains inferior to animal protein. Genetically engineered microorganisms may overcome this deficiency. (See also FOOD CHAIN; HUNGER; MEAT; PHOTOSYNTHESIS.)

skeleton The collection of bones that provides the framework and protective covering for many organs of the body including the brain, heart, and spinal cord. Unlike the NERVOUS SYSTEM, the IMMUNE SYSTEM or the ENDOCRINE SYSTEM, the skeletal system plays a passive role in maintaining normal body function (HOMEOSTASIS). The skeletal system protects internal organs; vertebrae protect the spinal column; the cranium, the brain; the rib cage, the heart, and the lungs; the pelvic bones, the reproductive organs. Bones store calcium and phosphorus, which can be released and distributed to other parts of the body via the bloodstream. Red bone marrow in certain bones yields blood cells; RED BLOOD CELLS, some white cells and blood PLATELETS required for blood clotting. Fat in bone marrow represents stored ENERGY. The human skeleton contains 206 bones and is held together by tough connective tissue and cartilage. Skeletal muscles adhere to bones via tendons to promote movement.

Bones range in size from the robust femur to the delicate, intricate bones of the wrist and ankle. Physical growth during maturation from infancy to adulthood entails a dramatic increase in bone mass and size. Nearly 67 percent of bone represents a mineral matrix, the compound calcium phosphate, composed of the nutrients CALCIUM and PHOSPHORUS. Many other nutrients are required in the growth and maintenance of the skeletal system. MAGNESIUM and FLUORIDE are also complexed with calcium phosphate to help harden the bone matrix. BORON may reduce calcium and magnesium losses from bone in post-menopausal women. The skeleton requires a healthy connective tissue. MANGANESE is required for the formation of mucopolysaccharides, while COPPER and VITAMIN C are required for the formation of COLLAGEN and ELASTIN, proteins of connective tissue and tendon, respectively. Bone-forming cells are maintained by VITAMIN A among other nutrients. VITAMIN D, together with ample calcium, phosphorus, and magnesium, promotes normal skeletal development and prevents RICKETS in children. In adults, vitamin D prevents bone thinning and softening. (See also OSTEOMALACIA; OSTEOPOROSIS.)

skim milk See MILK.

skin The outer surface of the body and its largest organ. The skin of an adult covers a surface area of 2 square meters and forms the primary physical barrier to the external environment, bacteria, and other microorganisms. The skin also helps regulate body temperature through heat lost by the evaporation of sweat and by changes in blood flow to the skin. A limited amount of body wastes and chemical toxic load can also be eliminated through sweat. The skin supports the sense of touch via sensory nerve endings embedded there. These nerves react to temperature, pressure, pain, and touch. The skin is responsible for synthesizing vitamin D_3 from a stored precursor when exposed to ultraviolet light. Finally, certain types of cells embedded in underlying layers are important components of immunity, the ability to ward off disease.

Nutrient Support

The chief constituent of the skin is COLLAGEN, a structural protein requiring vitamin C. Collagen and ELASTIN are fibers of connective tissue that keep the skin smooth and toned. VITAMIN C and COPPER are trace nutrients that support the synthesis of elastin proteins. Vitamin C and VITAMIN E together with SELENIUM are required for a healthy skin. They are powerful scavengers of FREE RADICALS, the highly reactive chemicals formed by sunlight and oxygen, smog, pollutants, and other factors. Essential fatty acids, LINOLEIC ACID and ALPHA LINOLENIC ACID, which occur in seed oils, are important in maintaining a lustrous skin. Sebaceous glands secrete an oily material called sebum, which is a mixture of oils, cholesterol, protein, and inorganic salts. This oily film protects hair and skin from drying out; prevents excessive evaporation from the skin; keeps the skin soft and pliable; and blocks the growth of certain bacteria. It forms a water-impermeable barrier and prevents the skin from becoming saturated with water.

AGING brings marked changes in the skin. The skin appears rougher, drier, and thinner, and the cushioning layer of fat beneath the skin diminishes. There are fewer melanocytes, cells that produce pigment to protect against sunlight's ultraviolet damage, and there is less collagen and elastin and that which remains may be damaged.

All structures in the skin can be affected by chronic exposure to U.V. light. U.V. light reacts with cells by initiating free radical reactions. Free radicals attack cells and damage their DNA, which accounts for most skin damage. Sunburn is an injury to the skin due to ultraviolet rays that may lead to cell death and mutations. The skin becomes leathery, with wrinkles, lines, sagging skin areas, wart-like or scaly precancerous growths, yellow discoloration, and abnormal elastic tissue.

The first line of IMMUNE SYSTEM defense in the skin are Langerhans cells. These sentries can detect the intrusion of foreign materials and quickly signal other components of the immune system to counterattack. U.V. light whether from tanning parlors or from sunlight suppresses these cells.

Photosensitivity can aggravate the reaction to the sun's rays. Certain foods (citrus fruits, for example), deodorant soaps, Retin-A, antibiotics, tranquilizers, and DIURETICS (water pills) contain materials that can accentuate a reaction to sunlight such as burning and development of age spots. By minimizing ultraviolet exposure, new connective tissue can replace the old with adequate nutrition.

Vitamin E, vitamin C, and B complex vitamins promote repair and cellular growth. These antioxidants also function as an anti-inflammatory agents that aid in the repair of cell damage. Flaxseed oil, borage oil, and EVENING PRIMROSE OIL provide essential fatty acids also needed for skin maintenance. COLLAGEN has a moisturizing effect when applied in skin lotion, but it is not absorbed or used by the skin when applied topically. Whether the skin can be nourished by external vitamin application remains unclear. Manufacturers often add antioxidants to skin lotions, and there is some evidence that fat-soluble vitamins and other oily (lipophilic) derivatives of vitamins do penetrate the skin. A 2 percent to 10 percent concentration of these substances may be needed to be effective; often, skin preparations contain low amounts. Some manufacturers incorporate materials in liposomes, microscopic sacs prepared from lipids, to aid the absorption of a variety of substances. Preparation of microscopic droplets (called micelles) also helps materials penetrate the upper dead layers of skin to reach cells of the dermis. (See also ACNE.)

Xue, L. "Influence of Dietary Calcium and Vitamin D on Diet-Induced Epithelial Cell Hyperproliferation in Mice," *Journal of the National Cancer Institute* 91 (1991): 176–181.

skin fold test See FAT FOLD TEST.

skin test See ALLERGY, FOOD.

small intestine (small bowel) The tube extending from the stomach to the large intestine (COLON). Typically, the small intestine is 1 in. (2.5 cm) in diameter and 21 ft. (6.35 m) long. It is divided into three regions; the first 10 inches is called the DUODENUM; the JEJUNUM represents the next 8 feet; and the ILEUM occupies the lower reaches of the small intestine. The intestine carries out two distinct functions: It selectively absorbs nutrients and important materials from food and beverages, and at the same time, it excludes a vast amount of foreign substances, ranging from microorganisms and food particles to pollutants and bacterial by-products. To carry out its absorptive function, the surface is highly convoluted and is covered with small projections about 1 mm high, called VILLI, giving it a velvet appearance. Within each villus is a capillary network and lymphatic vessel to aid the uptake and distribution of nutrients. The surfaces of villi are lined with absorptive cells; each cell possesses many microscopic projections called microvilli. The number of villi decreases in the ileum; most absorption occurs in the duodenum and jejunum. The total surface area of the intestine is huge. If the microvilli and villi were flattened out, the surface would be about the size of a tennis court.

The small intestine is the major site of DIGESTION. Pancreatic enzymes efficiently digest fat, protein, and starch. The intestinal lining secretes fluid (intestinal juice) containing electrolytes (ions) and mucus to protect the wall of the intestine from digestive enzymes. The volume is substantial. The small intestine secretes two to three liters of juice per day. Most of the ions and water are reabsorbed and recycled.

Intestinal enzymes complete the final stages of digestion. They include MALTASE to digest maltose, the sugar released from starch digestion; SUCRASE to digest SUCROSE (table sugar); and LACTASE to digest LACTOSE (milk sugar). A milk intolerance often reflects LACTOSE INTOLERANCE that is an impaired ability to digest lactose due to inadequate lactase. Undigested lactose passes on to the colon where bacteria rapidly ferment it, often producing gas, bloating, and diarrhea. The small intestine also produces peptidases to degrade small protein fragments to amino acids.

Partially digested food (chyme) moves down the intestine by localized muscle contraction, creating a mixing action. PERISTALSIS refers to the wave-like contractions moving down the gastrointestinal tract. Chyme moves at the rate of 1 cm/min; consequently, food remains in the small intestine three to five hours. The small intestine produces an array of hormones to regulate digestion. CHOLECYSTOKININ stimulates contraction of the gallbladder to release bile, and it stimulates pancreatic enzyme secretion. SECRETIN reduces gastric and duodenal motility and promotes bicarbonate secretion by the pancreas. Gastric inhibitory protein blocks stomach acid release, while stimulating insulin secretion. To exclude foreigners, the intestine maintains a physical barrier. The mucus coating is constantly being replaced as it is washed away, limiting penetration. Underlying cells are tightly bonded together to limit the leakage of unwanted substances into the body. The movement of food through the digestive tract and the presence of powerful digestive enzymes limit uptake of foreign materials. The major immune barrier is a secreted antibody called secretory IgA. This defensive protein is secreted by immune cells embedded within the intestinal wall and can bind to specific antigens (foreign substances) and prevent their adhering to the intestinal surface. Like all antibodies, specific types of IgA are produced against specific antigens.

Cells lining the intestine replenish themselves in one to two days, thus the nutrient needs of this rapidly dividing tissue are unusually high. Ample zinc and the B complex vitamins, especially FOLIC ACID, are essential for maintaining a healthy intestine. GLUTAMINE helps maintain enterocytes, the epithelial cells lining the small intestine, while butyrate (BUTYRIC ACID) is essential for the help of colonocytes, lining the colon.

If the intestine become inflamed, it can become more "leaky" and foreign substances can enter the body. The influx of foreign materials can trigger multiple food allergies, joint pain, skin conditions, and autoimmune disease in which the body's defenses attack itself. LEAKY GUT syndrome can be caused by alcoholism, overuse of pain medication (nonsteroidal anti-inflammatory drugs), inadequate pancreatic output, infection, AIDS, or Crohn's disease (ulcerated small intestine), among others. With chronic constipation, low stomach acid and aging, colon bacteria may creep upward into the small intestine, leading to a condition known as bacterial overgrowth of the small bowel. Symptoms include sensitivity to starchy food and refined carbohydrate—leading to bloating, gas, diarrhea and other discomfort. Bacterial overgrowth often leads to maldigestion and to malabsorption of vitamins, such as VITAMIN B_{12}. Eradicating the offending bacteria, while remedying the underlying cause, together with dietary modification can alleviate this condition. (See also AMINO ACID METABOLISM; CARBOHYDRATE METABOLISM; FAT METABOLISM.)

smell The olfactory sense and one of the five basic senses. Smell is a chemical sense, providing a direct link with the environment. It evolved primarily to determine which substances are acceptable. When molecules escape into the air, they travel up the nose to a small region of moist tissue called the olfactory membrane. The sense of smell relies on the binding of volatile (gaseous) compounds to cell membranes. Gaseous compounds penetrate the mucus covering the olfactory cells and bind to hair-like extension (cilia) like tassels. Signals are sent along a nerve to olfactory bulbs at the base of the brain, where they radiate out to regions of the brain concerned with mood, strong emotions, memory, and thought. There are about 1,000 different receptors or docking sites that are able to recognize some 10,000 different odors. Flavors of foods are often based on odors rather than mouth (taste) sensations. Unique flavors usually reflect a combination of smell and TASTE. When foods are placed in the mouth, odor molecules travel to the olfactory neurons up the passage linking the inside of the nose and throat. A serious loss of smell affects about two million Americans (a condition known as anosmia). Most commonly this is a result of allergies, certain medications, and head injury.

Axel, Richard. "The Molecular Logic of Smell," *Scientific American* 273 (October 1995): 154–159.

sodium The major positively charged ion in body fluids. Due to their chemical nature, metallic elements such as sodium exist in solutions and in compounds as cations, positively charged ions, where they counterbalance negatively charged ions, such as CHLORIDE. Sodium, therefore, functions in maintaining ELECTROLYTE balance, that is, the balance between negatively and positively charged ions and among complex ions such as proteins in the blood. Sodium predominates in the extracellular fluid, while POTASSIUM, another cation, concentrates within cells. Normally, chloride and sodium tends to leak into cells, while potassium tends to leak out. Sodium is pumped out of cells, while potassium is pumped inward by means of an energy-dependent process called "active transport." Maintaining normal cell volume (and shape) depends on sodium and potassium pumping. The active transport of sodium and potassium is a predominant energy-consuming process of the cells, accounting for a large percentage of the total energy expenditure of the body.

Sodium plays a vital role in controlling osmotic pressure, the pressure that develops between the blood and cells due to ionic concentration differences. The total volume of extracellular fluid is determined by its sodium level, which the body maintains under tight control by means of the endocrine and nervous systems. By balancing charges of negatively charged ions like chloride, BICARBONATE and phosphate, sodium assists in maintaining the proper balance between acidic and alkaline substances (acid-base balance).

Sodium works with potassium in nerve function. To transmit a nerve impulse, the nerve cell membrane is temporarily "depolarized"; potassium temporarily leaks outside and sodium and chloride leak in. This generates a decrease in electrical potential, which triggers a voltage-dependent increase in sodium penetration. Restoration of the potential differences to the resting state allows the impulse to be transmitted as a self-propagating wave down a nerve cell. Muscles, especially heart muscles, require an interplay of sodium and potassium by similar mechanisms.

The kidney normally reabsorbs sodium that was filtered out into the urine to maintain electrolyte balance. Water follows sodium back into the blood, thus hormones that increase sodium retention by the kidney also increase water retention. Sodium concentration and water balance are controlled by an interplay of the kidney and several hormones: When the level of sodium drops, the enzyme RENIN is released by the kidney. Renin catalyzes the conversion of a blood protein to ANGIOTENSIN. In turn, this hormone stimulates the adrenal gland to release ALDOSTERONE, a hormone that causes the kidney to increase the rate of sodium reabsorption from filtered fluid to correct the original sodium depletion. On the other hand, when dietary sodium intake is high, the kidney rapidly excretes sodium. Through the operation of these homeostatic (body balancing) mechanisms, the amount of sodium excreted is adjusted to equal the amount consumed. Ninety percent of ingested sodium is excreted; some is lost through sweat and feces. Excessive sodium intake and retention can cause swelling (EDEMA).

Sources

Most vegetables, fruits, and legumes contain only low levels of sodium, unless pickled. Although the U.S. FDA estimates that processed food contributes 25 percent to 50 percent of the sodium in the typical U.S. diet, other studies of sample diets indicate that an estimate of 60 percent to 75 percent is more realistic. Ninety percent of dietary sodium comes from sodium chloride (table salt); only 15 percent of dietary sodium comes from the salt shaker. There are several explanations for the prevalence of sodium in foods. Salt is a very inexpensive way to flavor PROCESSED FOOD, in place of more expensive herbs and spices. Sometimes companies are not aware of the sodium content in their products. The amount of sodium in the same type of food, produced by different manufacturers, can differ by 50 percent to 300 percent. Salt is also used in recipes dating to a time when salt was not known to be potentially harmful.

The only way to detect salty food is by taste, yet this is an unreliable indicator of sodium content. For example, FRENCH FRIES may have only one-quarter the amount of sodium in an equal serving (weight) of cherry pie because sugar masks the taste of salt. Hidden salt occurs in gelatin desserts, milk shakes, cheese, canned soups, packaged and frozen dinners, and foods at fast-food restaurants; in cured ham and bacon, cured fish, corned beef, smoked herring, and soy sauce. Processed meat like BOLOGNA and HOT DOGS, tomato KETCHUP, many cold BREAKFAST CEREALS, pickled foods, and salad dressings provide high levels of sodium. Sodium occurs in other food additives such as baking soda and sodium aluminum sulfate (in baked goods), sodium caseinate (a milk product), sodium phosphate (the major contributor of sodium in cheese), sodium nitrite and sodium benzoate (preservatives), and MONOSODIUM GLUTAMATE (flavor enhancer). LAXATIVES and ANTACIDS can account for a large percentage of sodium for some people, especially elderly persons. Human milk contains 161 mg of sodium per liter, while cow's milk provides 483 mg per liter; therefore, cow's milk provides considerably more sodium.

Soft water contains high levels of sodium. The amount depends upon the hardness of natural water. A glass of tap water usually contains less than 3 mg of sodium. However, salt from the de-icing of roads and ion exchange resins can raise sodium levels in inland areas. Sodium from seawater can leach into the water supplies of coastal areas.

Requirements

There is no RECOMMENDED DIETARY ALLOWANCE (RDA) for sodium. A safe and adequate level was proposed by the Food and Nutrition Board as 1,100 to 3,300 mg per day in 1980. The 1989 RDA recommendations list the minimum requirements for healthy persons (adults 18 or older) as 500 mg of sodium daily. The sodium requirements of infants and small children are estimated to be about 58 mg daily. The amount of sodium required to maintain sodium equilibrium for most adults may be less than 200 mg under normal circumstances, equivalent to one-tenth a teaspoon of salt per day. The overall consensus is that Americans generally consume too much salt. The typical adult intake is 6 g to 25 g of salt, with a mean of 10 g/day, equivalent to 4 g of sodium, 20 times as much as the listed minimum. The maximum recommended daily intake of sodium chloride is 6 g (2.4 g).

Few people in the United States are sodium deficient. Relatively heavy sweating is now associated with a need for extra salt, and the primary concern should be fluid replacement. Athletes undergoing strenuous physical exercise do not need salt until they have lost approximately three quarts of water by sweating. The kidney adapts to sodium losses in hot weather, so that less sodium, hence less water, is excreted. One typical meal will more than make up for sodium lost in sweat through moderate exercise. Chronic diarrhea, kidney disease, or other medical conditions can limit the body's ability to retain sodium and thus increase sodium requirements. Excessive sodium can be toxic to infants because their kidneys are not fully developed; it may also be toxic to those with kidney disease or those who have adjusted to a chronically low-sodium diet.

Sodium and High Blood Pressure

Sodium has been linked to high blood pressure (HYPERTENSION) in extensive studies spanning decades. Perhaps 10 percent to 20 percent of Americans experience increased blood pressure when they eat excess sodium. High blood pressure increases the risk of STROKE, HEART ATTACK, and kidney disease. Worldwide, a low sodium intake matches a lowered risk of hypertension. Certainly OBESITY, genetic makeup, lack of exercise, and excessive alcohol are risk factor for developing hypertension. Salt sensitivity increases with age. As people grow older, their kidneys excrete less sodium, and an increased sodium intake is more likely to raise blood pressure in susceptible people. Cutting back on salt intake may lower blood pressure by a small amount; however, even relatively small decreases in blood pressure readings could mean a significant decreases in the risk of death due to coronary heart disease. Excessive sodium increases urinary losses of calcium and can contribute to the risk of osteoporosis. Additionally, a high-salt diet is a dominant risk factor for stomach cancer. Governmental dietary guidelines recommend moderate sodium consumption, and individuals with hypertension or who have a family history of hypertension may be advised to curtail sodium consumption.

To cut back on salt, do not add salt to foods. Season with herbs or sauces instead. Cut back on processed, convenience foods. Read food labels to determine the sodium content and avoid foods with high sodium. Do not take salt tablets without consulting a doctor. Reducing high blood pressure can mean, in addition to cutting back on sodium, limiting alcohol consumption to one or two drinks per day; engaging in regular aerobic exercise; getting enough calcium, potassium, and magnesium; and losing weight.

Sodium on Food Labels

Sodium must be listed on the label of any foods that list nutritional content, and on those that make nutritional claims as being "low fat" or "enriched." (Exempt foods are those made with meat or poultry.)

- "Sodium free" means less than 5 mg of sodium per serving.
- "Very low sodium" foods contain at most 140 mg per serving.
- "Low sodium" foods contain at most 140 mg per serving.
- "Reduced sodium" means the food has been processed to reduce normal sodium levels by at least 75 percent.
- "No sodium" and "no salt" alternatives: Several cold breakfast cereals, canned vegetables, and herbal salt substitutes have been introduced to meet consumer demands.

SODIUM CONTENT OF COMMON FOODS

Food	Sodium (mg) per 100 g (3 oz.)
Canadian bacon	2,555
Green olives	2,400
Corned beef	1,740
Cheese	1,430
Bologna	1,300
Cold cereal (oats)	1,267
Cured ham	1,100
Wheatflake cereal	1,032
Potato chips	1,000
Sausage	958

(See also FOOD ADDITIVES; MINERALS.)

sodium alginate See ALGINATE.

sodium ascorbate See VITAMIN C.

sodium benzoate A food preservative that retards growth of microorganisms under acidic conditions. Foods and beverages can contain up to 0.1 percent sodium benzoate. Soft drinks, salad dressing, and fruit juices often contain this preservative. Sodium benzoate also occurs naturally in vegetables and fruit, for example, in prunes and cranberries. Sodium benzoate is a product of metabolism as well. Extensive studies indicate it is a safe additive.

sodium chloride See SODIUM.

sodium erythroborate See ERYTHROBORIC ACID.

sodium nitrate See NITRATE.

sodium nitrite See NITRITE.

soft drinks Carbonated, nonalcoholic beverages that contain dissolved CARBON DIOXIDE (carbonation), sweeteners, flavoring agents, edible acids, and food coloring. Soft drink consumption in the United States has doubled since 1974. Increased soft drink consumption means increased consumption of PHOSPHOROUS, ARTIFICIAL FOOD COLORS, and ARTIFICIAL SWEETENERS, and sugar. In contrast, water contains none of these additives.

In 2001 a team of U.S. researchers published an article in the British medical journal *Lancet* linking soft drink consumption among children and adolescents with the rise in obesity rates among U.S. teens. The researchers found that for every additional serving of soft drink consumed each day, the risk of becoming obese increased by 50 percent. Some researchers also blame increased soft drink consumption with a rise in calcium deficiency among young people. According to the American Academy of Orthopedic Surgeons, children from birth to age 11 and teenage boys consume only half the amount of calcium they need daily. Teenage girls are meeting only 14 percent to 20 percent of their daily calcium requirements.

STANDARDS OF IDENTITY define certain aspects of the composition of foods and beverages. Soft drinks are classified as soda water and must contain more carbon dioxide than can be absorbed at normal air pressure. Alcohol content, if contributed by a flavoring agent, cannot exceed 0.5 percent of the weight. CAFFEINE can be added to any soda water to a final concentration of 0.02 percent by weight. Optional ingredients include sweeteners (synthetic and nonsynthetic), edible acids, flavors, colors, preservatives, emulsifying agents to prevent ingredients from separating, thickening agents to create cloudiness and "mouth feel," and foaming agents.

SUCROSE (table sugar) is among the most common NATURAL SWEETENERS used in soft drinks. Also approved are dextrose (GLUCOSE), INVERT SUGAR, FRUCTOSE, CORN SYRUP, high FRUCTOSE CORN SYRUP (now a general soft drink sweetener), and glucose syrup. The artificial sweetener ASPARTAME is used extensively in diet soft drinks. SACCHARIN, another noncaloric sweetener, is used in soft drinks as well. Phosphoric acid is added to acidify soft drinks. Other acids used in soft drinks include ACETIC ACID, fumaric acid, LACTIC ACID, and gluconic acid, an acid of glucose. The phosphate in soft drinks increases the overall phosphate consumption. This can be detrimental because a high phosphate intake is linked to an overactive thyroid gland and bone loss (OSTEOPOROSIS). Furthermore, drinking large amounts of diet soda (eight to 10 cans a day) is a cause of tooth erosion.

Types of Soft Drinks

Colas These contain extract of the cola nut and caffeine. The coloring agent is typically caramel (brown sugar) and the sugar content can be 11 percent to 13 percent.

Orange Soft Drinks Artificial colors, orange oil, or orange juice may be added. The sugar content resembles colas and the edible acid is usually CITRIC ACID. These are not substitutes for orange juice.

Ginger Ale Ginger root extract, ginger, and lime oil may be the flavoring agents in these soft drinks. Caramel may be used as a coloring and citric acid is the edible acid. The sugar content ranges from 7 percent to 11 percent.

Grape-flavor Soft Drinks Synthetic grape flavor or grape juice may be used in flavoring and artificial coloring is used. The sugar content is generally between 11 percent and 13 percent, and the edible acid is TARTARIC ACID. (See also CONVENIENCE FOOD; EMPTY CALORIES; JUNK FOOD.)

Ludwig, David S. et al. "Relation Between Consumption of Sugar-Sweetened Drinks and Childhood Obesity: A Prospective, Observational Analysis," *Lancet* 357 (2001): 505–508.

Wyshak, G. "Teenaged Girls Carbonated Beverage Consumption, and Bone Fractures," *Archives of Pediatric Adolescent Medicine* 154 (2000): 610–613.

solanine An ALKALOID that acts as a plant's defensive agent against insects. Solanine is found in very low levels in apples, tomatoes, eggplant, and sugar beets. POTATOES contain the highest concentration of solanine, which contributes to their characteristic flavor. Solanine acts as a nerve poison by blocking the action of NEUROTRANSMITTERS, brain chemicals required for transmitting nerve impulses. Most American-growth varieties of potatoes contain low levels of solanine, so that a person would have to consume 4.5 lb. (2 kg) of unbruised, nonsprouted potatoes to ingest 200 mg of solanine, a dose that could cause drowsiness, cramps, neck itchiness and DIARRHEA. However, the content of solanine in potatoes increases dramatically with bruising or sprouting, or when the skin turns green due to exposure to too much sunlight after harvest. Damaged or green-skinned potatoes should be discarded for this reason.

somatotropin See MEAT CONTAMINANTS.

sorbic acid (potassium sorbate) A food PRESERVATIVE used to inhibit the growth of molds, yeast, and fungi, but not bacteria. Sorbic acid is used in CHEESE manufacture, allowing bacteria to ferment milk products while inhibiting yeast and mold growth. Because sorbic acid is effective over a wide range of pH, it is used in a variety of foods, including MAYONNAISE, cake, MARGARINE, dried fruit, SOFT DRINKS, and syrup at concentrations up to 0.03 percent. It breaks down at high temperature and cannot be pasteurized. The body metabolizes sorbic acid like a fatty acid; consequently, it is an energy source. It is considered a safe FOOD ADDITIVE.

sorbitol (hexitol) A naturally occurring sugar ALCOHOL. Sorbitol is 60 percent as sweet as SUCROSE (table sugar) although it is not a carbohydrate. It is used in chewing gum, confections, icing, food toppings, meat products, milk products, and beverages. It reduces the rate of sugar crystal formation, maintains moisture, and sequesters (binds) food ingredients.

Sorbitol occurs in many fruits, including berries, CHERRIES, PEARS, PLUMS, and APPLES and in SEAWEED. Both apple juice and pear juice contain a high concentration. Sorbitol in apple juice is not absorbed well by infants and small children; it can ferment in the large intestine, producing gas, cramps, and DIARRHEA. Large doses of sorbitol (50 g) can cause diarrhea in adults.

Sorbitol is synthesized by hydrogenation of the simple sugar GLUCOSE (dextrose). Sorbitol contains the same number of four calories per gram as carbohydrate and is burned completely to carbon dioxide. However, it does not form glucose in the body, thus it does not raise BLOOD SUGAR. Therefore, sorbitol is used as a sweetener in certain dietetic foods. Sorbitol-containing foods and chewing gums are not calorie-free, although they carry a "sugarless" or "sugar free" label. Sorbitol formation in cells occurs as a side effect of DIABETES MELLITUS. Since it cannot leak out of cells, sorbitol can gradually accumulate, leading eventually to osmotic imbalances and tissue damage. (See also ARTIFICIAL SWEETENERS; FOOD ADDITIVES; NATURAL SWEETENERS.)

sorghum (*Sorghum vulgare;* Guinea corn, kaffir corn) A major cereal GRAIN that is a staple in Africa and Asia. Sorghum ranks in the top five most important cereal grains worldwide. Well adapted to climates too hot and dry for CORN and WHEAT, sorghum has been grown in regions of Africa and Asia since 2000 B.C. The People's Republic of China, the United States, India, and Argentina provide much of the world's production. In the United States sorghum is used primarily as animal fodder. Only 1 percent to 2 percent of U.S. sorghum is used for food or alcoholic fermentation.

Though related to MILLET, nutritionally sorghum resembles corn. Both grains are deficient in the essential AMINO ACID, LYSINE. In Africa and Asia, sorghum is used as a flour or a porridge. Sweet sorghum is used to make an unrefined syrup, more sour than molasses. As with all refined sweeteners, the amounts are too low to be reliable sources of minerals or B complex vitamins. The nutrient content of 1 cup (3 oz., 100 g) of sorghum is: 366 calories; protein, 11.0 g; carbohydrate, 73 g; fat, 3.3 g; thiamin, 0.38 mg; riboflavin, 0.15 mg; niacin, 3.9 mg.

soul food A cuisine originating in the southern United States, where, in the antebellum era, slaves developed eating practices from their West African roots. Soul food has been modified by later generations, but typically includes collard greens, mustard greens, turnip greens, fried chicken, sweet potato pie, and corn bread. Traditionally, these high-salt, high-fat foods pose a potential health problem, especially among blacks who are experiencing an epidemic of high blood pressure in the United States. As with other ethnic dishes, the use of spices and herbs for seasoning is recommended to cut down on salt. Recipes can be adapted to use less FAT in cooking, such as the substitution of VEGETABLE OIL for LARD to reduce consumption of SATURATED FAT. Modifications can help make soul food dishes nutritious and heart healthy, while still tasty and appetizing. (See also DIETARY GUIDELINES FOR AMERICANS; FOOD PYRAMID; HYPERTENSION.)

soybean (*Glycine max;* soya, soy pea) The oil-rich seed of a bushy LEGUME; a food staple in Asia. The soybean originated in eastern Asia and was cultivated in ancient China. American and Canadian cooperative agricultural projects in the 1930s yielded soybean varieties with increased yield and oil content, making soybeans more appealing as a crop. Today, soybeans are the leading U.S. cash crop, ahead of WHEAT and CORN, and the United States is the world's major supplier of soybeans. Illinois, Iowa, Missouri, Minnesota, and Ohio are among the top producers of soybeans, which represent the largest domestic source of VEGETABLE OIL. Dried soybeans can be cooked like dried beans and served in salads or casseroles. Roasted soybeans are a high-fat snack food.

Soybeans contain about 20 percent to 25 percent oil, 30 percent to 50 percent protein and 14 percent to 21 percent carbohydrate, but little STARCH. Processing soybeans has traditionally separated oil and protein. Soybean oil is one of the most widely used vegetable oils. Over 90 percent of the oil is used for food processing, cooking oil, and MARGARINE. Solvents are generally used to extract oil from cracked seeds after heating. The oil must first be degummed, then bleached, partially hydrogenated to increase stability and extend its shelf life, and finally deodorized. Because of its high content of polyunsaturated FATTY ACIDS (with multiple hydrogen-deficient linkages), soybean oil is classified as a polyunsaturated oil. Soybean oil contains LINOLEIC ACID, an essential fatty acid, up to 55 percent; OLEIC ACID, a monounsaturate and fatty acid, up to 25 percent. The saturated fatty acids represent about 15 percent. Soybean oil is often used in cooking and in processed foods.

Soybean protein is used as a meat substitute because its protein is unusually well balanced for a plant protein. The NET PROTEIN UTILIZATION (NPU) is 65, comparable to animal protein in quality. Soy protein contains substantial amounts of LYSINE, an essential amino acid, and sulfur-containing amino acids, especially METHIONINE, often deficient in legumes and grains. Soy-based infant formulas may be appropriate for babies who are allergic to cow's milk protein, and soy protein can increase the nutritive value of baby cereals and canned baby foods. Soy protein is used to fortify pasta products, hot cereals, and various breakfast or granola bars. Because of its low cost, soy protein is often used in institutional settings. The National SCHOOL LUNCH PROGRAM is permitted to offer vegetable protein products in place of meat products.

Soy Products

Processed soy protein, TEXTURIZED VEGETABLE PROTEIN, soybean flour, and soybean grits contain 40 percent to 50 percent protein. They are used in baked goods like bread, rolls, cakes, pancake and waffle mixes, crackers, and cookies; in meat products like SAUSAGE, hot dogs, soy burgers, MEAT LOAF, meat patties, canned meats; in breakfast cereals and confections; in infant and children's foods; and in dietetic foods.

Soy protein hydrolyzate (hydrolyzed vegetable protein) is a mixture produced by degrading soy protein by any of a variety of agents: enzymes, yeast, molds, bacteria, acids, or alkali. It is used in soy sauce, and as a flavoring, foaming, or whipping agent.

Soy milk is prepared by first soaking beans in water, grinding the moistened beans and then filtering to remove the particles. The milk is used in soy-based infant formulas. Commercial products contain water, homogenized soybeans, vegetables, oils, and sometimes kelp. Unless specified otherwise, soy milk is not fortified with vitamins A or D or minerals. Nutritionally, fortified soy milk can be a good source of vitamin B_{12}.

TOFU (soybean curd) can be coagulated from soy protein by boiling or by adding lime water. The precipitating protein is pressed into blocks to prepare tofu. Tofu can be seasoned or converted to foods ranging from eggless egg salad to tofu burgers and stir-fries.

Soy sauce (shoyu, chiang-yu) is a salty sauce prepared by fermenting a mixture of wheat and soybeans and water. It contains relatively high levels of free amino acids and protein fermentation products. It is generally a high-salt seasoning. Reduced salt and varieties without wheat are available.

A variety of population studies link the consumption of soy protein with reduced risk of heart disease. As soy protein replaces animal protein in the diet, elevated blood cholesterol levels decline. Individuals with blood cholesterol levels greater than 250 and who substitute soy for animal protein may be able to lower their cholesterol by up to 25 percent by consuming about 40 g of soy protein daily. The reasons behind this reduction are not known; several possibilities are being examined. Soy contains complex substances called ISO-

FLAVONES, such as GENISTEIN which may prevent the formation of fatty deposits in arteries (plaque) by blocking the formation of oxidized LOW-DENSITY LIPOPROTEIN (LDL), believed to be the promoter of plaque formation. Isoflavones block the formation of blood clots in plaque in partially blocked arteries and to increase the flexibility of hardened (atherosclerotic) arteries. Also in experiments on animals, genistein inhibits the regrowth of plaque after balloon angioplasty. On the other hand, soy contains fiber that may bind bile salts, derived from cholesterol, and help excrete them, thus helping to flush cholesterol out of the blood. Soy may alter hormone levels: Thyroxine, a thyroid hormone, is higher in the blood of people on soy-based diets. Thyroxine may lower cholesterol levels.

A growing number of laboratory studies indicate that genistein and cholesterol analogs called saponins can block cancer development in experimental animals. Soy isoflavones and saponins may mimic the female hormone estrogen (PHYTOESTROGENS), which promotes breast and cervical cancer. By inhibiting estrogen production, isoflavones may convince the body to make less estrogen, thus lowering the cancer risk. Population studies support the protective role of soy. Asian women, who traditionally consume eight times more soy than American women, have half the rate of breast cancer. How much genistein is required to offer a protective effect is not known. The estrogen-like effects of genistein and similar isoflavones may help prevent bone loss associated with osteoporosis and they may lessen the symptoms of menopause. (See also PROTEIN QUALITY; RANCIDITY.)

Anderson, J. W., B. M. Johnstone, and M. E. Cook-Newell. "Meta-analysis of the Effects of Soy Protein Intake on Serum Lipids," *New England Journal of Medicine* 333 (August 3, 1995): 276–282.

soy milk See SOYBEAN.

soy sauce See SOYBEAN.

spastic colon See IRRITABLE BOWEL SYNDROME.

specific dynamic effect (SDE; specific dynamic activity, SDA) The ENERGY used by the body to digest and process foods. The secretion of ENZYMES and HORMONES and the uptake of nutrients by the INTESTINE are energy-requiring processes. Smooth muscles are activated to move food through the digestive system (PERISTALSIS), and the rate of degradation of enzymes increases. The SDE amounts to an increase of 6 percent to 10 percent in energy expenditure above the fasting or basal level. This stimulation of cell processes is also called diet-induced thermogenesis because increased metabolism inevitably produces more heat. (See also CALORIES.)

spelt (*Triticum spelta*) A GRAIN closely related to WHEAT (*Triticum sativum*). Spelt has been cultivated in Europe and the Middle East since ancient times. The protein content ranges from 13.1 percent to 14.3 percent, comparable to durum wheat (hard wheat) but significantly greater than soft wheat. Spelt protein contains somewhat more of the essential amino acid METHIONINE than wheat. This amino acid is deficient in most grains. The whole grain contains higher levels of B complex vitamins than most other grains. The nutrient content of 100 g of spelt flour is: 382 calories; protein, 14.3 g carbohydrate, 74.5 g; fat, 2.94 g; iron, 4.2 mg; thiamin, 0.649 mg; riboflavin, 0.227 mg; niacin, 8.46 mg. For comparison, white bleached flour (100 g), enriched, provides: thiamin, 0.64 mg; riboflavin, 0.40 mg; niacin, 5.22 mg; and corn, 4.35 mg. Whole wheat flour provides: thiamin, 0.57 mg; riboflavin, 0.12 mg; niacin, 0.44 mg; and iron, 4.44 mg.

spice Seasonings prepared mainly from tropical plants. Spices are generally more pungent than herbs and have a strong flavor. They may represent seeds, roots, stems, or bark, depending on which part of the plant is the most aromatic (spicy). In contrast, herbs generally utilize most of the plant. The following are representative: Allspice and red PEPPER come from the dried fruits; CLOVES from dried flower buds; cinnamon from bark; MUSTARD from seeds; black pepper from dried berries; GINGER and horseradish from roots; SAFFRON from dried flower stigmas. Spices are among the oldest FOOD ADDITIVES; the amounts used to flavor food are too small to contribute significant nutrients, although they stimulate digestion. Certain oils possess preservative or antioxidants effects. (See also APPETITE.)

spina bifida A severe neural tube BIRTH DEFECT in which the spinal cord is exposed. About 1,500 to 2,000 infants are born each year in the United States with this condition. A related defect is anencephaly, an absence of part or all of the brain. NEURAL TUBE DEFECTS may occur in the first month of pregnancy, before women realize they are pregnant. Genetic as well as environmental factors affect the probability of this condition.

Current studies link a deficiency of the B vitamin FOLIC ACID, to this defect. Women at risk for Neural tube defects who take multivitamin pills containing folic acid around the time of conception have fewer babies with neurological birth defects. In 1998 the U.S. FDA began requiring all enriched grain products, including flour, to be fortified with folic acid at the rate of 140 mcg per 100 g of grain. This action was taken based on studies that showed that only about 25 percent of women of childbearing age regularly consumed enough folic acid. Women who consume at least 400 mcg daily have a significantly lower risk of bearing children with neural tube defects such as spina bifida. The U.S. Public Health Service contends that folic acid intake should not exceed 1 mg daily because it could mask or aggravate ANEMIA. Folic acid occurs in dark green leafy vegetables, citrus fruit, whole grain bread, and beans, and women who eat at least five servings daily can meet the guidelines. (See also HOMOCYSTEINE.)

spinach (*Spinacia oleracea*) A dark green leafy VEGETABLE related to chard and beets. Spinach is believed to have originated in south western Asia. Although Moors brought spinach to Europe about A.D. 1000, it was not cultivated in northern Europe until the 1700s. The United States is a major producer of spinach, and much of the domestic crop is grown in California and Texas. As much as 75 percent is processed by canning or freezing.

There are three basic types of spinach: Savoy spinach with curly leaves; flat or smooth-leaf spinach, usually frozen or canned; and semi-Savoy, with slightly crinkled leaves. Spinach is an excellent source of BETA-CAROTENE (provitamin A) and VITAMIN K (required for normal blood clotting) and the B vitamin folacin. Spinach is used in fillings or stuffings, souffles, casseroles, soups, and salads. Spinach contains oxalates, salts of OXALIC ACID. Oxalates bind CALCIUM and IRON, two minerals that are high in spinach, so that these minerals cannot be completely used. Consequently, spinach is not the wonder food popularized by cartoons. Other vegetarian sources such as kale and turnip greens provide more of these minerals. Various studies indicate that the oxalate content of spinach does not appreciably decrease calcium uptake from other foods. Only massive amounts of spinach can create a nutritional problem. The nutrient content of 1 cup (cooked, drained, 180 g) is: 41 calories; protein, 5.3 g; carbohydrate, 6.8 g; fiber, 5.8 g; fat, 0.5 g; calcium, 244 mg; iron, 6.4 mg; potassium, 838 mg; vitamin A, 1,474 retinol equivalents; thiamin, 0.17 mg; riboflavin, 0.42 mg; niacin, 0.88 mg. (See also BIOAVAILABILITY; TRACE MINERALS.)

spirulina A form of microscopic blue-green algae used as a food supplement. Spirulina is a rich source of BETA-CAROTENE (provitamin A), a blue pigment called phycocyanin, and CHLOROPHYLL, the green plant pigment. Spirulina contains 65 percent protein, 18 percent carbohydrate, 5 percent fat, and 7 percent minerals. Spirulina contains appreciable IRON and B complex vitamins. Although claimed to be a good source of VITAMIN B_{12}, spirulina contains vitamin B_{12} analogs or other substances that prevent its use in the body. Spirulina provides GAMMA LINOLENIC ACID, a polyunsaturated FATTY ACID. This lipid is a parent compound of a hormone-like family of lipids called PROSTAGLANDINS, which possess anti-inflammatory activity.

Spirulina is added to soups, salads, pasta, fruit dishes, and vegetable juices. The nutrient content of a 10 g (1/3 oz.) serving is: protein, 6.5 g; carbohydrate, 1.8 g; fat, 0.5 g; calcium, 100 mg; iron, 15 mg; vitamin A, 2,300 retinol equivalents; thiamin, 0.31 mg; riboflavin, 0.35 mg; niacin, 1.46 mg.

Splenda See SUCRALOSE.

spoilage A change in food that makes it unsuitable for human consumption. Spoilage can alter the texture, odor, color, taste, and nutrient content of a food, changes that are usually readily detected. Microbial spoilage is caused by growth of YEAST, MOLDS, and bacteria and is favored by warm, moist conditions. Bacteria can degrade MEAT, dairy products, and canned foods, while mold and yeast can grow on BREAD, CHEESE, FRUIT, VEGETABLES, and sugary foods like jelly and jam.

Enzymes in foods can also lead to spoilage. Alternatively, insect pests can infest foods, making them unfit. Softening and ripening of fruit and vegetables are caused by enzymatic changes. Enzymes may survive processing and create "off" flavors.

Spontaneous chemical reactions due to oxygen, light and metal ion contaminants can lead to rancidity (breakdown) of fat and oil-containing foods. Heat can increase the rate of chemical reactions leading to degradation, whether affected by enzymes or not. Alternatively, extreme cold can crack fresh foods or alter their texture. Modern food processing and preservation aims to minimize food spoilage. Canning, drying, freezing or chilling, and the use of FOOD PRESERVATIVES, as well as sanitation, play a role in preventing spoilage up to the time of purchase. As an example, food manufacturers can limit oxidation by minimizing exposure to air (vacuum-sealed containers); by adding preservatives like CITRIC ACID to bind metal ion contaminants; or by adding synthetic ANTIOXIDANTS like BHA and BHT. (See also FOOD POISONING.)

sport drinks Electrolyte replacement beverages popular among athletes to replace water lost during exercise. It is important to drink plenty of fluids during strenuous EXERCISE, especially during hot weather, because the body requires water for efficient cooling and for efficient operation of the kidneys in moving wastes from the blood. GLUCOSE-sodium sport drinks provide extra sugar and sodium, which also promote rapid fluid uptake by the small intestine. Some beverages contain glucose polymers (maltodextrins), small fragment of STARCH. Glucose polymer beverages may be more effective than glucose drinks in replacing carbohydrates and in increasing BLOOD SUGAR during endurance events (more than two hours in duration). They do not slow the passage of liquid through the stomach as a high-glucose concentration does.

Simple carbohydrates seem to provide their greatest benefit when exercise exceeds 60 minutes. A potential benefit of consuming glucose replacements during exercise is that fluid intake may increase if the taste is more appealing than plain water. The carbohydrate-electrolyte sport drink should be mixed so that the carbohydrate concentration is less than 10 percent to minimize retention by the stomach. On the other hand, the carbohydrate concentration should be at least 6 percent to improve endurance. When fluid loss is reduced by a cold environment such as in cross-country skiing, fluids with a carbohydrate concentration greater than 10 percent are appropriate.

Sport drinks often contain more sugar and salt than are needed for optimal absorption of fluids, and they often contain less POTASSIUM than a glass of ORANGE juice. Plain water, which is both easily absorbed and palatable, effectively replaces water lost with strenuous exercise. In general, there does not seem to be any need to replace electrolytes lost through sweating by consuming expensive beverages. Sport drinks appear likely to improve performance only in endurance exercise or day-long events.

Diluted fruit juices are usually adequate electrolyte replacements. Fruit juices should be diluted at least twofold from standard preparations to prevent delayed gastric emptying. Electrolytes and carbohydrates are readily replenished by eating a banana, fruit, or crackers with water. Many commercial soft drinks contain CAFFEINE, which acts as a diuretic. Therefore, athletes are advised to limit their intake of such beverages. (See also DEHYDRATION.)

sprue A digestive disorder typically characterized by weight loss, weakness, bloating and gas, loss of appetite, greasy, frothy stools, DIARRHEA, and malabsorption. Poor absorption of SUGAR, fat-soluble vitamins (A, D, E, and K), and MINERALS by the small intestine is responsible for the weight loss. Malabsorption of vitamin D and calcium promotes bone thinning. The intestinal surface becomes damaged, leading to nutrient malabsorption. Sprue occurs sporadically without any known cause, although FOOD SENSITIVES have been implicated in some individuals. Inadequate uptake of VITAMIN B_{12}, FOLIC ACID, and IRON can lead to anemia. Vitamin B_{12} and folic acid shots can be given to overcome deficiencies because they cannot be taken up efficiently if given orally to these patients. Fiber supplements should not be used with any acute gastrointestinal disease (DIVERTICULITIS, CELIAC DISEASE, or ulcerative COLITIS). Foods that provoke symptoms should be avoided.

Celiac Sprue

Celiac disease refers to damaged intestine due to an inherited immunologic sensitivity to wheat protein and GLUTEN. This is one of the most common malabsorption syndromes in the United States. This disease is characterized by a marked loss in flattening of the villi—the small, hairlike projections that increase the absorptive surface of the small intestine. Celiac sprue is usually diagnosed in childhood and can be cured by placing the patient on a gluten-free diet. Celiac disease increases the risk of gastric intestinal cancer, especially of the small intestine.

Tropical Sprue

Like celiac sprue, this malabsorption syndrome is also characterized by atrophy of the villi, drastically reducing the surface area. Intestinal enzyme deficiencies lead to carbohydrate and fat maldigestion and malabsorption. Anemia often develops as a consequence of vitamin B_{12} and folic acid deficiencies. Tropical sprue affects populations living in Asia, Central America, and the West Indies or people who have visited the tropics. Administration of vitamin B_{12} and folic acid may successfully treat macrocytic anemia (anemia characterized by large, pale red blood cells). Substitutions of fat and oils by MEDIUM-CHAIN TRIGLYCERIDES (fats with smaller fatty acids) can increase fat absorption, correct fatty stools and assist with weight gain. The cause of this disease is unknown, although there are hints that specific disease-producing strains of the bacterium *ESCHERICHIA COLI* are involved. Response to a wheat-free (glutein free) diet is minimal but administration of broad-spectrum antibiotics may be effective. (See also IRRITABLE BOWEL SYNDROME.)

squash (Cucurbita genus) A gourd native to North and South America related to MELONS, PUMPKINS, and CUCUMBERS used as food in Mexico and Guatemala about 8000 B.C. Aztec, Inca, and Mayan civilizations cultivated squash, corn, and beans, which spread throughout Native American populations. Hundreds of varieties of squash now exist. Summer squash is a quick-growing bushy squash that produces many fruit, which are usually harvested in the summer months while still immature. They have soft shells and tender flesh. Summer squashes are about 95 percent water, and so are very low in calories. Examples include pattypan, scallop, chayote, cocozelle, zucchini, yellow crookneck, yellow straightneck, and Caserta.

Winter squashes are harvested in the fall when fully mature. They have a tough, coarse rind that is dark green or orange, and their flesh is darker than that of summer varieties. Winter squash is easily stored. Acorn or Danish, butternut, spaghetti, Warren turban, Hubbard, and sugar squash are common winter squashes. Squash blossom can be eaten, as well as the dried seeds. Summer squash is usually cooked unpeeled. It can be stuffed or grated and cooked as patties; or fried or baked in casseroles. Winter squash is cut in half and the seeds removed. It is then microwaved, baked, broiled, or steamed. All winter squashes are excellent sources of BETA-CAROTENE (provitamin A). The nutrient content of 1 cup (cooked, 180 g) of crookneck squash is: 36 calories; protein, 1.6 g; carbohydrate, 7.8 g; fiber, 3.2 g; fat, 0.6 g; iron, 0.63 mg; potassium, 455 mg; vitamin A, 43 retinol equivalents; thiamin, 0.07 mg; riboflavin, 0.07 mg; niacin, 0.77 mg.

One cup (205 g) of baked and mashed butternut winter squash provides: 83 calories; protein, 1.8 g; carbohydrate, 21.5 g; fiber, 4.9 g; iron, 1.23 mg; potassium, 583 mg; vitamin A, 1,435 retinol equivalents; thiamin, 0.15 mg; riboflavin, 0.04 mg; niacin, 2.0 mg. (See also VEGETABLES.)

stabilizers Food additives used as thickening agents in processing to avoid watery or lumpy products. Examples are CARRAGEENAN, DEXTRIN, KARAYA GUM, LECITHIN, LOCUST BEAN GUM, TRAGACANTH GUM, and XANTHAN GUM.

Carrageenan comes from a SEAWEED known as Irish moss. It is used to keep cocoa butter suspended in chocolate milk and fat suspended in evaporated milk, canned milk, instant breakfasts, and infant formulas. It thickens SOFT DRINKS, ICE CREAM, frozen whipped topping, and YOGURT. Carrageenan appears to be safe, except for premature infants.

Dextrin is partially hydrolyzed STARCH. It finds use in candy, powdered mixes of various kinds, and in soups and gravy and other foods. Dextrin is considered a safe food additive.

Karaya gum comes from India. Food manufacturers use this complex carbohydrate to stabilize whipped products, salad dressing, processed meat products like SAUSAGE, and ice cream. Long-term studies on its safety have not been carried out.

Lecithin is a nutrient and a constituent of all plant and animal food. As a FOOD ADDITIVE it stabilizes MARGARINE, CHOCOLATE, baked goods like rolls and bread, and ice cream. It is classified as a safe additive.

Locust bean gum (carob seed gum) comes from the bean of the carob tree. It is used to stabilize ice cream, salad dressing, pie filling, cakes, and biscuits. It often is used together with carrageenan to improve the qualities and thickening properties of that additive. Locust bean gum is considered safe.

Tragacanth gum is a product of the Middle East. It is especially useful in acidic foods, such as salad dressing, because it does not break down under acidic conditions. The safety of this additive has not been studied.

Xanthan gum is produced by a bacterium. It is widely used because it is stable in acidic media and because it thickens even at high temperatures. Xanthan gum stabilizes salad dressing, syrup, pie fillings, pudding, and processed foods. It is a safe additive. (See also EMULSIFIERS.)

standards of identity The Federal Food, Drug and Cosmetic Act defined the standard formulations of commercial "recipes" now available for about 400 common foods and condiments, such as ketchup, HAMBURGER, ICE CREAM, jelly, MAYONNAISE, PEANUT BUTTER, SAUSAGE, cheese, frankfurters, and bread. Manufacturers of these items do not have to list the ingredients on labels. These standards were established to ensure consistent quality and composition and to prevent fraud. The standards of identity for foods specify required levels of ingredients. As an example, ice cream must contain at least 10 percent milkfat, otherwise it must be renamed as frozen dessert or labeled as imitation. Low fat and reduced fat now have specific meanings on food labels. The use of artificial sweeteners in standard formulations is also being explored. (See also FOOD ADDITIVES; FOOD LABELING; PROCESSED FOOD.)

staphylococcal food poisoning An infectious type of FOOD POISONING induced by toxins released from Staphylococcus bacteria. The bacteria form toxins in improperly stored or cooked food, which are not easily destroyed by cooking. Staphylococci are common in the environment and are present in secretions from the nose and throat, as well as from skin infections. Therefore, food exposed to air and to infected food handlers can become contaminated. Staphylococcus can rapidly multiply in certain foods stored at room temperature. They can hibernate in the food when refrigerated, and then begin reproduction when warmed to room temperature. A variety of foods are implicated, including HAM and other meats, POULTRY and chicken salad, cream-filled desserts, custards and custard-filled baked desserts, pasta salad, and cheese products.

Staph-infected food does not taste different from normal food, thus there is no change in flavor to serve as a warning. Staphylococcus is destroyed by boiling, but toxins developed before heating may resist this treatment. Prevention of staph food poisoning requires cleanliness in food preparation, elimination of flies from the kitchen area, education of food handlers in personal hygiene, and refrigeration of all perishable foods. (See also BOTULISM; SALMONELLA.)

staple A food that is consumed in large amounts and provides a large percentage of total daily calories. Staples anchor traditional diets; POTATOES, BREAD, RICE, and MILK fall into this category. Staples can significantly affect health because they provide much more than calories. As whole foods—that is, foods that have been minimally processed—they provide MINERALS, VITAMINS, ESSENTIAL FATTY ACIDS, FIBER, and certain non-nutrient materials that have less well-defined functions in the body. Thus, consuming ample amounts of whole GRAINS and VEGETABLES can lower the risk of CARDIOVASCULAR

DISEASE, CANCER and GASTROINTESTINAL disease in populations throughout the world.

starch The storage carbohydrate that occurs in granules in seeds, stems, and roots of higher plants. Starch consists of long chains of GLUCOSE, a simple sugar, formed during PHOTOSYNTHESIS. Starch accounts for 50 percent to 75 percent of the weight of cereal GRAIN and 75 percent of the weight of POTATOES. Unripened apples and bananas contain starch; as these fruits ripen, much of the starch is converted to glucose. With moist heat, starch granules absorb water and rupture, releasing starch to an easily digested, water-soluble form.

Starch is classified as a COMPLEX CARBOHYDRATE because of its complex structure, which requires DIGESTION to be assimilated. Starch occurs either as long, unbranched chains (AMYLOSE) or as highly branched chains (AMYLOPECTIN). The ratio of these two types varies with the source; an average composition is 27 percent amylose and 73 percent amylopectin.

As a carbohydrate, starch produces four calories per gram when burned for ENERGY. Starchy foods are dietary staples throughout the world. These foods are economical and contribute a large percentage of daily calories. Examples include RICE in Asian countries, CORN in Mexico, roots, tubers, and SORGHUM in Africa. Contrary to old ideas, starch is not fattening nor is starch the major villain in the standard American diet. Fat contains more than twice the number of calories per gram as carbohydrate, and because a high-fat intake is common, fat calories are more critical in controlling weight and maintaining long-term health. Excessive dietary fat, particularly saturated fat, no starch, increases the risk of heart disease and some forms of cancer.

Starch represents the most important source of carbohydrate in the American diet where it occurs as the main ingredient of rice, WHEAT, RYE, MILLET, corn, BARLEY, and OATS. Pasta and baked goods are common sources of starch from wheat. Cornstarch and potato starch are used as thickening agents in prepared foods. Starch occurs in high amounts also in LEGUMES, dried BEANS, kidney beans, black-eyed peas, CHICKPEAS, and SOYBEANS. Cornstarch is converted to high FRUCTOSE CORN SYRUP, which is extensively used as a sweetener in SOFT DRINKS.

Starch Digestion

Starch digestion produces glucose. Digestion begins in the mouth with an enzyme (AMYLASE) in SALIVA; it is completed in the intestine by the combined action of pancreatic amylase, and yields fragments containing a pair of glucose units (maltose) and dextrins, composed of several glucose units. Intestinal enzymes (MALTASE, dextrinase) degrade these fragments to glucose, which is then rapidly absorbed by the small intestine. Depending on the form of starch and other ingredients of the meal, starch can be more or less completely converted to blood glucose from one to four hours after a meal.

The rate at which food liberates glucose and increases blood sugar can be compared to the rate from eating the sugar alone. Processed starches such as white bread, white rice, and instant mashed potatoes send blood glucose soaring almost as fast as sugar does. On the other hand, starch in whole foods like legumes is more slowly digested and does not cause a surge of blood sugar. Consequently, the pancreas does not need to release such a large amount of the hormone INSULIN to stimulate glucose utilization. Chronic high insulin levels can increase blood lipids.

Starch as an Additive

Corn is the primary source for commercial starch, followed by sorghum, wheat and rice, potato and ARROWROOT, among others. Waxy hybrid strains of corn and sorghum yield starches that range from almost completely amylose to those that are almost completely amylopectin, which have different uses. The tendency to gel upon cooking is caused by the presence of amylose. Some starches form gels that are more translucent than usual; others make puddings stiffer and give baked goods a velvety texture that stays fresh longer.

Starches can be modified chemically to create useful FOOD ADDITIVES. Treatment with alkali or acid yields GUMS and DEXTRINS, which are partially degraded starch. Cross-linked starches, chemically stabilized against acid and mechanical agitation, were discontinued voluntarily as food additives by the food industry when questions arose about their safety. "Derivatized" starches contain acidic groups such as ACETIC ACID, SUCCINIC ACID, or phosphate, which prevent starch molecules from clumping or crystallizing. Solutions of these starches are clearer and more viscous then untreated starch and are used in frozen foods as thickening agents. Most derivatized starches have not been exhaustively studied by lifetime feeding experiments. Previously, manufacturers of baby foods used modified starches extensively to improve consistency of product and to increase the nutrient value, but they have gradually moved away from adding starches. (See also CARBOHYDRATE METABOLISM; DIETARY GUIDELINES FOR AMERICANS; GLYCEMIC INDEX; STAPLE.)

Cummings, J. H. et al. "A New Look at Dietary Carbohydrate: Chemistry, Physiology and Health," *European Journal of Clinical Nutrition* 52 (1997): 1–7.

Hudnall, Marsha. "Pasta Makes You Fat Furor Raises the Question of Insulin Resistance," *Environmental Nutrition* 18, no. 5 (May 1995): 1, 6.

starch blockers Kidney bean proteins believed to curtail STARCH digestion in the INTESTINE. Starch blockers were marketed according to the belief that by eating them with meals, dieters could eat starchy foods without adding calories. In 1982 the U.S. Food and Drug Administration (FDA) classified starch blockers as drugs; tests indicated that starch blockers are not effective and cause gas, bloating, and DIARRHEA, and their sale was banned by the FDA in 1987. (See also CARBOHYDRATE METABOLISM; DIETING.)

starvation A condition due to chronic food deprivation characterized by tissue wasting. Starvation can occur due to unavailability of food; self-denial of food (FASTING); institutional restriction of food intake; or anorexia. Protein-calorie malnutrition ranges from MARASMUS, in which people do not get adequate calories, to KWASHIORKOR, in which they lack adequate protein although their diet supplies adequate calories. Anorexia may be caused by severe thiamin deficiency; KETOSIS (excessive KETONE BODIES in the blood); kidney failure; or an emotional aversion to food (ANOREXIA NERVOSA). Ketone bodies are water-soluble acid derivatives of fat, produced when massive fat breakdown occurs. Disorders of the digestive tract that can lead to starvation include: severe DIARRHEA, MALABSORPTION (such as CROHN'S DISEASE), vomiting, or surgical removal of part of the digestive tract. Severe malnutrition may accompany metabolic disorders such as DIABETES, wasting diseases like CANCER, or severe physical trauma.

Vulnerability to famine rests upon the degree of civil tranquility, adequacy of trained personnel, institutions and infrastructure for the production, distribution and storage of food, as well as the state of general economic development. When starvation affects entire populations, the result is a famine. Historically, war or crop failure due to poor weather or both have caused most famines. The unavailability of food due to natural catastrophes such as drought, flood, and earthquake, as well as to human causes such as war, civil disruption, and governmental mismanagement, reduces the food supply and leads to a decline in an entitlement to food. High food prices, unemployment, and loss of assets are symptoms of underlying problems. In a typical scenario experienced in regions of Africa, sequential years of crop failure produce increased agricultural prices, less farming activity, and a decline in employment of workers and farm laborers. The financially privileged class may hoard food from the poor, who are then forced to sell assets. HUNGER follows poverty with the ultimate outcome of increased mortality.

Effects of Starvation

Children, infants, and the elderly are the most susceptible to the effects of starvation because of their high rates of growth and/or small reserves of energy and tissue. Impaired mental development is particularly pronounced for children starved during the first years of life, and their growth may be permanently retarded. Many nutrients are required to support the normal function of the IMMUNE SYSTEM, and adults and children who have starved are more susceptible to infectious disease due to reduced immunity.

Signs and symptoms of starvation include weight loss and muscle wasting, ketosis, ketone body excretion in the urine, low blood pressure, edema, diarrhea, irritability, and smaller than normal growth and body weight.

Metabolic adaptations to starvation include an increased utilization of fat stores to spare muscle, and decreased BASAL METABOLIC RATE (metabolism required to maintain the body at rest) as the body adapts to lowered nutrient intake. Body temperature may be abnormally low. Muscle protein degradation continues at a slow rate to provide amino acids that are converted to BLOOD SUGAR. The brain and nervous system cannot use FAT as a fuel and rely upon this glucose for energy. Accumulated fatty acids in the liver are converted to ketone bodies, acids that are released into the bloodstream. As levels rise, ketone bodies can enter the brain, which then uses them to meet some of its energy needs. High blood levels of ketone bodies acidify the blood; when they are excreted in the urine this causes dehydration and loss of critical minerals (ELECTROLYTES). (See also ACIDOSIS; GLUCONEOGENESIS.)

stearic acid A common saturated FATTY ACID in animal fat. Stearic acid is classified as "saturated" because its carbon atoms cannot take up more hydrogen and it lacks double bonds. Stearic acid with 18 carbon atoms is a solid at room temperature and contributes to the hardness of animal fat. Unlike palmitic acid, stearic acid alone does not appear to raise blood CHOLESTEROL. However, stearic acid may promote blood clots more than other saturated fats; consequently, its relative safety has not been determined. In addition, food occurs as fatty acid mixtures, not isolated nutrients. Thus, saturated fats like BUTTER, SHORTENING, and even chocolate tend to raise cholesterol levels due to their content of saturated fatty acids. Additionally, fat is a calorie-rich nutrient, and excessive calories in processed foods contribute to problems of WEIGHT MANAGEMENT and OBESITY, said to be an American epidemic. Dietary recommendations generally call for decreasing fat consumption, especially saturated fat. (See also DIETARY GUIDELINES FOR AMERICANS; FAT METABOLISM; FOOD GUIDE PYRAMID; HEART DISEASE; VEGETABLE OIL.)

steatorrhea Smelly, fatty stools that may be tan or light colored. Steatorrhea indicates severe fat MALABSORPTION and/or fat maldigestion. Inadequate digestive enzymes from the pancreas or a blocked bile duct can lead to fatty stools because both pancreatic lipase and bile are needed for fat breakdown and absorption. Alternatively, fat malabsorption can be produced by conditions affecting the health of the small intestine, like CELIAC DISEASE and CROHN'S DISEASE. Deficiencies of fat-soluble vitamins may develop with fat malabsorption. Further weight loss and malnutrition can develop, leading to worsening malabsorption and malnutrition. (See also FAT DIGESTION.)

steroids A family of hormones related to CHOLESTEROL. Steroid HORMONES are produced by the ADRENAL GLANDS. Steroids are LIPIDS and, such as cholesterol, have an affinity for fatty materials. Steroid hormones include sex hormones, TESTOSTERONE and ESTROGEN; GLUCOCORTICOIDS, which regulate carbohydrate metabolism; and mineralocorticoids, like ALDOSTERONE, which regulate sodium and water excretion. Calcitriol, activated vitamin D_3, is another type of steroid hormone. (See also BILE; ENDOCRINE SYSTEM; FAT METABOLISM.)

sterol A family of fat-soluble materials (LIPIDS), of which CHOLESTEROL is the most prominent member. Cholesterol is a primary component of all membranes and is therefore essential for cell function and metabolism. Its metabolites (metabolic products) also serve important functions. BILE salts are made by the LIVER from cholesterol to aid FAT DIGESTION. In terms of chemical structure, sterols consist of interlocking rings and possess a hydroxyl group, making them ALCOHOLS. Ergosterol is a plant sterol that forms vitamin D_2, ERGOCALCIFEROL, when exposed to ultraviolet light. (See FORTIFICATION; MILK.)

Saint-John's-wort (*Hypericum perforatum*) A perennial herb native to Europe, North Africa, and Asia with oblong leaves and yellow flowers that bloom in midsummer. Saint-John's-wort has long been used for medicinal purposes in Europe, where its flowers were harvested around the time of a festival celebrating St. John the Baptist. It is thought that this is the derivation of the plant's name; *wort* means "plant" in Old English.

Ancient Romans used the herb to treat battle wounds. Medieval healers used it to treat people who suffered hallucinations and other mental disorders. In modern times the herb has been used to treat depression. Several European clinical studies indicated regular supplements of the herb were superior to placebo and as effective as antidepressant drugs such as Prozac in treating mild to moderate depression.

Saint-John's-wort first appeared in the United States as an herbal antidepressant in the mid-1990s, and its popularity soared amid reports of its mood enhancing abilities. There have been conflicting reports about the herb's effectiveness in treating major depression. A recent study found that Saint-John's-wort could interfere with the effectiveness of other drugs, including some that are used to lower blood cholesterol and treat cancer and AIDS. There is also some concern that the herb can interfere with general anesthesia. Before undergoing surgery, patients should always tell their doctors if they have been using Saint-John's-wort. This herb may be unsafe for pregnant or breast-feeding women.

Linde, K. et al. "St John's Wort for Depression: An Overview and Meta-analysis of Randomized Clinical Trials," *British Medical Journal* 313 (1996): 258–261.

stock Extracts of foods that form the basis of soups, gravies, and sauces. Traditionally, MEAT from older animals and mature vegetables like CARROTS, CABBAGE, TURNIPS, or BEANS are heated to extract juices and flavors. Meat is trimmed of excess fat, vegetables are cleaned and even blended. Bones with marrow are used for gravies and sauces. Appropriate spices include allspice, peppercorn, coriander, celery seed, and bay leaf.

stomach A long J-shaped pouch that receives swallowed, masticated food from the MOUTH via the ESOPHAGUS. The stomach lies in the upper part of the abdominal cavity under the diaphragm. Muscles encircle the stomach and run lengthwise and obliquely to make the stomach one of the strongest internal organs. The muscles squeeze and churn the pulverized food and mix it thoroughly with digestive juices. Stomach muscle contraction produces PERISTALSIS, a movement that propels food down the DIGESTIVE TRACT. Without food, the stomach compresses to the size of a large sausage with large folds called rugae, which allow the stomach to expand after a large meal.

Glands in the stomach wall secrete a mixture of stomach acid, a strong mineral acid called hydrochloric acid, and a DIGESTIVE ENZYME called PEPSIN to begin protein DIGESTION. Stomach acid creates a low pH required for optimal activity of this enzyme. Chief cells produce an inactive form of pepsin, which is activated by stomach acid. Acid-producing cells are called parietal cells. Stomach acid softens and denatures proteins, easing their digestion, and it sterilizes food, killing many potentially dangerous microorganisms. The stomach's thick mucus forms a layer that protects the lining against stomach acid, which maintains a strongly acidic environment. The stomach wall is impermeable to most nutrients, and usually they do not reach the blood until they reach the intestine. The stomach can absorb water, alcohol, electrolytes, aspirin, and certain drugs. An alcohol oxidizing system in men's stomachs is more prevalent than in women's, which partially explains why men are more often able to drink more alcohol than women without ill effects. Parietal cells also produce INTRINSIC FACTOR, a vitamin B_{12}-binding protein that is required for intestinal absorption of this vitamin.

The lower part of the stomach is called the pylorus. Here, hormone-producing (enteroendocrine) cells secrete GASTRIN, a hormone that stimulates and increases gastrointestinal tract peristalsis. A pyloric sphincter (valve) retains food long enough for partial digestion to occur in the stomach, then waves of contraction squeeze small amounts of liquefied food (CHYME) into the upper region of the small intestine (DUODENUM).

Secretion of gastric juice is regulated by gastrin and by nerve stimulation. In the "reflex phase" (cephalic phase) of nerve stimulation, the sight, taste, smell, or thought of food can initiate a nerve impulse via the feeding center of the brain (HYPOTHALAMUS); this in turn activates the PARASYMPATHETIC NERVOUS SYSTEM to prepare the body for feeding. In the "gastric phase," foods that fill the stomach will activate regions in the stomach wall, which relay nerve signals back to the brain that, in turn, activate gastric secretion. Partially digested protein and CAFFEINE also stimulate gastrin production. Secretion of gastrin stops when the pH drops to 2 (more acidic). This "feedback" system normally maintains the acidic pH in the stomach without over-producing acid.

The net effect of food in the small intestine is inhibition of gastrin secretion. Certain intestinal hormones can block gastrin secretion. The stomach empties its contents into the duodenum in one to four hours. Carbohydrate-rich foods leave more quickly than fat-containing foods. The rate is limited by the amount of chyme the small intestine can process. A high sugar content in beverages (greater than 10 percent glucose) slows gastric emptying. This is a consideration when attempting to consume fluids to rehydrate the body. (See also EXERCISE; *HELICOBACTER PYLORI;* SPORT DRINKS.)

stomach acid (hydrochloric acid) The very strong mineral acid, hydrochloric acid, produced by the stomach. Stomach acid is secreted by parietal cells of the gastric glands lining the wall of the stomach. Hydrochloric acid normally maintains stomach pH between 1.5 and 2.5, an acidic environment that can sterilize food and activate pepsinogen, the inactive form of PEPSIN. This enzyme initiates protein digestion in the stomach. Stomach acid also maintains an acidic environment required for pepsin activity. The mixture of food particles, digestive enzymes, and acid forms an acidic mixture called CHYME, which is released into the upper small intestine (DUODENUM). Chyme stimulates secretion of alkaline BICARBONATE to neutralize the acid. Enzymes produced further down the gastrointestinal tract do not break down food (to release bound minerals like CALCIUM and IRON) efficiently when there is inadequate stomach acid. Chewing food stimulates stomach acid production via the nervous system. The process requires 15 to 30 minutes to be fully activated. Gulping down a meal does not provide adequate time to digest food completely.

Low stomach acid production is called HYPOCHLORHYDRIA. Stomach acid production declines with age; low stomach acidity is associated with diabetes mellitus, thyroid imbalance, ECZEMA, gallbladder disease, OSTEOPOROSIS, RHEUMATOID ARTHRITIS, food allergy, and FOOD SENSITIVITY. Without adequate stomach acid, intestinal flora can become imbalanced, which increases susceptibility to disease-producing microorganisms like yeast (candida) or parasites. The stomach possesses a protective mucous layer to prevent damage to the lining. Rarely, acid can break through the barrier and cause sores (ULCERS). The precise mechanisms are not known. (See also ACHLORHYDRIA; AGING; DIGESTION.)

stone age diet (paleolithic diet) Studies of hunter-gatherer societies as well as studies of paleolithic sites have yielded information regarding the diet of our ancestors long before the domestication of plants and animals. These studies are prompted by the observation that modern hunter-gatherers are apparently free of HYPERTENSION, HEART DISEASE, DIABETES MELLITUS, and certain CANCERS, diseases all too common in industrialized nations.

Evidence suggests that paleolithic peoples foraged and hunted, and ate nuts, fruits, berries, and roots that are available by season. GRAINS and dairy products like MILK and CHEESE were unavailable. These became a major part of the diet only when agriculture and animal husbandry began, between 5,000 to 10,000 years ago. The stone age diet probably consisted of about 35 percent MEAT and 65 percent VEGETABLES. This diet was rich in PROTEIN, but the meat was lean and contained essential fatty acids. The FAT of game animals contains two to five times more polyunsaturated fat per gram than livestock. The opposite is true for the typical U.S. diet. The fat of game animals contains a higher percentage of the essential fatty acids of the omega-3 family, which help protect against clogged arteries and the formation of blood clots. The omega-3 fatty acids therefore lower the risk of cardiovascular disease; long-chain omega-3 fatty acids like EICOSAPENTAENOIC ACID are especially low in domestic animals.

Paleolithic people probably ate a greater variety of vegetables and plant products than obtainable in industrialized societies until the development of post-World War II supermarkets and modern food production distribution networks. The stone age diet contributed many nutrients and a high percentage of FIBER. Consequently, prehistoric people are believed to have consumed more VITAMINS, especially VITAMIN C, more CALCIUM and other minerals, more high-quality protein, and more polyunsaturated fats and oils than are in the diets of industrialized societies. The diet provided adequate IRON, FOLIC ACID, and VITAMIN B_{12}, and the amount of CHOLESTEROL was about the same as in present day Western diets. (See also FOOD GUIDE PYRAMID; WHEAT.)

strawberry (*Fragaria spp.*) The juicy fruit of a herbaceous plant and a member of the rose family. Strawberries are native to both the Old World and the New World. Strawberries lead the world production of berries and berry-like fruit. The United States remains a leading producer of strawberries, and nearly 80 percent of the U.S. crop comes from California. Strawberries are grown in all states and are the most popular berries, containing more VITAMIN C than most other berries. About one-third of the crop is frozen. Strawberries are also processed as jam, fruit-flavored beverages and other products. They are added fresh to cereals, cheesecake, fruit salads, custards, crepes, puddings, ice cream, and milkshakes. The nutrient content of 1 cup (149 g) of fresh strawberries is: 45 calories; protein, 0.9 g; carbohydrate, 10.5 g; fiber, 3.3 g; fat, 0.6 g; vitamin C, 85 mg; thiamin, 0.03 mg; riboflavin, 0.1 mg; niacin, 0.34 mg.

stress The adjustment of the body's mechanisms to adverse conditions or changes in the environment. Stimuli ("stressors") run the gamut of disturbances from heat, cold, injury, and environmental pollutants, to glare from video screens and bacterial toxins. Psychological stress relates to coping with demands of work, relationships, and the demands of life in general. Coping with stress relies on the NERVOUS SYSTEM and the closely-linked ENDOCRINE SYSTEM (hormone secreting system).

Alarm Reaction

The alarm reaction or FIGHT OR FLIGHT RESPONSE is the first reaction to a stressor. Stimuli rapidly mobilize the body to defend against danger. The brain and nervous system regulate fast responses of the body to changes in the environment within seconds; the endocrine system regulates longer responses (minutes to hours) by releasing hormones. The region of the brain called the HYPOTHALAMUS activates the sympathetic nervous system, the portion of the nervous system that controls involuntary response to stress, to adapt the body to meet a challenge. The brain also stimulates the adrenal glands to release hormones like EPINEPHRINE (adrenaline) that support adaptation by increasing ENERGY and by decreasing nonessential functions such as DIGESTION and urine production.

The heart rate increases to supply oxygen and GLUCOSE (blood sugar) to the muscles and the brain, which must be very alert. Epinephrine and norepinephrine, hormones from the adrenal medulla, stimulate the breakdown of carbohydrate reserves (GLYCOGEN) in the liver to increase BLOOD SUGAR. Sympathetic nerve impulses, supplemented by hormones, prolong typical responses of the sympathetic nervous system-constricted blood vessels in skin and viscera; dilated blood vessels of the heart and skeletal muscle; increased sweating; expanded bronchial tubes; decreased production of digestive enzymes; and increased rate of breathing to bring additional oxygen to muscle.

Resistance Reaction

The second stage of the stress response is called the resistance reaction. The resistance reaction represents a long-term adjustment to stress, after the flight or fight response has worn off, in order to meet emotional crises and perform tasks. It is initiated by hormones secreted by the hypothalamus. Chronic stress causes higher than normal levels of stress hormones. Energy stockpiles are broken down to provide blood glucose, and long-term building and maintenance are slowed. The hypothalamus secretes corticotropin-releasing hormone (CRH), growth hormone-releasing hormone and thyrotropin-releasing hormone (TRH).

CRH stimulates the pituitary to increase the secretion of ADRENOCORTICOTROPIC HORMONE (ACTH), the hormone that stimulates the adrenal cortex to secrete steroid hormones. MINERALOCORTICOIDS increase sodium conservation by the kidneys, leading to water retention and elevated blood pressure. GLUCOCORTICOIDS increase protein degradation and amino acid conversion to blood glucose; reduce INFLAMMATION; and inhibit the immune response, especially production of antibodies like secretory IgA. This antibody, when released by the small intestine, protects against the onslaught of foreign materials presented in foods daily. Chronic overexposure to glucocorticoids leads to fatigue and muscle wasting, fragile bones, ulcers, impotence, infertility, and lowered resistance to disease. It may worsen neurological disorders. Growth hormone stimulates the liver to increase the concentration of blood sugar and to increase fat degradation. TRH stimulates the thyroid gland to secrete thyroxine, which increases the basal metabolic rate and energy production.

The excessive activity of adrenal glands over time can lead to fatigue, susceptibility to food allergies, high blood pressure, elevated blood cholesterol and blood sugar. If the resistance stage fails to combat a stressor, the adrenal glands may become "exhausted" due to constant demands. Prolonged, excessive stress places a high demand on the endocrine system, the circulatory system, and the immune system. In this situation there may be little reserve capacity to meet additional challenges. When glucocorticoids are depleted, blood glucose levels fall and the body cannot receive enough energy. Loss of potassium also contributes to exhaustion. CHRONIC FATIGUE can result, as well as DEPRESSION and anxiety.

Health Consequences of Chronic Stress

Stress is linked to a number of diseases, among them are angina (heart pain due to limited oxygen supply); GASTRITIS (inflamed stomach); ulcerative COLITIS (ulcerated and inflamed colon); irritable bowel syndrome; PEPTIC ULCERS; ASTHMA; autoimmune disease (such as RHEUMATOID ARTHRITIS); migraine headaches; CARDIOVASCULAR DISEASE; adult onset diabetes; depression; and PREMENSTRUAL SYNDROME. Stress hormones may damage arterial linings and may also temporarily increase blood cholesterol and blood pressure. Psychological stress is a risk factor for developing viral respiratory infections and for developing symptoms of the common cold. Hypotheses explaining these phenomena hinge upon the interaction of the central nervous system and the immune system.

Stress Management and Recovery from Stress

In the recovery stage, the body readjusts to normal functioning. Hormonal and metabolic equilibrium is reestablished. Lifestyle changes incorporating sound nutrition can significantly speed this stage by lowering the effects of stress on the body. Relaxation methods such as meditation, biofeedback, guided imagery, prayer, yoga, and self-hypnosis can be important components of a stress management program. Such strategies favor the dominance of the parasympathetic nervous system, which counterbalances the sympathetic nervous system. Expressing feelings and pent up emotions can help maintain health. Writing in a notebook or recording thoughts/feelings on a tape can improve immune function. Relaxation methods tend to normalize digestion, breathing, blood pressure, heart rate, and nervous respiration, and return blood sugar levels to a normal physiologic range. Acknowledgment of emotions seems important in improving the lives of some cancer patients. Psychological intervention may help cancer patients deal with stress, enhance their immune system and thus improve long-term survival.

EXERCISE is a physical stressor, although regular exercise reduces the risk of chronic stress-related disease and inability to cope with stress. Exercise improves cardiovascular function and oxygen delivery to tissues and reduces epinephrine secretion in response to stress; it improves nutrient utilization by tissues and increases endocrine function; it also elevates mood.

There is agreement that physical stress—injury, surgery or extreme temperatures—increases nutrient needs. Whether psychological stress increases nutrient needs is controversial. Stress creates a greater turnover of water-soluble vitamins. The level of vitamin C can fluctuate depending on the degree of physical and emotional stress. A variety of nutrients support adrenal gland function. Vitamin C, VITAMIN B_6, ZINC, MAGNESIUM and PANTOTHENIC ACID, and the amino acid TYROSINE are required to synthesize adrenal hormones. A deficiency of pantothenic acid causes adrenal atrophy. This vitamin occurs in whole grains, legumes like lentils, vegetables like sweet potatoes, tomatoes, broccoli, salmon, and liver. Adequate POTASSIUM is important in maintaining normal adrenal function. Bovine glandular extracts have been used therapeutically to control the physiologic imbalances of chronic stress. Chinese GINSENG seems to help balance the body in the face of challenges by stressors. (See also HOMEOSTASIS; PLACEBO; TOLERANCE TO TOXIC MATERIALS.)

Bremner, J. D. "Does Stress Damage the Brain?" *Society of Biological Psychiatry* 45 (1999): 797–805.

stroke Damage to the brain due to interrupted blood flow. Loss of consciousness is often followed by more or less severe paralysis, depending upon the severity of oxygen deprivation to brain tissue. Strokes can usually be traced to preexisting conditions such as HYPERTENSION (high blood pressure) and diseases of the arterial walls. In cerebral thrombosis, normal blood circulation in the brain is blocked by a blood clot. ATHEROSCLEROSIS leads to clogged arteries where blood clots can form. Cerebral embolism refers to arterial blockage due to a traveling blood clot or a trapped air bubble. A leaking or burst artery can cause cerebral hemorrhage. An aneurysm or bulge in an arterial wall can burst with overexertion, overeating, extreme stress, or violent coughing. A complete physical checkup may detect underlying conditions, including hypertension.

The risk for stroke increases with advanced age, heavy cigarette smoking, diabetes, present angina or history of HEART ATTACK, use of oral contraceptives in susceptible women, in addition to high blood pressure. Warning episodes of stroke include sudden dizziness, unsteadiness, numbness, and difficulty in speaking. Typically, these symptoms come and go quickly, indicative of temporary insufficient blood flow to the brain. The following symptoms may indicate an impending stroke: sudden temporary weakness of face, arm, or leg; temporary loss of speech, or the understanding of speech; bouts of double vision; loss of vision or dimness in one eye; momentary blackout; confusion; personality changes. There are many variations. A person may experience many transient episodes (ischemia) without ever getting a stroke, while another may have a single episode followed by a permanent, serious attack. A person who has experienced transient ischemia needs a complete medical checkup.

Reducing overall fat intake and increasing unsaturated fats is recommended, especially for people with elevated blood CHOLESTEROL, high blood pressure or a family history of CARDIOVASCULAR DISEASE, especially stroke. Fatty fish like SALMON provide OMEGA-3 FATTY ACIDS, EICOSAPENTAENOIC ACID (EPA) and docosahex aenoic acid (DHA), which can reduce BLOOD CLOTTING and reduce the risk of heart attack and cerebral thrombosis. Inuits who consume large amounts of marine lipids have a low incidence of heart attack, although they experience a higher incidence of cerebral hemorrhage, likely due to decreased blood clotting ability. Adequate POTASSIUM can lessen the tendency for SODIUM to raise blood pressure in susceptible people. The addition of potassium-rich foods such as fruit and vegetables can reduce the risk of fatal stroke. MAGNESIUM deficiency is linked to sudden heart attack, angina, arrhythmia (irregular heartbeat), high blood pressure, and stroke. Fruits and vegetables, as well as whole grains, supply ANTIOXIDANTS, such as VITAMIN C, VITAMIN E, and FLAVONOIDS, which reduce damage to the nervous system caused by temporary interruption of blood flow to the brain (STROKE). In general, population studies indicate that people who eat more fruits and vegetables suffer fewer coronary problems and strokes. (See also AGING; CARDIOVASCULAR DISEASE; CORONARY ARTERY DISEASE.)

strontium A metallic element, in the same chemical family as CALCIUM and MAGNESIUM. The biological behavior of strontium resembles that of calcium. Strontium occurs in high-calcium foods like MILK and milk products. It is stored in BONES and TEETH. Notoriety surrounding strontium focuses on the radioactive isotope, strontium-90, a product of nuclear fallout. This radioactive element is stored in the bones of all vertebrates.

Strontium is considered a nonessential nutrient for humans. Omission of strontium from a purified diet for experimental animals led to slowed growth. The incidence of dental caries has been found to be lower in areas with high strontium levels in drinking water. Chronic consumption of highly refined foods, deficient in strontium and other nutrients, correlates with decreased bone strength. Ingesting pharmacologic doses (gram amounts) of strontium for periods up to three years has been reported to reduce bone pain and increase bone density in a group of osteoporotic patients. Typical U.S. consumption is several milligrams daily. (See also OSTEOPOROSIS.)

subclinical nutrient deficiency A mild form of a nutrient deficiency that is not readily detected by usual clinical means because of the lack of well-defined signs and symptoms. Suboptimal nutrition contributes to decreased organ reserve. With less reserves, nutrient supply may be inadequate to mount a defense. The IMMUNE SYSTEM, the NERVOUS SYSTEM, and the ENDOCRINE SYSTEM (hormone-producing system) rely on many vitamins and minerals for maintenance and optimal functioning. The table on page 606 lists *possible* subclinical nutrient deficiencies and chronic conditions and diseases.

The recognition of subclinical nutrient deficiencies forms a basis for preventative intervention through dietary modification and lifestyle changes. Long before the appearance of a full-blown nutritional disease or conditions related to severe nutrient deficiency like SCURVY, RICKETS, PELLAGRA ANEMIA, or EMACIATION, a variety of subtle indicators warn of impending problems. Anemia is the last stage of iron deficiency. Certain lab tests can detect these early signs of iron deficiency: elevated serum TRANSFERRIN, low serum iron (total iron binding capacity), and low iron saturation. An early symptom of a nutrient deficiency could be fatigue.

The development of accurate methods of measuring nutrient status (nutritional adequacy) has become a major focus of nutritional medicine. Serum folic acid, vitamin B_{12}, and vitamin E can be measured. Functional tests for red blood cell enzymes can be used to assess thiamin, and selenium status. Measurement of minerals such as magnesium, ZINC, and MANGANESE in white blood cells and potassium and COPPER in red blood cells are often useful parameters. (See also MALNUTRITION; NUTRITIONAL STATUS; SIGNS.)

subcutaneous fat The layer of fatty tissue lying directly under the SKIN. A subcutaneous FAT layer is present in all well-nourished people where it serves as an insulation to protect individuals from heat loss in cold environments. The degree of fat deposition varies with gender, dietary choices, metabolic efficiency in converting nutrients to fat, as well as in overall body build. (See also ADIPOSE TISSUE.)

substrate A substance that is converted by an ENZYME to its product. Substrates can be simple molecules or as complex as POLYSACCHARIDES, PROTEINS, LIPIDS, and DNA, the genetic material of the cell. (See also METABOLITE.)

succinic acid A food additive and common intermediate in the KREB'S CYCLE, major energy-producing pathway of the body. Succinic acid is present in vegetables like beets and broccoli, fruit like rhubarb, and in meat and cheese. It is sometimes added to foods to impart a distinctive flavor. When ingested, succinic acid is readily used as fuel and is considered a safe additive. There is no evidence that supplemental forms of succinic acid (succinates) increase energy production or boost athletic performance as sometimes claimed. (See also FOOD ADDITIVES.)

succistearin A synthetic FOOD ADDITIVE used as an EMULSIFIER in VEGETABLE SHORTENING. Succistearin contains SUCCINIC ACID and the fatty acid STEARIC ACID. Succistearin is broken down to its components, which are burned for ENERGY. It is considered a safe additive.

sucrase An enzyme of the small intestine that digests SUCROSE (table sugar) to its simple sugar components, GLUCOSE and FRUCTOSE. This enzyme is necessary because sucrose cannot be absorbed by the intestine, while each of these simple sugars is readily assimilated. (See also CARBOHYDRATE METABOLISM; DIGESTION.)

sucrose (table sugar) The most common dietary SUGAR and SWEETENER. Chemically, sucrose is classified as a disaccharide, a chemical combination of the simple sugars GLUCOSE and FRUCTOSE, and represents the broad family of sugars, the simple CARBOHYDRATE. Sucrose is widely distributed among higher plants, but it is obtained commercially from sugar beets and sugarcane. More than 60 percent of refined sucrose comes from sugarcane (*Saccharum officinarum*), a jointed grass cultivated in tropical and semitropical regions of the world. Sugarcane may have originated in New Guinea. Currently, India, Brazil, Cuba, China, and Mexico are major producers of canesugar. At harvest, sugarcane contains about 15 percent sucrose. The sugar beet (*Beta vulgaris*) is a biennial that produces a root containing 13 percent to 22 percent sugar. Regions of the former Soviet Union, the United States, France, Germany, and Poland are major producers of sugar beets.

Types of Sugar Products

Raw sugar contains about 96 percent sucrose. It is produced by juice obtained from either sugarcane or sugar beets. The remaining syrup after sugar crystallization is called MOLASSES. A crude molasses can be recrystallized to remove more sugar. The remaining syrup is called BLACKSTRAP MOLASSES, a by-product of sugar manufacture. Repeated crystallization and decolorization ultimately yields highly purified sucrose as table sugar.

Granulated table sugar is the final product of sugar refining and contains 99.9 percent pure sucrose. Powdered sugar represents finely ground crystals such as confectioner's sugar. Powdered sugar is usually packaged with cornstarch to prevent caking.

Brown sugar represents the sugar that can be crystallized from syrup once the white sugar has been removed. Some brown sugar is made by adding molasses to white sugar. Brown sugar is not usually made from sugar beet molasses because it has a strong flavor.

TURBINADO SUGAR is partially refined sugar resembling raw sugar with large and coarse granules. It is about 95 percent pure sucrose and is no more natural than table sugar because it has gone through all but the last steps in refining.

CARAMELIZED SUGAR is used as a coloring agent. It is prepared by heating sucrose without water until it turns brown, then water is added to create a syrup.

INVERT SUGAR is the product of hydrolysis of sucrose. It contains equal amounts of fructose (levulose) and glucose (dextrose). It resists crystallization and prolongs freshness of baked goods and confectionery items.

Consumption

From 1970 to 1995 sugar consumption in the United States increased by about 22 percent. According to the U.S. Department of Agriculture, people who consume 2,000 calories a day should eat no more than about 10 teaspoons of added sugar. Recent surveys show that the average American consumes about 20 teaspoons of sugar each day. Sugar now accounts for 16 percent of the calories consumed by the average American and 20 percent of the calories taken in by teenagers.

A sharp increase in the consumption of soft drinks, which contain about 12 teaspoons of sugar per 12 oz. can, is one of the reasons sugar consumption has risen so dramatically. The per capita consumption of soft drinks has doubled since 1974.

Current dietary guidelines recommend eating sugars only in moderation. The FOOD GUIDE PYRAMID recommends eating sugar and sugary foods sparingly. The U.S. Dietary Goals for Healthy Americans (1972) called for reducing by one-half the amount of sugar consumed in the typical American diet and substituting complex carbohydrate as found in whole grains, vegetables, bread, and pasta. The more recent Dietary Guidelines for Americans recommended avoiding too much sugar, including sweets and soft drinks.

Effects on Health

As with any nutrient, whether sugar is desirable or not depends upon the amount eaten, the types of other foods eaten, and the general state of health of the individual. On one hand many people can tolerate sugar, and moderate amounts of sugar are safe for people in good health. Although diabetics have shunned sugar, recent research suggests that a little sugar eaten with high complex carbohydrates as part of a low-fat meal can be tolerated if it replaces other calories.

On the other hand, table sugar is highly purified and contributes only calories to the diet; other nutrients like FIBER, VITAMINS, or MINERALS are not present. Because table sugar is one of the most common FOOD ADDITIVES, it is partially responsible for the low nutrient density of convenience and fast foods, processed foods, and soft drinks. Sucrose is hidden in spaghetti, frozen dinners, BREAKFAST CEREALS, bread, KETCHUP, and canned goods. It pushes out nutrient-rich food from the diet and therefore can contribute to overnutrition and excess weight. There is general agreement that sugar consumption increases tooth decay. Bacteria in the mouth live on carbohydrate and produce acids that erode tooth enamel.

Sugar can increase blood fat. Perhaps 20 percent of Americans are sensitive to sugar, that is, sugar will increase their risk of heart disease because of elevated serum TRIGLYCERIDES (fat). Diabetics often have a weight problem, and eating table sugar will not help dealing with this issue. In addition, blood fat tends to increase in some patients with non-insulin-dependent diabetes with increased carbohydrate intake. Such patients should avoid table sugar.

POSSIBLE SUBCLINICAL NUTRIENT DEFICIENCIES ASSOCIATED WITH CHRONIC CONDITIONS

Condition	Possible Deficiency
Cardiovascular Disease	Magnesium, vitamin E, selenium, essential fatty acids, carnitine, folic acid, taurine
Hypertension	Magnesium, coenzyme Q_{10}
Osteoporosis	Copper, magnesium, manganese, folic acid, boron, calcium, zinc, vitamin B_6, vitamin C, vitamin K, vitamin D
Cancer (various forms)	Vitamin E, selenium, vitamin C, carotenoids, folic acid, thiamin, vitamin A, vitamin B_6, vitamin E, calcium, copper
Diabetes	Chromium, niacin, thiamin, vitamin B_6, vitamin E, calcium, magnesium, manganese, zinc, coenzyme Q_{10}, essential fatty acids
Hypertension	Magnesium, coenzyme Q_{10}, potassium, vitamin C, calcium, essential fatty acids
Chronic Infection	B complex, vitamin C, vitamin A, vitamin E, zinc, copper, iron
Depression	Folic acid, vitamin B_6, riboflavin, thiamin, vitamin C, vitamin B_{12}, calcium, copper, iron, magnesium, potassium
Cataract (macular degeneration)	Vitamin E, vitamin C, carotenoids, zinc
Neuropathy	Vitamin B_{12}, folic acid, thiamin, niacin, vitamin B_6, vitamin E, zinc
Birth Defects	Folic acid
Chronic Fatigue	Vitamin B_{12} and other B vitamins, magnesium, zinc, copper, chromium, manganese, iron, essential fatty acids

Sugar is not a leading cause of obesity. Studies have found that lean people tend to eat more sugar but less fat than obese people. Fat contains more calories per teaspoon (36 vs. 16 for sucrose), and dietary fat is more efficiently converted to body fat than carbohydrate. Surplus calories, regardless of source, increase body weight. Cakes, pies, ice cream, chocolate, and other sweets derive most of their calories from fat, not sugar, and surplus calories, not sugar per se, cause weight gain.

Craving of sweet foods is a common phenomena, perhaps genetically determined. Craving sweet, high-fat foods could involve a similar mechanism as addictive drugs. Baby rats tolerate pain better after eating fatty, sweet foods. While some individuals crave sugar and carbohydrate, more frequently people crave sweet-fat foods like ice cream, chocolate, or cookies. The most uncontrollable food cravings affect bulimics. When some people eat sugar and carbohydrate, they often feel calm and become sleepy. Ingestion of sugar may raise the level of a brain chemical called SEROTONIN, which diminishes pain and has a calming effect. Thus, sugar could theoretically operate as an antidepressant. According to this hypothesis, overeating sweets can be a method of coping with stressful situations and emotional issues.

The relationship between sugar and hyperactivity is a controversial area. A number of earlier reports pointed to a relationship between consumption of sugary foods and hyperactivity or disruptive behavior in susceptible children. However, several studies have shown there is little or no connection between sugar consumption and behavior. Nevertheless, limiting children's consumption of sugary foods such as doughnuts and drinks such as sweetened fruit juices can have many positive effects: reducing tooth decay, lowering the risk of obesity, and increasing the consumption of more nutritious foods that offer a variety of vitamins and minerals, not just fats and sugars.

Food Labels

The terms *sugar free* and *no sugar added* on food labels may not mean "low calorie." These terms mean that table sugar (sucrose) has not been used in making the product. Other calorie-containing sweeteners have been used: SORBITOL, fructose, HONEY, and CORN SYRUP are possibilities. Sorbitol can affect blood sugar, though at a slower rate than sucrose. Diabetics should obtain professional advice before switching to sorbitol-sweetened foods. Sugar-free products may be sweetened with artificial sweeteners such as ACESULFAME-K, SACCHARIN, and ASPARTAME to lower the calorie content. Only diabetics have a justifiable medical need for artificial sweeteners.

Sucrose in Typical Sugar-rich Foods

12 oz. sugar-containing cola drink	8 tsp
12 oz. chocolate malt shake	18 tsp
8 oz. eggnog	6 tsp
average cinnamon roll	8 tsp
brownie	4 tsp
chocolate cupcake with fudge icing	14 tsp
small serving sugar-containing fruit gelatin dessert	4.5 tsp
cup vanilla ice cream	7.5 tsp
piece apple pie	15 tsp
2 oz. candy bar	9 tsp
2 oz. milk chocolate	8 tsp
cup sugar-coated cereal	8 tsp
baking-powder biscuit, small	4 tsp
white flour pancake, plain	2.5 tsp
hard roll	4.5 tsp

(See also BULEMIA NERVOSA; CARBOHYDRATE METABOLISM; DIABETES MELLITUS; DIGESTION; OBESITY; PROCESSED FOOD; TEETH).

Wolraich, M. L. et al. "Effects of Diets High in Sucrose or Aspartame on the Behavior and Cognitive Performance of Children," *New England Journal of Medicine* 330 (1994): 301–307.

sucralose (Splenda) A "high intensity" artificial sweetener approved by the U.S. Food and Drug Administration (FDA) in April 1998. Splenda, a white crystalline powder that dissolves in water, is 600 times sweeter than sugar. Splenda is produced in the lab by replacing parts of the sugar molecule with chlorine atoms, so that the vast majority of the resulting compound is not absorbed by the body. Unlike other sweeteners, it passes straight through the body without being digested—somewhat like the OLESTRA product Olean.

The FDA has approved Splenda for use in almost every kind of processed food, including soda, ice cream, baked goods, jellies, chewing gum, puddings, and fillings. It also can be used by consumers as a tabletop sweetener to add directly to foods. The new sweetener is also safe for diabetics, the FDA says, after it spent more than a decade deciding whether to approve the new sweetener. The FDA reviewed 110 studies in animals and people to verify its safety and reported that long-term studies of extremely high doses found no evidence of cancer, birth defects, or immune system problems. Splenda is sold in more than 25 countries, including Canada; millions of consumers around the world have been using the product since 1991.

sucrose polyester See OLESTRA.

sugar See NATURAL SWEETENERS; SUCROSE.

sugar beet See SUCROSE.

sugarcane See SUCROSE.

sugar-free foods See SUCROSE.

sugarless gum See CHEWING GUM.

sulfites (sulfiting agents, sodium sulfite, potassium and sodium metabisulfite, potassium-sodium bisulfite, sulfur dioxide) Sulfur based FOOD ADDITIVES used as PRESERVATIVES added to prevent discoloration and spoilage of FRUIT and vegetables as well as PROCESSED FOODS. Restaurant foods and salad bars previously treated raw vegetables and fruits with sulfites, but this is now forbidden by federal regulations because so many consumers are allergic to the preservative. Because sulfites can still be added to canned products, salad bars may still serve canned foods containing sulfites. Sulfites also occur in many medications.

Foods that may legally contain sulfites include POTATOES (raw, frozen, or as potato chips); MUSHROOMS (canned or raw); salad mixes (unless specifically noted otherwise); vegetables and fruits (canned, frozen, or dried); canned, frozen or dried shrimp, fish, clams, crabs, lobster, and oysters; and vinegar and cider. Grapes are gassed with sulfur dioxide approximately once a week after they are picked, so they may contain significant sulfites.

Condiments may contain sulfites (relishes, salad dressing, pickled pepper, sauerkraut and avocado dips). Sulfites may also be present in beverages (wine, wine coolers, beer, cordials, cocktail mixes, and lemon and grape juices) and baked goods (pizzas, cookies, crackers, pie crusts, and tortillas). About one in every 100 Americans is sensitive to sulfites; most of these people have asthma and allergies. Symptoms of sulfite sensitivity include nausea, headache, skin rash, swelling, flushing, and diarrhea. Severe reaction can lead to asthmatic attacks and unconsciousness. Sulfites are risky additives; they have killed highly sensitive individuals by anaphylactic shock. Patients should notify their dentists if they have experienced problems with sulfites because they are often used to preserve local anesthetics. Some sulfite sensitive people find relief of their symptoms with the supplemented trace mineral molybdenum.

Lester, M. R. "Sulfite Sensitivity: Significance in Human Health," *Journal of the American College of Nutrition,* 14:3 (1995): 229–232.

sulforaphane A sulfur-containing compound found in the cabbage family and in other vegetables that helps protect against cancer-causing agents. Sulforaphane is classified as an ISOTHIOCYANATE. These compounds occur in BROCCOLI, CAULIFLOWER, mustard greens, green ONIONS, and BRUSSELS SPROUTS as well as in horseradish. Population studies have shown that vegetables of the cabbage family afford protection against some forms of cancer. In general the mechanisms are not known. Isothiocyanates and sulforaphane in particular guard against cancer. Recent research suggests that sulforaphane increases the production of enzyme systems (called phase 2 enzymes) in the liver that detoxify reactive, potentially damaging molecules so that they can be flushed out of the body, thus blocking cancer induction and tumor formation. Sulforaphane is classified as a monofunctional inducer of liver enzymes, meaning that this substance increases the levels of the second stage of enzymatic detoxication (phase 2) and not those of the first stage (phase 1). Bifunctional inducers increase both phase 1 and phase 1 enzymes. Monofunctional inducers are safer than bifunctional inducers because activating phase 1 enzymes can produce reactive chemicals that can be mutagens and carcinogens (cancer-causing agents). Identification of other nonnutrients and the roles they play are actively being investigated. Researchers have discovered that sulforaphane kills *HELICOBACTER PYLORI*, a bacteria that causes stomach ulcers and stomach cancer, in mice. Scientists hope to duplicate these results in human studies. Current dietary guidelines recommend daily consumption of five or more servings of fruit and vegetables every day. Green and yellow vegetables are particularly important (See also BETA-CAROTENE; CRUCIFEROUS VEGETABLES; FOOD PYRAMID.)

sulfur A nonmetal element essential for life. The body contains 140 g of sulfur, primarily in the form of the sulfur-containing amino acids, METHIONINE and CYSTEINE, which function as essential protein building blocks. Proteins that require large amounts of these amino acids occur in hair, nails, and skin, whose toughness is largely due to strands of KERATIN, a protein that contains 6 percent sulfur. In proteins cysteine often links up with an adjacent cysteine unit to yield CYSTINE, an important structural crosslink in many proteins.

The oxidized (inorganic) form of sulfur is sulfate. Dietary sulfate is poorly absorbed. Instead sulfate is produced in the body primarily by oxidation of the sulfur-containing amino acids. There is no RECOMMENDED DIETARY ALLOWANCE for sulfur or its derivatives. Methionine is an essential amino acid which is converted to cysteine by the body. Thus cysteine is not a dietary essential amino acid when the diet supplies adequate methionine. The sulfur content of most animal proteins varies from 0.4 percent to 1.6 percent. Good sources of sulfur-containing amino acids include EGGS, CHEESE, MEAT, POULTRY, nuts and legumes.

The liver uses sulfate to process waste materials. It adds sulfate to a variety of foreign compounds and metabolic end products to inactivate them and to increase their water solubility to help flush them out of the body. For example, the industrial chemical phenol is excreted as phenol sulfate, and the hormone PROGESTERONE is excreted as progesterone sulfate.

Sulfate is a component of GLYCOSAMINOGLYCANS (mucopolysaccharides). These polysaccharide molecules are long chains of sulfated carbohydrate derivatives that provide slippery surfaces, a resilient framework in the connective TISSUE, and a lubricant for joints and other surfaces of the body. Sulfur occurs in COENZYME A, the enzyme helper derived from the B vitamin PANTOTHENIC ACID and cysteine, which assists in the burning of fat and carbohydrate in energy metabolism. Cysteine is a constituent of GLUTATHIONE, a predominant cellular

ANTIOXIDANT that protects cell membranes against oxidative damage. Cysteine is metabolized to TAURINE, an important sulfur compound that helps regulate nerves and muscles. Sulfur also appears in the B vitamins, THIAMIN and BIOTIN.

Another form of sulfur occurs frequently in the diet. SULFITE, a common food PRESERVATIVE, is not a nutrient. It is believed to be broken down by an enzyme called sulfite oxidase, which requires the trace mineral nutrient MOLYBDENUM for activity. Sulfite can trigger ASTHMA and food and chemical sensitivities. (See also GLUTATHIONE PEROXIDASE; MINERALS.)

sulfur dioxide See SULFITES.

Sunett See ACESULFAME-K.

sunflower (*Helianthus annus*) An annual that produces an oily seed. The sunflower is native to North America and it was cultivated first in the United States, Mexico, and Peru. High-oil varieties of sunflower were developed in the Soviet Union; oilseed varieties produce seeds containing about 40 percent oil. Sunflower oil is second among vegetable oils worldwide. The United States is a major producer of sunflowers, together with regions of the former Soviet Union, Argentina, Romania, Turkey, and Spain, among others. Non-oil varieties of North American origin produce large seeds used in salads and baked goods.

Sunflower oil typically contains 47.3 percent monounsaturates, 42 percent polyunsaturates and 10.7 percent saturated FATTY ACIDS. Most of the polyunsaturated fatty acid is the essential fatty acid, LINOLEIC ACID. Sunflower seeds contain more iron than raisins, a popular source of this nutrient. Sunflower seeds are used as a snack food. The nutrient contents of a quarter-cup (34 g) of oil-roasted seeds (edible portion) is: 208 calories; protein, 7.2 g; carbohydrate, 5 g; fiber, 1.8 g; fat, 19.4 g; iron, 2.3 mg; sodium, 205 mg; thiamin, 0.11 mg; riboflavin, 0.1 mg; niacin, 1.4 mg.

supermarkets Large, self-service retail stores offering a wide variety of foods, beverages, and household items. Grocery stores expanded in the 1950s to meet divergent consumer needs in addition to the staples like BREAD, EGGS, MILK, flour, and meat products. Modern supermarkets offer exotic fruit, snack foods, fish markets, take-out foods, salad bars, bakery, deli, and even pizza booths. Of all retail stores, Americans visit supermarkets most often: The average U.S. consumer visits a supermarket more than twice weekly, and shopping times range between 35 and 45 minutes per trip. The majority of trips to the supermarket occur on weekends.

superoxide dismutase (SOD) An antioxidant enzyme that destroys a reactive form of OXYGEN called superoxide. Superoxide (O_2^-) is a type of FREE RADICAL. As such it is very reactive chemically. Stimulated neutrophils and macrophages, two types of immune cells responsible for eliminating foreign materials, release superoxide to kill bacteria. A mechanism that enhances the destruction of virus-infected cells also operates through superoxide. Superoxide can also occur in MITOCHONDRIA, the powerhouses of cells. They consume most of the oxygen used by cells in order to burn fuels for energy; they can produce superoxide as a by-product. Superoxide can react with cellular metal ions to produce hydroxyl radicals, an extremely reactive free radical that can attack DNA and cause mutations. Oxidative damage is believed to underlie degenerative conditions including cardiovascular disease, premature aging, cancer, and even senility.

Three variants of superoxide dismutase require COPPER, and ZINC or MANGANESE. Consequently, these trace mineral nutrients are classified as ANTIOXIDANTS. Copper and zinc SOD are the major forms in the body and they are essential in protecting cells against damage due to inflammation. Injected SOD has been used to treat ARTHRITIS, CROHN'S DISEASE, LUPUS ERYTHEMATOSUS, and other conditions related to an imbalanced immune system and severe inflammation.

Superoxide dismutase is sold as a supplement in health food stores. The idea behind these pills is to bolster the body's enzymes. Generally, the levels of superoxide dismutase in the blood have not been shown to increase after SOD supplementation. Plant-based SOD seems to resist the rigors of the digestive tract, increasing the possibility of its absorption. (See also CATALASE.)

Hsieh, Y. et al. "Probing the Active Site of Human Manganese Superoxide Dismutase: the Role of Glutamine 143," *Biochemistry* 37 (1998): 4,731.

supplements See VITAMIN.

surfactant A food additive that acts as an antifoaming agent. Surfactants decrease the surface tension of water solutions, thus decreasing foaming. In PROCESSED FOODS, surfactants act as stabilizers to avoid watery mixtures, lumpy preparations, and oil-water separation as in chocolate milk and salad dressings. There are three categories of surfactant: detergents, wetting agents and EMULSIFIERS. Emulsifiers are used to form stable mixtures of normally incompatible materials—the polar (water attracting or HYDROPHILIC) and the nonpolar (lipid, water repelling, or HYDROPHOBIC). Examples include BILE acids in bile to emulsify FAT for DIGESTION; and the FOOD ADDITIVES, LECITHIN, DIGLYCERIDES, POLYSORBATES, SUCCISTEARIN, and XANTHAN GUM. (See also MICELLE.)

surimi Imitation shellfish prepared from fish paste. The Japanese developed a process for preparing fish paste from inexpensive bottom fish such as POLLOCK. Whitefish is soaked extensively, mashed into a paste that looks like mashed potatoes, and then molded into the desired shape and flavored. Surimi appears as artificial crabmeat, scallops, shrimp, and lobster tails. The usual imitation shellfish contains 50 percent to 60 percent surimi and only 5 percent to 10 percent of the authentic shellfish, and restaurants can profit by substituting surimi for shellfish. Surimi is popular because it provides shellfish flavor at low cost.

Surimi contains high amount of SODIUM, MONOSODIUM GLUTAMATE, and ARTIFICIAL FOOD COLORS and is blended with phosphates, sugar, and sorbitol. The product is low in VITAMINS and MINERALS due to extensive processing. Although the U.S. FDA requires that surimi be labeled as "artificial seafood," the packaging may mislead consumers by saying "sealegs" or the word "imitation" may be in small print. (See also FOOD ADDITIVES; IMITATION FOOD; PROCESSED FOOD.)

sushi See SEAFOOD.

sweeteners See NATURAL SWEETENERS.

sweetness Refers to sweet-tasting foods. The brain has taste centers that receive input from taste receptors on the tongue. Theoretically, all materials that taste sweet have a common molecular shape that can make contact with a receptor docking site. This brief contact may activate a chemical or electrical signal that is relayed to the brain. Individual taste sensitivity varies immensely. A person's tongue can have as few as 500 taste buds to as many as 10,000. Quite likely, as food is homogenized and mixed with SALIVA, flavor components interact with different receptors and together convey the identity of a food. (See also NATURAL SWEETENERS; SMELL; TASTE.)

sweet potato (*Ipomoea batatas*) A tropical plant that forms edible tubers. Sweet potatoes originated in Mexico or northern regions of South America. Europeans spread sweet potatoes to the Philippines, Africa, India, and Southeast Asia. The sweet potato ranks third among leading crop vegetables worldwide; only POTATOES and CASSAVA are more popular. China and Indonesia are among the major producers. Sweet potatoes have a reddish or gray skin and their flesh may be pink, orange, or purple. There are several varieties, including the Virginia (yellow flesh) and Malaga (pink flesh). Moist, orange-fleshed sweet potatoes are frequently called YAMS in the United States. However, true yams belong to a different plant family and are very large, starchy root vegetables grown in Asia and Africa. Although sweet potatoes taste sweeter than white potatoes, they don't contain more calories. Sweet potatoes are canned, dehydrated, frozen, or processed for starch, sugar, and syrup. Sweet potatoes may be baked, cooked in their skins, pureed, or candied. Sweet potatoes are excellent sources of provitamin A (BETA-CAROTENE) and other carotenoids. The nutrient contents of one potato (baked with skin, 11 g) is: 118 calories; protein, 2 g; carbohydrate, 27.7 g; fiber, 3 g; vitamin A, 2,575 retinol equivalents; thiamin, 0.08 mg; riboflavin, 0.21 mg; niacin, 1 mg.

sweets Foods that contain a high level of SUGAR. CANDY, CHOCOLATE, cake, cookies, ICE CREAM, jam, jelly, marshmallows, pastries, pie, tarts, sweetened gelatin desserts, and SOFT DRINKS sweetened with sugar are sugary foods. The sweetener may be TABLE SUGAR, HONEY, or another NATURAL SWEETENER. Often sweets contain a high percentage of FAT. The fat content may account for more calories than the sugar in such foods. The FOOD PYRAMID for consumers recommends using sweets sparingly because such foods contain fewer nutrients than vegetables, whole grains and fresh fruits, lentils, and beans. (See also DIETARY GUIDELINES FOR AMERICANS; TEETH.)

systemic Pertaining to most or all organ systems of the body. A systemic disease can affect the NERVOUS SYSTEM, the IMMUNE SYSTEM, musculature, gastrointestinal tract, or CIRCULATORY SYSTEM or a combination of these systems. (See also ALLERGY, FOOD; LUPUS ERYTHEMATOSUS.)

T

table salt See SODIUM.

table sugar See SUCROSE.

tahini A butter prepared from ground, hulled SESAME seeds. Tahini prepared from untoasted seeds has a mild flavor and is easily spreadable. Toasting sesame seeds yields a more oily mixture and adds a stronger flavor. Most commercial production of sesame seeds occurs in Mexico and Guatemala. Like sesame seed, tahini is a vegetarian source of iron. One tablespoon (15 g) provides 91 calories; protein, 2.7 g; carbohydrate, 2.7 g; fiber, 2.2 g; fat, 8.5 g; iron, 0.95 mg; thiamin, 0.24 mg; riboflavin, 0.02; mg niacin, 0.85 mg.

tallow FAT extracted from fatty tissue of sheep and cattle. Tallow hardens at room temperature, reflecting its relatively high content of saturated FATTY ACIDS; it contains about 46 percent saturated fatty acids and only 4 percent polyunsaturated fatty acids. Beef tallow is used in prepared foods such as chili and refried beans and french fries. It is also used industrially in soap and candle manufacture. Fat regardless of its source yields nine calories per gram, more than double the amount of calories in carbohydrate. (See also FAT METABOLISM; LARD.)

tamari (natural shoyu, Japanese soy sauce) A soy sauce prepared from the formation of SOYBEANS and cracked, roasted WHEAT. Tamari is fermented slowly and no preservatives are added. Tamari is a salty food containing 16 percent salt. Tamari contains little vitamin B_{12} activity.

tangelo A citrus fruit that is a result of cross-breeding a grapefruit and a tangerine. They have fewer seeds than tangerines but retain most of that fruit's flavor and sweetness. They are generally easier to peel and eat because the skin is somewhat loose around the pulpy flesh. The fruit has existed for several thousand years, probably originating in Southeast Asia from an accidental cross-breeding of mandarin oranges and pomelos (an ancestor of the modern grapefruit). Like other citrus fruits, tangelos are rich in vitamin C. One medium tangelo provides 60 calories; fiber, 3 g; potassium, 240 mg.

tangerine A smallish, tart CITRUS FRUIT. Tangerine is a descendant of the mandarin ORANGE and originated in China. The fruit has a thin, easily peeled skin and segments separate readily. Unlike oranges, which can be stored at room temperature for several weeks, tangerines need to be refrigerated if kept longer than a couple of days. They are eaten raw or used in fruit or gelatin-based salads. Tangerines provide less vitamin C than oranges. The edible portion of one raw tangerine (84 g) provides 37 calories; protein, 0.5 g; carbohydrate, 9.4 g; fiber, 1.6 g; fat, 0.2 g; potassium, 132 mg; vitamin C, 26 mg; thiamin, 0.09 mg; riboflavin, 0.02 mg; niacin, 0.13 mg.

tannins A family of complex compounds that occur in the bark or leaves of certain plants and trees. Tannins are classified chemically as flavonoids they are composed of two or more aromatic ring structures that act as antioxidants to quench oxidative damage due to FREE RADICALS. Polyphenols block the ability of certain compounds to cause mutations in test tube experiments and inhibit lung and skin tumors in experimental animals. Tannins are classified as hydrolyzable or condensed. Hydrolyzable tannins such as ellagic acid, gallic acid, and related compounds, are often complexed with glucose. Hydrolyzable tannins could serve as anticancer agents, increasing the liver's ability to "detoxify" potential cancer-causing agents by increasing their water-solubility, thus speeding up their removal (excretion). A second type, condensed tannins (flavolans), are chains of polyphenol units that do not break down readily and combine with iron and other metals.

Individuals consuming COFFEE, TEA, COCOA, and CHOCOLATE may ingest on the order of 1,000 mg of tannins daily. Tannins occur in all coffees, even decaffeinated coffee. A child consuming chocolate milk together with chocolate candy could consume 160 mg of cocoa tannin per kilogram of body weight per day. Brewed teas supply tannins. Some population studies suggest that tea drinkers have a reduced risk of dying from coronary heart disease. High levels of tannic acid can bind protein and limit digestion, limit the uptake of GLUCOSE and METHIONINE, and bind iron from vegetable sources. Acute toxicity tests with adult animals did not indicate toxicity.

tapioca A form of starch derived from the CASSAVA, a tropical root vegetable. Tapioca is prepared by drying pulped roots after fibers have been removed. Special grinding and sieving is required to produce the type of tapioca used in popular puddings. Like most starches, tapioca swells and thickens when cooked in water. It is often used to thicken soups, pies, and puddings. High-grade tapioca forms milky beads with a brilliant white luster. The nutrient content of 1 cup (165 g) of tapioca cream pudding is: 221 calories; protein, 8.3 g; carbohydrate, 28.2 g; fat, 8.4 g; sodium, 257 mg; calcium, 173 mg; thiamin, 0.07 mg; riboflavin, 0.30 mg; niacin, 0.2 mg. (See also FLOUR.)

tardive dyskinesia A disabling disorder sometimes produced by the long-term use of antipsychotic drugs and neuroleptic drugs (tranquilizers). Tardive dyskinesia occurs in 10 percent to 20 percent of patients treated with these drugs. Symptoms include involuntary twitching of mouth and face, hand trembling, spasms, and speech disturbances. Sometimes these drug-induced effects are irreversible.

Supplements of the nitrogen-containing nutrient CHOLINE and of LECITHIN, the PHOSPHOLIPID from which choline is derived, reduce the abnormal movements of tardive dyskinesia, and lecithin remains an important treatment option. TRYPTOPHAN, together with NIACINAMIDE and VITAMIN B_6, may relieve symptoms of tardive dyskinesia. Large-scale studies have suggested that patients who supplement with NIACIN, MANGANESE, and ZINC concomitantly with drug treatment experience decreased symptoms of tardive dyskinesia. The American Psychiatric Association concluded (1991) that the general clinical value of such nutrients should be confirmed with long-term, large-scale studies before acceptance. Preliminary clinical studies suggest that VITAMIN E may also decrease the severity of symptoms. (See also NERVOUS SYSTEM; PARKINSON'S DISEASE.)

Dannon, P. N. et al. "Vitamin E Treatment in Tardive Dyskinesia," *Human Psychopharmacology* 12 (1997): 217–220.

target heart rate See EXERCISE.

taro *(Colocasia esculenta)* A tropical, tuber-bearing plant native to Southeast Asia. Taro cultivation gradually spread to Japan, China, the eastern Mediterranean region, Polynesia, New Zealand, West Africa, and South America. Taro root is a high-carbohydrate food. Poi, a staple food of Polynesia, is made from the taro root. A common variety of taro produces a brown-skinned root with a pale purple or white flesh. Taro root is sold in Asian markets and specialty shops. Taro leaves should not be consumed raw because some varieties contain high levels of OXALIC ACID (calcium oxalate) that can be toxic when large amounts are consumed. Taro root can be used like potatoes; it is boiled, baked, or steamed. The vegetable becomes very sticky upon cooling. The tuber has a nutrient value similar to the Irish POTATO.

tarragon (*Artemesia dracunculus*) A small perennial shrub with a dark green, narrow leaf that is used as a culinary HERB. The name comes from the French *estragon*, meaning "little dragon," because the twisted roots resemble dragons. Tarragon is used fresh or dried to create a somewhat anise-like flavor in chicken, veal, and turkey dishes; in broiled fish and shellfish; omelet and egg dishes; MUSTARD; and MAYONNAISE. Tarragon is used in bearnaise sauce. Tarragon can overwhelm other seasonings, and it is not recommended in recipes calling for a blend of herbs. (See also ANISE; SPICE.)

tartaric acid An acidic FOOD ADDITIVE used to create a tart taste. Tartaric ACID occurs widely in plants, especially in fruits and ripe grapes. Commercially, tartaric acid is a by-product of wine production. Tartaric acid is used with grape flavors and other flavoring agents in SOFT DRINKS, CANDY, gelatin-based desserts, and YOGURT.

The potassium salt of tartaric acid (potassium tartrate) is called "cream of tartar." This compound is used as a leavening agent and as an anticaking agent in baking. A mixture of sodium tartrate and sodium-potassium tartrate, "Rochelle salt," is used to control acidity and to emulsify ingredients of processed foods (CHEESE and jam, among others). Intestinal bacteria produce most of the tartaric acid people ingest, and it is considered a safe food additive. (See also CITRIC ACID.)

tartrazine (FD&C yellow no. 5) One of the most widely used artificial colorings in the United States. Low levels of tartrazine are used in beverages like SOFT DRINKS; higher levels are used in BREAKFAST CEREALS, baked goods and snack foods. Health concerns have been raised because tartrazine causes allergic reactions in certain people, particularly if they are sensitive to ASPIRIN. Asthma, hives and typical "hay fever" symptoms can occur, although more severe symptoms have been reported. Tartrazine sensitivity was estimated to be prevalent in less than 100,000 Americans in the late 1970s. In 1981 the U.S. FDA required that ingredient labels on foods disclose the presence of tartrazine rather than simply noting "artificial coloring." Several European countries have banned this dye from food use. Coloring from TURMERIC and ANNATTO can be used in place of this yellow food coloring. (See also ALLERGY, FOOD; FOOD ADDITIVES; FOOD SENSITIVITY.)

taste The flavor sensation of substances placed in the mouth. The sensation of taste relies on the stimulation of receptors (taste buds) by substances dissolved in SALIVA. An adult possesses about 2,000 taste buds located chiefly on the tongue. They occur also on the soft palate and in the throat. Typically, taste buds occur in small protuberances called papillae, which give the upper surface of the tongue a rough appearance. Taste buds possess external cells with hair-like extensions that project through a central taste pore. When a dissolved substance enters a taste pore and contacts the hair-like projections, it can generate a nerve impulse that is relayed to the brain.

Of all the seemingly endless different flavors and subtle tastes, there are only four basic taste sensations: sweet, sour, salt, and bitter. Most other tastes are combinations of these modified by odors. When a person has a cold, the olfactory sensations (SMELL) do not operate normally, although the taste sensations may be normal. The olfactory system (sense of smell) is much more sensitive to stimulation than the gustatory system for a given concentration of a substance.

Taste buds located in different areas possess different sensitivities to taste sensations. Thus, the tip of the tongue reacts with all primary taste sensations, but it is highly sensitive to salty and sweet materials. The edges of the tongue respond more readily to sour substances, while the back of the tongue responds most to bitter substances.

Foods that taste bitter are generally rejected. This may be part of a protective mechanism in human evolution, because many poisonous plants contain toxic substances that produce a bitter taste. A degree of saltiness is often considered pleasant but very salty foods will be rejected. The preference for salty foods in most people is acquired. Gradually, reducing the amount of salt in foods will uncover the subtle, rich flavors of minimally processed foods. Sweet tasting foods create pleasurable feelings. ARTIFICIAL SWEETENERS have been developed that will trigger the sweet receptors without contributing calories. A sour taste may be either objectionable or desirable. Dilute acid solutions such as VINEGAR can create tangy, zestful foods and beverages, while excessive acidity is not palatable. The taste threshold varies for each primary taste. Bitter substances possess the lowest taste threshold, that is, they can be distinguished at low concentrations; the threshold for sour substances is higher; and the thresholds for salt and sweet materials are higher than for sour or bitter foods. Adding sugar to highly seasoned dishes increases the ability to sense hot spices.

Children up to the age of five have more taste buds than adults, so foods taste richer to them. Babies explore their environment by tasting everything they can reach. Possible reasons for a decrease in the sense of taste include: cigarette smoking, eating excessively salty foods or drinking alcoholic beverages, and a ZINC deficiency. Elderly persons gradually lose some of their sense of taste; food tends to taste bland to them.

Adler, E. et al. "A Novel Family of Mammalian Taste Receptors," *Cell* 100 (March 17, 2000): 693.

Fackelmann, K. A. "The Bitter Truth," *Science News* 152 (July 12, 1997): 24.

taurine A sulfur-containing compound produced by the liver. Taurine serves multiple functions. The liver uses taurine to convert CHOLESTEROL to BILE salts, required to digest FAT and to modify toxic chemicals to help flush them out of the body. Taurine helps regulate nerves and muscles and supports SODIUM and POTASSIUM transport across cell membranes. It is required for normal function of the heart, brain, eyes, and vascular system. Taurine is the most prevalent free amino acid in the heart, where it contributes to muscle contraction. With chronic stress and when the oxygen supply to the heart drops (ischemia), taurine levels in the heart decrease. In Japan, taurine is used in treating HEART DISEASE and congestive heart failure. Taurine administered to experimental animals can prevent induced heart muscle damage. In the brain, taurine acts as a NEUROTRANSMITTER, a chemical released by a nerve cell (neuron) to help carry a nerve impulse to an adjacent cell. Taurine seems to be inhibitory, that is, it depresses the brain. Therefore, it is being studied as an anticonvulsant in the treatment of epilepsy. Taurine is also involved in calcium metabolism of the brain.

The body possesses a limited capacity to produce taurine, and certain individuals may require dietary taurine, depending on their nutritional status. Pre-term and full-term infants do not synthesize appreciable taurine, which is the most abundant amino acid in breast milk. With time the taurine content of breast milk declines as the infant grows and begins to manufacture taurine. Taurine was once omitted from infant formulas; now it is added routinely. Taurine is concentrated in animal protein, especially organ meats, fish, and milk, but is absent from plant foods.

Taurine is a nerve depressant and when used as a supplement it may affect short-term memory. Its use is considered experimental. (See also METHIONINE; NERVOUS SYSTEM.)

tea (*Camellia sinensis*) The dried leaves of a tropical evergreen that grows as a small tree or shrub. Brewed tea is the most popular beverage worldwide. The origin of tea is obscure, though it probably originated in regions of Tibet, western China, and northern India. India, Sri Lanka, and China are the leading tea growing countries. Flower, leaf, bark, roots, and seeds of various plants are used in herbal teas but these are not derived from *Camellia sinensis.*

Differences in color and aroma among various types of tea reflect primarily differences in tea processing. Nearly 75 percent of tea ends up as black tea, in which leaves are crushed to release enzymes that oxidize substances in leaves (polyphenols) that create the rich flavor. The leaves are then dried in hot air to develop a brown/black color. For green tea, fresh leaves are steamed to destroy the oxidizing enzymes, then rolled and dried. Instant tea was developed in the United States in 1948. It is prepared by brewing a strong tea and removing water to leave a dried concentrate, which can be added to water. Oolong tea is partially fermented to create a green-brown leaf.

Brewed tea is prepared by pouring boiling water over dried tea leaves. Generally, the best flavor is obtained when tea has steeped (soaked) in boiled water for up to five minutes for black tea, one to two minutes for green tea. Longer steeping creates tea with more TANNIN and increased bitterness. Black tea, and to a lesser extent, green tea bind iron because of the tannin content. Tannins contribute to the pungency of tea. Tea is a mild stimulant because it contains CAFFEINE. A cup of black tea provides about 90 mg, about half the amount in COFFEE (160 mg/cup). Green tea contains up to 30 mg per cup. Caffeine increases urination and is responsible for the diuretic effect of tea.

Brewed tea contains other substances as well. Tea is a source of FLUORIDE; a cup of tea provides about 0.3 mg. Green tea yields more fluoride and less caffeine than black tea. Green tea provides vitamin C; on the average, one cup of green tea provides as much vitamin C as half a cup of orange juice. Tea also contains tannin and catechin (classified as FLAVONOIDS), widely distributed among plants. Cancer of the esophagus, stomach, and intestine are rare in regions of Japan and China where large amounts of green tea are consumed. They possess ANTIOXIDANT properties. Epigallocatechin is the most potent catechin in tea. It is reported to be 200 times stronger antioxidant than vitamin E. Antioxidants have been proposed as anti-cancer agents. Studies have shown that green tea extracts can inhibit the growth of bladder, stomach, and esophageal cancer cells. Population studies suggest that regularly drinking green or black tea can lower the risk of developing cancer. Other studies link tea consumption with a lowered risk of dying from heart disease. In one study, people who drank more than two cups of tea daily reduced the risk of death following heart attack by 44 percent. Tea flavonoids may limit the oxidation of LOW-DENSITY LIPOPROTEIN (LDL) cholesterol, believed to be an early event in atherosclerosis. Other studies suggest that tea can increase bone density, inhibit the bacterium responsible for tooth decay, improve the growth of beneficial gut bacteria, and inhibit flu virus and boost the immune system. However, the mechanism of action of tea flavonoids is still being investigated.

Imai, K. "Cross-sectional Study of Effects of Drinking Green Tea on Cardiovascular and Liver Diseases," *British Medical Journal* 310 (1995): 693–696.

teeth Bony projections from the upper and lower jaws used for chewing food. Each tooth possesses an exposed crown and one or more roots that anchor the tooth in the jawbone. Each jaw has 16 teeth. A child may develop up to 20 teeth that are replaced with permanent teeth. Incisors and cuspids (canines) are for biting off pieces of food. Bicuspids (premolars) and molars provide grinding surfaces to pulverize food.

The outer coating of the tooth is called the enamel, the hardest part of the tooth. This protective layer resists the wear of chewing and the action of bacteria. A hardened type of bone covers the roots. Dentine, a hard, mineralized layer, lies beneath the enamel. Dentine surrounds a central cavity of the tooth, filled with nerves and blood vessels. The gums (gingivae) bridge the gap between the tooth and bone. Tooth sockets are lined with a periodontal ligament and elastic connective tissue, which both anchor the tooth and act as a shock absorber.

FLUORIDE is incorporated into teeth during their formation in the first years of life. Fluoride enters the mineral structure, increasing its resistance to microbial degradation. Fluoride has its greatest effect before and during the emergence of teeth, and it is recommended in the diet until all teeth are in place. Fluoride has been recommended in drinking water up to a concentration of 1 mg per milliliter as a supplement during tooth formation.

Most adults over 50 exhibit symptoms of GINGIVITIS (inflamed gums) due to dental plaque accumulation. Plaque is the sticky mass of bacterial deposit, which can harden and become tartar. In certain cases, bacterial infection spreads to deep tissues (periodontitis) and can cause tooth and bone loss. Flossing, brushing, and professional cleaning are the foundation for oral health and best defense against plaque formation. Topical application of fluoride as toothpaste or oral antiseptic rinse further reduces tooth decay. (See also PERIODONTAL DISEASE.)

tempeh A type of fermented soybean cake and a meat substitute. Tempeh is a food staple in Indonesia, New Guinea, and, to a lesser degree, in Malaysia. Soaked soybeans are boiled, usually with grains, then fermented (aged) with a mold, *Rhizopus oligosporus.* Mold growth forms a mat around the cooked beans that binds the mixture into a firm cake, which can be fried, baked, roasted, or diced and served in soups. Tempeh contains somewhat more protein than soybean curd (TOFU).

teratogen An agent that causes BIRTH DEFECTS. The placenta acts as a barrier to many potentially damaging substances in maternal blood. However, a number of fat-soluble compounds and drugs can penetrate the placenta and can damage the embryo or fetus. In the United States alone nearly 150,000 infants are born with malformations and developmental defects that require medical treatment. About 60 percent of all birth defects have an unknown cause. The other 40 percent are caused by either genetic factors or environmental exposures, or both.

The catalog of teratogenic agents lists all chemicals that have been reported to be teratogenic in humans or in animals. Americans are exposed to approximately 5 million chemicals; 1,600 of these have been tested in lab animals and about 50 percent are known teratogens. A number of these are related to nutrients. Retinoids, a family of lipids related to VITAMIN A, affect the development of body shape, and overdoses can lead to severe malformation. Retinoic acid (C_{13} cis—retinoic acid), a vitamin A derivative used in skin treatment for severe ACNE, is a human teratogen. Some investigators believe that ETHANOL, the alcohol in alcoholic beverages, could be responsible for as much as 20 percent of cases of mental retardation in the United States. About one-third of all children born to alcoholic mothers are affected by FETAL ALCOHOL SYNDROME, a condition characterized by long-term growth retardation, nervous system irregularities, small head size, and facial anomalies. Maternal alcohol consumption during pregnancy is also associated with cleft palate and congenital head defects. Excessive consumption of selenium can cause a condition called selenosis in which very high levels of selenium accumulate in maternal tissues. Animal studies indicate that selenium under these extreme conditions can be a teratogen. A variety of drugs are teratogens. The general recommendation is to avoid alcohol and drugs during pregnancy.

terpenoid (terpene) A large family of compounds produced by plants and animals that are classified as LIPIDS. Lipids are fat-soluble (hydrophobic) compounds that dissolve oils and organic solvents. Terpenoids are ring structures assembled from acetyl COENZYME A, the activated form of ACETIC ACID derived from the degradation of CARBOHYDRATE and FAT. Terpenoids include a large number of plant and animal materials such as VITAMIN A, VITAMIN D, VITAMIN E, VITAMIN K, CHOLESTEROL, steroid hormones, BILE salts; plant oils like limonene from oil of LEMON and ORANGE; pinene from turpentine; geraniol from flowers; menthol from PEPPERMINT; zingiberene from oil of GINGER; B-selinene from oil of CELERY; and squalene from fish liver oil. (See also CARBOHYDRATE METABOLISM; FAT METABOLISM; HORMONE; STEROIDS.)

testosterone The predominant male sex HORMONE. Testosterone is the major androgenic hormone (hormones that guide the development and maintenance of male organs and secondary male characteristics, including facial hair, male musculature, with widened shoulders and narrowed hips, among others). Testosterone stimulates the accumulation of muscle and the maturation of sperm and stimulates bone growth. Testosterone, like other STEROID hormones, is synthesized from CHOLESTEROL and is secreted by the testicles. Illicit use of synthetic androgens by athletes and body builders has led to increased muscle mass above the level induced by workouts, with often disastrous side effects.

In females, testosterone is synthesized by the ovaries and adrenal glands; the blood levels of testosterone in women are about 10 percent of a typical male. The role of androgens in female development is unclear. The effects of excessive male hormones are better documented with increased risk of diabetes, high blood pressure, heart disease, breast cancer, irregular periods and endometrial cancer. (See also ANABOLIC STEROIDS.)

tetrahydrofolic acid (THF) The biologically active form of the B vitamin, FOLIC ACID. THF functions as a coenzyme, that is, an enzyme helper. It differs from folic acid because it possesses extra hydrogen atoms and GLUTAMIC ACID units. THF figures predominantly in the transfer of single carbon units. It helps catalyze the synthesis of the amino acid SERINE from the simplest amino acid, GLYCINE; helps catalyze the nitrogen-containing bases, PURINE and THYMINE, which are used as building blocks of genetic material, DNA; and helps catalyze EPINEPHRINE, a stress hormone released by the adrenal gland, among others. (See also COENZYME.)

texture The sensation produced in the mouth by a food or beverage, often referred to as "mouth feel." Adjectives such as chewy, sticky, creamy, hard, lumpy, soft, rough, smooth, gritty, crisp, and the like describe food textures. The physical and chemical properties of a food form the basis for acceptance or rejection. Experience teaches associations between certain foods and textures. If food has a texture that differs from expectations it is judged as of lower quality. A rejected food may be stringy, slimy, gritty, greasy, or contain hard to chew pieces or fragments. (See also FOOD PROCESSING; TASTE.)

texturized vegetable protein (TVP) SOYBEAN protein that has been processed to resemble meat. Protein is isolated from soybeans, chemically treated, combined with additives and further processed to create colored granules, chunks, or strips. TVP is made by cooking soybean flour with other ingredients and extruding the mixture to form hamburger extenders, bacon bits, and the like. Spun forms are made by spinning fibers and adding flavor and color. TVP can be formed to resemble meat, fish, or poultry. Imitation meat products contain many additives to create a desired texture and flavor, including MONOSODIUM GLUTAMATE, salt, ARTIFICIAL FOOD COLORS, flavors, flavor enhancers, EMULSIFIERS, and various types of VEGETABLE OIL. Although low in cholesterol, imitation meat can be a high-fat option because of the added hydrogenated vegetable oil.

TVP is an inexpensive, versatile imitation meat used in a large number of manufactured foods, including simulated CHICKEN, simulated HAMBURGER, simulated HAM and BACON, simulated pepperoni, and even imitation nuts. Soybean protein finds its way into casseroles, pizza toppings, stews, snacks, other CONVENIENCE FOODS, and institutionalized cooking. The amount used in soy products is up to the discretion of the manufacturer. TVP is considered a safe food additive. (See also IMITATION FOOD; PROCESSED FOOD.)

thermogenesis (nonshivering thermogenesis) The generation of heat by the body in response to cold. Brown fat tissue (adipose tissue) is geared to produce heat. Brown adipose is most predominant in newborn infants and decreases with age. It is much less abundant in the body than white fat, and occurs in only a few regions, especially the back of the neck and the upper back in adults. The amount of brown fat can increase with exposure to low temperatures. Fat cells in brown adipose tissue can switch over to burn fat and produce heat in response to thyroid hormone. Released heat can then warm the body. This response is more prominent in babies than in adults. (See also FAT METABOLISM; SPECIFIC DYNAMIC EFFECT.)

thiamin (vitamin B_1) A water-soluble vitamin and a member of the B complex. Thiamin is essential for the energy production from carbohydrate and fat. The active form (coenzyme), thiamin pyrophosphate, serves as an enzyme helper in the breakdown of glucose (blood sugar) and in the Kreb's cycle, the central energy-yielding pathway of the body. Thiamin is also required in the PENTOSE phosphate pathway, a sequence of enzymes that converts glucose to the smaller sugars and energy and liberates hydrogen atoms for biosynthesis. These energy-yielding pathways are critical for normal function of peripheral nerves, skeletal muscle and heart muscle, among others.

Severe thiamin deficiency causes BERIBERI. Although rare in the United States, this disease occurs all too frequently in malnourished populations in developing nations who rely on white flour and white rice that are not enriched with thiamin. When beriberi affects primarily the nervous system, it is called "dry" beriberi. Degeneration of insulation (myelin sheath) around nerves of the central nervous system occurs, leading to nerve irritation, pain, numbness, and, in extreme cases, paralysis and muscle wasting. Beriberi produces a staggering gait, numbness of legs, and retarded growth. Mental symptoms such as disorientation, hallucinations and depression occur as well. These symptoms usually respond to thiamin supplementation, and thiamin is also important in treating polyneuritis (nerve inflammation) associated with pregnancy and ALCOHOLISM. Thiamin deficiency can masquerade as SENILITY. Alcoholics may exhibit the mental confusion typical of beriberi. Thiamin supplementation alone does not seem to affect mental processes and memory if thiamin deficiency is not involved.

An alternate course results in "wet" beriberi, seen as problems with the heart and circulation (abnormal heart rhythm, low blood pressure, elevated levels of blood lactic acid, edema [water retention] of the legs, heart muscle weakness, and, ultimately, heart failure). This form of beriberi usually responds quickly and dramatically to thiamin supplementation.

Requirements

The RECOMMENDED DIETARY ALLOWANCE (RDA) for thiamin for men is 1.5 mg and for nonpregnant women 1.1 mg, and based on an allowance of 0.5 mg per 1,000 calories consumed daily. The requirement increases with pregnancy and lactation. Because of the prevalence of alcoholism in the United States, thiamin deficiency is not uncommon. Symptoms of moderate deficiency include FATIGUE, apathy, nausea, irritability, depression, slowed wound healing, loss of appetite, indigestion, and constipation. Moderate deficiency symptoms can be caused by crash dieting, alcohol abuse, or liver disease. People relying on highly processed foods are at risk, for example, elderly people; low-income persons; teenagers relying on sweets, soft drinks, and low-nutrient foods; and pregnant women. Consuming large amounts of sugar as found in sweets and soft drinks increases the need for thiamin. Also at risk are patients on kidney dialysis or who are sustained for long periods by intravenous nutrients.

Factors That Increase Thiamin Requirements

- Alcohol. Thiamin assimilation is blocked by alcohol consumption. Alcohol use also injures the small intestine and reduces its ability to absorb thiamin. Alcohol decreases thiamin conversion to thiamin pyrophosphate and depletes tissues of this coenzyme.
- Thiamin antagonists. Raw SEAFOOD, such as shrimp, carp, herring, mussels, and clams, and YEAST contain thiaminase, an enzyme that degrades thiamin. Eating a large amount of live yeast can reduce thiamin ABSORPTION. Cooking seafood destroys this enzyme.
- Heat-stable anti-thiamin factors have been isolated from several sources. Fermented fish contain factors that limit thiamin uptake. Tea, coffee, and even decaffeinated coffee reduce thiamin absorption.
- Baking soda. Cooking with baking soda destroys thiamin.
- Cigarette smoking. Smoking adversely affects thiamin uptake and use by tissues.
- Medications. Antacids and barbiturates may interfere with thiamin uptake.

Foods that contain ample thiamin are wheat germ; meats (pork, beef, ham, organ meats); nuts (pecans, peanuts, walnuts); brewer's yeast; fortified cereals and grain products. Thiamin is used to enrich flour, breads, and cereals, a practice that has eliminated the widespread thiamin deficiency that existed prior to enrichment programs. Heating food and processing destroys this fragile vitamin. The higher the cooking temperature, the greater the loss. However, microwave cooking does not seem to increase thiamin loss. Thiamin is relatively nontoxic. Very high doses rarely lead to headaches, mental instability, irritability or weakness. Some people are allergic to thiamin injections. (See also CARBOHYDRATE METABOLISM.)

Brady, J. A. "Thiamin Status, Diuretic Medications, and the Management of Congestive Heart Failure," *Journal of the American Dietetic Association* 95 (1995): 541–544.

thickening agents (thickeners) Food additives used to modify the consistency of ice cream, yogurt, pudding, soft drinks, soups, salad dressing, and baby food, among other products. They stabilize complex mixtures in manufactured foods to prevent a lumpy or watery consistency or crystallization or to prevent oils, coloring agents, and nutrients from separating. Many thickeners are naturally occurring polysaccharides (AGAR, CARRAGEENAN, PECTIN, and the like). Chemically modified starches, called "derivatized starches," cellulose gums, and other chemically modified materials are frequently used for this purpose. (See also GUAR GUM; GUM; SEAWEED.)

thiourea A small sulfur compound analog that occurs in vegetables like TURNIPS and CABBAGE and other cruciferous vegetables. Thiourea inhibits the synthesis of thyroxine (thyroid hormone) and can cause goiter formation in lab animals. These vegetables nonetheless add considerable nutritional value and variety to the diet. Vegetables high in thiourea theoretically could cause a potential health problem for people with iodine-deficient diets who rely on turnips—not a likely circumstance in the United States.

thirst A craving for WATER. Thirst sensation is caused by cells in the HYPOTHALAMUS, a small region of the brain that controls both drinking and excreting water and processes information about the external environment in order to maintain an optimal internal environment (HOMEOSTASIS). Certain cells detect the concentration of SODIUM in the blood. When the concentration increases above 310 to 340 mg per 100 ml (136 to 145 milli-equivalents per liter), cells of the thirst center begin to shrink, triggering nerve impulses that evoke the sensation of being thirsty. A 1 percent increase in effective ion concentration (osmolarity) can trigger this response. Intracellular DEHYDRATION can also stimulate thirst. Another nerve center of the hypothalamus triggers the release of ANTIDIURETIC HORMONE from the PITUITARY GLAND. This hormone causes the KIDNEYS to decrease urine output, effectively conserving water. (See also ELECTROLYTES.)

threonine (Thr, L-threonine) A dietary essential AMINO ACID that serves as a building block of PROTEIN. Threonine resembles SERINE, which is a simple amino acid that can be synthesized by tissues. Severe threonine deficiency in experimental animals causes neurologic dysfunction and lameness. In addition to being a raw material for protein synthesis, animal studies suggest that threonine stimulates the THYMUS GLAND and supports the IMMUNE SYSTEM. Adults need an estimated 7 mg/kg of body weight per day. Animal protein like meat, fish, poultry, and dairy products are good dietary sources of this amino acid. (See also AMINO ACID METABOLISM.)

thrombin The enzyme derived from the serum protein prothrombin that catalyzes the final step in the BLOOD CLOTTING cascade. VITAMIN K is required in the maturation of prothrombin, and hence is indirectly responsible for thrombin formation. Hemorrhagic (bleeding) disease in newborn infants due to inadequate blood clotting may respond to vitamin K supplementation because vitamin K stores are low at birth, and the sterile gut lacks the beneficial bacteria that normally produce vitamin K in adults. Breast milk contains little vitamin K, and the American Academy of Pediatrics recommends administration of vitamin K at birth to promote normal thrombin formation and clotting.

thrombosis The obstruction of a blood vessel by a blood clot. Detachment of a fixed blood clot (thrombus) produces a traveling blood clot (embolus) that can block a vessel at a distant site. Blockages of arteries feeding the brain lead to STROKES, while blockage of arteries feeding the heart contribute to HEART ATTACKS. (See also ATHEROSCLEROSIS; CARDIOVASCULAR DISEASE.)

thyme (*Thymus vulgaris*) A fragrant culinary HERB. Thyme was known to Egyptians, Greeks, and Romans and traditionally was used to instill courage. There are many varieties of this plant. Garden thyme is a small bushy perennial. Thyme is a powerful herb with a distinctive aroma. It can be mixed with PARSLEY and bay leaves as a seasoning, and is used in marinades and sauces. It is used sparingly with veal, pork, poultry and poultry stuffing, vegetable soups, chowders, summer squash, and gumbo dishes. Thyme is also used in custards and jellies. Thyme tea has been used in folk medicine for coughs, colds, and sore throats. It has antibacterial properties and can boost the immune system. Thyme possesses powerful antifungal properties. (See also SAGE.)

thymine A nitrogen-containing base that functions as raw material for DNA. Thymine is easily made by the body and is not a dietary necessity. However, synthesis of thymine requires FOLIC ACID, a B vitamin. Thymine consists of a six-membered ring containing four nitrogen atoms and two carbon atoms. Thymine and other bases of DNA contribute to the unique properties of DNA. DNA exists as two parallel chains linked side by side as a helix. This association relies on a linkage of bases between the two strands; thus thymine in one DNA chain binds to a base called ADENINE on the adjacent chain. It is this specificity of base-pairing that underlies the genetic code and DNA replication during cell division. Thymine is readily broken down by the body and does not yield URIC ACID, a general waste product of DNA and RNA degradation. (See also PURINE; PYRIMIDINE.)

thymus gland A component of the IMMUNE SYSTEM that produces HORMONES to support the development of the immune cells. The thymic hormones include thymosin, thymic humoral factor, thymic factor, and thymopoietin. Together they promote the proliferation and maturation of various types of T cells, lymphocytes (white blood cells) that help defend the body against foreign invaders. Helper T cells (which activate other lymphocytes), cytotoxic T cells (which attack cells) and suppressor T cells (which limit lymphocyte activity) represent the major class of T cells.

The thymus shrinks as people age. At birth, thymic tissue represents 0.4 percent of body weight. At the age of 70, the thymus accounts for only 0.0007 percent. This atrophy correlates with a gradual weakening of the immune system. Orally administered extracts of beef thymus have been used to support the function of the thymus gland. Antioxidants like VITAMIN C, VITAMIN E, BETA-CAROTENE, and SELENIUM are nutrients that enhance T-cell function and may retard thymic shrinkage because the gland is susceptible to oxidative damage. The amino acids ORNITHINE and ARGININE can also stimulate the thymus gland. ZINC, VITAMIN B_6, and vitamin C seem crucial to support thymic hormone production and cell-dependent immune function. *Echinacea angustifolia* and licorice enhance immune function performed by the thymus gland. Thymic factors are being studied as therapeutic agents for AIDS patients and cancer patients. (See also AGING; ENDOCRINE SYSTEM.)

thyroid gland The gland responsible for the formation of thyroid HORMONES and calcitonin. The most plentiful thyroid hormone is thyroxine (T4), which is converted to triiodothyronine (T3), which is more potent but is present in smaller amounts in the blood. This conversion takes place in the liver and lungs. Thyroxine consists of the amino acid TYROSINE, to which iodine is bound. Tyrosine is a building block of the protein thyroglobulin, to which IODINE is added during its processing. Thyroxine is released from thyroglobulin when the thyroid gland is stimulated, for instance, by other hormone signals.

T3 and T4 increase the rate of oxygen uptake, the rate of oxidation of fat and carbohydrate for ENERGY, and the BASAL METABOLIC RATE, the rate at which energy maintains body function. Thyroid hormones also increase carbohydrate uptake by the intestine; regulate lipid metabolism; help regulate normal growth, brain development, and skeletal maturation in children; and help regulate the central nervous system as well as the function of peripheral nerves. In children, thyroid hormones help regulate growth and development by working together with GROWTH HORMONE. Furthermore, thyroid hormones regulate the activity of the nervous system, which in turn increases blood flow, increases heartbeat and blood pressure, and increases movement of the gastrointestinal tract (PERISTALSIS).

Calcitonin operates differently. This hormone lowers the level of CALCIUM and phosphate in the blood by inhibiting BONE breakdown (demineralization) and by increasing calcium and phosphate incorporation into bones. This appears to take place by inhibiting bone-destroying cells called osteoclasts.

The HYPOTHALAMUS regulates the activity of the thyroid gland. This portion of the brain regulates responses to changes in blood chemistry such as lowered blood sugar and decreased body temperature. It releases a hormone called thyrotropin releasing hormone which stimulates the pituitary to secrete thyroid stimulating hormone (TSH) into the bloodstream. In turn, TSH then stimulates the thyroid gland to release its hormones to speed up metabolism.

In decreased thyroid gland function (HYPOTHYROIDISM), body temperature decreases, reaction time is decreased and thought processes are slowed. Low basal temperature, depression, FATIGUE, dry skin, dry hair, low blood pressure and difficulty in losing weight also characterize hypothyroidism. In extreme cases, a GOITER develops (enlarged thyroid gland). Iodine, ZINC, VITAMIN E and VITAMIN A, RIBOFLAVIN, NIACIN, VITAMIN B_6, and vitamin C are required for the formation of thyroid hormone. Exercise stimulates the thyroid gland. On the other hand, an overactive thyroid gland (hyperthyroidism) is characterized by a high metabolic rate, nervousness, weight loss, heat intolerance, excessive sweating, and increased heart rate. This metabolic disorder can mimic IRRITABLE BOWEL SYNDROME. (See also CATABOLISM; ENDOCRINE SYSTEM.)

Weetman, A. P. "Graves' Disease," *New England Journal of Medicine* 343, no. 17 (2000): 1,236–1,248.

tin A heavy metal. There is weak evidence that it is a required nutrient in animals, although it has no known metabolic function. Rigorous exclusion of tin from diets of laboratory animals impaired reproduction and caused other abnormal growth. If it functions as a nutrient in humans, typical daily ingestion of 1.5 to 5 mg per day more than meets requirements. Tin is used to line certain cans, and acidic foods like canned PINEAPPLE and canned TOMATOES can leach out tin from the inside of a can. However, there is little evidence to indicate that tin can be toxic. (See also HEAVY METALS.)

tissue A level of cellular organization in which groups of similar cells perform similar functions. Cells of tissues adhere to each other through intercellular materials (connective tissue) and tight bonding (tight junctions). The epithelial tissue of the intestine is representative of this layer of cells and contains mucus-secreting cells and enzyme-secreting cells. Other tissues include nervous tissue, muscle tissue, connective tissue, and ADIPOSE TISSUE. Nerve tissue is composed of nerve cells (neurons) and their supporting cell types (neuroglial cells). Muscle tissue contains muscle fibers assembled from muscle cells (myoblasts). Connective tissue contains fibroblasts, cells that secrete materials from an extracellular matrix, including the structural protein, COLLAGEN, together with GLYCOSAMINOGLYCANS (MUCOPOLYSACCHARIDES), consisting of long chains of modified sugars. Mucopolysaccharides absorb water and are slippery. They form a gel-like environment for connective tissue cells called ground substance. Adipose tissue is fatty connective tissue that contains fat cells (ADIPOCYTES). Reticular tissue is a fibrous connective tissue that forms the support for internal organs like the liver, spleen, lymph glands, and lungs. (See also BONE; SKIN.)

tocopherol See VITAMIN E.

tocotrienols Members of the vitamin E family. The four tocotrienols—alpha, beta, gamma, and delta—are one of the two families of compounds that make up what experts call vitamin E. The other family is tocopherols, which are more common in the diet. Preliminary research has revealed that tocotrienols' ANTIOXIDANT properties show promise in treating a variety of illnesses including cancer, cardiovascular disease, and memory deterioration associated with aging. Tocotrienols are found in most vegetable oils.

Packer, L. et al. "Molecular Aspects of alpha Tocotrienol Antioxidant Action and Cell Signaling," *Journal of Nutrition* 131 (2001): 369S–373S.

tofu A SOYBEAN curd prepared by coagulations of the PROTEIN in soybean milk with calcium or magnesium salts. Tofu is a white semisolid containing 88 percent water, 6 percent protein, and 3 percent fat. It is shaped into blocks and kept moistened and refrigerated in plastic tubs. In much of Asia, tofu is the most common soy-based food. Tofu appears as deep-fried cakes, pouches, and puffs; tofu pudding; fermented tofu (bean curd cheese); tofu burgers and grilled tofu; bean curd sheets (dried yuba); Chinese-style pressed tofu; and savory pressed tofu. Tofu offers a number of advantages as a protein source. Soy protein is a high-quality protein, approaching the value of MEAT because it is rich in essential amino acids. Furthermore, soy protein is inexpensive and contains no CHOLESTEROL. Tofu supplies CALCIUM when soy milk is coagulated with lime. Such tofu contains 130 mg of calcium per 3.5-oz. serving, a substantial part of the daily calcium requirement. (If tofu is prepared with magnesium, the calcium content is negligible.) Nutrient content of one piece of tofu measuring two in. by three in. by one in. (120 g) is: 86 calories; protein, 9.4 g; carbohydrate, 2.9 g; fiber, 2.2 g; fat, 5 g; calcium, 108 mg; iron, 2.2 mg; thiamin, 0.18 mg; riboflavin, 0.08 mg; niacin, 0.1 mg.

tolerance to toxic materials (specific adaptive response) Refers to the body's adaptation to harmful substances. The first reactions to addictive substances or toxic materials are usually uncomfortable—gagging, choking, chest pains, and/or sneezing. After repeated exposure to harmful materials, the body may adapt to tolerate the material (maladaptation). In this stage, the body stops sending obvious distress signals. A CRAVING for the substance in question can develop, and when again ingested or taken up, the provoking substance can provide an emotional "high" or euphoria and decreased awareness of pain. Tolerance to the addictive or toxic material increases the risk of lowered immunity, weakened ADRENAL GLANDS, and physical exhaustion. These factors in turn set the stage for DEGENERATIVE DISEASES like CANCER and heart disease. Minimizing exposure or avoidance of active agents, preventive nutrition, and EXERCISE may counteract these effects. (See also ADDICTION; STRESS.)

tomato (*Lycopersicon esculentum*) A vegetable from an annual vine. Botanically speaking, the tomato is a fruit and is related to capsicum peppers, eggplant, and potatoes (members of the NIGHTSHADE FAMILY). The modern tomato apparently originated from an ancestor in the region of Peru and Ecuador and was first domesticated in Mexico. Tomatoes were long regarded by Europeans as poisonous and used only as a decorative plant. It was not until the 1800s that tomatoes were generally accepted as food. Tomatoes are now a leading vegetable crop in the United States. It ranks second to potatoes, when the consumption of processed tomatoes is included.

Tomatoes come in many shapes and sizes such as ribbed, pear-shaped or cherry-shaped. Colors range from the best known red varieties to green, yellow, or vari-colored. They range in size from less than an inch in diameter to five or six inches in diameter. Supermarket varieties fall into three categories: Cherry or grape tomatoes are small and less juicy; plum tomatoes are egg-shaped and less juicy and have a firmer flesh; round (slicing) tomatoes (also known as beefsteak tomatoes) are large, round varieties.

One reason for the tomato's popularity is that it combines well with so many foods. Large red tomatoes and small cherry or grape tomatoes are used for salads and sauces, while pear-shaped tomatoes are used in tomato pastes. Tomatoes are a traditional ingredient in dishes such as Italian pasta, gazpacho soup, guacamole, shrimp (seafood) cocktail, Spanish rice, stuffed tomatoes, and CHUTNEY. The United States is the major producer of tomatoes. Nearly 75 percent of the crop is processed as canned tomatoes, KETCHUP, chili sauce, tomato juice, tomato paste, tomato powder, salad dressings, and soups. Vegetable juice cocktails are usually tomato-based.

Fresh tomatoes are a good source of VITAMIN C, although the vitamin C content varies with the time of year. Because the consumption is so high, tomatoes are a major dietary source of vitamin C in the United States. Tomatoes also provide beta-carotene, although their intense orange-red color is due to another carotenoid called LYCOPENE, which lacks vitamin A activity. Lycopene acts as an antioxidant and, like beta-carotene, offers protection against the damaging effects of free radicals, highly reactive molecules that can attack cells. Free radical damage is linked to cancer and aging. Tomatoes contain courmaric acid and chlorogenic acid, compounds that block nitrosoamines. Nitrosoamines are cancer-causing agents that can form in the digestive tract from nitrites in cured meat. The nutrient content of one raw tomato (123 g) is: 29 calories; protein, 1.1 g; carbohydrate, 5.3 g; fiber, 2.2 g; fat, 0.3 g; potassium, 255 mg; vitamin A, 139 retinol equivalents; vitamin C, 22 mg; thiamin, 0.07 mg; riboflavin, 0.06 mg; niacin, 0.74 mg. One cup of tomato paste (262 g) provides 220 calories; protein, 9.9 g; carbohydrate, 49.3 g; fiber, 6.2 g; fat, 2.3 g; iron, 7.8 mg; potassium, 2,442 mg; sodium, 170 mg (if salted, sodium is 2,070 mg); vitamin A, 647 retinol equivalents; thiamin, 0.41 mg; riboflavin, 0.5 mg; niacin, 8.4 mg.

tongue This muscular organ is located in the MOUTH and partially in the PHARYNX. The tongue assists mastication, swallowing, speech, and taste functions. It pushes food into the teeth for grinding; once the food is masticated, the tongue forms a ball of food (bolus) and pushes it into the throat. The upper surface of the tongue is covered by small projections called papillae. TASTE buds are located on the papillae; they are responsible for the sense of taste. Taste receptors located at the tip of the tongue are most responsive to sweet and salty foods but respond to sour and bitter-tasting substances as well. The taste buds along the sides of the tongue respond to sour (acidic) substances, while the back of the tongue senses bitter materials more readily. (See also DEGLUTITION; SALIVA; TEETH.)

tooth See TEETH.

tooth decay See TEETH.

torula yeast (*Torulopsis utilis*) A very hardy YEAST cultured as a food for human consumption and livestock feed. Torula can be grown using molasses, carbohydrates from wood processing, fruit wastes, and citrus pulp extract. The dried yeast is tasteless and contains 50 percent to 62 percent protein. It is a source of the B vitamins, including vitamin B_{12}. (See also B COMPLEX.)

toxemia A potentially dangerous condition that may occur after the 20th week of pregnancy. Pre-eclampsia and ECLAMPSIA represent early and late stages of toxemia. Nearly 7 percent of pregnant women develop a degree of toxemia, characterized by elevated blood pressure, swollen neck and ankles, nausea, anorexia, puffy face, and kidney problems. Eclampsia indicates an intensification of symptoms with protein in urine, severe high blood pressure, blurred vision, and a sudden weight gain in the last trimester. If not corrected, toxemia of pregnancy can lead to circulatory failure, convulsions, and coma at time of labor. Although the cause of toxemia is not known, women who are young and pregnant for the first time, who lack prenatal care, and who may be nutrient deficient are at greatest risk.

Kidney disturbances, endocrine and metabolic irregularities, and compromised nutrient status have been implicated as risk factors in toxemia. PROTEIN, CALCIUM, CALORIE, and VITAMIN B_6 deficiencies may have a role. Studies of pregnant women suggest that oxidative damage may be related to the development of pre-eclampsia. Clinical studies suggest that CALCIUM may be beneficial and MAGNESIUM has been used to decrease complications of pregnancy, including toxemia. While well-balanced diets afford protection against complications, sodium restriction is discouraged in managing this condition. Delivery terminates the condition. Toxemia requires prompt medical attention.

toxicity The degree to which a substance can cause injury. In toxicology, toxicity refers to doses at which a large fraction of the exposed population would be expected to die. For example, LD50 is the dose of a substance that is lethal to 50 percent of a population of experimental animals. Toxicity can be distinguished from side effects. Side effects refer to the action or effect of a substance beyond that which is desired. Undesirable consequences include headache, nausea, dizziness, and sleepiness.

Toxicity can be the result of nutrient excess. Trace mineral nutrients like FLUORIDE, IODINE, SELENIUM, COPPER, IRON, ZINC, VITAMIN A, VITAMIN D, and VITAMIN B_6 cause a variety of symptoms of toxicity when sufficiently high levels are consumed. Even water, which is required in volumes of 1.5 to 2 liters daily, becomes toxic when large volumes are ingested because the blood becomes so diluted that it exceeds the ability of the kidneys to excrete water rapidly enough. Toxicity can occur with exposure to naturally occurring plant and microbial poisons (toxins) in foods, like aflatoxin in moldy peanuts and poisonous MUSHROOMS. Heavy metals like LEAD, CADMIUM, and MERCURY have no known biological roles and are toxic when present in sufficiently high concentrations. Toxic exposure may be due to synthetic chemicals like PESTICIDES, fertilizers, FOOD ADDITIVES, fuel additives, household chemicals, and industrial solvents.

A hazardous material is one that poses a health RISK. Hazardous materials can produce toxic symptoms under conditions of actual or realistic use. Thus, a food additive would be considered a hazard when amounts people usually consume can cause toxic signs and symptoms. The use of oyster shell and bone meal as calcium supplements is believed to be hazardous because they can be contaminated with lead. These effects on health may be subtle, such as lowered resistance to disease, increased risk of CANCER and of emphysema (due to cigarette smoking).

Margin of Safety

Food additives are generally permitted at levels several orders of magnitude lower than those at which they are believed to have no effect in order to create a "safety cushion." More generally, the margin of safety is the range between the level usually used and that which could create a hazard. The margin of safety for vitamin D is 1/40. Thus 40 times the common usage of vitamin D could cause toxic symptoms in susceptible people. Drugs may have lower margins of safety. Toxic effects of drugs and side effects with normal usage are commonplace among medications. Risks must be balanced against benefits.

The science of toxicology is imprecise for several reasons. Most information is generated from animal studies that may not relate to human risk. Most food additives have been tested for acute toxicity, but few have been tested for carcinogenicity, for long-range toxicity on the nervous system, or for additive or cumulative effects with pollutants, drugs or pesticides. Food additives react with each other and with other ingredients, and combinations can reveal unpredictable properties. This continues to be a critical area of research because people eat mixtures of chemicals in foods, rather than isolated chemicals. (See also ANTIBIOTIC RESISTANT BACTERIA IN FOOD; PESTICIDES; DIOXIN; HEAVY METALS.)

Seawright, A. A. "Directly Toxic Effects of Plants and Chemicals Which May Occur in Human and Animal Foods," *Natural Toxins* 3 (1995): 227–232.

toxic metals See HEAVY METALS.

toxin See AFLATOXIN; ENTEROTOXIN.

toxoplasmosis A type of FOOD POISONING caused by a disease-producing microorganism that can contaminate raw MEAT and POULTRY. Toxoplasmosis affects the eyes, lungs, and brain, sometimes leading to convulsions. The parasite can be transmitted via cat feces. About 40 percent of Americans have been exposed to toxoplasm from the family cat but have no symptoms because their IMMUNE SYSTEM destroys the invader. However, if a woman is exposed during her pregnancy, toxoplasmosis can affect the fetus. Infants exposed to toxoplasm during their fetal development may suffer from epilepsy, mental retardation, and blindness. Toxoplasmosis may affect one in 1,000 births—much more often than German measles, PHENYLKETONURIA, or syphilis in infants. U.S. physicians rarely check for toxoplasmosis in pregnant women, though this is commonly done in Europe. Healthy women who are exposed before pregnancy have antibodies that combat the parasite. Toxoplasmosis encephalitis (brain inflammation) is the most common opportunistic infection among AIDS patients, affecting 5 percent to 10 percent of them. Toxoplasmosis can also become a problem after treatment with immunosuppressant drugs (drugs that slow down the immune system). To prevent toxoplasmosis, patients should:

- Wear gloves when handling raw meat or poultry if they have cuts on their hands.
- Cook meat and poultry thoroughly (at 150° F).
- Avoid nibbling raw HAMBURGER and avoid eating raw steak (tartare). Cook eggs well.
- Pet owners should use gloves when cleaning the litter box and when gardening to minimize exposure from cat feces.

(See also GIARDIASIS.)

trace minerals (trace elements) Nutrients that are required in minute levels, ranging from micrograms (millionths of a gram) to milligrams (thousandths of a gram). Trace MINERALS include BORON, CHROMIUM, COPPER, FLUORIDE, IODINE, IRON, MANGANESE, MOLYBDENUM, SELENIUM, SILICON, and ZINC. RECOMMENDED DIETARY ALLOWANCES (RDAs) have been established for iodine, iron, selenium, and zinc. "Estimated safe and adequate" dietary intakes have been recommended for chromium, copper, fluoride, manganese, and molybdenum. Cobalt functions only as a constituent of VITAMIN B_{12} and has no other known function in animals. Selenium usually is ingested in organic form (selenomethionine and selenocysteine) rather than as the inorganic (uncombined) form.

The trace minerals vary in their function. A number aid ENZYMES (biological catalysts) by functioning as COFACTORS. Thus, iron and copper function in oxidation reactions and help enzymes burn

FAT and CARBOHYDRATES for energy. Cell division and growth require copper, zinc, iron, and other minerals. Iron serves to transport oxygen as part of the red blood cell protein (HEMOGLOBIN). Zinc assists enzymes responsible for the synthesis of genetic machinery, DNA and RNA. Chromium assists INSULIN to regulate BLOOD SUGAR. Iodine is required in the synthesis of thyroid hormones. Manganese assists enzymes, notably in the formation of GLUCOSE from noncarbohydrate precursors and in protection against chemical damage. Fluoride is a constituent of bones and teeth. Selenium as well as zinc, copper, and manganese function as ANTIOXIDANTS. Molybdenum assists various oxidases such as the enzyme that destroys SULFITE, a preservative. Silicon seems to be incorporated into bone and connective tissue. ARSENIC, NICKEL, and boron are essential nutrients in animals. Boron may help in bone building and may prevent calcium losses in post-menopausal women. The roles of other minerals are generally not known. Vanadium is present in tissues, although it is not known whether it is required for health. (See also NUTRIENT; VITAMIN.)

Blostein-Fujii, A. et al. "Short-Term Zinc Supplementation in Women with Non-Insulin-Dependent Diabetes Mellitus: Effects on Plasma 5-Nucleotidase Activities Insulin-Like Growth Factor I Concentrations and Lysoprotein Oxidation Rates in Vitro," *American Journal of Clinical Nutrition* 66, no. 3 (1997): 639–642.

tragacanth gum A gum obtained from the bark of a tragalus, a small bush that grows in the Middle East. Among vegetable gums, tragacanth gum is among the most resistant to acidic solutions, making it ideal for thickening salad dressings. There is little known regarding its chemical composition, and long-term feeding experiments to evaluate its safety are lacking. Because some people are allergic to tragacanth gum, it is no longer used in any of the leading fast-food hamburger franchises. (See also FOOD ADDITIVES.)

transamination The ENZYME-catalyzed transfer of nitrogen from AMINO ACIDS. Transamination is the first step in the degradation of most of the 20 amino acids used as protein-building blocks. The two exceptions are LYSINE and THREONINE, dietary essential amino acids. Transamination removes an amino group and transfers it to an acceptor molecule (KETO ACID), which is then converted to a new amino acid. This process frees the donor amino acid of its carbon skeleton, a new organic acid. Thus, ALANINE yields PYRUVIC ACID; GLUTAMIC ACID, alpha ketoglutaric acid; ASPARTIC ACID, OXALOACETIC ACID. Each of these acids is readily broken down for energy. Alternatively, these acids can be converted to blood glucose during fasting or STARVATION to supply fuel for the brain.

Enzymes that carry out transamination are called transaminases or aminotransferases. This class of enzyme is unique in its requirement for VITAMIN B_6 as the COENZYME, pyridoxal phosphate. Coenzymes are vitamin-derived enzyme helpers. Transaminases catalyze completely reversible reactions. This has important dietary implications because many amino acids can be formed simply by adding nitrogen to a keto acid with the appropriate carbon skeleton, thus, they are not dietary essentials (nonessential amino acids). As examples, nitrogen can be transferred to pyruvic acid to form alanine; alpha ketoglutaric acid reforms to glutamic acid; and oxaloacetic acid reforms to aspartic acid. In certain diseases transaminases may leak out of cells into the blood, and elevated blood levels of several transaminases are used in the clinical diagnosis of heart disease, liver disease, and other conditions. (See also AMINO ACID METABOLISM; PROTEIN QUALITY.)

trans-fatty acids By-products of the processing of polyunsaturated vegetable oils. Trans-fatty acids occur in safflower, corn, sunflower seed oils, and soybean oil, as well as in hardened fats like SHORTENING and MARGARINE.

Fatty acids are long chains of carbon atoms with hydrogen atoms attached. Fatty acids with fewer hydrogen-B atoms (double bonds) are called unsaturated. Manufacturers create trans-fatty acids as a by-product of chemical process called partial hydrogenation, which fills in some of the empty spaces for hydrogen and makes the fatty acid less saturated. Hydrogenation of vegetable oils extends their shelf life, cuts costs, and makes vegetable oils firmer and more spreadable. During the process, some of the unsaturated fatty acids are flipped from their bent shape to a straightened form, called trans-fatty acids. The resulting trans-fat possesses many properties of saturated fats.

Trans-fatty acids possess higher melting points than unaltered unsaturates and are solids at room temperature. The trans-fatty acid content of partially hydrogenated vegetable oil ranges between 5 percent and 16 percent. By comparison, canola oil and olive oil do not contain trans-fatty acids. Butter contains about 5 percent trans-fatty acids naturally. Margarine contains 10 percent to 27 percent, while stick margarine and shortening contain the most trans-fats. Vegetable shortening is sometimes used by food manufacturers in place of highly saturated tropical oils (coconut and palm). Fast foods are often cooked in shortening that has a high content of trans-fatty acids. For example, french fries may contain up to 38 percent trans-fatty acids. Food manufacturers frequently vary the oils and fats and the degree of hydrogenation in processed foods. Restaurant foods and commercially baked goods like cookies and crackers prepared with vegetable shortening represent other major sources of trans-fatty acids in the American diet. Low levels of trans-fatty acids are a normal part of the diet. However, the U.S. diet typically provides 20 times the intake of trans-fatty acids obtained from natural sources. Estimates of trans-fat intake range from 8 g to 20 g per day, reflecting an increased consumption of vegetable fat and processed foods.

Trans-fatty fats do not substitute for ESSENTIAL FATTY ACIDS, and they may worsen symptoms of essential fatty acid deficiency. They seem to antagonize the conversion of essential fatty acids to PROSTAGLANDINS, hormone-like lipids that regulate pain, smooth muscle contraction, raise or lower blood pressure depending on the type, and perform many other functions. Diets that incorporate high levels of trans-fatty acid are associated with an increased risk of coronary artery disease (heart disease). Trans-fatty acids may raise blood CHOLESTEROL as LOW-DENSITY LIPOPROTEIN (LDL, the less desirable form) while reducing the beneficial form of cholesterol, HIGH-DENSITY LIPOPROTEIN (HDL). In contrast, untreated polyunsaturated oils lower LDL. They may alter normal cell function in the heart muscle in lab animals when consumed at high levels. Experiments with animals indicate that trans-fatty acids can interfere with the function of insulin receptors, making insulin less effective and forcing the pancreas to produce more insulin to dispose of blood sugar. Such an effect on humans would increase the risk of diabetes. Whether trans-fatty acids impair the immune system or cause tumors in humans remains to be proven. Some animal studies show no effects with high trans-fatty acid consumption. The National Academy of Sciences concluded that currently consumed levels of trans-fatty acids are safe because small amounts are consumed.

Food labels will soon indicate the amount of trans-fatty acids in a food. Until then, when a food label lists the amount of unsaturated (monounsaturated and polyunsaturated fat), it cannot include trans-fats. When a product label claims a food is "saturated fat free," the food cannot contain more than half a gram of trans-fat.

Current dietary guidelines recommend cutting back on all fats and oils, including butter and margarine. Small amounts of butter or margarine are probably safe for most healthy people. Trans-fats in margarine do not mean that it is better to overindulge in butter. Tub margarine or liquid margarine are better than stick margarine because they are less hydrogenated and contain less trans-fat. In baking it is preferable to use liquid vegetable oil rather than margarine (which has trans-fats) or butter (which has more saturated fat plus cholesterol). Nonhydrogenated vegetable oils like olive oil and canola oil are better than margarine for cooking; they do not contain trans-fats. "Diet" margarine or "light" margarine contain more water and fewer calories than regular margarine. (See also FAT METABOLISM; FOOD GUIDE PYRAMID.)

Holmes, M. D. "Association of Dietary Intake of Fat and Fatty Acids with Risk of Breast Cancer," *Journal of the American Medical Association* 281, no. 10 (1999): 914–920.

transferrin A protein that transports IRON in the bloodstream. This protein can be measured by immunologic methods. Iron deficiency, pregnancy, low oxygen supply and chronic blood losses raise serum transferrin levels. Decreased transferrin occurs in PERNICIOUS ANEMIA, long-term infections, liver disease and excessive iron load. Transferrin levels respond quickly to changes in dietary protein, and low levels can reflect MALNUTRITION. The ability of transferrin to bind iron is called total iron binding capacity of serum (the straw-colored fluid remaining after blood has clotted). Depletion of iron stores is indicated by an increased total iron-binding capacity. (See also FERRITIN.)

trichinosis A disease caused by a parasitic worm, *Trichinela spiralis,* which can infect meat. Trichinosis remains an important disease in the United States and Latin America and results from consuming infected, raw or partially cooked pork. In addition to pigs, wild carnivorous animals such as bears may carry the parasite. Symptoms of trichinosis include fever, gastrointestinal upset, swelling of infected muscles, and severe muscular pain. Unusually high white cell count, recovery of larvae from blood, and immunologic tests are used for clinical diagnosis.

Prevention is best achieved by thoroughly cooking pork (137° F, 58° C) or by freezing pork continuously for at least 20 days at or below 5° F (–15° C) or for 24 hours at 2° F (–17° C). The same precautions apply to bear meat. Smoking or salting meat does not necessarily destroy this parasite. Infection in pigs can be minimized by cooking all garbage and offal from slaughterhouses used as feed. All states have laws requiring that garbage be cooked before feeding to pigs.

Pork Tapeworm

In Asia, Africa, and Latin America, infection by pork tapeworm (*Taenia solium*) is common. Microscopic tapeworm eggs follow an oral-fecal route of infection. Infection can be spread by eating food when infected food handlers do not wash their hands before meal preparation. The larvae infect the brain, which causes inflammation and seizures. In the United States, infection most frequently appears in communities populated by recent immigrants, for example, from Latin America. An immunologic test can detect parasite antibodies if present. Scrupulous hygienic practice and thorough cooking to avoid consumption of contaminated food are important preventative measures. (See also FOOD POISONING.)

triglycerides (triacylglycerols) Fats and oils. Triglycerides are the most energy-rich nutrients; they provide nine calories per gram, more than twice the amount in protein and carbohydrate. Triglycerides are digested in the intestine by lipases, enzymes that specifically degrade fat. Triglyceride digestion and absorption requires bile to free fatty acids and monoglycerides (fat fragments). These digestion products are reassembled into triglycerides within intestinal cells, then are packaged as CHYLOMICRONS (sub-microscopic particles that carry triglycerides) and released into the circulatory system. An enzyme in capillaries releases fatty acids from chylomicrons, to be absorbed by fat cells and stored as fat, or to be absorbed by muscle cells and burned for energy.

Triglycerides are classified as LIPIDS, because they are insoluble in water. Chemically, they are combinations of three FATTY ACIDS with a molecule of GLYCEROL, a fragment of glucose with three attachment points. Physical properties of triglycerides differ according to the types of fatty acids attached to glycerol. Thus, fats solidify at room temperature while oils remain liquid. This difference in physical properties reflects the relative amounts of saturated FATTY ACIDS and unsaturated fatty acids, which contain double bonds (bonds deficient in hydrogen atoms). Most naturally occurring triglycerides contain mixtures of fatty acids, and oils generally contain more unsaturated fatty acids. Synthetic triglycerides can contain a single type of fatty acid; in this case, the triglyceride is named after the fatty acid, e.g., tripalmitin contains only PALMITIC ACID (a fatty acid with 16 carbon atoms) and tristearin contains only STEARIC ACID (a fatty acid with 18 carbon atoms). MEDIUM-CHAIN TRIGLYCERIDES occur in COCONUT OIL and palm kernel oil and BUTTER. They contain shorter saturated fatty acids such as lauric acid (with eight to 12 carbon atoms). Medium-chain fatty acids are taken up directly by the intestine and processed by the liver. They are used in treating conditions with fat MALABSORPTION: SPRUE, STEATORRHEA, and other conditions.

Triglycerides are measured in a lab test of serum lipids. High levels of blood triglycerides increase the likelihood of blood clots and may indirectly contribute to processes leading to clogged arteries. High serum triglyceride levels have been found to increase the risk of coronary heart disease associated with high LOW-DENSITY LIPOPROTEIN (LDL, the less desirable form of cholesterol) and low HIGH-DENSITY LIPOPROTEIN (HDL). Fasting triglyceride levels in the range of 100 mg/dl are considered normal; 200 to 400 mg/dl are considered borderline high, and levels above 400 mg/dl are high. People with triglycerides over 150 and HDL levels lower than 40 can be considered at risk for heart attack, even while LDL is normal. Serum triglyceride levels temporarily increase after a meal due to digested fat. Alcohol consumption and vigorous exercise 24 hours before testing can also affect triglyceride readings. Exercising, losing weight, lowering fat intake, and limiting alcohol consumption can help lower serum triglycerides. (See also ATHEROSCLEROSIS; DIGESTION; FAT METABOLISM.)

Avins, A. L. et al. "Do Triglycerides Provide Meaningful Information About Heart Disease Risk?" *Archives of Internal Medicine* 160 (2000): 1,937–1,944.

triiodothyronine (T3) See THYROID GLAND.

triticale (*Triticum secale*) A hybrid cereal GRAIN derived from WHEAT (Triticum) and RYE (Secale). Extensive Canadian research has led to the development of more satisfactory varieties for milling and baking. In general, triticale has a higher PROTEIN content, a somewhat better balance of essential AMINO ACIDS and is more resistant to cold than wheat. Much of current production is used for animal feed.

tropical oils (coconut oil and palm oils) Saturated VEGETABLE OILS and common FOOD ADDITIVES. The most common tropical oils are COCONUT OIL and PALM OIL, mainstays of PROCESSED FOODS. They provide a rich taste and pleasing flavor to granola, cold BREAKFAST CEREALS, CRACKERS, cookies, and other products. Tropical oils are among the most saturated FATS, even more saturated than lard and beef tallow. Coconut oil is 92 percent saturated; palm kernel oil is 86 percent saturated; while palm oil is 52 percent saturated. For comparison, BUTTER is 65 percent saturated and LARD is 41 percent saturated. Unlike unsaturated vegetable oils such as OLIVE OIL, CORN OIL, SAFFLOWER oil, or CANOLA OIL, which lower blood CHOLESTEROL, tropical oils seem to increase blood cholesterol levels among Americans. Consumption of tropical oils may increase the risk of clogged arteries and HEART DISEASE.

Tropical oil can be disguised by food labeling. Over half the products with added vegetable oil use "multiple choice labeling." The manufacturer can use the least expensive oil available and add the following descriptions on food labels. "100 percent vegetable oil"; "partially hydrogenated vegetable oil (may contain one or more of the following: coconut, soybean, corn oils)"; "hydrogenated vegetable shortening (soybean, palm, and/or palm kernel oil)"; or "contains one or more of the following: palm, palm kernel, cottonseed, peanut, soybean, and safflower oil." These phrases on food labels are too vague to allow consumers to determine the exact types of oils present. Several food producers are changing their formulations and are in the process of gradually phasing out tropical oils in fast foods such as french fries. (See also DIETARY GUIDELINES FOR AMERICANS.)

tropical sprue See SPRUE.

trout A large group of mainly freshwater fish related to salmon. Several species are marine fish and ascend rivers to breed. Trout are primarily a sport fish; trout are raised commercially in pens for food use. The most widely known species of trout include rainbow trout, *Salmo gairdneri;* brook trout, *Salvelinus fontinalis;* steelhead or salmon trout, a variety of rainbow trout; cutthroat trout, *Salmo clarki;* and Dolly Varden, *Salvelinus malma.* Steelhead trout is an ocean-going rainbow trout. Lake trout is a large deep-lake trout found in Canada, the Great Lakes, and in deep lakes of the Northeast. Lake trout from the Great Lakes is likely to be contaminated with industrial pollutants such as PBBs, PCBS, and PESTICIDES. Great Lakes states have set limits for weekly consumption of game fish from these lakes. It is recommended that pregnant women avoid eating contaminated fish regardless of their source. Trout is sauteed, grilled, baked, or poached. It can be substituted for salmon in recipes. The nutrient content of a 3-oz. (85 g) trout is: 126 calories; protein, 17.7 g; fat, 5.6 g; cholesterol, 49 mg; thiamin, 0.28 mg; riboflavin, 0.26 mg; niacin, 7.6 mg (See also POLYBROMINATED BIPHENYLS; POLYCHLORINATED BIPHENYLS; PREGNANCY AND NUTRITIONAL REQUIREMENTS.)

trypsin An important protein-digesting enzyme produced by the PANCREAS. Trypsin is initially synthesized as an inactive form called trypsinogen and is released as such into the pancreatic duct, together with other inactive precursors of other digestive enzymes. Once in the small intestine, an intestinal enzyme (ENTEROPEPTIDASE) converts trypsinogen to trypsin. Trypsin then activates other protein-digesting enzymes such as CHYMOTRYPSIN and CARBOXYPEPTIDASE. Premature activation of these enzymes in the pancreas or duct can lead to localized inflammation and tissue destruction (PANCREATITIS).

Proteins consist of long chains of amino acids. Trypsin digests proteins by breaking (hydrolyzing) amino acid linkages within the protein chain. Trypsin is highly specific: It hydrolyzes bonds adjacent only at two amino acids, ARGININE and LYSINE. Another digestive enzyme, chymotrypsin, is less specific; it hydrolyzes bonds next to PHENYLALANINE, METHIONINE, TYROSINE, TRYPTOPHAN, and LEUCINE. The combined activities of these and other digestive enzymes efficiently degrades most food proteins to simple amino acids. (See also DIGESTION; PROTEASE; ZYMOGEN.)

tryptophan (Trp, L-tryptophan) A dietary essential amino acid and a building block of proteins. Tryptophan must be consumed daily because the body cannot synthesize it. In addition to serving as a raw material for proteins, tryptophan is required for the synthesis of SEROTONIN, a neurotransmitter that helps conduct nerve impulses between cells. Serotonin is also released by mast cells, defensive cells embedded in tissues, and by blood platelets. Serotonin causes smooth muscle to contract; it functions as a vasoconstrictor to constrict blood vessels. Dietary sources of tryptophan include PINEAPPLE, TURKEY, CHICKEN, YOGURT, unripened CHEESE, and BANANAS. The usual diet provides 1 to 2 g daily spread out over time, rather than as a single dose.

Tryptophan supplementation has been used with the following conditions:

Depression DEPRESSION is a facet of many diseases and tryptophan, together with painkillers, may help unresponsive depression in some cases. Tryptophan supplements in combination with VITAMIN B_6 have been tested as antidepressants. The effects of tryptophan on mania and aggressive behavior have also been examined clinically. Its use has been criticized as being less effective than standard drugs.

Food Cravings Administering a combination of tryptophan and TYROSINE has been used to help with depression and CRAVING during withdrawal from addictive substances.

Difficulty in Sleeping The effectiveness of tryptophan for inducing sleep is well established. Tryptophan has been used for many years in Great Britain to treat insomnia. For certain people, it enhances relaxation and sleepiness. Tryptophan seems more effective when taken before bedtime with a carbohydrate-rich food.

Side Effects from Oral Contraceptives Women taking oral contraceptives may metabolize tryptophan abnormally, which may be helped by taking vitamin B_6.

Chronic Pain Research suggests that tryptophan partially reduces sensitivity to pain. Administration of small doses of tryptophan throughout the day with a high carbohydrate, low-fat, low-protein diet and appropriate medication can decrease symptoms in some people. More research in this area is needed.

Toxicity and Side Effects

Amino acids are powerful agents in the body. Amino acid research in humans is still considered preliminary, and the long-term effects and safe dosages are not known for many situations. The Centers for Disease Control linked large doses of tryptophan supplements to a rare, painful blood disorder called eosinophilia-myalgia syndrome (EMS) that became an epidemic in 1989. Subsequently, the U.S. FDA issued a nationwide recall of all tryptophan products in which this amino acid is the sole or the major constituent. The only products containing tryptophan not recalled include certain protein supplements, infant formula, and special dietary foods that contain small amounts of tryptophan for nutrient fortification. No cases of EMS have been reported from this use. EMS is marked by severe muscle pain, joint pain, difficulty in breathing, swollen limbs, and fever. In severe cases there are signs of congestive heart failure and paralysis. Most cases were associated with a tryptophan from a single manufacturer; it was contaminated with a related product. Moderate doses of tryptophan (as low as 1 g/day in certain individuals) may cause liver abnormalities. When used with antidepressants, side effects may worsen.

tuna ***(Thunnus)*** A marine food fish that is a member of the mackerel family that inhabits temperate waters throughout the world. Some varieties of this fish can reach up to 1,500 lb. Albacore, bluefin, skipjack, and yellow fin are common varieties. Tuna has a red, dense flesh that lightens when cooked.

Tuna is the most popular fish in the United States based on annual consumption, and serves as a source of OMEGA-3 FATTY ACIDS, a group of FATTY ACIDS that reduce serum cholesterol and decrease the risk of blood clotting and hence heart attacks. Tuna is a large predatory fish at the top of its food chain. Like other such fish, tuna is more likely to be contaminated with pollutants like MERCURY.

In July 2002, an advisory panel to the U.S. Food and Drug Administration recommended that pregnant women eat no more than two cans of tuna a week. If they eat other fish, they should limit consumption to just one can of tuna.

Ninety-five percent of tuna that is consumed in the United States is canned. Canned tuna in oil is a high-calorie food. Oil-packed tuna contains 23 g of fat and 1,400 calories per 3-oz. serving, while water-packed tuna contains 1 g of fat and a total of 135 calories. Fresh tuna is usually sold as steaks, which can be broiled, poached, baked, or sauteed. The nutrient content of 3 oz. (85 g) of tuna packed in oil and drained is: 165 calories; protein, 24 g; fat, 7 g; cholesterol, 55 mg; calcium, 7 mg; iron, 1.6 mg; sodium, 303 mg; thiamin, 0.04 mg; riboflavin, 0.09 mg; niacin, 10.1 mg. The same size serving, water packed, provides fewer calories (135); more protein (30 g); less fat (1 g); more sodium, (468 mg); and comparable amounts of other nutrients. (See also FISH OIL; HEAVY METALS; SEAFOOD.)

turbinado sugar See SUCROSE.

turkey (*Meleagris gallopavo*) A large native American bird related to the pheasant. The domestic turkey was derived from a Mexican variety of wild turkey. The United States remains the largest producer of turkeys and accounts for over 55 percent of the world turkey production. Fast growing, broad-breasted, large white turkeys are typical of new varieties raised for their flesh. Turkey produces a higher proportion of edible meat per live weight than any other POULTRY. The time needed to raise a 25-lb. tom (male) turkey is 20 weeks. Fryer-roaster turkeys are young, immature turkeys under 16 weeks of age and of either sex. Young hen or tom turkeys are usually five to seven months of age. Grading by the USDA is voluntary. Unlike the grading of red meat, poultry grading is based on appearance, not fat content. Graded birds should be free of feathers and blemishes.

Turkey meat is lower in fat than most red meat, and brown meat contains more fat than light meat. Almost all of the fat lies under the skin and can be trimmed off. White meat, without skin, is a low-fat protein and is the leanest meat. Turkey white meat contains 14 percent calories as fat, dark meat contains 30 percent fat calories, while lean steak provides 37 percent fat calories. Turkey fat provides 40 percent saturated fatty acids and 35 percent polyunsaturated fatty acids; in contrast, beef fat provides 45 percent to 46 percent saturates and only 3.6 percent to 4.4 percent polyunsaturates. Self-basting turkeys contain much more fat than unbasted birds, and often the injected fat is saturated (butter or coconut oil).

Ground turkey combines both white and dark meat and may include fat and skin. The amounts of skin and fat vary because there are no official standards for fat content for ground turkey. The food label may indicate the percentage of fat content: Supermarkets may provide products listed as "not more than 15 percent fat" or "not more than 20 percent fat." Turkey is also processed into hot dogs, turkey ham, turkey pastrami, and turkey sausage. Turkey has become more popular than just a Thanksgiving meal, with the availability of turkey parts and turkey products and an increased consumer awareness of health problems associated with high saturated fat.

Turkey is perishable; frozen turkey should be stored frozen, then thawed in the refrigerator or under cold running water. The sell date on fresh turkeys is one week after the bird has been processed. Perhaps a third of CHICKENS and turkeys are contaminated with salmonella due to fecal exposure during processing. To prevent food poisoning, all items that come into contact with raw meat should be washed, including the cutting board and one's hands. Turkey should be cooked thoroughly. Stuffing should either be cooked separately or it should be added just before roasting.

Turkey is a good source of the B vitamins niacin, vitamin B_6 and vitamin B_{12} as well as minerals—iron, zinc, and magnesium. Like most meat, it is not a good source of calcium. The nutrient content of 3 oz. (85 g) of dark, roasted turkey meat is: 159 calories; protein, 24.3 g; fat, 6.1 g; cholesterol, 72 mg; iron, 2.0 mg; thiamin, 0.05 mg; riboflavin, 0.11 mg; niacin, 5.8 mg. Light meat, roasted (3 oz., 85 g) provides 133 calories; protein, 25.4 g; fat, 2.7 g; cholesterol, 59 mg; iron, 1.1 mg; thiamin, 0.09 mg; riboflavin, 0.26 mg; niacin, 7.6 mg.

turmeric (*Curcuma longa*) A natural yellow food coloring. Turmeric is obtained from the underground stem of an East Indian herb related to GINGER. When turmeric is cooked and dried, it possesses a mustard-like taste and a brilliant yellow color. Turmeric is used extensively in Indian, Spanish, Mediterranean, and Middle Eastern cuisine as a flavoring and coloring agent. It is used in commercial MUSTARD and is a traditional ingredient of curry. Turmeric is used with meat, poultry, fish, deviled eggs, shellfish, egg salad, and potato salad. As with most natural coloring agents, there is little information on its long-term effects from clinical studies. Turmeric is classified as a "generally recognized as safe" food additive.

Turmeric contains materials that can decrease inflammation and it is a potent antioxidant. It contains curcumin, a substance that blocks free radicals, extremely reactive molecules that can attack all cell components. Curcumin has strong anti-inflammatory effects, equivalent to typical non-steroidal anti-inflammatory drugs although it does not reduce pain. It seems to inhibit neutrophil response (defensive white cells) that triggers inflammation and to block the formation of leukotrienes, powerful stimulants of inflammation. In folk medicine turmeric poultices are applied to relieve pain and inflammation.

Recent research suggests curcumin has anticancer properties. In animal studies and laboratory tests curcumin was shown to slow or stop the growth of cancer cells. Curcumin and curcuminoid blends of curcumin and other ingredients are sold as a DIETARY SUPPLEMENT. Because dietary supplements are not tested by the U.S. government for safety or efficacy, the claims of companies making these supplements have not been substantiated. Large amounts of turmeric and curcumin are probably unsafe for pregnant women. Safety data for breast-feeding women are inadequate. (See also ARTIFICIAL FOOD COLORS; FOOD COLORING, NATURAL.)

Han, S-S. et al. "Curcumin Causes the Growth Arrest and Apoptosis of B Cell Lymphoma by Downregulation of egr-1, C-myc, Bcl-X_L, NF-kB, and p53," *Clinical Immunology* 93, no. 2 (1999): 152–161.

turnip (*Brassica rapa*) A member of the cabbage family (CRUCIFEROUS VEGETABLE) with edible leaves and root. Turnips are related to the RUTABAGA. Turnips were first cultivated about 2000 B.C. in the Near East. California, Colorado, and Indiana account for most of U.S. production. Turnips may be shaped like carrots, round or flat and broad. They can weigh up to 40 pounds. Turnips planted in the fall may be left in the ground until the following spring. Most of the U.S. crop is processed (frozen). Turnip roots are served with mashed potatoes, served with sauces, and cooked in casseroles, soups, and stews. Turnip greens are a rich source of calcium: 1 cup of cooked greens provides 198 mg of calcium, about 68 percent of a cup of milk. The nutrient content of 1 cup (156 g) of cooked turnips is: 28 calories; protein, 1.2 g; carbohydrate, 7.6 g; fiber, 2.8 g; vitamin C, 18 mg; thiamin, 0.04 mg; riboflavin, 0.04 mg; niacin, 0.46 mg.

tyramine An AMINE present in fermented or aged foods. Tyramine is produced by the degradation of the AMINO ACID, TYROSINE, either by FERMENTATION or by chemical action. This nitrogen-containing compound increases blood pressure dramatically. It can cause migraine headaches in sensitive people. Normally, tyramine is destroyed in the body by monoamine oxidase (MAO), the enzyme that degrades the hormone EPINEPHRINE. However, certain antidepressant drugs like isocarboxazid and phenelzine are classified as MAO INHIBITORS. By inhibiting this enzyme, they interfere with the disposal of tyramine, which can lead to headache, nausea, and high blood pressure when tyramine-containing foods are eaten. In extreme cases, a normal-sized serving of a tyramine-containing food or beverage taken with such medications causes life-threatening elevated blood pressure. The tyramine content of specific foods per 100 g is as follows: pickled herring, 303 mg; cheddar cheese, 141 mg; Gruyère cheese, 52 mg; Brie, 18 mg; chianti wine, 2.5 mg; sherry, 0.4 mg; beer, 0.3 mg; beef liver, 0.5 mg. Bananas, soft drinks, pineapples, yeast extract, yogurt, anchovies, canned figs, chicken liver, chocolate, mushrooms, pastrami, peanuts, sausage, soy sauce, coffee, and tea also contain significant amounts. Cottage cheese and processed cheese contain little tyramine. (See also DRUG-NUTRIENT INTERACTION.)

tyrosine (Tyr, L-tyrosine) A nonessential AMINO ACID required to build proteins and other important compounds. Tyrosine is readily synthesized by the body from the essential amino acid PHENYLALANINE. Tyrosine in the diet decreases the requirement of phenylalanine because less needs to be shunted to tyrosine synthesis. In addition to serving as a raw material for proteins, tyrosine is converted by the nervous system into a family of NEUROTRANSMITTERS, chemicals that help transmit nerve impulses between cells. These "catecholamines" include DOPAMINE, norepinephrine, and EPINEPHRINE. They play a role in sensitivity to pain and in feeling alert. In addition, the ADRENAL GLANDS convert tyrosine to epinephrine (adrenaline) and norepinephrine, which are released as hormones to gear up the body to respond to STRESS. The THYROID GLAND combines iodine with tyrosine to form the thyroid hormone thyroxine, which regulates basal metabolism. Tyrosine also forms melanin, the pigment of SKIN. Normal transformations of tyrosine require NIACIN, COPPER, and VITAMIN C.

In humans, tyrosine appears to increase performance under stress. Under stress nerve cells release norepinephrine more rapidly. Tyrosine supplements could theoretically increase norepinephrine formation and indirectly help maintain vigilance. Tyrosine may help reduce DEPRESSION and FATIGUE associated with PREMENSTRUAL SYNDROME (PMS). TRYPTOPHAN and tyrosine have been used to minimize cravings and depression during withdrawal from addictive substances. In lab animals, administration of tyrosine can increase brain uptake and increase brain production of neurotransmitters. One hypothesis of schizophrenia proposes that dopamine is increased in certain individuals. Some antipsychotic medications are designed to block the conversion of tyrosine to dopamine. Tyrosine seems to be most effective for nerve cells that fire frequently, therefore supplements can affect an aspect of physiology differently depending on the conditions. For example, certain brain cells fire rapidly in HYPERTENSION (high blood pressure); thus, giving tyrosine to hypertensive rats lowers the blood pressure. With low blood pressure, sympathetic nerves outside the brain are being triggered in order to raise blood pressure. Administration of tyrosine in this case helps raise blood pressure. Liver CIRRHOSIS can lead to a brain condition called encephalopathy (hepatic encephalopathy). Unusually high blood levels of phenylalanine and tyrosine could increase brain formation of TYRAMINE, and this could disrupt normal nerve function. In any event, cirrhosis alters tyrosine formation from phenylalanine as well as altering tyrosine degradation.

Tyrosine supplements can either raise or lower blood pressure depending on the individual, and migraine headaches can worsen, depending on the conditions. Tyrosine and phenylalanine supplements should not be taken at the same time as antidepressant drugs containing monoamine oxidase inhibitors. Taken together they can raise blood pressure to fatal levels. (See also AMINO ACID METABOLISM.)

U

ubiquinone See COENZYME Q.

ulcerative colitis See COLITIS.

ulcers See DUODENAL ULCER; PEPTIC ULCER.

ultraviolet light (UV light) A form of radiant energy that lies between visible light and X rays in the electromagnetic spectrum. Ultraviolet light has a shorter wavelength than visible light and therefore has more energy than visible light. In fact, UV light can induce chemical reactions in the body and in manufacturing processes. UV light from the sun converts a cholesterol product in the skin called 7-dehydrocholesterol to vitamin D_1. Commercial treatment of the plant STEROL, ERGOSTEROL, with UV light produces vitamin D_2. UV light is used to sterilize milk and foods and has other industrial uses because it can destroy viruses and bacteria.

UV light is potentially harmful to eyes and SKIN. Lifelong exposure increases the risk of CATARACTS due to damage to the lens of the eye. UV exposure is also implicated in damage to the cornea and the retina. Sunburn is an immediate symptom of the dangers of overexposure to UV light. Prolonged exposure to UV light in sunlight can cause premature aging of the skin; loss of the skin's elasticity causes wrinkles. Long-term exposure to sunlight can cause rough, brownish, scaly growth on the skin, a precancerous condition called actinic keratosis. Tanning increases the risk of skin cancer, the most common type of cancer; malignant melanoma is the most serious form. A second type of skin cancer, basal cell carcinoma, does not spread to other parts of the body and is more prevalent. Above 1 million new cases were diagnosed in 2001. Those at greatest risk are fair-skinned people with light-colored eyes; those who have a high incidence of moles or who have a family history of cancer; and people who spend long periods of time out of doors.

Preventing skin cancer involves protection from direct exposure to sunlight. Specialists recommend wearing UV-absorbing sunglasses and using appropriate sunscreen lotion whenever individuals are out in the sun. Nutrition seems to play an important role in limiting the effects of long-term UV exposure. The reason for this lies in the nature of the damage induced by UV light. UV light causes the formation of free radicals, highly reactive chemical fragments that randomly attack cell components like protein. When free radicals attack DNA, they can cause mutations, which can be a prelude to cancer. Nutritional ANTIOXIDANTS are agents that counter the effects of free radicals by either squelching them or by preventing their formation. Included in the family of antioxidants are VITAMIN C, VITAMIN E, and BETA-CAROTENE. Certain trace minerals like selenium and zinc can also effectively protect cells against oxidative damage. (See also MACULAR DEGENERATION; CARCINOGEN.)

undernutrition See MALNUTRITION.

unsaturated fat FAT that contains a relatively high percentage of FATTY ACIDS containing chains of carbon atoms that are deficient in hydrogen atoms and possess double bonds. Each double bond lacks two hydrogen atoms:

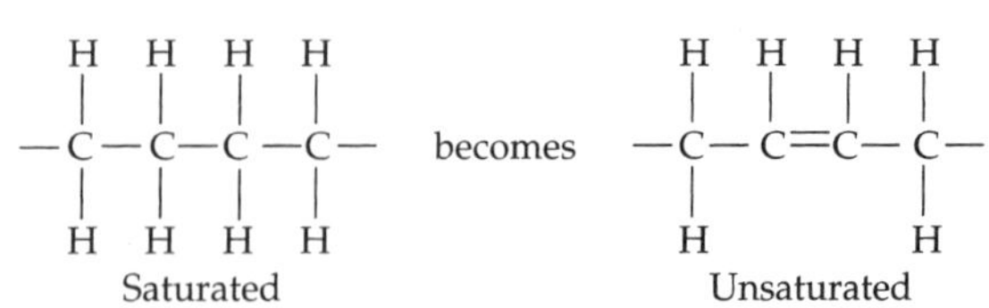

Fish oils and most vegetable oils are unsaturates. In contrast, animal fat and shortening are saturated fats, enriched in saturated fatty acids whose carbon atom chains are filled up with hydrogen atoms. These important chemical differences govern the physical and chemical properties of fats. Unsaturated fats are liquids at room temperature and are sensitive to attack by OXYGEN, which can lead to RANCIDITY (decomposition), while saturated fats are solid at room temperature and are more stable to heat and oxidation.

Unsaturated fats fall into two groups. MONOUNSATURATED OILS are rich in the monounsaturated fatty acid, OLEIC ACID; this building block lacks a single pair of hydrogen atoms. Such oils are called "monounsaturates" or "oleic-rich" oils; OLIVE OIL is a typical example. Monounsaturates seem to lower the risk of HEART DISEASE by lowering blood CHOLESTEROL (a desirable effect) without lowering HIGH-DENSITY LIPOPROTEIN (HDL), the beneficial form of cholesterol. Monounsaturates are not usually partially hydrogenated.

Polyunsaturates are the second type of unsaturated fats. These oils are rich in polyunsaturated fatty acids, which lack many hydrogen atoms. Because they are less saturated, polyunsaturated are more susceptible to oxidation. Vitamin E protects polyunsaturates against oxidation, and the requirement for vitamin E increases with increased consumption of polyunsaturates.

An industrial process called hydrogenation is used to harden unsaturated fats by adding hydrogen atoms and making the fatty acids more saturated. Partially hydrogenated vegetable oils maintain some of their unsaturated character and possess some double bonds; such oils are less susceptible to rancidity and have a longer shelf life than untreated oils.

Polyunsaturates provide varying amounts of ESSENTIAL FATTY ACIDS, required in the diet because they cannot be manufactured by the body. Most vegetable oils like soybean oil, corn oil, and safflower oil provide the essential fatty acid, LINOLEIC ACID, a polyunsaturated fatty acid of the omega-6 family, the most prevalent in the diet. These polyunsaturated oils seem to lower blood cholesterol (a desirable effect), but in large amounts they also lower the beneficial HDL. Polyunsaturates lower the risk of HEART ATTACK and STROKE because they block the formation of dangerous blood clots. On the other hand, in excess they may increase the risk of CANCER and lower immunity, at least in lab animals.

Certain seed oils like FLAXSEED OIL and fish oil supply the second essential fatty acid, ALPHA LINOLENIC ACID, and other omega-3 polyunsaturated fatty acids. Fish oils supply large polyunsaturated fatty acids that may help prevent or decrease the symptoms of heart disease and HYPERTENSION and of inflammatory conditions like RHEUMATOID ARTHRITIS.

Unsaturated fats produce essentially the same number of calories as saturated fats when burned for energy, nine calories per gram—more than twice the amount derived from carbohydrate or protein. Both saturated and unsaturated fats when consumed in excess can lead to weight gain. Current dietary guidelines call for selecting a diet that is lower in total fat (less than 30 percent of total daily calories, with saturated fat representing less than 10 percent of calories) in order to lower the risk of cancer and heart disease. (See also FAT METABOLISM.)

Judd, J. T. et al. "Effects of Margarine Compared with Those of Butter on Blood Lipid Profiles Related to Cardiovascular Disease Risk Factors in Normolipidemic Adults Fed Controlled Diets," *American Journal of Clinical Nutrition* 68, no. 4. (1998): 768–777.

urea The major nitrogen-containing waste produced by the body. Urea production is the body's way of safely disposing of ammonia, the potentially dangerous product released when AMINO ACIDS are broken down. Urea is nontoxic; it accounts for 60 percent to 90 percent of total excreted nitrogen.

Urea production occurs in the LIVER as part of the body's detoxification function; the amount produced is proportional to the amount of protein consumed. The liver uses a group of specialized enzymes (the UREA CYCLE) to produce urea. Urea is released into the bloodstream and transported to the kidney for excretion in the urine. Normally 20 to 35 g of urea are excreted each day. Blood urea nitrogen (BUN) refers to the measurement of blood urea levels and is used as a diagnostic tool to assess liver and kidney function. The amount of urea nitrogen in a 24-hour urine sample can be multiplied by 6.25 to estimate the amount of protein used per day. (See also AMINO ACID METABOLISM.)

urea cycle A collection of enzymes responsible for transforming AMMONIA to UREA. Ammonia is a toxic by-product of amino acid breakdown (AMINO ACID METABOLISM) that is released into the bloodstream. The brain is extremely sensitive to ammonia; therefore, its disposal is important. To detoxify this substance and simplify its elimination from the body, ammonia is efficiently removed from the blood by the liver, where it is combined with bicarbonate to create a safe product, urea, to be excreted by the kidneys. The liver also disposes of ammonia produced by gut bacteria and absorbed by the intestine. ORNITHINE, a nonprotein amino acid that accepts ammonia, is regenerated when ammonia is released. It is worth noting that the urea cycle produces the amino acid ARGININE. However, the production of this amino acid can be limited during illness and periods of rapid growth, and dietary sources are important. (See also GLUTAMINE; KREB'S CYCLE.)

urethane A cancer-causing agent in alcoholic beverages. Urethane has been found to form spontaneously in WINE, BEER, and hard liquors. Bourbon whiskey, fruit brandies, and some desserts and table wines sold in the United States may contain high levels, exceeding levels permitted in a number of countries, including Canada. Research is underway to lessen urethane contamination of alcoholic beverages. Because the PRESERVATIVE DEPC (diethylpyrocarbonate) spontaneously breaks down into urethane, it was banned by the FDA in 1972. (See also CANCER.)

uric acid A waste product form the degradation of RNA and DNA. Uric acid is a nitrogen-containing carbon compound derived from PURINES, which are building blocks of DNA, the genetic material of the cell, and of RNA, which directs the manufacture of proteins. Because the body cannot decompose the purine ring system, enzymes convert purines to uric acid instead. Between 0.5 and 1.0 g of uric acid is secreted in the urine daily.

A high blood level of uric acid is associated with GOUT, a form of ARTHRITIS that is characterized by deposits of uric acid in joints. The risk of gout increases with a high protein diet, a family history of gout and an acidic blood pH. Uric acid can form kidney stones, particularly in patients with gout. People with gout should minimize their consumption of foods with a high purine content: liver and organ meats; fish like anchovies, MACKEREL, and SARDINES; and yeast. Excessive alcohol can raise blood uric acid levels and increase the risk of kidney stones and gout. Extra fluid, 10 to 12 glasses of nonalcoholic, noncaffeinated beverages daily, can minimize uric acid deposits.

Uric acid performs a useful function for the body: It is a powerful ANTIOXIDANT that can destroy dangerous free radicals, which are linked to degenerative diseases and AGING. Evolution may have favored humans' ability to accumulate relatively high blood levels of uric acid in order to assure the presence of an antioxidant that is unrelated to diet. (See also VITAMIN C; VITAMIN E.)

urinary tract A system made up of two kidneys, two ureters (tubes leading to the urinary bladder) and a single urethra, the duct that conveys urine to outside the body. The primary function of the urinary tract is to assist the body in maintaining a constant internal environment (homeostasis) by controlling the composition and volume of the BLOOD. Kidneys aid in eliminating toxic materials, drugs, normal waste products, and even excesses of essential nutrients as urine. Kidneys assume a role in red blood cell production by secreting erythropoietin, stimulatory protein. They help regulate blood pH and form RENIN, a hormone to regulate BLOOD PRESSURE. Finally, the kidneys activate VITAMIN D to its hormone form, dihydroxycalciferol (calcitriol).

The two kidneys are located in the back just above the waistline. Usually each kidney is encased in a heavy cushion of fat for protection. An extremely thin person may lack this fatty support, and the kidneys may drop, placing a kink in the ureter. The rate of blood flow through the kidney is extremely high; about 10 percent of the total blood pumped each minute enters the kidneys. This high volume, together with a normal blood pressure, is required to filter the blood and to form urine.

Each kidney contains more than a million microscopic functional units called NEPHRONS. A nephron resembles a tiny funnel with an extremely long, twisted stem. Nephrons filter blood: some materials, like water, pass into the tubules, small tubes that drain the kidney. Others stay in the blood. Useful nutrients like GLUCOSE and minerals (ELECTROLYTES) are reabsorbed into the blood. The sum of these activities is urine.

Filtration usually occurs at a rate of 7,500 ml per hour, equivalent to 190 quarts of fluid filtered per day. Normally between 97 percent and 99 percent of the water is reabsorbed, together with all of the glucose because this nutrient, the primary brain fuel, is too precious to waste. However, in DIABETES MELLITUS the blood glucose concentration may exceed the rate at which it can be reabsorbed by kidney cells and is excreted in urine. Glucose in the urine (glucosuria) is a sign of uncontrolled diabetes.

Sodium reabsorption by the kidneys varies with blood pressure: When the sodium concentration in the blood is low, blood pressure drops and renin is released. This enzyme activates ANGIOTENSIN, a hormone that constricts minute arteries located at the nephron, increasing blood pressure. Angiotensin further stimulates the ADRENAL GLAND to release ALDOSTERONE, which increases sodium and water reabsorption by the tubules. Conditions that limit urine output are inadequate fluid consumption, stress, kidney disease, and CARDIOVASCULAR DISEASE.

Usually urine is sterile; the closer it gets to the urethra, the greater the possibility of bacterial contamination. The daily flow of urine out of the body and the immune defenses are usually adequate to assure a sterile urinary tract. However, bladder infections are common among women. Because over half of these infections involve the kidneys, they can be serious. Partial blockage of the urinary tract, for example by stone formation or scarring, can reduce urine flow and favor infection. Cranberry juice contains materials that prevent bacteria from sticking to the walls of the bladder or urethra, thus inhibiting bacterial infection. Garlic and onions also contain substances that limit bacterial growth. Sugar and sweetened juice can help promote bacterial growth, however. Drinking plenty of water (5 pints daily) is recommended.

Stone formation is a second frequent problem of the urinary tract; 10 percent of men and 5 percent of women in the United States will experience stone formation. Calcium as calcium carbonate or calcium oxalate can become insoluble and form crystalline deposits when water consumption is inadequate. Alternatively, uric acid can form stones when certain anti-cancer drugs are taken, or when excessive purines (yeast sardines, organ meats like liver, caviar) are part of the diet. Stone formation correlates with inadequate water intake and fiber consumption; high intake of foods like cocoa, spinach, parsley, rhubarb, and certain nuts containing oxalate, can favor stone formation in the urinary tract. (See also AMINO ACID METABOLISM; ERYTHROPOIESIS; KIDNEY STONES; UREA CYCLE.)

urticaria The medical term for hives, welts that form in response to irritation or allergy. Urticaria is typical of an immediate allergy reaction (immediate hypersensitivity) and is often accompanied by ASTHMA, itchy eyes, and runny nose. Animal dander, pollen, house dust, and certain foods can cause urticaria in susceptible people. (See also ALLERGY, IMMEDIATE.)

USDA (U.S. Department of Agriculture) A federal agency responsible for regulating food quality and safety. The USDA operates under the authority of the Federal Meat Inspection Act and the Poultry Products Act, which assign the USDA the responsibility for assuring the safety of MEAT and POULTRY. The USDA inspects meat and meat products, as well as poultry and poultry products destined for human consumption. It inspects slaughtering and processing practices. State laws for meat and poultry inspection must equal USDA standards.

The USDA sets guidelines for meat labeling and grades beef according to eating quality for food companies that pay for this service. Programs for health and nutrition, nutrition education and research are carried out by the eight divisions of the USDA. These divisions are the Agricultural Research Service; Consumer and Marketing Service; Cooperative State Research Service; Annual and Plant Health Inspection Service; Federal Extension Service; Cooperative State Research Service; Food and Nutrition Service; Veterinary Services;

Labeling and Registration Section. (See also PROCESSED FOOD.)

USRDA (U.S. recommended daily allowances) A standard for nutrient intake for healthy people, designed by the U.S. Department of Agriculture (USDA) for use on food labels through 1994. The USRDAs represent the highest RECOMMENDED DIETARY ALLOWANCES (RDAs), which were developed by the Food and Nutrition Board of the National Academy of Sciences for several nutrients in 1968. The USRDAs are not to be confused with the RDAs, which are not used on food labels. The list of RDAs is much more extensive now, and several values differ from those specified in 1968.

The USRDA was replaced in 1994 by the RDI or REFERENCE DAILY INTAKE (RDI) on food labels. For the time being, the RDI is identical to the USRDA. Individual USRDAs were condensed into just four population groupings: adults and children over four years; infants up to one year; children under four years; and pregnant or lactating women. Generally the highest values for a given age group were used. Thus the USRDAs for adults and children over four years generally were the dietary allowances recommended for a teenage male.

When nutritional claims about a food were made on a food label, or if the food was labeled "enriched," or if extra nutrients were added, the manufacturer was required to list the content of several nutrients as percentages of the USRDAs. The values food manufacturers used for the most common category, adults and children over four, are shown in the accompanying table.

Nutrient	USRDA
Vitamin A	1,000 mcg
Vitamin C	60 mg
Calcium	1,000 mg
Iron	18 mg
Vitamin D	10 mcg
Vitamin E	30 IU
Thiamin	1.5 mg
Riboflavin	1.7 mg
Niacin	20 mg
Vitamin B_6	2.0 mg
Folate	400 mcg
Vitamin B_{12}	6 mcg
Biotin	300 mcg
Pantothenic Acid	10 mg
Phosphorus	1,000 mg
Magnesium	400 mg
Zinc	15 mg
Iodine	150 mcg
Selenium	N/A
Copper	2 mg

For this category the protein value is 45 g of high-quality protein (equivalent to milk protein, CASEIN), or 65 g of lower quality protein (less than casein). (See also FOOD LABELING.)

National Research Council. *Recommended Dietary Allowances,* 10th ed. Washington, D.C.: 1989.

V

valerian root (*Valerian officinalis;* garden heliotrope; setwall) The root of a perennial herb native to Europe, North America, and northern Asia that has been used as a sleep aid and antianxiety treatment for more than 1,000 years. The plant is inconspicuous except for its small white or pink flowers and an unusual odor that some have described as reminiscent of aged cheese. According to legend, the Pied Piper used valerian to lure rats from the village of Hamelin.

Valerian is a popular dietary supplement in the United States and in Europe whose supporters claim it has a calming effect and can induce sleep. Reliable research to support these claims does not yet exist, but the herb does appear to have some effect on the neurotransmitter gamma-aminobutyric acid (GABA). Small studies suggest effectiveness in promoting sleep compared to placebo. People with nerve disorders that causes uncontrollable spasms or who suffer from TARDIVE DYSKINESIA have been found to have low levels of GABA in their brains. Because of the herb's reputation as an antispasmodic, it has been used for centuries by women seeking relief from menstrual cramps. As a food, valerian is classified "generally recognized as safe."

Because valerian root is available in the United States as an herb, its safety and efficacy have not been tested by the U.S. Food and Drug Administration (FDA). However, in high doses valerian root rarely can cause liver damage with long-term use or high doses. Some patients who have taken the supplements have suffered chest pain, heart arrhythmia, tremors, insomnia, headache, and blurred vision. With long-term high doses, suddenly stopping valerian may be associated with a withdrawal syndrome. A few reports suggest possible decreased alertness after valerian use. Women who are pregnant or nursing should not take this supplement due to inadequate safety data.

Garges, P. et al. "Cardiac Complications and Delirium Associated with Valerian Root Withdrawal," *Journal of the American Medical Association* 280 (November 1998): 1,566–1,567.

valine (Val, L-valine) A dietary essential AMINO ACID that serves as an important protein building block. Valine is classified as a BRANCHED CHAIN AMINO ACID, along with ISOLEUCINE and LEUCINE. The daily requirement for valine is estimated to be 10 mg per kilograms of body weight, similar to the other branched chain amino acids. Infused branched chain amino acids are selectively used for energy by skeletal muscle rather than by the LIVER. Branched chain amino acids may help restore muscles in patients with liver disease or in patients who have undergone physical trauma such as surgery. However, it is not established that these amino acids have an anabolic (muscle enhancing) effect when used as supplements for healthy people.

Valine and other branched chain amino acids are useful in treating liver damage associated with ALCOHOLISM (hepatic encephalopathy). They seem to limit muscle wasting and reduce some of the neurologic effects related to this disease. Valine and branched chain amino acids may be useful in treating amyotrophic lateral sclerosis (Lou Gehrig's disease). Levels of these amino acids are low in these patients. On the other hand, animal studies indicate that an excess of one branched chain amino acid antagonizes the other two. (See also AMINO ACID METABOLISM.)

vanadium A TRACE MINERAL required by animals for normal growth and development. Deprivation of this element causes slowed growth, reproductive problems and blood abnormalities in rats and chicks. Vanadium in the form of vanadate and vanadyl sulfate improves the effect of insulin in diabetic animals; and artificially induced diabetes in rats can be reversed by vanadate. Large doses also affect serum FAT and CHOLESTEROL levels, although more research in this area is needed.

There is no RECOMMENDED DIETARY ALLOWANCE for vanadium, and the amounts required for optimal health are unknown. Nutritional requirements would likely be met by levels present in food. Black pepper and dill seeds are the richest sources. Whole grains, seafood, milk products, and meat are fair sources, while beverages, vegetables, and fruits contain the lowest amounts. The average daily intake in the United States is about 20 mcg, quite low in comparison to known essential trace elements. Elevated vanadium is associated with bipolar disorder, and high levels of vanadium may be toxic.

vanilla (*Vanilla planifolia*) A tropical plant that produces pods containing vanilla, an aromatic ingredient used as a food flavoring. Vanilla is a member of a group of tropical orchids, native to Central America and Mexico. The active ingredient, ethyl vanillin, is chemically synthesized and marketed as "vanillin." Ethyl vanillin has 3.5 times the flavor intensity of vanilla bean extract. Because it lacks minor ingredients found in the extract, the taste is not identical. Vanilla is used to flavor ice cream, beverages, chocolate, candy, and gelatin. Vanilla is considered a safe additive. (See also FLAVORS; FOOD ADDITIVES.)

variant Creutzfeldt-Jakob disease (vCJD) See BEEF.

varicose veins Bulging, sinuous veins that are close to the surface of the skin. Usually the term varicose veins refers to distended leg veins in which blood vessels become weakened, permitting blood to flow backward instead of forward to the heart. This condition affects an estimated 25 percent of American women, 10 percent of men, and 50 percent of people over the age of 50. Often, varicose veins are only a cosmetic issue with no symptoms. However, symptoms like aching legs can develop after a person has been standing for a long time. Leg cramps, swollen ankles, intense pain or tenderness along the vein at the end of the day can occur.

Occupations that require extended periods of standing increase the risk of varicose leg veins. Pregnancy also increases venous pressure in the legs and may lead to the development of varicose veins. Standing places heavy pressure against leg veins, and the extra weight of the blood stretches the walls of the vessels, which pulls apart vessel valves, causing blood to pool in the veins. This pressure can cause surface vein walls to bulge out into varicose veins.

Varicose veins can occur anywhere in the body. Hemorrhoids are a common example; they can be aggravated in straining during bowel movements because intense abdominal pressure is transmitted to all veins, even leg veins. Defective, deeper veins can become inflamed (phlebitis) and create a blood clot, resulting in a more serious condition. If the clot dislodges, it can cause blockage in vessels of the lung, the heart (HEART ATTACK or myocardial infarction), or the brain (STROKE).

In addition to inheritance, lifestyle and diet are believed to be predominant factors in the development of varicose veins. They seldom occur in populations relying on a diet high in unrefined, fiber-rich foods. EXERCISE such as walking and bike riding contract leg muscles that push blood along the venous system. Increasing the strength of vessel walls may minimize the risk of varicose veins. Blue-red berry pigments called anthocyanidins and proanthocyanins can strengthen vessel walls, reduce capillary fragility and help protect the venous connective tissue. BLACKBERRIES, CHERRIES, and BLUEBERRIES are rich sources. People who have varicose veins may also be less able to break down FIBRIN, a clotting protein that is often deposited near varicose veins and increases the risk of clot formation. CAPSICUM (cayenne pepper), GINGER, GARLIC, and ONIONS increase fibrin breakdown. (See also CIRCULATORY SYSTEM; DIET, HIGH COMPLEX CARBOHYDRATE; FIBER.)

vasoconstriction Reducing the diameter of blood vessels. Both environmental and physiologic factors can constrict vessels. For example, a drop in temperature causes vasoconstriction, an adaptation that helps conserve body heat. All blood vessels except capillaries and venules are regulated by the NERVOUS SYSTEM. Thus fear and other emotions can reduce blood flow. At wound sites, SEROTONIN and other products are liberated by blood PLATELETS, cells that stick to the walls of damaged vessels to form clots. Serotonin helps reduce blood loss by acting as a vasoconstrictor. Certain hormones act as vasoconstrictors: EPINEPHRINE and norepinephrine (released by the ADRENAL GLANDS in response to stress) and ANGIOTENSIN II (formed in the KIDNEYS in response to a drop in blood pressure).

vasodilation Increasing the diameter of blood vessels. Vasodilation increases blood flow and removes waste products while replenishing oxygen and nutrients. Decreased oxygen concentration and the accumulation of metabolic waste products help expand blood vessel walls. The accumulation of LACTIC ACID, decreased pH (more acidic blood), the buildup of carbon dioxide, and increased blood ion concentration (osmolarity) dilate blood vessels. Increased body temperature exerts a vasodilator effect to help cool the body. During inflammation, HISTAMINE is released from damaged cells and from immune cells called mast cells. Histamine is known to increase capillary leakiness, and fluid leakage out of capillaries accounts for swelling in areas of inflammation.

An important family of vasodilators is the kinins, which represent peptides, whose parents occur in the blood and in tissues. Kinins resemble histamine: They relax the smooth muscles around vessels and increase capillary leakiness and blood flow through the kidneys. Kinins occur in sweat glands, salivary glands, and the PANCREAS. Kinin release is inhibited by GLUCOCORTICOIDS, hormones produced by the adrenal glands. A high protein diet also increases blood flow in the kidneys. PROSTAGLANDINS, hormone-like substances made from essential fatty acids, can have similar effects. (See also EDEMA; NITRIC OXIDE.)

vasopressin See ANTIDIURETIC HORMONE.

veal BEEF from male dairy calves, ranging in age from four to 18 weeks. Subtherapeutic doses of drugs may be used when veal calves are very young; this treatment is discontinued as the animal's immune system matures. Veal, like most red MEAT, is a good source of ZINC and other trace minerals. The nutrient content of a 3-oz. (85 g) braised veal cutlet is: 185 calories; protein, 23 g; fat, 9.4 g; cholesterol, 109 mg; calcium, 9 mg; iron, 0.8 mg; thiamin, 0.06 mg; riboflavin, 0.21 mg; niacin, 4.6 mg.

vegan See VEGETARIAN.

vegetable oil Edible oil extracted from seeds or nuts. Plant oils provide ENERGY, VITAMIN E, and polyunsaturated FATTY ACIDS. No vegetable oil contains CHOLESTEROL because plants do not synthesize it. Vegetable oils classified as TRIGLYCERIDES; like animal FAT, they contain three fatty acids and GLYCEROL (glycerin) and contain just as many calories as animal fat (nine calories per gram).

Vegetable oils fall into three classes: saturated, monounsaturated, and polyunsaturated:

1. Saturated vegetable oils are solid at room temperature. The so-called TROPICAL OILS, palm kernel oil and COCONUT OIL, and VEGETABLE SHORTENING, a chemically hardened vegetable fat, are saturated and are solids at room temperatures. These saturated fats resemble saturated animal fat, as in LARD, BUTTERFAT, and beef TALLOW. The excessive consumption of SATURATED FAT regardless of its source is believed to increase the risk of CARDIOVASCULAR DISEASE.
2. Monounsaturated oils including OLIVE OIL are rich in a fatty acid called OLEIC ACID, which lacks two hydrogen atoms and contains a single double bond. Olive oil apparently lowers blood LOW-DENSITY LIPOPROTEIN (LDL) cholesterol, the less desirable form, without lowering the "good" kind of cholesterol HIGH-DENSITY LIPOPROTEIN (HDL), and probably lowers the risk of cardiovascular disease.
3. Polyunsaturated oils such as CORN OIL, SAFFLOWER oil, SUNFLOWER oil, and SOYBEAN oil contain a preponderance of polyunsaturated fatty acids. These fat building blocks lack many hydrogen atoms and contain two or more dou-

ble bonds. High consumption of polyunsaturated vegetables oils apparently lowers LDL cholesterol levels, a desirable result, but also lowers HDL levels, which is undesirable. High consumption of polyunsaturated oils increases the need for the antioxidant vitamin E.

Extraction of Oils

The first step in oil extraction involves crushing or grinding oil-bearing tissue to release oil from cells. The second step involves pressing to squeeze oil from crushed tissue. Residues from pressing are usually extracted with solvents such as hexane to remove the remaining oil. The solvent is then removed. To purify these oils, they are further extracted with alkali and heated, degummed, deodorized by steam treatment, and decolorized by treatment with charcoal or clay. Since these procedures remove or destroy vitamin E, synthetic antioxidants like BHT, BHA, and PROPYL GALLATE are often added to retard RANCIDITY. Oils may be "winterized" by removing particulate matter that form upon chilling.

The assumption that cold-pressed oils have been extracted from the seeds under mild conditions and contain more vitamin E and polyunsaturated fatty acids may not be valid. Cold-pressed oils are often heated between 120° F and 150° F, then refined, bleached, and deodorized, processes that can involve further heating, possibly at temperatures as high as 450° F.

Certain "unrefined oils" are available. In the preparation of these oils, processors do nothing to the oils after heating ground seeds and pressing them to extract the oils. Because such oils are less pure, they have distinctive flavors and colors.

Hydrogenation

Unsaturated vegetable oils can be hardened and stabilized by chemically adding hydrogen atoms to reduce the degree of polyunsaturation. Hydrogenation increases the shelf-life of an oil by making it more resistant to rancidity. Heating vegetable oils at high temperatures does not hydrogenate oils, nor does it convert them to saturated fat. "Partially hydrogenated" vegetable oils retain some of their polyunsaturated fatty acids and remain oils at room temperature, while completely hydrogenated (saturated) oils are solid at room temperature (vegetable shortening). Hydrogenated vegetable oils as well as partially hydrogenated oils contain chemically altered fatty acids called TRANS-FATTY ACIDS; their long-term safety has been questioned.

Americans generally consume too much fat and oil, which increases the risk of HEART ATTACK, STROKE, OBESITY, and certain forms of CANCER. A person with high blood cholesterol may be advised to reduce saturated fat intake. Total fat should account for less than 30 percent of daily calories, perhaps as low as 20 percent of calories according to some authorities. To reduce the decomposition and rancidity of vegetable oils, store oils in the refrigerator in sealed dark containers. Do not heat oils any more than is necessary and limit cooking with oils at high temperatures. Discard cooking oils after use.

vegetables Cultivated plants that generally provide leaves, stems, roots, and flowers used as foods. Leafy vegetables include SPINACH, CHARD, CABBAGE, and LETTUCE. Stem vegetables are CELERY and ASPARAGUS; BEETS, TURNIPS, YAMS, POTATOES, and CARROTS are roots and tubers as opposed to stems. Vegetables like pumpkin, squash, BROCCOLI, and CAULIFLOWER are flowers. GARLIC and ONIONS are bulbs. Corn is a seed vegetable. Vegetables include several botanical classes, including TOMATOES (fruit); PEAS and BEANS (legumes); and MUSHROOMS (FUNGI).

Most regions of the world have contributed vegetables, as indicated by the following examples:

- Europe, the origin of beets, broccoli, BRUSSELS SPROUTS, cabbage, CHIVE, MUSTARD GREEN, pea, and turnip; the Mediterranean region: ARTICHOKE, asparagus, celery, chard, CHICKPEA, ENDIVE, KALE, KOHLRABI, OLIVE, PARSLEY, PARSNIP.
- Africa: the BROAD BEAN, CRESS, OKRA, yam; the Middle East: broad bean, cabbage, carrot, cauliflower, CUCUMBER, LENTIL, lettuce, mustard green, RADISH, SPINACH
- India: EGGPLANT, MUNG BEAN; China: Chinese cabbage, SOYBEAN, water chestnut
- Central Asia: beet, chive, carrot, DANDELION, garlic, LEEK, onion, pea, shallot, turnip
- Central America: bean, corn, jicama, green PEPPER, PUMPKIN, SQUASH, SWEET POTATO, tomato

- South America: cassava, corn, lima bean, pepper potato, sweet potato, tomato

Root vegetables and tubers like yams, sweet potatoes, carrots, and potatoes are by far the leading vegetable crops. They provide starch, fiber, minerals, and some vitamins. Orange-colored vegetables like sweet potato and carrot provide BETA-CAROTENE. Several of the most popular vegetables in the United States provide minimal nutrient content: celery, lettuce, cucumbers. The greener the vegetable, the more the beta-carotene (provitamin A) and CAROTENOIDS it contains. Spinach, collard greens, dandelion greens, kale, and Swiss chard are excellent sources and they provide vitamin C, iron, and calcium.

The consumption of fresh vegetables in the United States has steadily increased since 1980 from about 115 lb. per person per year to over 190 lb. per year (1990). Nonetheless, fewer than 10 percent to 20 percent of U.S. citizens report eating the minimum recommended five daily servings of vegetables and fruits. Potatoes represent nearly 37 percent of all fresh vegetables, and their popularity accounts in part for this increased vegetable consumption. Much of this increase represents french fries and baked potatoes eaten away from home; french fries and baked potatoes with fatty sauces are high-fat foods, in comparison with baked potatoes without toppings. Lettuce, broccoli, tomatoes, carrots, and cauliflower show increased popularity, probably a reflection of the increased availability of salad bars in fast-food restaurants.

There is a growing awareness that vegetables provide materials besides vitamins and minerals that are important for long-term health. Some plant substances (PHYTOCHEMICALS) are not considered essential nutrients, yet their consumption can have long-term effects on reducing the risk of CARDIOVASCULAR DISEASES, CANCER, CATARACTS, AUTOIMMUNE DISEASES like rheumatoid arthritis, premature senility, and other chronic problems associated with AGING. Plants of the cabbage family, including broccoli, cabbage, and brussels sprouts, produce materials called ISOTHIOCYNATES and indoles, which seem to lower the risk of cancer. Sulfur compounds of onions, garlic, leeks, and chives seem to boost the immune system and inhibit tumors. Many plants including vegetables produce FLAVONOIDS, a broad family of substances that can function as antioxidants to block the oxidative damage to cells due to free radicals. Free radical-induced damage is now believed to be a factor in some degenerative diseases, like heart disease, associated with aging. For example, dark green leafy and orange vegetables and some fruits are a rich source of CAROTENOIDS, including beta-carotene. These phytochemicals function as antioxidants and they enhance the immune system. As a group they reduce the risk of some forms of cancer.

Rather than a simple ingredient, vegetables provide a wide array of known phytochemicals; undoubtedly, many more remain to be discovered. Phytochemicals appear to be most effective when supplied in combination with a range of substances as found in minimally processed foods, including vegetables. Their effects are often synergistic, that is, the overall effect of a combination is more beneficial than any one isolated ingredient.

Vegetable Processing

Although fresh vegetables are available year round due to large refrigerated warehouses and fast transportation systems, processed vegetables remain an important part of the American diet. A variety of methods are used to prepare or to preserve vegetables. Several of the more common methods include:

Canning Developed in the 19th century in France, canning remains a major food preservation strategy. This process involves heating vegetables in metal or glass containers to a sufficiently high temperature to destroy microorganisms that cause spoilage or disease. Heat-treated contents are sealed against air to prevent oxidation.

Drying Drying food in the sun for preservation has been carried out for thousands of years. Drying must be carried out rapidly to avoid changes in nutrients, flavor, or texture. The action of plant enzymes that darken produce, destroy nutrients and alter flavor can be limited by blanching (a brief heat treatment) or by treatment with preservatives like sulfites or antioxidants such as VITAMIN C.

Freezing Commercial techniques for rapid cooling and freezing allow many vegetables to retain most qualities of fresh vegetables for periods lasting up to eight to 12 months. Blanching slows alterations in flavor, color, and texture of frozen vegetables.

Pickling Vegetables can be preserved in a salt solution (brine) or in VINEGAR, or a combination of the two. Pickled cucumber and relishes are common food items. Commercially pickled products require heating to destroy microorganisms and to inactivate plant enzymes that alter vegetables properties.

Raw or Cooked Vegetables?

There are certain advantages to eating cooked vegetables. Cooking a vegetable can increase the availability of beta-carotene because it is released from storage sites in plant cells. Cooking starchy vegetables breaks down starch granules so they can be digested. On the other hand there are advantages to eating vegetables raw. Raw vegetables may contain higher levels of heat-sensitive nutrients because cooking decreases the content of water-soluble vitamins. For example, baked potatoes and sweet potatoes lose about 20 percent of the B vitamins and vitamin C. Boiling causes lower losses. Boiling leaches B vitamins and minerals out of vegetables. Losses may be as high as 80 percent. Steaming and microwave cooking of vegetables greatly reduces this loss. Boiling also removes vitamins and minerals. Note that keeping foods warm on a steam table increases the loss of vitamins such as vitamin C, thiamin, and riboflavin.

On the other hand, vegetables that have not been stored properly, or have been handled carelessly, can suffer similar nutrient losses. Slicing, mashing, dicing, mincing, and grating break vegetable cells and expose vitamins to oxygen and degradative enzymes. Vitamin C is especially sensitive to oxygen exposure. The longer the storage period for sliced vegetables, the greater the loss of vitamin C. (See also BALANCED DIET; DIETARY GUIDELINES FOR AMERICANS; FOOD PRESERVATION; FOOD PROCESSING; FOOD GUIDE PYRAMID; ORGANIC FOODS.)

Graziano, J. M. et al. "A Prospective Study of Consumption of Carotenoids in Fruits and Vegetables and Decreased Cardiovascular Mortality in the Elderly," *Annals of Epidemiology* 5 (1995): 225–260.

vegetable shortening A form of saturated fat, prepared from vegetable oil, that resembles animal fat. A major advantage of vegetable shortening is that, unlike lard, butter, or beef fat, it does not contain CHOLESTEROL. Vegetable shortening does contain the same high calories as butter or lard, however. Vegetable shortening is a product of the chemical processing called hydrogenation. This process adds hydrogen atoms to unsaturated FATTY ACIDS, thereby converting naturally liquid fat (oils) to materials with varying degrees of stiffness. Usually several different fats are blended to achieve the desired consistency of a shortening. CORN OIL, COTTONSEED OIL, SOYBEAN oil, OLIVE OIL, PALM OIL, PEANUT oil, SAFFLOWER oil, and SESAME oil may be combined. Shortening, like other hydrogenated vegetable oils, contains TRANS-FATTY ACIDS as a by-product of manufacture. The long-term safety of trans-fatty acids has been questioned. A diet high in saturated fat is linked to an increased risk of HEART DISEASE and CANCER. (See also HYDROGENATED VEGETABLE OIL; VEGETABLE OIL.)

vegetarian One who eats predominantly VEGETABLES, FRUITS, GRAINS, and NUTS and either limits or excludes animal products, including MEAT, FISH, SEAFOOD, and dairy products from the diet. With a thoughtful selection of a variety of foods, vegetarians can easily meet all their nutrient needs. People choose vegetarianism for a variety of reasons. Vegetarianism may be related to religious or philosophical beliefs. Ecologically, vegetarianism represents a more efficient use of energy than relying on meat and meat products. From a health perspective, plant products do not contain the growth promoters and antibiotics used in poultry and meat production nor do they contain cholesterol. Plants are excellent sources of FIBER and ESSENTIAL FATTY ACIDS.

There are varying degrees of vegetarianism:

- Vegans rely on foods of plant origin and omit all meat, poultry, fish, and eggs, as well as milk and meat products.
- Fruitarians rely on dry or raw fruits, together with nuts, honey, grains, LEGUMES, and OLIVE OIL while excluding animal products.
- Semivegetarians occasionally eat some meat, fish, or poultry, eggs and milk or cheese while relying on cereals, grains, fruit, and vegetables.

Most "heart healthy" diets are semivegetarian diets. There are a variety of such diets.

- Ovo-vegetarians include eggs with foods of plant origin in the diet.
- Lactovegetarians include milk and milk products, together with foods of plant origin.
- Lacto-ovo-vegetarians include both milk products and eggs with grains, fruits, and vegetables. Vegetarians who eat dairy products tend to have higher blood cholesterol levels than those who do not.
- Pescovegetarians include fish and seafood, together with foods derived from plants.

Vegetarians may have a reduced risk of obesity, type II (adult onset) diabetes, GALLSTONES, and CORONARY ARTERY DISEASE. There is evidence that vegetarian diets reduce the risk of breast CANCER, DIVERTICULOSIS, colonic cancer, hemorrhoids, OSTEOPOROSIS, and dental caries.

Nutrient Needs

Vegans who are pregnant or lactating, children of vegans, and people who are ill run the greatest risk for certain nutrient deficiencies because these individuals have high nutrient needs that may not be readily met by eating a limited variety of plant foods.

Minerals The amounts of many TRACE MINERALS are low in plant products, and the body's ability to absorb them from plant sources is often low. Milk and milk products provides the most of the calcium and meat provides the most iron and zinc in the usual diet. Vegans may have difficulties in obtaining minerals such as:

- CALCIUM. Major plant sources are: BROCCOLI, KALE, COLLARD greens, kelp, PARSLEY, prunes, SESAME seeds, fortified TOFU, and fortified soymilk.
- ZINC. Sources are: whole grains, BREWER'S YEAST, LIMA BEANS, SOYBEANS, sunflower seeds, PEAS, LENTILS, and wheat germ.
- IRON. This nutrient occurs in dried beans and peas, dried fruit, fortified cereals, and bread. Iron uptake can be significantly increased by eating iron-rich vegetable foods with vitamin C-rich foods (citrus fruit, berries, dark green leafy vegetables).
- COPPER. Copper occurs in AVOCADOS, BARLEY, BEANS, broccoli, BEETS, PECANS, RAISINS, and soybeans.
- MANGANESE. This nutrient occurs in avocados, NUTS, seeds, whole grains, legumes, dried peas, and dark green leafy vegetables.

Energy The energy demands of infants and growing children are quite relative to their body size. Fat is a calorie-dense food that is an important part of a child's diet. Often vegetarian foods offer high fiber but low energy (fat) content. When the diet provides inadequate calories, a muscle protein is degraded for energy, not a desirable situation in a young, growing body.

Protein Dietary protein must supply adequate essential AMINO ACIDS (the amino acids that cannot be fabricated in amounts to meet the body's requirements). Plant proteins may be less easily digested depending on the meal preparation. Their amino acid compositions are usually not as well balanced as animal protein. Consequently, vegetarian diets based on a single grain like corn can contribute to MALNUTRITION. Plant proteins from different sources can complement each other, so that the net amino acid intake of a mixture of plant protein can adequately meet the daily requirement for essential amino acids. For example, combining whole grain foods with legumes is a traditional practice (rice and beans, corn and beans, wheat and lentils, for example).

Vitamin D The best sources of this vitamin are fatty fish, egg yolk, liver, and milk and milk products—all of which are eliminated from a strictly vegetarian diet. Exposure to sunlight may meet individual needs; however, supplementation may be necessary for people living in northern regions of the United States during the winter months, as well as for institutionalized people.

B Vitamins A number of cereal grain products are enriched with RIBOFLAVIN, THIAMIN, and NIACIN. Legumes and whole grains can provide significant riboflavin. VITAMIN B_{12} deficiency is a major concern for strict vegetarians. There is probably no very good plant source, other than nutritional YEAST. The amounts provided in sea vegetables, fermented soy, and algae may be inadequate. The best sources are animal products such as meat; thus a strict vegetarian may need a supplement, fortified soy milk, or fortified meat analog. Once vitamin B_{12} deficiency has occurred, the resulting nerve degeneration may not be reversible.

Strict vegetarian diets are not recommended for infants or children. Pregnant women should plan their diet very carefully to maximize nutrient-dense foods and:

1. emphasize unrefined, whole foods;
2. use protein-rich sources like legumes, seeds, and nuts;
3. eat a variety of fruits, vegetables, legumes, and whole grains to assure adequate protein complementation;
4. eat fruit and vitamin C-rich foods with each meal to enhance iron uptake;
5. consider supplemental sources of vitamin B_{12}, vitamin D, calcium, and trace minerals or properly fortified sources;
6. eat enough food to provide adequate protein and energy.

(See also CHOLESTEROL-LOWERING DRUGS; COMPLETE PROTEIN.)

Appleby, P. N. et al. "The Oxford Vegetarian Study: An Overview," *American Journal of Clinical Nutrition* 70, suppl. (1999): 525S–531S.

Key, T. J. et al. "Health Benefits of a Vegetarian Diet," *Proceedings of the Nutrition Society* 58 (1999): 271–275.

very low-density lipoprotein (VLDL) A lipid-protein particle that transports FAT from the LIVER to other tissues via the bloodstream. After a carbohydrate meal, the liver absorbs glucose from the blood and converts it to fat (TRIGLYCERIDES). The liver packages fat to export it to other parts of the body via the bloodstream in the form of VLDL. In composition, VLDL resembles chylomicrons, the fat transport vesicles from the intestine. VLDL contains triglycerides, a low amount of CHOLESTEROL, and two types of protein designated B-100 and C-II.

When VLDL reaches the capillaries, its triglycerides are broken down by an enzyme in the walls of the capillaries called lipoprotein lipase. Tissues then absorb the released fatty acids. After releasing their fat, VLDL remnants follow an unusual pathway: They become enriched in cholesterol as they are transformed in the blood to LOW-DENSITY LIPOPROTEIN (LDL)—the particle that carries cholesterol to tissues.

The blood levels of both chylomicrons and VLDL increase for several hours after eating. Therefore, lab tests that measure triglycerides in serum, the clear cell-free fluid remaining after blood clots, are usually performed after an overnight fast when levels have stabilized. Middle-aged white males with high levels of serum triglycerides (essentially VLDL) and high LDL appear to be more likely to have heart attacks than men with normal levels, even in the people with somewhat elevated serum cholesterol levels. The risk of heart attack may decrease by lowering serum triglycerides and raising HIGH-DENSITY LIPOPROTEIN (HDL), the "desirable cholesterol." (See also CARDIOVASCULAR DISEASE; FAT METABOLISM.)

villi Microscopic, fuzzy layer coating the inner side of the wall of the SMALL INTESTINE like a shag carpet. Cells that line the surface of villi possess numerous, tiny projections called MICROVILLI. If all of the intestinal folds, villi, and microvilli were flattened out, the total surface area would be about the size of a tennis court. Thus villi dramatically increase the absorptive area of the intestinal surface and facilitate efficient nutrient uptake. CELIAC DISEASE, CROHN'S DISEASE, and intestinal parasitic diseases (like GIARDIASIS) can lead to a loss of the villi and subsequent MALABSORPTION and maldigestion syndromes. With appropriate treatment and dietary modification, the villi can grow back and digestion can improve. (See also DIGESTION; DIGESTIVE TRACK.)

villikinin A hormone produced by the SMALL INTESTINE that stimulates the movement of VILLI, microscopic hair-like projections that coat the inner surface of the small intestine. This action serves to mix chewed food and digestive juice (CHYME) and to increase nutrient absorption by the intestine. (See also DIGESTION; ENDOCRINE SYSTEM.)

vinegar A dilute solution of ACETIC ACID. The term is derived from the French *vinaigre,* which means sour wine. Vinegar has been used in food preservation and medicine for thousands of years. Typically vinegar contains 4 percent to 12 percent acetic ACID, which is produced by the bacterial oxidation of alcohol formed by the fermentation of sugars and fruits. Apples yield cider vinegar; grapes, wine vinegar; and sugar and hydrolyzed starches from corn and wheat, white vinegar. Depending upon the nature of the fruit fermented, the resulting vinegar will have a unique flavor without adding significant calories. Vinegar provides only two calories per teaspoon. Because it is so acidic, vinegar is used to preserve foods in pickling. In salad dressing, MAYONNAISE, MUSTARD, and tomato sauce, vinegar helps retard spoilage. Vinegar contains traces of minerals but it is not a significant food source. (See also FOOD PROCESSING.)

vitamin An essential organic nutrient. Minute amounts of vitamins participate in three general functions of the body: growth, protection, and energy regulation. There are a total of 13 vitamins. Four are fat-soluble vitamins A, D, E, and K. The rest are water-soluble. Eight vitamins are in the B complex: RIBOFLAVIN (B_1), THIAMIN (B_2), NIACIN (B_3), VITAMIN B_6, vitamin B_{12}, FOLIC ACID, PANTOTHENIC ACID, and biotin. VITAMIN C is also water-soluble but is not considered a B vitamin, which function as enzyme helpers (coenzymes).

Vitamins either cannot be synthesized by the body or they cannot be made in adequate amounts, so they must be supplied by the diet. As examples of the latter, vitamin D can be made in the skin when exposed to sunlight, while some niacin can be made from the amino acid tryptophan. The intestine is a source of BIOTIN, pantothenic acid, and VITAMIN K; these are supplied by "friendly" intestinal bacteria, though the exact amounts supplied are difficult to assess.

The term *vitamin* dates from 1912, and the first vitamin to be isolated was vitamin A in 1913. Thiamin was discovered in 1926, vitamin K in 1929, and vitamin C in 1932. Vitamin B_{12} was the most recent vitamin to be discovered (1948). Before a compound can be classified as a vitamin, it must be proven that animals must obtain the compound from their diet. Typically, scientists test lab animals such as mice with a diet free of the test substance, together with a dose of antibiotics to eliminate intestinal bacteria.

Vitamins originate chiefly from plant sources. Except for vitamin D and vitamin C, vitamins are present in animal tissue only if the animal consumes foods containing them or harbors microorganisms capable of synthesizing them. B vitamins are universally distributed; fat-soluble vitamins may be absent from some types of organisms. Each of the vitamins plays a specific role in the body; a deficiency of one vitamin cannot be eliminated by consuming an excess of another.

Fat-Soluble Vitamins

VITAMIN A, VITAMIN D, VITAMIN E, and vitamin K are oily materials and dissolve in fats and oils, not in water. Unlike the B complex, these vitamins generally do not serve as enzyme helpers, nor are they involved in energy production; each has an entirely different function, ranging from acting as an ANTIOXIDANT (E), to producing a visual pigment for night vision (A), to blood clothing (K), and to bone formation (D).

Fat-soluble vitamins are absorbed best when they are eaten with fats and oils. These vitamins are stored in the body, so they do not need to be consumed daily. Because they are stored, excessive consumption can lead to high tissue levels resulting in toxic side effects, especially for vitamins A and D. For example, 50,000 international units of vitamin A over several months can cause toxic symptoms in adults. Symptoms of toxicity, such as achy joints, fatigue, headaches, and nausea, disappear when the high intake stops. What represents an excessive intake depends on many factors, including the type of vitamin, individual tolerance, which varies with age, and the length of time for which the supplement is taken.

Water-Soluble Vitamins

B complex vitamins help convert food into energy; they include THIAMIN (B_1), RIBOFLAVIN (B_2), NIACIN (B_3), VITAMIN B_6, pantothenic acid, and biotin. FOLIC ACID and vitamin B_{12} are involved in building new cells, while vitamin C serves as an antioxidant and helps build healthy capillaries, gums, and joints. Except for vitamin B_{12}, water-soluble vitamins are not stored well in the body and must be replenished daily. Excesses are generally excreted in the urine.

Vitamin Deficiencies

Long-term vitamin deficiencies often lead to serious illness. Deficiencies can be due to an inadequate diet (MALNUTRITION); inability to digest food (maldigestion); inability to absorb vitamins due to damage to the intestine or to competition with another material such as a drug (MALABSORPTION); increased physiological need as during pregnancy; growth, injury, choice of lifestyle, or other environmental factors.

Physicians may use lab tests to diagnose vitamin deficiencies. Most tests involve blood analyses, even though these are not always reliable. For example, a common antibody test for serum vitamin B_{12} detects both vitamin B_{12} together with inactive derivatives. Measurement of enzyme levels or levels of metabolic products can provide useful information. Dietary analysis can reveal levels of nutrients in the diet and guide a nutritional evaluation and assessment of individual needs complementing the physical examination and health history.

Natural vs. Synthetic Vitamins

Natural vitamins are those occurring in food. All substances classified as vitamins have been isolated from animal or plant sources, and most have been chemically synthesized in the lab to establish their structures. In other words, synthetic vitamins are usually identical to the product in cells. As an example, vitamin C in cells is defined chemically as L-ascorbic acid, identical to synthetic L-ascorbic acid. Most vitamins found in supplements are chemically synthesized, because there simply is not enough of most vitamins extracted from plant materials to meet world demand. Most vitamin C comes from a few major commercial sources worldwide.

A few synthetic vitamins differ from the natural forms. Synthetic vitamin E, called d, 1-alpha-tocopherol, is a mixture of both left- and right-handed molecules, while the natural alpha tocopherol is a single form called d-tocopherol. The synthetic product is adjusted to provide the same biological activity as the natural form. Certain vitamins like vitamin B_{12} possess structures that are too complex for a convenient lab synthesis. Microbial sources have been selected to produce large amounts.

Vitamin Supplements

Nutritionists often recommend obtaining vitamins from foods for several reasons.

Foods supply mixtures of vitamins, minerals, and other materials that may have beneficial effects. Mixtures are what the body uses. Foods supply materials that are not vitamins, yet are important. In this class are FLAVONOIDS, which work together with vitamin C to build strong capillaries and serve as antioxidants and as anti-inflammatory agents. Substances with anticancer properties have recently been isolated from vegetables of the cabbage family; they include isothiocyanates and indoles, in addition to the flavonoids.

Recent surveys show that about 158 million consumers take supplements and spend about $8.5 billion yearly on vitamins, minerals, and other supplements. One explanation for this widespread practice is that many people have subclinical deficiencies. They are not sick, but they are not well, either. They may want to feel more energetic and to have more stable moods. Others want to take supplements as insurance in preventing certain diseases if they live in a polluted environment or if their genetic makeup, medical history, and lifestyle choices warrant it. A growing number of consumers want to promote optimal health. Although there is a natural tendency to search for an easy solution to health problems, there are limits regarding what vitamins can do for health. No single supplement can compensate for overindulgence, physical inactivity, or genetic predisposition.

Deciding who needs vitamin supplements and how much should be taken is a controversial area. Conventional wisdom says that by following DIETARY GUIDELINES FOR AMERICANS and using a recommended plan such as the FOOD PYRAMID, an individual should be assured of an adequate supply of nutrients. Thus, if an individual is healthy and is eating a BALANCED DIET, vitamin supplements would not be needed. There is general agreement that individuals with well recognized needs may require supplements. These people include:

- women with heavy menstrual bleeding (extra IRON)

- women taking oral contraceptives (may need extra vitamin B_6)
- pregnant women (extra iron, folic acid, and CALCIUM)
- malnourished individuals, including dieters, elderly people with a low caloric intake, chronic alcoholics, and those with other chemical dependencies
- strict vegetarians (many need extra iron, zinc, calcium, and vitamin B_{12})
- newborn infants (may be deficient in vitamin E and vitamin K)
- individuals with chronic disorders, such as patients with OSTEOPOROSIS (may need extra vitamin D, calcium, magnesium, and trace minerals)
- hospitalized patients. Patients in hospitals and institutionalized people may become deficient in one or more vitamin.
- people who smoke (extra vitamin C)

Another viewpoint is that many people who live in modern industrial societies and are exposed to environmental stressors and rely on refined foods, often can benefit from supplements for optimal health and maximal longevity. However, the optimal amounts for any vitamin are merely estimates. Other individuals may benefit from supplements when their nutrient consumption is below normal although they lack symptoms of serious deficiency diseases. It has been proposed that nutrient needs increase with:

- exposure to pollution
- physical and mental stress
- frequent skipping of meals
- increased reliance on highly processed foods
- inadequate exercise and rest
- use of recreational drugs and alcohol
- widespread chemical and food sensitivities
- increased prevalence of conditions characterized by suppressed immunity, including AIDS
- dieting

There are many advantages in obtaining nutrients from food: It is practically impossible to get an overdose. Food supplies mixtures of nutrients and mixtures are what the body needs; food supplies other substances that may have beneficial effects and are not found in a pill or capsule. But supplements can be used as part of a wellness program to prevent illness and promote well-being. Such a program should include physical exercise, eating wholesome meals, maintaining psychological fitness and emotional stability.

Any patient who is considering taking dietary supplements should:

- Consult with a knowledgeable health professional about possible contraindications, adverse side effects, or interference with other medications or treatments the patient is receiving.
- Avoid taking any supplements while pregnant or nursing unless under the advice or supervision of a doctor.
- Focus on individual needs—more does not necessarily mean better.
- Tell their doctors what supplements they are taking, especially before submitting to a blood or urine test, as the results can be affected by some supplements.
- Be aware of sensitivities to wheat, soy, yeast, corn, milk, artificial coloring, starch, or preservatives—many supplements contain these products.
- Select supplements with multiple nutrients—many nutrients work best in tandem with others.
- Test supplements for their ability to dissolve (a sign that they will be effective) by placing them in a cup of warm water with a teaspoon of vinegar to see if they disintegrate within 45 minutes.
- Keep vitamins and minerals out of children's reach.
- Monitor the effect of the supplement to ensure it is providing a health benefit.

(See also ORTHOMOLECULAR MEDICINE; SUBCLINICAL NUTRIENT DEFICIENCY.)

Hathcock, J. N. "Vitamins and Minerals: Efficacy and Safety," *American Journal of Clinical Nutrition* 66, no. 2 (1997): 427–437.

vitamin A (retinol) A fat-soluble vitamin and one of the first vitamins to be discovered. Vitamin A is required for a healthy immune system, vision, growth, and reproduction. Vitamin A supports normal tissue development, which accounts for its influence on taste and hearing. The liver stores 90 percent or more of this vitamin. Many plants produce a parent compound of vitamin A called BETA-CAROTENE, also called "provitamin A." This orange-yellow pigment is stored in fat tissue and other tissues, but comparatively little is stored in the liver, unlike vitamin A. Beta-carotene is cleaved to form retinol and an inactive molecule called retinoic acid, which lacks vitamin A activity.

Vitamin A and Vision Perhaps the best known role for vitamin A is its effect on vision. Vitamin A forms a pigment in the eye called visual purple, required for night vision, and outright deficiency causes NIGHT BLINDNESS. Large amounts of vitamin A taken daily can delay blindness caused by retinitis pigmentosa, an inherited disease that leads to degeneration of the retina. It is worth noting that vitamin A has no effect on defective vision from other causes, and most vision problems do not involve vitamin A.

Wound Healing Both vitamin A and beta-carotene speed wound healing in lab animals. The effect is quite pronounced when the animals are vitamin-A deficient.

Resistance to Infection Population studies in developing nations have demonstrated that vitamin A reduces death by increasing resistance to infections, such as measles. This is not surprising because vitamin A supports a healthy IMMUNE SYSTEM, including increased production of antibodies and various lymphocytes (disease-fighting cells). Beta-carotene, which is nontoxic, increases T-helper cells even in normal people. Lowered immunity due to surgery has been blocked in patients given large amounts of vitamin A, and it increases the resistance of the digestive system and the respiratory tract to infection. Vitamin A can minimize decreased immunity due to radiation and chemotherapy.

Cancer Vitamin A and beta-carotene possess anticancer properties. Vitamin A can block cancer cells in cultures, and even block malignancy in animals exposed to cancer-causing agents (CARCINOGENS). A diet rich in beta-carotene and other carotenoids may lower the risk of lung, bladder, larynx, esophagus, stomach, prostate, and colon cancer.

Vitamin A, a product of vitamin A called retinoic acid, and beta-carotene may be able to prevent or eliminate precancerous sores (leukoplakia) in the mouths of smokers. Retinoic acid may also prevent recurring tumors of the head and neck. Another derivative of vitamin A, tretinoin (retin A), may be able to combat precancerous cervical conditions.

Skin Conditions Vitamin A can clear up ACNE but extremely large doses are required to do so, increasing the risk of toxicity. Derivatives are more effective; for example, tretinoin clears up the most common form of acne, acne vulgaris, and another derivative (etretinate) may be useful for psoriasis. Tretinoin helps with sun-damaged skin, although long-term effects on aging skin are not clear.

Other Conditions Vitamin A supports the maintenance and healing of lung tissue and the intestine, and it has been used to treat peptic ulcers and inflammatory bowel disease. Vitamin A deficiency associated with AIDS is linked to decreased T-helper lymphocytes and a higher rate of mortality due to HIV. Because retinoic acid may increase HIV replication, beta-carotene could be the preferred form for supplementation.

Sources

Vitamin A is either supplied as such in food, or it is formed from beta-carotene in the body. Fish liver oil and liver are rich in vitamin A. Milk is fortified with vitamin A. Vitamin A palmitate is often the form of the vitamin found in supplements. Its advantage is that it is easily suspended in water, therefore it is easily absorbed by the body. Beta-carotene occurs in yams, winter SQUASH, carrots, and CANTALOUPE, as well as in dark green leafy vegetables like KALE and SPINACH.

Requirements

The amount of vitamin A in a food can be given in terms of retinol equivalents (RE). One RE is defined as 1 mcg of retinol or 6 mcg of beta-carotene. The uptake of beta-carotene is less than retinol and its conversion to retinol is incomplete. Vitamin A activity may also be expressed in international units (IU). One IU of vitamin A activity equals 0.3 mcg of retinol or 0.6 mcg of beta-carotene. Put another way, 1 retinol equivalent equals 3.33 IU of retinol (preformed vitamin A from animal sources) or 10 IU of beta-carotene (plant sources).

The RECOMMENDED DIETARY ALLOWANCE (RDA) for vitamin A for men (25 to 50 years) is 1,000 mcg of retinol or retinol equivalents and 800 mcg (RE) for nonpregnant women. In pregnancy, the requirement increases to 1,300 mcg. Vitamin A deficiency is common in nonindustrialized societies, but a significant number of Americans might also be deficient in vitamin A, particularly young children and others consuming highly processed foods. Factors that increase the need for vitamin A include a high-fiber diet, chronic fat MALABSORPTION, stress, and high alcohol consumption. Symptoms of deficiency include coarse dry skin, slow growth, night blindness, frequent infections, and anemia.

Safety

Women who are pregnant should not take vitamin A supplements. Amounts greater than 10,000 IU (3,000 RE) increase the risk of birth defects. On the other hand, there is no evidence that beta-carotene produces birth defects. Vitamin A is stored by the body and it is possible to accumulate too much, leading to toxicity (HYPERVITAMINOSIS). The response to high doses of vitamin A is quite variable. A high intake of 50,000 IU daily (15,000 RE) may be tolerated by some; others may have a reaction with 20,000 IU (6,000 RE). Symptoms of vitamin A overdose include headache, fatigue, dry skin, weakness, nausea, hair loss, blurred vision, bone aches, and loss of appetite. Jaundice and liver damage are possible. These symptoms usually disappear rapidly when vitamin A supplementation is stopped. In contrast, beta-carotene is relatively safe because it is converted to vitamin A only as needed.

Tretinoin, accutane, and etretinate should not be taken by pregnant women or by women who do not use birth control because of the high risk of BIRTH DEFECTS. Vitamin A may cause bone disease in individuals with chronic kidney problems.

Bates, C. J. "Vitamin A," *Lancet* 345 (January 7, 1995): 31–35.

vitamin B_1 See THIAMIN.

vitamin B_2 See RIBOFLAVIN.

vitamin B_3 See NIACIN.

vitamin B_6 (pyridoxine) An essential water-soluble nutrient and a member of the B COMPLEX. The term "vitamin B_6" pertains to two forms, pyridoxine and pyridoxamine, which can be converted back and forth. Vitamin B_6 is required by the body to produce nonessential AMINO ACIDS, to break down most amino acids, and to support healthy immune systems, normal immunity, and nerve function. However, before it can help enzymes, vitamin B_6 like other B complex vitamins must be activated. The enzyme helper (COENZYME) in this case is pyridoxal phosphate, employed by a family of enzymes called transaminases required in the first stage of amino acid utilization by the body.

Chemicals known as hydrazides and hydrazines interfere with the functions of vitamin B_6. These chemicals are widely used in industry and contaminate the food supply. Derivatives of hydrazines appear in cigarette smoke and food additives, thus, the environmental burden could deplete this nutrient.

Possible Roles in Maintaining Health

Red Blood Cells Vitamin B_6 is essential for the production of RED BLOOD CELLS. Vitamin B_6 plays a role in protein synthesis as well as in the synthesis of DNA and RNA, and it is required to make HEME, the red pigment of the oxygen transport protein of blood (HEMOGLOBIN). A deficiency can cause anemia.

Nervous System The formation of certain brain chemicals (NEUROTRANSMITTERS) from amino acids requires this vitamin, hence it affects the NERVOUS SYSTEM. Certain inherited metabolic disorders lead to convulsions in infants, and B_6 supplementation usually abolishes their seizures.

Immune System Vitamin B_6 is one of the most important B vitamins in maintaining a robust IMMUNE SYSTEM. Vitamin B_6 supplements can boost immunity in older people who may not consume enough of this important vitamin. Vitamin B_6 deficiency decreases immune function in humans and lab animals, and low vitamin B_6 levels are common in people with weakened immunity, including people with CANCER and AIDS. Vitamin B_6 also protects against certain types of cancer in lab animals.

Premenstrual Syndrome (PMS) Vitamin B_6 has long been claimed to relieve an array of symptoms occurring in the week to 10 days prior to menstruation. PMS affects the synthesis of several hormones believed to be involved in the cycle. Vitamin B_6 has been used to correct for some of the imbalances caused by estrogen-type birth control pills. Some clinical studies suggest that vitamin B_6 can improve certain symptoms of PMS, such as breast tenderness and PMS-related depression. Lower doses, 50–100mg/day are apparently as effective as large amounts.

Carpal Tunnel Syndrome Vitamin B_6 supplementation is apparently ineffective in providing short-term relief of symptoms, based on evaluation of randomized, controlled clinical trials.

High Blood Sugar Vitamin B_6 has been used to help treat diabetic patients whose condition can be attributed in part to a deficiency of this vitamin.

Cardiovascular Disease Vitamin B_6 may decrease the stickiness of platelets, cell fragments in the blood needed for clot formation, and thus the tendency to form blood clots. A deficiency of this vitamin has been linked to ATHEROSCLEROSIS in some instances, due to an accumulation of excessive amounts of an amino acid breakdown product homocysteine. Vitamin B_6 combined with folic acid and vitamin B_{12} can reduce blood levels of homocysteine, a potential risk factor for cardiovascular disease. It is uncertain whether reducing homocysteine prevents death from heart disease, however.

Senility Vitamin B_6 deficiency is linked to long-term memory loss in some elderly patients.

Other Conditions Some forms of arthritis and joint pain respond to extra vitamin B_6. In combination with magnesium this vitamin can lower the risk of calcium oxalate kidney stones, the most common kind. Vitamin B_6 deficiency is common among patients with asthma.

Sources

Vitamin B_6 occurs in FISH; MEAT, including liver and kidneys; BLACKSTRAP MOLASSES; NUTS and whole GRAINS; BREWER'S YEAST; and many VEGETABLES.

Requirements

The Recommended Dietary Allowances (RDA) for adults (25 to 50 years) is 2.0 mg for men and 1.6 mg for women. Many people do not obtain adequate amounts of this vitamin and it is one of the most common deficiencies. Those most at risk are older persons; it has been found that 61- to 71-year-olds need more vitamin B_6 than the RDA. Others who may not consume enough vitamin B_6 include adolescent women and pregnant and lactating women, alcoholics, and those with other chemical dependencies.

Factors that may increase the need for vitamin B_6 include alcohol consumption, several medications (L-dopa, penicillamine, hydralazine isoniazid), smoking, a high protein diet, deficiencies of magnesium, ZINC, and RIBOFLAVIN. A mild deficiency is sometimes associated with lowered immunity and nervous disorders. Severe deficiency causes depression, confusion, convulsions, inflamed mouth, and tongue, and skin disorders. The optimal amount for maximal health and longevity is not known.

Safety

There is general agreement that amounts up to 50 mg per day are relatively safe. Higher levels should be taken only with professional advice. Excessive consumption of vitamin B_6 can damage the nervous system and lead to numbness of hands and feet (peripheral neuropathy). Insomnia and anxiety are possible symptoms of excessive intake. Vitamin B_6 reduces the effectiveness of levodopa, a drug used to treat PARKINSON'S DISEASE. (See also AMINO ACID METABOLISM; DIABETES MELLITUS; TRANSAMINATION.)

Siri, P. W. "Vitamins B_6, B_{12}, and Folate: Association with Plasma Total Homocysteine and Risk of Coronary Atherosclerosis," *Journal of the American College of Nutrition* 17 (1998): 435–441.

vitamin B_{12} (cyanocobalamin) An essential water-soluble nutrient belonging to the B COMPLEX that is required in extremely minute amounts for cell division and growth. Vitamin B_{12} is unique in several respects: It is the only B vitamin stored in the body and the only known nutrient to contain the trace mineral COBALT. Like all B vitamins, vitamin B_{12} must be chemically modified to form a coenzyme (enzyme helper) before it can participate in metabolism. Vitamin B_{12} has important, though very limited, roles in metabolism. It assists in the utilization of single carbon (methyl) groups transfer from the amino acid, methionine, to donors, including thymin, a building block for DNA. Vitamin B_{12} also helps to oxidize certain fatty acids and it supports the maintenance of healthy nerves. With deficiencies, irreversible brain damage and nervous disorders can occur.

The body has evolved an efficient mechanism to absorb this vitamin. To begin the process, the stomach normally secretes INTRINSIC FACTOR, a protein that binds vitamin B_{12} and carries it to the INTESTINE where it aids B_{12} absorption. An estimated 20 percent of people in their 60s and 40 percent of people in their 80s develop atrophic gastritis, in which the stomach does not produce enough acid and intrinsic factor. With inadequate stomach acid to sterilize the stomach, certain bacteria can grow, consuming the vitamin that otherwise would be absorbed by the intestine. Vitamin B_{12}, together with another B vitamin, FOLIC ACID, functions in DNA synthesis and cell division, and supports red blood cell production. A large dose of folic acid to treat anemia can mask a vitamin B_{12} deficiency; folic acid often is administered with B_{12}.

Possible Roles in Maintaining Health

Anemia A deficiency of intrinsic factor causes PERNICIOUS ANEMIA, a disease caused by inadequate B_{12} absorption despite adequate dietary supplies. B_{12} injections clear up the problem.

Vitamin B_{12} Deficiency Signs of B_{12} deficiency include weakness in arms and legs, walking problems and paralysis, and irreversible nerve damage. Prolonged deficiency causes anemia and neurological symptoms. Vitamin B_{12} deficiency is particularly a concern for strict vegetarians; older adults; pregnant women; patients with bleeding, cancer, kidney or liver disease; alcoholics; patients with malabsorption syndromes, such as Crohn's disease; people with severe food sensitivities; those with a family history of anemia, or who have undergone stomach surgery.

Nervous Disorders An estimated 10 percent of elderly persons have marked vitamin B_{12} deficiencies, and many patients with senile dementia are B_{12}-deficient. Mental deterioration, SENILITY, and neuropsychiatric disorders—including dementia, DEPRESSION, and loss of balance—may respond to extra vitamin B_{12}. About 5 percent of adults over the age of 50 have low vitamin B_{12} levels. Half of these may have difficulty in absorbing the vitamin from food.

Cigarette Smoking Smokers have low vitamin B_{12} and folic acid levels. Preliminary clinical studies suggest that supplementation with both vitamins may reduce the amount of precancerous bronchial tissue.

Chronic Pain Vitamin B_{12} has been used to treat bronchial spasm (ASTHMA), bursitis, and bone spur pain. Neuralgia pain radiating along nerves may respond to intramuscular infections of vitamin B_{12}.

Sources

Vitamin B_{12} occurs mainly in animal products—MEAT, POULTRY, FISH, EGGS, and SHELLFISH. Some fortified foods like nutritional yeast contain vitamin B_{12}. Tamari, tempeh, and miso were found to be essentially lacking in this vitamin, although sometimes these foods are claimed to be rich sources of the vitamin. SPIRULINA contains fewer usable vitamins than formerly believed; the amount in seaweed is variable. Part of the problem seems to be that seaweed contains B_{12} analogs that do not form coenzymes in the body. Therefore, strict vegetarians (those who eat no animal products) may need to support their diet with vitamin B_{12} supplements.

Requirements

The RECOMMENDED DIETARY ALLOWANCE (RDA) for vitamin B_{12} for normal adults is 2 mcg daily. Severe vitamin B_{12} deficiency is rare. Newer, more sensitive laboratory blood tests and metabolic indicators have turned up low-level B_{12} deficiencies with surprising frequency. Low folic acid intake and some antibiotics interfere with Vitamin B_{12} uptake. People suffering from anxiety or depression who take antidepressants (tricyclics and chloromazine) may block vitamin B_{12} uptake.

Vitamin B_{12} is not toxic when taken orally. Nasal or sublingual (under the tongue) vitamin B_{12} gels or vitamin injections are effective for vegetarians and for those with malabsorption problems. There is no known toxicity associated with this vitamin when taken orally. Often, elevated vitamin B_{12} in the blood is most readily obtained through B_{12} injections. Some people are allergic to injections. (See also ACHLORHYDRIA; AGING; DIGESTION; MALABSORPTION.)

Naurath, Hans J. et al. "Effects of Vitamin B_{12}, Folate and Vitamin B_6 Supplements in Elderly People with Normal Serum Vitamin Concentrations," *Lancet* 346 (July 8, 1995): 85–89.

vitamin C (ascorbic acid, sodium ascorbate, calcium ascorbate) A water-soluble vitamin that promotes wound healing and healthy blood vessels, joints, gums, and connective tissue. Vitamin C helps in the synthesis of COLLAGEN, a structural protein that provides strength to bones and tissues. Most animals make ample vitamin C; exceptions include guinea pigs, humans and other primates, and certain bats.

Vitamin C occurs in high levels in endocrine (hormone-secreting) glands. It is needed by the ADRENAL GLANDS to make hormones: EPINEPHRINE (adrenaline), a stress hormone, plus the steroids regulating BLOOD SUGAR and the hormones regulating blood minerals, and assists in the activation of other hormones. Vitamin C also occurs in high levels in the brain, and it plays a role in nerve transmission through the production of SEROTONIN and norepinephrine, brain chemicals called NEUROTRANSMITTERS. Neurotransmitters are chemicals synthesized by nerve cells to conduct impulses between cells. Vitamin C is involved in the metabolism of folic acid.

Vitamin C serves as a powerful antioxidant and helps to prevent oxidative damage in the body. It can block many types of highly reactive chemical species called FREE RADICALS, including superoxide and hydroxyl radicals in blood and body fluids, as well as regenerating VITAMIN E, the free radical scavenger of cell membranes and lipids. As a versatile antioxidant, vitamin C offers protection against airborne pollutants and supports drug detoxication by the liver. Dietary vitamin C can increase the absorption of heme iron (the form in meat) two- to fourfold. Vitamin C suppresses the formation of NITROSOAMINES and quinones, known to cause cancer (carcinogens). On the other hand, it is possible that vitamin C can participate in the BHA-induced tissue growth in the stomach of rats, thus enhancing carcinogenesis. However, a higher consumption of vitamin C contributes to higher plasma levels of other antioxidants, including vitamin E.

Possible Role of Vitamin C in Disease

The functions of vitamin C in the body and the amounts required for optimal health remain one of the most controversial areas in nutrition. The following topics have been the focus of recent research.

Scurvy This full-blown vitamin C deficiency disease is characterized by swollen joints, poor wound healing, muscle wasting, bleeding gums and susceptibility to infection. In scurvy, defective COLLAGEN is formed, leading to diseased connective tissue. Vitamin C is required to synthesize collagen building blocks, hydroxylysine and hydroxyproline, for normal collagen formation. Scurvy has largely been eradicated from industrialized nations, though it continues to affect certain populations: the elderly, alcoholics, and chronically ill people. When large amounts of vitamin C are consumed, the body adapts by accelerating excretion and metabolism. When consumption suddenly drops, a person may experience a short-term vitamin C deficiency until the body readapts ("rebound scurvy"). Infants born to mothers who have taken large amounts of vitamin C may experience rebound scurvy after birth unless they are supplemented.

Infection and Colds Whether vitamin C can cure the common cold has remained a controversial issue since Dr. Linus Pauling first suggested it in 1970. The research that has been conducted since that time has yielded mixed results, possibly reflecting flaws in experiment design. There is general agreement that vitamin C can decrease the duration and severity of colds. The vitamin can affect the outcome by blocking viruses, as well as by helping the IMMUNE SYSTEM. White cells that devour bacteria and abnormal cells require vitamin C for normal functioning; vitamin C levels decline in these cells during infection and exposure to drugs, medications, alcohol, and cigarette smoking.

Cancer A variety of population studies suggest that a low vitamin C intake correlates with a higher rate of CANCER and that vitamin C from dietary sources has a protective effect for cancer of the oral cavity, larynx, esophagus, colon, lung, and stomach. Data supporting a beneficial relationship between vitamin C and bladder, cervix, endometrium, and breast cancer are not as convincing, although suggestive. Vitamin C supplementation reduces the rate of precancerous changes in the stomach. It protects against cervical dysplasia, a predisposing condition to cervical cancer, and it inhibits human leukemia cells in culture. Vitamin C can block the formation of cancer-causing agents like NITROSOAMINES, and it is a powerful blocker of free radicals, which can be carcinogenic. Whether vitamin C does more than prevent certain cancers, and whether it can extend the lives of terminally ill cancer patients, remains controversial. More research is needed to resolve these issues.

Cardiovascular Disease A popular hypothesis for the origin of atherosclerosis (cholesterol clogged arteries) states that the oxidation of LDL promotes the disease process. Vitamin C may help prevent oxidative damage to LOW-DENSITY LIPOPROTEIN (LDL), lipid-transport particles implicated in clogging arteries. Vitamin C can increase HIGH-DENSITY LIPOPROTEIN (HDL), the beneficial form of cholesterol, and it may lower total cholesterol values. However, epidemiologic studies did not detect a correlation between vitamin C intake and the risk of cardiovascular disease, and there as yet have not been randomized clinical studies of vitamin C supplements in reducing cardiovascular risk.

The Physicians Health Study found that taking vitamin C or multivitamins was not associated with a significant decrease in death rates from cardiovascular disease. The study included 83,639 male physicians in the United States who had no history of heart disease at baseline and were followed for an average of 5.5 years. Population studies have found an increased risk of elevated blood pressure with low vitamin C intake or low vitamin C plasma levels. Vitamin C together with usual antihypertensive drugs may decrease high blood pressure. Increased consumption of foods rich in vitamin C may decrease the risk of stroke. In combination with vitamin E, vitamin C may also slow the progression of atherosclerosis in men. Studies of treatment of hypertension with vitamin C have not been conclusive. Mortality from all causes of death was strongly inversely related to vitamin C intake, but other studies of vitamin C in preventing cardiovascular disease have yielded negative results.

Aging Free radical damage is implicated in aging, which can be viewed as the result of accumulated damaged protein and DNA and of damaged repair mechanisms. Population studies suggest that the consumption of ample fruits and vegetables, including those that are rich sources of vitamin C, decrease the risks of degenerative diseases associated with aging. Of the multitude of beneficial substances in these foods with antioxidant activity, vitamin C appears likely to play a central role.

Allergies Vitamin C can help reduce asthma in certain asthmatics, and it may reduce the severity of allergy symptoms by alleviating stuffy sinuses, achy joints and puffy eyes. Vitamin C helps detoxify HISTAMINE, which promotes these inflammation symptoms.

Eye Disease Free radicals probably promote cataracts and macular degeneration with aging. Thus, animals fed vitamin E-deficient diets develop macular degeneration and people with low-levels of antioxidants in their blood have a higher risk of cataracts. Adequate vitamin C, carotenoids, and vitamin E consumption are related to a decreased risk of cataracts associated with aging. Several studies have suggested that antioxidant supplements, including vitamin C, decrease the risk of cataract formation. Vitamin C supplementation may halt or retard cataract development. Together with zinc and other antioxidants vitamin C may slow the progression of intermediate and advanced stages of age-related macular degeneration according to a clinical trial.

Other Conditions A variety of studies suggest that supplements of vitamin C can: decrease the risk of PERIODONTAL DISEASE, help diabetics maintain healthy gums; help overcome infertility in male smokers; and ease muscle soreness in athletes. Some clinical evidence suggests that vitamin C from foods can slow the progression of osteoarthritis. This vitamin may prevent nitrate tolerance in patients taking nitroglycerin. When used with vitamin E, vitamin C may prevent preeclampsia in high risk women.

Sources

Fresh vegetables and fresh food are the best sources of vitamin C, including CITRUS FRUIT, CANTALOUPE, green PEPPERS, BROCCOLI, PAPAYA, berries, and green leafy vegetables. Grains lack vitamin C. Vitamin C is the most unstable vitamin: In food it is destroyed by heat and by exposure to air, and cooking and processing of foods leads to extensive destruction. Microwave cooking minimizes losses. Destruction in fruit and vegetables is faster at room temperature than in the refrigerator, and is fastest if the vegetable is chopped or peeled. Ascorbic acid powder is stable indefinitely if kept dry.

Requirements

The RECOMMENDED DIETARY ALLOWANCE (RDA) for vitamin C is 75 mg for adult women and 90 mg for adult men. Many nutritional scientists believe the RDA should be 200 mg. In one study, state plasma and tissue concentrations of vitamin C were measured at varying doses in healthy volunteers, after first being depleted with a vitamin C-deficient diet. Bioavailability was maximal at 200 mg of vitamin C per day, higher levels of vitamin C did not appreciably change tissue saturation. Vitamin C needs are highly individualistic and exposure to pollutants, drugs, medications, smoking, infections, recovery from injury or surgery, high stress levels and heavy drinking often increase the need for vitamin C above the usual intake. The elderly or people who rely on medications like aspirin, barbiturates, L-dopa, phenacetin, and cortisone need more vitamin C.

Safety

Vitamin C may have a dark side. Vitamin C increases iron uptake and hypothetically this could lead to iron accumulation in those with an inherited tendency to store iron. Iron and vitamin C spontaneously form free radicals (prooxidant effect). Excessive vitamin C supplementation together with excessive iron storage may be detrimental. However, under usual physiologic conditions, the amount of free iron would likely be very small; it would be stored in the iron binding protein FERRITIN. With injury or inflammation some iron could be released and could react with hydrogen peroxide to produce damaging free radicals. In susceptible people, large amounts of vitamin C could promote the appearance of oxalate in the urine, thus increasing the risk of kidney stones. Supplementing with magnesium and extra vitamin B_6 can diminish this risk.

The latest RDA, published in 2000, set a tolerable upper intake level (UL) for the first time at 2 g. Most patients who do not exceed this amount will avoid diarrhea and other gastrointestinal problems associated with consuming excessive amounts of vitamin C. Over time this could promote MALABSORPTION. Chewable vitamin C can erode tooth enamel, and taking aspirin with vitamin C can aggravate gastric bleeding caused by aspirin. Extremely high intakes of vitamin C may increase the need for COPPER, and may increase the risk of GOUT in individuals who are genetically susceptible to those conditions. Patients who are prone to gout or kidney stones or who are pregnant, should not supplement with vitamin C without first consulting a physician.

Vitamin C interferes with the effectiveness of amphetamines, blood thinning drugs, and tricyclic antidepressants like ritalin, and it can alter lab tests like urinary glucose and occult blood for bowel cancer. Patients should tell their doctors they are taking vitamin C supplements before undergoing diagnostic laboratory tests. They should also avoid abruptly quitting daily supplementation of 500 mg or more, as this can cause short-term scurvylike symptoms and temporarily lowered resistance to infections. (See also DETOXICATION; MEGADOSE.)

Bendich, Adrianne, and Langseth, L. "The Health Effects of Vitamin C Supplementation: a Review," *Journal of the American College of Nutrition* 14, no. 2 (1995): 124–136.

Carr, A. C. "Toward a New Recommended Dietary Allowance for Vitamin C Based on Antioxidant and Health Effects in Humans," *American Journal of Clinical Nutrition* 69, no. 6 (1999): 1,086–1,107.

Muntwyler, J. et al. "Vitamin Supplement Use in a Low-Risk Population of US Male Physicians and Subsequent Cardiovascular Mortality," *Archives of Internal Medicine* 162 (2002): 1,472–1,476.

vitamin D A fat-soluble trace nutrient required for healthy BONES and teeth. Vitamin D_2 (ERGOCAL-

CIFEROL) occurs in plants, yeast, and fungi. Commercially, vitamin D_2 is produced by exposing a plant sterol, ergosterol, to UV light. Vitamin D_3, cholecalciferol (25-hydroxy cholecalciferol), is the form found in animal tissue and in the oil of fatty fish, and it is also synthesized in the skin from a cholesterol derivative when exposed to sunlight (UV light). Vitamin D is the only VITAMIN to be formed in this manner. This fat-soluble vitamin is stored in fatty tissue as well as in the LIVER, bones, skin, and muscle. Vitamin D is required for calcium uptake, and so is linked to the formation of bones and teeth.

Vitamin D is the only vitamin that is converted to a HORMONE. Vitamin D is transported to the KIDNEYS, where it is again oxidized, yielding calcitriol (1,25 dihydroxy cholecalciferol), which is a hormone. Calcitriol in the bloodstream travels to the intestine where it stimulates the formation of calcium transport proteins. In addition calcitriol can increase bone rebuilding by working together with parathyroid hormone. It also stimulates calcium reabsorption by the kidney.

Vitamin D as calcitriol influences many glands and tissues. This hormone affects the PANCREAS (insulin secretion), the PARATHYROID GLANDS, PITUITARY GLAND, ovaries, testes, COLON, placenta, uterus, heart, THYMUS, mammary tissue, and brain (cerebellum). In a very real sense calcitriol is an immune enhancer. Calcitriol stimulates WHITE BLOOD CELLS, especially macrophages, and influences B and T lymphocytes—major classes of cells responsible for antibody production and the surveillance mechanism of the IMMUNE SYSTEM.

Possible Roles in Maintaining Health

Chronic vitamin D deficiency in children leads to RICKETS, characterized by abnormal calcification of bones. As a result, bones are soft and become deformed. Teeth do not develop normally and are subject to decay. Rickets is rare in Western societies owing to the prevalent practice of food FORTIFICATION with forms of vitamin D.

The adult equivalent of rickets is OSTEOMALACIA. In this disease bones become depleted of calcium and phosphorus. Osteomalacia is more common during pregnancy and lactation, as well as during old age. Supplementation with vitamin D can reduce the risk of osteomalacia. Although vitamin D is necessary for normal calcium metabolism, it does not seem to protect against OSTEOPOROSIS in postmenopausal women. Osteoporosis is mitigated by MAGNESIUM, CALCIUM, and possibly FLUORIDE, BORON, MANGANESE, and VITAMIN K.

Population studies suggest that vitamin D and calcium deficiencies account in part for the high rate of colorectal cancer and breast cancer worldwide. CALCIFEROL inhibits cancer cells in the test tube and inhibits chemically induced cancer in mice. Vitamin D applied to the skin or taken orally may clear up psoriasis, a condition characterized by scaly, itchy red patches of skin.

Sources

There are few good food sources of vitamin D, which is the least prevalent vitamin in the food supply. Vitamin D occurs in fatty fish, fish liver oils, egg yolk, and liver. Vitamin D is used to fortify MILK, and either vitamin D_3 or vitamin D_2 are used. Whole milk, low-fat milk, nonfat milk, and nonfat dry milk are fortified with 400 IUs, equivalent to 10 mcg of vitamin D per quart, although spotchecks have revealed variations in this level. Other foods may be fortified with vitamin D: breakfast cereal, infant cereal, bread, chocolate beverages, and margarine.

Requirements

Human requirements are difficult to establish because varying levels of this vitamin are synthesized by the skin. The National Institutes of Health have determined that there is insufficient evidence to establish a RDA for vitamin D. Instead, scientists have set an adequate intake (AI), a level of intake sufficient to maintain healthy blood levels in adults. For adults between 19 and 50 the AI is 5 mcg. For adults between the ages of 51 and 69 the amount is 10 mcg, and for people over 70 the AI is 15 mcg. Factors that increase the risk of vitamin D deficiency include: gallbladder removal, severe food allergies, poor fat absorption (for instance, due to CELIAC DISEASE) and liver disease. Several medications can interfere with vitamin D uptake: certain anticonvulsant agents, barbiturates and cortisone. Mineral oil blocks the uptake of this and other fat-soluble vitamins. People with kidney disease or diabetes may not be able to activate vitamin

D. Institutionalized people who get little exposure to sunlight, strict vegetarians, and elderly persons are more at risk for vitamin D deficiency. The efficiency of the skin's production of this vitamin declines with age.

Safety

Vitamin D can be toxic, due to high blood calcium levels (hypercalcemia) and the calcification of soft tissue. Symptoms include constipation, vomiting, fatigue, drowsiness, lack of appetite, and, in severe cases, high blood pressure, kidney stones, and even kidney failure and coma. Doses at two or three times the RDA seem unlikely to cause toxicity. Young children are more susceptible, and as little as 1,800 IU of vitamin D per day may cause toxicity. Moderately high consumption over a long period of time may increase the risk of atherosclerosis. Those with elevated blood calcium levels should not supplement with vitamin D without medical supervision. (See also ENRICHMENT; HYPERVITAMINOSIS.)

Fraser, D. R. "Vitamin D," *Lancet* 345 (January 14, 1995): 104–107.

vitamin E (tocopherol) A fat-soluble essential nutrient that stabilizes cell membranes. Naturally occurring tocopherols are a mixture of closely related compounds (isomers) designated alpha-tocopherol, beta-tocopherol, gamma-tocopherol, and delta-tocopherol. Alpha-tocopherol has the greatest vitamin E activity in the body. Synthetic vitamin E, designated as dl-tocopherol or rac-tocopherol, is less active. Supplements usually incorporate vitamin E bound to simple acids to prevent its oxidation. Alpha-tocopherol acetate and succinate are common forms; the acetate and succinate are forms broken down by intestinal enzymes to release vitamin E.

Free Radicals Vitamin E is the major lipid antioxidant in the body, the property for which it is best known. It squelches free radicals, highly reactive molecules that can attack neighboring molecules and damage polyunsaturated fatty acids in membrane lipids, proteins, and DNA, damaging cells and leading to disease. Free radical damage is linked to CANCER, HEART DISEASE, CATARACTS, and aging. This vitamin plays important roles in the immune system, the nervous system and the endocrine (hormonal) system.

Possible Roles in Maintaining Health

Cancer Studies to determine whether vitamin E is effective in the treatment or prevention of cancer have been inconclusive. Some studies have shown that patients who take supplements of vitamin E decrease their risk of colon cancer while in others supplementation had no effect on this cancer. Population studies and a clinical trial concluded that a high intake of vitamin E was related to a decreased incidence of prostate cancer. Population studies suggest that low blood levels of vitamin E and BETA-CAROTENE correlate with an increased risk of lung cancer.

Cardiovascular Disease Population studies suggest that increased vitamin E intake from foods may reduce the risk of heart disease. Protection against free radical damage by this vitamin is an attractive hypothesis. For example, the Physicians Health Study found that taking vitamin E, vitamin C, or multivitamins was not associated with a significant decrease in death rates from cardiovascular disease. The study included 83,639 male physicians in the United States who had no history of heart disease at baseline and were followed for an average of 5.5 years. The Heart Outcomes Prevention Evaluation (HOPE) Study followed almost 10,000 patients who were at high risk for heart attack or stroke for more than fours years. Participants who received a daily dose of 265 mg of vitamin E daily experienced no fewer cardiovascular events or hospitalizations for heart failure or chest pain than did those participants who were given a sugar pill (placebo). This study is ongoing, and with additional time researchers should have a better idea whether vitamin E is helpful in preventing cardiovascular disease.

Gamma-tocopherol Alpha tocopherol is the form of vitamin found in highest concentration in blood and tissues due to selection by the intestines and liver. However, gamma-tocopherol is the most common form of vitamin E in the diet of typical Americans. Some studies suggest that alpha-tocopherol, the form of vitamin E prevalent in SUPPLEMENTS, alone, may be ineffective in reducing the risk of heart disease. However, according to one study gamma-tocopherol alone does not seem to protect against heart disease at all. Other studies have shown that gamma-tocopherol is more beneficial in slowing or stopping the growth of prostate cancer cells than are other vitamin E compounds. In the test tube, vitamin E is a potent inhibitor of LDL oxidation. Oxidation of LDL by free radicals and its uptake by cells in arterial walls may initiate the development of ATHEROSCLEROSIS. However, most controlled clinical trials found that vitamin E supplements do not protect against cardiovascular disease.

Neurologic Disorders Vitamin E plays an important role in maintaining normal nerve function. Vitamin E deficiency is usually associated with symptoms of peripheral NEUROPATHY. Some studies suggest that low vitamin E content in nerves precedes nerve degeneration. Vitamin E has been found to be beneficial in reducing the severity of symptoms of TARDIVE DYSKINESIA, a side effect of long-term use of tranquilizers (phenothiazines) that produces involuntary movements.

Eye Diseases Population studies indicate that cataract-free people consume more vitamin E and vitamin C than those with cataracts. Premature infants can develop vitamin E deficiencies because they possess almost no FAT, hence fat-soluble vitamin stores are marginal. Premature infants receive vitamin E to prevent anemia and retinopathy. In another study cigarette smoking seemed to counter any beneficial effects of taking vitamin E to prevent cataracts. Together with vitamin C, zinc, and beta-carotene, vitamin E can decrease the progression of moderate to severe age-related macular degeneration.

Immune System Moderate amounts of vitamin E seem to increase the ability of macrophages to destroy bacteria and to boost activity of T lymphocytes, the foot-soldiers and generals of the IMMUNE SYSTEM. Vitamin E may alter production of certain PROSTAGLANDINS, hormone-like substances derived from essential fatty acids that promote INFLAMMATION. It has been used to manage autoimmune conditions like LUPUS ERYTHEMATOSUS. Healthy elderly men and women supplemented with moderate amounts of vitamin E can show greater immune responsiveness than those who do not supplement with this vitamin. On the other hand, very high levels of vitamin E may inhibit immune function.

Age-related Dementia Two studies showed that vitamin E may play an important role in maintaining mental function in the elderly. Participants in one four-year study who took high amounts of vitamin E had a 70 percent reduction in the risk of developing ALZHEIMER'S DISEASE. In another study researchers tracked 2,800 men and women between the ages of 65 and 102 for an average of three years. During that time 61 percent of the subjects showed some decline in mental functioning. The rest either showed no decline or improved. Those who had the best results were taking the highest amounts of vitamin E, and those who showed the sharpest decline were taking the lowest amounts of the vitamin.

Other Conditions Vitamin E has been used to treat tardive dyskinesia. It seems to be more effective for people who have had this condition for less than five years. The vitamin may normalize retinal blood flow in type 1 diabetes, and it may control red blood cell loss with some inherited diseases such as glucose-6 phosphate dehydrogenase deficiency, which produces fragile red blood cells. In combination with vitamin C, vitamin E seems to reduce the risk of pre-eclampsia in high risk women. There is some evidence that the vitamin can also reduce some symptoms of PMS, including anxiety, cravings, and PMS-related depression. Case studies support claims that vitamin E promotes wound healing and minimizes scar tissue formation. Vitamin E supplementation has been suggested to reduce symptoms of PREMENSTRUAL SYNDROME. Most careful studies on the effects of vitamin E supplementation on muscular strength, maximum oxygen consumption, or endurance have failed to demonstrate benefits. It is possible vitamin E can reduce oxygen debt and increase maximum oxygen consumption in adapting to high elevations.

Diabetes Sometimes supplementation with vitamins can improve glucose tolerance and insulin sensitivity in diabetic patients, and reduce the level of secondary damage due to the buildup of glucose-bound proteins.

Osteoarthritis Vitamin E possesses mild and inflammatory activity, which may explain why it can help lessen pain associated with osteoarthritis.

Skin Conditions A variety of skin conditions such as Raynaud's phenomenon and polymitosis have been treated with vitamin E.

Sources

The highest levels of vitamin E occur in VEGETABLE OILS (safflower, soybean, and sunflower oils), BUTTER and MARGARINE, NUTS, wheat germ, whole-grain CEREALS, EGGS, and green leafy vegetables. Most fruits and white bread contain negligible vitamin E. To obtain 100 IU of vitamin E, a level found to reduce the risk of heart disease, a person would have to eat six cups of kale, or 4.5 cups of sweet potatoes. Vitamin E supplements should not be taken together with iron because they interfere with each other.

Requirements

The RECOMMENDED DIETARY ALLOWANCE (RDA) for vitamin E is 15 mg of alpha tocopherol equivalents. In a 2000 report the Institutes of Medicine concluded that most adult Americans get enough vitamin E from their diets to meet daily requirements. Premature infants, individuals on very-low-calorie/low-fat diets or who do not absorb fat very well (including some elderly people) may be deficient. Chronic malabsorption of fat and fat-soluble vitamins, including vitamin E, can accompany cystic fibrosis, SPRUE and nontropical sprue, chronic PANCREATITIS, CELIAC DISEASE, and bile duct inflammation or blockage, among other conditions.

Symptoms of severe vitamin E deficiency include ANEMIA and neurologic disorders. Newborn infants, especially premature infants with vitamin E deficiency, experience EDEMA and blood abnormalities. The requirement for vitamin E increases with increased consumption of polyunsaturated oils due to the increased susceptibility to peroxidation. However, the optimal ratio is unclear. In extreme situations, the requirement may exceed the RDA.

Safety

Vitamin E is one of the least toxic fat-soluble vitamins when administered orally, and most healthy adults can tolerate 100 to 800 mg daily. Excessive vitamin E may cause fatigue, muscle weakness, stomach upset, headache, nausea, and skin disorders. In certain patients with high blood pressure, vitamin E may elevate blood pressure. Those with HYPERTENSION, rheumatic heart disease, or diabetes should seek medical advice before supplementing with vitamin E. People taking anticoagulant medications or who are deficient in VITAMIN K, or who have blood clots, should follow their physician's advice regarding vitamin E supplements to avoid the potential problem with increased bleeding. Iron and oral contraceptives can interfere with absorbing vitamin E. (See also AGING; DEGENERATIVE DISEASES; TOCOTRIENOLS.)

Engelhart, M. J. et al. "Dietary Intake of Antioxidants and the Risk of Alzheimer Disease," *JAMA* 287 (2002): 3,223–3,229.

The Heart Outcomes Prevention Evaluation Study Investigators. "Vitamin E Supplementation and Cardiovascular Events in High-risk Patients," *New England Journal of Medicine* 342 (2000): 154–160.

Meydani, Mohsen. "Vitamin E," *Lancet* 345 (January 21, 1995): 170–175.

Morris, M. et al. "Dietary Intake of Antioxidant Nutrients and the Risk of Incident Alzheimer Disease in a Biracial Community," *Journal of the American Medical Association* 287 (2002): 3,230–3,237.

Muntwyler, J. et al. "Vitamin Supplement Use in a Low-Risk Population of US Male Physicians and Subsequent Cardiovascular Mortality," *Archives of Internal Medicine* 162 (2002): 1,472–1,476.

vitamin F See ESSENTIAL FATTY ACIDS.

vitamin H See BIOTIN.

vitamin K A fat-soluble vitamin required for normal BLOOD CLOTTING. As with VITAMIN E and VITAMIN B_6, the term vitamin K represents several closely related forms: the most prevalent, naturally occurring forms are vitamin K_1 (philloquinone or hytonadione) and vitamin K_2 (menaquinone). Vitamin K_3 is MENADIONE, a synthetic form that can be activated in the LIVER.

Vitamin K serves as a cofactor for the processing of six proteins required in the complex chain of reactions that regulates blood clotting. One of these proteins is prothrombin, the inactive precursor of the enzyme that creates fibrin clots from fibrinogen, and vitamin K has been used to treat clotting disorders due to vitamin K deficiency. Vitamin K also assists in the synthesis of osteocalcin, a bone protein that forms the matrix for mineralization and bone building.

Possible Roles in Maintaining Health

Vitamin K is required for healing fractured bone and in the maintenance of normal bone. Elderly patients with osteoporosis (thin bone disease) may be low in vitamin K. Vitamin K supplementation may decrease calcium excretion and help protect against osteoporosis. A deficiency of vitamin K causes hemorrhaging. Pediatricians administer vitamin K to newborn infants to reduce their risk of spontaneous bleeding. Infants also run the risk of being permanently brain damaged by vitamin K deficiency in the first six months of life. There may be other important functions of this vitamin; vitamin K-dependent modified proteins occur in kidneys and other tissues as well, though their function is unclear.

Sources

Vitamin K occurs in highest levels in green leafy vegetables. Dairy products are good sources, and small amounts occur in cereals, meats, and other vegetables. Bacteria colonizing the mature small intestine produce vitamin K; LACTOBACILLUS ACIDOPHILUS is an example of such a beneficial gut bacteria. Vitamin K_3 is prescribed to treat vitamin K deficiencies.

Requirements

The adequate intake for normal adults is 120 mcg/day for men and 90 mcg/day for women. There are hints that optimal bone metabolism is more sensitive to inadequate vitamin K and the needs may be higher. Because vitamin K is widely distributed in food and is formed by normal gut flora, vitamin K deficiency is not believed to be common. Deficiency could occur in people who consume few vegetables, in people with lipid MALABSORPTION and in those with CELIAC DISEASE or bile duct obstruction. The prolonged use of oral antibiotics; certain medications like cholesterol lowering drugs, mineral oil, anticonvulsants (Dilantin), and some antibiotics (aphalosporins); and PARENTERAL NUTRITION (venous feeding) increase the risk. Vitamin K status needs to be monitored in patients being treated with anticoagulants (like coumadin). Symptoms of severe deficiency include a tendency to bleed and disturbed bone formation.

Safety

Naturally occurring forms of vitamin K are relatively nontoxic. The synthetic form may rarely cause liver problems. An allergic-type reaction can occur with high doses. A high intake of vitamin E may cause bleeding similar to vitamin K deficiency. Those who have a vitamin K deficiency need medical supervision. Patients taking anticoagulants should take vitamin K only with the advice of a physician. (See also VITAMIN A; VITAMIN D.)

vitamin P See FLAVONOIDS.

VLDL See VERY LOW-DENSITY LIPOPROTEIN.

W

walnut (*Juglans* spp.) A popular commercial nut with a hard, deeply furrowed shell surrounding the meat. The English walnut (*J. regia*) is the most important commercial walnut. It is native to southeastern Europe and western Asia and probably originated in Persia. The black walnut (*J. nigra*) is native to the Mississippi Valley and Appalachians of the United States; there is limited commercial production of black walnuts, however. The United States produces over half the world crop; most of it comes from California. About 40 percent of the walnut crop is marketed in shells, the remainder is processed. Machine-shelled nuts may be blanched to remove the inner skins, which give walnuts their somewhat bitter aftertaste. They may be blanched to even out the color.

Walnuts contain a large percentage of oil, with 66 percent of it as polyunsaturated fatty acids. It is a good source of alpha linolenic acid, an omega-3 fatty acid essential to the diet. Cholesterol-lowering diets in which meat and dairy products are substituted by walnuts may lower blood cholesterol levels because of their polyunsaturated fat. Shelled nuts are subject to rancidity; they should be vacuum-packed or stored in sealed plastic bags in the freezer. On the other hand, whole walnuts can be stored for months in a cool environment. If antioxidants are added to extend shelf life, they are listed on the food label. Walnuts are used in baking and confections. The nutrient content of 1 cup (120 g) of chopped English walnuts is: 770 calories; protein, 17.2 g; carbohydrate, 22 g; fiber, 8.4 g; fat, 74.2 g; iron, 2.8 mg; potassium, 602 mg; thiamine, 0.46 mg; riboflavin, 0.18 mg; niacin, 1.256 mg.

water A clear, colorless, odorless liquid that is essential for all life forms. Water is the most abundant nutrient in the body. More water is needed daily than any other nutrient because cells contain mainly water. A human embryo represents about 98 percent water; an infant's weight is about 75 percent water; and water accounts for 50 percent to 65 percent of an adult's weight. EXTRACELLULAR FLUID including blood and lymph accounts for 20 percent of body weight; INTRACELLULAR FLUID, the water within cells, accounts for 45 percent. Water represents 75 percent of muscle tissue and 92 percent of the cell-free fluid of blood (plasma). Excessive water can accumulate in tissues, a condition called EDEMA. Edema is caused by heart failure, low blood pressure due to low blood protein resulting from STARVATION, or to increased capillary leakiness due to INFLAMMATION.

Water serves many roles for the body. Water functions as a lubricant and is a major constituent of joint fluid. It helps internal organs slide by each other, for example, during PERISTALSIS, the muscular contraction that moves food down the digestive tract. Water comprises the major constituent of fluids important in digestion: SALIVA, MUCUS, gastric juice, BILE, pancreatic juices, and intestinal secretions. Because water is so prevalent in cells, most cellular macromolecules of the body like DNA, RNA, proteins, and polysaccharides function in a water environment. Water participates in many chemical reactions of the body. Thus DIGESTION refers to the hydrolysis of nutrients, that is, the breaking of chemical bonds by means of water molecules.

Because water is an excellent solvent, it readily transports nutrients and waste products in the bloodstream. Water also absorbs and releases heat slowly so that it can slow changes in body temperature as environmental temperatures fluctuate. Water possesses a high heat of vaporization; that is, a lot of heat is used up in evaporation. Thus when water evaporates as sweat, it provides an effective means of cooling the body. Gases dissolve readily in water, and moist tissue surfaces promote the absorption of gases like OXYGEN and the release of CARBON DIOXIDE in the lungs.

Water Balance

Water balance refers to the ability of the body to adjust water output to water intake. When a large volume of water is consumed, urine excretion increases; with limited water intake, urine production declines. Water is lost daily from the skin (450 ml), urine (1,400 ml), expired air from the lungs (350 ml) and in stools (200 ml). To make up for these losses, a typical adult uses 2 to 2.9 quarts (2 to 2.7 liters) of water daily. Beverages provide about 1.5 l; foods contribute about 0.70 l, and water from metabolism yields 0.20 l. RESPIRATION, the oxidation of nutrients to carbon dioxide, produces on the average 13 g of water per 100 calories with a typical diet. Thus oxidation of 100 g of carbohydrate yields 60 g of water; the oxidation of 100 g of protein, 42 g of water; and 100 g of fat, 110 g of water.

Water is also recycled. Each day the intestine receives 8 to 10 liters of secretions, including saliva, gastric juices and glandular products. Most water is reabsorbed; only 100 to 200 ml of water is lost through feces. Exceptions are DIARRHEA and vomiting. The kidneys play a major role in water conservation while removing waste materials in urine. Each day the kidneys filter nearly 2,000 liters of blood. Only 0.1 percent of this volume is released as urine.

Water balance is regulated by an elegant feedback system involving the brain and hormones. Nerve centers in the region of the brain called the HYPOTHALAMUS regulate hunger, thirst, and urine output. A loss of about 1 percent of body water creates the sensation of THIRST. Decreased water and elevated sodium in the blood are detected by osmoreceptor cells, regulatory cells located in the hypothalamus. As the effective ion concentration of blood increases, water leaves these cells and they shrink, generating nerve impulses that trigger thirst and stimulate the release of ANTIDIURETIC HORMONE (ADH) from the PITUITARY GLAND. ADH in turn increases the ability of NEPHRONS (the kidneys' filtration device) to absorb water that would otherwise be lost as urine. As a result, the sodium concentration of the blood decreases, cells of the hypothalamus regain water, and the thirst sensation diminishes.

Dehydration

DEHYDRATION can be caused by evaporation, diarrhea, blood losses, burns or excessive urine production, as in uncontrolled diabetes. Physical activity increases water loss through perspiration and breathing. Water depletion can become a serious problem with prolonged EXERCISE. With elevated temperatures, strenuous exercise can increase water losses three- to tenfold above normal. DIURETICS (water pills) increase urine output by increasing water and sodium excretion, as do CAFFEINE and related compounds like theophylline. ALCOHOL increases urination because it inhibits the release of ADH. Dehydration can cause discomfort, flushed skin, tingling in hands and feet, then increased heart rate, increased body temperature, weakness, confusion, spastic muscles, and decreased blood volume.

Overhydration

With excessive water intake, brain cells become swollen. This can cause drowsiness, lowered blood pressure, weakened heart, weakness, and even convulsions and coma. Patients administered excessive IV solutions too rapidly or who have impaired ADH production may develop symptoms of water intoxication.

Minerals in Drinking Water

All water except distilled water contains minerals, and domestic water supplies vary in their mineral content.

Hard water contains calcium and magnesium salts of bicarbonate and sulfate. The mineral content can be sufficiently high to contribute to daily requirements of these minerals. Boiling hard water converts bicarbonate to carbonate, and insoluble magnesium and calcium carbonate deposits form in tea kettles, hot water, and steam pipes. Calcium and magnesium in hard water also form solids with typical soaps.

Soft water contains sodium sulfate and sodium bicarbonate, which are soluble and do not form solids as water is boiled, nor do they react with soap. Soft water is associated with an increased risk of CARDIOVASCULAR DISEASE, possibly because low dietary calcium and magnesium increase the risk of heart disease. When drinking water contains more than 20 mg of sodium per liter, it represents a significant source of sodium for people on sodium-restricted diets. Soft water is more corrosive to plumbing and can dissolve CADMIUM and LEAD from galvanized pipes and soldered joints.

Water hardness is expressed in parts per million (ppm) equivalent to calcium carbonate, though magnesium or other minerals may be present. Water with a hardness less than 100 ppm of calcium carbonate is considered soft, while water with a hardness greater than 300 ppm is considered hard.

Over half of the municipal water supplies in the United States add FLUORIDE to reduce tooth decay. This has become a controversial issue because too much fluoride can cause health problems.

Demineralized water that is free of mineral ions, like calcium, magnesium, and carbonate, is prepared by ion exchange columns that replace calcium and magnesium with sodium and hydrogen ions, and replace carbonate with sulfate. Non-ionic materials such as pesticides are not removed.

Distillation, in which water is converted to steam and then condensed and collected, removes most organic residues as well as minerals. Volatile materials (those that readily vaporize) such as solvents may not be removed by distillation.

Disinfecting Drinking Water

Chlorination has long been used as a chemical treatment to disinfect water. In most industrialized countries, water treatment by chlorination has removed the threat of water-borne diseases like cholera, typhoid, dysentery, and gastroenteritis. However, inadequate treatment of sewage leads to periodic outbreaks of hepatitis A and other diseases. There are hints that chlorination by-products slightly increase the risk of cancer. Most public health officials agree that the health risks of not disinfecting water are very much greater than those posed by chlorination.

An alternative treatment to kill disease-causing microbes, chloramination, incorporates chlorine and ammonia to treat water supplies. It is as effective as chlorine, and this method is used by about 20 percent of the largest municipal water supplies. Ozonation disinfects water with ozone, with a follow-up chlorination or chloramination treatment to destroy microbes that may multiply after ozone wears off. Less than 1 percent of water systems use this method.

Parasites can contaminate water supplies in the United States. In 1993, an estimated 370,000 people in Milwaukee experienced diarrhea and flu-like symptoms due to water contamination by a parasite called *Cryptosporidium.* Elevated levels of particulate matter in drinking water in Washington, D.C., the same year caused the EPA to issue an alert to boil drinking water as a defense against *Cryptosporidium,* which resists chlorination. Although most people experience only mild discomfort with infection, *Cryptosporidium* can cause life-threatening illness in newborn infants and in people with impaired immune systems.

There are no standards for acceptable levels of this parasite in drinking water. *Giardia,* another intestinal parasite that can also cause intestinal distress, is larger than *Cryptosporidium* and is more easily removed by filtration in municipal water treatments. The presence of this parasite in water is essentially unacceptable to the EPA.

Suggestions for Water Purification When Camping

Boiling water up to 20 minutes is a tried and true method of disinfecting drinking water, and it is probably the safest. Using iodine to disinfect water may pose a hazard because excessive amounts of iodine can be toxic. Another form of iodine, hypoperiodide, is safer. Adding a couple of tablets of activated charcoal per quart can remove the unpleasant taste from sterilized water. Travelers should avoid drinking tap water and iced drinks when in countries where water quality is questionable. If water used to make ice cubes is contaminated, the iced beverage will be too.

Chemical Water Pollutants

Industrialization has introduced thousands of new chemicals into the environment, and about 700 chemical contaminants have been detected in drinking water in the United States including PESTICIDES; industrial solvents; toxic heavy metals like lead and MERCURY; NITRATES from fertilizer use; and radioactive contaminants like radon. Under the Safe Drinking Water Act of 1974, the Environmental Protection Agency is charged with setting standards of water quality for all local water systems and to make certain that states enforce the standards. According to the EPA more than 90 percent of the tap water supplied by public systems meets federal standards for safety.

Over 80 compounds and toxic substances are regulated in terms of maximum upper limits for concentrations in drinking water. The legal limits, called maximum contaminant levels (MCLs), are administered by individual states. Included are minerals like ARSENIC; nitrates; heavy metals like cadmium; lead; mercury; solvents like benzene and phenol; pesticides like Endrin, Diquat, Dalapon, and Simazine; products of incomplete combustion like BENZOPYRENE and DIOXIN. Antimony, NICKEL, pesticides like dinoseb (used on soybeans and other crops), atrazine (a herbicide used on corn), and halogenated hydrocarbons are among the most commonly found compounds in water supplies.

Halogenated hydrocarbons are quite stable in the environment and can contaminate the environment for decades. One class is called CHLORINATED HYDROCARBONS. As an example, trichloroethylene (TCE) and its degradation products are important contaminants of ground water. TCE was used as a degreasing agent. Since TCE is volatile, drinking water can be treated by air evaporation process (air stripping). Other regulated volatile chlorinated hydrocarbons include dichloromethane and trihalomethane, by-products of the reaction of chlorine with organic materials in drinking water. Because they evaporate easily, they may pose a hazard when taking a shower.

Home Water Treatment

No single device removes all contaminants. Water purifiers remove bacteria while water filters remove nonbacterial contaminants but not bacteria. The best systems can remove up to 99 percent of the chlorine and over 70 percent of other contaminants. Units should be certified by the nonprofit National Sanitation Foundation in Ann Arbor, Michigan. Water softeners or water treatment units to improve the taste or smell of drinking water may be certified by the Water Quality Association.

Activated carbon filtration units with high-quality carbon can absorb chlorine and organic compounds but are not very effective in removing minerals like IRON, lead, or fluoride. Carbon filters must be replaced about once a month. Some filters can become breeding grounds for harmful bacteria unless properly maintained. The best filters are solid blocks of activated charcoal with a diversion valve, so that unfiltered water can be used for dishes. Filters need to be changed regularly.

Reverse osmosis filtration forces water through a porous membrane at high pressures. Reverse osmosis effectively removes inorganic ions like fluoride and a few organic contaminants, but reverse osmosis also wastes about 75 percent of the water and the membranes need to be replaced periodically.

Water softener units incorporate ion exchangers, which will remove iron, calcium, and other minerals of hard water and replace them with sodium. Cooking with or drinking softened water is not advised due to the high sodium content.

Home distillation removes minerals and nonvolatile organic compounds (those that do not evaporate), but the process is slow and costly because of heating costs.

BOTTLED WATER is another alternative to tap water. Bottled water is classified as a food product by the U.S. FDA, but this is no guarantee that it will be safe or wholesome. Producers are not required to list the source of the water. Most bottled water comes from wells or springs, but it may be municipal water. Bottled water is less regulated than tap water, and spot checks have turned up traces of organic solvents, nitrates, and toxic heavy metals—and the sodium content can be high. Tests of domestic bottled water have seldom turned up harmful levels of chemical contaminants, though sampled bottled water may only meet, not exceed, health department standards. Bottled water is disinfected by ozone, not chlorine treatment, and it is not fluoridated.

Recommendations

To minimize chemical contaminants, use cold tap water for drinking because hot water tends to dissolve metals from pipes. Let the cold tap run until the water gets cold. This water contains the least amount of contaminants leached from metal pipes.

Water suppliers must provide the results of annual water tests for regulated contaminants to their customers.

Though bottled water generally appears to be good quality it may be prudent to request the latest chemical analysis from the bottler, or have a sample tested independently. To minimize the RISK of exposure to contaminants, vary your water supply from time to time.

"Over 50 Million Drink Water Failing Health Standards," *Nutrition Week* 25, no. 22 (June 9, 1995): 6.

watermelon (*Citrullus vulgaris*) The fruit of an annual vine belonging to the squash and melon family. This round or cylindrical fruit can weigh from 5 lb. to 85 lb. (2.3 to 38.3 kg). There are more than 50 varieties, including seedless watermelons. The juicy flesh may be red, pink, orange, yellow, or white. Watermelons originated in Africa and have been cultivated since ancient times in the Mediterranean region, Egypt, and India. Watermelons are now cultivated throughout the world from tropical to temperate regions. Florida, Texas, and California lead domestic production. The fruit is eaten fresh. Watermelon is a good source of vitamin C; it contains about 90 percent water and 8 percent sugar. The nutrient content of a slice of raw watermelon that is 1 in. thick and 10 in. in diameter, without refuse (480 g), is: 152 calories; protein, 3 g; carbohydrate, 34.6 g; fiber, 2.4 g; fat, 2.1 g; iron, 0.82 g; potassium, 560 mg; vitamin A, 176 retinol equivalents; vitamin C, 47 mg; thiamin, 0.3 mg; riboflavin, 0.1 mg; niacin, 0.96 mg.

water pills See DIURETICS.

water-soluble vitamins See VITAMIN.

wax A family of water resistant compounds that are solids or thick (viscous) liquids. Waxes consist of long chains of carbon atoms, and are obtained from petroleum products (paraffin), fat, beeswax, synthetic resins, and palm oil derivatives. Only insect-based waxes and vegetable waxes are applied on domestic produce, although imported produce may contain animal-based waxes. Commercially, waxes are generally sprayed as a thin film on produce to prevent loss of moisture and to enhance consumer appeal after polishing. Naturally occurring protective waxes on fruits and vegetables are generally washed off when the produce is harvested. Producers commonly wax APPLES, AVOCADOS, BEETS, green PEPPERS, CUCUMBERS, EGGPLANT, MELONS, certain nuts, PAPAYAS, PEACHES, PINEAPPLES, POTATOES, SQUASH, TANGERINES, TOMATOES, SWEET POTATOES, and WATERMELONS.

Waxes are classified as PRESERVATIVES, and the U.S. FDA regulations specify that waxes must be identified where the consumer purchases the produce. The type of wax applied is not specified, a concern for those following dietary laws or making dietary choices such as KOSHER, Muslim, Seventh-day Adventist, or vegetarian diets.

FUNGICIDES are generally applied before waxing or are mixed with waxes before application, and waxed produce cannot be washed free of fungicides. Benomyl, thiabendazole, phenol, captan, folpet, dicloran, and others are permitted to be used with waxes. The U.S. National Academy of Sciences estimates that 90 percent of fungicides are potential cancer-causing agents (carcinogens). Specifically, benomyl, captan, and folpet increase the risk of cancer. (See also DELANEY CLAUSE; FOOD ADDITIVES; ORGANIC FOODS; PESTICIDES; PRODUCE WASH.)

weight management Generally, programs designed to assist individuals to lose weight or to maintain a desired body weight. Americans who diet to lose weight frequently participate in weight management programs for many reasons. Statistics show that meeting external expectations motivates most dieters. Current American images of attractiveness and success place a premium on being slender, especially for women.

A second motivation to manage weight is an awareness of the ramifications of being excessively overweight. OBESITY, defined as having a BODY MASS INDEX of 25 or higher, carries increased risks for diabetes, HYPERTENSION, and CARDIOVASCULAR DISEASE. Certain people tend to gain excess fat on their upper body, and upper body fat increases the waist to hip ratio, which correlates with a greater risk of heart disease.

Strategies for Weight Loss

Short-term weight loss readily can be attained by extreme measures: a drastic reduction in caloric intake (semi-starvation); CRASH DIETING; unbalanced diets emphasizing high fat and high protein with little or no CARBOHYDRATE. However, most of this lost weight represents WATER and muscle protein loss rather than fat loss. Without a commitment to changing long-term behavior, pounds lost will be rapidly regained; frequently lost muscle is replaced by fat at the termination of the weight loss program. Several popular, doctor-supervised, very low-calorie programs are available. There is little published data on the success rates of most weight management programs. The limited information available suggests that only 2 percent to 10 percent of people who have enrolled in such programs successfully keep off lost pounds for a year or more. These strategies can lead to weight losses of several pounds per week and often employ liquid protein meal replacements. Current liquid formula diets are much improved over 1970s versions. Regular food allotments plus three meal replacements can bring the total calories up to 1,200 per day, and with supervision they are often safe for several weeks. A major disadvantage: They often reinforce the unhealthy pattern of eating lightly at breakfast and lunch, and eating heavily at dinner or later.

Under starvation or semi-starvation conditions, usually less than 1,200 calories per day, the body's metabolism compensates for decreased caloric intake by gearing down the rate at which calories are burned. In other words the BASAL METABOLIC RATE declines as a protective adaptation. Furthermore, the body preferentially breaks down protein in the early stages of semi-starvation to meet energy requirements; paradoxically, the body can therefore become proportionately fatter during this period. Programs that incorporate medications to curb CRAVING as well as increased exercise and restricted caloric intake have been recommended for obese people.

Recommendations for Weight Management

People who have lost weight permanently and have maintained a desired weight for a number of years share certain characteristics that permit several generalizations for managing weight successfully.

Committing to Exercising for Life Daily exercises can temporarily increase the basal metabolic rate and thus increase the efficiency of burning calories, even when calories are restricted. Even a daily half-hour of vigorous walking will help maintain weight. Regular exercise is often sufficient to lose a small amount of weight and to become leaner. Moderate exercise is more effective for weight management because it preferentially burns fat, and intense exercise burns carbohydrate (glycogen), which is easily replenished.

Committing to Changing Eating Habits High-calorie, high-fat foods make up a large percentage of the American diet. Fat provides more than twice as many calories per gram as carbohydrate or protein, and fat calories are more readily converted to body fat. Eating less fat will help bring about weight loss. High dietary fat correlates with increased risk of disease; generally, dietary guidelines call for consuming less saturated fat while increasing fresh fruits and vegetables, whole grains, and legumes. Foods containing high levels of refined carbohydrate, like sugar, white flour, and fat, provide few other nutrients. People relying on such foods need to select extra nutrient-rich foods to make up for this deficiency, not a usual pattern in the United States. A combination of exercise and improved food selection is often adequate to lose 10 to 20 pounds a year without dieting.

Dieting and Exercising Combined To lose up to 50 pounds, dieting combined with exercise is recommended. Patients should:

- Lose weight gradually, no more than a pound per week. Conditions that promote rapid weight loss cause the body's METABOLISM to switch to favor loss of muscle protein and water and, less rapidly, fat. Severe caloric restriction reduces thyroid gland activity, slowing the metabolism and slowing fat loss.
- Consume at least 1,200 calories daily with adequate intake of high-quality protein, vitamins, and minerals to meet daily needs in order to accomplish gradual weight loss. Generally 45 to 60 g of FISH, POULTRY, lean MEAT, soy protein, or other complete protein will meet daily requirements of all essential amino acids. This step will assure an adequate supply of all essential amino

acids and will help prevent loss of muscle. Diets supplying less than 1,500 calories per day require supplementation—for example, with calcium—to achieve adequate intake. VITAMIN C, the B COMPLEX, and TRACE MINERALS are known to help metabolize fat, and adequate intakes are important.

- Eat adequate FIBER: Both soluble fiber, as found in fresh FRUITS, VEGETABLES, LEGUMES, and certain grains, and insoluble fiber, as found in whole grains and bran. Fiber contributes to normal digestion, maintenance of the digestive tract, and a feeling of satiety.
- Drink plenty of water. The kidneys require water to excrete metabolic wastes and fat breakdown products.

Seeking Out Emotional Support Overeating usually is symptomatic of deeper emotional issues. Until these are dealt with, long-term changes in eating behavior are difficult to achieve. When people substitute eating for self-acceptance or for avoiding emotional pain, weight management becomes increasingly difficult. Overeaters Anonymous and other support groups can help nurture self-esteem and self-forgiveness. (See also ANOREXIA NERVOSA; BULIMIA NERVOSA; DIETARY GUIDELINES FOR AMERICANS; DIETING; EATING DISORDERS.)

Gibbs, W. W. "Gaining on Fat," *Scientific American* 275, no. 2 (1996): 88–94.

weights and measures See MEASURES.

Wernicke's disease (Wernicke-Korsakoff syndrome) A disorder of the NERVOUS SYSTEM usually associated with a deficiency of the B vitamin, THIAMIN. Typical symptoms include: poor balance and uncoordinated walk, double vision, confusion, delusion, and psychosis. It can occur in chronic ALCOHOLISM, BERIBERI, and STARVATION. Some alcoholics apparently possess enzymes that require higher than normal levels of thiamin for energy production from carbohydrate. When the diet is depleted in B vitamins and the need for B vitamins increases, these individuals are more prone to thiamin deficiency symptoms. Wernicke's disease represents a medical emergency. Massive doses of thiamin are used therapeutically. (See also MALNUTRITION; NEUROPATHY; PERIPHERAL.)

wheat A cereal GRAIN that serves as a staple for one-third of the world's population. Wheat accounts for 40 percent to 60 percent of the calorie and protein intake in many developing countries. Wheat is related to other true grains including RICE, CORN, BARLEY, and RYE. Wheat apparently developed from a wild grass in southwestern Asia, and it was cultivated as early as 6000 B.C. in the regions of China, Egypt, and Iraq. The United States, southeastern European nations, India, Canada, and Australia rank among the leading wheat-producing countries. In the United States, wheat ranks second to corn in terms of total grain production and is still the most important cereal grain for human consumption. The general trend in grain consumption since the early 1900s has been a gradual decline as processed sugar and fat have become more prominent carbohydrates.

During the 1960s, new high-yield strains of wheat and rice were developed and cultivated in the Philippines, Mexico, India, and Pakistan. These advances, together with increased use of pesticides and irrigation, ushered in the GREEN REVOLUTION, which dramatically increased grain production. Despite the Green Revolution, domestic food production remains critical in many regions of the world.

Efforts continue to develop new strains of wheat. In the past, development of new wheat strains required up to 10 years. Now biotechnology offers new techniques for screening different strains and for breeding wheat. A new wheat strain is likely to be profitable for only an estimated 10 years before it is improved upon or becomes susceptible to pests and disease. Efforts are being directed toward breeding pesticide-resistant strains. Nonetheless, food production alone cannot eradicate hunger in countries disrupted by civil strife, breakdown of government services, drought, poverty, illiteracy, and high birth rates.

Types of Wheat

Thousands of varieties of wheat exist today; about 100 varieties are cultivated in the United States. Wheat varieties fall into two broad categories: winter wheat and spring wheat. Winter wheat is planted in the fall and harvested the following summer in the midwestern United States. Spring wheat is planted in the spring in regions where winters are severe and harvested later in the summer. Most bread is made from hard, red winter wheat grown in the United States. As an example, durum wheat is grown mainly for PASTA, like spaghetti and noodles. Hard wheats contain a higher protein content than spring wheat. Soft, white winter wheat is best suited for pastries and Asian noodles.

Wheat Products

Wheat berries are kernels after the chaff (husk) has been removed by threshing. The wheat kernel has a tough outer layer with FIBER (BRAN); a soft, oily, nutrient-rich section (germ); and a starchy endosperm or inner core that represents about 80 percent of the kernel. The endosperm is the source of wheat flour.

Wheat germ represents 2.5 percent of the kernel. It contains many nutrients, including essential fatty acids and high-quality protein. Wheat germ can be used to supplement cereals, breads, cookies, and hot dishes. Because wheat germ can become rancid, it should be refrigerated after opening the container or frozen for long-term storage.

The kernel is surrounded with a tough outer coating called bran. Milling or grinding wheat kernels separates the starchy endosperm from the germ and bran to produce flour. Stone ground flour is thought to be more nutritious because the flour is not heated as much as it is in conventional milling. Different types of wheat yield flour with different properties. For example, bakery flour with a higher protein concentration creates doughs strong enough to permit extensive mechanical kneading.

Wheat flour contains a protein fraction called GLUTEN, consisting of GLIADEN and glutenin. When mixed with water they form an elastic dough that traps the carbon dioxide released by LEAVENING AGENTS. This accounts for the unique leavening properties of wheat doughs. The use of leavening agents is credited to the Egyptians who introduced yeast. Beating or kneading dough traps air bubbles in the mixture to give baked goods a lighter texture. Starch yields glucose, which is broken down by the yeast enzymes to carbon dioxide. Bubbles of carbon dioxide are trapped in elastic doughs. Alternatively, BAKING POWDER can be used as a leavening agent; it contains chemicals that yield carbon dioxide upon mixing and heating the dough.

White bleached flour accounts for more than 95 percent of the wheat flour used in the United States. In terms of nutrients, the annual consumption of 120 lb. of refined wheat products per year is comparable to consuming 30 lb. of whole wheat plus 90 lb. of pure starch. White flour is aged to increase its elasticity as a dough, using several oxidizing agents to modify gluten. It may contain phosphate and other additives to shorten kneading time. All-purpose flour was developed in the 1960s for greater convenience in home cooking. The flour does not form clumps readily, it is dust free, and it disperses in cold water. Special flours have also been developed for cakes, pastries, Italian and French breads, and rolls. The food label will indicate whether the flour has been bleached.

REPRESENTATIVE NUTRIENT CONTENTS OF WHEAT

Nutrient	Whole Wheat	White Flour*
Energy, calories	300	355
Crude fiber	2.3 g	0.3 g
Linoleic acid	1.5 g	0.75 g
Protein	13 g	11 g
Biotin	0.010 mg	0.002 mg
Vitamin B_6	0.30 mg	0.05 mg
Calcium	35 mg	17 mg
Choline	170 mg	80 mg
Chromium	0.06 mg	0.02 mg
Copper	0.5 mg	0.1 mg
Vitamin E	1.5 IU	0.03 IU
Fluoride	0.1 mg	0.06 mg
Folic acid	0.04 mg	0.01 mg
Vitamin K	0.017 mg	0.004 mg
Iron	3.0 mg	0.6 (3.0) mg
Magnesium	140 mg	25 mg
Manganese	3 mg	0.3 mg
Molybdenum	0.05 mg	0.025 mg
Niacin	5 mg	1.0 (5.3) mg
Pantothenic acid	1.0 mg	0.5 mg
Phosphorus	350 mg	90 mg
Potassium	400 mg	90 mg
Riboflavin	0.12 mg	0.04 (0.4) mg
Selenium	0.04 mg	0.03 mg
Thiamin	0.5 mg	0.09 (0.64) mg
Zinc	3 mg	0.6 mg

* Based on 60 percent to 72 percent extraction white flour, per 100 g (13 percent moisture basis). Values in parentheses are after U.S. enrichment and are valid only for iron, niacin, riboflavin, and thiamin. Amounts are representative of U.S. samples, which may vary widely in composition especially for minerals.

Whole wheat flour represents 95 percent of the whole kernel contents. It provides all common nutrients except VITAMIN A, VITAMIN B_{12}, VITAMIN C, and IODINE. Whole wheat also contains trace minerals like tin and nickel for which there is no established role in the body. The amounts of nutrients vary according to the variety of wheat and the soil conditions where it was grown. Whole wheat flour is less stable than bleached white flour because it contains wheat germ oils and can become rancid when stored. Whole wheat flour should be used soon after purchase and refrigerated to preserve freshness.

White flour represents a refined or purified carbohydrate with lesser amounts of key nutrients than whole wheat flour. The production of white flour requires about two dozen different steps that remove or destroy substantial amounts of nutrients found in whole wheat. White flour retains starch and about 70 percent of the protein, but losses of other nutrients average 70 percent to 80 percent. In order to partially remedy this deficiency, an enrichment program increases the levels of IRON, THIAMIN, and NIACIN to those approximating whole wheat. RIBOFLAVIN is increased threefold; CALCIUM is often added. Canada and Britain have similar enrichment programs. Other nutrients—including FOLIC ACID, VITAMIN B_6, VITAMIN E, BIOTIN, CHROMIUM, COPPER, MAGNESIUM, MANGANESE, ZINC, and fiber—are not added back. All white flour produced in the United States is enriched, as are about 90 percent of commercial baked goods prepared from white flour. The accompanying table compares the nutrient contents of whole wheat, nonenriched white flour and enriched flour. (See also BREAKFAST CEREAL.)

whey protein High quality, nutritious dairy protein found in milk that is a complete protein containing all the essential amino acids required by the body. Proponents of whey protein take it as a supplement to boost the immune system; build strong, lean muscles; and lower elevated cholesterol and high blood pressure. It is also being researched as a possible preventive treatment for cancer in laboratory animals.

When cheese is produced, liquid whey separates from the curd (casein); whey proteins are then separated from the liquid whey and purified to various concentrations. Whey protein is not a single protein but includes a number of individual protein components, many of which are commercially available in isolated form. Individual components in whey protein include beta-lactoglobulin, glycomacropeptide, alpha-lactalbumin, lactoferrin, immunoglobulins, lactoperoxidase, bovine serum albumin, and lysozyme. The composition of specific whey protein products varies based on several factors including source of the milk, method of production, type of cheese being produced, and individual manufacturer specifications.

Groziak S. M., and Miller G. D. "Natural Bioactive Substances in Milk and Colostrum: Effects on the Arterial Blood Pressure System," *British Journal of Nutrition* Suppl. 84, no. 1 (2000): S119–S125.

Lemon, W. R. "Effects of Exercise on Dietary Protein Requirements," *International Journal of Sport Nutrition and Exercise Metabolism* 8, no. 4: 426–447.

white blood cells See LEUKOCYTES.

WIC (Supplemental Food Program for Women, Infants, Children) A federal program initiated in 1972 to improve pregnant women's health and the health of their children by providing them with a good diet. Since 1972 WIC has assisted state agencies in giving food to impoverished women and children. Due to sharp increases in food prices and a scarcity of funding, thousands of recipients in many states were dropped from assistance programs in 1990, when a House Select Committee on Hunger found at least 50,000 people were dropped in 27 states. In 2002 the program had more than 7 million participants and cost $4.39 billion.

The original philosophy was preventative, rather than therapeutic. Full disclosure of a comprehensive study of its efficacy revealed that between 1972 and 1980 WIC reduced infant mortality. There is a possibility that WIC food supplements might have increased skull growth and mental development in poor children. Other studies since 1980 have shown that adequate prenatal nutrition helps prevent low birth weight babies and reduces long-term medical expenses that would otherwise be publicly financed. The U.S. General Accounting Office reported that the WIC funding of $2.6 billion for 1992 paid for itself in a year due to reduced health costs.

Each state WIC program authorizes food that will be redeemable with WIC checks. WIC clients are provided with coupons to obtain fresh fruit and vegetables, in addition to milk, eggs, cheese, cereal, juice, and infant formula. WIC actively promotes breast-feeding, but the program supplies formula for infants up to one year of age. For any new food to be authorized, in general the food manufacturer must submit a request for authorization, the product must meet state requirements in packaging, the food must be available statewide, and the product must be consistent with the WIC program promotion of healthy, economic food purchasing practices. (See also PREGNANCY AND NUTRITIONAL REQUIREMENTS; SCHOOL LUNCH PROGRAM.)

Auruch, S., and A. P. Cackley. "Savings Achieved by Giving WIC Benefits to Women Prenatally," *Public Health Report* 110, no. 7 (January–February 1995): 27–34.

wild rice (*Zizania aquatica;* Indian rice) The only native cereal GRAIN domesticated in North America. Wild RICE grows in Minnesota and Wisconsin in the United States, and in Manitoba, Canada. Harvesting has traditionally been performed by hand because kernels of wild rice fall off the stalks as they ripen. Improved varieties can be harvested mechanically like wheat and barley, and 90 percent of the annual wild rice crop in Minnesota is grown in paddies and harvested by combines.

Wild rice is cooked like regular rice: The larger the kernel and the darker its color, the longer the required cooking time. Its protein content is higher than typical grains. The nutrient content of a half-cup (100 g) of cooked wild rice is: 92 calories; protein, 3.6 g; carbohydrate, 11 g; fiber, 2.6 g; fat, 0.2 g; iron, 1.1 mg; thiamin, 0.11 mg; riboflavin, 0.16 mg; niacin, 1.6 mg.

wine The fermented juice of grapes. When other fruit juices are fermented, the name of the fruit is given, as in blackberry wine or plum wine. Archaeological evidence indicates that wine was prepared between 6000 and 5000 B.C. in the Middle East. Wine making was described in Egypt by 2500 B.C. American grapes, *Vitus labrusca,* are pest-resistant, and European varieties, *V. vinifera,* are grafted onto American root stocks. The Concord grape, developed in 1852 in Massachusetts, yields a full-bodied wine. Grapes grown in cooler regions of California, Oregon, and Washington yield grapes with the higher acid content and the low to medium alcohol content of typical table wines. Dessert wines require grapes with a high sugar content.

To prepare wine, grapes are crushed and treated with sulfur dioxide to kill wild yeasts on the grapes. Additional dextrose (glucose) may be added if the sugar content is inadequate and the mixture is inoculated with a culture of a pure yeast strain. Fermentation is then carried out in temperature-controlled vats. Red wines are produced by fermenting grape pulp with skins; white wines are fermented with only minimal contact with skin. After fermentation, the wine is clarified by adding gelatin or egg white protein to coagulate suspended materials. After settling, the mixture is filtered. Most wine is mellowed by aging from several months to several years to remove bitter or harsh flavors. Among the many chemical changes that occur, acidic substances slowly form fragrant compounds called esters. Wooden barrels have traditionally been used for aging because they absorb astringent substances and contribute their own subtle flavors. Wine is filtered and usually treated with sulfur dioxide to prevent spoilage. Aging continues after the wine is bottled.

Drinking red wine may lower LOW-DENSITY LIPOPROTEINS (LDL), the less desirable form of blood cholesterol. During fermentation of grape skins, a compound called resveratrol leaches out of the skin. Resveratrol is responsible in part for the cholesterol-lowering effect of red wine in experimental animals. It occurs naturally in grapes and offers natural protection against fungus. Heat treatment of Concord grapes, used to prepare red grape juice, releases resveratrol also. The cholesterol lowering effect of alcoholic beverages declines rapidly after more than one or two drinks are consumed daily. Alcohol is inappropriate for people with a history of ALCOHOLISM, HYPERTENSION, liver disease, smoking, DIABETES, OBESITY, or PEPTIC ULCERS.

Red wine contains substantial amounts of IRON. However, the amounts of most nutrients found in grapes are quite low. Red wine also contains a mixture of FLAVONOIDS, complex plant substances that can function as ANTIOXIDANTS. Test-tube experiments demonstrated that red wine flavonoids can protect LDL-cholesterol, the most prevalent form of cholesterol in blood, from oxidation. Whether this occurs in the body remains unclear. The so-called "French Paradox" describes the phenomenon of those who consume wine, together with substantial animal fat and meat, yet have lower rates of heart disease than those who do not consume wine. Moderate consumption of alcoholic beverages, regardless of the source, raise HDL cholesterol, the beneficial form. In addition, the MEDITERRANEAN DIET entails a higher consumption of fruits, legumes, and vegetables than in the typical U.S. diet. These factors also decrease the risk of heart disease. Wine like all alcoholic beverages has a low nutrient density and displaces more nutrient-rich sources of calories when consumed in excess. An estimated 4 percent of domestic and imported wines contain 0.3 parts per million of LEAD. The lead cap can leach a lead residue that dissolves as the wine is poured. The nutrient contents of 3.5 fl oz. of wine is: 74 calories; protein, 0.2 g; carbohydrate, 1.8 g; iron, 0.44 mg; potassium, 115 mg; riboflavin, 0.03 mg; niacin, 0.08 mg; and about 10 ml of pure ethanol. (See also BEER; CARDIOVASCULAR DISEASE.)

Vinson, Joe L., and Barbara A. Hontz. "Phenol Antioxidant Index: Comparative Antioxidant Effectiveness of Red and White Wines," *Journal of Agriculture and Food Chemistry* 43 (1995): 401–403.

World Health Organization (WHO) A specialized agency of the United Nations founded in 1948 to promote international cooperation to improve health. Member governments finance WHO with annual contributions on the basis of their relative ability to pay. WHO works in conjunction with the FOOD AND AGRICULTURAL ORGANIZATION to focus on three areas:

1. International sanitary regulations. WHO provides current information regarding such matters as control of drug addicts, vaccination practices, advances in nutrition, cancer research, and hazards of nuclear radiation. It standardizes quarantine measures.
2. Support of member health programs. Upon request, WHO provides technical advice, assists in setting up health centers, and aids in training of medical personnel.
3. Control of epidemics. WHO promotes nationwide vaccination programs, clinics for disease prevention, clean water supplies, and modern sanitation systems, health education, antibiotic use and insecticide application. It has helped wage campaigns against tuberculosis, smallpox, malaria, and, more recently, the AIDS epidemic.

(See also GREEN REVOLUTION.)

X

xanthan gum A food additive used as an emulsifier in salad dressing, syrup, and pie fillings where viscous mixtures are desired. Xanthan gum is stable to heat and acidic conditions, making it a versatile stabilizer. A water-soluble POLYSACCHARIDE, xanthan gum is produced by bacteria and is considered a safe additive.

As a supplement, xanthan gum is a source of water-soluble FIBER, and it improves the body's ability to use glucose (BLOOD SUGAR), decreasing the need for INSULIN, the hormone responsible for lowering blood sugar. Xanthan gum improves GLUCOSE TOLERANCE in diabetics, apparently by slowing starch digestion and preventing glucose from being dumped into the bloodstream. Xanthan gum may also help lower blood CHOLESTEROL. (See also DIABETES MELLITUS; FOOD ADDITIVES.)

xanthophyll A yellow pigment related to BETA-CAROTENE that cannot be converted to vitamin A. XANTHOPHYLL belongs to the family of CAROTENOIDS, widely distributed yellow-orange pigments found in many plants. It is often added to poultry feed to color poultry skin yellow and to deepen the color of egg yolks. Consumers often associate these color changes with quality.

xenobiotic Any compound found in the body that originated from the external environment. Xenobiotics represent a diverse group of chemicals, ranging from PESTICIDES to drugs, industrial solvents and cigarette tar. Xenobiotics are either stored in fatty tissues, such as adipose (fat) tissue and nerves, or they are processed by enzymes and eliminated through the bile, urine, and, to a certain extent, in sweat. However, long-term exposure to environmental chemicals in the home or the workplace can lead to their buildup in the body, ultimately leading to illness.

Chemical modification of xenobiotics occurs chiefly in the LIVER; lungs, kidneys, and intestines also play a role. Enzymes of these organs convert foreign compounds to more water-soluble forms, so that they can be excreted. To accomplish this feat, the body employs a battery of oxidizing enzymes, called Phase 1 enzymes. These enzymes require IRON, NIACIN, and RIBOFLAVIN for their activity. A second battery of enzymes, called Phase 2 enzymes, then attaches compounds—including amino acids, sulfate, and sugar acids—to the modified xenobiotic. The "conjugated" product is generally much more soluble in body fluids, is more easily excreted and is less harmful than the unprocessed *xenobiotic.* Key nutrients support Phase 2 processes: the sulfur-containing amino acid CYSTEINE, VITAMIN C, PANTOTHENIC ACID and niacin. (See also CANCER; DETOXICATION; GLUTATHIONE.)

McFadden, S. A. "Phenotypic Variation in Zenobiotic Metabolism and Adverse Environmental Response: Focus on Sulfur-Dependent Detoxification Pathways," *Toxicology* 111 (1996): 43–65.

xylitol A sugar alcohol used as a sweetener. Xylitol is a derivative of a common pentose (small sugar) that is as sweet as SUCROSE (table sugar). Small amounts occur naturally in PLUMS, RASPBERRIES, STRAWBERRIES, and vegetables like CAULIFLOWER and EGGPLANT. The commercial source is birch bark. Xylitol is used in sugar-free gum and diet foods like jams and jellies. It has little effect on BLOOD SUGAR.

Like other sugar alcohols, such as MANNITOL and SORBITOL, xylitol resists fermentation by oral bacteria. Early studies indicated that chewing sugarless gum sweetened with xylitol after eating sugar-rich foods reduced the rate of dental cavities. More recently, children given xylitol daily seemed to develop less tooth decay. Xylitol may interfere with decay-causing bacteria by blocking their utilization of other sugars. However, the safety of this additive is questionable. Bladder and adrenal gland tumors can form and organs can be damaged when animals consume xylitol for long periods. (See also ARTIFICIAL SWEETENERS; NATURAL SWEETENERS; TEETH.)

Y

yam (*Dioscorea* spp.) A starchy tuber of a tropical plant. Yams are unrelated to the rich SWEET POTATOES sold in the United States, which they resemble. Yams were cultivated in Africa and Asia as early as 8000 B.C. and are now a staple among people living in tropical regions. They are produced in West Africa, Southeast Asia, and the Polynesian islands. The cush cush yam (*D. trifida*), the Asiatic yam (*D. alata*), and the white yam (*D. rotunda*) are important food yams. Yams can be baked, broiled, roasted, or fried. Unlike sweet potatoes, true yams contain little BETA-CAROTENE. Compared to POTATOES, yams contain the same amount of protein, but 50 percent more starch. They contain half as much vitamin C as potatoes.

Several varieties of yams contain ALKALOIDS, plant substances that possess powerful physiologic effects. The Asiatic bitter yam, *D. hispida,* contains diosorine, a toxin that can be removed by soaking or boiling it in water. Chinese yams, *D. opposita* and *D. batatas,* are used in Oriental medicine. Certain wild types of yams yield STEROIDS, hormone-like substances that have been used to prepare oral contraceptives and arthritis medications.

yeast See BAKER'S YEAST; BREWER'S YEAST; *CANDIDA ALBICANS.*

yellow no. 5 and no. 6 See ARTIFICIAL FOOD COLORS.

yogurt A fermented milk product. Yogurt is one of the oldest cultured dairy foods. Commercially, a mixture of fresh, skimmed, and nonfat dry MILKS are inoculated with bacteria that ferment milk sugar to LACTIC ACID, which both curdles the milk and acts as a PRESERVATIVE.

In terms of nutrients, yogurt resembles the milk from which it was prepared, including the calcium content. The nutritional quality varies with the type of milk, type of lactic acid cultures, fermentation conditions, storage conditions, and additives. Producers may add thickeners (CARRAGEENAN, modified starch, PECTIN, or AGAR), nonfat dry milk solids and SUGAR, as well as fruit flavor, to yogurt. Acid-producing bacteria such as *LACTOBACILLUS ACIDOPHILUS, L. bulgaricus,* and *Streptococcus thermophilus* are sometimes added as well.

Various claims have been made regarding the possible health benefits of yogurt. Studies have shown that yogurt with live cultures of lactic acid-producing bacteria is tolerated by lactose-sensitive people, presumably due to the presence of bacterial enzymes capable of degrading LACTOSE (milk sugar) to simple sugars. The conjecture that yogurt offers protection against coronary heart disease by lowering blood CHOLESTEROL arose from observations of Masai tribesmen of East Africa who consume large amounts of yogurt-like foods, yet maintain low blood cholesterol levels. Subsequent studies have failed to support this hypothesis. Data on the effects of yogurt on gastrointestinal infections are conflicting. Yogurt's role in increasing longevity remains unproven.

Yogurt has become popular in the United States since the 1960s due to its convenience, variety of flavors, and its image as a health food. Many varieties of yogurt are available: fat and nonfat, plain and flavored, frozen yogurts, and yogurt drinks. Yogurt may be pasteurized, so the live bacteria are destroyed. Manufacturers may add back acid-producing bacteria. Nonfat yogurt contains 6 percent of its calories as fat; low-fat yogurt, 24 percent; and whole milk yogurt, 48 percent. The nutrient content of 1 cup (227 g) of nonfat yogurt is: 127

calories; protein, 13 g; carbohydrate, 17.4 g; fat, 0.41 g; cholesterol, 4 mg; calcium, 452 mg; potassium, 579 mg; thiamin, 0.11 mg; riboflavin, 0.53 mg; niacin, 0.28 mg. One cup of yogurt made from whole milk (227 g) provides 138 calories; protein, 7.9 g; carbohydrate, 10.6 g; fat, 7.6 g; cholesterol, 29 mg; calcium, 275 mg; potassium, 216 mg; thiamin, 0.07 mg; riboflavin, 0.32 mg; niacin, 0.17 mg.

Shalev, E. et al. "Ingestion of Yogurt Containing Lactobacillus Acidophilus Compared with Pasteurized Yogurt as Prophylaxis for Recurrent Candidal Vaginitis and Bacterial Vaginosis," *Archives of Family Medicine* 5 (1996): 593–596.

yo-yo dieting (diet-induced obesity) A pattern of repeated losing and regaining of weight. This pattern of weight fluctuation may carry added health risks for overweight people. People whose weight fluctuates repeatedly suffer increased mortality from heart disease as well as other causes. With on-again off-again DIETING, some people may gradually adapt to using food more efficiently, possibly making weight loss more difficult with repeated dieting cycles, although there is no consensus on the long-term consequences.

There are other possibilities: Yo-yo dieting may increase a dieter's desire for fatty foods and it may lower self-esteem, leading to other ineffective weight-loss strategies. Fat regained after drastic weight loss tends to cluster in the upper body and the abdominal cavity. The so-called android pattern, with a waist to hip ratio greater than 1.0, increases the risk of CARDIOVASCULAR DISEASE. The National Task Force on the Prevention and Treatment of Obesity concluded that yo-yo dieting may not pose serious health risks (1994). OBESITY is a complex phenomenon due to many factors, including inheritance and environmental influences. More study is needed to define long-term health effects of repeated dieting. (See also WEIGHT MANAGEMENT.)

Z

zeaxanthin A yellow-pigmented XANTHOPHYLL derived from BETA-CAROTENE. This CAROTENOID has powerful ANTIOXIDANT properties and is plentiful in corn and dark green leafy vegetables such as spinach and collard greens. It is typically found in combination with lutein, a closely-related carotenoid. Neither zeaxanthin nor lutein can be converted to vitamin A. Recent studies have linked consumption of zeaxanthin and LUTEIN, from foods, with reduced risk of eye diseases such as macular degeneration and cataracts. It is believed that these carotenoids protect delicate eye tissue from damage by FREE RADICALS and that they may act as light filters, preventing harmful blue light from the sun from reaching inner eye structures.

zein A protein from CORN. Zein is deficient in two dietary essential AMINO ACIDS, LYSINE, and TRYPTOPHAN. High lysine varieties of corn have been developed to partially remedy this deficiency. Zein is commercially produced by treating cornmeal with alcohol. It is used as an edible coating for CANDY and shelled nuts and finds many industrial uses, ranging from paper coating to microencapsulation. (See also GLUTEN.)

Zen macrobiotic diet See MACROBIOTIC DIET.

zinc An essential trace mineral nutrient required for a wide array of metabolic processes. The body contains about 2.2 g of zinc, more than any trace mineral except iron. The highest concentrations occur in the skin, prostate gland, eyes, nails, and hair, although it is widely distributed among tissues. Over 100 different ENZYMES (biological catalysts) require zinc. For example, zinc is required by DNA polymerase, an enzyme required for the synthesis of DNA (responsible for inheritance), and by RNA polymerase, an enzyme required for the synthesis of RNA. RNA guides the synthesis of proteins using the genetic information stored in DNA. Gene activators that regulate the expression of genetic information often utilize proteins containing zinc to bind to specific regions on the DNA molecule.

Possible Roles in Maintaining Health

Other roles range from protection against oxidation to digestion and BLOOD SUGAR regulation. Thus zinc is classified as an ANTIOXIDANT when it functions as a cofactor for SUPEROXIDE DISMUTASE, the enzyme that disarms a particularly reactive form of oxygen. In digestion, the pancreatic PROTEASE, CARBOXYPEPTIDASE, requires zinc for its protein-degrading action. Furthermore, the hormone INSULIN is processed and packaged as a zinc complex. Zinc also aids the interaction of insulin with its target tissues to facilitate the uptake of blood sugar.

Zinc supports normal cell division and growth, the function of cell membranes, the IMMUNE SYSTEM, BONE calcification and the development and function of male reproductive organs. Many trace minerals and vitamins, including zinc, are required for normal growth and development. Zinc deficiency can cause birth defects, complicated deliveries and low birth weight, as well as impaired learning and delayed sexual development.

Immune System It is well established that zinc stimulates the IMMUNE SYSTEM. Zinc activates T-lymphocytes, the soldiers and generals of the immune system. Furthermore, zinc deficiency in the womb can lead to a weakened immune system at birth and enhanced risk of infection in newborn infants. Furthermore, zinc deficiency may be partially responsible for the weakened immunity that so frequently accompanies AGING. Zinc supplementation can improve white cell counts and antibody production in healthy, elderly people. There are intriguing hints that the zinc status of some AIDS patients is marginal; these patients have a severely imbalanced immune system. Zinc may help lessen symptoms of such autoimmune diseases as RHEUMATOID ARTHRITIS, when the body begins to attack its own tissues. Zinc's role in combating the common cold is controversial. Some studies have shown that zinc supplements can reduce the length and severity of cold symptoms, while other studies have been inconclusive. Additional research is needed to determine whether zinc can help cold sufferers lessen their misery.

Cancer A healthy immune system helps prevent cancer, and zinc-deficient animals are more sensitive to carcinogens (cancer-causing agents). Patients with prostate cancer have significantly lower zinc levels, as do those with esophageal cancer. Whether zinc supplementation alone corrects prostate enlargement or slows prostate cancer is unproven.

Male Fertility Zinc is implicated in normal prostate functions and male infertility. The male sex hormone, TESTOSTERONE, may regulate zinc metabolism in the prostate, and zinc, in turn, may affect testosterone metabolism in the prostate. Zinc deficiency leads to a lowered sperm count as well as impotence, and initial studies suggest that zinc can be used therapeutically in these cases.

Vision Zinc plays a role in vision. Conversion of VITAMIN A to its biologically active form, retinal, requires zinc. Zinc-deficient alcoholics may suffer from night blindness, and zinc has been used in this situation. Aging frequently brings blindness. In certain cases, zinc supplementation may slow the progress of vision loss due to this condition.

Tissue Repair Zinc seems to promote wound healing, particularly in zinc-deficient individuals. Zinc is necessary for tissue repair and growth. Zinc ointments have been used to treat ACNE.

Taste Zinc deficiency leads to altered taste and smell sensitivity; diminished taste acuity may respond to zinc.

Requirements The RECOMMENDED DIETARY ALLOWANCE for adult men is 11 mg and for adult women is 8 mg. Pregnancy and lactation increase a woman's requirements.

Sources The best sources of zinc are animal products. SEAFOODS, MEAT, and POULTRY provide readily absorbed forms of zinc. BREWER'S YEAST, whole GRAINS, and BRAN contain zinc. Zinc in vegetables and grains is tightly bound, limiting its BIOAVAILABILITY. Recently zinc has been added to parenteral (IV) nutrient formulations and to breakfast cereals.

Marginal (subclinical) zinc deficiency can be a problem for many Americans. Early symptoms of a subclinical deficiency include loss of appetite, altered taste and smell, decreased appetite, as well as slow growth in children. Lethargy, white spots on fingernails, slow wound healing, impotence, and delayed sexual development may follow. Chronic dieters, alcoholics, strict vegetarians, and young children with diets compromised by junk food often consume inadequate zinc and other trace nutrients. Some patients with EATING DISORDERS may be zinc deficient. Zinc may help patients recovering from injury or infection. Pregnant and lactating women require zinc and other trace minerals. Elderly people may rely on zinc-deficient foods, a situation that is compounded by their reduced ability to absorb trace minerals like zinc. Strenuous exercise increases zinc loss through sweating and increased excretion, consequently an athlete's need for zinc increases.

Factors that increase the need for zinc include kidney disease, diabetes, cystic fibrosis, INFLAMMATORY BOWEL DISEASE, inherited zinc deficiency, and the use of diuretics and laxatives. A high-fiber diet and foods containing PHYTIC ACID can bind trace minerals and limit zinc uptake when large amounts are taken. Likewise, excessive COPPER, IRON, or CALCIUM displace zinc and limit its uptake.

Safety Zinc is relatively nontoxic, and modest zinc supplementation for insurance may be appropriate particularly when the diet is compromised or there is maldigestion or malabsorption. The ratio of zinc to copper should be about seven to one, the ratio of the RDAs. Symptoms of zinc excess include nausea, bloating, abdominal cramps, diarrhea, and fever. A high zinc intake (100 to 300 mg daily) may suppress the immune system, lower HIGH-DENSITY LIPOPROTEIN (HDL, believed to protect against heart disease) and block the absorption of copper, creating a copper deficiency. Copper deficiency in turn can increase blood CHOLESTEROL, LOW-DENSITY LIPOPROTEIN (LDL, the undesirable form) and lower HDL, thus increasing the risk of CARDIOVASCULAR DISEASE. (See also ATHEROSCLEROSIS.)

Mares-Perlman, J. A. et al. "Zinc Intake and Sources in the U.S. Adult Population 1976–1980," *Journal of the American College of Nutrition* 14, no. 4 (1995): 349–357.

Mossad, S. B. et al. "Zinc Gluconate Lozenges for Treating the Common Cold," *Annals of Internal Medicine* 125 (1996): 81–88.

zymogen (proenzyme) An inactive form of an enzyme that is converted in the body to an active enzyme. Examples include pepsinogen, secreted by the STOMACH to form PEPSIN for protein digestion in the stomach; chymotrypsinogen and trypsinogen secreted by the PANCREAS to form CHYMOTRYPSIN and TRYPSIN for protein DIGESTION in the intestine. Secretion of these DIGESTIVE ENZYMES as zymogens normally assures their safe transit through the cell before activation so they do not attack the tissue that is their source.

GLOSSARY

amino acids Nitrogen-containing compounds that are the building blocks of protein. There are 22 different amino acids from which all the proteins in the human body are made. Nine "essential amino acids" are not manufactured by the body and must come from food.

anorexia Loss or lack of appetite.

calcium A mineral that makes bones and teeth strong, helps muscles work, and aids in proper blood clotting.

calorie A unit of food energy (the energy the body needs to maintain itself). Carbohydrates, fat, and protein provide the energy from food.

carbohydrate Sugars and starches that are the most efficient source of food energy. The most basic carbohydrate is a simple sugar (such as glucose or fructose), which serves as a building block for complex carbohydrates (starchy foods like pastas, whole grains, and potatoes).

cholesterol Waxy substance made by the body and obtained from food. Blood cholesterol circulates in the bloodstream and is a combination of cholesterol obtained from food and that which the body makes. HDL-cholesterol and LDL-cholesterol are forms of lipoproteins, which help transport cholesterol throughout the body. HDL (high-density lipoprotein) is the "good" cholesterol and LDL (low-density lipoprotein) is the "bad" cholesterol. HDL participates in removing excess blood cholesterol from the body; LDL is the form that can build up in artery walls and thus is a serious risk factor for heart disease.

chronic Lasting months or years. In medicine, a condition or illness of long duration, in contrast with acute conditions. The degenerative diseases of aging are typical chronic diseases. Thus, arthritis, osteoporosis, periodontal disease, cardiovascular disease are slow to develop and they may go on for years before becoming debilitating.

electrolytes Minerals (such as sodium or potassium) that regulate body functions.

emaciation An extensive loss of body fat and muscle mass.

enzymes Proteins necessary to trigger biochemical reactions.

fat Caloric energy found in food that is essential for many body functions. Dietary fats can be either saturated (butter, meat, fried foods) or unsaturated (vegetable oils). Unsaturated fats are considered to be healthier. Fat also provides essential fatty acids, is an important component of cell structure, and transports vitamins A, D, E, and K.

fatty acids Basic units of fat molecules that are mixtures of different fatty acids, including monounsaturated, polyunsaturated, saturated, omega-3, and trans-fatty acids.

fiber A form of carbohydrate that the body cannot digest. Dietary fiber can be either soluble (dissolves in water) or insoluble (such as bran). Fiber is important in maintaining intestinal health.

folate Also called folic acid, this B vitamin helps the body make nucleic acids (RNA and DNA), amino acids, and red blood cells.

glucose The form of sugar in which all carbohydrates are used by the body for energy.

glycogen A form of glucose that is stored in the liver and muscles.

hormone A chemical substance that is secreted into body fluids and transported to another organ where it affects metabolism.

insulin A hormone secreted by the pancreas that helps regulate carbohydrate metabolism.

iron A mineral that is an important part of hemoglobin, the blood's oxygen-carrying molecule. Iron also helps the body resist infection and use energy from food.

metabolism The chemical and physiological process by which the body builds and maintains itself and breaks down food and nutrients to produce energy.

nutrient A substance derived from food that is needed by the body to supply energy and maintain normal cell functioning, repair, and growth.

protein A major component of all body tissue that helps the body grow and repair itself. Protein is also a necessary component of hormones, enzymes, and hemoglobin.

triglyceride A type of stored fat.

INDEX

Page numbers in **boldface** indicate extensive treatment of a topic. Page numbers followed by the letter *t* indicate tables.

I

M

N

Q

R

T